ICD·10·PCS

International Classification of Diseases
10th Revision

Procedure Coding System

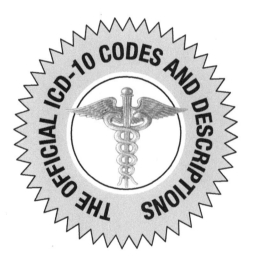

THE OFFICIAL ICD-10 CODES AND DESCRIPTIONS

2014

Transition & Training Edition

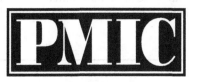

ISBN: 978-1-939852-03-8 (print)
        978-1-939852-06-9 (e-Book)

Practice Management Information Corporation (PMIC)
4727 Wilshire Boulevard
Los Angeles, California 90010
http://www.pmiconline.com

Printed in the United States of America

On October 1, 2014 a key element of the data foundation of the United States' health care system will undergo a major transformation. We will transition from the decades-old Ninth Edition of the International Classification of Diseases (ICD-9) set of diagnosis and inpatient procedure codes to the far more contemporary, vastly larger, and much more detailed Tenth Edition of those code sets—or ICD-10—used by most developed countries throughout the world. This transition will have a major impact on anyone who uses health care information that contains a diagnosis and/or inpatient procedure code, including:

- Hospitals
- Health care practitioners and institutions
- Health insurers and other third-party payers
- Electronic-transaction clearinghouses
- Hardware and software manufacturers and vendors
- Billing and practice-management service providers
- Health care administrative and oversight agencies
- Public and private health care research institutions

All "covered entities"—as defined by the Health Insurance Portability and Accountability Act of 1996 (HIPAA)—are required to adopt ICD-10 codes for use in all HIPAA transactions with dates of service on or after the October 1, 2013 compliance date for HIPAA inpatient claims, ICD-10 diagnosis and procedure codes are required for all inpatient stays with discharge dates on or after October 1, 2014 (or subsequently revised implementation date). Please note that the transition to ICD-10 does not directly affect provider use of the Current Procedural Terminology (CPT) and Healthcare Common Procedure Coding System (HCPCS) codes.

Unlike the annual revisions of an existing code set, for example ICD-9 2014 replacing ICD-9 2013 on October 1, 2013, this is not a revision, but a complete replacement of an entire code set. The ICD-10 code set is different from the ICD-9 code set in format and the number of possible digits, and also has many more codes to choose from. The draft ICD-10-PCS code set includes 69,370 codes excluding the potential for placeholders and 7th digits. The draft ICD-10-PCS code set includes 72,083 codes. That's a total of 141,453 (even more with 7th digits and placeholders) codes in the ICD-10 system compared to 22,202 codes in the ICD-9 coding system.

The transition will require business and systems changes throughout the health care industry. Everyone who is covered by the Health Insurance Portability and Accountability Act (HIPAA) must make the transition, not just those who submit Medicare or Medicaid claims.

This edition of ICD-10-CM includes all official codes, descriptions and guidelines. A new edition is available approximately mid-September of each year. New editions may be purchased from:

Practice Management Information Corporation
4727 Wilshire Boulevard
Los Angeles, CA 90010
1-800-MED-SHOP
http://pmiconline.com

DISCLAIMER

This publication is designed to offer basic information regarding the ICD-10 coding system. The information presented is based upon extensive review of existing literature and the experience and interpretations of the author. Though all of the information has been carefully researched and checked for accuracy and completeness, neither the authors nor the publisher accepts any responsibility or liability with regard to errors, omissions, misuse or misinterpretation.

CONTENTS

TERMINOLOGY

Acute Conditions – The medical conditions characterized by sudden onset, severe change, and/or short duration.

Additional Diagnosis – The secondary diagnosis code used, if available, to provide a more complete picture of the primary diagnosis..

Alteration -- Modifying the anatomic structure of a body part without affecting the function of the body part

Applied mapping – Distillation of a reference mapping to conform to the needs of a particular application (e.g., data quality, research).

Approach (5th character) – Defines the technique used to reach the site of the procedure.

Backward mapping – mapping that proceeds from a newer code set to an older code set, for example from ICD-10-CM to ICD-9-CM.

Bilateral – For bilateral sites, the final character of the codes in the ICD-10-CM indicates laterality. An unspecified side code is also provided should the side not be identified in the medical record. If no bilateral code is provided and the condition is bilateral, assign separate codes for both the left and right side.

Body Part or Region (4th character) – Defines the specific anatomical site where the procedure is performed.

Body System (2nd character) – Defines the general physiological system on which the procedure is performed or anatomical region where the procedure is performed.

Bypass -- Altering the route of passage of the contents of a tubular body part.

Category – The three-digit diagnosis code classifications that broadly define each condition (e.g., 250 for diabetes mellitus).

Centers for Disease Control and Prevention (CDC) – A federal health data organization that helps maintain several code sets included in the HIPAA standards, including the ICD-9-CM codes.

Centers for Medicare & Medicaid Services (CMS) – The federal agency that runs the Medicare program. In addition, CMS works with the States to run the Medicaid program. CMS works to make sure that the beneficiaries in these programs are able to get high quality healthcare.

Change -- Taking out or off a device from a body part and putting back an identical or similar device in or on the same body part without cutting or puncturing the skin or a mucous membrane

Character – One of the seven components that comprise an ICD-10-PCS procedure code.

Chronic Conditions – Medical conditions characterized by long duration, frequent recurrence over a long period of time, and/or slow progression over time.

Cluster – in a combination entry, one instance where a code is chosen from each of the choice lists in the target system entry, that when combined satisfies the equivalent meaning of the corresponding code in the source system

Combination Codes – A single code used to classify any of the following: two diagnoses; a diagnosis with an associated secondary process (manifestation); or a diagnosis with an associated complication.

Control -- Stopping, or attempting to stop, postprocedural bleeding.

Conventions of ICD-10 – The general rules for use of the classification independent of guidelines. These conventions are incorporated within the Index and Tabular of the ICD-10-CM as instructional notes.

Creation -- Making a new genital structure that does not take over the function of a body part.

Crosswalk/mapping – A new test is determined to be similar to an existing test, multiple existing test codes, or a portion of an existing test code. The new test code is then assigned to the related existing local fee schedule amounts and resulting national limitation amount. In some instances, a test may only equate to a portion of a test, and, in those instances, payment at an appropriate percentage of the payment for the existing test is assigned.

Destruction -- Physical eradication of all or a portion of a body part by the direct use of energy, force or a destructive agent.

Detachment -- Cutting off all or a portion of the upper or lower extremities.

Dilation -- Expanding an orifice or the lumen of a tubular body part.

Division -- Cutting into a body part without draining fluids and/or gases from the body part in order to separate or transect a body part.

Drainage -- Taking or letting out fluids and/or gases from a body part.

Excision -- Cutting out or off, without replacement, a portion of a body part.

External (approach) -- Procedures performed directly on the skin or mucous membrane and procedures performed indirectly by the application of external force through the skin or mucous membrane.

Extirpation -- Taking or cutting out solid matter from a body part.

Extraction -- Pulling or stripping out or off all or a portion of a body part by the use of force.

Federal Register – The "Federal Register" is the official daily publication for rules, proposed rules and notices of federal agencies and organizations, as well as Executive Orders and other Presidential documents.

Forward mapping – mapping that proceeds from an older code set to a newer code set, for example from ICD-9-CM Volume 3 to ICD-10-PCS.

Fragmentation -- Breaking solid matter in a body part into pieces.

Fusion -- Joining together portions of an articular body part rendering the articular body part immobile.

GEMs - This reference mapping attempts to include all valid relationships between the codes in the ICD-9-CM diagnosis classification and the ICD-10-CM diagnosis classification.

General Equivalence Map (GEM) – reference mapping that attempts to include all valid relationships between the codes in the ICD-9- CM diagnosis classification and the ICD-10-CM diagnosis classification

Health Insurance Portability & Accountability Act (HIPAA) – A law passed in 1996 which is also sometimes called the "Kassebaum-Kennedy" law. This law expands healthcare coverage for patients who have lost or changed jobs, or have pre-existing conditions. HIPAA does not replace the states' roles as primary regulators of insurance.

HIPAA 4010 – The original healthcare transactions version of HIPAA (officially known as Version 004010 of the ASC X12 transaction implementation guides) named as part of HIPAA's Electronic Transaction Standards regulation. Version 4010 was required to be used by HIPAA covered healthcare entities by Oct. 16, 2003.

HIPAA 5010 – Required by Jan. 1, 2012 to be the new version of the HIPAA healthcare transactions. Officially known as Version 005010 of the ASC X12 transaction Technical Report Type 3. This new version was required as a result of Department of Health and Human Services (HHS) final rules published on Jan. 6, 2009.

ICD-10 – The mortality and morbidity classification coding system implemented by WHO in 1993 to replace ICD-9.

ICD-10-CM – The updated version of the clinical modification coding set defined by the National Center for Health Statistics that will replace ICD-9-CM on Oct. 1, 2013.

ICD-10-PCS – The updated procedural coding system defined by CMS that will replace Volume 3 of ICD-9-CM for hospital inpatient services.

ICD-9 – The mortality and morbidity classification coding system that is currently used throughout most of the world, including the United States. The ICD-9 classification of death and disease is based a series of classifications systems first adopted in 1893.

ICD-9-CM – The "clinical modification" to the ICD-9 code set that is currently used in America to report medical diagnoses. The "Clinical Modification" refers to the base WHO defined ICD-9 code set that has been defined for use in United State by the National Center for Health Statistics (NCHS) division of the Centers for Disease Control (CDC).

ICD-9-PCS – The procedural coding system currently used in America primarily for hospital inpatient services. It is contained in Volume 3 of ICD-9-CM.

Index (to diseases) – The ICD-10-CM is divided into the Alphabetic Index, an alphabetical list of terms and their corresponding code, and the Tabular List, a chronological list of codes divided into chapters based on body system or condition. The Alphabetic Index consists of the following parts: the Index of Diseases and Injury, the Index of External Causes of Injury, the Table of Neoplasms and the Table of Drugs and Chemicals.

Insertion -- Putting in a nonbiological device that monitors, assists, performs or prevents a physiological function but does not physically take the place of a body part.

Inspection -- Visually and/or manually exploring a body part.

International Classification of Diseases (ICD) – A medical code set maintained by the World Health Organization (WHO). The primary purpose of this code set is to classify both causes of death or mortality and diseases or morbidity. A U.S. extension, known as ICD-CM, "Clinical Modification," is maintained by the NCHS within the CDC to more precisely define ICD use in the U.S.

Manifestation Codes – Certain conditions have both an underlying etiology and multiple body system manifestations due to the underlying etiology. For such conditions, the ICD-10-CM has a coding convention that requires the underlying condition be sequenced first followed by the manifestation. Wherever such a combination exists, there is a "use additional code" note at the etiology code, and a "code first" note at the manifestation code. These instructional notes indicate the proper sequencing order of the codes, etiology followed by manifestation.

Map -- Locating the route of passage of electrical impulses and/or locating functional areas in a body part.

Medical Necessity – Services or supplies that: are proper and needed for the diagnosis or treatment of a medical condition; are provided for the diagnosis, direct care, and treatment of a medical condition; meet the standards of good medical practice in the local area; and are not mainly for the convenience of the patient or doctor.

Morbidity – Term refers to the disease rate or number of cases of a particular disease in a given age range, gender, occupation, or other relevant population based grouping.

Mortality –Term refers to the death rate reflected by the population in a given region, age range, or other relevant statistical grouping

National Center for Health Statistics (NCHS) – A federal organization within the CDC that collects, analyzes, and distributes healthcare statistics. The NCHS helps maintain the ICD-CM codes.

No Map Flag – attribute in a GEM that when turned on indicates that a code in the source system is not linked to any code in the target system .

Occlusion -- Completely closing an orifice or the lumen of a tubular body part.

Open (approach) -- Cutting through the skin or mucous membrane and any other body layers necessary to expose the site of the procedure.

Percutaneous (approach) -- Entry, by puncture or minor incision, of instrumentation through the skin or mucous membrane and any other body layers necessary to reach the site of the procedure.

Percutaneous Endoscopic (approach) -- Entry, by puncture or minor incision, of instrumentation through the skin or mucous membrane and any other body layers necessary to reach and visualize the site of the procedure.

Principle Diagnosis – First-listed/primary diagnosis code. The code sequenced first on a medical record defines the primary reason for the encounter as determined at the end of the encounter.

Procedure – The complete specification of the ICD-10-PCS seven characters.

Reattachment -- Putting back in or on all or a portion of a separated body part to its normal location or other suitable location.

Release -- Freeing a body part from an abnormal physical constraint by cutting or by use of force.

Removal -- Taking out or off a device from a body part.

Repair -- Restoring, to the extent possible, a body part to its normal anatomic structure and function.

Replacement -- Putting in or on biological or synthetic material that physically takes the place and/or function of all or a portion of a body part.

Reposition -- Moving to its normal location, or other suitable location, all or a portion of a body part.

Resection -- Cutting out or off, without replacement, all of a body part.

Restriction -- Partially closing an orifice or the lumen of a tubular body part.

Reverse lookup – using a GEM by looking up a target system code to see all the codes in the source system that translate to it.

Revision -- Correcting, to the extent possible, a portion of a malfunctioning device or the position of a displaced device.

Root Operation/Type (3rd character) – Defines the objective of the procedure.

Section (1st character) – Defines the general type of procedure.

Sequelae – A late effect is the residual effect (condition produced) after the acute phase of an illness or injury has terminated. There is no time limit on when a late effect code can be used. The residual may be apparent early, such as in cerebral infarction, or it may occur months or years later, such as that due to a previous injury.

Signs/Symptoms – Codes that describe symptoms and signs, as opposed to diagnoses, are acceptable for reporting purposes when a related definitive diagnosis has not been established (confirmed) by the provider.

Source system -- code set of origin in the mapping; the set being mapped 'from'

Supplement -- Putting in or on biological or synthetic material that physically reinforces and/or augments the function of a portion of a body part

Tabular List – It is essential to use both the Alphabetic Index and Tabular List when locating and assigning a code. The Alphabetic Index does not always provide the full code. Selection of the full code, including laterality and any applicable 7th character can only be done in the Tabular List. A dash (-) at the end of an Alphabetic Index entry indicates that additional characters are required. Even if a dash is not included at the Alphabetic Index entry, it is necessary to refer to the Tabular List to verify that no 7th character is required.

Target system – destination code set in the mapping; the set being mapped 'to'.

Transfer -- Moving, without taking out, all or a portion of a body part to another location to take over the function of all or a portion of a body part.

Transplantation -- Putting in or on all or a portion of a living body part taken from another individual or animal to physically take the place and/or function of all or a portion of a similar body part.

Uniform Hospital Discharge Data Set (UHDDS) – The UHDDS definitions are used by hospitals to report inpatient data elements in a standardized manner. These data elements and their definitions can be found in the July 31, 1985, Federal Register (Vol. 50, No, 147), pp. 31038-40.

Value – Individual units defined for each character of ICD-10-PCS and represented by a number or letter.

Via Natural or Artificial Opening (approach) -- Entry of instrumentation through a natural or artificial external opening to reach the site of the procedure.

Via Natural or Artificial Opening Endoscopic (approach) -- Entry of instrumentation through a natural or artificial external opening to reach and visualize the site of the procedure.

Via Natural or Artificial Opening With Percutaneous Endoscopic Assistance (approach) -- Entry of instrumentation through a natural or artificial external opening and entry, by puncture or minor incision, of instrumentation through the skin or mucous membrane and any other body layers necessary to aid in the performance of the procedure.

Volume I – The detailed, tabular list of diagnosis codes in the ICD-9-CM manual.

Volume II – The alphabetical index to diseases in the ICD-9-CM diagnosis coding manual.

Volume III – The ICD-9/ICD-10 list of procedure codes, used in inpatient settings.

World Health Organization (WHO) – An organization that maintains the International Classification of Diseases (ICD) medical code set.

INTRODUCTION TO ICD-10-PCS

The International Classification Of Diseases Tenth Revision Procedure Coding System (ICD-10-PCS) was created to accompany the World Health Organization's (WHO) ICD-10 diagnosis classification. The new procedure coding system was developed to replace ICD-9-CM procedure codes for reporting inpatient procedures.

Unlike the ICD-9-CM classification, ICD-10-PCS was designed to enable each code to have a standard structure and be very descriptive, and yet flexible enough to accommodate future needs. Information about the structure, organization, and application of ICD-10-PCS codes, along with reference material for coding with ICD-10-PCS, is provided in this manual.

WHAT IS ICD-10-PCS?

ICD-10-PCS is a procedure coding system that will be used to collect data, determine payment, and support the electronic health record for all inpatient procedures performed in the United States.

HISTORY OF ICD-10-PCS

The World Health Organization has maintained the International Classification of Diseases (ICD) for recording cause of death since 1893. It has updated the ICD periodically to reflect new discoveries in epidemiology and changes in medical understanding of disease.

The International Classification of Diseases Tenth Revision (ICD-10), published in 1992, is the latest revision of the ICD. The WHO authorized the National Center for Health Statistics (NCHS) to develop a clinical modification of ICD-10 for use in the United States. This version of ICD-10 is called ICD-10-CM. ICD-10-CM is intended to replace the previous U.S. clinical modification, ICD-9-CM, that has been in use since 1979. ICD-9-CM contains a procedure classification; ICD-10-CM does not.

The Centers for Medicare and Medicaid Services, the agency responsible for maintaining the inpatient procedure code set in the U.S., contracted with 3M Health Information Systems in 1993 to design and then develop a procedure classification system to replace Volume 3 of ICD-9-CM. ICD-10-PCS is the result.

ICD-10-PCS was initially released in 1998. It has been updated annually since that time.

ICD-9-CM VOLUME 3 COMPARED TO ICD-10-PCS

With ICD-10 implementation, the U.S. clinical modification of the ICD will not include a procedure classification based on the same principles of organization as the diagnosis classification. Instead, a separate procedure coding system has been developed to meet the rigorous and varied demands that are made of coded data in the healthcare industry. This represents a significant step toward building a health information infrastructure that functions optimally in the electronic age.

The following table highlights basic differences between ICD-9-CM Volume 3 and ICD-10-PCS.

ICD-9-CM VOLUME 3	ICD-10-PCS
Follows ICD structure (designed for diagnosis coding)	Designed/developed to meet healthcare needs for a procedure code system
Codes available as a fixed/finite set in list form	Codes constructed from flexible code components (values) using tables
Codes are numeric	Codes are alphanumeric
Codes are 3 through 4 digits long	All codes are seven characters long

ICD-10-PCS CODE STRUCTURE

Undergirding ICD-10-PCS is a logical, consistent structure that informs the system as a whole, down to the level of a single code. This means that the process of constructing codes in ICD-10-PCS is also logical and consistent: individual letters and numbers, called "values," are selected in sequence to occupy the seven spaces of the code, called "characters."

CHARACTERS

All codes in ICD-10-PCS are seven characters long. Each character in the seven-character code represents an aspect of the procedure, as shown in the following diagram of characters from the main section of ICD-10-PCS, called Medical and Surgical.

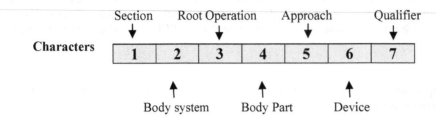

An ICD-10-PCS code is best understood as the result of a process rather than as an isolated, fixed quantity. The process consists of assigning values from among the valid choices for that part of the system, according to the rules governing the construction of codes.

VALUES

One of 34 possible values can be assigned to each character in a code: the numbers 0 through 9 and the alphabet (except I and O, because they are easily confused with the numbers 1 and 0). A finished code looks like the example below.

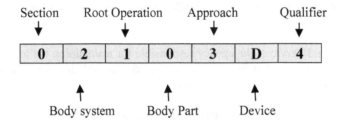

This code is derived by choosing a specific value for each of the seven characters. Based on details about the procedure performed, values for each character specifying the section, body system, root operation, body part, approach, device, and qualifier are assigned.

Because the definition of each character is a function of its physical position in the code, the same value placed in a different position in the code means something different. The value 0 in the first character means something different than 0 in the second character, or 0 in the third character, and so on.

CODE STRUCTURE: MEDICAL AND SURGICAL SECTION

The following pages define each character using the code 0LB50ZZ, "Excision of right lower arm and wrist tendon, open approach" as an example. This example comes from the Medical and Surgical section of ICD-10-PCS.

CHARACTER 1: SECTION

The first character in the code determines the broad procedure category, or section, where the code is found. In this example, the section is Medical and Surgical. 0 is the value that represents Medical and Surgical in the first character. The sample code looks like this so far:

Character 1 Section	Character 2 Body System	Character 3 Root Operation	Character 4 Body Part	Character 5 Approach	Character 6 Device	Character 7 Qualifier
Medical and Surgical						
0						

CHARACTER 2: BODY SYSTEM

The second character defines the body system—the general physiological system or anatomical region involved. Examples of body systems include Lower Arteries, Central Nervous System, and Respiratory System. In this example, the body system is Tendons, represented by the value L.

Character 1 Section	Character 2 Body System	Character 3 Root Operation	Character 4 Body Part	Character 5 Approach	Character 6 Device	Character 7 Qualifier
Medical and Surgical	Tendons					
0	**L**					

CHARACTER 3: ROOT OPERATION

The third character defines the root operation, or the objective of the procedure. Some examples of root operations are Bypass, Drainage, and Reattachment. In the sample code below, the root operation is Excision. When used in the third character of the code, the value B represents Excision.

Character 1 Section	Character 2 Body System	Character 3 Root Operation	Character 4 Body Part	Character 5 Approach	Character 6 Device	Character 7 Qualifier
Medical and Surgical	Tendons	Excision				
0	**L**	**B**				

CHARACTER 4: BODY PART

The fourth character defines the body part, or specific anatomical site where the procedure was performed. The body system (second character) provides only a general indication of the procedure site. The body part and body system values together provide a precise description of the procedure site.

Examples of body parts are Kidney, Tonsils, and Thymus. In this example, the body part value is 5, Lower Arm and Wrist, Right. when the second character is L, the value 5 when used in the fourth character of the code represents the right lower arm and wrist tendon.

Character 1 Section	Character 2 Body System	Character 3 Root Operation	Character 4 Body Part	Character 5 Approach	Character 6 Device	Character 7 Qualifier
Medical and Surgical	Tendons	Excision	Lower Arm and Wrist, Right			
0	**L**	**B**	**5**			

CHARACTER 5: APPROACH

The fifth character defines the approach, or the technique used to reach the procedure site. Seven different approach values are used in the Medical and Surgical section to define the approach. Examples of approaches include Open and Percutaneous Endoscopic.

In the sample code below, the approach is Open and is represented by the value 0.

Character 1 Section	Character 2 Body System	Character 3 Root Operation	Character 4 Body Part	Character 5 Approach	Character 6 Device	Character 7 Qualifier
Medical And Surgical	Tendons	Excision	Lower Arm And Wrist, Right	Open		
0	**L**	**B**	**5**	**0**		

CHARACTER 6: DEVICE

Depending on the procedure performed, there may or may not be a device left in place at the end of the procedure. The sixth character defines the device. Device values fall into four basic categories:

- Grafts and Prostheses
- Implants
- Simple or Mechanical Appliances
- Electronic Appliances

In this example, there is no device used in the procedure. The value Z is used to represent NO DEVICE, as shown below.

	Character 2 Body System	Character 3 Root Operation	Character 4 Body Part	Character 5 Approach	Character 6 Device	Character 7 Qualifier
Medical And Surgical	Tendons	Excision	Lower Arm And Wrist, Right	Open	No Device	
0	**L**	**B**	**5**	**0**	**Z**	

CHARACTER 7: QUALIFIER

The seventh character defines a qualifier for the code. A qualifier specifies an additional attribute of the procedure, if applicable.

Examples of qualifiers include Diagnostic and Stereotactic. Qualifier choices vary depending on the previous values selected. in this example, there is no specific qualifier applicable to this procedure, so the value is No Qualifier, represented by the letter Z.

	Character 2 Body System	Character 3 Root Operation	Character 4 Body Part	Character 5 Approach	Character 6 Device	Character 7 Qualifier
Medical And Surgical	Tendons	Excision	Lower Arm And Wrist, Right	Open	No Device	No Qualifier
0	**L**	**B**	**5**	**0**	**Z**	**Z**

0LB50ZZ is the complete specification of the procedure "Excision of right lower arm and wrist tendon, open approach."

ICD-10-PCS SYSTEM ORGANIZATION

ICD-10-PCS is composed of 16 sections, represented by the numbers 0 through 9 and the letters B through D and F.

- Medical and Surgical
- Obstetrics
- Placement
- Administration
- Measurement and Monitoring
- Extracorporeal Assistance and Performance
- Extracorporeal Therapies
- Osteopathic
- Other Procedures
- Chiropractic
- Imaging
- Nuclear Medicine
- Radiation Oncology
- Physical Rehabilitation and Diagnostic Audiology
- Mental Health

- Substance Abuse Treatment

MEDICAL AND SURGICAL SECTION

The first section, Medical and Surgical, contains the great majority of procedures typically reported in an inpatient setting. As shown in the previous section discussing ICD-10-PCS code structure, all procedure codes in the Medical and Surgical section begin with the section value 0.

	Character 2 Body System	Character 3 Root Operation	Character 4 Body Part	Character 5 Approach	Character 6 Device	Character 7 Qualifier
Medical and Surgical	Tendons	Excision	Lower arm and Wrist, right	Open	No device	No qualifier
0	**L**	**B**	**5**	**0**	**Z**	**Z**

Sections 1 through 9 of ICD-10-PCS comprise the Medical and Surgical-related sections. These sections include obstetrical procedures, administration of substances, measurement and monitoring of body functions, and extracorporeal therapies, as listed in the table below.

Section Value	Description
1	Obstetrics
2	Placement
3	Administration
4	Measurement and Monitoring
5	Extracorporeal Assistance and Performance
6	Extracorporeal Therapies
7	Osteopathic
8	Other Procedures
9	Chiropractic

In sections 1 and 2, all seven characters define the same aspects of the procedure as in the Medical and Surgical section.

Codes in sections 3 through 9 are structured for the most part like their counterparts in the Medical and Surgical section, with a few exceptions. For example, in sections 5 and 6, the fifth character is defined as duration instead of approach, as in this code for intra-aortic balloon pump (IABP):

Additional differences include these uses of the sixth character:

- Section 3 defines the sixth character as substance.
- Sections 4 and 5 define the sixth character as function.
- Sections 7 through 9 define the sixth character as method.

	Character 2 Body System	Character 3 Root Operation	Character 4 Body system	Character 5 Duration	Character 6 Function	Character 7 Qualifier
Extracorporeal Assist. And Performance	Physiological Systems	Assistance	Cardiac	Continuous	Output	Balloon Pump
5	**A**	**0**	**2**	**2**	**1**	**0**

ANCILLARY SECTIONS

Sections B through D and F through H comprise the ancillary sections of ICD-10-PCS. These six sections include imaging procedures, nuclear medicine, and substance abuse treatment, as listed in the following table.

Section Value	Description
B	Imaging
C	Nuclear Medicine
D	Radiation Oncology

F	Physical Rehabilitation and Diagnostic Audiology
G	Mental Health
H	Substance Abuse Treatment

The definitions of some characters in the ancillary sections differs from that seen in previous sections. In the Imaging section, the third character is defined as type, and the fifth and sixth characters define contrast and contrast/qualifier respectively, as in the CT scan example below.

	Character 2 Body System	Character 3 Type	Character 4 Body Part	Character 5 Contrast	Character 6 Qualifier	Character 7 Qualifier
Imaging	Central Nervous	Computerized Tomography	Brain	High Osmolar	Unenhanced and Enhanced	None
B	**0**	**2**	**0**	**0**	**0**	**Z**

Additional differences include:

- Section C defines the fifth character as radionuclide.
- Section D defines the fifth character as modality qualifier and the sixth character as isotope.
- Section F defines the fifth character as type qualifier and the sixth character as equipment.

TABLES

The complete ICD-10-PCS is presented in three parts: the Tables, the Index, and the List of Codes.

The Tables are organized in a series, beginning with section 0, Medical and Surgical, and body system 0, Central Nervous, and proceeding in numerical order. Sections 0 through 9 are followed by sections B through D and F through H. The same convention is followed within each table for the second through the seventh characters—numeric values in order first, followed by alphabetical values in order.

The following examples use the Medical and Surgical section to describe the organization and format of the ICD-10-PCS Tables.

The Medical and Surgical section (first character 0) is organized by its 31 body system values. Each body system subdivision in the Medical and Surgical section contains tables that list the valid root operations for that body system. These are the root operation tables that form the system. These tables provide the valid choices of values available to construct a code.

The root operation tables consist of four columns and a varying number of rows, as in the following example of the root operation Bypass, in the Central Nervous body system.

Section	0	Medical And Surgical
Body System	0	Central Nervous
Operation	1	Bypass: Altering the route of passage of the contents of a tubular body part (Root operation)

Body Part (Character 4)	Approach (Character 5)	Device (Character 6)	Qualifier (Character 7)
6 Cerebral Ventricle	0 Open	7 Autologous Tissue Substitute J Synthetic Substitute K Nonautologous Tissue Substitute	0 Nasopharynx 1 Mastoid Sinus 2 Atrium 3 Blood Vessel 4 Pleural Cavity 5 Intestine 6 Peritoneal Cavity 7 Urinary Tract 8 Bone Marrow B Cerebral Cisterns
U Spinal Canal	0 Open	7 Autologous Tissue Substitute J Synthetic Substitute K Nonautologous Tissue Substitute	4 Pleural Cavity 6 Peritoneal Cavity 7 Urinary Tract 9 Fallopian Tube

The values for characters 1 through 3 are provided at the top of each table. Four columns contain the applicable values for characters 4 through 7, given the values in characters 1 through 3.

A table may be separated into rows to specify the valid choices of values in characters 4 through 7. A built using values from more than one row of a table is not a valid code.

INDEX

The ICD-10-PCS Index can be used to access the Tables. The Index mirrors the structure of the Tables, so it follows a consistent pattern of organization and use of hierarchies.

The Index is organized as an alphabetic lookup. Two types of main terms are listed in the Index:

- Based on the value of the third character
- Common procedure terms

MAIN TERMS

For the medical and surgical and related sections, the root operation values are used as main terms in the index. in other sections, the values representing the general type of procedure performed, such as nuclear medicine or imaging type, are listed as main terms.

For the medical and surgical and related sections, values such as excision, bypass, and transplantation are included as main terms in the index. the applicable body system entries are listed beneath the main term, and refer to a specific table. for the ancillary sections, values such as fluoroscopy and positron emission tomography are listed as main terms.

In the example below, the index entry "bypass" refers to the medical and surgical section tables for all applicable body systems, including anatomical regions and central nervous system.

Bypass
    by Body System
        Anatomical Regions 0W1....
            Central Nervous System 001....

The body system listings may be followed by entries for specific body parts, as in the excerpt below. In the root operations CHANGE, INSERTION, REMOVAL, and REVISION, the device entries follow the body system listings.

    by Body Part
        Artery
            Aorta, Abdominal 0410...
            Aorta, Thoracic 021W...
            Axillary 031....
            Brachial 031....
            Common Carotid 031....

COMMON PROCEDURE TERMS

The second type of term listed in the Index uses procedure names, such as "appendectomy" or "fundoplication." These entries are listed as main terms, and refer to a table or tables from which a valid code can be constructed, as shown in the following example.

Cholecystectomy

- see Excision, Hepatobiliary System & Pancreas 0FB....
- see Resection, Hepatobiliary System & Pancreas 0FT....

LIST OF CODES

The ICD-10-PCS List of Codes is a resource that displays all valid codes in alphanumeric order. Each entry begins with the seven-character code, followed by the full text description.

The code descriptions are generated using rules that produce standardized, complete, and easy-to-read code descriptions.

ICD-10-PCS DESIGN

ICD-10-PCS is fundamentally different from ICD-9-CM in its structure, organization, and capabilities. It was designed and developed to adhere to recommendations made by the National Committee on Vital and Health Statistics (NCVHS). It also incorporates input from a wide range of organizations, individual physicians, healthcare professionals, and researchers.

Several structural attributes were recommended for a new procedure coding system. These attributes include

- Multiaxial structure
- Completeness
- Expandability

MULTIAXIAL STRUCTURE

The key attribute that provides the framework for all other structural attributes is multiaxial code structure. Multiaxial code structure makes it possible for the ICD-10-PCS to be complete, expandable, and to provide a high degree of flexibility and functionality. ICD-10-PCS codes are composed of seven characters. Each character represents a category of information that can be specified about the procedure performed. A character defines both the category of information and its physical position in the code.

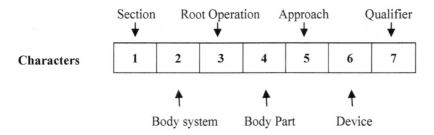

A character's position can be understood as a semi-independent axis of classification that allows different specific values to be inserted into that space, and whose physical position remains stable. Within a defined code range, a character retains the general meaning that it confers on any value in that position. For example, the fifth character retains the general meaning "approach" in sections 0 through 4 and 7 through 9 of the system. Any specific value in the fifth character will define a specific approach, such as Open.

Each group of values for a character contains all of the valid choices in relation to the other characters of the code, giving the system completeness. in the fifth character, for example, each significantly distinct approach is assigned its own approach value and all applicable approach values are included to represent the possible versions of a procedure.

Each group of values for a character can be added to as needed, giving the system expandability. if a significantly distinct approach is used to perform procedures, a new approach value can be added to the system.
Each group of values is confined to its own character, giving ICD-10-PCS a stable, predictable readability across a wide range of codes. In sections 0 through 4 and 7 through 9 of the system, for example, the fifth character always represents the approach.

ICD-10-PCS' multiaxial structure houses its capacity for completeness, expandability, and flexibility, giving it a high degree of functionality for multiple uses.

COMPLETENESS

Completeness is considered a key structural attribute for a new procedure coding system. The specific recommendation for completeness includes these characteristics:

- A unique code is available for each significantly different procedure.
- Each code retains its unique definition. Codes are not reused.

In Volume 3 of ICD-9-CM, procedures performed on many different body parts using different approaches or devices may be assigned to the same procedure code. In ICD-10-PCS, a unique code can be constructed for every significantly different procedure.

Within each section, a character defines a consistent component of a code, and contains all applicable values for that character. The values define individual expressions (open, percutaneous) of the character's general meaning (approach) that are then used to construct unique procedure codes.

Because all approaches by which a procedure is performed are assigned a separate approach value in the system, every procedure which uses a different approach will have its own unique code. This is true of the other characters as well. The same procedure performed on a different body part has its own unique code, the same procedure performed using a different device has its own unique code, and so on.

In the case of the coronary artery bypass graft (CABG), ICD-9-CM contains a total of nine codes to describe different versions of the procedure. These codes specify the version based on one aspect of the procedure, and the aspect defined is not consistent for all nine codes. Four of the codes specify the number of coronary arteries bypassed, four specify the source of the new blood flow, and one is an "unspecified" choice.

By contrast, ICD-10-PCS components can be combined to produce 34 unique codes defining all significantly different versions of the comparable CABG procedure. All 34 codes specify the same four aspects of the procedure: the number of coronary artery sites bypassed, i.e., the approach to the procedure site, the type of graft if used, and the origin of the bypass (source of the new blood flow). The differences are summarized in the table below.

ICD-9-CM VOLUME 3 CODE & DESCRIPTION		ICD-10-PCS CODE & DESCRIPTION	
36.11	Aortocoronary bypass of one coronary artery (1 of 4)	021009W	Bypass coronary artery, one site to aorta with autologous venous tissue, open approach(1 of 8)
36.15	Single internal mammary- coronary artery bypass (1 of 2)	02100Z8	Bypass coronary artery, one site to right internal mammary, open approach (1 of 16)
36.17	Abdominal-coronary artery bypass (1 of 2)	02100AF	Bypass coronary artery, one site to abdominal artery with autologous arterial tissue, open approach (1 of 10)
36.10	Aortocoronary bypass for heart revascularization, not otherwise specified (1 of 1)	No Equivalent	ICD-10-PCS codes all contain a minimum level of specificity

UNIQUE DEFINITIONS

Because ICD-10-PCS codes are constructed of individual values rather than lists of fixed codes and text descriptions, the unique, stable definition of a code in the system is retained. New values may be added to the system to represent a specific new approach or device or qualifier, but whole codes by design cannot be given new meanings and reused.

EXPANDABILITY

Expandability was also recommended as a key structural attribute. The specific recommendation for expandability includes these characteristics:

- Accommodate new procedures and technologies
- Add new codes without disrupting the existing structure

ICD-10-PCS is designed to be easily updated as new codes are required for new procedures and new techniques. Changes to ICD-10-PCS can all be made within the existing structure, because whole codes are not added. Instead, one of two possible changes is made to the system:

- A new value for a character is added as needed to the system.
- An existing value for a character is added to a table(s) in the system.

ICD-10-PCS UPDATE: PICVA

An example of how the updating of ICD-10-PCS works can be seen in the coronary artery bypass procedure called Percutaneous in-situ coronary venous arterialization (PICVA). This procedure is no more invasive than a percutaneous coronary angioplasty, but achieves the benefits of a bypass procedure by placing a specialized stent into the diseased coronary artery, through its wall into the adjacent coronary vein, and diverting blood flow through the stent into the artery past the blockage.

ICD-10-PCS was updated in 2004 to include an appropriate range of codes for the PICVA procedure (16 possible codes). This was accomplished simply by adding another row to the relevant table (see table 021, Bypass, Heart and Great Vessels) containing two approach values for the non-invasive approach, two device values for the possible types of stent, and a single qualifier.

0: MEDICAL AND SURGICAL **2: HEART AND GREAT VESSELS** **1: BYPASS:** Altering the route of passage of the contents of a tubular body part			
Body Part (Character 4)	**Approach (Character 5)**	**Device (Character 6)**	**Qualifier (Character 7)**
0 Coronary Artery, One Site **1** Coronary Artery, Two Sites **2** Coronary Artery, Three Sites **4** Coronary Artery, Four or More Sites	**3** Percutaneous **4** Percutaneous Endoscopic	**4** Drug-eluting Intraluminal Device **D** Intraluminal Device	**D** Coronary Vein

STRUCTURAL INTEGRITY

As shown in the previous example, ICD-10-PCS can be easily expanded without disrupting the structure of the system.

In the PICVA example, one new value—the qualifier value Coronary Vein—was added to the system to effect this change. All other values in the new row are existing values used to create unique, new codes.

This type of updating can be replicated anywhere in the system when a change is required. ICD-10-PCS allows unique new codes to be added to the system because values for the seven characters that make up a code can be combined as needed. The system can evolve as medical technology and clinical practice evolve, without disrupting the ICD-10-PCS structure.

ICD-10-PCS ADDITIONAL CHARACTERISTICS

ICD-10-PCS possesses several additional characteristics in response to government and industry recommendations. These characteristics are

- Standardized terminology within the coding system
- Standardized level of specificity
- No diagnostic information
- No explicit "not otherwise specified" (NOS) code options
- Limited use of "not elsewhere classified" (NEC) code options

STANDARDIZED TERMINOLOGY

Words commonly used in clinical vocabularies may have multiple meanings. This can cause confusion and result in inaccurate data. ICD-10-PCS is standardized and self-contained. Characters and values used in the system are defined in the system.

For example, the word "excision" is used to describe a wide variety of surgical procedures. In ICD-10-PCS, the word "excision" describes a single, precise surgical objective, defined as "Cutting out or off, without replacement, a portion of a body part."

NO EPONYMS OR COMMON PROCEDURE NAMES

The terminology used in ICD-10-PCS is standardized to provide precise and stable definitions of all procedures performed. This standardized terminology is used in all ICD-10-PCS code descriptions.

As a result, ICD-10-PCS code descriptions do not include eponyms or common procedure names. Two examples from ICD-9-CM are 22.61, "Excision of lesion of maxillary sinus with Caldwell-Luc approach," and 51.10, "Endoscopic retrograde cholangiopancreatography [ERCP]." In ICD-10-PCS, physicians' names are not included in a code description, nor are procedures identified by common terms or acronyms such as appendectomy or CABG. Instead, such procedures are coded to the root operation that accurately identifies the objective of the procedure.

The procedures described in the preceding paragraph by ICD-9-CM codes are coded in ICD-10-PCS according to the root operation that matches the objective of the procedure. Here the ICD-10-PCS equivalents would be Excision and Inspection respectively. By relying on the universal objectives defined in root operations rather than eponyms or specific procedure titles that change or become obsolete, ICD-10-PCS preserves the capacity to define past, present, and future procedures accurately using stable terminology in the form of characters and values.

NO COMBINATION CODES

With rare exceptions, ICD-10-PCS does not define multiple procedures with one code. This is to preserve standardized terminology and consistency across the system. Procedures that are typically performed together but are distinct procedures may be defined by a single "combination code" in ICD-9-CM. An example of a combination code in ICD-9-CM is 28.3, "Tonsillectomy with adenoidectomy."
A procedure that meets the reporting criteria for a separate procedure is coded separately in ICD-10-PCS. This allows the system to respond to changes in technology and medical practice with the maximum degree of stability and flexibility.

STANDARDIZED LEVEL OF SPECIFICITY

In ICD-9-CM, one code with its description and includes notes may encompass a vast number of procedure variations while another code defines a single specific procedure. ICD-10-PCS provides a standardized level of specificity for each code, so that each code represents a single procedure variation.

The ICD-9-CM code 39.31, "Suture of artery," does not specify the artery, whereas the code range 38.40 through 38.49, "Resection of artery with replacement," provides a fourth-digit subclassification for specifying the artery by anatomical region (thoracic, abdominal, etc.).

In ICD-10-PCS, the codes identifying all artery suture and artery replacement procedures possess the same degree of specificity. The ICD-9-CM examples above coded to their ICD-10-PCS equivalents would use the same artery body part values in all codes identifying the respective procedures.

In general, ICD-10-PCS code descriptions are much more specific than their ICD-9-CM counterparts, but sometimes an ICD-10-PCS code description is actually less specific. In most cases this is because the ICD-9-CM code contains diagnosis information. The standardized level of code specificity in ICD-10-PCS cannot always take account of these fluctuations in ICD-9-CM level of specificity. Instead, ICD-10-PCS provides a standardized level of specificity that can be predicted across the system.

DIAGNOSIS INFORMATION EXCLUDED

Another key feature of ICD-10-PCS is that information pertaining to a diagnosis is excluded from the code descriptions.

ICD-9-CM often contains information about the diagnosis in its procedure codes. Adding diagnosis information limits the flexibility and functionality of a procedure coding system. It has the effect of placing a code "off limits" because the diagnosis in the medical record does not match the diagnosis in the procedure code description. The code cannot be used even though the procedural part of the code description precisely matches the procedure performed.

Diagnosis information is not contained in any ICD-10-PCS code. The diagnosis codes, not the procedure codes, will specify the reason the procedure is performed.

NOS CODE OPTIONS RESTRICTED

ICD-9-CM often designates codes as "unspecified" or "not otherwise specified" codes. By contrast, the standardized level of specificity designed into ICD-10-PCS restricts the use of broadly applicable NOS or unspecified code options in the system. A minimal level of specificity is required to construct a valid code.

In ICD-10-PCS, each character defines information about the procedure and all seven characters must contain a specific value obtained from a single row of a table to build a valid code. Even values such as the sixth-character value Z, No Device and the seventh-character value Z, No Qualifier, provide important information about the procedure performed.

LIMITED NEC CODE OPTIONS

ICD-9-CM often designates codes as "not elsewhere classified" or "other specified" versions of a procedure throughout the code set. NEC options are also provided in ICD-10-PCS, but only for specific, limited use.

In the Medical and Surgical section, two significant "not elsewhere classified" options are the root operation value Q, Repair and the device value Y, Other Device.

The root operation Repair is a true NEC value. It is used only when the procedure performed is not one of the other root operations in the Medical and Surgical section.

Other Device, on the other hand, is intended to be used to temporarily define new devices that do not have a specific value assigned, until one can be added to the system. No categories of medical or surgical devices are permanently classified to Other Device.

ICD-10-PCS APPLICATIONS

ICD-10-PCS code structure results in qualities that optimize the performance of the system in electronic applications, and maximize the usefulness of the coded healthcare data. These qualities include:

- Optimal search capability
- Consistent character definitions
- Consistent values wherever possible
- Code readability

Some have argued that, in the world of the electronic health record, the classification system as we know it is outmoded, that classification doesn't matter because a computer is able to find a code with equal ease whether the code has been generated at random or is part of a classification scheme. While this may be true from an IT perspective, assignment of randomly generated code numbers makes it impossible to aggregate data according to related ranges of codes. This is a critical capability for providers, payers, and researchers to make meaningful use of the data.

OPTIMAL SEARCH CAPABILITY

ICD-10-PCS is designed for maximum versatility in the ability to aggregate coded data. Values belonging to the same character as defined in a section or sections can be easily compared, since they occupy the same position in a code. This provides a high degree of flexibility and functionality for data mining.

For example, the body part value 6, Stomach, retains its meaning for all codes in the Medical and Surgical section that define procedures performed on the stomach. Because the body part value is dependent for its meaning on the body system in which it is found, the body system value D, Gastrointestinal, must also be included in the search.

A person wishing to examine data regarding all medical and surgical procedures performed on the stomach could do so simply by searching the code range below.

0D*6***

CONSISTENT CHARACTERS AND VALUES

In the previous example, the value 6 means Stomach only when the body system value is D, Gastrointestinal. In many other cases, values retain their meaning across a much broader range of codes. This provides consistency and readability.

For example, the value 0 in the fifth character defines the approach Open and the value 3 in the fifth character defines the approach Percutaneous across sections 0 through 4 and 7 through 9, where applicable. As a result, all open and percutaneous procedures represented by codes in sections 0-4 and 7-9 can be compared based on a single character—approach—by conducting a query on the code ranges below.

[0 through 4,7 through 9]***0** vs. [0 through 4,7through 9]***3**

Searches can be progressively refined by adding specific values. For example, one could search on a body system value or range of body system values, plus a body part value or range of body part values, plus a root operation value or range of root operation values.

To refine the search above, one could add the body system value for Gastrointestinal and the body part value for Stomach to limit the search to open vs. percutaneous procedures performed on the stomach:

0D*60** vs. 0D*63"

To refine the search even further and limit the comparison to open and percutaneous biopsies of the stomach, one could add the third-character value for the root operation Excision and the seventh-character qualifier Diagnostic, as below.

0DB60*X vs. 0DB63*X

Stability of characters and values across vast ranges of codes provides the maximum degree of functionality and flexibility for the collection and analysis of data. The search capabilities demonstrated above function equally well for all uses of healthcare data: investigating quality of care, resource utilization, risk management, conducting research, determining reimbursement, and many others.

Because the character definition is consistent, and only the individual values assigned to that character differ as needed, meaningful comparisons of data over time can be conducted across a virtually infinite range of procedures.

CODE READABILITY

ICD-10-PCS resembles a language in the sense that it is made up of semi-independent values combined by following the rules of the system, much the way a sentence is formed by combining words and following the rules of grammar and syntax. As with words in their context, the meaning of any single value is a combination of its position in the code and any preceding values on which it may be dependent.

For example, in the Medical and Surgical section, a body part value is always dependent for its meaning on the body system in which it is found. It cannot stand alone as a letter or a number and be meaningful. A fourth-character value of 6 by itself can mean 31 different things, but a fourth-character value of 6 in the context of a second-character value of D means one thing only—Stomach.

On the other hand, a root operation value is not dependent on any character but the section for its meaning, and identifies a single consistent objective wherever the third character is defined as root operation. For example, the third-character value T identifies the root operation Resection in both the Medical and Surgical and Obstetrics sections.

The approach value also identifies a single consistent approach wherever the fifth character is defined as approach. The fifth-character value 3 identifies the approach Percutaneous in the Medical and Surgical section, the Obstetrics section, the Administration section, and others.

The sixth-character device value or seventh-character qualifier value identifies the same device or qualifier in the context of the body system where it is found. Although there may be consistencies across body systems or within whole sections, this is not true in all cases.

Values in their designated context have a precise meaning, like words in a language. As seen in the code example which began this chapter, 0LB50ZZ represents the text description of the specific procedure "Excision of right lower arm and wrist tendon, open approach." Since ICD-10-PCS values in context have a single, precise meaning, a complete, valid code can be read and understood without its accompanying text description, much like one would read a sentence.

ICD-10-PCS PROCEDURES IN THE MEDICAL AND SURGICAL SECTION

This chapter provides reference material for the root operations in the Medical and Surgical section of ICD-10-PCS. The vast majority of codes reported in an inpatient setting are found in this section.

First, a table presents all root operations in the Medical and Surgical section, organized into logical groups. Following the table are definitions of each root operation, presented in the order shown in the table. Material on each root operation includes

- Definition, explanation, and examples of the root operation
- Coding notes as needed
- A representative procedure excerpt for each root operation, followed by the correct code for the procedure. The code is provided in table excerpt format, along with explanatory notes as needed.
- Coding exercises that provide example procedures and their corresponding ICD-10-PCS codes, with explanatory notes as needed

ROOT OPERATION GROUPS

The Medical and Surgical root operations are divided into groups that share similar attributes. These groups, and the root operations in each, are listed in the table below. Subsequent pages of this chapter provide a definition of each root operation in a group.

Root Operation	What Operation Does	Objective Of Procedure	Procedure Site	Example
Excision	Takes out some/all of a body part	Cutting out/off without replacement	Some of a body part	Breast lumpectomy
Resection	Takes out some/all of a body part	Cutting out/off without replacement	All of a body part	Total mastectomy
Detachment	Takes out some/all of a body part	Cutting out/off without replacement	Extremity only, any level	Amputation above elbow
Destruction	Takes out some/all of a body part	Eradicating without replacement	Some/all of a body part	Fulguration of endometrium
Extraction	Takes out some/all of a body part	Pulling out or off without replacement	Some/all of a body part	Suction D & C
Drainage	Takes out solids/fluids/ gases from a body part	Taking/letting out fluids/ gases	Within a body part	Incision and Drainage
Extirpation	Takes out solids/fluids/ gases from a body part	Taking/cutting out solid matter	Within a body part	Thrombectomy
Fragmentation	Takes out solids/fluids/ gases from a body part	Breaking solid matter into pieces	Within a body part	Lithotripsy
Division	Involves cutting or separation only	Cutting into/separating a body part	Within a body part	Neurotomy
Release	Involves cutting or separation only	Freeing a body part from constraint	Around a body part	Adhesiolysis
Transplantation	Puts in/puts back or move some/all of a body part	Putting in a living body part from a person/animal	Some/all of a body part	Kidney transplant
Reattachment	Puts in/puts back or move some/all of a body part	Putting back a detached body part	Some/all of a body part	Reattach severed finger
Transfer	Puts in/puts back or move some/all of a body part	Moving, to function for a similar body part	Some/all of a body part	Skin transfer flap
Reposition	Puts in/puts back or move some/all of a body part	Moving, to normal or other suitable location	Some/all of a body part	Move undescended testicle
Restriction	Alters the diameter/route of a tubular body part	Partially closing orifice/ lumen	Tubular body part	Gastroesophageal fundoplication
Occlusion	Alters the diameter/route of a tubular body part	Completely closing orifice/ lumen	Tubular body part	Fallopian tube ligation
Dilation	Alters the diameter/route of a tubular body part	Expanding orifice/lumen	Tubular body part	Percutaneous transluminal coronary angioplasty (PTCA)

Bypass	Alters the diameter/route of a tubular body part	Altering route of passage	Tubular body part	Coronary artery bypass graft (CABG)
Insertion	Always involve a device	Putting in non-biological device	In/on a body part	Central line insertion
Replacement	Always involve a device	Putting in device that replaces a body part	Some/all of a body part	Total hip replacement
Supplement	Always involve a device	Putting in device that reinforces or augments a body part	In/on a body part	Abdominal wall herniorrhaphy using mesh
Change	Always involve a device	Exchanging device w/out cutting/puncturing	In/on a body part	Drainage tube change
Removal	Always involve a device	Taking out device	In/on a body part	Central line removal
Revision	Always involve a device	Correcting a malfunctioning/displaced device	In/on a body part	Revision of pacemaker insertion
Inspection	Involves examination only	Visual/manual exploration	Some/all of a body part	Diagnostic cystoscopy
Map	Involves examination only	Locating electrical impulses/functional areas	Brain/cardiac conduction mechanism	Cardiac mapping
Repair	Includes other repairs	Restoring body part to its normal structure	Some/all of a body part	Suture laceration
Control	Includes other repairs	Stopping/attempting to stop postprocedural bleed	Anatomical region	Post-prostatectomy bleeding
Fusion	Includes other objectives	Rendering joint immobile	Joint	Spinal fusion
Alteration	Includes other objectives	Modifying body part for cosmetic purposes without affecting function	Some/all of a body part	Face lift
Creation	Includes other objectives	Making new structure for sex change operation	Perineum	Artificial vagina/ penis

ROOT OPERATIONS THAT TAKE OUT SOME OR ALL OF A BODY PART

Five root operations represent procedures for taking out or otherwise eradicating some or all of a body part. These root operations are listed in the table below and described in detail in the pages that follow.

Root Operation	Objective of Procedure	Site of Procedure	Example
Excision	Cutting out/off without replacement	Some of a body part	Breast lumpectomy
Resection	Cutting out/off without replacement	All of a body part	Total mastectomy
Detachment	Cutting out/off without replacement	Extremity only, any level	Amputation above elbow
Destruction	Eradicating without replacement	Some/all of a body part	Fulguration of endometrium
Extraction	Pulling out or off without replacement	Some/all of a body part	Suction D&C

EXCISION—ROOT OPERATION B

Excision **B**	Definition	Cutting out or off, without replacement, a portion of a body part
	Explanation	The qualifier **Diagnostic** is used to identify excision procedures that are biopsies
	Examples	Partial nephrectomy, liver biopsy

Excision is coded when a portion of a body part is cut out or off using a sharp instrument. All root operations that employ cutting to accomplish the objective allow the use of any sharp instrument, including but not limited to

- Scalpel
- Wire
- Scissors
- Bone saw
- Electrocautery tip

CODING NOTE	**BONE MARROW AND ENDOMETRIAL BIOPSIES** are not coded to the root operation excision. They are coded to Extraction, with the qualifier Diagnostic.

Example: Excision of sebaceous cyst (right buttock)

...the patient was brought in the room and placed on the table in jack knife, prone position and a spinal block was used for anesthesia. She was prepped and draped in the usual sterile manner. A digital rectal examination was performed and we did not notice any communication between mass and rectum. The mass was palpated and a radial transverse incision was made over the mass.

Using blunt and sharp dissection the top of the mass was identified and shown to be a sebaceous cyst. The sebaceous cyst was freed from the surrounding tissue using blunt dissection. The entire cyst was removed. Hemostasis was obtained and the skin was closed using 5-0 Dexon interrupted sutures...

Character 1 Section	Character 2 Body System	Character 3 Root Operation	Character 4 Body Part	Character 5 Approach	Character 6 Device	Character 7 Qualifier
Medical and Surgical	Skin	Excision	Buttock	External	No Device	No Qualifier
0	**H**	**B**	**8**	**X**	**Z**	**Z**

RESECTION—ROOT OPERATION T

Resection **T**	Definition	Cutting out or off, without replacement, all of a body part
	Explanation	N/A
	Examples	Total nephrectomy, total lobectomy of lung

Resection is similar to Excision *(seepage 2.9)*, except Resection includes all of a body part, or any subdivision of a body part that has its own body part value in ICD-10-PCS, while Excision includes only a portion of a body part.

CODING NOTE	**LYMPH NODES.** When an entire lymph node chain is cut out, the appropriate root operation is Resection. When a lymph node(s) is cut out, the root operation is Excision.

Example: Right hemicolectomy

...a vertical midline incision was used to enter the abdominal cavity. There was noted to be a mass in the region of the cecum. The mass was easily mobilized and it was felt that a right hemicolectomy was indicated. The right colon was mobilized by incising the white line of Toldt and reflecting colon medially. The loose tissue was taken down bluntly with a hand and adhesions were taken down sharply.

The colon was mobilized to the left end up to the level of the hepatic flexure. The mesentery was incised sharply with a knife and down to the level of the root of the mesentery. The mesentery of the right colon and the distal ileum was then taken down between Kelly's and tied with 2-0 silk, down to the level of the takeoff vessels.

After removing the right colon specimen off the field, a primary anastomosis was planned...

Character 1 Section	Character 2 Body System	Character 3 Root Operation	Character 4 Body Part	Character 5 Approach	Character 6 Device	Character 7 Qualifier
Medical and Surgical	Gastro-intestinal system	Resection	Large Intestine, Right	Open	No Device	No Qualifier
0	**D**	**T**	**F**	**0**	**Z**	**Z**

CODING NOTE	**ANASTOMOTIC.** Adjunct information about the anastomotic technique used to *technique* complete a colectomy procedure (e.g., side to end) is not specified in ICD-10-PCS. Only the specific Excision or Resection code is assigned.

DETACHMENT—ROOT OPERATION 6

Detachment represents a narrow range of procedures; it is used exclusively for amputation procedures.

Detachment 6	Definition	Cutting off all or part of the upper or lower extremities
	Explanation	The body part value is the site of the detachment, with a qualifier if applicable to further specify the level where the extremity was detached
	Examples	Below knee amputation, disarticulation of shoulder

Detachment procedure codes are found only in body systems X Anatomical Regions, Upper Extremities and Y Anatomical Regions, Lower Extremities, because amputations are performed on the extremities, across overlapping body layers, and so could not be coded to a specific musculoskeletal body system such as the bones or joints.

Detachment Qualifiers

The specific qualifiers used for Detachment are dependent on the body part value in the upper and lower extremities body systems. The table below defines the meaning of the qualifiers used in both the upper and lower extremities.

Body Part	Qualifier Value	Definition
Upper arm and upper leg	1	High: Amputation at the proximal portion of the shaft of the humerus or femur
	2	Mid: Amputation at the middle portion of the shaft of the humerus or femur
	3	Low: Amputation at the distal portion of the shaft of the humerus or femur
Hand and foot	0	Complete
	4	Complete 1st Ray
	5	Complete 2nd Ray
	6	Complete 3rd Ray
	7	Complete 4th Ray
	8	Complete 5th Ray
	9	Partial 1st Ray
	B	Partial 2nd Ray
	C	Partial 3rd Ray
	D	Partial 4th Ray
	F	Partial 5th Ray
		Complete: Amputation through the carpometacarpal joint of the hand, or through the tarsal-metatarsal joint of the foot Partial: Amputation anywhere along the shaft or head of the metacarpal bone of the hand, or of the metatarsal bone of the foot
Thumb, finger, or toe	0	Complete: Amputation at the metacarpophalangeal/metatarsal-phalangeal joint
	1	High: Amputation anywhere along the proximal phalanx
	2	Mid: Amputation through the proximal interphalangeal joint or anywhere along the middle phalanx

Character 1 Section	Character 2 Body System	Character 3 Root Operation	Character 4 Body Part	Character 5 Approach	Character 6 Device	Character 7 Qualifier
Medical and Surgical	Lower Extremities	Detachment	Foot, Left	Open	No Device	Partial 5th Ray
0	Y	6	N	0	Z	f

CODING NOTE	QUALIFIER VALUE. The surgeon uses the word "toe" to describe the amputation, but the operative report says he extends the amputation to the midshaft of the fifth metatarsal, which is the foot, so the qualifier is Partial 5th Ray.

ROOT OPERATIONS THAT TAKE OUT SOME OR ALL OF A BODY PART

DESTRUCTION—ROOT OPERATION 5

Destruction 5	Definition	Physical eradication of all or a portion of a body part by the direct use of energy, force or a destructive agent
	Explanation	None of the body part is physically taken out
	Examples	Fulguration of rectal polyp, cautery of skin lesion

Destruction "takes out" a body part in the sense that it obliterates the body part so it is no longer there. This root operation defines a broad range of common procedures, since it can be used anywhere in the body to treat a variety of conditions, including:

- Skin and genital warts
- Nasal and colon polyps
- Esophageal varices
- Endometrial implants
- Nerve lesions

Example: Radiofrequency coagulation of the trigeminal nerve

...The right cheek was infiltrated dermally with Xylocaine, and a small nick in the skin 2.5 cm lateral to the corner of the mouth was performed with an 18 gauge needle. The radiofrequency needle with 2 mm exposed tip was then introduced using the known anatomical landmarks and under lateral fluoroscopy guidance into the foramen ovale.

Confirmation of the placement of the needle was done by the patient grimacing to pain and by the lateral x-ray. The first treatment, 90 seconds in length, was administered with the tip of the needle 3 mm below the clival line at a temperature of 75 degrees C.

The needle was then advanced further to the mid clival line and another treatment of similar strength and duration was also administered. Finally the third and last treatment was administered with the tip of the needle about 3 cm above the line. The needle was removed. The patient tolerated the procedure well...

Character 1 Section	Character 2 Body System	Character 3 Root Operation	Character 4 Body Part	Character 5 Approach	Character 6 Device	Character 7 Qualifier
Medical And Surgical	Central Nervous	Destruction	Trigeminal Nerve	Percutaneous	No Device	No Qualifier
0	**0**	**5**	**K**	**3**	**Z**	**Z**

CODING **NOTE**	**APPROACH VALUE.** The small nick in the skin does not constitute an open approach. it was made to accommodate the radiofrequency needle. The needle was advanced all the way to the operative site, so the correct approach value is Percutaneous.

ROOT OPERATIONS THAT TAKE OUT SOME OR ALL OF A BODY PART

EXTRACTION—ROOT OPERATION D

Extraction **D**	Definition	Pulling or stripping out or off all or a portion of a body part by the use of force
	Explanation	The qualifier Diagnostic is used to identify extraction procedures that are biopsies
	Examples	Dilation and curettage, vein stripping

Extraction is coded when the method employed to take out the body part is pulling or stripping. Minor cutting, such as that used in vein stripping procedures, is included in Extraction if the objective of the procedure is nevertheless met by pulling or stripping. As with all applicable ICD-10-PCS codes, cutting used to reach the procedure site is specified in the approach value.

Example: Suction dilation & curettage

...after induction of general anesthesia the patient was placed in the dorsal lithotomy position and appropriately prepped and draped. Successive dilators were placed until the cervix was adequate for insertion of the suction cannula. Suction cannula was placed and suction curettage performed with no residual endometrial lining. The tissue was sent to pathology to rule out endometrial cancer...

	Character 2 Body System	Character 3 Root Operation	Character 4 Body Part	Character 5 Approach	Character 6 Device	Character 7 Qualifier
Medical and Surgical	Female Reproductive	Extraction	Endometrium	Via Natural/ Artificial Opening	No Device	Diagnostic
0	**U**	**D**	**B**	**7**	**Z**	**X**

ROOT OPERATIONS THAT TAKE OUT SOLIDS/FLUIDS/GASES FROM A BODY PART

The table below lists the root operations that take out solids, fluids, or gases from a body part. Each is described in detail in the pages that follow.

Root Operation	Objective of Procedure	Site of Procedure	Example
Drainage	Taking/letting out fluids/gases	Within a body part	Incision and drainage
Extirpation	Taking/cutting out solid matter	Within a body part	Thrombectomy
Fragmentation	Breaking solid matter into pieces	Within a body part	Lithotripsy

DRAINAGE---ROOT OPERATION 9

Drainage 9	Definition	Taking or letting out fluids and/or gases from a body part
	Explanation	The qualifier Diagnostic is used to identify drainage procedures that are biopsies
	Examples	Thoracentesis, incision and drainage

The root operation Drainage is coded for both diagnostic and therapeutic drainage procedures. When drainage is accomplished by putting in a catheter, the device value Drainage Device is coded in the sixth character.

Example: Urinary nephrostomy catheter placement
...using fluoroscopy and sterile technique a needle was placed through the skin into a markedly dilated right renal collecting system. Guidewire was inserted and an 8 French locking catheter was positioned with the dilated right renal pelvis. It was attached to a bag and immediate drainage of urine was evident...

	Character 2 Body System	Character 3 Root Operation	Character 4 Body Part	Character 5 Approach	Character 6 Device	Character 7 Qualifier
Medical and Surgical	Urinary	Drainage	Kidney Pelvis, Right	Percutaneous	Drainage Device	No Qualifier
0	**T**	**9**	**3**	**3**	**0**	**Z**

ROOT OPERATIONS THAT TAKE OUT SOLIDS/FLUIDS/GASES FROM A BODY PART

EXTIRPATION—ROOT OPERATION C

Extirpation C	Definition	Taking or cutting out solid matter from a body part
	Explanation	The solid matter may be an abnormal byproduct of a biological function or a foreign body; it may be imbedded in a body part or in the lumen of a tubular body part. The solid matter may or may not have been previously broken into pieces.
	Examples	Thrombectomy, endarterectomy, choledocholithotomy

Extirpation represents a range of procedures where the body part itself is not the focus of the procedure. Instead, the objective is to remove solid material such as a foreign body, thrombus, or calculus from the body part.

Example: De-clotting of AV dialysis graft

...the right upper extremity was properly prepped and draped. Local anesthesia was used to explore the graft. A transverse incision in the previous site of the incision, 1 cm below the elbow crease, was performed. The venous limb of the graft was dissected free up to the venous anastomosis. A small incision on the graft was performed. Then a 3 Fogarty catheter was passed on the venous side. The cephalic vein was found obstructed, not on the anastomotic site, but about 4 cm proximal to the anastomosis. A large number of clots were extracted. After the embolectomy a good back flow from the venous side was obtained. Then the embolectomy was performed throughout the limb on the arterial side. More clots were extracted and a good arterial flow was obtained. The procedure was concluded, closing the incision on the graft with 6-0prolene...

	Character 2 Body System	Character 3 Root Operation	Character 4 Body Part	Character 5 Approach	Character 6 Device	Character 7 Qualifier
Medical and Surgical	Upper Veins	Extirpation	Cephalic Vein, Right	Open	No Device	No Qualifier
0	**5**	**C**	**D**	**0**	**Z**	**Z**

CODING NOTE	**BODY PART VALUE.** Do not code separate body parts based on the words "venous side" and "arterial side" in the procedure report. They refer to the two ends of the cephalic vein used to create the fistula.

ROOT OPERATIONS THAT TAKE OUT SOLIDS/FLUIDS/GASES FROM A BODY PART

FRAGMENTATION—ROOT OPERATION F

Fragmentation F	Definition	Breaking solid matter in a body part into pieces
	Explanation	The Physical force (e.g., manual, ultrasonic) applied directly or indirectly is used to break the solid matter into pieces. The solid matter may be an abnormal byproduct of a biological function or a foreign body. The pieces of solid matter are not taken out.
	Examples	Extracorporeal shockwave lithotripsy, transurethral lithotripsy

Fragmentation is coded for procedures to break up, but not remove, solid material such as a calculus or foreign body. This root operation includes both direct and extracorporeal Fragmentation procedures.

Example: ESWL of left kidney

With the patient having been identified, under satisfactory IV sedation and using the MFL 1000 for extracorporeal shock wave lithotripsy, 1000 shocks were delivered to the stone in the lower pole of the left kidney, and 800 shocks were delivered to the stone in the upper pole of the same, with change in shape and density of the stone indicating fragmentation. The patient tolerated the procedure well...

Character 1 Section	Character 2 Body System	Character 3 Root Operation	Character 4 Body Part	Character 5 Approach	Character 6 Device	Character 7 Qualifier
Medical and Surgical	Urinary	Fragment.	Kidney Pelvis, Left	External	No Device	No Qualifier
0	**T**	**F**	**4**	**X**	**Z**	**Z**

ROOT OPERATIONS INVOLVING CUTTING OR SEPARATION ONLY

The table below lists the root operations that cut or separate a body part. Each is described in detail in the pages that follow.

Root Operation	Objective of Procedure	Site of Procedure	Example
Division	Cutting into/separating a body part	Within a body part	Neurotomy
Release	Freeing a body part from constraint	Around a body part	Adhesiolysis

DIVISION---ROOT OPERATION 8

Division	Definition	Cutting into a body part without draining fluids and/or gases from the body part in order to separate or transect a body part
8	Explanation	All or a portion of the body part is separated into two or more portions
	Examples	Spinal cordotomy, osteotomy

The root operation Division is coded when the objective of the procedure is to cut into, transect, or otherwise separate all or a portion of a body part. When the objective is to cut or separate the area around a body part, the attachments to a body part, or between subdivisions of a body part that are causing abnormal constraint, then the root operation Release is coded instead.

Example: Anal sphincterotomy

Manual examination of the rectum and anus was done, and examination showed that the patient has an anterior anal fissure. For that reason, lateral sphincterotomy was done at the 3 o'clock position using the closed approach, dividing only the internal sphincter using the 11 blade...

	Character 2 Body System	Character 3 Root operation	Character 4 Body Part	Character 5 Approach	Character 6 Device	Character 7 Qualifier
Medical and Surgical	Gastro-intestinal System	Division	Anal Sphincter	Percutaneous	No Device	No Qualifier
0	**D**	**8**	**R**	**3**	**Z**	**Z**

CODING NOTE	**APPROACH VALUE.** This is coded to the Percutaneous approach, because the procedure report says that the sphincterotomy was done using the closed approach, dividing only the internal sphincter.

ROOT OPERATIONS INVOLVING CUTTING OR SEPARATION ONLY

RELEASE—ROOT OPERATION N

Release	Definition	Freeing a body part from an abnormal physical constraint by cutting or by use of force
N	Explanation	Some of the restraining tissue may be taken out but none of the body part is taken out
	Examples	Adhesiolysis, carpal tunnel release

The objective of procedures represented in the root operation Release is to free a body part from abnormal constraint. Release procedures are coded to the body part being freed. The procedure can be performed on the area around a body part, on the attachments to a body part, or between subdivisions of a body part that are causing the abnormal constraint.

Example: Release of median nerve

...the right arm was scrubbed with Betadine and prepped and draped in the usual sterile fashion. A well-padded tourniquet was fixed to the right proximal arm but not inflated until after draping. After draping, the right arm was exsanguinated with a combination of elevation and an Esmarch bandage, placing a sponge in the palm. The tourniquet was inflated to 250.

A transverse incision was made at the level of the proximal wrist crease between the palmaris longus and the flexor carpi ulnaris sharply through the skin with a knife, and subcutaneous tissue was dissected by blunt spreading.

The volar fascia was identified and a transverse incision was made sharply with a knife. The flat synovial retractor was pushed through the underneath of the transverse carpal ligament, removing synovium from beneath the ligament.

The entire carpal tunnel and the fat pad distally was visualized. The blade was inserted into the carpal tunnel, was elevated at the distal edge of the transverse carpal ligament, and was pulled proximally, spreading and cutting through the transverse carpal ligament.

It was visualized that the entire median nerve had been released, and that configuration of the end of the transverse carpal ligament was a rectangle, denoting that both the deep and the superficial fibers had been cut.
The wound was then copiously irrigated with saline...

Character 1 Section	Character 2 Body System	Character 3 Root Operation	Character 4 Body Part	Character 5 Approach	Character 6 Device	Character 7 Qualifier
Medical and Surgical	Peripheral Nervous	Release	Median Nerve	Open	No Device	No Qualifier
0	1	N	5	0	Z	Z

CODING NOTE	BODY PART VALUE. The body part value assigned is the structure released and not the structure cut to obtain the release, where the two differ. The transverse carpal ligament was cut to release the median nerve and not for its own sake.

ROOT OPERATIONS THAT PUT IN/PUT BACK OR MOVE SOME/ALL OF A BODY PART

The table below lists the root operations that put in, put back, or move some or all of a body part. Each is described in detail in the pages that follow.

Root Operation	Objective of Procedure	Site of Procedure	Example
Transplantation	Putting in a living body part from a person/ animal	Some/all of a body part	Kidney transplant
Reattachment	Putting back a detached body part	Some/all of a body part	Reattach finger
Transfer	Moving a body part to function for a similar body part	Some/all of a body part	Skin transfer flap
Reposition	Moving a body part to normal or other suitable location	Some/all of a body part	Move undescended testicle

TRANSPLANTATION---ROOT OPERATION Y

Transplantation Y	Definition	Putting in or on all or a portion of a living body part taken from another individual or animal to physically take the place and/or function of all or a portion of a similar body part
	Explanation	The native body part may or may not be taken out, and the transplanted body part may take over all or a portion of its function
	Examples	Kidney transplant, heart transplant

A small number of procedures is represented in the root operation Transplantation and includes only the body parts currently being transplanted. Qualifier values specify the genetic compatibility of the body part transplanted.

Example: Right kidney transplant (syngeneic)

...the abdomen was sterilely prepped and draped in the usual fashion and incision in the right flank, the Gibson technique, performed. In doing so the right pelvis was entered and Book- Walter retractor appropriately positioned to provide exposure of the external iliac artery and vein.

The artery was placed on vessel loop retraction. We then proceeded with the kidney transplant, and the kidney which was trimmed on the back table was brought into the field. The right renal vein was cut short without reconstruction of the inferior vena cava, and single ureter was identified. Kidney was brought up in an ice chest and an end-to-end anastomosis was performed in the usual fashion with 5-0 Prolene between donor renal vein and external iliac vein on the right.

The long renal artery was brought into view, and end-to-side anastomosis performed in the usual fashion with 5-0 Prolene.

We then turned our attention to performing the neoureterocystostomy after appropriate positioning of the graft and evaluation of the vessels.

After the anastomosis was completed there was no evidence of leak. A Blake drain was brought out through a stab incision and the tip of the drain placed near the neoureterocystostomy and both wounds were closed. The infrainguinal wound was closed with running 3-0 Vicryl and the kidney transplant wound was closed with 1 PDS...

Character 1 Section	Character 2 Body System	Character 3 Root Operation	Character 4 Body Part	Character 5 Approach	Character 6 Device	Character 7 Qualifier
Medical and Surgical	Urinary	Transplant.	Kidney, Right	Open	No Device	Syngeneic
0	**T**	**Y**	**0**	**0**	**Z**	**1**

CODING **NOTE**	**BONE MARROW TRANSPLANT PROCEDURES** are coded in section 3 Transplant Administration to the root operation 2 Transfusion.

REATTACHMENT---ROOT OPERATION M

Reattachment **M**	Definition	Putting back in or on all or a portion of a separated body part to its normal location or other suitable location
	Explanation	Vascular circulation and nervous pathways may or may not be reestablished
	Examples	Reattachment of hand, reattachment of avulsed kidney

Procedures coded to Reattachment include putting back a body part that has been cut off or avulsed. Nerves and blood vessels may or may not be reconnected in a Reattachment procedure.

Example: Complex reattachment, left index finger

A sharp debridement of grossly contaminated tissue was carried out. It was noted that the extensor mechanism distal to the PIP joint had been lost. There were circumferential lacerations about the finger, save for a cutaneous bridge and ulnar vascular pedicle present at the PIP level.

Nonviable bony fragments were removed and then the distal portion of the PIP joint was reshaped with removal of cartilage using double- rongeurs. It was noted that the fractures through the proximal phalanx extended longitudinally. Stabilization was then carried out, with 0.062 K-wire brought down through the distal finger, out through the fingertip, and then back into the proximal phalanx centrally.

The A2 pulley was restored, using figure of eight interrupted sutures of 4 and 5-0 Vicryl, reapproximating the flexor tendons. The extensor mechanisms and tendons were repaired using 4 and 5-0 Vicryl, and anchored to the periosteum on the middle phalanx. A digital nerve was then carried out on the radial aspect of the digit at the PIP joint level using interrupted sutures of 9-0 Ethilon beneath the microscope.

At this point, the skin was trimmed, removing skin margins, and then multiple lacerations were closed with 5-0 Prolene...

Character 1 Section	Character 2 Body System	Character 3 Root Operation	Character 4 Body Part	Character 5 Approach	Character 6 Device	Character 7 Qualifier
Medical and Surgical	Upper Extremities	Reattachment	Index Finger, Left	Open	No Device	No Qualifier
0	**X**	**M**	**P**	**0**	**Z**	**Z**

TRANSFER---ROOT OPERATION X

Transfer **X**	Definition	Moving, without taking out, all or a portion of a body part to another location to take over the function of all or a portion of a body part
	Explanation	The body part transferred remains connected to its vascular and nervous supply
	Examples	Tendon transfer, skin pedicle flap transfer

The root operation Transfer is used to represent procedures where a body part is moved to another location without disrupting its vascular and nervous supply. In the body systems that classify the subcutaneous tissue, fascia and muscle body parts, qualifiers can be used to specify when more than one tissue layer was used in the transfer procedure, such as a musculocutaneous flap transfer.

Example: Fasciocutaneous flap from scalp to cheek

...development of the plane of dissection was completed into the superficial temporal fascia.
Development of subgaleal dissection posteriorly was then completed, a distance of 7-8 cm, with hemo- stasis by electrocautery.
The flaps were advanced to the cheek defect and secured with 2-0 inverted PDS sutures and3-0 inverted Monocryl...

	Character 2 Body System	Character 3 Root Operation	Character 4 Body Part	Character 5 Approach	Character 6 Device	Character 7 Qualifier
Medical and Surgical	Subcut Tissue and Fascia	Transfer	Scalp	Open	No Device	Skin, Subcut And Fascia
0	**J**	**X**	**0**	**0**	**Z**	**C**

CODING NOTE	**BODY SYSTEM VALUE.** The body system value describes the deepest tissue layer in the flap. The qualifier can be used to describe the other tissue layers, if any, being transferred.

REPOSITION---ROOT OPERATION S

Reposition **S**	Definition	Moving to its normal location or other suitable location all or a portion of a body part
	Explanation	The body part is moved to a new location from an abnormal location, or from a normal location where it is not functioning correctly. The body part may or may not be cut out or off to be moved to the new location
	Examples	Reposition of undescended testicle, fracture reduction

Reposition represents procedures for moving a body part to a new location. The range of Reposition procedures includes moving a body part to its normal location, or moving a body part to a new location to enhance its ability to function.

Example: Reposition of undescended right testicle from pelvic region to scrotum

...Following satisfactory induction of general anesthesia, an incision was made in the inguinal region and dissection carried down to the pelvic cavity, where the right testis was located and mobilized.
The spermatic cord was located and freed from surrounding tissue, and its length judged to be sufficient.
A one centimeter incision was made in the scrotum and a pouch created in the usual fashion. The right testicle was mobilized down through the inguinal canal into the scrotum, and stitched in place.
Meticulous hemostasis was obtained, and the incisions closed in layers...

Character 1 Section	Character 2 Body System	Character 3 Root Operation	Character 4 Body Part	Character 5 Approach	Character 6 Device	Character 7 Qualifier
Medical and Surgical	Male Reproductive	Reposition	Testis, Right	Open	No Device	No Qualifier
0	**V**	**S**	**9**	**0**	**Z**	**Z**

ROOT OPERATIONS THAT ALTER THE DIAMETER/ROUTE OF A TUBULAR BODY PART

The table below lists the root operations that alter the diameter or route of a tubular body part. Tubular body parts are defined in ICD-10-PCS as those hollow body parts that provide a route of passage for solids, liquids, or gases. They include the cardiovascular system, and body parts such as those contained in the gastrointestinal tract, genitourinary tract, biliary tract, and respiratory tract. Each root operation is described in detail in the pages that follow.

Root Operation	Objective of Procedure	Site of Procedure	Example
Restriction	Partially closing orifice/ lumen	Tubular body part	Gastroesophageal fundoplication
Occlusion	Completely closing orifice/ lumen	Tubular body part	Fallopian tube ligation
Dilation	Expanding orifice/lumen	Tubular body part	Percutaneous transluminal coronary angioplasty (PTCA)
Bypass	Altering route of passage	Tubular body part	Coronary artery bypass graft (CABG)

ROOT OPERATIONS THAT ALTER THE DIAMETER/ROUTE OF A TUBULAR BODY PART

RESTRICTION—ROOT OPERATION V

Restriction	Definition	Partially closing an orifice or the lumen of a tubular body part
V	Explanation	The orifice can be a natural orifice or an artificially created orifice
	Examples	Esophagogastric fundoplication, cervical cerclage

The root operation Restriction is coded when the objective of the procedure is to narrow the diameter of a tubular body part or orifice. Restriction includes both intraluminal or extraluminal methods for narrowing the diameter.

Example: Laparoscopic gastroesophageal fundoplication

...Insufflation was accomplished through a 5 infraumbilical incision. Five separate 5 mm ports were placed under direct visualization other than the initial port. Laparoscopy revealed a large hiatal hernia. Electrocautery was used to free up adhesions from the hernia sac to the stomach.

Next, the fundus which had been mobilized was brought down into the stomach and it was felt there was enough mobilization to perform a fundoplication. A generous loose fundoplication was then performed by wrapping the fundus around the esophagus. Interrupted 0 Ethibond sutures were used to secure the stomach in this fashion.

There was generally good hemostasis throughout the case. All instruments were removed and ports closed.

Character 1 Section	Character 2 Body System	Character 3 Root Operation	Character 4 Body Part	Character 5 Approach	Character 6 Device	Character 7 Qualifier
Medical And Surgical	Gastro-intestinal System	Restriction	Esophago-gastric Junction	Percutaneous Endoscopic	No Device	No Qualifier
0	**D**	**V**	**4**	**4**	**Z**	**Z**

ROOT OPERATIONS THAT ALTER THE DIAMETER/ROUTE OF A TUBULAR BODY PART

OCCLUSION—ROOT OPERATION L

Occlusion	Definition	Completely closing an orifice or the lumen of a tubular body part
L	Explanation	The orifice can be a natural orifice or an artificially created orifice
	Examples	Fallopian tube ligation, ligation of inferior vena cava

The root operation Occlusion is coded when the objective of the procedure is to close off a tubular body part or orifice. Occlusion includes both intraluminal or extraluminal methods of closing off the body part. Division of the tubular body part prior to closing it is an integral part of the Occlusion procedure.

Example: Uterine artery embolization

... catheter was advanced over a 0.18 Terumo gold guidewire and advanced several centimeters super selectively into the left uterine artery. Contrast injection was performed here, confirming filling of the uterine artery and subsequent opacification of large vascular structures in the uterus compatible with uterine fibroids.

A syringe and a half of 500-700 micron biospheres was then instilled slowly through the catheter, and at the conclusion of this infusion there was cessation of flow through the uterine artery.

The catheter was then removed and hemostasis achieved...

Character 1 Section	Character 2 Body System	Character 3 Root Operation	Character 4 Body Part	Character 5 Approach	Character 6 Device	Character 7 Qualifier
Medical And Surgical	Lower Arteries	Occlusion	Internal Iliac Artery, Left	Percutaneous	Intraluminal Device	Uterine Artery, Left
0	**4**	**L**	**F**	**3**	**D**	**U**

ROOT OPERATIONS THAT ALTER THE DIAMETER/ROUTE OF A TUBULAR BODY PART

DILATION—ROOT OPERATION 7

Dilation 7	Definition	Expanding an orifice or the lumen of a tubular body part
	Explanation	The orifice can be a natural orifice or an artificially created orifice. Accomplished by stretching a tubular body part using intraluminal pressure or by cutting part of the orifice or wall of the tubular body part
	Examples	Percutaneous transluminal angioplasty, pyloromyotomy

The root operation Dilation is coded when the objective of the procedure is to enlarge the diameter of a tubular body part or orifice. Dilation includes both intraluminal or extraluminal methods of enlarging the diameter. A device placed to maintain the new diameter is an integral part of the Dilation procedure, and is coded to a sixth-character device value in the Dilation procedure code.

> ### Example: PTCA of left anterior descending
> ...under 1% Lidocaine local anesthesia, the right femoral artery was entered by the Seldinger technique and a 7French sheath was placed. A Judkins left guiding catheter was advanced to the left coronary ostium and using a .014 Entree wire and a 2.5 x 30 mm Panther balloon, it was easily placed across the lesion in the left anterior descending.
>
> The balloon was inflated times two for five minutes for up to 9 atmospheres. Angiography demonstrated an excellent result...

Character 1 Section	Character 2 Body System	Character 3 Root Operation	Character 4 Body Part	Character 5 Approach	Character 6 Device	Character 7 Qualifier
Medical and Surgical	Heart and Great Vessels	Dilation	Coronary Art., One Site	Percutaneous	No Device	No Qualifier
0	**2**	**7**	**0**	**3**	**Z**	**Z**

ROOT OPERATIONS THAT ALTER THE DIAMETER/ROUTE OF A TUBULAR BODY PART

BYPASS—ROOT OPERATION 1

Bypass 1	Definition	Altering the route of passage of the contents of a tubular body part
	Explanation	Rerouting contents of a body part to a downstream area of the normal route, to a similar route and body part, or to an abnormal route and dissimilar body part. Includes one or more anastomoses, with or without the use of a device
	Examples	Coronary artery bypass, colostomy formation

> ### Example: Aorto-bifemoral bypass graft
> ...the patient was prepped and draped, and groin incisions were opened. The common femoral vein and its branches were isolated and Teflon tapes were placed around the vessels.
>
> The aorta and iliacs were mobilized. Bleeding points were controlled with electrocautery and Liga clips. Tapes were placed around the vessel, the vessel measured, and the aorta was found to be 12 mm. A 12 x 7 bifurcated microvelour graft was then preclotted with the patient's own blood.
>
> An end-to-end anastomosis was made on the aorta and the graft using a running suture of 2-0 Prolene. The limbs were taken down through tunnels noting that the ureters were anterior, and at this point an end-to-side anastomosis was made between the graft and the femoral arteries with running suture of 4-0 Prolene.
>
> The inguinal incisions were closed.

Bypass is coded when the objective of the procedure is to reroute the contents of a tubular body part. The range of Bypass procedures includes normal routes such as those made in coronary artery bypass procedures, and abnormal routes such as those made in colostomy formation procedures.

Character 1 Section	Character 2 Body System	Character 3 Root Operation	Character 4 Body Part	Character 5 Approach	Character 6 Device	Character 7 Qualifier
Medical And Surgical	Lower Arteries	Bypass	Abdominal Aorta	Open	Synthetic Substitute	Bilat Femoral Arteries
0	4	1	0	0	J	K

ROOT OPERATIONS THAT ALWAYS INVOLVE A DEVICE

The table below lists the root operations that always involve a device. Each is described in detail in the pages that follow.

Root Operation	Objective of Procedure	Site of Procedure	Example
Insertion	Putting in non-biological device	In/on a body part	Central line insertion
Replacement	Putting in device that replaces a body part	Some/all of a body part	Total hip replacement
Supplement	Putting in device that reinforces or augments a body part	In/on a body part	Abdominal wall herniorrhaphy using mesh
Change	Exchanging device w/out cutting/ puncturing	In/on a body part	Drainage tube change
Removal	Taking out device	In/on a body part	Central line removal
Revision	Correcting a malfunctioning/ displaced device	In/on a body part	Revision of pacemaker insertion

INSERTION---ROOT OPERATION H

Insertion **H**	Definition	Putting in a non-biological device that monitors, assists, performs or prevents a physiological function but does not physically take the place of a body part
	Explanation	N/A
	Examples	Insertion of radioactive implant, insertion of central venous catheter

The root operation Insertion represents those procedures where the sole objective is to put in a device without doing anything else to a body part. Procedures typical of those coded to Insertion include putting in a vascular catheter, a pacemaker lead, or a tissue expander.

Example: Port-a-cath placement

...the right chest and neck were prepped and draped in the usual manner and 10 cc's of 1% Lidocaine were injected in the right infraclavicular area.

The right subclavian vein was then punctured and a wire was passed through the needle into the superior vena cava. This was documented by fluoroscopy. Introducer kit was introduced into the subclavian vein and the Port-a-cath was placed through the introducer and by fluoroscopy was placed down to the superior vena cava.

The pocket was then made over the right pectoralis major muscle, superior to the breast, and the Port-a-cath reservoir was placed into this pocket and tacked down with 0 Prolene sutures.

The catheter was then tunneled through a subcutaneous tunnel to this receptacle. Hemostasis was achieved and the subcutaneous tissue closed.

Character 1 Section	Character 2 Body System	Character 3 Root Operation	Character 4 Body Part	Character 5 Approach	Character 6 Device	Character 7 Qualifier
Medical and Surgical	Heart and Gr. Vessels	Insertion	Superior Vena Cava	Percutaneous	Vascular Access Device	No Qualifier
0	2	H	V	3	X	Z

Character 1 Section	Character 2 Body System	Character 3 Root Operation	Character 4 Body Part	Character 5 Approach	Character 6 Device	Character 7 Qualifier
Medical and Surgical	Subcut Tissue and Fascia	Insertion	Chest	Open	Reservoir	No Qualifier
0	J	H	6	0	W	Z

REPLACEMENT---ROOT OPERATION R

Replacement	Definition	Putting in or on biological or synthetic material that physically takes the place and/or function of all or a portion of a body part
R	Explanation	The body part may have been taken out or replaced, or may be taken out, physically eradicated, or rendered nonfunctional during the Replacement procedure. A Removal procedure is coded for taking out the device used in a previous replacement procedure.
	Examples	Total hip replacement, bone graft, free skin graft

The objective of procedures coded to the root operation Replacement is to put in a device that takes the place of some or all of a body part. Replacement encompasses a wide range of procedures, from joint replacements to grafts of all kinds.

Character 1 Section	Character 2 Body System	Character 3 Root Operation	Character 4 Body Part	Character 5 Approach	Character 6 Device	Character 7 Qualifier
Medical And Surgical	Eye	Replacement	Lens, Left	Percutaneous	Synthetic Substitute	No Qualifier
0	**8**	**R**	**K**	**3**	**J**	**Z**

Example: Prosthetic lens implantation

...a superior peritomy was made on the left eye and adequate hemostasis was achieved using eraser cautery. A posterior one-half thickness groove was placed posterior to the blue line. This was beveled forward toward clear cornea.

The anterior chamber was entered at the 11:30position with a blade. The eye was filled with viscoelastic substance. A can-opener type capsulotomy was performed with a cystotome. Hydrodissection was carried out and the lens was rocked gently with a cystotome to loosen it from the cortex.

The wound was then opened with corneal scleral scissors. The lens was prolapsed in the anterior chamber and removed. The anterior chamber was then temporarily closed with 8-0 Vicryl sutures and cortical clean-up was performed.

One of the sutures was removed and a posterior chamber intraocular lens (Alcon model MZ50BD) was inspected, rinsed, and placed into a capsular bag. Miochol was then instilled into the anterior chamber. The conjunctiva was pulled over the incision and cauterized into place...

SUPPLEMENT---ROOT OPERATION U

Supplement	Definition	Putting in or on biologic or synthetic material that physically reinforces and/ or augments the function a portion of a body part
U	Explanation	The biological material is non-living, or is living and from the same individual. The body part may have been previously replaced, and the Supplement procedure is performed to physically reinforce and/or augment the function of the replaced body part.
	Examples	Herniorrhaphy using mesh, free nerve graft, mitral valve ring annuloplasty, put a new acetabular liner in a previous hip replacement

The objective of procedures coded to the root operation Supplement is to put in a device that reinforces or augments the functions of some or all of a body part. The body part may have been taken out during a previous procedure, but is not taken out as part of the Supplement procedure. Supplement includes a wide range of procedures, from hernia repairs using mesh reinforcement to heart valve annuloplasties and grafts such as nerve grafts that supplement but do not physically take the place of the existing body part.

Example: Posterior colporrhaphy with Gynemesh

...attention was then turned to the posterior wall. Two Allis clamps were placed at the mucocutaneous junction in the region of the fourchette, and another clamp was placed at the apex of the rectocele.

The tissue between the distal clamps and the fourchette was excised, and carefully measured so that the introitus would be a 3-finger introitus The posterior vaginal mucosa was then incised in the midline by sharp and blunt dissection. The mucosa was then dissected to the level at the Allis clamp at the apex of the rectocele, and dissected with blunt and sharp dissection from the underlying tissue. The rectocele was then imbricated using mattress sutures of 2-0 Vicryl, and the area of the levator ani reinforced with Gynemesh.

Two sutures of 2-0 Vicryl were taken in the levator ani muscle, the excess posterior vaginal mucosa excised, and then closed with interrupted sutures of 2-0 Vicryl.

The perineal muscles were then approximated in the midline in layers, using 2-0 Vicryl, after which the perineal skin was approximated using interrupted sutures of 2-0 Vicryl...

Character 1 Section	Character 2 Body System	Character 3 Root Operation	Character 4 Body Part	Character 5 Approach	Character 6 Device	Character 7 Qualifier
Medical and Surgical	Female Reproductive	Supplement	Vagina	Open	Synthetic Substitute	No Qualifier
0	**U**	**U**	**G**	**0**	**J**	**Z**

CHANGE---ROOT OPERATION 2

Change **2**	Definition	Taking out or off a device from a body part and putting back an identical or similar device in or on the same body part without cutting or puncturing the skin or a mucous membrane
	Explanation	All Change procedures are coded using the approach External
	Examples	Urinary catheter change, gastrostomy tube change

The root operation Change represents only those procedures where a similar device is exchanged without making a new incision or puncture. Typical Change procedures include exchange of drainage devices and feeding devices.

CODING NOTE	**CHANGE.** In the root operation Change, general body part values are used when the specific body part value is not in the table

Example: Percutaneous endoscopic gastrostomy (PEG) tube exchange

Character 1 Section	Character 2 Body System	Character 3 Root Operation	Character 4 Body Part	Character 5 Approach	Character 6 Device	Character 7 Qualifier
Medical and Surgical	Gastro-intestinal System	Change	Upper Intestinal Tract	External	Feeding Device	No Qualifier
0	**D**	**2**	**0**	**X**	**U**	**Z**

ROOT OPERATIONS THAT ALWAYS INVOLVE A DEVICE

REMOVAL—ROOT OPERATION P

Removal **P**	Definition	Taking out or off a device from a body part
	Explanation	If a device is taken out and a similar device put in without cutting or puncturing the skin or mucous membrane, the procedure is coded to the root operation Change. Otherwise, the procedure for taking out a device is coded to the root operation Removal.
	Examples	Drainage tube removal, cardiac pacemaker removal

Removal represents a much broader range of procedures than those for removing the devices contained in the root operation Insertion. A procedure to remove a device is coded to Removal if it is not an integral part of another root operation, and regardless of the approach or the original root operation by which the device was put in.

CODING NOTE	REMOVAL. In the root operation Removal, general body part values are used when the specific body part value is not in the table.

Example: Removal of right forearm external fixator

...the right upper extremity was prepped and draped in a sterile fashion. A tourniquet was placed at 250 mm of pressure.

The external fixator was removed using the appropriate wrench. The four pins in the ulna were then removed manually, as well as with the drill. The wounds were irrigated with antibiotic solution and a sterile dressing applied...

Character 1 Section	Character 2 Body System	Character 3 Root Operation	Character 4 Body Part	Character 5 Approach	Character 6 Device	Character 7 Qualifier
Medical and Surgical	Upper Bones	Removal	Ulna, Right	External	External Fixation	No Qualifier
0	**P**	**P**	**K**	**X**	**5**	**Z**

ROOT OPERATIONS THAT ALWAYS INVOLVE A DEVICE

REVISION—ROOT OPERATION W

Revision W	Definition	Correcting, to the extent possible, a malfunctioning or displaced device
	Explanation	Revision can include correcting a malfunctioning device by taking out and/or putting in part of the device
	Examples	Adjustment of pacemaker lead, adjustment of hip prosthesis

Revision is coded when the objective of the procedure is to correct the position or function of a previously placed device, without taking the entire device out and putting a whole new device in its place. A complete re-do of a procedure is coded to the root operation performed.

CODING NOTE	REVISION. In the root operation Revision, general body part values are used when the specific body part value is not in the table.

Example: Revision of artificial anal sphincter

...Proceeding through a suprapubic incision, this was then extended after injecting local anesthetic, thereby exposing the underlying tubing, which was then delivered through the suprapubic region.

Meticulous hemostasis was achieved using electrocautery. At that point the pump device was then repositioned in the left lower quadrant abdominal wall region. The tubing was reinserted using dilators, and the skin reapproximated using 2-0 Vicryl sutures. Sterile dressing was then applied...

Character 1 Section	Character 2 Body System	Character 3 Root Operation	Character 4 Body Part	Character 5 Approach	Character 6 Device	Character 7 Qualifier
Medical and Surgical	Gastrointestinal System	Revision	Anus	Open	Artificial Sphincter	No Qualifier
0	**D**	**W**	**Q**	**0**	**L**	**Z**

ROOT OPERATIONS INVOLVING EXAMINATION ONLY

The table below lists the root operations that involve examination of a body part. Each is described in detail in the pages that follow.

Root operation	Objective of Procedure	Site of Procedure	Example
Inspection	Visual/manual exploration	Some/all of a body part	Diagnostic cystoscopy
Map	Location electrical impulses/ functional areas	Brain/cardiac conduction mechanism	Cardiac mapping

ROOT OPERATIONS INVOLVING EXAMINATION ONLY

INSPECTION—ROOT OPERATION J

Inspection	Definition	Visually and/or Manually Exploring A Body Part
J	Explanation	Visual Exploration May Be Performed With Or Without Optical Instrumentation. Manual Exploration May Be Performed Directly Or Through Intervening Body Layers
	Examples	Diagnostic Arthroscopy, Exploratory Laparotomy

The root operation Inspection represents procedures where the sole objective is to examine a body part. Procedures that are discontinued without any other root operation being performed are also coded to Inspection.

Example: *Diagnostic colposcopy with examination of cervix*
...Colposcopy was done which revealed pseudo-white areas at 2 o'clock and 6o'clock on the cervix, with abnormal cells and irregular white borders noted on both...

Character 1 Section	Character 2 Body System	Character 3 Root Operation	Character 4 Body Part	Character 5 Approach	Character 6 Device	Character 7 Qualifier
Medical And Surgical	Female Reproductive	Inspection	Uterus And Cervix	Via Natural/ Artificial Opening Endo	No Device	No Qualifier
0	**U**	**J**	**D**	**8**	**Z**	**Z**

MAP---ROOT OPERATION K

Map	Definition	Locating the route of passage of electrical impulses and/or locating functional areas in a body part
K	Explanation	Applicable only to the cardiac conduction mechanism and the central nervous system
	Examples	Cardiac mapping, cortical mapping

Mapping represents a very narrow range of procedures. Procedures include only cardiac mapping and cortical mapping.

Example: *Cardiac mapping*
. ..under sterile technique arterial sheath was placed in the right femoral artery. The electrical catheter was advanced up the aorta and into the left atrium under fluoroscopic guidance and mapping commenced. After adequate recordings were obtained the catheter was withdrawn and hemostasis achieved with manual pressure on the right femoral artery...

Character 1 Section	Character 2 Body System	Character 3 Root Operation	Character 4 Body Part	Character 5 Approach	Character 6 Device	Character 7 Qualifier
Medical and Surgical	Heart & Great Vessels	Map	Conduction Mechanism	Percutaneous	No Device	No Qualifier
0	**2**	**K**	**8**	**3**	**Z**	**Z**

ROOT OPERATIONS THAT DEFINE OTHER REPAIRS

The table below lists the root operations that define other repairs. CONTROL describes the effort to locate and stop

Root Operation	Objective of Procedure	Site of Procedure	Example
Control	Stopping/attempting to stop postprocedural bleed	Anatomical region	Post-prostatectomy bleeding control
Repair	Restoring body part to its normal structure	Some/all of a body part	Suture laceration

postprocedural hemorrhage. Repair is described in detail in the pages that follow.

CONTROL---ROOT OPERATION 3

Control	Definition	Stopping, or attempting to stop, postprocedural bleeding
3	Explanation	The site of the bleeding is coded as an anatomical region and not to a specific body part
	Examples	Control of post-prostatectomy hemorrhage, control of post-tonsillectomy hemorrhage

CONTROL is used to represent a small range of procedures performed to treat postprocedural bleeding. If performing Bypass, Detachment, Excision, Extraction, Reposition, Replacement, or Resection is required to stop the bleeding, then Control is not coded separately.

CODING NOTE	CONTROL includes irrigation or evacuation of hematoma done at the operative site. Both irrigation and evacuation may be necessary to clear the operative field and effectively stop the bleeding.

Example: Re-opening of laparotomy site with ligation of arterial bleeder

Character 1 Section	Character 2 Body System	Character 3 Root Operation	Character 4 Body Part	Character 5 Approach	Character 6 Device	Character 7 Qualifier
Medical and Surgical	Anatomical Regions, Gen.	Control	Peritoneal Cavity	Open	No Device	No Qualifier
0	**W**	**3**	**g**	**0**	**Z**	**Z**

ROOT OPERATIONS THAT DEFINE OTHER REPAIRS

REPAIR—ROOT OPERATION Q

Repair Q	Definition	Restoring, to the extent possible, a body part to its normal anatomic structure and function
	Explanation	Used only when the method to accomplish the repair is not one of the other root operations
	Examples	Herniorrhaphy, suture of laceration

The root operation Repair represents a broad range of procedures for restoring the anatomic structure of a body part such as suture of lacerations. Repair also functions as the "not elsewhere classified (NEC)" root operation, to be used when the procedure performed does not meet the definition of one of the other root operations. Fixation devices are included for procedures to repair the bones and joints.

> ## Example: Left open inguinal herniorrhaphy
> *...an incision in the left groin extending on the skin from the internal to the external inguinal ring was made. The external oblique aponeurosis was exposed.*
>
> *The hernia sac was then ligated at the internal ring with non-dissolving sutures. A hernia repair was then performed. The internal oblique fascia was sutured in interrupted stitches to the ilio-pubic fascia. The spermatic cord was then returned to its anatomical position.*
>
> *The external oblique aponeurosis was then repaired in interrupted sutures. Complete hemostasis was obtained, and the skin closed...*

Character 1 Section	Character 2 Body System	Character 3 Root Operation	Character 4 Body Part	Character 5 Approach	Character 6 Device	Character 7 Qualifier
Medical and Surgical	Lower Extremities	Repair	Inguinal Region, Left	Open	No Device	No Qualifier
0	**Y**	**Q**	**6**	**0**	**Z**	**Z**

ROOT OPERATIONS THAT DEFINE OTHER OBJECTIVES

The last three root operations in the Medical and Surgical section, Fusion, Alteration, and Creation, describe procedures performed for three distinct reasons. Beyond that they have little in common. A Fusion procedure puts a dysfunctional joint out of service rather than restoring function to the joint. Alteration encompasses a whole range of procedures that share only the fact that they are done to improve the way the patient looks. Creation represents only two very specific sex change operations.

Root operation	Objective of procedure	Site of procedure	Example
Fusion	Rendering joint immobile	Joint	Spinal fusion
Alteration	Modifying body part for cosmetic purposes without affecting function	Some/all of a body part	Face lift
Creation	Making new structure for sex change operation	Perineum	Artificial vagina/penis

FUSION---ROOT OPERATION G

Fusion **G**	Definition	Joining together portions of an articular body part rendering the articular body part immobile
	Explanation	The body part is joined together by fixation device, bone graft, or other means
	Examples	Spinal fusion, ankle arthrodesis

A limited range of procedures is represented in the root operation Fusion, because fusion procedures are by definition only performed on the joints. Qualifier values are used to specify whether a vertebral joint fusion uses an anterior or posterior approach, and whether the anterior or posterior column of the spine is fused.

> ### Example: Anterior cervical fusion C-2 through C-4 with bone bank graft
>
> ...after skull tong traction was applied, incision was made in the left neck, and Gardner retractors placed to separate the intervertebral muscles at the C-2 through C-4 levels.
>
> Using the drill, a trough was incised on the anterior surface of the C-2 vertebra, and the C-2/C-3 space evacuated with a rongeur, and the accompanying cartilage removed. This procedure was then repeated at the C-3/C-4 level.
>
> Bone bank patella strut graft was trimmed with a saw and fashioned to fit the C-2/C-3 interspace. After adequate adjustments in the size and shape had been made, the graft was tapped securely into place. The procedure was repeated for the C-3/C-4 level.
>
> X-rays revealed good alignment and final position. Traction was gradually decreased to maintain position. Retractors were removed and the fascia was reapproximated with 0 Vicryl...

Character 1 Section	Character 2 Body System	Character 3 Root Operation	Character 4 Body part	Character 5 Approach	Character 6 Device	Character 7 Qualifier
Medical and Surgical	Upper Joints	Fusion	Cervical Joint, 2 or More	OPEN	Nonautologous Tissue Substance	Ant Approach Ant Column
0	**R**	**G**	**2**	**0**	**K**	**0**

ALTERATION---ROOT OPERATION 0

Alteration **0**	Definition	Modifying the natural anatomic structure of a body part without affecting the function of the body part
	Explanation	Principal purpose is to improve appearance
	Examples	Face lift, breast augmentation

Alteration is coded for all procedures performed solely to improve appearance. All methods, approaches, and devices used for the objective of improving appearance are coded here.

CODING NOTE	**ALTERATION.** Because some surgical procedures can be performed for either medical or cosmetic purposes, coding for Alteration requires diagnostic confirmation that the surgery is in fact performed to improve appearance.

Example: Cosmetic blepharoplasty
...attention was turned to the redundant upper eyelid skin. The ellipse of skin as marked preoperatively was excised bilaterally.
The medial and lateral fat compartments were open bilaterally. The medial compartment had severe fatty excess and periorbital fat herniation. This was resected. The lateral fat compartment was opened and the lateral fat tailored as well. Subdermal closure was performed with interrupted 3-0 sutures bilaterally. The skin was closed.

Character 1 Section	Character 2 Body System	Character 3 Root Operation	Character 4 Body Part	Character 5 Approach	Character 6 Device	Character 7 Qualifier
Medical And Surgical	Eye	Alteration	Upper Eyelid, Left	Open	No Device	No Qualifier
0	8	0	P	0	Z	Z

Character 1 Section	Character 2 Body System	Character 3 Root Operation	Character 4 Body Part	Character 5 Approach	Character 6 Device	Character 7 Qualifier
Medical And Surgical	Eye	Alteration	Upper Eyelid, Right	Open	No Device	No Qualifier
0	8	0	N	0	Z	Z

CREATION---ROOT OPERATION 4

Creation	Definition	Making a new genital structure that does not physically take the place of a body part
4	Explanation	Used only for sex change operations
	Examples	Creation of vagina in a male, creation of penis in a female

Creation is used to represent a very narrow range of procedures. Only the procedures performed for sex change operations are included here.

CODING NOTE	**HARVESTING.** If a separate procedure is performed to harvest autograft tissue, *autograft tissue* it is coded to the appropriate root operation in addition to the primary procedure.

Example: Creating a vagina in a male patient using autograft

Character 1 Section	Character 2 Body System	Character 3 Root Operation	Character 4 Body Part	Character 5 Approach	Character 6 Device	Character 7 Qualifier
Medical and Surgical	Anatomical Regions, Gen.	Creation	Perineum, Male	Open	Autologous Tissue Subst.	Vagina
0	W	4	M	0	7	0

ICD-10-PCS PROCEDURES IN THE MEDICAL AND SURGICAL-RELATED SECTIONS

This chapter provides reference material for procedure codes in sections 1 through 9 of ICD-10-PCS. These nine sections define procedures related to the Medical and Surgical section. Codes in these sections contain characters not previously defined, such as substance, function, and method.

First, a table is provided, listing the sections in order. Following the table, reference material is provided for each section, and includes

- General description of the section
- A table listing each root operation in the section, with its corresponding definition
- Coding notes as needed
- Representative examples of procedures coded in that section, in table excerpt format, with explanatory notes as needed
- Coding exercises that provide example procedures and their corresponding ICD-10-PCS codes, with explanatory notes as needed

LIST OF MEDICAL AND SURGICAL-RELATED SECTIONS OF ICD-10-PCS

Nine additional sections of ICD-10-PCS include procedures related to the Medical and Surgical section, such as obstetrical procedures, administration of substances, and extracorporeal procedures.

Section Value	Description
1	Obstetrics
2	Placement
3	Administration
4	Measurement and Monitoring
5	Extracorporeal Assistance and Performance
6	Extracorporeal Therapies
7	Osteopathic
8	Other Procedures
9	Chiropractic

OBSTETRICS—SECTION 1

The Obstetrics section follows the same conventions established in the Medical and Surgical section, with all seven characters retaining the same meaning, as shown in this example of a low forceps extraction.

Character 1 Section	Character 2 Body System	Character 3 Root Operation	Character 4 Body Part	Character 5 Approach	Character 6 Device	Character 7 Qualifier
Obstetrics	Pregnancy	Extraction	Products of Conception	Via Nat./Artificial Opening	No Device	Low Forceps
1	**0**	**D**	**0**	**7**	**Z**	**3**

ROOT OPERATIONS

There are twelve root operations in the Obstetrics section. Ten of these are also found in the Medical and Surgical section.

The two root operations unique to Obstetrics are defined below.

Value	Description	Definition
A	Abortion	Artificially terminating a pregnancy
E	Delivery	Assisting the passage of the products of conception from the genital canal

CODING NOTE	ABORTION is subdivided according to whether an additional device such as a laminaria or abortifacient is used, or whether the abortion was performed by mechanical means.
	If either a laminaria or abortifacient is used, then the approach is Via Natural or Artificial Opening. All other abortion procedures are those done by mechanical means (the products of conception are physically removed using instrumentation), and the device value is Z, No Device.

Example: Transvaginal abortion using vacuum aspiration technique

	Character 2 Body System	Character 3 Root Operation	Character 4 Body Part	Character 5 Approach	Character 6 Device	Character 7 Qualifier
Obstetrics	Pregnancy	Abortion	Products Of Conception	Via Nat/Artificial Opening	No Device	Vacuum
1	**0**	**A**	**0**	**7**	**Z**	**6**

CODING NOTE	DELIVERY applies only to manually-assisted, vaginal delivery and is defined as assisting the passage of the products of conception from the genital canal. Cesarean deliveries are coded in this section to the root operation Extraction.

Example: Manually-assisted delivery

	Character 2 Body System	Character 3 Root Operation	Character 4 Body Part	Character 5 Approach	Character 6 Device	Character 7 Qualifier
Obstetrics	Pregnancy	Delivery	Products Of Conception	External	No Device	No Qualifier
1	**0**	**E**	**0**	**X**	**Z**	**Z**

OTHER OBSTETRICS CODING EXAMPLES

Procedure	Code
Abortion by dilation and evacuation following laminaria insertion	10A07ZW
Manually assisted spontaneous abortion	10E0XZZ Since the pregnancy was not artificially terminated, this is coded to DELIVERY, because it captures the procedure objective. The fact that it was an abortion will be identified in the diagnosis code.
Abortion by abortifacient insertion	10A07ZX
Bimanual pregnancy examination	10J07ZZ
Extraperitoneal c-section, low transverse incision	10D00Z2
Fetal spinal tap, percutaneous	10903ZA
Fetal kidney transplant, laparoscopic	10Y04ZS
Open in utero repair of congenital diaphragmatic hernia	10Q00ZK Diaphragm is classified to the RESPIRATORY body system in the MEDICAL AND SURGICAL section.
Laparoscopy with total excision of tubal pregnancy	10T24ZZ
Transvaginal removal of fetal monitoring electrode	10P073Z

PLACEMENT—SECTION 2

The Placement section follows the same conventions established in the Medical and Surgical section, with all seven characters retaining the same meaning, as in the example of cast change on the right forearm below.

	Character 2 Body System	Character 3 Root Operation	Character 4 Body Part	Character 5 Approach	Character 6 Device	Character 7 Qualifier
Placement	Anatomical Regions	Change	Lower Arm, Right	External	Cast	No Qualifier
2	**W**	**0**	**C**	**X**	**2**	**Z**

ROOT OPERATIONS

The root operations in the Placement section include only those procedures performed without making an incision or a puncture.

Value	Description	Definition
0	Change	Taking out or off a device from a body region and putting back an identical or similar device in or on the same body region without cutting or puncturing the skin or a mucous membrane
1	Compression	Putting pressure on a body region
2	Dressing	Putting material on a body region for protection
3	Immobilization	Limiting or preventing motion of a body region
4	Packing	Putting material in a body region
5	Removal	Taking out or off a device from a body region
6	Traction	Exerting a pulling force on a body region in a distal direction

Example: Change of vaginal packing

Character 1 Section	Character 2 Body System	Character 3 Root Operation	Character 4 Body Part	Character 5 Approach	Character 6 Device	Character 7
Placement	Anatomical Orifices	Change	Female Genital Tract	External	Packing Material	No Qualifier
2	**Y**	**0**	**4**	**X**	**5**	**Z**

Example: Placement of pressure dressing on abdominal wall

	Character 2 Body System	Character 3 Root operation	Character 4 Body Region	Character 5 Approach	Character 6 Device	Character 7 Qualifier
Placement	Anatomical Regions	Compression	Abdominal Wall	External	Pressure Dressing	No Qualifier
2	**W**	**1**	**3**	**X**	**6**	**Z**

Example: Application of sterile dressing to head wound

Character 1 Section	Character 2 Body System	Character 3 Root operation	Character 4 Body Region	Character 5 Approach	Character 6 Device	Character 7 Qualifier
Placement	Anatomical Regions	Dressing	Head	External	Bandage	No Qualifier
2	**W**	**2**	**0**	**X**	**4**	**Z**

CODING NOTE	**IMMOBILIZATION:** The procedures to fit a device, such as splints and braces, as described in F0DZ6EZ and F0DZ7EZ, apply only to the rehabilitation setting. splints and braces placed in other inpatient settings are coded to Immobilization, table 2X3 in the Placement section.

Example: Placement of splint on left finger

	Character 2 Body System	Character 3 Root operation	Character 4 Body Region	Character 5 Approach	Character 6 Device	Character 7 Qualifier
Placement	Anatomical Regions	Immobilization	Finger, Left	External	Splint	No Qualifier
2	**W**	**3**	**K**	**X**	**1**	**Z**

Example: Placement of nasal packing

Character 1 Section	Character 2 Body System	Character 3 Root operation	Character 4 Body Region	Character 5 Approach	Character 6 Device	Character 7 Qualifier
Placement	Anatomical Orifices	Packing	Nasal	External	Packing Material	No Qualifier
2	**Y**	**4**	**1**	**X**	**5**	**Z**

Example: Removal of stereotactic head frame

Character 1 Section	Character 2 Body System	Character 3 Root operation	Character 4 Body Region	Character 5 Approach	Character 6 Device	Character 7 Qualifier
Placement	Anatomical Regions	Removal	Head	External	Stereotactic Apparatus	No Qualifier
2	**W**	**5**	**0**	**X**	**8**	**Z**

CODING NOTE	TRACTION in this section includes only the task performed using a mechanical traction apparatus. Manual traction performed by a physical therapist is coded to Manual Therapy Techniques in section F, Physical Rehabilitation and Diagnostic Audiology.

Example: Lumbar traction using motorized split-traction table

	Character 2 Body System	Character 3 Root Operation	Character 4 Body Part	Character 5 Approach	Character 6 Device	Character 7 Qualifier
Placement	Anatomical Regions	Traction	Back	External	Traction Apparatus	No Qualifier
2	**W**	**6**	**5**	**X**	**0**	**Z**

OTHER PLACEMENT CODING EXAMPLES

Procedure	Code
Placement of packing material, right ear	2Y42X5Z
Mechanical traction of entire left leg	2W6MX0Z
Removal of splint, right shoulder	2W5AX1Z
Placement of neck brace	2W32X3Z
Change of vaginal packing	2Y04X5Z
Packing of wound, chest wall	2W44X5Z
Sterile dressing placement to left groin region	2W27X4Z
Removal of packing material from pharynx	2Y50X5Z
Placement of intermittent pneumatic compression device, covering entire right arm	2W18X7Z
Exchange of pressure dressing to left thigh	2W0PX6Z

ADMINISTRATION—SECTION 3

The Administration section includes infusions, injections, and transfusions, as well as other related procedures, such as irrigation and tattooing. All codes in this section define procedures where a diagnostic or therapeutic substance is given to the patient, as in the platelet transfusion example below.

	Character 2 Body System	Character 3 Root Operation	Character 4 Body System	Character 5 Approach	Character 6 Substance	Character 7 Qualifier
Administration	Circulatory	Transfusion	Central Vein	Percutaneous	Platelets	Non-auto logous
3	**0**	**2**	**4**	**3**	**R**	**1**

ROOT OPERATIONS

Root operations in this section are classified according to the broad category of substance administered. If the substance given is a blood product or a cleansing substance, then the procedure is coded to Transfusion and Irrigation respectively. All the other substances administered, such as anti-neoplastic substances, are coded to the root operation Introduction.

Value	Description	Definition
0	Introduction	Putting in or on a therapeutic, diagnostic, nutritional, physiological, or prophylactic substance except blood or blood products
1	Irrigation	Putting in or on a cleansing substance
2	Transfusion	Putting in blood or blood products

Example: Nerve block injection to median nerve

Character 1 Section	Character 2 Body System	Character 3 Root operation	Character 4 Body System	Character 5 Approach	Character 6 Substance	Character 7 Qualifier
Administration	Phys. Sys. & Anat. Regions	Introduction	Peripheral Nerves	Percutaneous	Regional Anesthetic	No Qualifier
3	**E**	**0**	**T**	**3**	**C**	**Z**

Example: Flushing of eye

Character 1 Section	Character 2 Body System	Character 3 Root operation	Character 4 Body System	Character 5 Approach	Character 6 Substance	Character 7 Qualifier
Administration	Phys. Sys. & Anat. Regions	Irrigation	Eye	External	Irrigating Substance	No Qualifier
3	**E**	**1**	**C**	**X**	**8**	**Z**

Example: Transfusion of cell saver red cells into central venous line

Character 1 Section	Character 2 Body System	Character 3 Root operation	Character 4 Body System	Character 5 Approach	Character 6 Substance	Character 7 Qualifier
Administration	Circulatory	Transfusion	Central Vein	Percutaneous	Red Blood Cells	Autologous
3	**0**	**2**	**4**	**3**	**N**	**0**

OTHER ADMINISTRATION CODING EXAMPLES

Procedure	Code
Peritoneal dialysis via indwelling catheter	3E1M39Z
Transvaginal artificial insemination	3E0P7LZ
Infusion of total parenteral nutrition via central venous catheter	3E0436Z
Esophagogastroscopy with Botox injection into esophageal sphincter	3E0G8GC Botulinum toxin is a paralyzing agent with temporary effects; it does not sclerose or destroy the nerve.
Percutaneous irrigation of knee joint	3E1U38Z
Epidural injection of mixed steroid and local anesthetic for pain control	3E0S33Z This is coded to the substance value ANTI-INFLAMMATORY. The anesthetic is only added to lessen the pain of the injection.
Chemical pleurodesis using injection of tetracycline	3E0L3TZ
Transfusion of antihemophilic factor, (nonautologous) via arterial central line	30263V1
Transabdominal in-vitro fertilization, implantation of donor ovum	3E0P3Q1

| Autologous bone marrow transplant via central venous line | 30243G0 |
| Implantation of anti-microbial envelope with cardiac defibrillator placement, open | 3E0102A |

MEASUREMENT AND MONITORING—SECTION 4

There are two root operations in this section, and they differ in only one respect: Measurement defines one procedure and Monitoring defines a series of procedures.

ROOT OPERATIONS

Measurement describes a single level taken, while Monitoring describes a series of levels obtained at intervals. For example,

- A single temperature reading is considered Measurement.
- Temperature taken every half hour for 8 hours is considered Monitoring. Instead of defining a device, the sixth character defines the physiological or physical function being tested.

Value	Description	Definition
0	Measurement	Determining the level of a physiological or physical function at a point in time
1	Monitoring	Determining the level of a physiological or physical function repetitively over a period of time

Example: External electrocardiogram (EKG), single reading

Character 1 Section	Character 2 Body System	Character 3 Root Operation	Character 4 Body System	Character 5 Approach	Character 6 Function	Character 7 Qualifier
Measurement & Monitoring	Physiological Systems	Measurement	Cardiac	External	Electrical Activity	No Qualifier
4	A	0	2	X	4	Z

Example: Urinary pressure monitoring

Character 1 Section	Character 2 Body System	Character 3 Root operation	Character 4 Body System	Character 5 Approach	Character 6 Device	Character 7 Qualifier
Measurement & Monitoring	Physiological Systems	Monitoring	Urinary	Via Nat./Artificial Opening	Pressure	No Qualifier
4	A	1	D	7	B	Z

OTHER MEASURING AND MONITORING CODING EXAMPLES

Procedure	Code
Cardiac stress test, single measurement	4A02XM4
EGD with biliary flow measurement	4A0C85Z
Right and left heart cardiac catheterization with bilateral sampling and pressure measurements	4A023N8
Peripheral venous pulse, external, single measurement	4A04XJ1
Holter monitoring	4A12X45
Respiratory rate, external, single measurement	4A09XCZ
Fetal heart rate monitoring, transvaginal	4A1H7CZ
Visual mobility test, single measurement	4A07X7Z
Pulmonary artery wedge pressure monitoring from Swan-Ganz catheter	4A133B3
Olfactory acuity test, single measurement	4A08X0Z

EXTRACORPOREAL ASSISTANCE AND PERFORMANCE— SECTION 5

This section includes procedures performed in a critical care setting, such as mechanical ventilation and cardioversion. It also includes other procedures, such as hemodialysis and hyper- baric oxygen treatment. These procedures all use equipment to support a physiological function in some way, whether it is breathing, circulating the blood, or restoring the natural rhythm of the heart.

The fifth and sixth characters in this section define duration and function respectively. These characters describe the duration of the procedure and the body function being acted upon, rather than the approach and device used.

Root operations

Assistance and Performance are two variations of the same kinds of procedures, varying only in the degree of control exercised over the physiological function.

Value	Description	Definition
0	Assistance	Taking over a portion of a physiological function by extracorporeal means
1	Performance	Completely taking over a physiological function by extracorporeal means
2	Restoration	Returning, or attempting to return, a physiological function to its original state by extracorporeal means

CODING NOTE	**ASSISTANCE** defines procedures that support a physiological function but do not take complete control of it, such as intra-aortic balloon pump to support cardiac output and hyperbaric oxygen treatment.

Example: Hyperbaric oxygenation of wound

Character 1 Section	Character 2 Body System	Character 3 Root Operation	Character 4 Body System	Character 5 Duration	Character 6 Function	Character 7 Qualifier
Extracorporeal Assistance & Performance	Physiological Systems	Assistance	Circulatory	Intermittent	Oxygenation	Hyperbaric
5	**A**	**0**	**5**	**1**	**2**	

CODING NOTE	**PERFORMANCE** defines procedures where complete control is exercised over a physiological function, such as total mechanical ventilation, cardiac pacing, and cardiopulmonary bypass.

Example: Cardiopulmonary bypass in conjunction with CABG

Character 1 Section	Character 2 Body System	Character 3 Root Operation	Character 4 Body System	Character 5 Duration	Character 6 Function	Character 7 Qualifier
Extracorporeal Assistance & Performance	Physiological Systems	Performance	Cardiac	Continuous	Output	No Qualifier
5	**A**	**1**	**2**	**2**	**1**	**Z**

Character 1 Section	Character 2 Body System	Character 3 Root Operation	Character 4 Body System	Character 5 Duration	Character 6 Function	Character 7 Qualifier
Extracorporeal Assistance & Performance	Physiological Systems	Performance	Respiratory	Less Than 24 Consecutive Hrs	Ventilation	No Qualifier
5	**A**	**1**	**9**	**3**	**5**	**Z**

CODING NOTE	RESTORATION defines only external cardioversion and defibrillation procedures. Failed cardioversion procedures are also included in the definition of Restoration, and are coded the same as successful procedures.

Example: Attempted cardiac defibrillation, unsuccessful

Character 1 Section	Character 2 Body System	Character 3 Root Operation	Character 4 Body System	Character 5 Duration	Character 6 Function	Character 7 Qualifier
Extracorporeal Assist. And Performance	Physiological Systems	Restoration	Cardiac	Single	Rhythm	No Qualifier
5	**A**	**2**	**2**	**0**	**4**	**Z**

OTHER EXTRACORPOREAL ASSISTANCE AND PERFORMANCE CODING EXAMPLES

Procedure	Code
Intermittent mechanical ventilation, 16 hours	5A1935Z
Liver dialysis, single encounter	5A1C00Z
Cardiac countershock with successful conversion to sinus rhythm	5A2204Z
IPPB (intermittent positive pressure breathing) for mobilization of secretions, 22 hours	5A09358
Renal dialysis, series of encounters	5A1D60Z
IABP (intra-aortic balloon pump) continuous	5A02210 The procedure to insert the balloon pump is coded to the root operation INSERTION in the MEDICAL AND SURGICAL section.
Intra-operative cardiac pacing, continuous	5A1223Z
ECMO (extracorporeal membrane oxygenation), continuous	5A15223
Controlled mechanical ventilation (CMV), 45 hours	5A1945Z The endotracheal tube associated with the mechanical ventilation procedure is considered a component of the equipment used in performing the procedure and is not coded separately.
Pulsatile compression boot with intermittent inflation	5A02115 This is coded to the function value CARDIAC OUTPUT, because the purpose of such compression devices is to return blood to the heart faster

EXTRACORPOREAL THERAPIES—SECTION 6

Section 6, Extracorporeal Therapies, describes other extracorporeal procedures that are not defined by Assistance and Performance in section 5 *(see page 3 16)*. Examples are bili-lite phototherapy, apheresis, and whole body hypothermia.

The second character contains a single general body system choice, Physiological Systems, as in the phototherapy example below. The sixth character is defined as a qualifier, but contains no specific qualifier values. The seventh-character qualifier identifies various blood components separated out in pheresis procedures.

Character 1 Section	Character 2 Body System	Character 3 Root Operation	Character 4 Body System	Character 5 Duration	Character 6 Function	Character 7 Qualifier
Extracorporeal Therapies	Physiological Systems	Phototherapy	Skin	Single	No Qualifier	No Qualifier
6	A	6	0	0	Z	Z

ROOT OPERATIONS

The meaning of each root operation is consistent with the term as used in the medical community. Decompression and Hyperthermia have a more specialized meaning. All are defined in the table below.

Value	Description	Definition
0	Atmospheric Control	Extracorporeal control of atmospheric pressure and composition
1	Decompression	Extracorporeal elimination of undissolved gas from body fluids
2	Electromagnetic Therapy	Extracorporeal treatment by electromagnetic rays
3	Hyperthermia	Extracorporeal raising of body temperature
4	Hypothermia	Extracorporeal lowering of body temperature
5	Pheresis	Extracorporeal separation of blood products
6	Phototherapy	Extracorporeal treatment by light rays
7	ultrasound Therapy	Extracorporeal treatment by ultrasound
8	Ultraviolet Light Therapy	Extracorporeal treatment by ultraviolet light
9	Shock Wave Therapy	Extracorporeal treatment by shock waves

CODING NOTE	**DECOMPRESSION** describes a single type of procedure—treatment for decompression sickness (the bends) in a hyperbaric chamber.

Example: Hyperbaric decompression treatment, single

Character 1 Body System	Character 2 Root Operation	Character 3 Body System	Character 4 Duration	Character 5 Qualifier	Character 6 Qualifier	Character 7 Qualifier
Extracorporeal Therapies	Physiological Systems	Decomp-ression	Circulatory	Single	No Qualifier	No Qualifier
6	A	1	5	0	Z	Z

CODING NOTE	**HYPERTHERMIA** is used both to treat temperature imbalance, and as an adjunct radiation treatment for cancer. When performed to treat temperature imbalance, the procedure is coded to this section. When performed for cancer treatment, whole-body hyperthermia is classified as a modality qualifier in section D, Radiation Oncology.

Example: Whole body hypothermia treatment for temperature imbalance, series

	Character 2 Body System	Character 3 Root Operation	Character 4 Body System	Character 5 Duration	Character 6 Qualifier	Character 7 Qualifier
Extracorporeal Therapies	Physiological Systems	Hypothermia	None	Multiple	No Qualifier	No Qualifier
6	A	4	Z	1	Z	Z

CODING NOTE	**PHERESIS** is used in medical practice for two main purposes: to treat diseases where too much of a blood component is produced, such as leukemia, or to remove a blood product such as platelets from a donor, for transfusion into a patient who needs them.

Example: Therapeutic leukapheresis, single treatment

Character 1 Section	Character 2 Body System	Character 3 Root Operation	Character 4 Body System	Character 5 Duration	Character 6 Qualifier	Character 7 Qualifier
Extracorporeal Therapies	Physiological Systems	Pheresis	Circulatory	Single	No Qualifier	Leukocytes
6	**A**	**5**	**5**	**0**	**Z**	**1**

Example: Phototherapy of circulatory system, series treatment

Character 1 Section	Character 2 Body System	Character 3 Root Operation	Character 4 Body System	Character 5 Duration	Character 6 Qualifier	Character 7 Qualifier
Extracorporeal Therapies	Physiological Systems	Phototherapy	Circulatory	Multiple	No Qualifier	No Qualifier
6	**A**	**6**	**5**	**1**	**Z**	**Z**

Example: Ultraviolet Light Phototherapy, Series Treatment

Character 1 Section	Character 2 Body System	Character 3 Root Operation	Character 4 Body System	Character 5 Duration	Character 6 Qualifier	Character 7 Qualifier
Extracorporeal Therapies	Physiological Systems	UV Light Phototherapy	Skin	Multiple	No Qualifier	No Qualifier
6	**A**	**8**	**0**	**1**	**Z**	**Z**

OTHER EXTRACORPOREAL THERAPIES CODING EXAMPLES

Procedure	Code
Donor thrombocytapheresis, single encounter	6A550Z2
Bili-lite UV phototherapy, series treatment	6A801ZZ
Whole body hypothermia, single treatment	6A4Z0ZZ
Circulatory phototherapy, single encounter	6A650ZZ
Shock wave therapy of plantar fascia, single treatment	6A930ZZ
Antigen-free air conditioning, series treatment	6A0Z1ZZ
TMS (transcranial magnetic stimulation), series treatment	6A221ZZ
Therapeutic ultrasound of peripheral vessels, single treatment	6A750ZZ
Plasmapheresis, series treatment	6A551Z3
Extracorporeal electromagnetic stimulation (EMS) for urinary incontinence, single treatment	6A210ZZ

OSTEOPATHIC—SECTION 7

Section 7, Osteopathic, is one of the smallest sections in ICD-10-PCS. There is a single body system, Anatomical Regions, and a single root operation, Treatment.

The sixth-character methods such as Lymphatic Pump and Fascial Release are not explicitly defined in ICD-10-PCS, and rely on the standard definitions as used in this specialty.

Value	Description	Definition
0	Treatment	Manual treatment to eliminate or alleviate somatic dysfunction and related disorders

Example: Fascial release of abdomen, osteopathic treatment

	Character 2 Body System	Character 3 Operation	Character 4 Body Region	Character 5 Approach	Character 6 Method	Character 7 Qualifier
Osteopathic	Anatomical Regions	Treatment	Abdomen	External	Fascial Release	No Qualifier
7	W	0	9	X	1	Z

Example: General osteopathic mobilization of legs

Character 1 Section	Character 2 Body System	Character 3 Operation	Character 4 Body Region	Character 5 Approach	Character 6 Method	Character 7
Osteopathic	Anatomical Regions	Treatment	Lower Extremities	External	General Mobilization	No Qualifier
7	W	0	6	X	2	Z

OTHER OSTEOPATHIC CODING EXAMPLES

PROCEDURES	CODE
Isotonic muscle energy treatment of right leg	7W06X8Z
Low velocity-high amplitude osteopathic treatment of head	7W00X5Z
Lymphatic pump osteopathic treatment of left axilla	7W07X6Z
Indirect osteopathic treatment of sacrum	7W04X4Z
Articulatory osteopathic treatment of cervical region	7W01X0Z

OTHER PROCEDURES—SECTION 8

The Other Procedures section contains codes for procedures not included in the other medical and surgical-related sections A single root operation, Other Procedures, is defined below.

Value	Description	Definition
0	Other Procedures	Methodologies which attempt to remediate or cure a disorder or disease

There are relatively few procedure codes in this section, for nontraditional, whole body therapies including acupuncture and meditation. There is also a code for the fertilization portion of an in-vitro fertilization procedure.

Example: Acupuncture

	Character 2 Body System	Character 3 Root Operation	Character 4 Body Region	Character 5 Approach	Character 6 Method	Character 7 Qualifier
Other Procedures	Phys. Sys. & Anat. Regions	Other Procedures	Integumentary Sys. & Breast	Percutaneous	Acupuncture	No Qualifier
8	E	0	H	3	0	Z

Example: Yoga therapy

Character 1 Section	Character 2 Body System	Character 3 Root Operation	Character 4 Body Region	Character 5 Approach	Character 6 Method	Character 7 Qualifier
Other Procedures	Phys. Sys. & Anat. Regions	Other Procedures	None	External	Other Method	Yoga Therapy
8	E	0	Z	X	Y	4

OTHER PROCEDURES CODING EXAMPLES

Procedure	Code
Near infrared spectroscopy of leg vessels	8E023DZ
CT computer assisted sinus surgery	8E09XBG The primary procedure is coded separately.
Suture removal, abdominal wall	8E0WXY8
Isolation after infectious disease exposure	8E0ZXY6
Robotic assisted open prostatectomy	8E0W0CZ The primary procedure is coded separately.

CHIROPRACTIC—SECTION 9

The Chiropractic section consists of a single body system, Anatomical Regions, and a single root operation, Manipulation, defined below.

Value	Description	Definition
B	Manipulation	Manual procedure that involves a directed thrust to move a joint past the physiological range of motion, without exceeding the anatomical limit

Example: Chiropractic treatment of cervical spine, short lever specific contact

	Character 2 Body System	Character 3 Root Operation	Character 4 Body Region	Character 5 Approach	Character 6 Method	Character 7 Qualifier
Chiropractic	Anatomical Regions	Manipulation	Cervical	External	Short Lever Sp. Contact	No Qualifier
9	**W**	**B**	**1**	**X**	**H**	**Z**

Example: Non-manual chiropractic manipulation of pelvis

Character 1 Section	Character 2 Body System	Character 3 Root Operation	Character 4 Body Region	Character 5 Approach	Character 6 Method	Character 7 Qualifier
Chiropractic	Anatomical Regions	Manipulation	Pelvis	External	Non-Manual	No Qualifier
9	**W**	**B**	**5**	**X**	**B**	**Z**

OTHER CHIROPRACTIC CODING EXAMPLES

Procedure	Code
Chiropractic treatment of lumbar region using long lever specific contact	9WB3XGZ
Chiropractic manipulation of abdominal region, indirect visceral	9WB9XCZ
Chiropractic extra-articular treatment of hip region	9WB6XDZ
Chiropractic treatment of sacrum using long and short lever specific contact	9WB4XJZ
Mechanically-assisted chiropractic manipulation of head	9WB0XKZ

PROCEDURES IN THE ANCILLARY SECTIONS

This section provides reference material for procedure codes in the six ancillary sections of ICD-10-PCS (B through D, F through H). Codes in these sections contain characters not previously defined, such as contrast, modality qualifier and equipment.

First, a table is provided, listing the sections in order. Following the table, reference material is provided for each section, and includes

- General description of the section
- A table listing each root type in the section, with its corresponding definition (sections B, C and F only)
- Coding notes as needed
- Representative examples of procedures coded in that section, in table excerpt format, with explanatory notes as needed
- Coding exercises that provide example procedures and their corresponding ICD-10-PCS codes, with explanatory notes as needed

LIST OF ANCILLARY SECTIONS IN ICD-10-PCS

Six ancillary sections of ICD-10-PCS include procedures such as imaging, radiation oncology, and rehabilitation.

Section Value	Description
B	Imaging
C	Nuclear Medicine
D	Radiation Oncology
F	Physical Rehabilitation and Diagnostic Audiology
G	Mental Health
H	Substance Abuse Treatment

IMAGING—SECTION B

Imaging follows the same conventions established in the Medical and Surgical section (*see chapter* 2), for the section, body system, and body part characters. However, the third and fourth characters introduce definitions not used in previous sections.

- Third character defines procedure by root type, instead of root operation.
- Fifth character defines contrast if used.
- Sixth character is a qualifier that specifies an image taken without contrast followed by one with contrast.
- Seventh character is a qualifier that is not specified in this section.

ROOT TYPES

The Imaging root types are defined in the following table.

Value	Description	Definition
0	Plain Radiography	Planar display of an image developed from the capture of external ionizing radiation on photographic or photoconductive plate
1	Fluoroscopy	Single plane or bi-plane real time display of an image developed from the capture of external ionizing radiation on a fluorescent screen. The image may also be stored by either digital or analog means
2	Computerized Tomography (CT scan)	Computer reformatted digital display of multiplanar images developed from the capture of multiple exposures of external ionizing radiation
3	Magnetic Resonance Imaging (MRI)	Computer reformatted digital display of multiplanar images developed from the capture of radio-frequency signals emitted by nuclei in a body site excited within a magnetic field
4	Ultrasonography	Real time display of images of anatomy or flow information developed from the capture of reflected and attenuated high frequency sound waves

Example: X-ray of right clavicle, limited study

Character 1 Section	Character 2 Body System	Character 3 Root Type	Character 4 Body Part	Character 5 Contrast	Character 6 Qualifier	Character 7 Qualifier
Imaging	Veins	Fluoroscopy	Dialysis Shunt/Fistula	Other Contrast	None	None
B	**5**	**1**	**W**	**Y**	**Z**	**Z**

Example: CT of brain without contrast followed by high osmolar contrast

Character 1 Section	Character 2 Body System	Character 3 Root Type	Character 4 Body Part	Character 5 Contrast	Character 6 Qualifier	Character 7 Qualifier
Imaging	Central Nervous	Computerized Tomography	Brain	High Osmolar	Unenhanced and Enhanced	None
B	**0**	**2**	**0**	**0**	**0**	**Z**

Example: MRI of liver using Gadoteridol

Character 1 Section	Character 2 Body System	Character 3 Root Type	Character 4 Body Part	Character 5 Contrast	Character 6 Qualifier	Character 7 Qualifier
Imaging	Hepatobiliary & Pancreas	Magnetic Resonance Imaging	Liver	Other Contrast	None	None
B	**F**	**3**	**5**	**Y**	**Z**	**Z**

Example: Ultrasound of prostate gland

Character 1 Section	Character 2 Body System	Character 3 Root Type	Character 4 Body Part	Character 5 Contrast	Character 6 Qualifier	Character 7 Qualifier
Imaging	Male Reproductive	Ultrasonography	Prostate and Seminal Vesicles	None	None	None
B	**V**	**4**	**9**	**Z**	**Z**	**Z**

Example: X-ray of right clavicle, limited study

Character 1 Section	Character 2 Body System	Character 3 Root Type	Character 4 Body Part	Character 5 Contrast	Character 6 Qualifier	Character 7 Qualifier
Imaging	Non-axial Upper Bones	Plain Radiography	Clavicle, Right	None	None	None
B	**P**	**0**	**4**	**Z**	**Z**	**Z**

OTHER IMAGING CODING EXAMPLES

Procedure	Code
Non-contrast CT of abdomen and pelvis	BW21ZZZ
Intravascular ultrasound, left subclavian artery	B342ZZ3
Fluoroscopic guidance for insertion of central venous catheter in SVC, low osmolar contrast	B5181ZA
Endoluminal ultrasound of gallbladder and bile ducts	BF43ZZZ
Left ventriculography using low osmolar contrast	B2151ZZ
Esophageal videofluoroscopy study with oral barium contrast	BD11YZZ
Portable X-ray study of right radius/ulna shaft, standard series	BP0JZZZ
Routine fetal ultrasound, second trimester twin gestation	BY4DZZZ
CT scan of bilateral lungs, high osmolar contrast with densitometry	BB240ZZ
Fluoroscopic guidance for percutaneous transluminal angioplasty (PTA) of left common femoral artery, low osmolar contrast	B41G1ZZ

NUCLEAR MEDICINE—SECTION C

Nuclear Medicine is organized like the Imaging section *(see page 4.5).* The only significant difference is that the fifth character defines the radionuclide instead of the contrast material used in the procedure, as described below.

- The fifth character specifies the radionuclide, the radiation source used in the procedure. Choices are applicable for the root procedure type.
- The sixth and seventh characters are qualifiers, and are not specified in this section.

ROOT TYPES

The third character classifies the procedure by root type instead of by root operation.

Value	Description	Definition
1	Planar Nuclear Medicine Imaging	Introduction of radioactive materials into the body for single plane display of images developed from the capture of radioactive emissions
2	Tomographic (Tomo) Nuclear Medicine Imaging	Introduction of radioactive materials into the body for three-dimensional display of images developed from the capture of radioactive emissions
3	Positron Emission Tomography (PET)	Introduction of radioactive materials into the body for three-dimensional display of images developed from the simultaneous capture, 180 degrees apart, of radioactive emissions
4	Nonimaging Nuclear Medicine Uptake	Introduction of radioactive materials into the body for measurements of organ function, from the detection of radioactive emissions
5	Nonimaging Nuclear Medicine Probe	Introduction of radioactive materials into the body for the study of distribution and fate of certain substances by the detection of radioactive emissions from an external source
6	Nonimaging Nuclear medicine Assay	Introduction of radioactive materials into the body for the study of body fluids and blood elements, by the detection of radioactive emissions
7	Systemic Nuclear Medicine Therapy	Introduction of unsealed radioactive materials into the body for treatment

Example: Adenosine sestamibi (technetium) planar scan of heart muscle at rest

Character 1 Section	Character 2 Body System	Character 3 Root Type	Character 4 Body Part	Character 5 Radionuclide	Character 6 Qualifier.	Character 7 Qualifier
Nuclear Medicine	Heart	Planar Nuclear Imaging	Myocardium	Technetium 99m	None	None
C	**2**	**1**	**G**	**1**	**Z**	**Z**

Example: Technetium tomo scan of liver

Character 1 Section	Character 2 Body System	Character 3 Root Type	Character 4 Body Part	Character 5 Radionuclide	Character 6 Qualifier	Character 7 Qualifier
Nuclear Medicine	Hepatobiliary And Pancreas	Tomo Nuclear Imaging	Liver	Technetium 99M	None	None
C	**F**	**2**	**5**	**1**	**Z**	**Z**

OTHER NUCLEAR MEDICINE CODING EXAMPLES

Procedure	Code
Tomo scan of right and left heart, unspecified radiopharmaceutical, qualitative gated rest	C226YZZ
Technetium pentetate assay of kidneys, ureters, and bladder	CT631ZZ
Uniplanar scan of spine using technetium oxidronate, with first pass study	CP151ZZ
Thallous chloride tomographic scan of bilateral breasts	CH22SZZ
PET scan of myocardium using rubidium	C23GQZZ
Gallium citrate scan of head and neck, single plane imaging	CW1BLZZ
Xenon gas non-imaging probe of brain	C050VZZ

Upper GI scan, radiopharmaceutical unspecified, for gastric emptying	CD15YZZ
Carbon 11 PET scan of brain with quantification	C030BZZ
Iodinated albumin nuclear medicine assay, blood plasma volume study	C763HZZ

RADIATION ONCOLOGY—SECTION D

Radiation Oncology contains the radiation procedures performed for cancer treatment. Character meanings are described below.

- Third character defines root type, which is the basic modality.
- Fifth character further specifies treatment modality.
- Sixth character defines the radioactive isotope used, if applicable.
- Seventh character is a qualifier, and is not specified in this section.

ROOT TYPE

The third character defines the treatment modality as root type.

Examples are Brachytherapy and Stereotactic Radiosurgery. Four different root types are used in this section, as listed in the table below.

Value	Description
0	Beam Radiation
1	Brachytherapy
2	Stereotactic Radiosurgery
Y	Other Radiation

Example: LDR Brachytherapy of cervix using Iridium 192

Character 1 Section	Character 2 Body System	Character 3 Root Type	Character 4 Body part	Character 5 Modal. Qualifier	Character 6 isotope	Character 7 Qualifier
Radiation Oncology	Female Reproductive	Brachytherapy	Cervix	LDR Brachy-therapy	Iridium 192	None
D	**U**	**1**	**1**	**B**	**8**	**Z**

Example: Intraoperative radiation therapy (IORT) of bladder

Character 1 Section	Character 2 Body Sys	Character 3 Root Type	Character 4 Body part	Character 5 Modal. Qualifier	Character 6 isotope	Character 7 Qualifier
Radiation Oncology	Urinary System	Other Radiation	Bladder	IORT	None	None
D	**T**	**Y**	**2**	**C**	**Z**	**Z**

OTHER RADIATION ONCOLOGY CODING EXAMPLES

Procedure	Code
Plaque radiation of left eye, single port	D8Y0FZZ
8 MeV photon beam radiation to brain	D0011ZZ
IORT of colon, 3 ports	DDY5CZZ
HDR Brachytherapy of prostate using Palladium 103	DV109BZ
Electron radiation treatment of right breast, custom device	DM013ZZ
Hyperthermia oncology treatment of pelvic region	DWY68ZZ
Contact radiation of tongue	D9Y57ZZ

Heavy particle radiation treatment of pancreas, four risk sites	DF034ZZ
LDR brachytherapy to spinal cord using iodine	D016B9Z
Whole body Phosphorus 32 administration with risk to hematopoietic system	DWY5GFZ

PHYSICAL REHABILITATION AND DIAGNOSTIC AUDIOLOGY—SECTION F

Physical Rehabilitation and Diagnostic Audiology contains character definitions unlike the other sections in ICD-10-PCS. The following table defines the special character definitions:

Value	Description	Definition
0	Speech Assessment	Measurement of speech and related functions
1	Motor and/or Nerve Function Assessment	Measurement of motor, nerve, and related functions
2	Activities of Daily Living Assessment	Measurement of functional level for activities of daily living
3	Hearing Assessment	Measurement of hearing and related functions
4	Hearing Aid Assessment	Measurement of the appropriateness and/or effectiveness of a hearing device
5	Vestibular Assessment	Measurement of the vestibular system and related functions
6	Speech Treatment	Application of techniques to improve, augment, or compensate for speech and related functional impairment
7	Motor Treatment	Exercise or activities to increase or facilitate motor function
8	Activities of Daily Living Treatment	Exercise or activities to facilitate functional competence for activities of daily living
9	Hearing Treatment	Application of techniques to improve, augment, or compensate for hearing and related functional impairment
B	Hearing Aid Treatment	Application of techniques to improve the communication abilities of individuals with cochlear implant
C	Vestibular Treatment	Application of techniques to improve, augment, or compensate for vestibular and related functional impairment
D	Device Fitting	Fitting of a device designed to facilitate or support achievement of a higher level of function
F	Caregiver Training	Training in activities to support patient's optimal level of function

- Second character is a section qualifier that specifies whether the procedure is a rehabilitation or diagnostic audiology procedure.
- Third character defines the general procedure root type.
- Fourth character defines the body system and body region combined, where applicable
- Fifth character further specifies the procedure type.
- Sixth character specifies the equipment used, if any.

ROOT TYPES

This section uses the third character to classify procedures into 14 root types. They are defined in the table below.

CODING NOTE	TREATMENT procedures include swallowing dysfunction exercises, bathing and showering techniques, wound management, gait training, and a host of activities typically associated with rehabilitation.

Example: Wound care treatment of left calf ulcer using pulsatile lavage

Character 1 Section	Character 2 Section Qualifier	Character 3 Root Type	Character 4 Body System & Region	Character 5 Type Qualifier	Character 6 Equipment	Character 7 Qualifier
Rehabilitation & Diagnostic Audiology	Rehabilitation	Activities Of Daily Living Treatment	Musculoskeletal Lower Extremity	Wound Management	Physical Agents	None
F	**0**	**8**	**L**	**5**	**B**	**Z**

CODING NOTE	ASSESSMENTS are further classified into more than 100 different tests or methods. The majority of these focus on the faculties of hearing and speech, but others focus on various aspects of body function, and on the patient's quality of life, such as muscle performance, neuromotor development, and reintegration skills.

Example: Articulation and phonology assessment using spectrograph

Character 1 Section	Character 2 Section Qualifier	Character 3 Root Type	Character 4 Body System & Region	Character 5 Type Qualifier	Character 6 Equipment	Character 7 Qualifier
Rehabilitation & Diagnostic Audiology	Rehabilitation	Speech Assessment	None	Articulation/ Phonology	Speech Analysis	None
F	0	0	Z	9	Q	Z

CODING NOTE	DEVICE FITTING. The fifth character used in Device Fitting describes the device being fitted rather than the method used to fit the device. Detailed descriptions of the devices are provided in the reference materials, the table specific to Device Fitting.

Example: Individual fitting of moveable brace, right knee

Character 1 Section	Character 2 Section Qualifier	Character 3 Root Type	Character 4 Body System & Region	Character 5 Type Qualifier	Character 6 Equipment	Character 7 Qualifier
Rehabilitation & Diagnostic Audiology	Rehabilitation	Device Fitting	None	Dynamic Orthosis	Orthosis	None
F	0	D	Z	6	E	Z

CODING NOTE	CAREGIVER TRAINING is divided into eighteen different broad subjects taught to help a caregiver provide proper patient care.

Example: Caregiver training in feeding, no special equipment used

Character 1 Section	Character 2 Section Qualifier	Character 3 Root Type	Character 4 Body System & Region	Character 5 Type Qualifier	Character 6 Equipment	Character 7 Qualifier
Rehabilitation & Diagnostic Audiology	Rehabilitation	Caregiver Training	None	Feeding and Eating	None	None
F	0	F	Z	2	Z	Z

OTHER PHYSICAL REHABILITATION AND DIAGNOSTIC AUDIOLOGY CODING EXAMPLES

Procedure	Code
Bekesy assessment using audiometer	F13Z31Z
Individual fitting of left eye prosthesis	F0DZ8UZ
Physical therapy for range of motion and mobility, patient right hip, no special equipment	F07L0ZZ
Bedside swallow assessment using assessment kit	F00ZHYZ
Caregiver training in airway clearance techniques	F0FZ8ZZ
Application of short arm cast in rehabilitation setting	F0DZ7EZ Inhibitory cast is listed in the equipment reference table under E, ORTHOSIS.
Verbal assessment of patient's pain level	F02ZFZZ

Caregiver training in communication skills using manual communication board	F0FZJMZ Manual communication board is listed in the equipment reference table under M, AUGMENTATIVE/ALTERNATIVE COMMUNICATION.
Group musculoskeletal balance training exercises, whole body, no special equipment	F07M6ZZ Balance training is included in the MOTOR TREATMENT reference table under THERAPEUTIC EXERCISE.
Individual therapy for auditory processing using tape recorder	F09Z2KZ Tape recorder is listed in the equipment reference table under AUDIOVISUAL EQUIPMENT.

MENTAL HEALTH—SECTION G

Mental Health contains specific values in the third and fourth characters to describe mental health procedures. The remaining characters function as placeholders only. Character meanings are described below.

- Third character describes the mental health procedure root type.
- Fourth character further specifies the procedure type as needed.
- Second, fifth, sixth, and seventh characters do not convey specific information about the procedure. The value Z functions as a placeholder in these characters.

ROOT TYPE

The third character describes the mental health root type. There are 11 root type values in this section, as listed in the table below.

Value	Description
1	Psychological Tests
2	Crisis Intervention
5	Individual Psychotherapy
6	Counseling
7	Family Psychotherapy
B	Electroconvulsive Therapy
C	Biofeedback
F	Hypnosis
G	Narcosynthesis
H	Group Therapy
J	Light Therapy

Example: Galvanic skin response (GSR) biofeedback

Character 1 Section	Character 2 Body System	Character 3 Root Type	Character 4 Type Qualifier	Character 5 Qualifier	Character 6 Qualifier	Character 7 Qualifier
Mental Health	None	Biofeedback	Other Biofeedback	None	None	None
G	**Z**	**C**	**9**	**Z**	**Z**	**Z**

Procedure	Code
Cognitive-behavioral psychotherapy, individual	GZ58ZZZ
Narcosynthesis	GZGZZZZ
Light therapy	GZJZZZZ
ECT (Electroconvulsive therapy), unilateral, multiple seizure	GZB1ZZZ
Crisis intervention	GZ2ZZZZ
Neuropsychological testing	GZ13ZZZ
Hypnosis	GZFZZZZ

Developmental testing	GZ10ZZZ
Vocational counseling	GZ61ZZZ
Family psychotherapy	GZ72ZZZ

SUBSTANCE ABUSE TREATMENT—SECTION H

Substance Abuse Treatment is structured like a smaller version of the Mental Health section. Character meanings are described below.

- Third character describes the root type.
- Fourth character is a qualifier that further classifies the root type
- Second, fifth, sixth, and seventh characters do not convey specific information about the procedure. The value Z functions as a placeholder in these characters.

ROOT TYPES

There are seven different root type values classified in this section, as listed in the following table.

Value	Description
2	Detoxification Services
3	Individual Counseling
4	Group Counseling
5	Individual Psychotherapy
6	Family Counseling
8	Medication Management
9	Pharmacotherapy

Example: Pharmacotherapy treatment with Antabuse for alcohol addiction

Character 1 Section	Character 2 Body System	Character 3 Root Type	Character 4 Type Qualifier	Character 5 Qualifier	Character 6 Qualifier	Character 7 Qualifier
Substance Abuse Treatment	None	Pharmaco-therapy	Antabuse	None	None	None
H	**Z**	**9**	**3**	**Z**	**Z**	**Z**

OTHER SUBSTANCE ABUSE CODING EXAMPLES

Procedure	Code
Naltrexone treatment for drug dependency	HZ94ZZZ
Substance abuse treatment family counseling	HZ63ZZZ
Medication monitoring of patient on methadone maintenance	HZ81ZZZ
Individual interpersonal psychotherapy for drug abuse	HZ54ZZZ
Patient in for alcohol detoxification treatment	HZ2ZZZZ
Group motivational counseling	HZ47ZZZ
Individual 12-step psychotherapy for substance abuse	HZ53ZZZ
Post-test infectious disease counseling for IV drug abuser	HZ3CZZZ
Psychodynamic psychotherapy for drug dependent patient	HZ5CZZZ
Group cognitive-behavioral counseling for substance abuse	HZ42ZZZ

ICD-10-PCS ROOT OPERATIONS AND APPROACHES

This section contains reference tables listing the root operations and approaches used in the Medical and Surgical section. The first table includes the definition of each root operation, with explanation and examples. The second table includes the definition of each approach.

The root operations are listed by name in alphabetical order. The approaches are listed by approach value, in numeric order followed by alphabetical order. For the full ICD-10-PCS definitions, please refer to the Definitions portion of the ICD-10 Procedure Coding System.

ROOT OPERATIONS		
Alteration	Definition	Modifying the anatomic structure of a body part without affecting the function of the body part
	Explanation	Principal purpose is to improve appearance
	Examples	Face lift, breast augmentation
Bypass	Definition	Altering the route of passage of the contents of a tubular body part
	Explanation	Rerouting contents of a body part to a downstream area of the normal route, to a similar route and body part, or to an abnormal route and dissimilar body part. Includes one or more anastomoses, with or without the use of a device
	Examples	Coronary artery bypass, colostomy formation
Change	Definition	Taking out or off a device from a body part and putting back an identical or similar device in or on the same body part without cutting or puncturing the skin or a mucous membrane
	Explanation	All CHANGE procedures are coded using the approach EXTERNAL
	Examples	Urinary catheter change, gastrostomy tube change
Control	Definition	Stopping, or attempting to stop, postprocedural bleeding
	Explanation	The site of the bleeding is coded as an anatomical region and not to a specific body part
	Examples	Control of post-prostatectomy hemorrhage, control of post-tonsillectomy hemorrhage
Creation	Definition	Making a new genital structure that does not take over the function of a body part
	Explanation	Used only for sex change operations
	Examples	Creation of vagina in a male, creation of penis in a female
Destruction	Definition	Physical eradication of all or a portion of a body part by the direct use of energy, force or a destructive agent
	Explanation	None of the body part is physically taken out
	Examples	Fulguration of rectal polyp, cautery of skin lesion
Detachment	Definition	Cutting off all or a portion of the upper or lower extremities
	Explanation	The body part value is the site of the detachment, with a qualifier if applicable to further specify the level where the extremity was detached
	Examples	Below knee amputation, disarticulation of shoulder
Dilation	Definition	Expanding an orifice or the lumen of a tubular body part
	Explanation	The orifice can be a natural orifice or an artificially created orifice. Accomplished by stretching a tubular body part using intraluminal pressure or by cutting part of the orifice or wall of the tubular body part
	Examples	Percutaneous transluminal angioplasty, pyloromyotomy
Division	Definition	Cutting into a body part without draining fluids and/or gases from the body part in order to separate or transect a body part
	Explanation	All or a portion of the body part is separated into two or more portions
	Examples	Spinal cordotomy, osteotomy
Drainage	Definition	Taking or letting out fluids and/or gases from a body part
	Explanation	The qualifier DIAGNOSTIC is used to identify drainage procedures that are biopsies
	Examples	Thoracentesis, incision and drainage

Excision	Definition	Cutting out or off, without replacement, a portion of a body part
	Explanation	The qualifier DIAGNOSTIC is used to identify excision procedures that are biopsies
	Examples	Partial nephrectomy, liver biopsy
Extirpation	Definition	Taking or cutting out solid matter from a body part
	Explanation	The solid matter may be an abnormal byproduct of a biological function or a foreign body; it may be imbedded in a body part or in the lumen of a tubular body part. The solid matter may or may not have been previously broken into pieces
	Examples	Thrombectomy, choledocholithotomy
Extraction	Definition	Pulling or stripping out or off all or a portion of a body part by the use of force
	Explanation	The qualifier DIAGNOSTIC is used to identify extraction procedures that are biopsies
	Examples	Dilation and curettage, vein stripping
Fragmentation	Definition	Breaking solid matter in a body part into pieces
	Explanation	Physical force (e.g., manual, ultrasonic) applied directly or indirectly is used to break the solid matter into pieces. The solid matter may be an abnormal byproduct of a biological function or a foreign body. The pieces of solid matter are not taken out
	Examples	Extracorporeal shockwave lithotripsy, transurethral lithotripsy
Fusion	Definition	Joining together portions of an articular body part rendering the articular body part immobile
	Explanation	The body part is joined together by fixation device, bone graft, or other means
	Examples	Spinal fusion, ankle arthrodesis
Insertion	Definition	Putting in a nonbiological device that monitors, assists, performs or prevents a physiological function but does not physically take the place of a body part
	Explanation	N/A
	Examples	Insertion of radioactive implant, insertion of central venous catheter
Inspection	Definition	Visually and/or manually exploring a body part
	Explanation	Visual exploration may be performed with or without optical instrumentation. Manual exploration may be performed directly or through intervening body layers
	Examples	Diagnostic arthroscopy, exploratory laparotomy
Map	Definition	Locating the route of passage of electrical impulses and/or locating functional areas in a body part
	Explanation	Applicable only to the cardiac conduction mechanism and the central nervous system
	Examples	Cardiac mapping, cortical mapping
Occlusion	Definition	Completely closing an orifice or the lumen of a tubular body part
	Explanation	The orifice can be a natural orifice or an artificially created orifice
	Examples	Fallopian tube ligation, ligation of inferior vena cava
Reattachment	Definition	Putting back in or on all or a portion of a separated body part to its normal location or other suitable location
	Explanation	Vascular circulation and nervous pathways may or may not be reestablished
	Examples	Reattachment of hand, reattachment of avulsed kidney
Release	Definition	Freeing a body part from an abnormal physical constraint by cutting or by use of force
	Explanation	Some of the restraining tissue may be taken out but none of the body part is taken out
	Examples	Adhesiolysis, carpal tunnel release
	Definition	Taking out or off a device from a body part

Removal	Explanation	If a device is taken out and a similar device put in without cutting or puncturing the skin or mucous membrane, the procedure is coded to the root operation CHANGE. Otherwise, the procedure for taking out a device is coded to the root operation REMOVAL
	Examples	Drainage tube removal, cardiac pacemaker removal
	Definition	Restoring, to the extent possible, a body part to its normal anatomic structure and function
Repair	Explanation	Used only when the method to accomplish the repair is not one of the other root operations
	Examples	Colostomy takedown, suture of laceration
	Definition	Putting in or on biological or synthetic material that physically takes the place and/or function of all or a portion of a body part
Replacement	Explanation	The body part may have been taken out or replaced, or may be taken out, physically eradicated, or rendered nonfunctional during the Replacement procedure. A Removal procedure is coded for taking out the device used in a previous replacement procedure
	Examples	Total hip replacement, bone graft, free skin graft
	Definition	Moving to its normal location, or other suitable location, all or a portion of a body part
Reposition	Explanation	The body part is moved to a new location from an abnormal location, or from a normal location where it is not functioning correctly. The body part may or may not be cut out or off to be moved to the new location
	Examples	Reposition of undescended testicle, fracture reduction
	Definition	Cutting out or off, without replacement, all of a body part
Resection	Explanation	N/A
	Examples	Total nephrectomy, total lobectomy of lung
	Definition	Partially closing an orifice or the lumen of a tubular body part
Restriction	Explanation	The orifice can be a natural orifice or an artificially created orifice
	Examples	Esophagogastric fundoplication, cervical cerclage
	Definition	Correcting, to the extent possible, a portion of a malfunctioning device or the position of a displaced device
Revision	Explanation	Revision can include correcting a malfunctioning or displaced device by taking out or putting in components of the device such as a screw or pin
	Examples	Adjustment of position of pacemaker lead, recementing of hip prosthesis
	Definition	Putting in or on biological or synthetic material that physically reinforces and/or augments the function of a portion of a body part
Supplement	Explanation	The biological material is non-living, or is living and from the same individual. The body part may have been previously replaced, and the Supplement procedure is performed to physically reinforce and/or augment the function of the replaced body part
	Examples	Herniorrhaphy using mesh, free nerve graft, mitral valve ring annuloplasty, put a new acetabular liner in a previous hip replacement
	Definition	Moving, without taking out, all or a portion of a body part to another location to take over the function of all or a portion of a body part
Transfer	Explanation	The body part transferred remains connected to its vascular and nervous supply
	Examples	Tendon transfer, skin pedicle flap transfer
	Definition	Putting in or on all or a portion of a living body part taken from another individual or animal to physically take the place and/or function of all or a portion of a similar body part
Transplantation	Explanation	The native body part may or may not be taken out, and the transplanted body part may take over all or a portion of its function
	Examples	Kidney transplant, heart transplant

APPROACHES	
Open	Cutting through the skin or mucous membrane and any other body layers necessary to expose the site of the procedure
Percutaneous	Entry, by puncture or minor incision, of instrumentation through the skin or mucous membrane and any other body layers necessary to reach the site of the procedure
Percutaneous Endoscopic	Entry, by puncture or minor incision, of instrumentation through the skin or mucous membrane and any other body layers necessary to reach and visualize the site of the procedure
Via Natural or Artificial Opening	Entry of instrumentation through a natural or artificial external opening to reach the site of the procedure
Via Natural or Artificial Opening Endoscopic	Entry of instrumentation through a natural or artificial external opening to reach and visualize the site of the procedure
Via Natural or Artificial Opening With Percutaneous Endoscopic Assistance	Entry of instrumentation through a natural or artificial external opening and entry, by puncture or minor incision, of instrumentation through the skin or mucous membrane and any other body layers necessary to aid in the performance of the procedure
External	Procedures performed directly on the skin or mucous membrane and procedures performed indirectly by the application of external force through the skin or mucous membrane

ICD-10-PCS OFFICIAL GUIDELINES
FOR CODING AND REPORTING

The Centers for Medicare and Medicaid Services (CMS) and the National Center for Health Statistics (NCHS), two departments within the U.S. Federal Government's Department of Health and Human Services (DHHS) provide the following guidelines for coding and reporting using the International Classification of Diseases, 10th Revision, Procedure Coding System (ICD-10-PCS). These guidelines should be used as a companion document to the official version of the ICD-10-PCS as published on the CMS website. The ICD-10-PCS is a procedure classification published by the United States for classifying procedures performed in hospital inpatient health care settings.

These guidelines have been approved by the four organizations that make up the Cooperating Parties for the ICD-10-PCS: the American Hospital Association (AHA), the American Health Information Management Association (AHIMA), CMS, and NCHS.

These guidelines are a set of rules that have been developed to accompany and complement the official conventions and instructions provided within the ICD-10-PCS itself. The instructions and conventions of the classification take precedence over guidelines. These guidelines are based on the coding and sequencing instructions in the Tables, Index and Definitions of ICD-10-PCS, but provide additional instruction. Adherence to these guidelines when assigning ICD-10-PCS procedure codes is required under the Health Insurance Portability and Accountability Act (HIPAA). The procedure codes have been adopted under HIPAA for hospital inpatient healthcare settings. A joint effort between the healthcare provider and the coder is essential to achieve complete and accurate documentation, code assignment, and reporting of diagnoses and procedures. These guidelines have been developed to assist both the healthcare provider and the coder in identifying those procedures that are to be reported. The importance of consistent, complete documentation in the medical record cannot be overemphasized. Without such documentation accurate coding cannot be achieved.

CONVENTIONS

A1   ICD-10-PCS codes are composed of seven characters. Each character is an axis of classification that specifies information about the procedure performed. Within a defined code range, a character specifies the same type of information in that axis of classification.

Example: The fifth axis of classification specifies the approach in sections 0 through 4 and 7 through 9 of the system.

A2   One of 34 possible values can be assigned to each axis of classification in the seven-character code: they are the numbers 0 through 9 and the alphabet (except I and O because they are easily confused with the numbers 1 and 0). The number of unique values used in an axis of classification differs as needed.

Example: Where the fifth axis of classification specifies the approach, seven different approach values are currently used to specify the approach.

A3   The valid values for an axis of classification can be added to as needed.

Example: If a significantly distinct type of device is used in a new procedure, a new device value can be added to the system.

A4   As with words in their context, the meaning of any single value is a combination of its axis of classification and any preceding values on which it may be dependent.

Example: The meaning of a body part value in the Medical and Surgical section is always dependent on the body system value. The body part value 0 in the Central Nervous body system specifies Brain and the body part value 0 in the Peripheral Nervous body system specifies Cervical Plexus.

A5   As the system is expanded to become increasingly detailed, over time more values will depend on preceding values for their meaning.

Example: In the Lower Joints body system, the device value 3 in the root operation Insertion specifies Infusion Device and the device value 3 in the root operation Replacement specifies Ceramic Synthetic Substitute.

A6   The purpose of the alphabetic index is to locate the appropriate table that contains all information necessary to construct a procedure code. The PCS Tables should always be consulted to find the most appropriate valid code.

A7   It is not required to consult the index first before proceeding to the tables to complete the code. A valid code may be chosen directly from the tables.

A8   All seven characters must be specified to be a valid code. If the documentation is incomplete for coding purposes, the physician should be queried for the necessary information.

A9   Within a PCS table, valid codes include all combinations of choices in characters 4 through 7 contained in the same row of the table. In the example below, 0JHT3VZ is a valid code, and 0JHW3VZ is *not* a valid code.

Section:	0	Medical and Surgical		
Body System:	J	Subcutaneous Tissue and Fascia		
Operation:	H	Insertion: Putting in a nonbiological appliance that monitors, assists, performs, or prevents a physiological function but does not physically take the place of a body part		

Body Part	Approach	Device	Qualifier
S Subcutaneous Tissue and Fascia, Head and Neck **V** Subcutaneous Tissue and Fascia, Upper Extremity **W** Subcutaneous Tissue and Fascia, Lower Extremity	**0** Open **3** Percutaneous	**1** Radioactive Element **3** Infusion Device	**Z** No Qualifier
T Subcutaneous Tissue and Fascia, Trunk	**0** Open **3** Percutaneous	**1** Radioactive Element **3** Infusion Device **V** Infusion Pump	**Z** No Qualifier

A10   "And," when used in a code description, means "and/or."

Example: Lower Arm and Wrist Muscle means lower arm and/or wrist muscle.

A11   Many of the terms used to construct PCS codes are defined within the system. It is the coder's responsibility to determine what the documentation in the medical record equates to in the PCS definitions. The physician is not expected to use the terms used in PCS code descriptions, nor is the coder required to query the physician when the correlation between the documentation and the defined PCS terms is clear.

Example: When the physician documents "partial resection" the coder can independently correlate "partial resection" to the root operation Excision without querying the physician for clarification.

MEDICAL AND SURGICAL SECTION GUIDELINES (SECTION 0)

B2. Body System

General guidelines

B2.1a   The procedure codes in the general anatomical regions body systems should only be used when the procedure is performed on an anatomical region rather than a specific body part (e.g., root operations Control and Detachment,

Drainage of a body cavity) or on the rare occasion when no information is available to support assignment of a code to a specific body part.

Example: Control of postoperative hemorrhage is coded to the root operation Control found in the general anatomical regions body systems.

B2.1b   Where the general body part values "upper" and "lower" are provided as an option in the Upper Arteries, Lower Arteries, Upper Veins, Lower Veins, Muscles and Tendons body systems, "upper" or "lower "specifies body parts located above or below the diaphragm respectively.

Example: Vein body parts above the diaphragm are found in the Upper Veins body system; vein body parts below the diaphragm are found in the Lower Veins body system.

B3. Root Operation

General guidelines

B3.1a   In order to determine the appropriate root operation, the full definition of the root operation as contained in the PCS Tables must be applied.

B3.1b   Components of a procedure specified in the root operation definition and explanation are not coded separately. Procedural steps necessary to reach the operative site and close the operative site, including anastomosis of a tubular body part, are also not coded separately. *Example*: Resection of a joint as part of a joint replacement procedure is included in the root operation definition of Replacement and is not coded separately. Laparotomy performed to reach the site of an open liver biopsy is not coded separately. In a resection of sigmoid colon with anastomosis of descending colon to rectum, the anastomosis is not coded separately.

Multiple procedures

B3.2   During the same operative episode, multiple procedures are coded if:

a.   The same root operation is performed on different body parts as defined by distinct values of the body part character.

Example: Diagnostic excision of liver and pancreas are coded separately.

b.   The same root operation is repeated at different body sites that are included in the same body part value.

Example: Excision of the sartorius muscle and excision of the gracilis muscle are both included in the upper leg muscle body part value, and multiple procedures are coded.

c.   Multiple root operations with distinct objectives are performed on the same body part.

Example: Destruction of sigmoid lesion and bypass of sigmoid colon are coded separately.

d.   The intended root operation is attempted using one approach, but is converted to a different approach.

Example: Laparoscopic cholecystectomy converted to an open cholecystectomy is coded as percutaneous endoscopic Inspection and open Resection.

Discontinued procedures

B3.3   If the intended procedure is discontinued, code the procedure to the root operation performed. If a procedure is discontinued before any other root operation is performed, code the root operation Inspection of the body part or anatomical region inspected. *Example*: A planned aortic valve replacement procedure is discontinued after the initial thoracotomy and before any incision is made in the heart muscle, when the patient becomes hemodynamically unstable. This procedure is coded as an open Inspection of the mediastinum.

Biopsy procedures

B3.4a   Biopsy procedures are coded using the root operations Excision, Extraction, or Drainage and the qualifier Diagnostic. The qualifier Diagnostic is used only for biopsies. Examples: Fine needle aspiration biopsy of lung is coded to the root operation Drainage with the qualifier Diagnostic. Biopsy of bone marrow is coded to the root operation Extraction with the qualifier Diagnostic. Lymph node sampling for biopsy is coded to the root operation Excision with the qualifier Diagnostic.

Biopsy followed by more definitive treatment

B3.4b   If a diagnostic Excision, Extraction, or Drainage procedure (biopsy) is followed by a more definitive procedure, such as Destruction, Excision or Resection at the same procedure site, both the biopsy and the more definitive treatment are coded.

Example: Biopsy of breast followed by partial mastectomy at the same procedure site, both the biopsy and the partial mastectomy procedure are coded.

Overlapping body layers

B3.5   If the root operations Excision, Repair or Inspection are performed on overlapping layers of the musculoskeletal system, the body part specifying the deepest layer is coded. *Example*: Excisional debridement that includes skin and subcutaneous tissue and muscle is coded to the muscle body part.

Bypass procedures

B3.6a   Bypass procedures are coded by identifying the body part bypassed "from" and the body part bypassed "to." The fourth character body part specifies the body part bypassed from, and the qualifier specifies the body part bypassed to.

Example: Bypass from stomach to jejunum, stomach is the body part and jejunum is the qualifier.

B3.6b   Coronary arteries are classified by number of distinct sites treated, rather than number of coronary arteries or anatomic name of a coronary artery (e.g., left anterior descending). Coronary artery bypass procedures are coded differently than other bypass procedures as described in the previous guideline. Rather than identifying the body part bypassed from, the body part identifies the number of coronary artery sites bypassed to, and the qualifier specifies the vessel bypassed from.

Example: Aortocoronary artery bypass of one site on the left anterior descending coronary artery and one site on the obtuse marginal coronary artery is classified in the body part axis of classification as two coronary artery sites and the qualifier specifies the aorta as the body part bypassed from.

B3.6c   If multiple coronary artery sites are bypassed, a separate procedure is coded for each coronary artery site that uses a different device and/or qualifier.

Example: Aortocoronary artery bypass and internal mammary coronary artery bypass are coded separately.

Control vs. more definitive root operations

B3.7   The root operation Control is defined as, "Stopping, or attempting to stop, postprocedural bleeding." If an attempt to stop postprocedural bleeding is initially unsuccessful, and to stop the bleeding requires performing any of the definitive root operations Bypass, Detachment, Excision, Extraction, Reposition, Replacement, or Resection, then that root operation is coded instead of Control.

Example: Resection of spleen to stop postprocedural bleeding is coded to Resection instead of Control.

Excision vs. Resection

B3.8   PCS contains specific body parts for anatomical subdivisions of a body part, such as lobes of the lungs or liver and regions of the intestine. Resection of the specific body part is coded whenever all of the body part is cut out or off, rather than coding Excision of a less specific body part.

Example: Left upper lung lobectomy is coded to Resection of Upper Lung Lobe, Left rather than Excision of Lung, Left.

Excision for graft

B3.9   If an autograft is obtained from a different body part in order to complete the objective of the procedure, a separate procedure is coded.

Example: Coronary bypass with excision of saphenous vein graft, excision of saphenous vein is coded separately.

Fusion procedures of the spine

B3.10a   The body part coded for a spinal vertebral joint(s) rendered immobile by a spinal fusion procedure is classified by the level of the spine (e.g. thoracic). There are distinct body part values for a single vertebral joint and for multiple vertebral joints at each spinal level.

Example: Body part values specify Lumbar Vertebral Joint, Lumbar Vertebral Joints, 2 or More and Lumbosacral Vertebral Joint.

B3.10b   If multiple vertebral joints are fused, a separate procedure is coded for each vertebral joint that uses a different device and/or qualifier.

Example: Fusion of lumbar vertebral joint, posterior approach, anterior column and fusion of lumbar vertebral joint, posterior approach, posterior column are coded separately.

B3.10c   Combinations of devices and materials are often used on a vertebral joint to render the joint immobile. When combinations of devices are used on the same vertebral joint, the device value coded for the procedure is as follows:

- If an interbody fusion device is used to render the joint immobile (alone or containing other material like bone graft), the procedure is coded with the device value Interbody Fusion Device
- If bone graft is the *only* device used to render the joint immobile, the procedure is coded with the device value Nonautologous Tissue Substitute or Autologous Tissue Substitute
- If a mixture of autologous and nonautologous bone graft (with or without biological or synthetic extenders or binders) is used to render the joint immobile, code the procedure with the device value Autologous Tissue Substitute

Examples: Fusion of a vertebral joint using a cage style interbody fusion device containing morselized bone graft is coded to the device Interbody Fusion Device. Fusion of a vertebral joint using a bone dowel interbody fusion device made of cadaver bone and packed with a mixture of local morsellized bone and demineralized bone matrix is coded to the device Interbody Fusion Device.

Fusion of a vertebral joint using both autologous bone graft and bone bank bone graft is coded to the device Autologous Tissue Substitute.

Inspection procedures

B3.11a   Inspection of a body part(s) performed in order to achieve the objective of a procedure is not coded separately.

Example: Fiberoptic bronchoscopy performed for irrigation of bronchus, only the irrigation procedure is coded.

B3.11b   If multiple tubular body parts are inspected, the most distal body part inspected is coded. If multiple non-tubular body parts in a region are inspected, the body part that specifies the entire area inspected is coded.

Examples: Cystoureteroscopy with inspection of bladder and ureters is coded to the ureter body part value.

Exploratory laparotomy with general inspection of abdominal contents is coded to the peritoneal cavity body part value.

B3.11c When both an Inspection procedure and another procedure are performed on the same body part during the same episode, if the Inspection procedure is performed using a different approach than the other procedure, the Inspection procedure is coded separately.

Example: Endoscopic Inspection of the duodenum is coded separately when open Excision of the duodenum is performed during the same procedural episode.

Occlusion vs. Restriction for vessel embolization procedures

B3.12 If the objective of an embolization procedure is to completely close a vessel, the root operation Occlusion is coded. If the objective of an embolization procedure is to narrow the lumen of a vessel, the root operation Restriction is coded.

Examples: Tumor embolization is coded to the root operation Occlusion, because the objective of the procedure is to cut off the blood supply to the vessel.

Embolization of a cerebral aneurysm is coded to the root operation Restriction, because the objective of the procedure is not to close off the vessel entirely, but to narrow the lumen of the vessel at the site of the aneurysm where it is abnormally wide.

Release procedures

B3.13 In the root operation Release, the body part value coded is the body part being freed and not the tissue being manipulated or cut to free the body part.

Example: Lysis of intestinal adhesions is coded to the specific intestine body part value.

Release vs. Division

B3.14 If the sole objective of the procedure is freeing a body part without cutting the body part, the root operation is Release. If the sole objective of the procedure is separating or transecting a body part, the root operation is Division.

Examples: Freeing a nerve root from surrounding scar tissue to relieve pain is coded to the root operation Release. Severing a nerve root to relieve pain is coded to the root operation Division.

Reposition for fracture treatment

B3.15 Reduction of a displaced fracture is coded to the root operation Reposition and the application of a cast or splint in conjunction with the Reposition procedure is not coded separately. Treatment of a nondisplaced fracture is coded to the procedure performed.

Examples: Putting a pin in a nondisplaced fracture is coded to the root operation Insertion.

Casting of a nondisplaced fracture is coded to the root operation Immobilization in the Placement section.

Transplantation vs. Administration

B3.16 Putting in a mature and functioning living body part taken from another individual or animal is coded to the root operation Transplantation. Putting in autologous or nonautologous cells is coded to the Administration section.

Example: Putting in autologous or nonautologous bone marrow, pancreatic islet cells or stem cells is coded to the Administration section.

B4. Body Part

General guidelines

B4.1a   If a procedure is performed on a portion of a body part that does not have a separate body part value, code the body part value corresponding to the whole body part.

Example: A procedure performed on the alveolar process of the mandible is coded to the mandible body part.

B4.1b   If the prefix "peri" is combined with a body part to identify the site of the procedure, the procedure is coded to the body part named.

Example: A procedure site identified as perirenal is coded to the kidney body part.

Branches of body parts

B4.2   Where a specific branch of a body part does not have its own body part value in PCS, the body part is coded to the closest proximal branch that has a specific body part value. *Example*: A procedure performed on the mandibular branch of the trigeminal nerve is coded to the trigeminal nerve body part value.

Bilateral body part values

B4.3   Bilateral body part values are available for a limited number of body parts. If the identical procedure is performed on contralateral body parts, and a bilateral body part value exists for that body part, a single procedure is coded using the bilateral body part value. If no bilateral body part value exists, each procedure is coded separately using the appropriate body part value.

Example: The identical procedure performed on both fallopian tubes is coded once using the body part value Fallopian Tube, Bilateral. The identical procedure performed on both knee joints is coded twice using the body part values Knee Joint, Right and Knee Joint, Left.

Coronary arteries

B4.4   The coronary arteries are classified as a single body part that is further specified by number of sites treated and not by name or number of arteries. Separate body part values are used to specify the number of sites treated when the same procedure is performed on multiple sites in the coronary arteries.
Examples: Angioplasty of two distinct sites in the left anterior descending coronary artery with placement of two stents is coded as Dilation of Coronary Arteries, Two Sites, with Intraluminal Device.

Angioplasty of two distinct sites in the left anterior descending coronary artery, one with stent placed and one without, is coded separately as Dilation of Coronary Artery, One Site with Intraluminal Device, and Dilation of Coronary Artery, One Site with no device.

Tendons, ligaments, bursae and fascia near a joint

B4.5   Procedures performed on tendons, ligaments, bursae and fascia supporting a joint are coded to the body part in the respective body system that is the focus of the procedure. Procedures performed on joint structures themselves are coded to the body part in the joint body systems.

Example: Repair of the anterior cruciate ligament of the knee is coded to the knee bursae and ligament body part in the bursae and ligaments body system. Knee arthroscopy with shaving of articular cartilage is coded to the knee joint body part in the Lower Joints body system.

Skin, subcutaneous tissue and fascia overlying a joint

B4.6   If a procedure is performed on the skin, subcutaneous tissue or fascia overlying a joint, the procedure is coded to the following body part:

- Shoulder is coded to Upper Arm
- Elbow is coded to Lower Arm
- Wrist is coded to Lower Arm
- Hip is coded to Upper Leg
- Knee is coded to Lower Leg
- Ankle is coded to Foot

Fingers and toes

B4.7   If a body system does not contain a separate body part value for fingers, procedures performed on the fingers are coded to the body part value for the hand. If a body system does not contain a separate body part value for toes, procedures performed on the toes are coded to the body part value for the foot.

Example: Excision of finger muscle is coded to one of the hand muscle body part values in the Muscles body system.

Upper and lower intestinal tract

B4.8   In the Gastrointestinal body system, the general body part values Upper Intestinal Tract and Lower Intestinal Tract are provided as an option for the root operations Change, Inspection, Removal and Revision. Upper Intestinal Tract includes the portion of the gastrointestinal tract from the esophagus down to and including the duodenum, and Lower Intestinal Tract includes the portion of the gastrointestinal tract from the jejunum down to and including the rectum and anus.

Example: In the root operation Change table, change of a device in the jejunum is coded using the body part Lower Intestinal Tract.

B5. Approach

Open approach with percutaneous endoscopic assistance

B5.2   Procedures performed using the open approach with percutaneous endoscopic assistance are coded to the approach Open.

Example: Laparoscopic-assisted sigmoidectomy is coded to the approach Open.

External approach

B5.3a   Procedures performed within an orifice on structures that are visible without the aid of any instrumentation are coded to the approach External.

Example: Resection of tonsils is coded to the approach External.

B5.3b   Procedures performed indirectly by the application of external force through the intervening body layers are coded to the approach External.

Example: Closed reduction of fracture is coded to the approach External.

Percutaneous procedure via device

B5.4   Procedures performed percutaneously via a device placed for the procedure are coded to the approach Percutaneous.

Example: Fragmentation of kidney stone performed via percutaneous nephrostomy is coded to the approach Percutaneous.

B6. Device

General guidelines

B6.1a   A device is coded only if a device remains after the procedure is completed. If no device remains, the device value No Device is coded.

B6.1b   Materials such as sutures, ligatures, radiological markers and temporary post-operative wound drains are considered integral to the performance of a procedure and are not coded as devices.

B6.1c   Procedures performed on a device only and not on a body part are specified in the root operations Change, Irrigation, Removal and Revision, and are coded to the procedure performed.

Example: Irrigation of percutaneous nephrostomy tube is coded to the root operation Irrigation of indwelling device in the Administration section.

Drainage device

B6.2   A separate procedure to put in a drainage device is coded to the root operation Drainage with the device value Drainage Device.

Obstetric Section Guidelines (section 1)

C. Obstetrics Section

Products of conception

C1   Procedures performed on the products of conception are coded to the Obstetrics section. Procedures performed on the pregnant female other than the products of conception are coded to the appropriate root operation in the Medical and Surgical section.

Example: Amniocentesis is coded to the products of conception body part in the Obstetrics section. Repair of obstetric urethral laceration is coded to the urethra body part in the Medical and Surgical section.

Procedures following delivery or abortion

C2   Procedures performed following a delivery or abortion for curettage of the endometrium or evacuation of retained products of conception are all coded in the Obstetrics section, to the root operation Extraction and the body part Products of Conception, Retained. Diagnostic or therapeutic dilation and curettage performed during times other than the postpartum or post-abortion period are all coded in the Medical and Surgical section, to the root operation Extraction and the body part Endometrium.

Selection of Principal Procedure

The following instructions should be applied in the selection of principal procedure and clarification on the importance of the relation to the principal diagnosis when more than one procedure is performed:

1. Procedure performed for definitive treatment of both principal diagnosis and secondary diagnosis

    a. Sequence procedure performed for definitive treatment most related to principal diagnosis as principal procedure.

2. Procedure performed for definitive treatment and diagnostic procedures performed for both principal diagnosis and secondary diagnosis

    a. Sequence procedure performed for definitive treatment most related to principal diagnosis as principal procedure

3. A diagnostic procedure was performed for the principal diagnosis and a procedure is performed for definitive treatment of a secondary diagnosis.

    a.   Sequence diagnostic procedure as principal procedure, since the procedure most related to the principal diagnosis takes precedence.

4.   No procedures performed that are related to principal diagnosis; procedures performed for definitive treatment and diagnostic procedures were performed for secondary diagnosis

    a.   Sequence procedure performed for definitive treatment of secondary diagnosis as principal procedure, since there are no procedures (definitive or nondefinitive treatment) related to principal diagnosis.

ICD-10-PCS DEVICE AND SUBSTANCE CLASSIFICATION

THIS APPENDIX DISCUSSES the distinguishing features of device, substance and equipment as classified in ICD-10-PCS, to provide further guidance for correct identification and coding. The appendix includes discussion of the ICD-10-PCS definitions and classification of device, substance and equipment, and is accompanied by specific coding instruction and examples.

ICD-10-PCS DEVICE CLASSIFICATION

In most ICD-10-PCS codes, the 6th character of the code is used to classify device. The 6th character device value "defines the material or appliance used to accomplish the objective of the procedure that remains in or on the procedure site at the end of the procedure." If the device is the means by which the procedural objective is accomplished, then a specific device value is coded in the 6th character. If no device is used to accomplish the objective of the procedure, the device value NO DEVICE is coded in the 6th character.

For example, an aortocoronary bypass that uses saphenous vein graft to accomplish the bypass is coded to the device value AUTOLOGOUS VENOUS TISSUE in the 6th character of the ICD-10-PCS code. A coronary bypass that uses the patient's internal mammary artery directly to accomplish the bypass uses the device value NO DEVICE in the 6th character of the ICD-10-PCS code

DEVICE AND PROCEDURAL OBJECTIVE

Whether or not the material used in a procedure should be coded using a specific ICD-10-PCS device value can be determined primarily by asking the question

* Is this material central to achieving the objective of the procedure, or does it only support the performance of the procedure?

For example, radiological markers are put in the procedure site to guide the performance of a primary procedure such as excision of a tumor, whereas radioactive brachytherapy seeds are put in the procedure site as an end in themselves, to treat a malignant tumor. The radiological marker is not classified as a device in ICD-10-PCS, but the brachytherapy seeds are classified to the device value RADIOACTIVE ELEMENT in the root operation INSERTION.

The same device coded as a specific device value for one procedure may not be coded at all for another procedure where it is not central to the procedural objective. For example, a procedure performed specifically to place a drain in a body part for diagnostic or therapeutic purposes is coded to the root operation DRAINAGE with the specific device value DRAINAGE DEVICE in the 6th character of the code. However, a wound drain placed at an incision site at the conclusion of the procedure to promote healing is not central to the procedural objective and therefore not coded separately as a device in ICD-10-PCS. For this reason, materials such as wound dressings and operative site drains that support the performance of the procedure are not coded separately.

Sutures and suture alternatives (e.g., fibrin glue, Dermabond, specialized vessel closures) are not coded as devices in ICD-10-PCS, because in most cases using material to bring the edges of a procedure site together is not central to the procedural objective, but is used to support the performance of the procedure (to close the site). For procedures where the sole objective is to close a wound created by trauma or other incident, the procedure is coded to the root operation REPAIR with the device value NO DEVICE in the 6th character of the ICD-10-PCS code.

DEVICE AND LOCATION

Whether material or an appliance is coded as a device cannot be determined by the size, shape or complexity of the object or material being used. A device may be too small to be seen with the naked eye (microcoils used to occlude a vessel) or two feet long (external fixator for a long bone). A device may be of a predetermined shape (prosthetic heart valve) or no particular shape (morselized bone graft). A device may be a highly complex machine (cardiac synchronization pacemaker/defibrillator) or a simple piece of hardware (internal fixation bone screw).

However, material that is classified as a ICD-10-PCS device is distinguished from material classified as a ICD-10-PCS substance by the fact that it has a specific location. A device is intended to maintain a fixed location at the procedure site where it was put, whereas a substance is intended to disperse or be absorbed in the body. Indeed, a device that does not stay where it was put may need to be "revised" in a subsequent procedure, to move the device back to its intended location.

DEVICE AND REMOVABILITY

Material that is classified as a ICD-10-PCS device is also distinguishable by the fact that it is removable. Although it may not be *practical* to remove some types of devices once they become established at the site, it is *physically possible* to remove a device for some time after the procedure. A skin graft, once it "takes," may be nearly indistinguishable from the surrounding skin and so is no longer clearly identifiable as a device. Nevertheless, procedures that involve material coded as a device can for the most part be "reversed" by removing the device from the procedure site.

DEVICE DISTRIBUTION IN ICD-10-PCS

The general distribution and use of the 6th character when specified as a device is summarized in the table below. The sections and root operations that specify device in the 6th character are listed. Also included are examples of 6th character values and corresponding procedure examples.

PCS Section	Root Operation	Device Value Example	Procedure Example
Medical and Surgical	Alteration	Autologous Tissue Substitute	Nasal tip elevation using fat autograft
Medical and Surgical	Bypass	Synthetic Substitute	Femoral-popliteal bypass using synthetic graft
Medical and Surgical	Change	Drainage Device	Foley catheter exchange
Medical and Surgical	Creation	Nonautologous Tissue Substitute	Sex change operation using tissue bank graft material
Medical and Surgical	Dilation	Intraluminal Device	Percutaneous coronary angioplasty using stent
Medical and Surgical	Drainage	Drainage Device	Drainage of pleural effusion using chest tube
Medical and Surgical	Fusion	Interbody Fusion Device	Spinal interbody fusion
Medical and Surgical	Insertion	Infusion Pump	Insertion of infusion pump for pain control
Medical and Surgical	Occlusion	Extraluminal Device	Fallopian tube ligation using clips
Medical and Surgical	Removal	Spacer	Removal of joint spacer
Medical and Surgical	Replacement	Autologous Tissue Substitute	Skin graft using patient's own skin
Medical and Surgical	Reposition	Internal Fixation Device	Fracture reduction with plate and screw fixation
Medical and Surgical	Restriction	Extraluminal Device	Laparoscopic gastric banding, adjustable band
Medical and Surgical	Revision	Neurostimulator Lead	Reposition of spinal neurostimulator lead
Medical and Surgical	Supplement	Zooplastic Tissue	Pulmonary artery patch graft using bovine pericardium
Obstetrics	Insertion, Removal	Monitoring Electrode	Insertion of fetal monitoring electrode
Placement	Change	Cast	Forearm cast change
Placement	Compression	Pressure Dressing	Application of pressure dressing to lower leg
Placement	Dressing	Bandage	Application of bandage to chest wall
Placement	Immobilization	Splint	Splint placement to wrist

Placement	Packing	Packing Material	Nasal packing
Placement	Removal	Brace	Removal of back brace
Placement	Traction	Traction Apparatus	Skin traction of lower leg using traction device

ICD-10-PCS SUBSTANCE CLASSIFICATION

The 6th character substance value "defines the blood component or other liquid put in or on the body to accomplish the objective of the procedure." The 6th character is defined as substance in the ADMINISTRATION section. Administration is the only section where a substance is classified as a separate code, and not included as information in a more definitive procedure.

SUBSTANCE AND PROCEDURAL OBJECTIVE

Many different substances are typically put in or on the body in the course of an inpatient hospital stay, both during surgical procedures and at the bedside. Only those which meet UHDDS and facility coding guidelines are coded separately. Most material classified as a substance in the ADMINISTRATION section is in liquid form and intended to be immediately absorbed by the body or, in the case of blood and blood products, disseminated in the circulatory system. An exception is the substance value ADHESION BARRIER. It is a non-liquid substance classified in the Administration section, and coded separately for tracking purposes.

SUBSTANCE AND REMOVABILITY

Most substances cannot be removed once they are administered, because the whole point of administering them is for them to be dispersed and/or absorbed by the body. Imaging contrast is sometimes extracted from the bloodstream at the conclusion of a procedure to minimize the possibility of adverse effects.

SUBSTANCE DISTRIBUTION IN ADMINISTRATION SECTION

The general distribution and use of the 6th character specified as a substance in the ADMINISTRATION section is summarized in the table below. All root operations that specify substance in the 6th character are listed. Also included are examples of 6th character values and corresponding procedure examples.

Root Operation	Substance Value Example	Procedure Example
Introduction	Nutritional substance	Infusion of total parenteral nutrition
Irrigation	Irrigating Substance	Irrigation of eye
Transfusion	Frozen Plasma	Transfusion of frozen plasma

CLASSIFICATION OF SUBSTANCE IN ANCILLARY SECTIONS

Three ancillary sections record their own specific substance values as part of the ICD-10-PCS code, where a substance is used to support the objective of the procedure. They are the IMAGING, NUCLEAR MEDICINE and RADIATION ONCOLOGY sections, and they specify CONTRAST, RADIONUCLIDE and RADIOISOTOPE respectively. However, these substance values are unambiguously included as part of a more definitive procedure code, to be recorded when the substance is used to support the objective of the procedure. Substances in these three ancillary sections are therefore not likely to be confused with separately coded substances in the ADMINISTRATION section.

SUBSTANCE DISTRIBUTION IN ANCILLARY SECTIONS

The three ancillary sections that specify a type of substance used in the procedure are summarized in the table below. The sections and the type of substance classified are listed along with the ICD-10-PCS character where this information is recorded. Also included are examples of the values used and corresponding procedure examples.

PCS Section	Substance Classified	Substance Value Example	Procedure Example
Imaging	Contrast (5th character)	Low Osmolar Contrast	Left heart ventriculography using low osmolar contrast
Nuclear Medicine	Radionuclide (5th character)	Fluorine 18	PET scan of brain using Fluorine 18
Radiation oncology	Isotope (6th character)	Iodine 125	HDR brachytherapy of thyroid using Iodine 125

EQUIPMENT AND ICD-10-PCS CODING

For the most part, equipment used to assist in the performance of the procedure is not coded in ICD-10-PCS.

The only exception to this rule occurs in the REHABILITATION AND DIAGNOSTIC AUDIOLOGY section, where the 6th character is specified as *equipment*. The 6th character values in the REHABILITATION AND DIAGNOSTIC AUDIOLOGY section are used to capture information about the machine, physical aid, or other equipment used to assist in performing the procedure.

EQUIPMENT AND PROCEDURAL OBJECTIVE

For all other sections in ICD-10-PCS, equipment is distinguished from a codeable device by the fact that equipment is a method used to support the performance of a procedure. For example, the machine used to maintain cardiovascular circulation during an open heart bypass procedure is equipment that performs the circulatory functions for the heart so that the heart bypass can be performed. This support procedure is coded to the root operation PERFORMANCE in the EXTRACORPOREAL ASSISTANCE AND PERFORMANCE section, and the type of equipment used is not captured in the code. The primary procedure is coded to the root operation BYPASS in the MEDICAL AND SURGICAL section, and any graft material used is coded to the appropriate 6th character device value.

EQUIPMENT AND LOCATION

Equipment is also distinguished from a codeable device in ICD-10-PCS by the fact that equipment resides primarily outside the body during the procedure. Cardiopulmonary circulatory support is coded to the EXTRACORPOREAL ASSISTANCE AND PERFORMANCE section and the type of equipment used is not recorded in the ICD-10-PCS code. With cardiovascular support equipment, the machinery resides primarily outside the body. The outtake and return cannulae are the only portions of the machine directly connected to the patient.

On the other hand, insertion of intra-aortic balloon pump is coded as a separate INSERTION procedure in ICD-10-PCS, in addition to the ICD-10-PCS code in the EXTRACORPOREAL ASSISTANCE AND PERFOR-MANCE section specifying assistance with cardiac output. The intra-aortic balloon pump resides principally in the patient's body. The balloon mechanism that supports cardiac output is in the aorta itself.

Mechanical ventilation is also coded to the EXTRACORPOREAL ASSISTANCE AND PERFORMANCE section and the equipment used is not recorded in the ICD-10-PCS code. As with cardiovascular support equipment, the mechanical ventilation machine resides primarily outside the body. The endotracheal tube is the only portion of the machine directly connected to the patient. Insertion of the endotracheal tube as part of a mechanical ventilation procedure is not coded as a separate device insertion procedure, because it is merely the interface between the patient and the equipment used to perform the procedure, rather than an end in itself.

On the other hand, insertion of an endotracheal tube in order to maintain an airway in patients who are unconscious or unable to breathe on their own is the central objective of the procedure. Therefore, insertion of an endotracheal tube as an end in itself is coded to the root operation INSERTION and the device ENDOTRACHEAL AIRWAY.

EQUIPMENT AND REMOVABILITY

Equipment used solely to support the performance of a procedure and therefore not coded in ICD-10-PCS can be further distinguished by the fact that the equipment is used only for the duration of the procedure. Once the procedure is completed, any portions of the equipment attached to the patient are disconnected. For example, a patient no longer requiring mechanical ventilation is "extubated," or disconnected from the equipment that provides ventilation support.

SUMMARY

Three distinguishing features have been identified to enable correct identification and coding of device, substance and equipment: procedural objective, location, and removability. The procedural objective alone is sufficient in most cases to determine whether material or an appliance used in a procedure should be coded in ICD-10-PCS. Once it is determined that the information should be coded in ICD-10-PCS, location and removability are useful in determining whether the item is classified as a device or substance. The following table summarizes the distinguishing features of device, substance, and equipment in relation to each other, along with examples.

PCS 6th Character	Procedural Objective	Location	Removability	Procedure Example
Device	Material or appliance put in or on the body is central to accomplishing the procedural objective	Resides at the site of the procedure, not intended to change location	Capable of being removed from the procedure site	Neurostimulator lead insertion
Substance	Liquid or blood component is central to accomplishing the procedural objective	No fixed position, intended to be absorbed or dispersed	Not removable, once dispersed or absorbed	Antibiotic injection
Equipment	Machinery or other aid used to perform a procedure	Resides primarily outside the body	Temporary, used for the duration of the procedure only	Mechanical ventilation

ICD-10-PCS CHANGES AND REVISIONS

SUMMARY OF CHANGES FOR CALENDAR YEAR 2014

Four codes added under new technology application, valid October 1, 2013

- **08H005Z** Insertion of Epiretinal Visual Prosthesis into Right Eye, Open Approach

- **08H105Z** Insertion of Epiretinal Visual Prosthesis into Left Eye, Open Approach

- **30280B1** Transfusion of Nonautologous 4-Factor Prothrombin Complex Concentrate into Vein, Open Approach

- **30283B1** Transfusion of Nonautologous 4-Factor Prothrombin Complex Concentrate into Vein, Percutaneous Approach

Three new codes added and three codes deleted, to correct body part value for temporary occlusion of abdominal aorta

- **04V00DJ** Restriction of Abdominal Aorta with Intraluminal Device, Temporary, Open Approach

- **04V03DJ** Restriction of Abdominal Aorta with Intraluminal Device, Temporary, Percutaneous Approach

- **04V04DJ** Restriction of Abdominal Aorta with Intraluminal Device, Temporary, Percutaneous Endoscopic Approach

(**02VW0DJ**) Restriction of Thoracic Aorta with Intraluminal Device, Temporary, Open Approach

(**02VW3DJ**) Restriction of Thoracic Aorta with Intraluminal Device, Temporary, Percutaneous Approach

(**02VW4DJ**) Restriction of Thoracic Aorta with Intraluminal Device, Temporary, Percutaneous Endoscopic Approach

Revised Section Title

Section title for Radiation Oncology section revised to Radiation Therapy in response to public comment

▲ Because the phrase "Radiation Oncology" is not used in code titles, no code titles were revised as a result of the section title change.

CENTRAL NERVOUS SYSTEM

Section	0	Medical and Surgical		
Body System	0	Central Nervous System		
Operation	1	Bypass: Altering the route of passage of the contents of a tubular body part		

Body Part (Character 4)	Approach (Character 5)	Device (Character 6)	Qualifier (Character 7)
6 Cerebral Ventricle	0 Open 3 Percutaneous	7 Autologous Tissue Substitute J Synthetic Substitute K Nonautologous Tissue Substitute	0 Nasopharynx 1 Mastoid Sinus 2 Atrium 3 Blood Vessel 4 Pleural Cavity 5 Intestine 6 Peritoneal Cavity 7 Urinary Tract 8 Bone Marrow B Cerebral Cisterns
U Spinal Canal	0 Open 3 Percutaneous	7 Autologous Tissue Substitute J Synthetic Substitute K Nonautologous Tissue Substitute	4 Pleural Cavity 6 Peritoneal Cavity 7 Urinary Tract 9 Fallopian Tube

Section	0	Medical and Surgical		
Body System	0	Central Nervous System		
Operation	2	Change: Taking out or off a device from a body part and putting back an identical or similar device in or on the same body part without cutting or puncturing the skin or a mucous membrane		

Body Part (Character 4)	Approach (Character 5)	Device (Character 6)	Qualifier (Character 7)
0 Brain E Cranial Nerve U Spinal Canal	X External	0 Drainage Device Y Other Device	Z No Qualifier

Section	0	Medical and Surgical		
Body System	0	Central Nervous System		
Operation	5	Destruction: Physical eradication of all or a portion of a body part by the direct use of energy, force, or al destructive agent		

Body Part (Character 4)	Approach (Character 5)	Device (Character 6)	Qualifier (Character 7)
0 Brain 1 Cerebral Meninges 2 Dura Mater 6 Cerebral Ventricle 7 Cerebral Hemisphere 8 Basal Ganglia 9 Thalamus A Hypothalamus B Pons C Cerebellum D Medulla Oblongata F Olfactory Nerve G Optic Nerve H Oculomotor Nerve J Trochlear Nerve K Trigeminal Nerve L Abducens Nerve M Facial Nerve N Acoustic Nerve P Glossopharyngeal Nerve Q Vagus Nerve R Accessory Nerve S Hypoglossal Nerve T Spinal Meninges W Cervical Spinal Cord X Thoracic Spinal Cord Y Lumbar Spinal Cord	0 Open 3 Percutaneous 4 Percutaneous Endoscopic	Z No Device	Z No Qualifier

Section	0	Medical and Surgical		
Body System	0	Central Nervous System		
Operation	8	Division: Cutting into a body part, without draining fluids and/or gases from the body part, in order to separate or transect a body part		

Body Part (Character 4)	Approach (Character 5)	Device (Character 6)	Qualifier (Character 7)
0 Brain 7 Cerebral Hemisphere 8 Basal Ganglia F Olfactory Nerve G Optic Nerve H Oculomotor Nerve J Trochlear Nerve K Trigeminal Nerve L Abducens Nerve M Facial Nerve N Acoustic Nerve P Glossopharyngeal Nerve Q Vagus Nerve R Accessory Nerve S Hypoglossal Nerve W Cervical Spinal Cord X Thoracic Spinal Cord Y Lumbar Spinal Cord	0 Open 3 Percutaneous 4 Percutaneous Endoscopic	Z No Device	Z No Qualifier

Section	0	Medical and Surgical		
Body System	0	Central Nervous System		
Operation	9	Drainage: Taking or letting out fluids and/or gases from a body part		

Body Part (Character 4)	Approach (Character 5)	Device (Character 6)	Qualifier (Character 7)
0 Brain 1 Cerebral Meninges 2 Dura Mater 3 Epidural Space 4 Subdural Space 5 Subarachnoid Space 6 Cerebral Ventricle 7 Cerebral Hemisphere 8 Basal Ganglia 9 Thalamus A Hypothalamus B Pons C Cerebellum D Medulla Oblongata F Olfactory Nerve G Optic Nerve H Oculomotor Nerve J Trochlear Nerve K Trigeminal Nerve L Abducens Nerve M Facial Nerve N Acoustic Nerve P Glossopharyngeal Nerve Q Vagus Nerve R Accessory Nerve S Hypoglossal Nerve T Spinal Meninges U Spinal Canal W Cervical Spinal Cord X Thoracic Spinal Cord Y Lumbar Spinal Cord	0 Open 3 Percutaneous 4 Percutaneous Endoscopic	0 Drainage Device	Z No Qualifier

Section	0	Medical and Surgical	
Body System	0	Central Nervous System	[continued]
Operation	9	Drainage: Taking or letting out fluids and/or gases from a body part	

Body Part (Character 4)	Approach (Character 5)	Device (Character 6)	Qualifier (Character 7)
0 Brain	0 Open	Z No Device	X Diagnostic
1 Cerebral Meninges	3 Percutaneous		Z No Qualifier
2 Dura Mater	4 Percutaneous Endoscopic		
3 Epidural Space			
4 Subdural Space			
5 Subarachnoid Space			
6 Cerebral Ventricle			
7 Cerebral Hemisphere			
8 Basal Ganglia			
9 Thalamus			
A Hypothalamus			
B Pons			
C Cerebellum			
D Medulla Oblongata			
F Olfactory Nerve			
G Optic Nerve			
H Oculomotor Nerve			
J Trochlear Nerve			
K Trigeminal Nerve			
L Abducens Nerve			
M Facial Nerve			
N Acoustic Nerve			
P Glossopharyngeal Nerve			
Q Vagus Nerve			
R Accessory Nerve			
S Hypoglossal Nerve			
T Spinal Meninges			
U Spinal Canal			
W Cervical Spinal Cord			
X Thoracic Spinal Cord			
Y Lumbar Spinal Cord			

Section	0	Medical and Surgical	
Body System	0	Central Nervous System	
Operation	B	Excision: Cutting out or off, without replacement, a portion of a body part	

Body Part (Character 4)	Approach (Character 5)	Device (Character 6)	Qualifier (Character 7)
0 Brain	0 Open	Z No Device	X Diagnostic
1 Cerebral Meninges	3 Percutaneous		Z No Qualifier
2 Dura Mater	4 Percutaneous Endoscopic		
6 Cerebral Ventricle			
7 Cerebral Hemisphere			
8 Basal Ganglia			
9 Thalamus			
A Hypothalamus			
B Pons			
C Cerebellum			
D Medulla Oblongata			
F Olfactory Nerve			
G Optic Nerve			
H Oculomotor Nerve			
J Trochlear Nerve			
K Trigeminal Nerve			
L Abducens Nerve			
M Facial Nerve			
N Acoustic Nerve			
P Glossopharyngeal Nerve			
Q Vagus Nerve			
R Accessory Nerve			
S Hypoglossal Nerve			
T Spinal Meninges			
W Cervical Spinal Cord			
X Thoracic Spinal Cord			
Y Lumbar Spinal Cord			

Section	0	Medical and Surgical		
Body System	0	Central Nervous System		
Operation	C	Extirpation: Taking or cutting out solid matter from a body part		
Body Part (Character 4)		Approach (Character 5)	Device (Character 6)	Qualifier (Character 7)
0 Brain		**0** Open	**Z** No Device	**Z** No Qualifier
1 Cerebral Meninges		**3** Percutaneous		
2 Dura Mater		**4** Percutaneous Endoscopic		
3 Epidural Space				
4 Subdural Space				
5 Subarachnoid Space				
6 Cerebral Ventricle				
7 Cerebral Hemisphere				
8 Basal Ganglia				
9 Thalamus				
A Hypothalamus				
B Pons				
C Cerebellum				
D Medulla Oblongata				
F Olfactory Nerve				
G Optic Nerve				
H Oculomotor Nerve				
J Trochlear Nerve				
K Trigeminal Nerve				
L Abducens Nerve				
M Facial Nerve				
N Acoustic Nerve				
P Glossopharyngeal Nerve				
Q Vagus Nerve				
R Accessory Nerve				
S Hypoglossal Nerve				
T Spinal Meninges				
W Cervical Spinal Cord				
X Thoracic Spinal Cord				
Y Lumbar Spinal Cord				

Section	0	Medical and Surgical		
Body System	0	Central Nervous System		
Operation	D	Extraction: Pulling or stripping out or off all or a portion of a body part by the use of force		
Body Part (Character 4)		Approach (Character 5)	Device (Character 6)	Qualifier (Character 7)
1 Cerebral Meninges		**0** Open	**Z** No Device	**Z** No Qualifier
2 Dura Mater		**3** Percutaneous		
F Olfactory Nerve		**4** Percutaneous Endoscopic		
G Optic Nerve				
H Oculomotor Nerve				
J Trochlear Nerve				
K Trigeminal Nerve				
L Abducens Nerve				
M Facial Nerve				
N Acoustic Nerve				
P Glossopharyngeal Nerve				
Q Vagus Nerve				
R Accessory Nerve				
S Hypoglossal Nerve				
T Spinal Meninges				

Section	0	Medical and Surgical		
Body System	0	Central Nervous System		
Operation	F	Fragmentation: Breaking solid matter in a body part into pieces		
Body Part (Character 4)		Approach (Character 5)	Device (Character 6)	Qualifier (Character 7)
3 Epidural Space		**0** Open	**Z** No Device	**Z** No Qualifier
4 Subdural Space		**3** Percutaneous		
5 Subarachnoid Space		**4** Percutaneous Endoscopic		
6 Cerebral Ventricle		**X** External		
U Spinal Canal				

Section	0	Medical and Surgical
Body System	0	Central Nervous System
Operation	H	Insertion: Putting in a nonbiological appliance that monitors, assists, performs, or prevents a physiological function but does not physically take the place of a body part

Body Part (Character 4)	Approach (Character 5)	Device (Character 6)	Qualifier (Character 7)
0 Brain 6 Cerebral Ventricle E Cranial Nerve U Spinal Canal V Spinal Cord	0 Open 3 Percutaneous 4 Percutaneous Endoscopic	2 Monitoring Device 3 Infusion Device M Neurostimulator Lead	Z No Qualifier

Section	0	Medical and Surgical
Body System	0	Central Nervous System
Operation	J	Inspection: Visually and/or manually exploring a body part

Body Part (Character 4)	Approach (Character 5)	Device (Character 6)	Qualifier (Character 7)
0 Brain E Cranial Nerve U Spinal Canal V Spinal Cord	0 Open 3 Percutaneous 4 Percutaneous Endoscopic	Z No Device	Z No Qualifier

Section	0	Medical and Surgical
Body System	0	Central Nervous System
Operation	K	Map: Locating the route of passage of electrical impulses and/or locating functional areas in a body part

Body Part (Character 4)	Approach (Character 5)	Device (Character 6)	Qualifier (Character 7)
0 Brain 7 Cerebral Hemisphere 8 Basal Ganglia 9 Thalamus A Hypothalamus B Pons C Cerebellum D Medulla Oblongata	0 Open 3 Percutaneous 4 Percutaneous Endoscopic	Z No Device	Z No Qualifier

Section	0	Medical and Surgical
Body System	0	Central Nervous System
Operation	N	Release: Freeing a body part from an abnormal physical constraint by cutting or by the use of force

Body Part (Character 4)	Approach (Character 5)	Device (Character 6)	Qualifier (Character 7)
0 Brain 1 Cerebral Meninges 2 Dura Mater 6 Cerebral Ventricle 7 Cerebral Hemisphere 8 Basal Ganglia 9 Thalamus A Hypothalamus B Pons C Cerebellum D Medulla Oblongata F Olfactory Nerve G Optic Nerve H Oculomotor Nerve J Trochlear Nerve K Trigeminal Nerve L Abducens Nerve M Facial Nerve N Acoustic Nerve P Glossopharyngeal Nerve Q Vagus Nerve R Accessory Nerve S Hypoglossal Nerve T Spinal Meninges W Cervical Spinal Cord X Thoracic Spinal Cord Y Lumbar Spinal Cord	0 Open 3 Percutaneous 4 Percutaneous Endoscopic	Z No Device	Z No Qualifier

Section	0	Medical and Surgical	
Body System	0	Central Nervous System	
Operation	P	Removal: Taking out or off a device from a body part	

Body Part (Character 4)	Approach (Character 5)	Device (Character 6)	Qualifier (Character 7)
0 Brain V Spinal Cord	0 Open 3 Percutaneous 4 Percutaneous Endoscopic	0 Drainage Device 2 Monitoring Device 3 Infusion Device 7 Autologous Tissue Substitute J Synthetic Substitute K Nonautologous Tissue Substitute M Neurostimulator Lead	Z No Qualifier
0 Brain V Spinal Cord	X External	0 Drainage Device 2 Monitoring Device 3 Infusion Device M Neurostimulator Lead	Z No Qualifier
6 Cerebral Ventricle U Spinal Canal	0 Open 3 Percutaneous 4 Percutaneous Endoscopic	0 Drainage Device 2 Monitoring Device 3 Infusion Device J Synthetic Substitute M Neurostimulator Lead	Z No Qualifier
6 Cerebral Ventricle U Spinal Canal	X External	0 Drainage Device 2 Monitoring Device 3 Infusion Device M Neurostimulator Lead	Z No Qualifier
E Cranial Nerve	0 Open 3 Percutaneous 4 Percutaneous Endoscopic	0 Drainage Device 2 Monitoring Device 3 Infusion Device 7 Autologous Tissue Substitute M Neurostimulator Lead	Z No Qualifier
E Cranial Nerve	X External	0 Drainage Device 2 Monitoring Device 3 Infusion Device M Neurostimulator Lead	Z No Qualifier

Section	0	Medical and Surgical	
Body System	0	Central Nervous System	
Operation	Q	Repair: Restoring, to the extent possible, a body part to its normal anatomic structure and function	

Body Part (Character 4)	Approach (Character 5)	Device (Character 6)	Qualifier (Character 7)
0 Brain 1 Cerebral Meninges 2 Dura Mater 6 Cerebral Ventricle 7 Cerebral Hemisphere 8 Basal Ganglia 9 Thalamus A Hypothalamus B Pons C Cerebellum D Medulla Oblongata F Olfactory Nerve G Optic Nerve H Oculomotor Nerve J Trochlear Nerve K Trigeminal Nerve L Abducens Nerve M Facial Nerve N Acoustic Nerve P Glossopharyngeal Nerve Q Vagus Nerve R Accessory Nerve S Hypoglossal Nerve T Spinal Meninges W Cervical Spinal Cord X Thoracic Spinal Cord Y Lumbar Spinal Cord	0 Open 3 Percutaneous 4 Percutaneous Endoscopic	Z No Device	Z No Qualifier

Section	0	Medical and Surgical		
Body System	0	Central Nervous System		
Operation	S	Reposition: Moving to its normal location, or other suitable location, all or a portion of a body part		

Body Part (Character 4)	Approach (Character 5)	Device (Character 6)	Qualifier (Character 7)
F Olfactory Nerve G Optic Nerve H Oculomotor Nerve J Trochlear Nerve K Trigeminal Nerve L Abducens Nerve M Facial Nerve N Acoustic Nerve P Glossopharyngeal Nerve Q Vagus Nerve R Accessory Nerve S Hypoglossal Nerve W Cervical Spinal Cord X Thoracic Spinal Cord Y Lumbar Spinal Cord	0 Open 3 Percutaneous 4 Percutaneous Endoscopic	Z No Device	Z No Qualifier

Section	0	Medical and Surgical		
Body System	0	Central Nervous System		
Operation	T	Resection: Cutting out or off, without replacement, all of a body part		

Body Part (Character 4)	Approach (Character 5)	Device (Character 6)	Qualifier (Character 7)
7 Cerebral Hemisphere	0 Open 3 Percutaneous 4 Percutaneous Endoscopic	Z No Device	Z No Qualifier

Section	0	Medical and Surgical		
Body System	0	Central Nervous System		
Operation	U	Supplement: Putting in or on biological or synthetic material that physically reinforces and/or augments the function of a portion of a body part		

Body Part (Character 4)	Approach (Character 5)	Device (Character 6)	Qualifier (Character 7)
1 Cerebral Meninges 2 Dura Mater T Spinal Meninges	0 Open 3 Percutaneous 4 Percutaneous Endoscopic	7 Autologous Tissue Substitute J Synthetic Substitute K Nonautologous Tissue Substitute	Z No Qualifier
F Olfactory Nerve G Optic Nerve H Oculomotor Nerve J Trochlear Nerve K Trigeminal Nerve L Abducens Nerve M Facial Nerve N Acoustic Nerve P Glossopharyngeal Nerve Q Vagus Nerve R Accessory Nerve S Hypoglossal Nerve	0 Open 3 Percutaneous 4 Percutaneous Endoscopic	7 Autologous Tissue Substitute	Z No Qualifier

Section	0	Medical and Surgical		
Body System	0	Central Nervous System		
Operation	W	Revision: Correcting, to the extent possible, a portion of a malfunctioning device or the position of a displaced device		

Body Part (Character 4)	Approach (Character 5)	Device (Character 6)	Qualifier (Character 7)
0 Brain V Spinal Cord	0 Open 3 Percutaneous 4 Percutaneous Endoscopic X External	0 Drainage Device 2 Monitoring Device 3 Infusion Device 7 Autologous Tissue Substitute J Synthetic Substitute K Nonautologous Tissue Substitute M Neurostimulator Lead	Z No Qualifier
6 Cerebral Ventricle U Spinal Canal	0 Open 3 Percutaneous 4 Percutaneous Endoscopic X External	0 Drainage Device 2 Monitoring Device 3 Infusion Device J Synthetic Substitute M Neurostimulator Lead	Z No Qualifier
E Cranial Nerve	0 Open 3 Percutaneous 4 Percutaneous Endoscopic X External	0 Drainage Device 2 Monitoring Device 3 Infusion Device 7 Autologous Tissue Substitute M Neurostimulator Lead	Z No Qualifier

Section	0	Medical and Surgical		
Body System	0	Central Nervous System		
Operation	X	Transfer: Moving, without taking out, all or a portion of a body part to another location to take over the function of all or a portion of a body part		

Body Part (Character 4)	Approach (Character 5)	Device (Character 6)	Qualifier (Character 7)
F Olfactory Nerve G Optic Nerve H Oculomotor Nerve J Trochlear Nerve K Trigeminal Nerve L Abducens Nerve M Facial Nerve N Acoustic Nerve P Glossopharyngeal Nerve Q Vagus Nerve R Accessory Nerve S Hypoglossal Nerve	0 Open 4 Percutaneous Endoscopic	Z No Device	F Olfactory Nerve G Optic Nerve H Oculomotor Nerve J Trochlear Nerve K Trigeminal Nerve L Abducens Nerve M Facial Nerve N Acoustic Nerve P Glossopharyngeal Nerve Q Vagus Nerve R Accessory Nerve S Hypoglossal Nerve

Section	0	Medical and Surgical		
Body System	1	Peripheral Nervous System		
Operation	2	Change: Taking out or off a device from a body part and putting back an identical or similar device in or on the same body part without cutting or puncturing the skin or a mucous membrane		

Body Part (Character 4)	Approach (Character 5)	Device (Character 6)	Qualifier (Character 7)
Y Peripheral Nerve	X External	0 Drainage Device Y Other Device	Z No Qualifier

Section	0	Medical and Surgical		
Body System	1	Peripheral Nervous System		
Operation	5	Destruction: Physical eradication of all or a portion of a body part by the direct use of energy, force, or a destructive agent		

Body Part (Character 4)	Approach (Character 5)	Device (Character 6)	Qualifier (Character 7)
0 Cervical Plexus 1 Cervical Nerve 2 Phrenic Nerve 3 Brachial Plexus 4 Ulnar Nerve 5 Median Nerve 6 Radial Nerve 8 Thoracic Nerve 9 Lumbar Plexus A Lumbosacral Plexus B Lumbar Nerve C Pudendal Nerve D Femoral Nerve F Sciatic Nerve G Tibial Nerve H Peroneal Nerve K Head and Neck Sympathetic Nerve L Thoracic Sympathetic Nerve M Abdominal Sympathetic Nerve N Lumbar Sympathetic Nerve P Sacral Sympathetic Nerve Q Sacral Plexus R Sacral Nerve	0 Open 3 Percutaneous 4 Percutaneous Endoscopic	Z No Device	Z No Qualifier

Section	0	Medical and Surgical		
Body System	1	Peripheral Nervous System		
Operation	8	Division: Cutting into a body part, without draining fluids and/or gases from the body part, in order to separate or transect a body part		

Body Part (Character 4)	Approach (Character 5)	Device (Character 6)	Qualifier (Character 7)
0 Cervical Plexus 1 Cervical Nerve 2 Phrenic Nerve 3 Brachial Plexus 4 Ulnar Nerve 5 Median Nerve 6 Radial Nerve 8 Thoracic Nerve 9 Lumbar Plexus A Lumbosacral Plexus B Lumbar Nerve C Pudendal Nerve D Femoral Nerve F Sciatic Nerve G Tibial Nerve H Peroneal Nerve K Head and Neck Sympathetic Nerve L Thoracic Sympathetic Nerve M Abdominal Sympathetic Nerve N Lumbar Sympathetic Nerve P Sacral Sympathetic Nerve Q Sacral Plexus R Sacral Nerve	0 Open 3 Percutaneous 4 Percutaneous Endoscopic	Z No Device	Z No Qualifier

Section	0	Medical and Surgical		
Body System	1	Peripheral Nervous System		
Operation	9	Drainage: Taking or letting out fluids and/or gases from a body part		

Body Part (Character 4)	Approach (Character 5)	Device (Character 6)	Qualifier (Character 7)
0 Cervical Plexus	0 Open	0 Drainage Device	Z No Qualifier
1 Cervical Nerve	3 Percutaneous		
2 Phrenic Nerve	4 Percutaneous Endoscopic		
3 Brachial Plexus			
4 Ulnar Nerve			
5 Median Nerve			
6 Radial Nerve			
8 Thoracic Nerve			
9 Lumbar Plexus			
A Lumbosacral Plexus			
B Lumbar Nerve			
C Pudendal Nerve			
D Femoral Nerve			
F Sciatic Nerve			
G Tibial Nerve			
H Peroneal Nerve			
K Head and Neck Sympathetic Nerve			
L Thoracic Sympathetic Nerve			
M Abdominal Sympathetic Nerve			
N Lumbar Sympathetic Nerve			
P Sacral Sympathetic Nerve			
Q Sacral Plexus			
R Sacral Nerve			

Section	0	Medical and Surgical		
Body System	1	Peripheral Nervous System		
Operation	9	Drainage: Taking or letting out fluids and/or gases from a body part		

Body Part (Character 4)	Approach (Character 5)	Device (Character 6)	Qualifier (Character 7)
0 Cervical Plexus	0 Open	Z No Device	X Diagnostic
1 Cervical Nerve	3 Percutaneous		Z No Qualifier
2 Phrenic Nerve	4 Percutaneous Endoscopic		
3 Brachial Plexus			
4 Ulnar Nerve			
5 Median Nerve			
6 Radial Nerve			
8 Thoracic Nerve			
9 Lumbar Plexus			
A Lumbosacral Plexus			
B Lumbar Nerve			
C Pudendal Nerve			
D Femoral Nerve			
F Sciatic Nerve			
G Tibial Nerve			
H Peroneal Nerve			
K Head and Neck Sympathetic Nerve			
L Thoracic Sympathetic Nerve			
M Abdominal Sympathetic Nerve			
N Lumbar Sympathetic Nerve			
P Sacral Sympathetic Nerve			
Q Sacral Plexus			
R Sacral Nerve			

Section	0	Medical and Surgical			
Body System	1	Peripheral Nervous System			
Operation	B	Excision: Cutting out or off, without replacement, a portion of a body part			

Body Part (Character 4)	Approach (Character 5)	Device (Character 6)	Qualifier (Character 7)
0 Cervical Plexus	0 Open	Z No Device	X Diagnostic
1 Cervical Nerve	3 Percutaneous		Z No Qualifier
2 Phrenic Nerve	4 Percutaneous Endoscopic		
3 Brachial Plexus			
4 Ulnar Nerve			
5 Median Nerve			
6 Radial Nerve			
8 Thoracic Nerve			
9 Lumbar Plexus			
A Lumbosacral Plexus			
B Lumbar Nerve			
C Pudendal Nerve			
D Femoral Nerve			
F Sciatic Nerve			
G Tibial Nerve			
H Peroneal Nerve			
K Head and Neck Sympathetic Nerve			
L Thoracic Sympathetic Nerve			
M Abdominal Sympathetic Nerve			
N Lumbar Sympathetic Nerve			
P Sacral Sympathetic Nerve			
Q Sacral Plexus			
R Sacral Nerve			

Section	0	Medical and Surgical			
Body System	1	Peripheral Nervous System			
Operation	C	Extirpation: Taking or cutting out solid matter from a body part			

Body Part (Character 4)	Approach (Character 5)	Device (Character 6)	Qualifier (Character 7)
0 Cervical Plexus	0 Open	Z No Device	Z No Device
1 Cervical Nerve	3 Percutaneous		
2 Phrenic Nerve	4 Percutaneous Endoscopic		
3 Brachial Plexus			
4 Ulnar Nerve			
5 Median Nerve			
6 Radial Nerve			
8 Thoracic Nerve			
9 Lumbar Plexus			
A Lumbosacral Plexus			
B Lumbar Nerve			
C Pudendal Nerve			
D Femoral Nerve			
F Sciatic Nerve			
G Tibial Nerve			
H Peroneal Nerve			
K Head and Neck Sympathetic Nerve			
L Thoracic Sympathetic Nerve			
M Abdominal Sympathetic Nerve			
N Lumbar Sympathetic Nerve			
P Sacral Sympathetic Nerve			
Q Sacral Plexus			
R Sacral Nerve			

Section	0	Medical and Surgical		
Body System	1	Peripheral Nervous System		
Operation	D	Extraction: Pulling or stripping out or off all or a portion of a body part by the use of force		
Body Part (Character 4)		**Approach (Character 5)**	**Device (Character 6)**	**Qualifier (Character 7)**
0 Cervical Plexus		0 Open	Z No Device	Z No Qualifier
1 Cervical Nerve		3 Percutaneous		
2 Phrenic Nerve		4 Percutaneous Endoscopic		
3 Brachial Plexus				
4 Ulnar Nerve				
5 Median Nerve				
6 Radial Nerve				
8 Thoracic Nerve				
9 Lumbar Plexus				
A Lumbosacral Plexus				
B Lumbar Nerve				
C Pudendal Nerve				
D Femoral Nerve				
F Sciatic Nerve				
G Tibial Nerve				
H Peroneal Nerve				
K Head and Neck Sympathetic Nerve				
L Thoracic Sympathetic Nerve				
M Abdominal Sympathetic Nerve				
N Lumbar Sympathetic Nerve				
P Sacral Sympathetic Nerve				
Q Sacral Plexus				
R Sacral Nerve				

Section	0	Medical and Surgical		
Body System	1	Peripheral Nervous System		
Operation	H	Insertion: Putting in a nonbiological appliance that monitors, assists, performs, or prevents a physiological function but does not physically take the place of a body part		
Body Part (Character 4)		**Approach (Character 5)**	**Device (Character 6)**	**Qualifier (Character 7)**
Y Peripheral Nerve		0 Open	2 Monitoring Device	Z No Qualifier
		3 Percutaneous	M Neurostimulator Lead	
		4 Percutaneous Endoscopic		

Section	0	Medical and Surgical		
Body System	1	Peripheral Nervous System		
Operation	J	Inspection: Visually and/or manually exploring a body part		
Body Part (Character 4)		**Approach (Character 5)**	**Device (Character 6)**	**Qualifier (Character 7)**
Y Peripheral Nerve		0 Open	Z No Device	Z No Qualifier
		3 Percutaneous		
		4 Percutaneous Endoscopic		

Section	0	Medical and Surgical		
Body System	1	Peripheral Nervous System		
Operation	N	Release: Freeing a body part from an abnormal physical constraint by cutting or by the use of force		

Body Part (Character 4)	Approach (Character 5)	Device (Character 6)	Qualifier (Character 7)
0 Cervical Plexus 1 Cervical Nerve 2 Phrenic Nerve 3 Brachial Plexus 4 Ulnar Nerve 5 Median Nerve 6 Radial Nerve 8 Thoracic Nerve 9 Lumbar Plexus A Lumbosacral Plexus B Lumbar Nerve C Pudendal Nerve D Femoral Nerve F Sciatic Nerve G Tibial Nerve H Peroneal Nerve K Head and Neck Sympathetic Nerve L Thoracic Sympathetic Nerve M Abdominal Sympathetic Nerve N Lumbar Sympathetic Nerve P Sacral Sympathetic Nerve Q Sacral Plexus R Sacral Nerve	0 Open 3 Percutaneous 4 Percutaneous Endoscopic	Z No Device	Z No Qualifier

Section	0	Medical and Surgical		
Body System	1	Peripheral Nervous System		
Operation	P	Removal: Taking out or off a device from a body part		

Body Part (Character 4)	Approach (Character 5)	Device (Character 6)	Qualifier (Character 7)
Y Peripheral Nerve	0 Open 3 Percutaneous 4 Percutaneous Endoscopic	0 Drainage Device 2 Monitoring Device 7 Autologous Tissue Substitute M Neurostimulator Lead	Z No Qualifier
Y Peripheral Nerve	X External	0 Drainage Device 2 Monitoring Device M Neurostimulator Lead	Z No Qualifier

Section	0	Medical and Surgical		
Body System	1	Peripheral Nervous System		
Operation	Q	Repair: Restoring, to the extent possible, a body part to its normal anatomic structure and function		

Body Part (Character 4)	Approach (Character 5)	Device (Character 6)	Qualifier (Character 7)
0 Cervical Plexus 1 Cervical Nerve 2 Phrenic Nerve 3 Brachial Plexus 4 Ulnar Nerve 5 Median Nerve 6 Radial Nerve 8 Thoracic Nerve 9 Lumbar Plexus A Lumbosacral Plexus B Lumbar Nerve C Pudendal Nerve D Femoral Nerve F Sciatic Nerve G Tibial Nerve H Peroneal Nerve K Head and Neck Sympathetic Nerve L Thoracic Sympathetic Nerve M Abdominal Sympathetic Nerve N Lumbar Sympathetic Nerve P Sacral Sympathetic Nerve Q Sacral Plexus R Sacral Nerve	0 Open 3 Percutaneous 4 Percutaneous Endoscopic	Z No Device	Z No Qualifier

Section	0	Medical and Surgical			
Body System	1	Peripheral Nervous System			
Operation	S	Reposition: Moving to its normal location, or other suitable location, all or a portion of a body part			

Body Part (Character 4)	Approach (Character 5)	Device (Character 6)	Qualifier (Character 7)
0 Cervical Plexus 1 Cervical Nerve 2 Phrenic Nerve 3 Brachial Plexus 4 Ulnar Nerve 5 Median Nerve 6 Radial Nerve 8 Thoracic Nerve 9 Lumbar Plexus A Lumbosacral Plexus B Lumbar Nerve C Pudendal Nerve D Femoral Nerve F Sciatic Nerve G Tibial Nerve H Peroneal Nerve Q Sacral Plexus R Sacral Nerve	0 Open 3 Percutaneous 4 Percutaneous Endoscopic	Z No Device	Z No Qualifier

Section	0	Medical and Surgical			
Body System	1	Peripheral Nervous System			
Operation	U	Supplement: Putting in or on biological or synthetic material that physically reinforces and/or augments the function of a portion of a body part			

Body Part (Character 4)	Approach (Character 5)	Device (Character 6)	Qualifier (Character 7)
1 Cervical Nerve 2 Phrenic Nerve 4 Ulnar Nerve 5 Median Nerve 6 Radial Nerve 8 Thoracic Nerve B Lumbar Nerve C Pudendal Nerve D Femoral Nerve F Sciatic Nerve G Tibial Nerve H Peroneal Nerve R Sacral Nerve	0 Open 3 Percutaneous 4 Percutaneous Endoscopic	7 Autologous Tissue Substitute	Z No Qualifier

Section	0	Medical and Surgical			
Body System	1	Peripheral Nervous System			
Operation	W	Revision: Correcting, to the extent possible, a portion of a malfunctioning device or the position of a displaced device			

Body Part (Character 4)	Approach (Character 5)	Device (Character 6)	Qualifier (Character 7)
Y Peripheral Nerve	0 Open 3 Percutaneous 4 Percutaneous Endoscopic X External	0 Drainage Device 2 Monitoring Device 7 Autologous Tissue Substitute M Neurostimulator Lead	Z No Qualifier

Section	0	Medical and Surgical			
Body System	1	Peripheral Nervous System			
Operation	X	Transfer: Moving, without taking out, all or a portion of a body part to another location to take over the function of all or a portion of a body part			

Body Part (Character 4)	Approach (Character 5)	Device (Character 6)	Qualifier (Character 7)
1 Cervical Nerve 2 Phrenic Nerve	0 Open 4 Percutaneous Endoscopic	Z No Device	1 Cervical Nerve 2 Phrenic Nerve
4 Ulnar Nerve 5 Median Nerve 6 Radial Nerve	0 Open 4 Percutaneous Endoscopic	Z No Device	4 Ulnar Nerve 5 Median Nerve 6 Radial Nerve
8 Thoracic Nerve	0 Open 4 Percutaneous Endoscopic	Z No Device	8 Thoracic Nerve
B Lumbar Nerve C Pudendal Nerve	0 Open 4 Percutaneous Endoscopic	Z No Device	B Lumbar Nerve C Perineal Nerve
D Femoral Nerve F Sciatic Nerve G Tibial Nerve H Peroneal Nerve	0 Open 4 Percutaneous Endoscopic	Z No Device	D Femoral Nerve F Sciatic Nerve G Tibial Nerve H Peroneal Nerve

Section	0	Medical and Surgical	
Body System	2	Heart and Great Vessels	
Operation	1	Bypass: Altering the route of passage of the contents of a tubular body part	

Body Part (Character 4)	Approach (Character 5)	Device (Character 6)	Qualifier (Character 7)
0 Coronary Artery, One Site 1 Coronary Artery, Two Sites 2 Coronary Artery, Three Sites 3 Coronary Artery, Four or More Sites	0 Open	9 Autologous Venous Tissue A Autologous Arterial Tissue J Synthetic Substitute K Nonautologous Tissue Substitute	3 Coronary Artery 8 Internal Mammary, Right 9 Internal Mammary, Left C Thoracic Artery F Abdominal Artery W Aorta
0 Coronary Artery, One Site 1 Coronary Artery, Two Sites 2 Coronary Artery, Three Sites 3 Coronary Artery, Four or More Sites	0 Open	Z No Device	3 Coronary Artery 8 Internal Mammary, Right 9 Internal Mammary, Left C Thoracic Artery F Abdominal Artery
0 Coronary Artery, One Site 1 Coronary Artery, Two Sites 2 Coronary Artery, Three Sites 3 Coronary Artery, Four or More Sites	3 Percutaneous	4 Intraluminal Device, Drug-eluting D Intraluminal Device	4 Coronary Vein
0 Coronary Artery, One Site 1 Coronary Artery, Two Sites 2 Coronary Artery, Three Sites 3 Coronary Artery, Four or More Sites	4 Percutaneous Endoscopic	4 Intraluminal Device, Drug-eluting D Intraluminal Device	4 Coronary Vein
0 Coronary Artery, One Site 1 Coronary Artery, Two Sites 2 Coronary Artery, Three Sites 3 Coronary Artery, Four or More Sites	4 Percutaneous Endoscopic	9 Autologous Venous Tissue A Autologous Arterial Tissue J Synthetic Substitute K Nonautologous Tissue Substitute	3 Coronary Artery 8 Internal Mammary, Right 9 Internal Mammary, Left C Thoracic Artery F Abdominal Artery W Aorta
0 Coronary Artery, One Site 1 Coronary Artery, Two Sites 2 Coronary Artery, Three Sites 3 Coronary Artery, Four or More Sites	4 Percutaneous Endoscopic	Z No Device	3 Coronary Artery 8 Internal Mammary, Right 9 Internal Mammary, Left C Thoracic Artery F Abdominal Artery
6 Atrium, Right	0 Open 4 Percutaneous Endoscopic	9 Autologous Venous Tissue A Autologous Arterial Tissue J Synthetic Substitute K Nonautologous Tissue Substitute	P Pulmonary Trunk Q Pulmonary Artery, Right R Pulmonary Artery, Left

Section	0	Medical and Surgical	
Body System	2	Heart and Great Vessels	
Operation	1	Bypass: Altering the route of passage of the contents of a tubular body part	

Body Part (Character 4)	Approach (Character 5)	Device (Character 6)	Qualifier (Character 7)
6 Atrium, Right	0 Open 4 Percutaneous Endoscopic	Z No Device	7 Atrium, Left P Pulmonary Trunk Q Pulmonary Artery, Right R Pulmonary Artery, Left
7 Atrium, Left V Superior Vena Cava	0 Open 4 Percutaneous Endoscopic	9 Autologous Venous Tissue A Autologous Arterial Tissue J Synthetic Substitute K Nonautologous Tissue Substitute Z No Device	P Pulmonary Trunk Q Pulmonary Artery, Right R Pulmonary Artery, Left
K Ventricle, Right L Ventricle, Left	0 Open 4 Percutaneous Endoscopic	9 Autologous Venous Tissue A Autologous Arterial Tissue J Synthetic Substitute K Nonautologous Tissue Substitute	P Pulmonary Trunk Q Pulmonary Artery, Right R Pulmonary Artery, Left
K Ventricle, Right L Ventricle, Left	0 Open 4 Percutaneous Endoscopic	Z No Device	5 Coronary Circulation 8 Internal Mammary, Right 9 Internal Mammary, Left C Thoracic Artery F Abdominal Artery P Pulmonary Trunk Q Pulmonary Artery, Right R Pulmonary Artery, Left W Aorta
W Thoracic Aorta	0 Open 4 Percutaneous Endoscopic	9 Autologous Venous Tissue A Autologous Arterial Tissue J Synthetic Substitute K Nonautologous Tissue Substitute Z No Device	B Subclavian D Carotid P Pulmonary Trunk Q Pulmonary Artery, Right R Pulmonary Artery, Left

Section	0	Medical and Surgical
Body System	2	Heart and Great Vessels
Operation	5	Destruction: Physical eradication of all or a portion of a body part by the direct use of energy, force, or a destructive agent

Body Part (Character 4)	Approach (Character 5)	Device (Character 6)	Qualifier (Character 7)
4 Coronary Vein 5 Atrial Septum 6 Atrium, Right 8 Conduction Mechanism 9 Chordae Tendineae D Papillary Muscle F Aortic Valve G Mitral Valve H Pulmonary Valve J Tricuspid Valve K Ventricle, Right L Ventricle, Left M Ventricular Septum N Pericardium P Pulmonary Trunk Q Pulmonary Artery, Right R Pulmonary Artery, Left S Pulmonary Vein, Right T Pulmonary Vein, Left V Superior Vena Cava W Thoracic Aorta	0 Open 3 Percutaneous 4 Percutaneous Endoscopic	Z No Device	Z No Qualifier
7 Atrium, Left	0 Open 3 Percutaneous 4 Percutaneous Endoscopic	Z No Device	K Left Atrial Appendage Z No Qualifier

Section	0	Medical and Surgical
Body System	2	Heart and Great Vessels
Operation	7	Dilation: Expanding an orifice or the lumen of a tubular body part

Body Part (Character 4)	Approach (Character 5)	Device (Character 6)	Qualifier (Character 7)
0 Coronary Artery, One Site 1 Coronary Artery, Two Sites 2 Coronary Artery, Three Sites 3 Coronary Artery, Four or More Sites	0 Open 3 Percutaneous 4 Percutaneous Endoscopic	4 Intraluminal Device, Drug-eluting D Intraluminal Device T Intraluminal Device, Radioactive Z No Device	6 Bifurcation Z No Qualifier
F Aortic Valve G Mitral Valve H Pulmonary Valve J Tricuspid Valve K Ventricle, Right P Pulmonary Trunk Q Pulmonary Artery, Right S Pulmonary Vein, Right T Pulmonary Vein, Left V Superior Vena Cava W Thoracic Aorta	0 Open 3 Percutaneous 4 Percutaneous Endoscopic	4 Intraluminal Device, Drug-eluting D Intraluminal Device Z No Device	Z No Qualifier
R Pulmonary Artery, Left	0 Open 3 Percutaneous 4 Percutaneous Endoscopic	4 Intraluminal Device, Drug-eluting D Intraluminal Device Z No Device	T Ductus Arteriosus Z No Qualifier

Section	0	Medical and Surgical
Body System	2	Heart and Great Vessels
Operation	8	Division: Cutting into a body part, without draining fluids and/or gases from the body part, in order to separate or transect a body part

Body Part Character 4	Approach Character 5	Device Character 6	Qualifier Character 7
8 Conduction Mechanism 9 Chordae Tendineae D Papillary Muscle	0 Open 3 Percutaneous 4 Percutaneous Endoscopic	Z No Device	Z No Qualifier

Section	0	Medical and Surgical		
Body System	2	Heart and Great Vessels		
Operation	B	Excision: Cutting out or off, without replacement, a portion of a body part		

Body Part (Character 4)	Approach (Character 5)	Device (Character 6)	Qualifier (Character 7)
4 Coronary Vein 5 Atrial Septum 6 Atrium, Right 8 Conduction Mechanism 9 Chordae Tendineae D Papillary Muscle F Aortic Valve G Mitral Valve H Pulmonary Valve J Tricuspid Valve K Ventricle, Right L Ventricle, Left M Ventricular Septum N Pericardium P Pulmonary Trunk Q Pulmonary Artery, Right R Pulmonary Artery, Left S Pulmonary Vein, Right T Pulmonary Vein, Left V Superior Vena Cava W Thoracic Aorta	0 Open 3 Percutaneous 4 Percutaneous Endoscopic	Z No Device	X Diagnostic Z No Qualifier
7 Atrium, Left	0 Open 3 Percutaneous 4 Percutaneous Endoscopic	Z No Device	K Left Atrial Appendage X Diagnostic Z No Qualifier

Section	0	Medical and Surgical		
Body System	2	Heart and Great Vessels		
Operation	C	Extirpation: Taking or cutting out solid matter from a body part		

Body Part (Character 4)	Approach (Character 5)	Device (Character 6)	Qualifier (Character 7)
0 Coronary Artery, One Site 1 Coronary Artery, Two Sites 2 Coronary Artery, Three Sites 3 Coronary Artery, Four or More Sites 4 Coronary Vein 5 Atrial Septum 6 Atrium, Right 7 Atrium, Left 8 Conduction Mechanism 9 Chordae Tendineae D Papillary Muscle F Aortic Valve G Mitral Valve H Pulmonary Valve J Tricuspid Valve K Ventricle, Right L Ventricle, Left M Ventricular Septum N Pericardium P Pulmonary Trunk Q Pulmonary Artery, Right R Pulmonary Artery, Left S Pulmonary Vein, Right T Pulmonary Vein, Left V Superior Vena Cava W Thoracic Aorta	0 Open 3 Percutaneous 4 Percutaneous Endoscopic	Z No Device	Z No Qualifier

Section	0	Medical and Surgical		
Body System	2	Heart and Great Vessels		
Operation	F	Fragmentation: Breaking solid matter in a body part into pieces		

Body Part (Character 4)	Approach (Character 5)	Device (Character 6)	Qualifier (Character 7)
N Pericardium	0 Open 3 Percutaneous 4 Percutaneous Endoscopic X External	Z No Device	Z No Qualifier

Section	0	Medical and Surgical
Body System	2	Heart and Great Vessels
Operation	H	Insertion: Putting in a nonbiological appliance that monitors, assists, performs, or prevents a physiological function but does not physically take the place of a body part

Body Part (Character 4)	Approach (Character 5)	Device (Character 6)	Qualifier (Character 7)
4 Coronary Vein 6 Atrium, Right 7 Atrium, Left K Ventricle, Right L Ventricle, Left	0 Open 3 Percutaneous 4 Percutaneous Endoscopic	0 Monitoring Device, Pressure Sensor 2 Monitoring Device 3 Infusion Device D Intraluminal Device J Cardiac Lead, Pacemaker K Cardiac Lead, Defibrillator M Cardiac Lead	Z No Qualifier
A Heart	0 Open 3 Percutaneous 4 Percutaneous Endoscopic	Q Implantable Heart Assist System	Z No Qualifier
A Heart	0 Open 3 Percutaneous 4 Percutaneous Endoscopic	R External Heart Assist System	S Biventricular Z No Qualifier
N Pericardium	0 Open 3 Percutaneous 4 Percutaneous Endoscopic	0 Monitoring Device, Pressure Sensor 2 Monitoring Device J Cardiac Lead, Pacemaker K Cardiac Lead, Defibrillator M Cardiac Lead	Z No Qualifier
P Pulmonary Trunk Q Pulmonary Artery, Right R Pulmonary Artery, Left S Pulmonary Vein, Right T Pulmonary Vein, Left V Superior Vena Cava W Thoracic Aorta	0 Open 3 Percutaneous 4 Percutaneous Endoscopic	0 Monitoring Device, Pressure Sensor 2 Monitoring Device 3 Infusion Device D Intraluminal Device	Z No Qualifier

Section	0	Medical and Surgical
Body System	2	Heart and Great Vessels
Operation	J	Inspection: Visually and/or manually exploring a body part

Body Part (Character 4)	Approach (Character 5)	Device (Character 6)	Qualifier (Character 7)
A Heart Y Great Vessel	0 Open 3 Percutaneous 4 Percutaneous Endoscopic	Z No Device	Z No Qualifier

Section	0	Medical and Surgical
Body System	2	Heart and Great Vessels
Operation	K	Map: Locating the route of passage of electrical impulses and/or locating functional areas in a body part

Body Part (Character 4)	Approach (Character 5)	Device (Character 6)	Qualifier (Character 7)
8 Conduction Mechanism	0 Open 3 Percutaneous 4 Percutaneous Endoscopic	Z No Device	Z No Qualifier

Section	0	Medical and Surgical
Body System	2	Heart and Great Vessels
Operation	L	Occlusion: Completely closing an orifice or the lumen of a tubular body part

Body Part (Character 4)	Approach (Character 5)	Device (Character 6)	Qualifier (Character 7)
7 Atrium, Left	0 Open 3 Percutaneous 4 Percutaneous Endoscopic	C Extraluminal Device D Intraluminal Device Z No Device	K Left Atrial Appendage
R Pulmonary Artery, Left	0 Open 3 Percutaneous 4 Percutaneous Endoscopic	C Extraluminal Device D Intraluminal Device Z No Device	T Ductus Arteriosus
S Pulmonary Vein, Right T Pulmonary Vein, Left V Superior Vena Cava	0 Open 3 Percutaneous 4 Percutaneous Endoscopic	C Extraluminal Device D Intraluminal Device Z No Device	Z No Qualifier

Section	0	Medical and Surgical		
Body System	2	Heart and Great Vessels		
Operation	N	Release: Freeing a body part from an abnormal physical constraint by cutting or by the use of force		
Body Part (Character 4)		Approach (Character 5)	Device (Character 6)	Qualifier (Character 7)
4 Coronary Vein 5 Atrial Septum 6 Atrium, Right 7 Atrium, Left 8 Conduction Mechanism 9 Chordae Tendineae D Papillary Muscle F Aortic Valve G Mitral Valve H Pulmonary Valve J Tricuspid Valve K Ventricle, Right L Ventricle, Left M Ventricular Septum N Pericardium P Pulmonary Trunk Q Pulmonary Artery, Right R Pulmonary Artery, Left S Pulmonary Vein, Right T Pulmonary Vein, Left V Superior Vena Cava W Thoracic Aorta		0 Open 3 Percutaneous 4 Percutaneous Endoscopic	Z No Device	Z No Qualifier

Section	0	Medical and Surgical		
Body System	2	Heart and Great Vessels		
Operation	P	Removal: Taking out or off a device from a body part		
Body Part (Character 4)		Approach (Character 5)	Device (Character 6)	Qualifier (Character 7)
A Heart		0 Open 3 Percutaneous 4 Percutaneous Endoscopic	2 Monitoring Device 3 Infusion Device 7 Autologous Tissue Substitute 8 Zooplastic Tissue C Extraluminal Device D Intraluminal Device J Synthetic Substitute K Nonautologous Tissue Substitute M Cardiac Lead Q Implantable Heart Assist System R External Heart Assist System	Z No Qualifier
A Heart		X External	2 Monitoring Device 3 Infusion Device D Intraluminal Device M Cardiac Lead	Z No Qualifier
Y Great Vessel		0 Open 3 Percutaneous 4 Percutaneous Endoscopic	2 Monitoring Device 3 Infusion Device 7 Autologous Tissue Substitute 8 Zooplastic Tissue C Extraluminal Device D Intraluminal Device J Synthetic Substitute K Nonautologous Tissue Substitute	Z No Qualifier
Y Great Vessel		X External	2 Monitoring Device 3 Infusion Device D Intraluminal Device	Z No Qualifier

Section	0	Medical and Surgical
Body System	2	Heart and Great Vessels
Operation	Q	Repair: Restoring, to the extent possible, a body part to its normal anatomic structure and function

Body Part (Character 4)	Approach (Character 5)	Device (Character 6)	Qualifier (Character 7)
0 Coronary Artery, One Site 1 Coronary Artery, Two Sites 2 Coronary Artery, Three Sites 3 Coronary Artery, Four or More Sites 4 Coronary Vein 5 Atrial Septum 6 Atrium, Right 7 Atrium, Left 8 Conduction Mechanism 9 Chordae Tendineae A Heart B Heart, Right C Heart, Left D Papillary Muscle F Aortic Valve G Mitral Valve H Pulmonary Valve J Tricuspid Valve K Ventricle, Right L Ventricle, Left M Ventricular Septum N Pericardium P Pulmonary Trunk Q Pulmonary Artery, Right R Pulmonary Artery, Left S Pulmonary Vein, Right T Pulmonary Vein, Left V Superior Vena Cava W Thoracic Aorta	0 Open 3 Percutaneous 4 Percutaneous Endoscopic	Z No Device	Z No Qualifier

Section	0	Medical and Surgical
Body System	2	Heart and Great Vessels
Operation	R	Replacement: Putting in or on biological or synthetic material that physically takes the place and/or function of all or a portion of a body part

Body Part (Character 4)	Approach (Character 5)	Device (Character 6)	Qualifier (Character 7)
5 Atrial Septum 6 Atrium, Right 7 Atrium, Left 9 Chordae Tendineae D Papillary Muscle J Tricuspid Valve K Ventricle, Right L Ventricle, Left M Ventricular Septum N Pericardium P Pulmonary Trunk Q Pulmonary Artery, Right R Pulmonary Artery, Left S Pulmonary Vein, Right T Pulmonary Vein, Left V Superior Vena Cava W Thoracic Aorta	0 Open 4 Percutaneous Endoscopic	7 Autologous Tissue Substitute 8 Zooplastic Tissue J Synthetic Substitute K Nonautologous Tissue Substitute	Z No Qualifier
F Aortic Valve G Mitral Valve H Pulmonary Valve	0 Open 4 Percutaneous Endoscopic	7 Autologous Tissue Substitute 8 Zooplastic Tissue J Synthetic Substitute K Nonautologous Tissue Substitute	Z No Qualifier
F Aortic Valve G Mitral Valve H Pulmonary Valve	3 Percutaneous	7 Autologous Tissue Substitute 8 Zooplastic Tissue J Synthetic Substitute K Nonautologous Tissue Substitute	H Transapical Z No Qualifier

Section	0	Medical and Surgical		
Body System	2	Heart and Great Vessels		
Operation	S	Reposition: Moving to its normal location, or other suitable location, all or a portion of a body part		

Body Part (Character 4)	Approach (Character 5)	Device (Character 6)	Qualifier (Character 7)
P Pulmonary Trunk **Q** Pulmonary Artery, Right **R** Pulmonary Artery, Left **S** Pulmonary Vein, Right **T** Pulmonary Vein, Left **V** Superior Vena Cava **W** Thoracic Aorta	**0** Open	**Z** No Device	**Z** No Qualifier

Section	0	Medical and Surgical		
Body System	2	Heart and Great Vessels		
Operation	T	Resection: Cutting out or off, without replacement, all of a body part		

Body Part (Character 4)	Approach (Character 5)	Device (Character 6)	Qualifier (Character 7)
5 Atrial Septum **8** Conduction Mechanism **9** Chordae Tendineae **D** Papillary Muscle **H** Pulmonary Valve **M** Ventricular Septum **N** Pericardium	**0** Open **3** Percutaneous **4** Percutaneous Endoscopic	**Z** No Device	**Z** No Qualifier

Section	0	Medical and Surgical		
Body System	2	Heart and Great Vessels		
Operation	U	Supplement: Putting in or on biological or synthetic material that physically reinforces and/or augments the function of a portion of a body part		

Body Part (Character 4)	Approach (Character 5)	Device (Character 6)	Qualifier (Character 7)
5 Atrial Septum **6** Atrium, Right **7** Atrium, Left **9** Chordae Tendineae **A** Heart **D** Papillary Muscle **F** Aortic Valve **G** Mitral Valve **H** Pulmonary Valve **J** Tricuspid Valve **K** Ventricle, Right **L** Ventricle, Left **M** Ventricular Septum **N** Pericardium **P** Pulmonary Trunk **Q** Pulmonary Artery, Right **R** Pulmonary Artery, Left **S** Pulmonary Vein, Right **T** Pulmonary Vein, Left **V** Superior Vena Cava **W** Thoracic Aorta	**0** Open **3** Percutaneous **4** Percutaneous Endoscopic	**7** Autologous Tissue Substitute **8** Zooplastic Tissue **J** Synthetic Substitute **K** Nonautologous Tissue Substitute	**Z** No Qualifier

Section	0	Medical and Surgical		
Body System	2	Heart and Great Vessels		
Operation	V	Restriction: Partially closing an orifice or the lumen of a tubular body part		

Body Part (Character 4)	Approach (Character 5)	Device (Character 6)	Qualifier (Character 7)
A Heart	**0** Open **3** Percutaneous **4** Percutaneous Endoscopic	**C** Extraluminal Device **Z** No Device	**Z** No Qualifier
P Pulmonary Trunk **Q** Pulmonary Artery, Right **S** Pulmonary Vein, Right **T** Pulmonary Vein, Left **V** Superior Vena Cava	**0** Open **3** Percutaneous **4** Percutaneous Endoscopic	**C** Extraluminal Device **D** Intraluminal Device **Z** No Device	**Z** No Qualifier
R Pulmonary Artery, Left	**0** Open **3** Percutaneous **4** Percutaneous Endoscopic	**C** Extraluminal Device **D** Intraluminal Device **Z** No Device	**T** Ductus Arteriosus **Z** No Qualifier
W Thoracic Aorta	**0** Open **3** Percutaneous **4** Percutaneous Endoscopic	**C** Extraluminal Device **Z** No Device	**Z** No Qualifier

Section	0	Medical and Surgical		
Body System	2	Heart and Great Vessels		
Operation	W	Revision: Correcting, to the extent possible, a portion of a malfunctioning device or the position of a displaced device		

Body Part (Character 4)	Approach (Character 5)	Device (Character 6)	Qualifier (Character 7)
5 Atrial Septum **M** Ventricular Septum	**0** Open **4** Percutaneous Endoscopic	**J** Synthetic Substitute	**Z** No Qualifier
A Heart	**0** Open **3** Percutaneous **4** Percutaneous Endoscopic **X** External	**2** Monitoring Device **3** Infusion Device **7** Autologous Tissue Substitute **8** Zooplastic Tissue **C** Extraluminal Device **D** Intraluminal Device **J** Synthetic Substitute **K** Nonautologous Tissue Substitute **M** Cardiac Lead **Q** Implantable Heart Assist System **R** External Heart Assist System	**Z** No Qualifier
F Aortic Valve **G** Mitral Valve **H** Pulmonary Valve **J** Tricuspid Valve	**0** Open **4** Percutaneous Endoscopic	**7** Autologous Tissue Substitute **8** Zooplastic Tissue **J** Synthetic Substitute **K** Nonautologous Tissue Substitute	**Z** No Qualifier
Y Great Vessel	**0** Open **3** Percutaneous **4** Percutaneous Endoscopic **X** External	**2** Monitoring Device **3** Infusion Device **7** Autologous Tissue Substitute **8** Zooplastic Tissue **C** Extraluminal Device **D** Intraluminal Device **J** Synthetic Substitute **K** Nonautologous Tissue Substitute	**Z** No Qualifier

Section	0	Medical and Surgical		
Body System	2	Heart and Great Vessels		
Operation	Y	Transplantation: Putting in or on all or a portion of a living body part taken from another individual or animal to physically take the place and/or function of all or a portion of a similar body part		

Body Part (Character 4)	Approach (Character 5)	Device (Character 6)	Qualifier (Character 7)
A Heart	**0** Open	**Z** No Device	**0** Allogeneic **1** Syngeneic **2** Zooplastic

Section	0	Medical and Surgical			
Body System	3	Upper Arteries			
Operation	1	Bypass: Altering the route of passage of the contents of a tubular body part			

Body Part (Character 4)	Approach (Character 5)	Device (Character 6)	Qualifier (Character 7)
7 Brachial Artery, Right	0 Open	9 Autologous Venous Tissue A Autologous Arterial Tissue J Synthetic Substitute K Nonautologous Tissue Substitute Z No Device	0 Upper Arm Artery, Right 3 Lower Arm Artery, Right D Upper Arm Vein F Lower Arm Vein
8 Brachial Artery, Left	0 Open	9 Autologous Venous Tissue A Autologous Arterial Tissue J Synthetic Substitute K Nonautologous Tissue Substitute Z No Device	1 Upper Arm Artery, Left 4 Lower Arm Artery, Left D Upper Arm Vein F Lower Arm Vein
9 Ulnar Artery, Right B Radial Artery, Right	0 Open	9 Autologous Venous Tissue A Autologous Arterial Tissue J Synthetic Substitute K Nonautologous Tissue Substitute Z No Device	3 Lower Arm Artery, Right F Lower Arm Vein
A Ulnar Artery, Left C Radial Artery, Left	0 Open	9 Autologous Venous Tissue A Autologous Arterial Tissue J Synthetic Substitute K Nonautologous Tissue Substitute Z No Device	4 Lower Arm Artery, Left F Lower Arm Vein
G Intracranial Artery S Temporal Artery, Right T Temporal Artery, Left	0 Open	9 Autologous Venous Tissue A Autologous Arterial Tissue J Synthetic Substitute K Nonautologous Tissue Substitute Z No Device	G Intracranial Artery
H Common Carotid Artery, Right	0 Open	9 Autologous Venous Tissue A Autologous Arterial Tissue J Synthetic Substitute K Nonautologous Tissue Substitute Z No Device	G Intracranial Artery J Extracranial Artery, Right
J Common Carotid Artery, Left	0 Open	9 Autologous Venous Tissue A Autologous Arterial Tissue J Synthetic Substitute K Nonautologous Tissue Substitute Z No Device	G Intracranial Artery K Extracranial Artery, Left

Section	0	Medical and Surgical			
Body System	3	Upper Arteries			
Operation	1	Bypass: Altering the route of passage of the contents of a tubular body part			

Body Part (Character 4)	Approach (Character 5)	Device (Character 6)	Qualifier (Character 7)
K Internal Carotid Artery, Right M External Carotid Artery, Right	0 Open	9 Autologous Venous Tissue A Autologous Arterial Tissue J Synthetic Substitute K Nonautologous Tissue Substitute Z No Device	J Extracranial Artery, Right
L Internal Carotid Artery, Left N External Carotid Artery, Left	0 Open	9 Autologous Venous Tissue A Autologous Arterial Tissue J Synthetic Substitute K Nonautologous Tissue Substitute Z No Device	K Extracranial Artery, Left

Section	0	Medical and Surgical		
Body System	3	Upper Arteries		
Operation	5	Destruction: Physical eradication of all or a portion of a body part by the direct use of energy, force, or a destructive agent		

Body Part (Character 4)	Approach (Character 5)	Device (Character 6)	Qualifier (Character 7)
0 Internal Mammary Artery, Right	**0** Open	**Z** No Device	**Z** No Qualifier
1 Internal Mammary Artery, Left	**3** Percutaneous		
2 Innominate Artery	**4** Percutaneous Endoscopic		
3 Subclavian Artery, Right			
4 Subclavian Artery, Left			
5 Axillary Artery, Right			
6 Axillary Artery, Left			
7 Brachial Artery, Right			
8 Brachial Artery, Left			
9 Ulnar Artery, Right			
A Ulnar Artery, Left			
B Radial Artery, Right			
C Radial Artery, Left			
D Hand Artery, Right			
F Hand Artery, Left			
G Intracranial Artery			
H Common Carotid Artery, Right			
J Common Carotid Artery, Left			
K Internal Carotid Artery, Right			
L Internal Carotid Artery, Left			
M External Carotid Artery, Right			
N External Carotid Artery, Left			
P Vertebral Artery, Right			
Q Vertebral Artery, Left			
R Face Artery			
S Temporal Artery, Right			
T Temporal Artery, Left			
U Thyroid Artery, Right			
V Thyroid Artery, Left			
Y Upper Artery			

Section	0	Medical and Surgical		
Body System	3	Upper Arteries		
Operation	7	Dilation: Expanding an orifice or the lumen of a tubular body part		

Body Part (Character 4)	Approach (Character 5)	Device (Character 6)	Qualifier (Character 7)
0 Internal Mammary Artery, Right	**0** Open	**4** Intraluminal Device, Drug-eluting	**Z** No Qualifier
1 Internal Mammary Artery, Left	**3** Percutaneous	**D** Intraluminal Device	
2 Innominate Artery	**4** Percutaneous Endoscopic	**Z** No Device	
3 Subclavian Artery, Right			
4 Subclavian Artery, Left			
5 Axillary Artery, Right			
6 Axillary Artery, Left			
7 Brachial Artery, Right			
8 Brachial Artery, Left			
9 Ulnar Artery, Right			
A Ulnar Artery, Left			
B Radial Artery, Right			
C Radial Artery, Left			
D Hand Artery, Right			
F Hand Artery, Left			
G Intracranial Artery			
H Common Carotid Artery, Right			
J Common Carotid Artery, Left			
K Internal Carotid Artery, Right			
L Internal Carotid Artery, Left			
M External Carotid Artery, Right			
N External Carotid Artery, Left			
P Vertebral Artery, Right			
Q Vertebral Artery, Left			
R Face Artery			
S Temporal Artery, Right			
T Temporal Artery, Left			
U Thyroid Artery, Right			
V Thyroid Artery, Left			
Y Upper Artery			

Section	0	Medical and Surgical
Body System	3	Upper Arteries
Operation	9	Drainage: Taking or letting out fluids and/or gases from a body part

Body Part (Character 4)	Approach (Character 5)	Device (Character 6)	Qualifier (Character 7)
0 Internal Mammary Artery, Right	**0** Open	**0** Drainage Device	**Z** No Qualifier
1 Internal Mammary Artery, Left	**3** Percutaneous		
2 Innominate Artery	**4** Percutaneous Endoscopic		
3 Subclavian Artery, Right			
4 Subclavian Artery, Left			
5 Axillary Artery, Right			
6 Axillary Artery, Left			
7 Brachial Artery, Right			
8 Brachial Artery, Left			
9 Ulnar Artery, Right			
A Ulnar Artery, Left			
B Radial Artery, Right			
C Radial Artery, Left			
D Hand Artery, Right			
F Hand Artery, Left			
G Intracranial Artery			
H Common Carotid Artery, Right			
J Common Carotid Artery, Left			
K Internal Carotid Artery, Right			
L Internal Carotid Artery, Left			
M External Carotid Artery, Right			
N External Carotid Artery, Left			
P Vertebral Artery, Right			
Q Vertebral Artery, Left			
R Face Artery			
S Temporal Artery, Right			
T Temporal Artery, Left			
U Thyroid Artery, Right			
V Thyroid Artery, Left			
Y Upper Artery			

Section	0	Medical and Surgical
Body System	3	Upper Arteries
Operation	9	Drainage: Taking or letting out fluids and/or gases from a body part

Body Part (Character 4)	Approach (Character 5)	Device (Character 6)	Qualifier (Character 7)
0 Internal Mammary Artery, Right	**0** Open	**Z** No Device	**X** Diagnostic
1 Internal Mammary Artery, Left	**3** Percutaneous		**Z** No Qualifier
2 Innominate Artery	**4** Percutaneous Endoscopic		
3 Subclavian Artery, Right			
4 Subclavian Artery, Left			
5 Axillary Artery, Right			
6 Axillary Artery, Left			
7 Brachial Artery, Right			
8 Brachial Artery, Left			
9 Ulnar Artery, Right			
A Ulnar Artery, Left			
B Radial Artery, Right			
C Radial Artery, Left			
D Hand Artery, Right			
F Hand Artery, Left			
G Intracranial Artery			
H Common Carotid Artery, Right			
J Common Carotid Artery, Left			
K Internal Carotid Artery, Right			
L Internal Carotid Artery, Left			
M External Carotid Artery, Right			
N External Carotid Artery, Left			
P Vertebral Artery, Right			
Q Vertebral Artery, Left			
R Face Artery			
S Temporal Artery, Right			
T Temporal Artery, Left			
U Thyroid Artery, Right			
V Thyroid Artery, Left			
Y Upper Artery			

Section	0	Medical and Surgical		
Body System	3	Upper Arteries		
Operation	B	Excision: Cutting out or off, without replacement, a portion of a body part		

Body Part (Character 4)	Approach (Character 5)	Device (Character 6)	Qualifier (Character 7)
0 Internal Mammary Artery, Right **1** Internal Mammary Artery, Left **2** Innominate Artery **3** Subclavian Artery, Right **4** Subclavian Artery, Left **5** Axillary Artery, Right **6** Axillary Artery, Left **7** Brachial Artery, Right **8** Brachial Artery, Left **9** Ulnar Artery, Right **A** Ulnar Artery, Left **B** Radial Artery, Right **C** Radial Artery, Left **D** Hand Artery, Right **F** Hand Artery, Left **G** Intracranial Artery **H** Common Carotid Artery, Right **J** Common Carotid Artery, Left **K** Internal Carotid Artery, Right **L** Internal Carotid Artery, Left **M** External Carotid Artery, Right **N** External Carotid Artery, Left **P** Vertebral Artery, Right **Q** Vertebral Artery, Left **R** Face Artery **S** Temporal Artery, Right **T** Temporal Artery, Left **U** Thyroid Artery, Right **V** Thyroid Artery, Left **Y** Upper Artery	**0** Open **3** Percutaneous **4** Percutaneous Endoscopic	**Z** No Device	**X** Diagnostic **Z** No Qualifier

Section	0	Medical and Surgical		
Body System	3	Upper Arteries		
Operation	C	Extirpation: Taking or cutting out solid matter from a body part		

Body Part (Character 4)	Approach (Character 5)	Device (Character 6)	Qualifier (Character 7)
0 Internal Mammary Artery, Right **1** Internal Mammary Artery, Left **2** Innominate Artery **3** Subclavian Artery, Right **4** Subclavian Artery, Left **5** Axillary Artery, Right **6** Axillary Artery, Left **7** Brachial Artery, Right **8** Brachial Artery, Left **9** Ulnar Artery, Right **A** Ulnar Artery, Left **B** Radial Artery, Right **C** Radial Artery, Left **D** Hand Artery, Right **F** Hand Artery, Left **G** Intracranial Artery **H** Common Carotid Artery, Right **J** Common Carotid Artery, Left **K** Internal Carotid Artery, Right **L** Internal Carotid Artery, Left **M** External Carotid Artery, Right **N** External Carotid Artery, Left **P** Vertebral Artery, Right **Q** Vertebral Artery, Left **R** Face Artery **S** Temporal Artery, Right **T** Temporal Artery, Left **U** Thyroid Artery, Right **V** Thyroid Artery, Left **Y** Upper Artery	**0** Open **3** Percutaneous **4** Percutaneous Endoscopic	**Z** No Device	**Z** No Qualifier

Section	0	Medical and Surgical		
Body System	3	Upper Arteries		
Operation	H	Insertion: Putting in a nonbiological appliance that monitors, assists, performs, or prevents a physiological function but does not physically take the place of a body part		

Body Part (Character 4)	Approach (Character 5)	Device (Character 6)	Qualifier (Character 7)
0 Internal Mammary Artery, Right 1 Internal Mammary Artery, Left 2 Innominate Artery 3 Subclavian Artery, Right 4 Subclavian Artery, Left 5 Axillary Artery, Right 6 Axillary Artery, Left 7 Brachial Artery, Right 8 Brachial Artery, Left 9 Ulnar Artery, Right A Ulnar Artery, Left B Radial Artery, Right C Radial Artery, Left D Hand Artery, Right F Hand Artery, Left G Intracranial Artery H Common Carotid Artery, Right J Common Carotid Artery, Left M External Carotid Artery, Right N External Carotid Artery, Left P Vertebral Artery, Right Q Vertebral Artery, Left R Face Artery S Temporal Artery, Right T Temporal Artery, Left U Thyroid Artery, Right V Thyroid Artery, Left	0 Open 3 Percutaneous 4 Percutaneous Endoscopic	3 Infusion Device D Intraluminal Device	Z No Qualifier
K Internal Carotid Artery, Right L Internal Carotid Artery, Left	0 Open 3 Percutaneous 4 Percutaneous Endoscopic	3 Infusion Device D Intraluminal Device M Stimulator Lead	Z No Qualifier
Y Upper Artery	0 Open 3 Percutaneous 4 Percutaneous Endoscopic	2 Monitoring Device 3 Infusion Device D Intraluminal Device	Z No Qualifier

Section	0	Medical and Surgical		
Body System	3	Upper Arteries		
Operation	J	Inspection: Visually and/or manually exploring a body part		

Body Part (Character 4)	Approach (Character 5)	Device (Character 6)	Qualifier (Character 7)
Y Upper Artery	0 Open 3 Percutaneous 4 Percutaneous Endoscopic X External	Z No Device	Z No Qualifier

Section	0	Medical and Surgical		
Body System	3	Upper Arteries		
Operation	L	Occlusion: Completely closing an orifice or the lumen of a tubular body part		

Body Part (Character 4)	Approach (Character 5)	Device (Character 6)	Qualifier (Character 7)
0 Internal Mammary Artery, Right 1 Internal Mammary Artery, Left 2 Innominate Artery 3 Subclavian Artery, Right 4 Subclavian Artery, Left 5 Axillary Artery, Right 6 Axillary Artery, Left 7 Brachial Artery, Right 8 Brachial Artery, Left 9 Ulnar Artery, Right A Ulnar Artery, Left B Radial Artery, Right C Radial Artery, Left D Hand Artery, Right F Hand Artery, Left R Face Artery S Temporal Artery, Right T Temporal Artery, Left U Thyroid Artery, Right V Thyroid Artery, Left Y Upper Artery	0 Open 3 Percutaneous 4 Percutaneous Endoscopic	C Extraluminal Device D Intraluminal Device Z No Device	Z No Qualifier

Section	0	Medical and Surgical		
Body System	3	Upper Arteries		[continued]
Operation	L	Occlusion: Completely closing an orifice or the lumen of a tubular body part		

Body Part (Character 4)	Approach (Character 5)	Device (Character 6)	Qualifier (Character 7)
G Intracranial Artery **H** Common Carotid Artery, Right **J** Common Carotid Artery, Left **K** Internal Carotid Artery, Right **L** Internal Carotid Artery, Left **M** External Carotid Artery, Right **N** External Carotid Artery, Left **P** Vertebral Artery, Right **Q** Vertebral Artery, Left	**0** Open **3** Percutaneous **4** Percutaneous Endoscopic	**B** Intraluminal Device, Bioactive **C** Extraluminal Device **D** Intraluminal Device **Z** No Device	**Z** No Qualifier

Section	0	Medical and Surgical		
Body System	3	Upper Arteries		
Operation	N	Release: Freeing a body part from an abnormal physical constraint by cutting or by the use of force		

Body Part (Character 4)	Approach (Character 5)	Device (Character 6)	Qualifier (Character 7)
0 Internal Mammary Artery, Right **1** Internal Mammary Artery, Left **2** Innominate Artery **3** Subclavian Artery, Right **4** Subclavian Artery, Left **5** Axillary Artery, Right **6** Axillary Artery, Left **7** Brachial Artery, Right **8** Brachial Artery, Left **9** Ulnar Artery, Right **A** Ulnar Artery, Left **B** Radial Artery, Right **C** Radial Artery, Left **D** Hand Artery, Right **F** Hand Artery, Left **G** Intracranial Artery **H** Common Carotid Artery, Right **J** Common Carotid Artery, Left **K** Internal Carotid Artery, Right **L** Internal Carotid Artery, Left **M** External Carotid Artery, Right **N** External Carotid Artery, Left **P** Vertebral Artery, Right **Q** Vertebral Artery, Left **R** Face Artery **S** Temporal Artery, Right **T** Temporal Artery, Left **U** Thyroid Artery, Right **V** Thyroid Artery, Left **Y** Upper Artery	**0** Open **3** Percutaneous **4** Percutaneous Endoscopic	**Z** No Device	**Z** No Qualifier

Section	0	Medical and Surgical		
Body System	3	Upper Arteries		
Operation	P	Removal: Taking out or off a device from a body part		

Body Part (Character 4)	Approach (Character 5)	Device (Character 6)	Qualifier (Character 7)
Y Upper Artery	**0** Open **3** Percutaneous **4** Percutaneous Endoscopic	**0** Drainage Device **2** Monitoring Device **3** Infusion Device **7** Autologous Tissue Substitute **C** Extraluminal Device **D** Intraluminal Device **J** Synthetic Substitute **K** Nonautologous Tissue Substitute **M** Stimulator Lead	**Z** No Qualifier
Y Upper Artery	**X** External	**0** Drainage Device **2** Monitoring Device **3** Infusion Device **D** Intraluminal Device **M** Stimulator Lead	**Z** No Qualifier

Section	0	Medical and Surgical		
Body System	3	Upper Arteries		
Operation	Q	Repair: Restoring, to the extent possible, a body part to its normal anatomic structure and function		

Body Part (Character 4)	Approach (Character 5)	Device (Character 6)	Qualifier (Character 7)
0 Internal Mammary Artery, Right **1** Internal Mammary Artery, Left **2** Innominate Artery **3** Subclavian Artery, Right **4** Subclavian Artery, Left **5** Axillary Artery, Right **6** Axillary Artery, Left **7** Brachial Artery, Right **8** Brachial Artery, Left **9** Ulnar Artery, Right **A** Ulnar Artery, Left **B** Radial Artery, Right **C** Radial Artery, Left **D** Hand Artery, Right **F** Hand Artery, Left **G** Intracranial Artery **H** Common Carotid Artery, Right **J** Common Carotid Artery, Left **K** Internal Carotid Artery, Right **L** Internal Carotid Artery, Left **M** External Carotid Artery, Right **N** External Carotid Artery, Left **P** Vertebral Artery, Right **Q** Vertebral Artery, Left **R** Face Artery **S** Temporal Artery, Right **T** Temporal Artery, Left **U** Thyroid Artery, Right **V** Thyroid Artery, Left **Y** Upper Artery	**0** Open **3** Percutaneous **4** Percutaneous Endoscopic	**Z** No Device	**Z** No Qualifier

Section	0	Medical and Surgical		
Body System	3	Upper Arteries		
Operation	R	Replacement: Putting in or on biological or synthetic material that physically takes the place and/or function of all or a portion of a body part		

Body Part (Character 4)	Approach (Character 5)	Device (Character 6)	Qualifier (Character 7)
0 Internal Mammary Artery, Right **1** Internal Mammary Artery, Left **2** Innominate Artery **3** Subclavian Artery, Right **4** Subclavian Artery, Left **5** Axillary Artery, Right **6** Axillary Artery, Left **7** Brachial Artery, Right **8** Brachial Artery, Left **9** Ulnar Artery, Right **A** Ulnar Artery, Left **B** Radial Artery, Right **C** Radial Artery, Left **D** Hand Artery, Right **F** Hand Artery, Left **G** Intracranial Artery **H** Common Carotid Artery, Right **J** Common Carotid Artery, Left **K** Internal Carotid Artery, Right **L** Internal Carotid Artery, Left **M** External Carotid Artery, Right **N** External Carotid Artery, Left **P** Vertebral Artery, Right **Q** Vertebral Artery, Left **R** Face Artery **S** Temporal Artery, Right **T** Temporal Artery, Left **U** Thyroid Artery, Right **V** Thyroid Artery, Left **Y** Upper Artery	**0** Open **4** Percutaneous Endoscopic	**7** Autologous Tissue Substitute **J** Synthetic Substitute **K** Nonautologous Tissue Substitute	**Z** No Qualifier

Section	0	Medical and Surgical
Body System	3	Upper Arteries
Operation	S	Reposition: Moving to its normal location, or other suitable location, all or a portion of a body part

Body Part (Character 4)	Approach (Character 5)	Device (Character 6)	Qualifier (Character 7)
0 Internal Mammary Artery, Right	**0** Open	**Z** No Device	**Z** No Qualifier
1 Internal Mammary Artery, Left	**3** Percutaneous		
2 Innominate Artery	**4** Percutaneous Endoscopic		
3 Subclavian Artery, Right			
4 Subclavian Artery, Left			
5 Axillary Artery, Right			
6 Axillary Artery, Left			
7 Brachial Artery, Right			
8 Brachial Artery, Left			
9 Ulnar Artery, Right			
A Ulnar Artery, Left			
B Radial Artery, Right			
C Radial Artery, Left			
D Hand Artery, Right			
F Hand Artery, Left			
G Intracranial Artery			
H Common Carotid Artery, Right			
J Common Carotid Artery, Left			
K Internal Carotid Artery, Right			
L Internal Carotid Artery, Left			
M External Carotid Artery, Right			
N External Carotid Artery, Left			
P Vertebral Artery, Right			
Q Vertebral Artery, Left			
R Face Artery			
S Temporal Artery, Right			
T Temporal Artery, Left			
U Thyroid Artery, Right			
V Thyroid Artery, Left			
Y Upper Artery			

Section	0	Medical and Surgical
Body System	3	Upper Arteries
Operation	U	Supplement: Putting in or on biological or synthetic material that physically reinforces and/or augments the function of a portion of a body part

Body Part (Character 4)	Approach (Character 5)	Device (Character 6)	Qualifier (Character 7)
0 Internal Mammary Artery, Right	**0** Open	**7** Autologous Tissue Substitute	**Z** No Qualifier
1 Internal Mammary Artery, Left	**3** Percutaneous	**J** Synthetic Substitute	
2 Innominate Artery	**4** Percutaneous Endoscopic	**K** Nonautologous Tissue Substitute	
3 Subclavian Artery, Right			
4 Subclavian Artery, Left			
5 Axillary Artery, Right			
6 Axillary Artery, Left			
7 Brachial Artery, Right			
8 Brachial Artery, Left			
9 Ulnar Artery, Right			
A Ulnar Artery, Left			
B Radial Artery, Right			
C Radial Artery, Left			
D Hand Artery, Right			
F Hand Artery, Left			
G Intracranial Artery			
H Common Carotid Artery, Right			
J Common Carotid Artery, Left			
K Internal Carotid Artery, Right			
L Internal Carotid Artery, Left			
M External Carotid Artery, Right			
N External Carotid Artery, Left			
P Vertebral Artery, Right			
Q Vertebral Artery, Left			
R Face Artery			
S Temporal Artery, Right			
T Temporal Artery, Left			
U Thyroid Artery, Right			
V Thyroid Artery, Left			
Y Upper Artery			

Section	0	Medical and Surgical		
Body System	3	Upper Arteries		
Operation	V	Restriction: Partially closing an orifice or the lumen of a tubular body part		

Body Part (Character 4)	Approach (Character 5)	Device (Character 6)	Qualifier (Character 7)
0 Internal Mammary Artery, Right **1** Internal Mammary Artery, Left **2** Innominate Artery **3** Subclavian Artery, Right **4** Subclavian Artery, Left **5** Axillary Artery, Right **6** Axillary Artery, Left **7** Brachial Artery, Right **8** Brachial Artery, Left **9** Ulnar Artery, Right **A** Ulnar Artery, Left **B** Radial Artery, Right **C** Radial Artery, Left **D** Hand Artery, Right **F** Hand Artery, Left **R** Face Artery **S** Temporal Artery, Right **T** Temporal Artery, Left **U** Thyroid Artery, Right **V** Thyroid Artery, Left **Y** Upper Artery	**0** Open **3** Percutaneous **4** Percutaneous Endoscopic	**C** Extraluminal Device **D** Intraluminal Device **Z** No Device	**Z** No Qualifier
G Intracranial Artery **H** Common Carotid Artery, Right **J** Common Carotid Artery, Left **K** Internal Carotid Artery, Right **L** Internal Carotid Artery, Left **M** External Carotid Artery, Right **N** External Carotid Artery, Left **P** Vertebral Artery, Right **Q** Vertebral Artery, Left	**0** Open **3** Percutaneous **4** Percutaneous Endoscopic	**B** Intraluminal Device, Bioactive **C** Extraluminal Device **D** Intraluminal Device **Z** No Device	**Z** No Qualifier

Section	0	Medical and Surgical		
Body System	3	Upper Arteries		
Operation	W	Revision: Correcting, to the extent possible, a portion of a malfunctioning device or the position of a displaced device		

Body Part (Character 4)	Approach (Character 5)	Device (Character 6)	Qualifier (Character 7)
Y Upper Artery	**0** Open **3** Percutaneous **4** Percutaneous Endoscopic **X** External	**0** Drainage Device **2** Monitoring Device **3** Infusion Device **7** Autologous Tissue Substitute **C** Extraluminal Device **D** Intraluminal Device **J** Synthetic Substitute **K** Nonautologous Tissue Substitute **M** Stimulator Lead	**Z** No Qualifier

Section	0	Medical and Surgical		
Body System	4	Lower Arteries		
Operation	1	Bypass: Altering the route of passage of the contents of a tubular body part		

Body Part (Character 4)	Approach (Character 5)	Device (Character 6)	Qualifier (Character 7)
0 Abdominal Aorta **C** Common Iliac Artery, Right **D** Common Iliac Artery, Left	**0** Open **4** Percutaneous Endoscopic	**9** Autologous Venous Tissue **A** Autologous Arterial Tissue **J** Synthetic Substitute **K** Nonautologous Tissue Substitute **Z** No Device	**0** Abdominal Aorta **1** Celiac Artery **2** Mesenteric Artery **3** Renal Artery, Right **4** Renal Artery, Left **5** Renal Artery, Bilateral **6** Common Iliac Artery, Right **7** Common Iliac Artery, Left **8** Common Iliac Arteries, Bilateral **9** Internal Iliac Artery, Right **B** Internal Iliac Artery, Left **C** Internal Iliac Arteries, Bilateral **D** External Iliac Artery, Right **F** External Iliac Artery, Left **G** External Iliac Arteries, Bilateral **H** Femoral Artery, Right **J** Femoral Artery, Left **K** Femoral Arteries, Bilateral **Q** Lower Extremity Artery **R** Lower Artery
4 Splenic Artery	**0** Open **4** Percutaneous Endoscopic	**9** Autologous Venous Tissue **A** Autologous Arterial Tissue **J** Synthetic Substitute **K** Nonautologous Tissue Substitute **Z** No Device	**3** Renal Artery, Right **4** Renal Artery, Left **5** Renal Artery, Bilateral
E Internal Iliac Artery, Right **F** Internal Iliac Artery, Left **H** External Iliac Artery, Right **J** External Iliac Artery, Left	**0** Open **4** Percutaneous Endoscopic	**9** Autologous Venous Tissue **A** Autologous Arterial Tissue **J** Synthetic Substitute **K** Nonautologous Tissue Substitute **Z** No Device	**9** Internal Iliac Artery, Right **B** Internal Iliac Artery, Left **C** Internal Iliac Arteries, Bilateral **D** External Iliac Artery, Right **F** External Iliac Artery, Left **G** External Iliac Arteries, Bilateral **H** Femoral Artery, Right **J** Femoral Artery, Left **K** Femoral Arteries, Bilateral **P** Foot Artery **Q** Lower Extremity Artery

Section	0	Medical and Surgical		
Body System	4	Lower Arteries		
Operation	1	Bypass: Altering the route of passage of the contents of a tubular body part		

Body Part (Character 4)	Approach (Character 5)	Device (Character 6)	Qualifier (Character 7)
K Femoral Artery, Right **L** Femoral Artery, Left	**0** Open **4** Percutaneous Endoscopic	**9** Autologous Venous Tissue **A** Autologous Arterial Tissue **J** Synthetic Substitute **K** Nonautologous Tissue Substitute **Z** No Device	**H** Femoral Artery, Right **J** Femoral Artery, Left **K** Femoral Arteries, Bilateral **L** Popliteal Artery **M** Peroneal Artery **N** Posterior Tibial Artery **P** Foot Artery **Q** Lower Extremity Artery **S** Lower Extremity Vein
M Popliteal Artery, Right **N** Popliteal Artery, Left	**0** Open **4** Percutaneous Endoscopic	**9** Autologous Venous Tissue **A** Autologous Arterial Tissue **J** Synthetic Substitute **K** Nonautologous Tissue Substitute **Z** No Device	**L** Popliteal Artery **M** Peroneal Artery **P** Foot Artery **Q** Lower Extremity Artery **S** Lower Extremity Vein

Section	0	Medical and Surgical		
Body System	4	Lower Arteries		
Operation	5	Destruction: Physical eradication of all or a portion of a body part by the direct use of energy, force, or a destructive agent		

Body Part (Character 4)	Approach (Character 5)	Device (Character 6)	Qualifier (Character 7)
0 Abdominal Aorta	0 Open	Z No Device	Z No Qualifier
1 Celiac Artery	3 Percutaneous		
2 Gastric Artery	4 Percutaneous Endoscopic		
3 Hepatic Artery			
4 Splenic Artery			
5 Superior Mesenteric Artery			
6 Colic Artery, Right			
7 Colic Artery, Left			
8 Colic Artery, Middle			
9 Renal Artery, Right			
A Renal Artery, Left			
B Inferior Mesenteric Artery			
C Common Iliac Artery, Right			
D Common Iliac Artery, Left			
E Internal Iliac Artery, Right			
F Internal Iliac Artery, Left			
H External Iliac Artery, Right			
J External Iliac Artery, Left			
K Femoral Artery, Right			
L Femoral Artery, Left			
M Popliteal Artery, Right			
N Popliteal Artery, Left			
P Anterior Tibial Artery, Right			
Q Anterior Tibial Artery, Left			
R Posterior Tibial Artery, Right			
S Posterior Tibial Artery, Left			
T Peroneal Artery, Right			
U Peroneal Artery, Left			
V Foot Artery, Right			
W Foot Artery, Left			
Y Lower Artery			

Section	0	Medical and Surgical		
Body System	4	Lower Arteries		
Operation	7	Dilation: Expanding an orifice or the lumen of a tubular body part		

Body Part (Character 4)	Approach (Character 5)	Device (Character 6)	Qualifier (Character 7)
0 Abdominal Aorta	0 Open	4 Intraluminal Device, Drug-eluting	Z No Qualifier
1 Celiac Artery	3 Percutaneous	D Intraluminal Device	
2 Gastric Artery	4 Percutaneous Endoscopic	Z No Device	
3 Hepatic Artery			
4 Splenic Artery			
5 Superior Mesenteric Artery			
6 Colic Artery, Right			
7 Colic Artery, Left			
8 Colic Artery, Middle			
9 Renal Artery, Right			
A Renal Artery, Left			
B Inferior Mesenteric Artery			
C Common Iliac Artery, Right			
D Common Iliac Artery, Left			
E Internal Iliac Artery, Right			
F Internal Iliac Artery, Left			
H External Iliac Artery, Right			
J External Iliac Artery, Left			
K Femoral Artery, Right			
L Femoral Artery, Left			
M Popliteal Artery, Right			
N Popliteal Artery, Left			
P Anterior Tibial Artery, Right			
Q Anterior Tibial Artery, Left			
R Posterior Tibial Artery, Right			
S Posterior Tibial Artery, Left			
T Peroneal Artery, Right			
U Peroneal Artery, Left			
V Foot Artery, Right			
W Foot Artery, Left			
Y Lower Artery			

Section	0	Medical and Surgical		
Body System	4	Lower Arteries		
Operation	9	Drainage: Taking or letting out fluids and/or gases from a body part		

Body Part (Character 4)	Approach (Character 5)	Device (Character 6)	Qualifier (Character 7)
0 Abdominal Aorta	**0** Open	**0** Drainage Device	**Z** No Qualifier
1 Celiac Artery	**3** Percutaneous		
2 Gastric Artery	**4** Percutaneous Endoscopic		
3 Hepatic Artery			
4 Splenic Artery			
5 Superior Mesenteric Artery			
6 Colic Artery, Right			
7 Colic Artery, Left			
8 Colic Artery, Middle			
9 Renal Artery, Right			
A Renal Artery, Left			
B Inferior Mesenteric Artery			
C Common Iliac Artery, Right			
D Common Iliac Artery, Left			
E Internal Iliac Artery, Right			
F Internal Iliac Artery, Left			
H External Iliac Artery, Right			
J External Iliac Artery, Left			
K Femoral Artery, Right			
L Femoral Artery, Left			
M Popliteal Artery, Right			
N Popliteal Artery, Left			
P Anterior Tibial Artery, Right			
Q Anterior Tibial Artery, Left			
R Posterior Tibial Artery, Right			
S Posterior Tibial Artery, Left			
T Peroneal Artery, Right			
U Peroneal Artery, Left			
V Foot Artery, Right			
W Foot Artery, Left			
Y Lower Artery			

Section	0	Medical and Surgical		
Body System	4	Lower Arteries		
Operation	9	Drainage: Taking or letting out fluids and/or gases from a body part		

Body Part (Character 4)	Approach (Character 5)	Device (Character 6)	Qualifier (Character 7)
0 Abdominal Aorta	**0** Open	**Z** No Device	**X** Diagnostic
1 Celiac Artery	**3** Percutaneous		**Z** No Qualifier
2 Gastric Artery	**4** Percutaneous Endoscopic		
3 Hepatic Artery			
4 Splenic Artery			
5 Superior Mesenteric Artery			
6 Colic Artery, Right			
7 Colic Artery, Left			
8 Colic Artery, Middle			
9 Renal Artery, Right			
A Renal Artery, Left			
B Inferior Mesenteric Artery			
C Common Iliac Artery, Right			
D Common Iliac Artery, Left			
E Internal Iliac Artery, Right			
F Internal Iliac Artery, Left			
H External Iliac Artery, Right			
J External Iliac Artery, Left			
K Femoral Artery, Right			
L Femoral Artery, Left			
M Popliteal Artery, Right			
N Popliteal Artery, Left			
P Anterior Tibial Artery, Right			
Q Anterior Tibial Artery, Left			
R Posterior Tibial Artery, Right			
S Posterior Tibial Artery, Left			
T Peroneal Artery, Right			
U Peroneal Artery, Left			
V Foot Artery, Right			
W Foot Artery, Left			
Y Lower Artery			

Section	0	Medical and Surgical		
Body System	4	Lower Arteries		
Operation	B	Excision: Cutting out or off, without replacement, a portion of a body part		

Body Part (Character 4)	Approach (Character 5)	Device (Character 6)	Qualifier (Character 7)
0 Abdominal Aorta	0 Open	Z No Device	X Diagnostic
1 Celiac Artery	3 Percutaneous		Z No Qualifier
2 Gastric Artery	4 Percutaneous Endoscopic		
3 Hepatic Artery			
4 Splenic Artery			
5 Superior Mesenteric Artery			
6 Colic Artery, Right			
7 Colic Artery, Left			
8 Colic Artery, Middle			
9 Renal Artery, Right			
A Renal Artery, Left			
B Inferior Mesenteric Artery			
C Common Iliac Artery, Right			
D Common Iliac Artery, Left			
E Internal Iliac Artery, Right			
F Internal Iliac Artery, Left			
H External Iliac Artery, Right			
J External Iliac Artery, Left			
K Femoral Artery, Right			
L Femoral Artery, Left			
M Popliteal Artery, Right			
N Popliteal Artery, Left			
P Anterior Tibial Artery, Right			
Q Anterior Tibial Artery, Left			
R Posterior Tibial Artery, Right			
S Posterior Tibial Artery, Left			
T Peroneal Artery, Right			
U Peroneal Artery, Left			
V Foot Artery, Right			
W Foot Artery, Left			
Y Lower Artery			

Section	0	Medical and Surgical		
Body System	4	Lower Arteries		
Operation	C	Extirpation: Taking or cutting out solid matter from a body part		

Body Part (Character 4)	Approach (Character 5)	Device (Character 6)	Qualifier (Character 7)
0 Abdominal Aorta	0 Open	Z No Device	Z No Qualifier
1 Celiac Artery	3 Percutaneous		
2 Gastric Artery	4 Percutaneous Endoscopic		
3 Hepatic Artery			
4 Splenic Artery			
5 Superior Mesenteric Artery			
6 Colic Artery, Right			
7 Colic Artery, Left			
8 Colic Artery, Middle			
9 Renal Artery, Right			
A Renal Artery, Left			
B Inferior Mesenteric Artery			
C Common Iliac Artery, Right			
D Common Iliac Artery, Left			
E Internal Iliac Artery, Right			
F Internal Iliac Artery, Left			
H External Iliac Artery, Right			
J External Iliac Artery, Left			
K Femoral Artery, Right			
L Femoral Artery, Left			
M Popliteal Artery, Right			
N Popliteal Artery, Left			
P Anterior Tibial Artery, Right			
Q Anterior Tibial Artery, Left			
R Posterior Tibial Artery, Right			
S Posterior Tibial Artery, Left			
T Peroneal Artery, Right			
U Peroneal Artery, Left			
V Foot Artery, Right			
W Foot Artery, Left			
Y Lower Artery			

Section	0	Medical and Surgical		
Body System	4	Lower Arteries		
Operation	H	Insertion: Putting in a nonbiological appliance that monitors, assists, performs, or prevents a physiological function but does not physically take the place of a body part		

Body Part (Character 4)	Approach (Character 5)	Device (Character 6)	Qualifier (Character 7)
0 Abdominal Aorta **Y** Lower Artery	**0** Open **3** Percutaneous **4** Percutaneous Endoscopic	**2** Monitoring Device **3** Infusion Device **D** Intraluminal Device	**Z** No Qualifier
1 Celiac Artery **2** Gastric Artery **3** Hepatic Artery **4** Splenic Artery **5** Superior Mesenteric Artery **6** Colic Artery, Right **7** Colic Artery, Left **8** Colic Artery, Middle **9** Renal Artery, Right **A** Renal Artery, Left **B** Inferior Mesenteric Artery **C** Common Iliac Artery, Right **D** Common Iliac Artery, Left **E** Internal Iliac Artery, Right **F** Internal Iliac Artery, Left **H** External Iliac Artery, Right **J** External Iliac Artery, Left **K** Femoral Artery, Right **L** Femoral Artery, Left **M** Popliteal Artery, Right **N** Popliteal Artery, Left **P** Anterior Tibial Artery, Right **Q** Anterior Tibial Artery, Left **R** Posterior Tibial Artery, Right **S** Posterior Tibial Artery, Left **T** Peroneal Artery, Right **U** Peroneal Artery, Left **V** Foot Artery, Right **W** Foot Artery, Left	**0** Open **3** Percutaneous **4** Percutaneous Endoscopic	**3** Infusion Device **D** Intraluminal Device	**Z** No Qualifier

Section	0	Medical and Surgical		
Body System	4	Lower Arteries		
Operation	J	Inspection: Visually and/or manually exploring a body part		

Body Part (Character 4)	Approach (Character 5)	Device (Character 6)	Qualifier (Character 7)
Y Lower Artery	**0** Open **3** Percutaneous **4** Percutaneous Endoscopic **X** External	**Z** No Device	**Z** No Qualifier

Section	0	Medical and Surgical
Body System	4	Lower Arteries
Operation	L	Occlusion: Completely closing an orifice or the lumen of a tubular body part

Body Part (Character 4)	Approach (Character 5)	Device (Character 6)	Qualifier (Character 7)
0 Abdominal Aorta **1** Celiac Artery **2** Gastric Artery **3** Hepatic Artery **4** Splenic Artery **5** Superior Mesenteric Artery **6** Colic Artery, Right **7** Colic Artery, Left **8** Colic Artery, Middle **9** Renal Artery, Right **A** Renal Artery, Left **B** Inferior Mesenteric Artery **C** Common Iliac Artery, Right **D** Common Iliac Artery, Left **H** External Iliac Artery, Right **J** External Iliac Artery, Left **K** Femoral Artery, Right **L** Femoral Artery, Left **M** Popliteal Artery, Right **N** Popliteal Artery, Left **P** Anterior Tibial Artery, Right **Q** Anterior Tibial Artery, Left **R** Posterior Tibial Artery, Right **S** Posterior Tibial Artery, Left **T** Peroneal Artery, Right **U** Peroneal Artery, Left **V** Foot Artery, Right **W** Foot Artery, Left **Y** Lower Artery	**0** Open **3** Percutaneous **4** Percutaneous Endoscopic	**C** Extraluminal Device **D** Intraluminal Device **Z** No Device	**Z** No Qualifier
E Internal Iliac Artery, Right	**0** Open **3** Percutaneous **4** Percutaneous Endoscopic	**C** Extraluminal Device **D** Intraluminal Device **Z** No Device	**T** Uterine Artery, Right **Z** No Qualifier
F Internal Iliac Artery, Left	**0** Open **3** Percutaneous **4** Percutaneous Endoscopic	**C** Extraluminal Device **D** Intraluminal Device **Z** No Device	**U** Uterine Artery, Left **Z** No Qualifier

Section	0	Medical and Surgical		
Body System	4	Lower Arteries		
Operation	N	Release: Freeing a body part from an abnormal physical constraint by cutting or by the use of force		

Body Part (Character 4)	Approach (Character 5)	Device (Character 6)	Qualifier (Character 7)
0 Abdominal Aorta	0 Open	Z No Device	Z No Qualifier
1 Celiac Artery	3 Percutaneous		
2 Gastric Artery	4 Percutaneous Endoscopic		
3 Hepatic Artery			
4 Splenic Artery			
5 Superior Mesenteric Artery			
6 Colic Artery, Right			
7 Colic Artery, Left			
8 Colic Artery, Middle			
9 Renal Artery, Right			
A Renal Artery, Left			
B Inferior Mesenteric Artery			
C Common Iliac Artery, Right			
D Common Iliac Artery, Left			
E Internal Iliac Artery, Right			
F Internal Iliac Artery, Left			
H External Iliac Artery, Right			
J External Iliac Artery, Left			
K Femoral Artery, Right			
L Femoral Artery, Left			
M Popliteal Artery, Right			
N Popliteal Artery, Left			
P Anterior Tibial Artery, Right			
Q Anterior Tibial Artery, Left			
R Posterior Tibial Artery, Right			
S Posterior Tibial Artery, Left			
T Peroneal Artery, Right			
U Peroneal Artery, Left			
V Foot Artery, Right			
W Foot Artery, Left			
Y Lower Artery			

Section	0	Medical and Surgical		
Body System	4	Lower Arteries		
Operation	P	Removal: Taking out or off a device from a body part		

Body Part (Character 4)	Approach (Character 5)	Device (Character 6)	Qualifier (Character 7)
Y Lower Artery	0 Open 3 Percutaneous 4 Percutaneous Endoscopic	0 Drainage Device 2 Monitoring Device 3 Infusion Device 7 Autologous Tissue Substitute C Extraluminal Device D Intraluminal Device J Synthetic Substitute K Nonautologous Tissue Substitute	Z No Qualifier
Y Lower Artery	X External	0 Drainage Device 1 Radioactive Element 2 Monitoring Device 3 Infusion Device D Intraluminal Device	Z No Qualifier

Section	0	Medical and Surgical		
Body System	4	Lower Arteries		
Operation	Q	Repair: Restoring, to the extent possible, a body part to its normal anatomic structure and function		

Body Part (Character 4)	Approach (Character 5)	Device (Character 6)	Qualifier (Character 7)
0 Abdominal Aorta 1 Celiac Artery 2 Gastric Artery 3 Hepatic Artery 4 Splenic Artery 5 Superior Mesenteric Artery 6 Colic Artery, Right 7 Colic Artery, Left 8 Colic Artery, Middle 9 Renal Artery, Right A Renal Artery, Left B Inferior Mesenteric Artery C Common Iliac Artery, Right D Common Iliac Artery, Left E Internal Iliac Artery, Right F Internal Iliac Artery, Left H External Iliac Artery, Right J External Iliac Artery, Left K Femoral Artery, Right L Femoral Artery, Left M Popliteal Artery, Right N Popliteal Artery, Left P Anterior Tibial Artery, Right Q Anterior Tibial Artery, Left R Posterior Tibial Artery, Right S Posterior Tibial Artery, Left T Peroneal Artery, Right U Peroneal Artery, Left V Foot Artery, Right W Foot Artery, Left Y Lower Artery	0 Open 3 Percutaneous 4 Percutaneous Endoscopic	Z No Device	Z No Qualifier

Section	0	Medical and Surgical		
Body System	4	Lower Arteries		
Operation	R	Replacement: Putting in or on biological or synthetic material that physically takes the place and/or function of all or a portion of a body part		

Body Part (Character 4)	Approach (Character 5)	Device (Character 6)	Qualifier (Character 7)
0 Abdominal Aorta 1 Celiac Artery 2 Gastric Artery 3 Hepatic Artery 4 Splenic Artery 5 Superior Mesenteric Artery 6 Colic Artery, Right 7 Colic Artery, Left 8 Colic Artery, Middle 9 Renal Artery, Right A Renal Artery, Left B Inferior Mesenteric Artery C Common Iliac Artery, Right D Common Iliac Artery, Left E Internal Iliac Artery, Right F Internal Iliac Artery, Left H External Iliac Artery, Right J External Iliac Artery, Left K Femoral Artery, Right L Femoral Artery, Left M Popliteal Artery, Right N Popliteal Artery, Left P Anterior Tibial Artery, Right Q Anterior Tibial Artery, Left R Posterior Tibial Artery, Right S Posterior Tibial Artery, Left T Peroneal Artery, Right U Peroneal Artery, Left V Foot Artery, Right W Foot Artery, Left Y Lower Artery	0 Open 4 Percutaneous Endoscopic	7 Autologous Tissue Substitute J Synthetic Substitute K Nonautologous Tissue Substitute	Z No Qualifier

Section	0	Medical and Surgical		
Body System	4	Lower Arteries		
Operation	S	Reposition: Moving to its normal location, or other suitable location, all or a portion of a body part		

Body Part (Character 4)	Approach (Character 5)	Device (Character 6)	Qualifier (Character 7)
0 Abdominal Aorta 1 Celiac Artery 2 Gastric Artery 3 Hepatic Artery 4 Splenic Artery 5 Superior Mesenteric Artery 6 Colic Artery, Right 7 Colic Artery, Left 8 Colic Artery, Middle 9 Renal Artery, Right A Renal Artery, Left B Inferior Mesenteric Artery C Common Iliac Artery, Right D Common Iliac Artery, Left E Internal Iliac Artery, Right F Internal Iliac Artery, Left H External Iliac Artery, Right J External Iliac Artery, Left K Femoral Artery, Right L Femoral Artery, Left M Popliteal Artery, Right N Popliteal Artery, Left P Anterior Tibial Artery, Right Q Anterior Tibial Artery, Left R Posterior Tibial Artery, Right S Posterior Tibial Artery, Left T Peroneal Artery, Right U Peroneal Artery, Left V Foot Artery, Right W Foot Artery, Left Y Lower Artery	0 Open 3 Percutaneous 4 Percutaneous Endoscopic	Z No Device	Z No Qualifier

Section	0	Medical and Surgical		
Body System	4	Lower Arteries		
Operation	U	Supplement: Putting in or on biological or synthetic material that physically reinforces and/or augments the function of a portion of a body part		

Body Part (Character 4)	Approach (Character 5)	Device (Character 6)	Qualifier (Character 7)
0 Abdominal Aorta 1 Celiac Artery 2 Gastric Artery 3 Hepatic Artery 4 Splenic Artery 5 Superior Mesenteric Artery 6 Colic Artery, Right 7 Colic Artery, Left 8 Colic Artery, Middle 9 Renal Artery, Right A Renal Artery, Left B Inferior Mesenteric Artery C Common Iliac Artery, Right D Common Iliac Artery, Left E Internal Iliac Artery, Right F Internal Iliac Artery, Left H External Iliac Artery, Right J External Iliac Artery, Left K Femoral Artery, Right L Femoral Artery, Left M Popliteal Artery, Right N Popliteal Artery, Left P Anterior Tibial Artery, Right Q Anterior Tibial Artery, Left R Posterior Tibial Artery, Right S Posterior Tibial Artery, Left T Peroneal Artery, Right U Peroneal Artery, Left V Foot Artery, Right W Foot Artery, Left Y Lower Artery	0 Open 3 Percutaneous 4 Percutaneous Endoscopic	7 Autologous Tissue Substitute J Synthetic Substitute K Nonautologous Tissue Substitute	Z No Qualifier

Section	0	Medical and Surgical		
Body System	4	Lower Arteries		
Operation	V	Restriction: Partially closing an orifice or the lumen of a tubular body part		

Body Part (Character 4)	Approach (Character 5)	Device (Character 6)	Qualifier (Character 7)
0 Abdominal Aorta	**0** Open **3** Percutaneous **4** Percutaneous Endoscopic	**C** Extraluminal Device **Z** No Device	**Z** No Qualifier
0 Abdominal Aorta	**0** Open **3** Percutaneous **4** Percutaneous Endoscopic	**D** Intraluminal Device	**J** Temporary **Z** No Qualifier
1 Celiac Artery **2** Gastric Artery **3** Hepatic Artery **4** Splenic Artery **5** Superior Mesenteric Artery **6** Colic Artery, Right **7** Colic Artery, Left **8** Colic Artery, Middle **9** Renal Artery, Right **A** Renal Artery, Left **B** Inferior Mesenteric Artery **C** Common Iliac Artery, Right **D** Common Iliac Artery, Left **E** Internal Iliac Artery, Right **F** Internal Iliac Artery, Left **H** External Iliac Artery, Right **J** External Iliac Artery, Left **K** Femoral Artery, Right **L** Femoral Artery, Left **M** Popliteal Artery, Right **N** Popliteal Artery, Left **P** Anterior Tibial Artery, Right **Q** Anterior Tibial Artery, Left **R** Posterior Tibial Artery, Right **S** Posterior Tibial Artery, Left **T** Peroneal Artery, Right **U** Peroneal Artery, Left **V** Foot Artery, Right **W** Foot Artery, Left **Y** Lower Artery			

Section	0	Medical and Surgical		
Body System	4	Lower Arteries		
Operation	W	Revision: Correcting, to the extent possible, a portion of a malfunctioning device or the position of a displaced device		

Body Part (Character 4)	Approach (Character 5)	Device (Character 6)	Qualifier (Character 7)
Y Lower Artery	**0** Open **3** Percutaneous **4** Percutaneous Endoscopic **X** External	**0** Drainage Device **2** Monitoring Device **3** Infusion Device **7** Autologous Tissue Substitute **C** Extraluminal Device **D** Intraluminal Device **J** Synthetic Substitute **K** Nonautologous Tissue Substitute	**Z** No Qualifier

Section	0	Medical and Surgical		
Body System	5	Upper Veins		
Operation	1	Bypass: Altering the route of passage of the contents of a tubular body part		

Body Part (Character 4)	Approach (Character 5)	Device (Character 6)	Qualifier (Character 7)
0 Azygos Vein 1 Hemiazygos Vein 3 Innominate Vein, Right 4 Innominate Vein, Left 5 Subclavian Vein, Right 6 Subclavian Vein, Left 7 Axillary Vein, Right 8 Axillary Vein, Left 9 Brachial Vein, Right A Brachial Vein, Left B Basilic Vein, Right C Basilic Vein, Left D Cephalic Vein, Right F Cephalic Vein, Left G Hand Vein, Right H Hand Vein, Left L Intracranial Vein M Internal Jugular Vein, Right N Internal Jugular Vein, Left P External Jugular Vein, Right Q External Jugular Vein, Left R Vertebral Vein, Right S Vertebral Vein, Left T Face Vein, Right V Face Vein, Left	0 Open 4 Percutaneous Endoscopic	7 Autologous Tissue Substitute 9 Autologous Venous Tissue A Autologous Arterial Tissue J Synthetic Substitute K Nonautologous Tissue Substitute Z No Device	Y Upper Vein

Section	0	Medical and Surgical		
Body System	5	Upper Veins		
Operation	5	Destruction: Physical eradication of all or a portion of a body part by the direct use of energy, force, or a destructive agent		

Body Part (Character 4)	Approach (Character 5)	Device (Character 6)	Qualifier (Character 7)
0 Azygos Vein 1 Hemiazygos Vein 3 Innominate Vein, Right 4 Innominate Vein, Left 5 Subclavian Vein, Right 6 Subclavian Vein, Left 7 Axillary Vein, Right 8 Axillary Vein, Left 9 Brachial Vein, Right A Brachial Vein, Left B Basilic Vein, Right C Basilic Vein, Left D Cephalic Vein, Right F Cephalic Vein, Left G Hand Vein, Right H Hand Vein, Left L Intracranial Vein M Internal Jugular Vein, Right N Internal Jugular Vein, Left P External Jugular Vein, Right Q External Jugular Vein, Left R Vertebral Vein, Right S Vertebral Vein, Left T Face Vein, Right V Face Vein, Left Y Upper Vein	0 Open 3 Percutaneous 4 Percutaneous Endoscopic	Z No Device	Z No Qualifier

Section	0	Medical and Surgical		
Body System	5	Upper Veins		
Operation	7	Dilation: Expanding an orifice or the lumen of a tubular body part		

Body Part (Character 4)	Approach (Character 5)	Device (Character 6)	Qualifier (Character 7)
0 Azygos Vein	0 Open	D Intraluminal Device	Z No Qualifier
1 Hemiazygos Vein	3 Percutaneous	Z No Device	
3 Innominate Vein, Right	4 Percutaneous Endoscopic		
4 Innominate Vein, Left			
5 Subclavian Vein, Right			
6 Subclavian Vein, Left			
7 Axillary Vein, Right			
8 Axillary Vein, Left			
9 Brachial Vein, Right			
A Brachial Vein, Left			
B Basilic Vein, Right			
C Basilic Vein, Left			
D Cephalic Vein, Right			
F Cephalic Vein, Left			
G Hand Vein, Right			
H Hand Vein, Left			
L Intracranial Vein			
M Internal Jugular Vein, Right			
N Internal Jugular Vein, Left			
P External Jugular Vein, Right			
Q External Jugular Vein, Left			
R Vertebral Vein, Right			
S Vertebral Vein, Left			
T Face Vein, Right			
V Face Vein, Left			
Y Upper Vein			

Section	0	Medical and Surgical		
Body System	5	Upper Veins		
Operation	9	Drainage: Taking or letting out fluids and/or gases from a body part		

Body Part (Character 4)	Approach (Character 5)	Device (Character 6)	Qualifier (Character 7)
0 Azygos Vein	0 Open	0 Drainage Device	Z No Qualifier
1 Hemiazygos Vein	3 Percutaneous		
3 Innominate Vein, Right	4 Percutaneous Endoscopic		
4 Innominate Vein, Left			
5 Subclavian Vein, Right			
6 Subclavian Vein, Left			
7 Axillary Vein, Right			
8 Axillary Vein, Left			
9 Brachial Vein, Right			
A Brachial Vein, Left			
B Basilic Vein, Right			
C Basilic Vein, Left			
D Cephalic Vein, Right			
F Cephalic Vein, Left			
G Hand Vein, Right			
H Hand Vein, Left			
L Intracranial Vein			
M Internal Jugular Vein, Right			
N Internal Jugular Vein, Left			
P External Jugular Vein, Right			
Q External Jugular Vein, Left			
R Vertebral Vein, Right			
S Vertebral Vein, Left			
T Face Vein, Right			
V Face Vein, Left			
Y Upper Vein			

Section	0	Medical and Surgical		
Body System	5	Upper Veins		
Operation	9	Drainage: Taking or letting out fluids and/or gases from a body part		

Body Part (Character 4)	Approach (Character 5)	Device (Character 6)	Qualifier (Character 7)
0 Azygos Vein	0 Open	Z No Device	X Diagnostic
1 Hemiazygos Vein	3 Percutaneous		Z No Qualifier
3 Innominate Vein, Right	4 Percutaneous Endoscopic		
4 Innominate Vein, Left			
5 Subclavian Vein, Right			
6 Subclavian Vein, Left			
7 Axillary Vein, Right			
8 Axillary Vein, Left			
9 Brachial Vein, Right			
A Brachial Vein, Left			
B Basilic Vein, Right			
C Basilic Vein, Left			
D Cephalic Vein, Right			
F Cephalic Vein, Left			
G Hand Vein, Right			
H Hand Vein, Left			
L Intracranial Vein			
M Internal Jugular Vein, Right			
N Internal Jugular Vein, Left			
P External Jugular Vein, Right			
Q External Jugular Vein, Left			
R Vertebral Vein, Right			
S Vertebral Vein, Left			
T Face Vein, Right			
V Face Vein, Left			
Y Upper Vein			

Section	0	Medical and Surgical		
Body System	5	Upper Veins		
Operation	B	Excision: Cutting out or off, without replacement, a portion of a body part		

Body Part (Character 4)	Approach (Character 5)	Device (Character 6)	Qualifier (Character 7)
0 Azygos Vein	0 Open	Z No Device	X Diagnostic
1 Hemiazygos Vein	3 Percutaneous		Z No Qualifier
3 Innominate Vein, Right	4 Percutaneous Endoscopic		
4 Innominate Vein, Left			
5 Subclavian Vein, Right			
6 Subclavian Vein, Left			
7 Axillary Vein, Right			
8 Axillary Vein, Left			
9 Brachial Vein, Right			
A Brachial Vein, Left			
B Basilic Vein, Right			
C Basilic Vein, Left			
D Cephalic Vein, Right			
F Cephalic Vein, Left			
G Hand Vein, Right			
H Hand Vein, Left			
L Intracranial Vein			
M Internal Jugular Vein, Right			
N Internal Jugular Vein, Left			
P External Jugular Vein, Right			
Q External Jugular Vein, Left			
R Vertebral Vein, Right			
S Vertebral Vein, Left			
T Face Vein, Right			
V Face Vein, Left			
Y Upper Vein			

Section	0	Medical and Surgical		
Body System	5	Upper Veins		
Operation	C	Extirpation: Taking or cutting out solid matter from a body part		

Body Part (Character 4)	Approach (Character 5)	Device (Character 6)	Qualifier (Character 7)
0 Azygos Vein	0 Open	Z No Device	Z No Qualifier
1 Hemiazygos Vein	3 Percutaneous		
3 Innominate Vein, Right	4 Percutaneous Endoscopic		
4 Innominate Vein, Left			
5 Subclavian Vein, Right			
6 Subclavian Vein, Left			
7 Axillary Vein, Right			
8 Axillary Vein, Left			
9 Brachial Vein, Right			
A Brachial Vein, Left			
B Basilic Vein, Right			
C Basilic Vein, Left			
D Cephalic Vein, Right			
F Cephalic Vein, Left			
G Hand Vein, Right			
H Hand Vein, Left			
L Intracranial Vein			
M Internal Jugular Vein, Right			
N Internal Jugular Vein, Left			
P External Jugular Vein, Right			
Q External Jugular Vein, Left			
R Vertebral Vein, Right			
S Vertebral Vein, Left			
T Face Vein, Right			
V Face Vein, Left			
Y Upper Vein			

Section	0	Medical and Surgical		
Body System	5	Upper Veins		
Operation	D	Extraction: Pulling or stripping out or off all or a portion of a body part by the use of force		

Body Part (Character 4)	Approach (Character 5)	Device (Character 6)	Qualifier (Character 7)
9 Brachial Vein, Right	0 Open	Z No Device	Z No Qualifier
A Brachial Vein, Left	3 Percutaneous		
B Basilic Vein, Right			
C Basilic Vein, Left			
D Cephalic Vein, Right			
F Cephalic Vein, Left			
G Hand Vein, Right			
H Hand Vein, Left			
Y Upper Vein			

Section	0	Medical and Surgical		
Body System	5	Upper Veins		
Operation	L	Occlusion: Completely closing an orifice or the lumen of a tubular body part		

Body Part (Character 4)	Approach (Character 5)	Device (Character 6)	Qualifier (Character 7)
0 Azygos Vein 1 Hemiazygos Vein 3 Innominate Vein, Right 4 Innominate Vein, Left 5 Subclavian Vein, Right 6 Subclavian Vein, Left 7 Axillary Vein, Right 8 Axillary Vein, Left 9 Brachial Vein, Right A Brachial Vein, Left B Basilic Vein, Right C Basilic Vein, Left D Cephalic Vein, Right F Cephalic Vein, Left G Hand Vein, Right H Hand Vein, Left L Intracranial Vein M Internal Jugular Vein, Right N Internal Jugular Vein, Left P External Jugular Vein, Right Q External Jugular Vein, Left R Vertebral Vein, Right S Vertebral Vein, Left T Face Vein, Right V Face Vein, Left Y Upper Vein	0 Open 3 Percutaneous 4 Percutaneous Endoscopic	C Extraluminal Device D Intraluminal Device Z No Device	Z No Qualifier

Section	0	Medical and Surgical		
Body System	5	Upper Veins		
Operation	N	Release: Freeing a body part from an abnormal physical constraint by cutting or by the use of force		

Body Part (Character 4)	Approach (Character 5)	Device (Character 6)	Qualifier (Character 7)
0 Azygos Vein 1 Hemiazygos Vein 3 Innominate Vein, Right 4 Innominate Vein, Left 5 Subclavian Vein, Right 6 Subclavian Vein, Left 7 Axillary Vein, Right 8 Axillary Vein, Left 9 Brachial Vein, Right A Brachial Vein, Left B Basilic Vein, Right C Basilic Vein, Left D Cephalic Vein, Right F Cephalic Vein, Left G Hand Vein, Right H Hand Vein, Left L Intracranial Vein M Internal Jugular Vein, Right N Internal Jugular Vein, Left P External Jugular Vein, Right Q External Jugular Vein, Left R Vertebral Vein, Right S Vertebral Vein, Left T Face Vein, Right V Face Vein, Left Y Upper Vein	0 Open 3 Percutaneous 4 Percutaneous Endoscopic	Z No Device	Z No Qualifier

Section	0	Medical and Surgical		
Body System	5	Upper Veins		
Operation	P	Removal: Taking out or off a device from a body part		
Body Part (Character 4)	Approach (Character 5)	Device (Character 6)	Qualifier (Character 7)
---	---	---	---
Y Upper Vein	0 Open 3 Percutaneous 4 Percutaneous Endoscopic	0 Drainage Device 2 Monitoring Device 3 Infusion Device 7 Autologous Tissue Substitute C Extraluminal Device D Intraluminal Device J Synthetic Substitute K Nonautologous Tissue Substitute	Z No Qualifier
Y Upper Vein	X External	0 Drainage Device 2 Monitoring Device 3 Infusion Device D Intraluminal Device	Z No Qualifier

Section	0	Medical and Surgical		
Body System	5	Upper Veins		
Operation	Q	Repair: Restoring, to the extent possible, a body part to its normal anatomic structure and function		
Body Part (Character 4)	Approach (Character 5)	Device (Character 6)	Qualifier (Character 7)
---	---	---	---
0 Azygos Vein 1 Hemiazygos Vein 3 Innominate Vein, Right 4 Innominate Vein, Left 5 Subclavian Vein, Right 6 Subclavian Vein, Left 7 Axillary Vein, Right 8 Axillary Vein, Left 9 Brachial Vein, Right A Brachial Vein, Left B Basilic Vein, Right C Basilic Vein, Left D Cephalic Vein, Right F Cephalic Vein, Left G Hand Vein, Right H Hand Vein, Left L Intracranial Vein M Internal Jugular Vein, Right N Internal Jugular Vein, Left P External Jugular Vein, Right Q External Jugular Vein, Left R Vertebral Vein, Right S Vertebral Vein, Left T Face Vein, Right V Face Vein, Left Y Upper Vein	0 Open 3 Percutaneous 4 Percutaneous Endoscopic	Z No Device	Z No Qualifier

Section	0	Medical and Surgical			
Body System	5	Upper Veins			
Operation	R	Replacement: Putting in or on biological or synthetic material that physically takes the place and/or function of all or a portion of a body part			

Body Part (Character 4)	Approach (Character 5)	Device (Character 6)	Qualifier (Character 7)
0 Azygos Vein 1 Hemiazygos Vein 3 Innominate Vein, Right 4 Innominate Vein, Left 5 Subclavian Vein, Right 6 Subclavian Vein, Left 7 Axillary Vein, Right 8 Axillary Vein, Left 9 Brachial Vein, Right A Brachial Vein, Left B Basilic Vein, Right C Basilic Vein, Left D Cephalic Vein, Right F Cephalic Vein, Left G Hand Vein, Right H Hand Vein, Left L Intracranial Vein M Internal Jugular Vein, Right N Internal Jugular Vein, Left P External Jugular Vein, Right Q External Jugular Vein, Left R Vertebral Vein, Right S Vertebral Vein, Left T Face Vein, Right V Face Vein, Left Y Upper Vein	0 Open 4 Percutaneous Endoscopic	7 Autologous Tissue Substitute J Synthetic Substitute K Nonautologous Tissue Substitute	Z No Qualifier

Section	0	Medical and Surgical			
Body System	5	Upper Veins			
Operation	S	Reposition: Moving to its normal location, or other suitable location, all or a portion of a body part			

Body Part (Character 4)	Approach (Character 5)	Device (Character 6)	Qualifier (Character 7)
0 Azygos Vein 1 Hemiazygos Vein 3 Innominate Vein, Right 4 Innominate Vein, Left 5 Subclavian Vein, Right 6 Subclavian Vein, Left 7 Axillary Vein, Right 8 Axillary Vein, Left 9 Brachial Vein, Right A Brachial Vein, Left B Basilic Vein, Right C Basilic Vein, Left D Cephalic Vein, Right F Cephalic Vein, Left G Hand Vein, Right H Hand Vein, Left L Intracranial Vein M Internal Jugular Vein, Right N Internal Jugular Vein, Left P External Jugular Vein, Right Q External Jugular Vein, Left R Vertebral Vein, Right S Vertebral Vein, Left T Face Vein, Right V Face Vein, Left Y Upper Vein	0 Open 3 Percutaneous 4 Percutaneous Endoscopic	Z No Device	Z No Qualifier

Section	0	Medical and Surgical		
Body System	5	Upper Veins		
Operation	U	Supplement: Putting in or on biological or synthetic material that physically reinforces and/or augments the function of a portion of a body part		

Body Part (Character 4)	Approach (Character 5)	Device (Character 6)	Qualifier (Character 7)
0 Azygos Vein	**0** Open	**7** Autologous Tissue Substitute	**Z** No Qualifier
1 Hemiazygos Vein	**3** Percutaneous	**J** Synthetic Substitute	
3 Innominate Vein, Right	**4** Percutaneous Endoscopic	**K** Nonautologous Tissue Substitute	
4 Innominate Vein, Left			
5 Subclavian Vein, Right			
6 Subclavian Vein, Left			
7 Axillary Vein, Right			
8 Axillary Vein, Left			
9 Brachial Vein, Right			
A Brachial Vein, Left			
B Basilic Vein, Right			
C Basilic Vein, Left			
D Cephalic Vein, Right			
F Cephalic Vein, Left			
G Hand Vein, Right			
H Hand Vein, Left			
L Intracranial Vein			
M Internal Jugular Vein, Right			
N Internal Jugular Vein, Left			
P External Jugular Vein, Right			
Q External Jugular Vein, Left			
R Vertebral Vein, Right			
S Vertebral Vein, Left			
T Face Vein, Right			
V Face Vein, Left			
Y Upper Vein			

Section	0	Medical and Surgical		
Body System	5	Upper Veins		
Operation	V	Restriction: Partially closing an orifice or the lumen of a tubular body part		

Body Part (Character 4)	Approach (Character 5)	Device (Character 6)	Qualifier (Character 7)
0 Azygos Vein	**0** Open	**C** Extraluminal Device	**Z** No Qualifier
1 Hemiazygos Vein	**3** Percutaneous	**D** Intraluminal Device	
3 Innominate Vein, Right	**4** Percutaneous Endoscopic	**Z** No Device	
4 Innominate Vein, Left			
5 Subclavian Vein, Right			
6 Subclavian Vein, Left			
7 Axillary Vein, Right			
8 Axillary Vein, Left			
9 Brachial Vein, Right			
A Brachial Vein, Left			
B Basilic Vein, Right			
C Basilic Vein, Left			
D Cephalic Vein, Right			
F Cephalic Vein, Left			
G Hand Vein, Right			
H Hand Vein, Left			
L Intracranial Vein			
M Internal Jugular Vein, Right			
N Internal Jugular Vein, Left			
P External Jugular Vein, Right			
Q External Jugular Vein, Left			
R Vertebral Vein, Right			
S Vertebral Vein, Left			
T Face Vein, Right			
V Face Vein, Left			
Y Upper Vein			

Section	0	Medical and Surgical			
Body System	5	Upper Veins			
Operation	W	Revision: Correcting, to the extent possible, a portion of a malfunctioning device or the position of a displaced device			

Body Part (Character 4)	Approach (Character 5)	Device (Character 6)	Qualifier (Character 7)
Y Upper Vein	**0** Open **3** Percutaneous **4** Percutaneous Endoscopic **X** External	**0** Drainage Device **2** Monitoring Device **3** Infusion Device **7** Autologous Tissue Substitute **C** Extraluminal Device **D** Intraluminal Device **J** Synthetic Substitute **K** Nonautologous Tissue Substitute	**Z** No Qualifier

Section	0	Medical and Surgical		
Body System	6	Lower Veins		
Operation	1	Bypass: Altering the route of passage of the contents of a tubular body part		
Body Part (Character 4)		**Approach (Character 5)**	**Device (Character 6)**	**Qualifier (Character 7)**
0 Inferior Vena Cava		0 Open 4 Percutaneous Endoscopic	7 Autologous Tissue Substitute 9 Autologous Venous Tissue A Autologous Arterial Tissue J Synthetic Substitute K Nonautologous Tissue Substitute Z No Device	5 Superior Mesenteric Vein 6 Inferior Mesenteric Vein Y Lower Vein
1 Splenic Vein		0 Open 4 Percutaneous Endoscopic	7 Autologous Tissue Substitute 9 Autologous Venous Tissue A Autologous Arterial Tissue J Synthetic Substitute K Nonautologous Tissue Substitute Z No Device	9 Renal Vein, Right B Renal Vein, Left Y Lower Vein
2 Gastric Vein 3 Esophageal Vein 4 Hepatic Vein 5 Superior Mesenteric Vein 6 Inferior Mesenteric Vein 7 Colic Vein 9 Renal Vein, Right B Renal Vein, Left C Common Iliac Vein, Right D Common Iliac Vein, Left F External Iliac Vein, Right G External Iliac Vein, Left H Hypogastric Vein, Right J Hypogastric Vein, Left M Femoral Vein, Right N Femoral Vein, Left P Greater Saphenous Vein, Right Q Greater Saphenous Vein, Left R Lesser Saphenous Vein, Right S Lesser Saphenous Vein, Left T Foot Vein, Right V Foot Vein, Left		0 Open 4 Percutaneous Endoscopic	7 Autologous Tissue Substitute 9 Autologous Venous Tissue A Autologous Arterial Tissue J Synthetic Substitute K Nonautologous Tissue Substitute Z No Device	Y Lower Vein

Section	0	Medical and Surgical		
Body System	6	Lower Veins		
Operation	1	Bypass: Altering the route of passage of the contents of a tubular body part		
Body Part (Character 4)		**Approach (Character 5)**	**Device (Character 6)**	**Qualifier (Character 7)**
8 Portal Vein		0 Open	7 Autologous Tissue Substitute 9 Autologous Venous Tissue A Autologous Arterial Tissue J Synthetic Substitute K Nonautologous Tissue Substitute Z No Device	9 Renal Vein, Right B Renal Vein, Left Y Lower Vein
8 Portal Vein		3 Percutaneous	D Intraluminal Device	Y Lower Vein
8 Portal Vein		4 Percutaneous Endoscopic	7 Autologous Tissue Substitute 9 Autologous Venous Tissue A Autologous Arterial Tissue J Synthetic Substitute K Nonautologous Tissue Substitute Z No Device	9 Renal Vein, Right B Renal Vein, Left Y Lower Vein
8 Portal Vein		4 Percutaneous Endoscopic	D Intraluminal Device	Y Lower Vein

Section	0	Medical and Surgical			
Body System	6	Lower Veins			
Operation	5	Destruction: Physical eradication of all or a portion of a body part by the direct use of energy, force, or a destructive agent			

Body Part (Character 4)	Approach (Character 5)	Device (Character 6)	Qualifier (Character 7)
0 Inferior Vena Cava 1 Splenic Vein 2 Gastric Vein 3 Esophageal Vein 4 Hepatic Vein 5 Superior Mesenteric Vein 6 Inferior Mesenteric Vein 7 Colic Vein 8 Portal Vein 9 Renal Vein, Right B Renal Vein, Left C Common Iliac Vein, Right D Common Iliac Vein, Left F External Iliac Vein, Right G External Iliac Vein, Left H Hypogastric Vein, Right J Hypogastric Vein, Left M Femoral Vein, Right N Femoral Vein, Left P Greater Saphenous Vein, Right Q Greater Saphenous Vein, Left R Lesser Saphenous Vein, Right S Lesser Saphenous Vein, Left T Foot Vein, Right V Foot Vein, Left	0 Open 3 Percutaneous 4 Percutaneous Endoscopic	Z No Device	Z No Qualifier
Y Lower Vein	0 Open 3 Percutaneous 4 Percutaneous Endoscopic	Z No Device	C Hemorrhoidal Plexus Z No Qualifier

Section	0	Medical and Surgical			
Body System	6	Lower Veins			
Operation	7	Dilation: Expanding an orifice or the lumen of a tubular body part			

Body Part (Character 4)	Approach (Character 5)	Device (Character 6)	Qualifier (Character 7)
0 Inferior Vena Cava 1 Splenic Vein 2 Gastric Vein 3 Esophageal Vein 4 Hepatic Vein 5 Superior Mesenteric Vein 6 Inferior Mesenteric Vein 7 Colic Vein 8 Portal Vein 9 Renal Vein, Right B Renal Vein, Left C Common Iliac Vein, Right D Common Iliac Vein, Left F External Iliac Vein, Right G External Iliac Vein, Left H Hypogastric Vein, Right J Hypogastric Vein, Left M Femoral Vein, Right N Femoral Vein, Left P Greater Saphenous Vein, Right Q Greater Saphenous Vein, Left R Lesser Saphenous Vein, Right S Lesser Saphenous Vein, Left T Foot Vein, Right V Foot Vein, Left Y Lower Vein	0 Open 3 Percutaneous 4 Percutaneous Endoscopic	D Intraluminal Device Z No Device	Z No Qualifier

Section	0	Medical and Surgical		
Body System	6	Lower Veins		
Operation	9	Drainage: Taking or letting out fluids and/or gases from a body part		
Body Part (Character 4)		Approach (Character 5)	Device (Character 6)	Qualifier (Character 7)
0 Inferior Vena Cava		0 Open	0 Drainage Device	Z No Qualifier
1 Splenic Vein		3 Percutaneous		
2 Gastric Vein		4 Percutaneous Endoscopic		
3 Esophageal Vein				
4 Hepatic Vein				
5 Superior Mesenteric Vein				
6 Inferior Mesenteric Vein				
7 Colic Vein				
8 Portal Vein				
9 Renal Vein, Right				
B Renal Vein, Left				
C Common Iliac Vein, Right				
D Common Iliac Vein, Left				
F External Iliac Vein, Right				
G External Iliac Vein, Left				
H Hypogastric Vein, Right				
J Hypogastric Vein, Left				
M Femoral Vein, Right				
N Femoral Vein, Left				
P Greater Saphenous Vein, Right				
Q Greater Saphenous Vein, Left				
R Lesser Saphenous Vein, Right				
S Lesser Saphenous Vein, Left				
T Foot Vein, Right				
V Foot Vein, Left				
Y Lower Vein				

Section	0	Medical and Surgical		
Body System	6	Lower Veins		
Operation	9	Drainage: Taking or letting out fluids and/or gases from a body part		
Body Part (Character 4)		Approach (Character 5)	Device (Character 6)	Qualifier (Character 7)
0 Inferior Vena Cava		0 Open	Z No Device	X Diagnostic
1 Splenic Vein		3 Percutaneous		Z No Qualifier
2 Gastric Vein		4 Percutaneous Endoscopic		
3 Esophageal Vein				
4 Hepatic Vein				
5 Superior Mesenteric Vein				
6 Inferior Mesenteric Vein				
7 Colic Vein				
8 Portal Vein				
9 Renal Vein, Right				
B Renal Vein, Left				
C Common Iliac Vein, Right				
D Common Iliac Vein, Left				
F External Iliac Vein, Right				
G External Iliac Vein, Left				
H Hypogastric Vein, Right				
J Hypogastric Vein, Left				
M Femoral Vein, Right				
N Femoral Vein, Left				
P Greater Saphenous Vein, Right				
Q Greater Saphenous Vein, Left				
R Lesser Saphenous Vein, Right				
S Lesser Saphenous Vein, Left				
T Foot Vein, Right				
V Foot Vein, Left				
Y Lower Vein				

Section	0	Medical and Surgical		
Body System	6	Lower Veins		
Operation	B	Excision: Cutting out or off, without replacement, a portion of a body part		

Body Part (Character 4)	Approach (Character 5)	Device (Character 6)	Qualifier (Character 7)
0 Inferior Vena Cava **1** Splenic Vein **2** Gastric Vein **3** Esophageal Vein **4** Hepatic Vein **5** Superior Mesenteric Vein **6** Inferior Mesenteric Vein **7** Colic Vein **8** Portal Vein **9** Renal Vein, Right **B** Renal Vein, Left **C** Common Iliac Vein, Right **D** Common Iliac Vein, Left **F** External Iliac Vein, Right **G** External Iliac Vein, Left **H** Hypogastric Vein, Right **J** Hypogastric Vein, Left **M** Femoral Vein, Right **N** Femoral Vein, Left **P** Greater Saphenous Vein, Right **Q** Greater Saphenous Vein, Left **R** Lesser Saphenous Vein, Right **S** Lesser Saphenous Vein, Left **T** Foot Vein, Right **V** Foot Vein, Left	**0** Open **3** Percutaneous **4** Percutaneous Endoscopic	**Z** No Device	**X** Diagnostic **Z** No Qualifier
Y Lower Vein	**0** Open **3** Percutaneous **4** Percutaneous Endoscopic	**Z** No Device	**C** Hemorrhoidal Plexus **X** Diagnostic **Z** No Qualifier

Section	0	Medical and Surgical		
Body System	6	Lower Veins		
Operation	C	Extirpation: Taking or cutting out solid matter from a body part		

Body Part (Character 4)	Approach (Character 5)	Device (Character 6)	Qualifier (Character 7)
0 Inferior Vena Cava **1** Splenic Vein **2** Gastric Vein **3** Esophageal Vein **4** Hepatic Vein **5** Superior Mesenteric Vein **6** Inferior Mesenteric Vein **7** Colic Vein **8** Portal Vein **9** Renal Vein, Right **B** Renal Vein, Left **C** Common Iliac Vein, Right **D** Common Iliac Vein, Left **F** External Iliac Vein, Right **G** External Iliac Vein, Left **H** Hypogastric Vein, Right **J** Hypogastric Vein, Left **M** Femoral Vein, Right **N** Femoral Vein, Left **P** Greater Saphenous Vein, Right **Q** Greater Saphenous Vein, Left **R** Lesser Saphenous Vein, Right **S** Lesser Saphenous Vein, Left **T** Foot Vein, Right **V** Foot Vein, Left **Y** Lower Vein	**0** Open **3** Percutaneous **4** Percutaneous Endoscopic	**Z** No Device	**Z** No Qualifier

Section	0	Medical and Surgical		
Body System	6	Lower Veins		
Operation	D	Extraction: Pulling or stripping out or off all or a portion of a body part by the use of force		
Body Part (Character 4)		**Approach (Character 5)**	**Device (Character 6)**	**Qualifier (Character 7)**
M Femoral Vein, Right N Femoral Vein, Left P Greater Saphenous Vein, Right Q Greater Saphenous Vein, Left R Lesser Saphenous Vein, Right S Lesser Saphenous Vein, Left T Foot Vein, Right V Foot Vein, Left Y Lower Vein		0 Open 3 Percutaneous 4 Percutaneous Endoscopic	Z No Device	Z No Qualifier

Section	0	Medical and Surgical		
Body System	6	Lower Veins		
Operation	H	Insertion: Putting in a nonbiological appliance that monitors, assists, performs, or prevents a physiological function but does not physically take the place of a body part		
Body Part (Character 4)		**Approach (Character 5)**	**Device (Character 6)**	**Qualifier (Character 7)**
0 Inferior Vena Cava		0 Open 3 Percutaneous	3 Infusion Device	T Via Umbilical Vein Z No Qualifier
0 Inferior Vena Cava		0 Open 3 Percutaneous	D Intraluminal Device	Z No Qualifier
0 Inferior Vena Cava		4 Percutaneous Endoscopic	3 Infusion Device D Intraluminal Device	Z No Qualifier
1 Splenic Vein 2 Gastric Vein 3 Esophageal Vein 4 Hepatic Vein 5 Superior Mesenteric Vein 6 Inferior Mesenteric Vein 7 Colic Vein 8 Portal Vein 9 Renal Vein, Right B Renal Vein, Left C Common Iliac Vein, Right D Common Iliac Vein, Left F External Iliac Vein, Right G External Iliac Vein, Left H Hypogastric Vein, Right J Hypogastric Vein, Left M Femoral Vein, Right N Femoral Vein, Left P Greater Saphenous Vein, Right Q Greater Saphenous Vein, Left R Lesser Saphenous Vein, Right S Lesser Saphenous Vein, Left T Foot Vein, Right V Foot Vein, Left		0 Open 3 Percutaneous 4 Percutaneous Endoscopic	3 Infusion Device D Intraluminal Device	Z No Qualifier
Y Lower Vein		0 Open 3 Percutaneous 4 Percutaneous Endoscopic	2 Monitoring Device 3 Infusion Device D Intraluminal Device	Z No Qualifier

Section	0	Medical and Surgical		
Body System	6	Lower Veins		
Operation	J	Inspection: Visually and/or manually exploring a body part		
Body Part (Character 4)		**Approach (Character 5)**	**Device (Character 6)**	**Qualifier (Character 7)**
Y Lower Vein		0 Open 3 Percutaneous 4 Percutaneous Endoscopic X External	Z No Device	Z No Qualifier

Section	0	Medical and Surgical
Body System	6	Lower Veins
Operation	L	Occlusion: Completely closing an orifice or the lumen of a tubular body part

Body Part (Character 4)	Approach (Character 5)	Device (Character 6)	Qualifier (Character 7)
0 Inferior Vena Cava	0 Open	C Extraluminal Device	Z No Qualifier
1 Splenic Vein	3 Percutaneous	D Intraluminal Device	
2 Gastric Vein	4 Percutaneous Endoscopic	Z No Device	
3 Esophageal Vein			
4 Hepatic Vein			
5 Superior Mesenteric Vein			
6 Inferior Mesenteric Vein			
7 Colic Vein			
8 Portal Vein			
9 Renal Vein, Right			
B Renal Vein, Left			
C Common Iliac Vein, Right			
D Common Iliac Vein, Left			
F External Iliac Vein, Right			
G External Iliac Vein, Left			
H Hypogastric Vein, Right			
J Hypogastric Vein, Left			
M Femoral Vein, Right			
N Femoral Vein, Left			
P Greater Saphenous Vein, Right			
Q Greater Saphenous Vein, Left			
R Lesser Saphenous Vein, Right			
S Lesser Saphenous Vein, Left			
T Foot Vein, Right			
V Foot Vein, Left			
Y Lower Vein	0 Open	C Extraluminal Device	C Hemorrhoidal Plexus
	3 Percutaneous	D Intraluminal Device	Z No Qualifier
	4 Percutaneous Endoscopic	Z No Device	

Section	0	Medical and Surgical
Body System	6	Lower Veins
Operation	N	Release: Freeing a body part from an abnormal physical constraint by cutting or by the use of force

Body Part (Character 4)	Approach (Character 5)	Device (Character 6)	Qualifier (Character 7)
0 Inferior Vena Cava	0 Open	Z No Device	Z No Qualifier
1 Splenic Vein	3 Percutaneous		
2 Gastric Vein	4 Percutaneous Endoscopic		
3 Esophageal Vein			
4 Hepatic Vein			
5 Superior Mesenteric Vein			
6 Inferior Mesenteric Vein			
7 Colic Vein			
8 Portal Vein			
9 Renal Vein, Right			
B Renal Vein, Left			
C Common Iliac Vein, Right			
D Common Iliac Vein, Left			
F External Iliac Vein, Right			
G External Iliac Vein, Left			
H Hypogastric Vein, Right			
J Hypogastric Vein, Left			
M Femoral Vein, Right			
N Femoral Vein, Left			
P Greater Saphenous Vein, Right			
Q Greater Saphenous Vein, Left			
R Lesser Saphenous Vein, Right			
S Lesser Saphenous Vein, Left			
T Foot Vein, Right			
V Foot Vein, Left			
Y Lower Vein			

Section	0	Medical and Surgical		
Body System	6	Lower Veins		
Operation	P	Removal: Taking out or off a device from a body part		

Body Part (Character 4)	Approach (Character 5)	Device (Character 6)	Qualifier (Character 7)
Y Lower Vein	**0** Open **3** Percutaneous **4** Percutaneous Endoscopic	**0** Drainage Device **2** Monitoring Device **3** Infusion Device **7** Autologous Tissue Substitute **C** Extraluminal Device **D** Intraluminal Device **J** Synthetic Substitute **K** Nonautologous Tissue Substitute	**Z** No Qualifier
Y Lower Vein	**X** External	**0** Drainage Device **2** Monitoring Device **3** Infusion Device **D** Intraluminal Device	**Z** No Qualifier

Section	0	Medical and Surgical		
Body System	6	Lower Veins		
Operation	Q	Repair: Restoring, to the extent possible, a body part to its normal anatomic structure and function		

Body Part (Character 4)	Approach (Character 5)	Device (Character 6)	Qualifier (Character 7)
0 Inferior Vena Cava **1** Splenic Vein **2** Gastric Vein **3** Esophageal Vein **4** Hepatic Vein **5** Superior Mesenteric Vein **6** Inferior Mesenteric Vein **7** Colic Vein **8** Portal Vein **9** Renal Vein, Right **B** Renal Vein, Left **C** Common Iliac Vein, Right **D** Common Iliac Vein, Left **F** External Iliac Vein, Right **G** External Iliac Vein, Left **H** Hypogastric Vein, Right **J** Hypogastric Vein, Left **M** Femoral Vein, Right **N** Femoral Vein, Left **P** Greater Saphenous Vein, Right **Q** Greater Saphenous Vein, Left **R** Lesser Saphenous Vein, Right **S** Lesser Saphenous Vein, Left **T** Foot Vein, Right **V** Foot Vein, Left **Y** Lower Vein	**0** Open **3** Percutaneous **4** Percutaneous Endoscopic	**Z** No Device	**Z** No Qualifier

Section	0	Medical and Surgical		
Body System	6	Lower Veins		
Operation	R	Replacement: Putting in or on biological or synthetic material that physically takes the place and/or function of all or a portion of a body part		

Body Part (Character 4)	Approach (Character 5)	Device (Character 6)	Qualifier (Character 7)
0 Inferior Vena Cava	0 Open	7 Autologous Tissue Substitute	Z No Qualifier
1 Splenic Vein	4 Percutaneous Endoscopic	J Synthetic Substitute	
2 Gastric Vein		K Nonautologous Tissue Substitute	
3 Esophageal Vein			
4 Hepatic Vein			
5 Superior Mesenteric Vein			
6 Inferior Mesenteric Vein			
7 Colic Vein			
8 Portal Vein			
9 Renal Vein, Right			
B Renal Vein, Left			
C Common Iliac Vein, Right			
D Common Iliac Vein, Left			
F External Iliac Vein, Right			
G External Iliac Vein, Left			
H Hypogastric Vein, Right			
J Hypogastric Vein, Left			
M Femoral Vein, Right			
N Femoral Vein, Left			
P Greater Saphenous Vein, Right			
Q Greater Saphenous Vein, Left			
R Lesser Saphenous Vein, Right			
S Lesser Saphenous Vein, Left			
T Foot Vein, Right			
V Foot Vein, Left			
Y Lower Vein			

Section	0	Medical and Surgical		
Body System	6	Lower Veins		
Operation	S	Reposition: Moving to its normal location, or other suitable location, all or a portion of a body part		

Body Part (Character 4)	Approach (Character 5)	Device (Character 6)	Qualifier (Character 7)
0 Inferior Vena Cava	0 Open	Z No Device	Z No Qualifier
1 Splenic Vein	3 Percutaneous		
2 Gastric Vein	4 Percutaneous Endoscopic		
3 Esophageal Vein			
4 Hepatic Vein			
5 Superior Mesenteric Vein			
6 Inferior Mesenteric Vein			
7 Colic Vein			
8 Portal Vein			
9 Renal Vein, Right			
B Renal Vein, Left			
C Common Iliac Vein, Right			
D Common Iliac Vein, Left			
F External Iliac Vein, Right			
G External Iliac Vein, Left			
H Hypogastric Vein, Right			
J Hypogastric Vein, Left			
M Femoral Vein, Right			
N Femoral Vein, Left			
P Greater Saphenous Vein, Right			
Q Greater Saphenous Vein, Left			
R Lesser Saphenous Vein, Right			
S Lesser Saphenous Vein, Left			
T Foot Vein, Right			
V Foot Vein, Left			
Y Lower Vein			

Section	0	Medical and Surgical		
Body System	6	Lower Veins		
Operation	U	Supplement: Putting in or on biological or synthetic material that physically reinforces and/or augments the function of a portion of a body part		

Body Part (Character 4)	Approach (Character 5)	Device (Character 6)	Qualifier (Character 7)
0 Inferior Vena Cava **1** Splenic Vein **2** Gastric Vein **3** Esophageal Vein **4** Hepatic Vein **5** Superior Mesenteric Vein **6** Inferior Mesenteric Vein **7** Colic Vein **8** Portal Vein **9** Renal Vein, Right **B** Renal Vein, Left **C** Common Iliac Vein, Right **D** Common Iliac Vein, Left **F** External Iliac Vein, Right **G** External Iliac Vein, Left **H** Hypogastric Vein, Right **J** Hypogastric Vein, Left **M** Femoral Vein, Right **N** Femoral Vein, Left **P** Greater Saphenous Vein, Right **Q** Greater Saphenous Vein, Left **R** Lesser Saphenous Vein, Right **S** Lesser Saphenous Vein, Left **T** Foot Vein, Right **V** Foot Vein, Left **Y** Lower Vein	**0** Open **3** Percutaneous **4** Percutaneous Endoscopic	**7** Autologous Tissue Substitute **J** Synthetic Substitute **K** Nonautologous Tissue Substitute	**Z** No Qualifier

Section	0	Medical and Surgical		
Body System	6	Lower Veins		
Operation	V	Restriction: Partially closing an orifice or the lumen of a tubular body part		

Body Part (Character 4)	Approach (Character 5)	Device (Character 6)	Qualifier (Character 7)
0 Inferior Vena Cava **1** Splenic Vein **2** Gastric Vein **3** Esophageal Vein **4** Hepatic Vein **5** Superior Mesenteric Vein **6** Inferior Mesenteric Vein **7** Colic Vein **8** Portal Vein **9** Renal Vein, Right **B** Renal Vein, Left **C** Common Iliac Vein, Right **D** Common Iliac Vein, Left **F** External Iliac Vein, Right **G** External Iliac Vein, Left **H** Hypogastric Vein, Right **J** Hypogastric Vein, Left **M** Femoral Vein, Right **N** Femoral Vein, Left **P** Greater Saphenous Vein, Right **Q** Greater Saphenous Vein, Left **R** Lesser Saphenous Vein, Right **S** Lesser Saphenous Vein, Left **T** Foot Vein, Right **V** Foot Vein, Left **Y** Lower Vein	**0** Open **3** Percutaneous **4** Percutaneous Endoscopic	**C** Extraluminal Device **D** Intraluminal Device **Z** No Device	**Z** No Qualifier

Section	0	Medical and Surgical		
Body System	6	Lower Veins		
Operation	W	Revision: Correcting, to the extent possible, a portion of a malfunctioning device or the position of a displaced device		

Body Part (Character 4)	Approach (Character 5)	Device (Character 6)	Qualifier (Character 7)
Y Lower Vein	**0** Open **3** Percutaneous **4** Percutaneous Endoscopic **X** External	**0** Drainage Device **2** Monitoring Device **3** Infusion Device **7** Autologous Tissue Substitute **C** Extraluminal Device **D** Intraluminal Device **J** Synthetic Substitute **K** Nonautologous Tissue Substitute	**Z** No Qualifier

Section	0	Medical and Surgical			
Body System	7	Lymphatic and Hemic Systems			
Operation	2	Change: Taking out or off a device from a body part and putting back an identical or similar device in or on the same body part without cutting or puncturing the skin or a mucous membrane			

Body Part (Character 4)	Approach (Character 5)	Device (Character 6)	Qualifier (Character 7)
K Thoracic Duct	X External	0 Drainage Device	Z No Qualifier
L Cisterna Chyli		Y Other Device	
M Thymus			
N Lymphatic			
P Spleen			
T Bone Marrow			

Section	0	Medical and Surgical			
Body System	7	Lymphatic and Hemic Systems			
Operation	5	Destruction: Physical eradication of all or a portion of a body part by the direct use of energy, force, or a destructive agent			

Body Part (Character 4)	Approach (Character 5)	Device (Character 6)	Qualifier (Character 7)
0 Lymphatic, Head	0 Open	Z No Device	Z No Qualifier
1 Lymphatic, Right Neck	3 Percutaneous		
2 Lymphatic, Left Neck	4 Percutaneous Endoscopic		
3 Lymphatic, Right Upper Extremity			
4 Lymphatic, Left Upper Extremity			
5 Lymphatic, Right Axillary			
6 Lymphatic, Left Axillary			
7 Lymphatic, Thorax			
8 Lymphatic, Internal Mammary, Right			
9 Lymphatic, Internal Mammary, Left			
B Lymphatic, Mesenteric			
C Lymphatic, Pelvis			
D Lymphatic, Aortic			
F Lymphatic, Right Lower Extremity			
G Lymphatic, Left Lower Extremity			
H Lymphatic, Right Inguinal			
J Lymphatic, Left Inguinal			
K Thoracic Duct			
L Cisterna Chyli			
M Thymus			
P Spleen			

Section	0	Medical and Surgical		
Body System	7	Lymphatic and Hemic Systems		
Operation	9	Drainage: Taking or letting out fluids and/or gases from a body part		

Body Part (Character 4)	Approach (Character 5)	Device (Character 6)	Qualifier (Character 7)
0 Lymphatic, Head	**0** Open	**0** Drainage Device	**Z** No Qualifier
1 Lymphatic, Right Neck	**3** Percutaneous		
2 Lymphatic, Left Neck	**4** Percutaneous Endoscopic		
3 Lymphatic, Right Upper Extremity			
4 Lymphatic, Left Upper Extremity			
5 Lymphatic, Right Axillary			
6 Lymphatic, Left Axillary			
7 Lymphatic, Thorax			
8 Lymphatic, Internal Mammary, Right			
9 Lymphatic, Internal Mammary, Left			
B Lymphatic, Mesenteric			
C Lymphatic, Pelvis			
D Lymphatic, Aortic			
F Lymphatic, Right Lower Extremity			
G Lymphatic, Left Lower Extremity			
H Lymphatic, Right Inguinal			
J Lymphatic, Left Inguinal			
K Thoracic Duct			
L Cisterna Chyli			
M Thymus			
P Spleen			
T Bone Marrow			

Section	0	Medical and Surgical		
Body System	7	Lymphatic and Hemic Systems		
Operation	9	Drainage: Taking or letting out fluids and/or gases from a body part		

Body Part (Character 4)	Approach (Character 5)	Device (Character 6)	Qualifier (Character 7)
0 Lymphatic, Head	**0** Open	**Z** No Device	**X** Diagnostic
1 Lymphatic, Right Neck	**3** Percutaneous		**Z** No Qualifier
2 Lymphatic, Left Neck	**4** Percutaneous Endoscopic		
3 Lymphatic, Right Upper Extremity			
4 Lymphatic, Left Upper Extremity			
5 Lymphatic, Right Axillary			
6 Lymphatic, Left Axillary			
7 Lymphatic, Thorax			
8 Lymphatic, Internal Mammary, Right			
9 Lymphatic, Internal Mammary, Left			
B Lymphatic, Mesenteric			
C Lymphatic, Pelvis			
D Lymphatic, Aortic			
F Lymphatic, Right Lower Extremity			
G Lymphatic, Left Lower Extremity			
H Lymphatic, Right Inguinal			
J Lymphatic, Left Inguinal			
K Thoracic Duct			
L Cisterna Chyli			
M Thymus			
P Spleen			
T Bone Marrow			

Section	0	Medical and Surgical		
Body System	7	Lymphatic and Hemic Systems		
Operation	B	Excision: Cutting out or off, without replacement, a portion of a body part		
Body Part (Character 4)		**Approach (Character 5)**	**Device (Character 6)**	**Qualifier (Character 7)**
0 Lymphatic, Head		0 Open	Z No Device	X Diagnostic
1 Lymphatic, Right Neck		3 Percutaneous		Z No Qualifier
2 Lymphatic, Left Neck		4 Percutaneous Endoscopic		
3 Lymphatic, Right Upper Extremity				
4 Lymphatic, Left Upper Extremity				
5 Lymphatic, Right Axillary				
6 Lymphatic, Left Axillary				
7 Lymphatic, Thorax				
8 Lymphatic, Internal Mammary, Right				
9 Lymphatic, Internal Mammary, Left				
B Lymphatic, Mesenteric				
C Lymphatic, Pelvis				
D Lymphatic, Aortic				
F Lymphatic, Right Lower Extremity				
G Lymphatic, Left Lower Extremity				
H Lymphatic, Right Inguinal				
J Lymphatic, Left Inguinal				
K Thoracic Duct				
L Cisterna Chyli				
M Thymus				
P Spleen				

Section	0	Medical and Surgical		
Body System	7	Lymphatic and Hemic Systems		
Operation	C	Extirpation: Taking or cutting out solid matter from a body part		
Body Part (Character 4)		**Approach (Character 5)**	**Device (Character 6)**	**Qualifier (Character 7)**
0 Lymphatic, Head		0 Open	Z No Device	Z No Qualifier
1 Lymphatic, Right Neck		3 Percutaneous		
2 Lymphatic, Left Neck		4 Percutaneous Endoscopic		
3 Lymphatic, Right Upper Extremity				
4 Lymphatic, Left Upper Extremity				
5 Lymphatic, Right Axillary				
6 Lymphatic, Left Axillary				
7 Lymphatic, Thorax				
8 Lymphatic, Internal Mammary, Right				
9 Lymphatic, Internal Mammary, Left				
B Lymphatic, Mesenteric				
C Lymphatic, Pelvis				
D Lymphatic, Aortic				
F Lymphatic, Right Lower Extremity				
G Lymphatic, Left Lower Extremity				
H Lymphatic, Right Inguinal				
J Lymphatic, Left Inguinal				
K Thoracic Duct				
L Cisterna Chyli				
M Thymus				
P Spleen				

Section	0	Medical and Surgical		
Body System	7	Lymphatic and Hemic Systems		
Operation	D	Extraction: Pulling or stripping out or off all or a portion of a body part by the use of force		
Body Part (Character 4)		**Approach (Character 5)**	**Device (Character 6)**	**Qualifier (Character 7)**
Q Bone Marrow, Sternum		0 Open	Z No Device	X Diagnostic
R Bone Marrow, Iliac		3 Percutaneous		Z No Qualifier
S Bone Marrow, Vertebral				

Section	0	Medical and Surgical
Body System	5	Upper Veins
Operation	H	Insertion: Putting in a nonbiological appliance that monitors, assists, performs, or prevents a physiological function but does not physically take the place of a body part

Body Part (Character 4)	Approach (Character 5)	Device (Character 6)	Qualifier (Character 7)
0 Azygos Vein 1 Hemiazygos Vein 3 Innominate Vein, Right 4 Innominate Vein, Left 5 Subclavian Vein, Right 6 Subclavian Vein, Left 7 Axillary Vein, Right 8 Axillary Vein, Left 9 Brachial Vein, Right A Brachial Vein, Left B Basilic Vein, Right C Basilic Vein, Left D Cephalic Vein, Right F Cephalic Vein, Left G Hand Vein, Right H Hand Vein, Left L Intracranial Vein M Internal Jugular Vein, Right N Internal Jugular Vein, Left P External Jugular Vein, Right Q External Jugular Vein, Left R Vertebral Vein, Right S Vertebral Vein, Left T Face Vein, Right V Face Vein, Left	0 Open 3 Percutaneous 4 Percutaneous Endoscopic	3 Infusion Device D Intraluminal Device	Z No Qualifier
Y Upper Vein	0 Open 3 Percutaneous 4 Percutaneous Endoscopic	2 Monitoring Device 3 Infusion Device D Intraluminal Device	Z No Qualifier

Section	0	Medical and Surgical
Body System	5	Upper Veins
Operation	J	Inspection: Visually and/or manually exploring a body part

Body Part (Character 4)	Approach (Character 5)	Device (Character 6)	Qualifier (Character 7)
Y Upper Vein	0 Open 3 Percutaneous 4 Percutaneous Endoscopic X External	Z No Device	Z No Qualifier

Section	0	Medical and Surgical			
Body System	7	Lymphatic and Hemic Systems			
Operation	H	Insertion: Putting in a nonbiological appliance that monitors, assists, performs, or prevents a physiological function but does not physically take the place of a body part			

Body Part (Character 4)	Approach (Character 5)	Device (Character 6)	Qualifier (Character 7)
K Thoracic Duct L Cisterna Chyli M Thymus N Lymphatic P Spleen	0 Open 3 Percutaneous 4 Percutaneous Endoscopic	3 Infusion Device	Z No Qualifier

Section	0	Medical and Surgical			
Body System	7	Lymphatic and Hemic Systems			
Operation	J	Inspection: Visually and/or manually exploring a body part			

Body Part (Character 4)	Approach (Character 5)	Device (Character 6)	Qualifier (Character 7)
K Thoracic Duct L Cisterna Chyli M Thymus T Bone Marrow	0 Open 3 Percutaneous 4 Percutaneous Endoscopic	Z No Device	Z No Qualifier
N Lymphatic P Spleen	0 Open 3 Percutaneous 4 Percutaneous Endoscopic X External	Z No Device	Z No Qualifier

Section	0	Medical and Surgical			
Body System	7	Lymphatic and Hemic Systems			
Operation	L	Occlusion: Completely closing an orifice or the lumen of a tubular body part			

Body Part (Character 4)	Approach (Character 5)	Device (Character 6)	Qualifier (Character 7)
0 Lymphatic, Head 1 Lymphatic, Right Neck 2 Lymphatic, Left Neck 3 Lymphatic, Right Upper Extremity 4 Lymphatic, Left Upper Extremity 5 Lymphatic, Right Axillary 6 Lymphatic, Left Axillary 7 Lymphatic, Thorax 8 Lymphatic, Internal Mammary, Right 9 Lymphatic, Internal Mammary, Left B Lymphatic, Mesenteric C Lymphatic, Pelvis D Lymphatic, Aortic F Lymphatic, Right Lower Extremity G Lymphatic, Left Lower Extremity H Lymphatic, Right Inguinal J Lymphatic, Left Inguinal K Thoracic Duct L Cisterna Chyli	0 Open 3 Percutaneous 4 Percutaneous Endoscopic	C Extraluminal Device D Intraluminal Device Z No Device	Z No Qualifier

Section	0	Medical and Surgical
Body System	7	Lymphatic and Hemic Systems
Operation	N	Release: Freeing a body part from an abnormal physical constraint by cutting or by the use of force

Body Part (Character 4)	Approach (Character 5)	Device (Character 6)	Qualifier (Character 7)
0 Lymphatic, Head 1 Lymphatic, Right Neck 2 Lymphatic, Left Neck 3 Lymphatic, Right Upper Extremity 4 Lymphatic, Left Upper Extremity 5 Lymphatic, Right Axillary 6 Lymphatic, Left Axillary 7 Lymphatic, Thorax 8 Lymphatic, Internal Mammary, Right 9 Lymphatic, Internal Mammary, Left B Lymphatic, Mesenteric C Lymphatic, Pelvis D Lymphatic, Aortic F Lymphatic, Right Lower Extremity G Lymphatic, Left Lower Extremity H Lymphatic, Right Inguinal J Lymphatic, Left Inguinal K Thoracic Duct L Cisterna Chyli M Thymus P Spleen	0 Open 3 Percutaneous 4 Percutaneous Endoscopic	Z No Device	Z No Qualifier

Section	0	Medical and Surgical
Body System	7	Lymphatic and Hemic Systems
Operation	P	Removal: Taking out or off a device from a body part

Body Part (Character 4)	Approach (Character 5)	Device (Character 6)	Qualifier (Character 7)
K Thoracic Duct L Cisterna Chyli N Lymphatic	0 Open 3 Percutaneous 4 Percutaneous Endoscopic	0 Drainage Device 3 Infusion Device 7 Autologous Tissue Substitute C Extraluminal Device D Intraluminal Device J Synthetic Substitute K Nonautologous Tissue Substitute	Z No Qualifier
K Thoracic Duct L Cisterna Chyli N Lymphatic	X External	0 Drainage Device 3 Infusion Device D Intraluminal Device	Z No Qualifier
M Thymus P Spleen	0 Open 3 Percutaneous 4 Percutaneous Endoscopic X External	0 Drainage Device 3 Infusion Device	Z No Qualifier
T Bone Marrow	0 Open 3 Percutaneous 4 Percutaneous Endoscopic X External	0 Drainage Device	Z No Qualifier

Section	0	Medical and Surgical		
Body System	7	Lymphatic and Hemic Systems		
Operation	Q	Repair: Restoring, to the extent possible, a body part to its normal anatomic structure and function		

Body Part (Character 4)	Approach (Character 5)	Device (Character 6)	Qualifier (Character 7)
0 Lymphatic, Head 1 Lymphatic, Right Neck 2 Lymphatic, Left Neck 3 Lymphatic, Right Upper Extremity 4 Lymphatic, Left Upper Extremity 5 Lymphatic, Right Axillary 6 Lymphatic, Left Axillary 7 Lymphatic, Thorax 8 Lymphatic, Internal Mammary, Right 9 Lymphatic, Internal Mammary, Left B Lymphatic, Mesenteric C Lymphatic, Pelvis D Lymphatic, Aortic F Lymphatic, Right Lower Extremity G Lymphatic, Left Lower Extremity H Lymphatic, Right Inguinal J Lymphatic, Left Inguinal K Thoracic Duct L Cisterna Chyli M Thymus P Spleen	0 Open 3 Percutaneous 4 Percutaneous Endoscopic	Z No Device	Z No Qualifier

Section	0	Medical and Surgical		
Body System	7	Lymphatic and Hemic Systems		
Operation	S	Reposition: Moving to its normal location, or other suitable location, all or a portion of a body part		

Body Part (Character 4)	Approach (Character 5)	Device (Character 6)	Qualifier (Character 7)
M Thymus P Spleen	0 Open	Z No Device	Z No Qualifier

Section	0	Medical and Surgical		
Body System	7	Lymphatic and Hemic Systems		
Operation	T	Resection: Cutting out or off, without replacement, all of a body part		

Body Part (Character 4)	Approach (Character 5)	Device (Character 6)	Qualifier (Character 7)
0 Lymphatic, Head 1 Lymphatic, Right Neck 2 Lymphatic, Left Neck 3 Lymphatic, Right Upper Extremity 4 Lymphatic, Left Upper Extremity 5 Lymphatic, Right Axillary 6 Lymphatic, Left Axillary 7 Lymphatic, Thorax 8 Lymphatic, Internal Mammary, Right 9 Lymphatic, Internal Mammary, Left B Lymphatic, Mesenteric C Lymphatic, Pelvis D Lymphatic, Aortic F Lymphatic, Right Lower Extremity G Lymphatic, Left Lower Extremity H Lymphatic, Right Inguinal J Lymphatic, Left Inguinal K Thoracic Duct L Cisterna Chyli M Thymus P Spleen	0 Open 4 Percutaneous Endoscopic	Z No Device	Z No Qualifier

Section	0	Medical and Surgical		
Body System	7	Lymphatic and Hemic Systems		
Operation	U	Supplement: Putting in or on biological or synthetic material that physically reinforces and/or augments the function of a portion of a body part		

Body Part (Character 4)	Approach (Character 5)	Device (Character 6)	Qualifier (Character 7)
0 Lymphatic, Head 1 Lymphatic, Right Neck 2 Lymphatic, Left Neck 3 Lymphatic, Right Upper Extremity 4 Lymphatic, Left Upper Extremity 5 Lymphatic, Right Axillary 6 Lymphatic, Left Axillary 7 Lymphatic, Thorax 8 Lymphatic, Internal Mammary, Right 9 Lymphatic, Internal Mammary, Left B Lymphatic, Mesenteric C Lymphatic, Pelvis D Lymphatic, Aortic F Lymphatic, Right Lower Extremity G Lymphatic, Left Lower Extremity H Lymphatic, Right Inguinal J Lymphatic, Left Inguinal K Thoracic Duct L Cisterna Chyli	0 Open 4 Percutaneous Endoscopic	7 Autologous Tissue Substitute J Synthetic Substitute K Nonautologous Tissue Substitute	

Section	0	Medical and Surgical		
Body System	7	Lymphatic and Hemic Systems		
Operation	V	Restriction: Partially closing an orifice or the lumen of a tubular body part		

Body Part (Character 4)	Approach (Character 5)	Device (Character 6)	Qualifier (Character 7)
0 Lymphatic, Head 1 Lymphatic, Right Neck 2 Lymphatic, Left Neck 3 Lymphatic, Right Upper Extremity 4 Lymphatic, Left Upper Extremity 5 Lymphatic, Right Axillary 6 Lymphatic, Left Axillary 7 Lymphatic, Thorax 8 Lymphatic, Internal Mammary, Right 9 Lymphatic, Internal Mammary, Left B Lymphatic, Mesenteric C Lymphatic, Pelvis D Lymphatic, Aortic F Lymphatic, Right Lower Extremity G Lymphatic, Left Lower Extremity H Lymphatic, Right Inguinal J Lymphatic, Left Inguinal K Thoracic Duct L Cisterna Chyli	0 Open 3 Percutaneous 4 Percutaneous Endoscopic	C Extraluminal Device D Intraluminal Device Z No Device	Z No Qualifier

Section	0	Medical and Surgical		
Body System	7	Lymphatic and Hemic Systems		
Operation	W	Revision: Correcting, to the extent possible, a portion of a malfunctioning device or the position of a displaced device		

Body Part (Character 4)	Approach (Character 5)	Device (Character 6)	Qualifier (Character 7)
K Thoracic Duct **L** Cisterna Chyli **N** Lymphatic	**0** Open **3** Percutaneous **4** Percutaneous Endoscopic **X** External	**0** Drainage Device **3** Infusion Device **7** Autologous Tissue Substitute **C** Extraluminal Device **D** Intraluminal Device **J** Synthetic Substitute **K** Nonautologous Tissue Substitute	**Z** No Qualifier
M Thymus **P** Spleen	**0** Open **3** Percutaneous **4** Percutaneous Endoscopic **X** External	**0** Drainage Device **3** Infusion Device	**Z** No Qualifier
T Bone Marrow	**0** Open **3** Percutaneous **4** Percutaneous Endoscopic **X** External	**0** Drainage Device	**Z** No Qualifier

Section	0	Medical and Surgical		
Body System	7	Lymphatic and Hemic Systems		
Operation	Y	Transplantation: Putting in or on all or a portion of a living body part taken from another individual or animal to physically take the place and/or function of all or a portion of a similar body part		

Body Part (Character 4)	Approach (Character 5)	Device (Character 6)	Qualifier (Character 7)
M Thymus **P** Spleen	**0** Open	**Z** No Device	**0** Allogeneic **1** Syngeneic **2** Zooplastic

Section	0	Medical and Surgical		
Body System	8	Eye		
Operation	0	Alteration: Modifying the anatomic structure of a body part without affecting the function of the body part		
Body Part (Character 4)		**Approach (Character 5)**	**Device (Character 6)**	**Qualifier (Character 7)**
N Upper Eyelid, Right P Upper Eyelid, Left Q Lower Eyelid, Right R Lower Eyelid, Left		0 Open 3 Percutaneous X External	7 Autologous Tissue Substitute J Synthetic Substitute K Nonautologous Tissue Substitute Z No Device	Z No Qualifier

Section	0	Medical and Surgical		
Body System	8	Eye		
Operation	1	Bypass: Altering the route of passage of the contents of a tubular body part		
Body Part (Character 4)		**Approach (Character 5)**	**Device (Character 6)**	**Qualifier (Character 7)**
2 Anterior Chamber, Right 3 Anterior Chamber, Left		3 Percutaneous	J Synthetic Substitute K Nonautologous Tissue Substitute Z No Device	4 Sclera
X Lacrimal Duct, Right Y Lacrimal Duct, Left		0 Open 3 Percutaneous	J Synthetic Substitute K Nonautologous Tissue Substitute Z No Device	3 Nasal Cavity

Section	0	Medical and Surgical		
Body System	8	Eye		
Operation	2	Change: Taking out or off a device from a body part and putting back an identical or similar device in or on the same body part without cutting or puncturing the skin or a mucous membrane		
Body Part (Character 4)		**Approach (Character 5)**	**Device (Character 6)**	**Qualifier (Character 7)**
0 Eye, Right 1 Eye, Left		X External	0 Drainage Device Y Other Device	Z No Qualifier

Section	0	Medical and Surgical		
Body System	8	Eye		
Operation	5	Destruction: Physical eradication of all or a portion of a body part by the direct use of energy, force, or a destructive agent		
Body Part (Character 4)		**Approach (Character 5)**	**Device (Character 6)**	**Qualifier (Character 7)**
0 Eye, Right 1 Eye, Left 6 Sclera, Right 7 Sclera, Left 8 Cornea, Right 9 Cornea, Left S Conjunctiva, Right T Conjunctiva, Left		X External	Z No Device	Z No Qualifier
2 Anterior Chamber, Right 3 Anterior Chamber, Left 4 Vitreous, Right 5 Vitreous, Left C Iris, Right D Iris, Left E Retina, Right F Retina, Left G Retinal Vessel, Right H Retinal Vessel, Left J Lens, Right K Lens, Left		3 Percutaneous	Z No Device	Z No Qualifier
A Choroid, Right B Choroid, Left L Extraocular Muscle, Right M Extraocular Muscle, Left V Lacrimal Gland, Right W Lacrimal Gland, Left		0 Open 3 Percutaneous	Z No Device	Z No Qualifier
N Upper Eyelid, Right P Upper Eyelid, Left Q Lower Eyelid, Right R Lower Eyelid, Left		0 Open 3 Percutaneous X External	Z No Device	Z No Qualifier
X Lacrimal Duct, Right Y Lacrimal Duct, Left		0 Open 3 Percutaneous 7 Via Natural or Artificial Opening 8 Via Natural or Artificial Opening Endoscopic	Z No Device	Z No Qualifier

Section	0	Medical and Surgical		
Body System	8	Eye		
Operation	7	Dilation: Expanding an orifice or the lumen of a tubular body part		
Body Part (Character 4)		**Approach (Character 5)**	**Device (Character 6)**	**Qualifier (Character 7)**
X Lacrimal Duct, Right **Y** Lacrimal Duct, Left		**0** Open **3** Percutaneous **7** Via Natural or Artificial Opening **8** Via Natural or Artificial Opening Endoscopic	**D** Intraluminal Device **Z** No **Device** **Character 6**	**Z** No Qualifier

Section	0	Medical and Surgical		
Body System	8	Eye		
Operation	9	Drainage: Taking or letting out fluids and/or gases from a body part		
Body Part (Character 4)		**Approach (Character 5)**	**Device (Character 6)**	**Qualifier (Character 7)**
0 Eye, Right **1** Eye, Left **6** Sclera, Right **7** Sclera, Left **8** Cornea, Right **9** Cornea, Left **S** Conjunctiva, Right **T** Conjunctiva, Left		**X** External	**0** Drainage Device	**Z** No Qualifier
0 Eye, Right **1** Eye, Left **6** Sclera, Right **7** Sclera, Left **8** Cornea, Right **9** Cornea, Left **S** Conjunctiva, Right **T** Conjunctiva, Left		**X** External	**Z** No Device	**X** Diagnostic **Z** No Qualifier
2 Anterior Chamber, Right **3** Anterior Chamber, Left **4** Vitreous, Right **5** Vitreous, Left **C** Iris, Right **D** Iris, Left **E** Retina, Right **F** Retina, Left **G** Retinal Vessel, Right **H** Retinal Vessel, Left **J** Lens, Right **K** Lens, Left		**3** Percutaneous	**0** Drainage Device	**Z** No Qualifier

Section	0	Medical and Surgical		
Body System	8	Eye		
Operation	9	Drainage: Taking or letting out fluids and/or gases from a body part		

Body Part (Character 4)	Approach (Character 5)	Device (Character 6)	Qualifier (Character 7)
2 Anterior Chamber, Right **3** Anterior Chamber, Left **4** Vitreous, Right **5** Vitreous, Left **C** Iris, Right **D** Iris, Left **E** Retina, Right **F** Retina, Left **G** Retinal Vessel, Right **H** Retinal Vessel, Left **J** Lens, Right **K** Lens, Left	**3** Percutaneous	**Z** No Device	**X** Diagnostic **Z** No Qualifier
A Choroid, Right **B** Choroid, Left **L** Extraocular Muscle, Right **M** Extraocular Muscle, Left **V** Lacrimal Gland, Right **W** Lacrimal Gland, Left	**0** Open **3** Percutaneous	**0** Drainage Device	**Z** No Qualifier
A Choroid, Right **B** Choroid, Left **L** Extraocular Muscle, Right **M** Extraocular Muscle, Left **V** Lacrimal Gland, Right **W** Lacrimal Gland, Left	**0** Open **3** Percutaneous	**Z** No Device	**X** Diagnostic **Z** No Qualifier
N Upper Eyelid, Right **P** Upper Eyelid, Left **Q** Lower Eyelid, Right **R** Lower Eyelid, Left	**0** Open **3** Percutaneous **X** External	**0** Drainage Device	**Z** No Qualifier
N Upper Eyelid, Right **P** Upper Eyelid, Left **Q** Lower Eyelid, Right **R** Lower Eyelid, Left	**0** Open **3** Percutaneous **X** External	**Z** No Device	**X** Diagnostic **Z** No Qualifier
X Lacrimal Duct, Right **Y** Lacrimal Duct, Left	**0** Open **3** Percutaneous **7** Via Natural or Artificial Opening **8** Via Natural or Artificial Opening Endoscopic	**0** Drainage Device	**Z** No Qualifier

Section	0	Medical and Surgical		
Body System	8	Eye		
Operation	9	Drainage: Taking or letting out fluids and/or gases from a body part		

Body Part (Character 4)	Approach (Character 5)	Device (Character 6)	Qualifier (Character 7)
X Lacrimal Duct, Right **Y** Lacrimal Duct, Left	**0** Open **3** Percutaneous **7** Via Natural or Artificial Opening **8** Via Natural or Artificial Opening Endoscopic	**Z** No Device	**X** Diagnostic **Z** No Qualifier

Section	0	Medical and Surgical			
Body System	8	Eye			
Operation	B	Excision: Cutting out or off, without replacement, a portion of a body part			

Body Part (Character 4)	Approach (Character 5)	Device (Character 6)	Qualifier (Character 7)
0 Eye, Right **1** Eye, Left **N** Upper Eyelid, Right **P** Upper Eyelid, Left **Q** Lower Eyelid, Right **R** Lower Eyelid, Left	**0** Open **3** Percutaneous **X** External	**Z** No Device	**X** Diagnostic **Z** No Qualifier
4 Vitreous, Right **5** Vitreous, Left **C** Iris, Right **D** Iris, Left **E** Retina, Right **F** Retina, Left **J** Lens, Right **K** Lens, Left	**3** Percutaneous	**Z** No Device	**X** Diagnostic **Z** No Qualifier
6 Sclera, Right **7** Sclera, Left **8** Cornea, Right **9** Cornea, Left **S** Conjunctiva, Right **T** Conjunctiva, Left	**X** External	**Z** No Device	**X** Diagnostic **Z** No Qualifier
A Choroid, Right **B** Choroid, Left **L** Extraocular Muscle, Right **M** Extraocular Muscle, Left **V** Lacrimal Gland, Right **W** Lacrimal Gland, Left	**0** Open **3** Percutaneous	**Z** No Device	**X** Diagnostic **Z** No Qualifier
X Lacrimal Duct, Right **Y** Lacrimal Duct, Left	**0** Open **3** Percutaneous **7** Via Natural or Artificial Opening **8** Via Natural or Artificial Opening Endoscopic	**Z** No Device	**X** Diagnostic **Z** No Qualifier

Section	0	Medical and Surgical			
Body System	8	Eye			
Operation	C	Extirpation: Taking or cutting out solid matter from a body part			

Body Part (Character 4)	Approach (Character 5)	Device (Character 6)	Qualifier (Character 7)
0 Eye, Right 1 Eye, Left 6 Sclera, Right 7 Sclera, Left 8 Cornea, Right 9 Cornea, Left S Conjunctiva, Right T Conjunctiva, Left	X External	Z No Device	Z No Qualifier
2 Anterior Chamber, Right 3 Anterior Chamber, Left 4 Vitreous, Right 5 Vitreous, Left C Iris, Right D Iris, Left E Retina, Right F Retina, Left G Retinal Vessel, Right H Retinal Vessel, Left J Lens, Right K Lens, Left	3 Percutaneous X External	Z No Device	Z No Qualifier
A Choroid, Right B Choroid, Left L Extraocular Muscle, Right M Extraocular Muscle, Left N Upper Eyelid, Right P Upper Eyelid, Left Q Lower Eyelid, Right R Lower Eyelid, Left V Lacrimal Gland, Right W Lacrimal Gland, Left	0 Open 3 Percutaneous X External	Z No Device	Z No Qualifier
X Lacrimal Duct, Right Y Lacrimal Duct, Left	0 Open 3 Percutaneous 7 Via Natural or Artificial Opening 8 Via Natural or Artificial Opening Endoscopic	Z No Device	Z No Qualifier

Section	0	Medical and Surgical			
Body System	8	Eye			
Operation	D	Extraction: Pulling or stripping out or off all or a portion of a body part by the use of force			

Body Part (Character 4)	Approach (Character 5)	Device (Character 6)	Qualifier (Character 7)
8 Cornea, Right 9 Cornea, Left	X External	Z No Device	X Diagnostic Z No Qualifier
J Lens, Right K Lens, Left	3 Percutaneous	Z No Device	Z No Qualifier

Section	0	Medical and Surgical			
Body System	8	Eye			
Operation	F	Fragmentation: Breaking solid matter in a body part into pieces			

Body Part (Character 4)	Approach (Character 5)	Device (Character 6)	Qualifier (Character 7)
4 Vitreous, Right 5 Vitreous, Left	3 Percutaneous X External	Z No Device	Z No Qualifier

Section	0	Medical and Surgical			
Body System	8	Eye			
Operation	H	Insertion: Putting in a nonbiological appliance that monitors, assists, performs, or prevents a physiological function but does not physically take the place of a body part			

Body Part (Character 4)	Approach (Character 5)	Device (Character 6)	Qualifier (Character 7)
0 Eye, Right 1 Eye, Left	0 Open	3 Epiretinal Visual Prosthesis	Z No Qualifier
0 Eye, Right 1 Eye, Left	3 Percutaneous X External	1 Radioactive Element 3 Infusion Device	Z No Qualifier

Section	0	Medical and Surgical		
Body System	8	Eye		
Operation	J	Inspection: Visually and/or manually exploring a body part		
Body Part (Character 4)		**Approach (Character 5)**	**Device (Character 6)**	**Qualifier (Character 7)**
0 Eye, Right **1** Eye, Left **J** Lens, Right **K** Lens, Left		**X** External	**Z** No Device	**Z** No Qualifier
L Extraocular Muscle, Right **M** Extraocular Muscle, Left		**0** Open **X** External	**Z** No Device	**Z** No Qualifier

Section	0	Medical and Surgical		
Body System	8	Eye		
Operation	L	Occlusion: Completely closing an orifice or the lumen of a tubular body part		
Body Part (Character 4)		**Approach (Character 5)**	**Device (Character 6)**	**Qualifier (Character 7)**
X Lacrimal Duct, Right **Y** Lacrimal Duct, Left		**0** Open **3** Percutaneous	**C** Extraluminal Device **D** Intraluminal Device **Z** No Device	**Z** No Qualifier
X Lacrimal Duct, Right **Y** Lacrimal Duct, Left		**7** Via Natural or Artificial Opening **8** Via Natural or Artificial Opening Endoscopic	**D** Intraluminal Device **Z** No Device	**Z** No Qualifier

Section	0	Medical and Surgical		
Body System	8	Eye		
Operation	M	Reattachment Putting back in or on all or a portion of a separated body part to its normal location or other suitable location		
Body Part (Character 4)		**Approach (Character 5)**	**Device (Character 6)**	**Qualifier (Character 7)**
N Upper Eyelid, Right **P** Upper Eyelid, Left **Q** Lower Eyelid, Right **R** Lower Eyelid, Left		**X** External	**Z** No Device	**Z** No Qualifier

Section	0	Medical and Surgical		
Body System	8	Eye		
Operation	N	Release: Freeing a body part from an abnormal physical constraint by cutting or by the use of force		
Body Part (Character 4)		**Approach (Character 5)**	**Device (Character 6)**	**Qualifier (Character 7)**
0 Eye, Right **1** Eye, Left **6** Sclera, Right **7** Sclera, Left **8** Cornea, Right **9** Cornea, Left **S** Conjunctiva, Right **T** Conjunctiva, Left		**X** External	**Z** No Device	**Z** No Qualifier
2 Anterior Chamber, Right **3** Anterior Chamber, Left **4** Vitreous, Right **5** Vitreous, Left **C** Iris, Right **D** Iris, Left **E** Retina, Right **F** Retina, Left **G** Retinal Vessel, Right **H** Retinal Vessel, Left **J** Lens, Right **K** Lens, Left		**3** Percutaneous	**Z** No Device	**Z** No Qualifier
A Choroid, Right **B** Choroid, Left **L** Extraocular Muscle, Right **M** Extraocular Muscle, Left **V** Lacrimal Gland, Right **W** Lacrimal Gland, Left		**0** Open **3** Percutaneous	**Z** No Device	**Z** No Qualifier
N Upper Eyelid, Right **P** Upper Eyelid, Left **Q** Lower Eyelid, Right **R** Lower Eyelid, Left		**0** Open **3** Percutaneous **X** External	**Z** No Device	**Z** No Qualifier
X Lacrimal Duct, Right **Y** Lacrimal Duct, Left		**0** Open **3** Percutaneous **7** Via Natural or Artificial Opening **8** Via Natural or Artificial Opening Endoscopic	**Z** No Device	**Z** No Qualifier

Section	0	Medical and Surgical			
Body System	8	Eye			
Operation	P	Removal: Taking out or off a device from a body part			

Body Part (Character 4)	Approach (Character 5)	Device (Character 6)	Qualifier (Character 7)
0 Eye, Right **1** Eye, Left	**0** Open **3** Percutaneous **7** Via Natural or Artificial Opening **8** Via Natural or Artificial Opening Endoscopic **X** External	**0** Drainage Device **1** Radioactive Element **3** Infusion Device **7** Autologous Tissue Substitute **C** Extraluminal Device **D** Intraluminal Device **J** Synthetic Substitute **K** Nonautologous Tissue Substitute	**Z** No Qualifier
J Lens, Right **K** Lens, Left	**3** Percutaneous	**J** Synthetic Substitute	**Z** No Qualifier
L Extraocular Muscle, Right **M** Extraocular Muscle, Left	**0** Open **3** Percutaneous	**0** Drainage Device **7** Autologous Tissue Substitute **J** Synthetic Substitute **K** Nonautologous Tissue Substitute	**Z** No Qualifier

Section	0	Medical and Surgical			
Body System	8	Eye			
Operation	Q	Repair: Restoring, to the extent possible, a body part to its normal anatomic structure and function			

Body Part (Character 4)	Approach (Character 5)	Device (Character 6)	Qualifier (Character 7)
0 Eye, Right **1** Eye, Left **6** Sclera, Right **7** Sclera, Left **8** Cornea, Right **9** Cornea, Left **S** Conjunctiva, Right **T** Conjunctiva, Left	**X** External	**Z** No Device	**Z** No Qualifier
2 Anterior Chamber, Right **3** Anterior Chamber, Left **4** Vitreous, Right **5** Vitreous, Left **C** Iris, Right **D** Iris, Left **E** Retina, Right **F** Retina, Left **G** Retinal Vessel, Right **H** Retinal Vessel, Left **J** Lens, Right **K** Lens, Left	**3** Percutaneous	**Z** No Device	**Z** No Qualifier
A Choroid, Right **B** Choroid, Left **L** Extraocular Muscle, Right **M** Extraocular Muscle, Left **V** Lacrimal Gland, Right **W** Lacrimal Gland, Left	**0** Open **3** Percutaneous	**Z** No Device	**Z** No Qualifier
N Upper Eyelid, Right **P** Upper Eyelid, Left **Q** Lower Eyelid, Right **R** Lower Eyelid, Left	**0** Open **3** Percutaneous **X** External	**Z** No Device	**Z** No Qualifier
X Lacrimal Duct, Right **Y** Lacrimal Duct, Left	**0** Open **3** Percutaneous **7** Via Natural or Artificial Opening **8** Via Natural or Artificial Opening Endoscopic	**Z** No Device	**Z** No Qualifier

Section	0	Medical and Surgical		
Body System	8	Eye		
Operation	R	Replacement: Putting in or on biological or synthetic material that physically takes the place and/or function of all or a portion of a body part		

Body Part (Character 4)	Approach (Character 5)	Device (Character 6)	Qualifier (Character 7)
0 Eye, Right **1** Eye, Left **A** Choroid, Right **B** Choroid, Left	**0** Open **3** Percutaneous	**7** Autologous Tissue Substitute **J** Synthetic Substitute **K** Nonautologous Tissue Substitute	**Z** No Qualifier
4 Vitreous, Right **5** Vitreous, Left **C** Iris, Right **D** Iris, Left **G** Retinal Vessel, Right **H** Retinal Vessel, Left	**3** Percutaneous	**7** Autologous Tissue Substitute **J** Synthetic Substitute **K** Nonautologous Tissue Substitute	**Z** No Qualifier
6 Sclera, Right **7** Sclera, Left **S** Conjunctiva, Right **T** Conjunctiva, Left	**X** External	**7** Autologous Tissue Substitute **J** Synthetic Substitute **K** Nonautologous Tissue Substitute	**Z** No Qualifier
8 Cornea, Right **9** Cornea, Left	**3** Percutaneous **X** External	**7** Autologous Tissue Substitute **J** Synthetic Substitute **K** Nonautologous Tissue Substitute	**Z** No Qualifier
J Lens, Right **K** Lens, Left	**3** Percutaneous	**0** Synthetic Substitute, Intraocular Telescope **7** Autologous Tissue Substitute **J** Synthetic Substitute **K** Nonautologous Tissue Substitute	**Z** No Qualifier
N Upper Eyelid, Right **P** Upper Eyelid, Left **Q** Lower Eyelid, Right **R** Lower Eyelid, Left	**0** Open **3** Percutaneous **X** External	**7** Autologous Tissue Substitute **J** Synthetic Substitute **K** Nonautologous Tissue Substitute	**Z** No Qualifier
X Lacrimal Duct, Right **Y** Lacrimal Duct, Left	**0** Open **3** Percutaneous **7** Via Natural or Artificial Opening **8** Via Natural or Artificial Opening Endoscopic	**7** Autologous Tissue Substitute **J** Synthetic Substitute **K** Nonautologous Tissue Substitute	**Z** No Qualifier

Section	0	Medical and Surgical		
Body System	8	Eye		
Operation	S	Reposition: Moving to its normal location, or other suitable location, all or a portion of a body part		

Body Part (Character 4)	Approach (Character 5)	Device (Character 6)	Qualifier (Character 7)
C Iris, Right **D** Iris, Left **G** Retinal Vessel, Right **H** Retinal Vessel, Left **J** Lens, Right **K** Lens, Left	**3** Percutaneous	**Z** No Device	**Z** No Qualifier
L Extraocular Muscle, Right **M** Extraocular Muscle, Left **V** Lacrimal Gland, Right **W** Lacrimal Gland, Left	**0** Open **3** Percutaneous	**Z** No Device	**Z** No Qualifier
N Upper Eyelid, Right **P** Upper Eyelid, Left **Q** Lower Eyelid, Right **R** Lower Eyelid, Left	**0** Open **3** Percutaneous **X** External	**Z** No Device	**Z** No Qualifier
X Lacrimal Duct, Right **Y** Lacrimal Duct, Left	**0** Open **3** Percutaneous **7** Via Natural or Artificial Opening **8** Via Natural or Artificial Opening Endoscopic	**Z** No Device	**Z** No Qualifier

Section	0	Medical and Surgical		
Body System	8	Eye		
Operation	T	Resection: Cutting out or off, without replacement, all of a body part		
Body Part (Character 4)		**Approach (Character 5)**	**Device (Character 6)**	**Qualifier (Character 7)**
0 Eye, Right 1 Eye, Left 8 Cornea, Right 9 Cornea, Left		X External	Z No Device	Z No Qualifier
4 Vitreous, Right 5 Vitreous, Left C Iris, Right D Iris, Left J Lens, Right K Lens, Left		3 Percutaneous	Z No Device	Z No Qualifier
L Extraocular Muscle, Right M Extraocular Muscle, Left V Lacrimal Gland, Right W Lacrimal Gland, Left		0 Open 3 Percutaneous	Z No Device	Z No Qualifier
N Upper Eyelid, Right P Upper Eyelid, Left Q Lower Eyelid, Right R Lower Eyelid, Left		0 Open X External	Z No Device	Z No Qualifier
X Lacrimal Duct, Right Y Lacrimal Duct, Left		0 Open 3 Percutaneous 7 Via Natural or Artificial Opening 8 Via Natural or Artificial Opening Endoscopic	Z No Device	Z No Qualifier

Section	0	Medical and Surgical		
Body System	8	Eye		
Operation	U	Supplement: Putting in or on biological or synthetic material that physically reinforces and/or augments the function of a portion of a body part		
Body Part (Character 4)		**Approach (Character 5)**	**Device (Character 6)**	**Qualifier (Character 7)**
0 Eye, Right 1 Eye, Left C Iris, Right D Iris, Left E Retina, Right F Retina, Left G Retinal Vessel, Right H Retinal Vessel, Left L Extraocular Muscle, Right M Extraocular Muscle, Left		0 Open 3 Percutaneous	7 Autologous Tissue Substitute J Synthetic Substitute K Nonautologous Tissue Substitute	Z No Qualifier
8 Cornea, Right 9 Cornea, Left N Upper Eyelid, Right P Upper Eyelid, Left Q Lower Eyelid, Right R Lower Eyelid, Left		0 Open 3 Percutaneous X External	7 Autologous Tissue Substitute J Synthetic Substitute K Nonautologous Tissue Substitute	Z No Qualifier
X Lacrimal Duct, Right Y Lacrimal Duct, Left		0 Open 3 Percutaneous 7 Via Natural or Artificial Opening 8 Via Natural or Artificial Opening Endoscopic	7 Autologous Tissue Substitute J Synthetic Substitute K Nonautologous Tissue Substitute	Z No Qualifier

Section	0	Medical and Surgical		
Body System	8	Eye		
Operation	V	Restriction: Partially closing an orifice or the lumen of a tubular body part		
Body Part (Character 4)		**Approach (Character 5)**	**Device (Character 6)**	**Qualifier (Character 7)**
X Lacrimal Duct, Right Y Lacrimal Duct, Left		0 Open 3 Percutaneous	C Extraluminal Device D Intraluminal Device Z No Device	Z No Qualifier
X Lacrimal Duct, Right Y Lacrimal Duct, Left		7 Via Natural or Artificial Opening 8 Via Natural or Artificial Opening Endoscopic	D Intraluminal Device Z No Device	Z No Qualifier

Section	0	Medical and Surgical		
Body System	8	Eye		
Operation	W	Revision: Correcting, to the extent possible, a portion of a malfunctioning device or the position of a displaced device		
Body Part (Character 4)	Approach (Character 5)		Device (Character 6)	Qualifier (Character 7)
0 Eye, Right 1 Eye, Left	0 Open 3 Percutaneous 7 Via Natural or Artificial Opening 8 Via Natural or Artificial Opening Endoscopic X External		0 Drainage Device 3 Infusion Device 7 Autologous Tissue Substitute C Extraluminal Device D Intraluminal Device J Synthetic Substitute K Nonautologous Tissue Substitute	Z No Qualifier
J Lens, Right K Lens, Left	3 Percutaneous X External		J Synthetic Substitute	Z No Qualifier
L Extraocular Muscle, Right M Extraocular Muscle, Left	0 Open 3 Percutaneous		0 Drainage Device 7 Autologous Tissue Substitute J Synthetic Substitute K Nonautologous Tissue Substitute	Z No Qualifier

Section	0	Medical and Surgical		
Body System	8	Eye		
Operation	X	Transfer: Moving, without taking out, all or a portion of a body part to another location to take over the function of all or a portion of a body part		
Body Part (Character 4)	Approach (Character 5)	Device (Character 6)	Qualifier (Character 7)
L Extraocular Muscle, Right M Extraocular Muscle, Left	0 Open 3 Percutaneous	Z No Device	Z No Qualifier

Section	0	Medical and Surgical
Body System	9	Ear, Nose, Sinus
Operation	0	Alteration: Modifying the anatomic structure of a body part without affecting the function of the body part

Body Part (Character 4)	Approach (Character 5)	Device (Character 6)	Qualifier (Character 7)
0 External Ear, Right **1** External Ear, Left **2** External Ear, Bilateral **K** Nose	**0** Open **3** Percutaneous **4** Percutaneous Endoscopic **X** External	**7** Autologous Tissue Substitute **J** Synthetic Substitute **K** Nonautologous Tissue Substitute **Z** No Device	**Z** No Qualifier

Section	0	Medical and Surgical
Body System	9	Ear, Nose, Sinus
Operation	1	Bypass: Altering the route of passage of the contents of a tubular body part

Body Part Character 4	Approach Character 5	Device Character 6	Qualifier
D Inner Ear, Right **E** Inner Ear, Left	**0** Open	**7** Autologous Tissue Substitute **J** Synthetic Substitute **K** Nonautologous Tissue Substitute **Z** No Device	**0** Endolymphatic

Section	0	Medical and Surgical
Body System	9	Ear, Nose, Sinus
Operation	2	Change: Taking out or off a device from a body part and putting back an identical or similar device in or on the same body part without cutting or puncturing the skin or a mucous membrane

Body Part (Character 4)	Approach (Character 5)	Device (Character 6)	Qualifier (Character 7)
H Ear, Right **J** Ear, Left **K** Nose **Y** Sinus	**X** External	**0** Drainage Device **Y** Other Device	**Z** No Qualifier

Section	0	Medical and Surgical
Body System	9	Ear, Nose, Sinus
Operation	5	Destruction: Physical eradication of all or a portion of a body part by the direct use of energy, force, or a destructive agent

Body Part (Character 4)	Approach (Character 5)	Device (Character 6)	Qualifier (Character 7)
0 External Ear, Right **1** External Ear, Left **K** Nose	**0** Open **3** Percutaneous **4** Percutaneous Endoscopic **X** External	**Z** No Device	**Z** No Qualifier
3 External Auditory Canal, Right **4** External Auditory Canal, Left	**0** Open **3** Percutaneous **4** Percutaneous Endoscopic **7** Via Natural or Artificial Opening **8** Via Natural or Artificial Opening Endoscopic **X** External	**Z** No Device	**Z** No Qualifier
5 Middle Ear, Right **6** Middle Ear, Left **9** Auditory Ossicle, Right **A** Auditory Ossicle, Left **D** Inner Ear, Right **E** Inner Ear, Left	**0** Open	**Z** No Device	**Z** No Qualifier
7 Tympanic Membrane, Right **8** Tympanic Membrane, Left **F** Eustachian Tube, Right **G** Eustachian Tube, Left **L** Nasal Turbinate **N** Nasopharynx	**0** Open **3** Percutaneous **4** Percutaneous Endoscopic **7** Via Natural or Artificial Opening **8** Via Natural or Artificial Opening Endoscopic	**Z** No Device	**Z** No Qualifier
B Mastoid Sinus, Right **C** Mastoid Sinus, Left **M** Nasal Septum **P** Accessory Sinus **Q** Maxillary Sinus, Right **R** Maxillary Sinus, Left **S** Frontal Sinus, Right **T** Frontal Sinus, Left **U** Ethmoid Sinus, Right **V** Ethmoid Sinus, Left **W** Sphenoid Sinus, Right **X** Sphenoid Sinus, Left	**0** Open **3** Percutaneous **4** Percutaneous Endoscopic	**Z** No Device	**Z** No Qualifier

Section	0	Medical and Surgical		
Body System	9	Ear, Nose, Sinus		
Operation	7	Dilation: Expanding an orifice or the lumen of a tubular body part		
Body Part (Character 4)		**Approach (Character 5)**	**Device (Character 6)**	**Qualifier (Character 7)**
F Eustachian Tube, Right G Eustachian Tube, Left		0 Open 7 Via Natural or Artificial Opening 8 Via Natural or Artificial Opening Endoscopic	D Intraluminal Device Z No Device	Z No Qualifier
F Eustachian Tube, Right G Eustachian Tube, Left		3 Percutaneous 4 Percutaneous Endoscopic	Z No Device	Z No Qualifier

Section	0	Medical and Surgical		
Body System	9	Ear, Nose, Sinus		
Operation	8	Division: Cutting into a body part, without draining fluids and/or gases from the body part, in order to separate or transect a body part		
Body Part (Character 4)		**Approach (Character 5)**	**Device (Character 6)**	**Qualifier (Character 7)**
L Nasal Turbinate		0 Open 3 Percutaneous 4 Percutaneous Endoscopic 7 Via Natural or Artificial Opening 8 Via Natural or Artificial Opening Endoscopic	Z No Device	Z No Qualifier

Section	0	Medical and Surgical		
Body System	9	Ear, Nose, Sinus		
Operation	9	Drainage: Taking or letting out fluids and/or gases from a body part		
Body Part (Character 4)		**Approach (Character 5)**	**Device (Character 6)**	**Qualifier (Character 7)**
0 External Ear, Right 1 External Ear, Left K Nose		0 Open 3 Percutaneous 4 Percutaneous Endoscopic X External	0 Drainage Device	Z No Qualifier
0 External Ear, Right 1 External Ear, Left K Nose		0 Open 3 Percutaneous 4 Percutaneous Endoscopic X External	Z No Device	X Diagnostic Z No Qualifier
3 External Auditory Canal, Right 4 External Auditory Canal, Left		0 Open 3 Percutaneous 4 Percutaneous Endoscopic 7 Via Natural or Artificial Opening 8 Via Natural or Artificial Opening Endoscopic X External	0 Drainage Device	Z No Qualifier
3 External Auditory Canal, Right 4 External Auditory Canal, Left		0 Open 3 Percutaneous 4 Percutaneous Endoscopic 7 Via Natural or Artificial Opening 8 Via Natural or Artificial Opening Endoscopic X External	Z No Device	X Diagnostic Z No Qualifier
5 Middle Ear, Right 6 Middle Ear, Left 9 Auditory Ossicle, Right A Auditory Ossicle, Left D Inner Ear, Right E Inner Ear, Left		0 Open	0 Drainage Device	Z No Qualifier
5 Middle Ear, Right 6 Middle Ear, Left 9 Auditory Ossicle, Right A Auditory Ossicle, Left D Inner Ear, Right E Inner Ear, Left		0 Open	Z No Device	X Diagnostic Z No Qualifier

Section	0	Medical and Surgical		
Body System	9	Ear, Nose, Sinus		
Operation	9	Drainage: Taking or letting out fluids and/or gases from a body part		

Body Part (Character 4)	Approach (Character 5)	Device (Character 6)	Qualifier (Character 7)
7 Tympanic Membrane, Right **8** Tympanic Membrane, Left **F** Eustachian Tube, Right **G** Eustachian Tube, Left **L** Nasal Turbinate **N** Nasopharynx	**0** Open **3** Percutaneous **4** Percutaneous Endoscopic **7** Via Natural or Artificial Opening **8** Via Natural or Artificial Opening Endoscopic	**0** Drainage Device	**Z** No Qualifier
7 Tympanic Membrane, Right **8** Tympanic Membrane, Left **F** Eustachian Tube, Right **G** Eustachian Tube, Left **L** Nasal Turbinate **N** Nasopharynx	**0** Open **3** Percutaneous **4** Percutaneous Endoscopic **7** Via Natural or Artificial Opening **8** Via Natural or Artificial Opening Endoscopic	**Z** No Device	**X** Diagnostic **Z** No Qualifier
B Mastoid Sinus, Right **C** Mastoid Sinus, Left **M** Nasal Septum **P** Accessory Sinus **Q** Maxillary Sinus, Right **R** Maxillary Sinus, Left **S** Frontal Sinus, Right **T** Frontal Sinus, Left **U** Ethmoid Sinus, Right **V** Ethmoid Sinus, Left **W** Sphenoid Sinus, Right **X** Sphenoid Sinus, Left	**0** Open **3** Percutaneous **4** Percutaneous Endoscopic	**0** Drainage Device	**Z** No Qualifier
B Mastoid Sinus, Right **C** Mastoid Sinus, Left **M** Nasal Septum **P** Accessory Sinus **Q** Maxillary Sinus, Right **R** Maxillary Sinus, Left **S** Frontal Sinus, Right **T** Frontal Sinus, Left **U** Ethmoid Sinus, Right **V** Ethmoid Sinus, Left **W** Sphenoid Sinus, Right **X** Sphenoid Sinus, Left	**0** Open **3** Percutaneous **4** Percutaneous Endoscopic	**Z** No Device	**X** Diagnostic **Z** No Qualifier

Section	0	Medical and Surgical
Body System	9	Ear, Nose, Sinus
Operation	B	Excision: Cutting out or off, without replacement, a portion of a body part

Body Part (Character 4)	Approach (Character 5)	Device (Character 6)	Qualifier (Character 7)
0 External Ear, Right **1** External Ear, Left **K** Nose	**0** Open **3** Percutaneous **4** Percutaneous Endoscopic **X** External	**Z** No Device	**X** Diagnostic **Z** No Qualifier
3 External Auditory Canal, Right **4** External Auditory Canal, Left	**0** Open **3** Percutaneous **4** Percutaneous Endoscopic **7** Via Natural or Artificial Opening **8** Via Natural or Artificial Opening Endoscopic **X** External	**Z** No Device	**X** Diagnostic **Z** No Qualifier
5 Middle Ear, Right **6** Middle Ear, Left **9** Auditory Ossicle, Right **A** Auditory Ossicle, Left **D** Inner Ear, Right **E** Inner Ear, Left	**0** Open	**Z** No Device	**X** Diagnostic **Z** No Qualifier
7 Tympanic Membrane, Right **8** Tympanic Membrane, Left **F** Eustachian Tube, Right **G** Eustachian Tube, Left **L** Nasal Turbinate **N** Nasopharynx	**0** Open **3** Percutaneous **4** Percutaneous Endoscopic **7** Via Natural or Artificial Opening **8** Via Natural or Artificial Opening Endoscopic	**Z** No Device	**X** Diagnostic **Z** No Qualifier
B Mastoid Sinus, Right **C** Mastoid Sinus, Left **M** Nasal Septum **P** Accessory Sinus **Q** Maxillary Sinus, Right **R** Maxillary Sinus, Left **S** Frontal Sinus, Right **T** Frontal Sinus, Left **U** Ethmoid Sinus, Right **V** Ethmoid Sinus, Left **W** Sphenoid Sinus, Right **X** Sphenoid Sinus, Left	**0** Open **3** Percutaneous **4** Percutaneous Endoscopic	**Z** No Device	**X** Diagnostic **Z** No Qualifier

Section	0	Medical and Surgical		
Body System	9	Ear, Nose, Sinus		
Operation	C	Extirpation: Taking or cutting out solid matter from a body part		

Body Part (Character 4)	Approach (Character 5)	Device (Character 6)	Qualifier (Character 7)
0 External Ear, Right 1 External Ear, Left K Nose	0 Open 3 Percutaneous 4 Percutaneous Endoscopic X External	Z No Device	Z No Qualifier
3 External Auditory Canal, Right 4 External Auditory Canal, Left	0 Open 3 Percutaneous 4 Percutaneous Endoscopic 7 Via Natural or Artificial Opening 8 Via Natural or Artificial Opening Endoscopic X External	Z No Device	Z No Qualifier
5 Middle Ear, Right 6 Middle Ear, Left 9 Auditory Ossicle, Right A Auditory Ossicle, Left D Inner Ear, Right E Inner Ear, Left	0 Open	Z No Device	Z No Qualifier
7 Tympanic Membrane, Right 8 Tympanic Membrane, Left F Eustachian Tube, Right G Eustachian Tube, Left L Nasal Turbinate N Nasopharynx	0 Open 3 Percutaneous 4 Percutaneous Endoscopic 7 Via Natural or Artificial Opening 8 Via Natural or Artificial Opening Endoscopic	Z No Device	Z No Qualifier
B Mastoid Sinus, Right C Mastoid Sinus, Left M Nasal Septum P Accessory Sinus Q Maxillary Sinus, Right R Maxillary Sinus, Left S Frontal Sinus, Right T Frontal Sinus, Left U Ethmoid Sinus, Right V Ethmoid Sinus, Left W Sphenoid Sinus, Right X Sphenoid Sinus, Left	0 Open 3 Percutaneous 4 Percutaneous Endoscopic	Z No Device	Z No Qualifier

Section	0	Medical and Surgical		
Body System	9	Ear, Nose, Sinus		
Operation	D	Extraction: Pulling or stripping out or off all or a portion of a body part by the use of force		

Body Part (Character 4)	Approach (Character 5)	Device (Character 6)	Qualifier (Character 7)
7 Tympanic Membrane, Right 8 Tympanic Membrane, Left L Nasal Turbinate	0 Open 3 Percutaneous 4 Percutaneous Endoscopic 7 Via Natural or Artificial Opening 8 Via Natural or Artificial Opening Endoscopic	Z No Device	Z No Qualifier
9 Auditory Ossicle, Right A Auditory Ossicle, Left	0 Open	Z No Device	Z No Qualifier
B Mastoid Sinus, Right C Mastoid Sinus, Left M Nasal Septum P Accessory Sinus Q Maxillary Sinus, Right R Maxillary Sinus, Left S Frontal Sinus, Right T Frontal Sinus, Left U Ethmoid Sinus, Right V Ethmoid Sinus, Left W Sphenoid Sinus, Right X Sphenoid Sinus, Left	0 Open 3 Percutaneous 4 Percutaneous Endoscopic	Z No Device	Z No Qualifier

Section	0	Medical and Surgical		
Body System	9	Ear, Nose, Sinus		
Operation	H	Insertion: Putting in a nonbiological appliance that monitors, assists, performs, or prevents a physiological function but does not physically take the place of a body part		

Body Part (Character 4)	Approach (Character 5)	Device (Character 6)	Qualifier (Character 7)
D Inner Ear, Right **E** Inner Ear, Left	**0** Open **3** Percutaneous **4** Percutaneous Endoscopic	**4** Hearing Device, Bone Conduction **5** Hearing Device, Single Channel Cochlear Prosthesis **6** Hearing Device, Multiple Channel Cochlear Prosthesis **S** Hearing Device	**Z** No Qualifier
N Nasopharynx	**7** Via Natural or Artificial Opening **8** Via Natural or Artificial Opening Endoscopic	**B** Intraluminal Device, Airway	**Z** No Qualifier

Section	0	Medical and Surgical		
Body System	9	Ear, Nose, Sinus		
Operation	J	Inspection: Visually and/or manually exploring a body part		

Body Part (Character 4)	Approach (Character 5)	Device (Character 6)	Qualifier (Character 7)
7 Tympanic Membrane, Right **8** Tympanic Membrane, Left **H** Ear, Right **J** Ear, Left	**0** Open **3** Percutaneous **4** Percutaneous Endoscopic **7** Via Natural or Artificial Opening **8** Via Natural or Artificial Opening Endoscopic **X** External	**Z** No Device	**Z** No Qualifier
D Inner Ear, Right **E** Inner Ear, Left **K** Nose **Y** Sinus	**0** Open **3** Percutaneous **4** Percutaneous Endoscopic **X** External	**Z** No Device	**Z** No Qualifier

Section	0	Medical and Surgical		
Body System	9	Ear, Nose, Sinus		
Operation	M	Reattachment Putting back in or on all or a portion of a separated body part to its normal location or other suitable location		

Body Part (Character 4)	Approach (Character 5)	Device (Character 6)	Qualifier (Character 7)
0 External Ear, Right **1** External Ear, Left **K** Nose	**X** External	**Z** No Device	**Z** No Qualifier

Section	0	Medical and Surgical			
Body System	9	Ear, Nose, Sinus			
Operation	N	Release: Freeing a body part from an abnormal physical constraint by cutting or by the use of force			

Body Part (Character 4)	Approach (Character 5)	Device (Character 6)	Qualifier (Character 7)
0 External Ear, Right **1** External Ear, Left **K** Nose	**0** Open **3** Percutaneous **4** Percutaneous Endoscopic **X** External	**Z** No Device	**Z** No Qualifier
3 External Auditory Canal, Right **4** External Auditory Canal, Left	**0** Open **3** Percutaneous **4** Percutaneous Endoscopic **7** Via Natural or Artificial Opening **8** Via Natural or Artificial Opening Endoscopic **X** External	**Z** No Device	**Z** No Qualifier
5 Middle Ear, Right **6** Middle Ear, Left **9** Auditory Ossicle, Right **A** Auditory Ossicle, Left **D** Inner Ear, Right **E** Inner Ear, Left	**0** Open	**Z** No Device	**Z** No Qualifier
7 Tympanic Membrane, Right **8** Tympanic Membrane, Left **F** Eustachian Tube, Right **G** Eustachian Tube, Left **L** Nasal Turbinate **N** Nasopharynx	**0** Open **3** Percutaneous **4** Percutaneous Endoscopic **7** Via Natural or Artificial Opening **8** Via Natural or Artificial Opening Endoscopic	**Z** No Device	**Z** No Qualifier
B Mastoid Sinus, Right **C** Mastoid Sinus, Left **M** Nasal Septum **P** Accessory Sinus **Q** Maxillary Sinus, Right **R** Maxillary Sinus, Left **S** Frontal Sinus, Right **T** Frontal Sinus, Left **U** Ethmoid Sinus, Right **V** Ethmoid Sinus, Left **W** Sphenoid Sinus, Right **X** Sphenoid Sinus, Left	**0** Open **3** Percutaneous **4** Percutaneous Endoscopic	**Z** No Device	**Z** No Qualifier

Section	0	Medical and Surgical			
Body System	9	Ear, Nose, Sinus			
Operation	P	Removal: Taking out or off a device from a body part			

Body Part (Character 4)	Approach (Character 5)	Device (Character 6)	Qualifier (Character 7)
7 Tympanic Membrane, Right **8** Tympanic Membrane, Left	**0** Open **7** Via Natural or Artificial Opening **8** Via Natural or Artificial Opening Endoscopic **X** External	**0** Drainage Device	**Z** No Qualifier
D Inner Ear, Right **E** Inner Ear, Left	**0** Open **7** Via Natural or Artificial Opening **8** Via Natural or Artificial Opening Endoscopic	**S** Hearing Device	**Z** No Qualifier
H Ear, Right **J** Ear, Left **K** Nose	**0** Open **3** Percutaneous **4** Percutaneous Endoscopic **7** Via Natural or Artificial Opening **8** Via Natural or Artificial Opening Endoscopic **X** External	**0** Drainage Device **7** Autologous Tissue Substitute **D** Intraluminal Device **J** Synthetic Substitute **K** Nonautologous Tissue Substitute	**Z** No Qualifier
Y Sinus	**0** Open **3** Percutaneous **4** Percutaneous Endoscopic **X** External	**0** Drainage Device	**Z** No Qualifier

Section	0	Medical and Surgical		
Body System	9	Ear, Nose, Sinus		
Operation	Q	Repair: Restoring, to the extent possible, a body part to its normal anatomic structure and function		

Body Part (Character 4)	Approach (Character 5)	Device (Character 6)	Qualifier (Character 7)
0 External Ear, Right 1 External Ear, Left 2 External Ear, Bilateral K Nose	0 Open 3 Percutaneous 4 Percutaneous Endoscopic X External	Z No Device	Z No Qualifier
3 External Auditory Canal, Right 4 External Auditory Canal, Left F Eustachian Tube, Right G Eustachian Tube, Left	0 Open 3 Percutaneous 4 Percutaneous Endoscopic 7 Via Natural or Artificial Opening 8 Via Natural or Artificial Opening Endoscopic X External	Z No Device	Z No Qualifier
5 Middle Ear, Right 6 Middle Ear, Left 9 Auditory Ossicle, Right A Auditory Ossicle, Left D Inner Ear, Right E Inner Ear, Left	0 Open	Z No Device	Z No Qualifier
7 Tympanic Membrane, Right 8 Tympanic Membrane, Left L Nasal Turbinate N Nasopharynx	0 Open 3 Percutaneous 4 Percutaneous Endoscopic 7 Via Natural or Artificial Opening 8 Via Natural or Artificial Opening Endoscopic	Z No Device	Z No Qualifier
B Mastoid Sinus, Right C Mastoid Sinus, Left M Nasal Septum P Accessory Sinus Q Maxillary Sinus, Right R Maxillary Sinus, Left S Frontal Sinus, Right T Frontal Sinus, Left U Ethmoid Sinus, Right V Ethmoid Sinus, Left W Sphenoid Sinus, Right X Sphenoid Sinus, Left	0 Open 3 Percutaneous 4 Percutaneous Endoscopic	Z No Device	Z No Qualifier

Section	0	Medical and Surgical		
Body System	9	Ear, Nose, Sinus		
Operation	R	Replacement: Putting in or on biological or synthetic material that physically takes the place and/or function of all or a portion of a body part		

Body Part (Character 4)	Approach (Character 5)	Device (Character 6)	Qualifier (Character 7)
0 External Ear, Right 1 External Ear, Left 2 External Ear, Bilateral K Nose	0 Open X External	7 Autologous Tissue Substitute J Synthetic Substitute K Nonautologous Tissue Substitute	Z No Qualifier
5 Middle Ear, Right 6 Middle Ear, Left 9 Auditory Ossicle, Right A Auditory Ossicle, Left D Inner Ear, Right E Inner Ear, Left	0 Open	7 Autologous Tissue Substitute J Synthetic Substitute K Nonautologous Tissue Substitute	Z No Qualifier
7 Tympanic Membrane, Right 8 Tympanic Membrane, Left N Nasopharynx	0 Open 7 Via Natural or Artificial Opening 8 Via Natural or Artificial Opening Endoscopic	7 Autologous Tissue Substitute J Synthetic Substitute K Nonautologous Tissue Substitute	Z No Qualifier
L Nasal Turbinate	0 Open 3 Percutaneous 4 Percutaneous Endoscopic 7 Via Natural or Artificial Opening 8 Via Natural or Artificial Opening Endoscopic	7 Autologous Tissue Substitute J Synthetic Substitute K Nonautologous Tissue Substitute	Z No Qualifier
M Nasal Septum	0 Open 3 Percutaneous 4 Percutaneous Endoscopic	7 Autologous Tissue Substitute J Synthetic Substitute K Nonautologous Tissue Substitute	Z No Qualifier

Section	0	Medical and Surgical		
Body System	9	Ear, Nose, Sinus		
Operation	S	Reposition: Moving to its normal location, or other suitable location, all or a portion of a body part		

Body Part (Character 4)	Approach (Character 5)	Device (Character 6)	Qualifier (Character 7)
0 External Ear, Right 1 External Ear, Left 2 External Ear, Bilateral K Nose	0 Open 4 Percutaneous Endoscopic X External	Z No Device	Z No Qualifier
7 Tympanic Membrane, Right 8 Tympanic Membrane, Left F Eustachian Tube, Right G Eustachian Tube, Left L Nasal Turbinate	0 Open 4 Percutaneous Endoscopic 7 Via Natural or Artificial Opening 8 Via Natural or Artificial Opening Endoscopic	Z No Device	Z No Qualifier
9 Auditory Ossicle, Right A Auditory Ossicle, Left M Nasal Septum	0 Open 4 Percutaneous Endoscopic	Z No Device	Z No Qualifier

Section	0	Medical and Surgical		
Body System	9	Ear, Nose, Sinus		
Operation	T	Resection: Cutting out or off, without replacement, all of a body part		

Body Part (Character 4)	Approach (Character 5)	Device (Character 6)	Qualifier (Character 7)
0 External Ear, Right 1 External Ear, Left K Nose	0 Open 4 Percutaneous Endoscopic X External	Z No Device	Z No Qualifier
5 Middle Ear, Right 6 Middle Ear, Left 9 Auditory Ossicle, Right A Auditory Ossicle, Left D Inner Ear, Right E Inner Ear, Left	0 Open	Z No Device	Z No Qualifier
7 Tympanic Membrane, Right 8 Tympanic Membrane, Left F Eustachian Tube, Right G Eustachian Tube, Left L Nasal Turbinate N Nasopharynx	0 Open 4 Percutaneous Endoscopic 7 Via Natural or Artificial Opening 8 Via Natural or Artificial Opening Endoscopic	Z No Device	Z No Qualifier
B Mastoid Sinus, Right C Mastoid Sinus, Left M Nasal Septum P Accessory Sinus Q Maxillary Sinus, Right R Maxillary Sinus, Left S Frontal Sinus, Right T Frontal Sinus, Left U Ethmoid Sinus, Right V Ethmoid Sinus, Left W Sphenoid Sinus, Right X Sphenoid Sinus, Left	0 Open 4 Percutaneous Endoscopic	Z No Device	Z No Qualifier

Section	0	Medical and Surgical		
Body System	9	Ear, Nose, Sinus		
Operation	U	Supplement: Putting in or on biological or synthetic material that physically reinforces and/or augments the function of a portion of a body part		

Body Part (Character 4)	Approach (Character 5)	Device (Character 6)	Qualifier (Character 7)
0 External Ear, Right **1** External Ear, Left **2** External Ear, Bilateral **K** Nose	**0** Open **X** External	**7** Autologous Tissue Substitute **J** Synthetic Substitute **K** Nonautologous Tissue Substitute	**Z** No Qualifier
5 Middle Ear, Right **6** Middle Ear, Left **9** Auditory Ossicle, Right **A** Auditory Ossicle, Left **D** Inner Ear, Right **E** Inner Ear, Left	**0** Open	**7** Autologous Tissue Substitute **J** Synthetic Substitute **K** Nonautologous Tissue Substitute	**Z** No Qualifier
7 Tympanic Membrane, Right **8** Tympanic Membrane, Left **N** Nasopharynx	**0** Open **7** Via Natural or Artificial Opening **8** Via Natural or Artificial Opening Endoscopic	**7** Autologous Tissue Substitute **J** Synthetic Substitute **K** Nonautologous Tissue Substitute	**Z** No Qualifier
L Nasal Turbinate	**0** Open **3** Percutaneous **4** Percutaneous Endoscopic **7** Via Natural or Artificial Opening **8** Via Natural or Artificial Opening Endoscopic	**7** Autologous Tissue Substitute **J** Synthetic Substitute **K** Nonautologous Tissue Substitute	**Z** No Qualifier
M Nasal Septum	**0** Open **3** Percutaneous **4** Percutaneous Endoscopic	**7** Autologous Tissue Substitute **J** Synthetic Substitute **K** Nonautologous Tissue Substitute	**Z** No Qualifier

Section	0	Medical and Surgical		
Body System	9	Ear, Nose, Sinus		
Operation	W	Revision: Correcting, to the extent possible, a portion of a malfunctioning device or the position of a displaced device		

Body Part (Character 4)	Approach (Character 5)	Device (Character 6)	Qualifier (Character 7)
7 Tympanic Membrane, Right **8** Tympanic Membrane, Left **9** Auditory Ossicle, Right **A** Auditory Ossicle, Left	**0** Open **7** Via Natural or Artificial Opening **8** Via Natural or Artificial Opening Endoscopic	**7** Autologous Tissue Substitute **J** Synthetic Substitute **K** Nonautologous Tissue Substitute	**Z** No Qualifier
D Inner Ear, Right **E** Inner Ear, Left	**0** Open **7** Via Natural or Artificial Opening **8** Via Natural or Artificial Opening Endoscopic	**S** Hearing Device	**Z** No Qualifier
H Ear, Right **J** Ear, Left **K** Nose	**0** Open **3** Percutaneous **4** Percutaneous Endoscopic **7** Via Natural or Artificial Opening **8** Via Natural or Artificial Opening Endoscopic **X** External	**0** Drainage Device **7** Autologous Tissue Substitute **D** Intraluminal Device **J** Synthetic Substitute **K** Nonautologous Tissue Substitute	**Z** No Qualifier
Y Sinus	**0** Open **3** Percutaneous **4** Percutaneous Endoscopic **X** External	**0** Drainage Device	**Z** No Qualifier

Section	0	Medical and Surgical
Body System	B	Respiratory System
Operation	1	Bypass: Altering the route of passage of the contents of a tubular body part

Body Part (Character 4)	Approach (Character 5)	Device (Character 6)	Qualifier (Character 7)
1 Trachea	0 Open	D Intraluminal Device	6 Esophagus
1 Trachea	0 Open	F Tracheostomy Device Z No Device	4 Cutaneous
1 Trachea	3 Percutaneous 4 Percutaneous Endoscopic	F Tracheostomy Device Z No Device	4 Cutaneous

Section	0	Medical and Surgical
Body System	B	Respiratory System
Operation	2	Change: Taking out or off a device from a body part and putting back an identical or similar device in or on the same body part without cutting or puncturing the skin or a mucous membrane

Body Part (Character 4)	Approach (Character 5)	Device (Character 6)	Qualifier (Character 7)
0 Tracheobronchial Tree K Lung, Right L Lung, Left Q Pleura T Diaphragm	X External	0 Drainage Device Y Other Device	Z No Qualifier
1 Trachea	X External	0 Drainage Device E Intraluminal Device, Endotracheal Airway F Tracheostomy Device Y Other Device	Z No Qualifier

Section	0	Medical and Surgical
Body System	B	Respiratory System
Operation	5	Destruction: Physical eradication of all or a portion of a body part by the direct use of energy, force, or a destructive agent

Body Part (Character 4)	Approach (Character 5)	Device (Character 6)	Qualifier (Character 7)
1 Trachea 2 Carina 3 Main Bronchus, Right 4 Upper Lobe Bronchus, Right 5 Middle Lobe Bronchus, Right 6 Lower Lobe Bronchus, Right 7 Main Bronchus, Left 8 Upper Lobe Bronchus, Left 9 Lingula Bronchus B Lower Lobe Bronchus, Left C Upper Lung Lobe, Right D Middle Lung Lobe, Right F Lower Lung Lobe, Right G Upper Lung Lobe, Left H Lung Lingula J Lower Lung Lobe, Left K Lung, Right L Lung, Left M Lungs, Bilateral	0 Open 3 Percutaneous 4 Percutaneous Endoscopic 7 Via Natural or Artificial Opening 8 Via Natural or Artificial Opening Endoscopic	Z No Device	Z No Qualifier
N Pleura, Right P Pleura, Left R Diaphragm, Right S Diaphragm, Left	0 Open 3 Percutaneous 4 Percutaneous Endoscopic	Z No Device	Z No Qualifier

Section	0	Medical and Surgical
Body System	B	Respiratory System
Operation	7	Dilation: Expanding an orifice or the lumen of a tubular body part

Body Part (Character 4)	Approach (Character 5)	Device (Character 6)	Qualifier (Character 7)
1 Trachea 2 Carina 3 Main Bronchus, Right 4 Upper Lobe Bronchus, Right 5 Middle Lobe Bronchus, Right 6 Lower Lobe Bronchus, Right 7 Main Bronchus, Left 8 Upper Lobe Bronchus, Left 9 Lingula Bronchus B Lower Lobe Bronchus, Left	0 Open 3 Percutaneous 4 Percutaneous Endoscopic 7 Via Natural or Artificial Opening 8 Via Natural or Artificial Opening Endoscopic	D Intraluminal Device Z No Device	Z No Qualifier

Section	0	Medical and Surgical		
Body System	B	Respiratory System		
Operation	9	Drainage: Taking or letting out fluids and/or gases from a body part		
Body Part (Character 4)		**Approach (Character 5)**	**Device (Character 6)**	**Qualifier (Character 7)**
1 Trachea 2 Carina 3 Main Bronchus, Right 4 Upper Lobe Bronchus, Right 5 Middle Lobe Bronchus, Right 6 Lower Lobe Bronchus, Right 7 Main Bronchus, Left 8 Upper Lobe Bronchus, Left 9 Lingula Bronchus B Lower Lobe Bronchus, Left C Upper Lung Lobe, Right D Middle Lung Lobe, Right F Lower Lung Lobe, Right G Upper Lung Lobe, Left H Lung Lingula J Lower Lung Lobe, Left K Lung, Right L Lung, Left M Lungs, Bilateral		0 Open 3 Percutaneous 4 Percutaneous Endoscopic 7 Via Natural or Artificial Opening 8 Via Natural or Artificial Opening Endoscopic	0 Drainage Device	Z No Qualifier

Section	0	Medical and Surgical		
Body System	B	Respiratory System		
Operation	9	Drainage: Taking or letting out fluids and/or gases from a body part		
Body Part (Character 4)		**Approach (Character 5)**	**Device (Character 6)**	**Qualifier (Character 7)**
1 Trachea 2 Carina 3 Main Bronchus, Right 4 Upper Lobe Bronchus, Right 5 Middle Lobe Bronchus, Right 6 Lower Lobe Bronchus, Right 7 Main Bronchus, Left 8 Upper Lobe Bronchus, Left 9 Lingula Bronchus B Lower Lobe Bronchus, Left C Upper Lung Lobe, Right D Middle Lung Lobe, Right F Lower Lung Lobe, Right G Upper Lung Lobe, Left H Lung Lingula J Lower Lung Lobe, Left K Lung, Right L Lung, Left M Lungs, Bilateral		0 Open 3 Percutaneous 4 Percutaneous Endoscopic 7 Via Natural or Artificial Opening 8 Via Natural or Artificial Opening Endoscopic	Z No Device	X Diagnostic Z No Qualifier
N Pleura, Right P Pleura, Left R Diaphragm, Right S Diaphragm, Left		0 Open 3 Percutaneous 4 Percutaneous Endoscopic	0 Drainage Device	Z No Qualifier
N Pleura, Right P Pleura, Left R Diaphragm, Right S Diaphragm, Left		0 Open 3 Percutaneous 4 Percutaneous Endoscopic	Z No Device	X Diagnostic Z No Qualifier

Section	0	Medical and Surgical		
Body System	B	Respiratory System		
Operation	B	Excision: Cutting out or off, without replacement, a portion of a body part		

Body Part (Character 4)	Approach (Character 5)	Device (Character 6)	Qualifier (Character 7)
1 Trachea 2 Carina 3 Main Bronchus, Right 4 Upper Lobe Bronchus, Right 5 Middle Lobe Bronchus, Right 6 Lower Lobe Bronchus, Right 7 Main Bronchus, Left 8 Upper Lobe Bronchus, Left 9 Lingula Bronchus B Lower Lobe Bronchus, Left C Upper Lung Lobe, Right D Middle Lung Lobe, Right F Lower Lung Lobe, Right G Upper Lung Lobe, Left H Lung Lingula J Lower Lung Lobe, Left K Lung, Right L Lung, Left M Lungs, Bilateral	0 Open 3 Percutaneous 4 Percutaneous Endoscopic 7 Via Natural or Artificial Opening 8 Via Natural or Artificial Opening Endoscopic	Z No Device	X Diagnostic Z No Qualifier
N Pleura, Right P Pleura, Left R Diaphragm, Right S Diaphragm, Left	0 Open 3 Percutaneous 4 Percutaneous Endoscopic	Z No Device	X Diagnostic Z No Qualifier

Section	0	Medical and Surgical		
Body System	B	Respiratory System		
Operation	C	Extirpation: Taking or cutting out solid matter from a body part		

Body Part (Character 4)	Approach (Character 5)	Device (Character 6)	Qualifier (Character 7)
1 Trachea 2 Carina 3 Main Bronchus, Right 4 Upper Lobe Bronchus, Right 5 Middle Lobe Bronchus, Right 6 Lower Lobe Bronchus, Right 7 Main Bronchus, Left 8 Upper Lobe Bronchus, Left 9 Lingula Bronchus B Lower Lobe Bronchus, Left C Upper Lung Lobe, Right D Middle Lung Lobe, Right F Lower Lung Lobe, Right G Upper Lung Lobe, Left H Lung Lingula J Lower Lung Lobe, Left K Lung, Right L Lung, Left M Lungs, Bilateral	0 Open 3 Percutaneous 4 Percutaneous Endoscopic 7 Via Natural or Artificial Opening 8 Via Natural or Artificial Opening Endoscopic	Z No Device	Z No Qualifier
N Pleura, Right P Pleura, Left R Diaphragm, Right S Diaphragm, Left	0 Open 3 Percutaneous 4 Percutaneous Endoscopic	Z No Device	Z No Qualifier

Section	0	Medical and Surgical		
Body System	B	Respiratory System		
Operation	D	Extraction: Pulling or stripping out or off all or a portion of a body part by the use of force		

Body Part (Character 4)	Approach (Character 5)	Device (Character 6)	Qualifier (Character 7)
N Pleura, Right P Pleura, Left	0 Open 3 Percutaneous 4 Percutaneous Endoscopic	Z No Device	X Diagnostic Z No Qualifier

Section	0	Medical and Surgical		
Body System	B	Respiratory System		
Operation	F	Fragmentation: Breaking solid matter in a body part into pieces		

Body Part (Character 4)	Approach (Character 5)	Device (Character 6)	Qualifier (Character 7)
1 Trachea 2 Carina 3 Main Bronchus, Right 4 Upper Lobe Bronchus, Right 5 Middle Lobe Bronchus, Right 6 Lower Lobe Bronchus, Right 7 Main Bronchus, Left 8 Upper Lobe Bronchus, Left 9 Lingula Bronchus B Lower Lobe Bronchus, Left	0 Open 3 Percutaneous 4 Percutaneous Endoscopic 7 Via Natural or Artificial Opening 8 Via Natural or Artificial Opening Endoscopic X External	Z No Device	Z No Qualifier

Section	0	Medical and Surgical		
Body System	B	Respiratory System		
Operation	H	Insertion: Putting in a nonbiological appliance that monitors, assists, performs, or prevents a physiological function but does not physically take the place of a body part		

Body Part (Character 4)	Approach (Character 5)	Device (Character 6)	Qualifier (Character 7)
0 Tracheobronchial Tree	0 Open 3 Percutaneous 4 Percutaneous Endoscopic 7 Via Natural or Artificial Opening 8 Via Natural or Artificial Opening Endoscopic	1 Radioactive Element 2 Monitoring Device 3 Infusion Device D Intraluminal Device	Z No Qualifier
1 Trachea	0 Open	2 Monitoring Device D Intraluminal Device	Z No Qualifier
1 Trachea	3 Percutaneous	D Intraluminal Device E Intraluminal Device, Endotracheal Airway	Z No Qualifier
1 Trachea	4 Percutaneous Endoscopic	D Intraluminal Device	Z No Qualifier
1 Trachea	7 Via Natural or Artificial Opening 8 Via Natural or Artificial Opening Endoscopic	2 Monitoring Device D Intraluminal Device E Intraluminal Device, Endotracheal Airway	Z No Qualifier
3 Main Bronchus, Right 4 Upper Lobe Bronchus, Right 5 Middle Lobe Bronchus, Right 6 Lower Lobe Bronchus, Right 7 Main Bronchus, Left 8 Upper Lobe Bronchus, Left 9 Lingula Bronchus B Lower Lobe Bronchus, Left	0 Open 3 Percutaneous 4 Percutaneous Endoscopic 7 Via Natural or Artificial Opening 8 Via Natural or Artificial Opening Endoscopic	G Intraluminal Device, Endobronchial Valve	Z No Qualifier
K Lung, Right L Lung, Left	0 Open 3 Percutaneous 4 Percutaneous Endoscopic 7 Via Natural or Artificial Opening 8 Via Natural or Artificial Opening Endoscopic	1 Radioactive Element 2 Monitoring Device 3 Infusion Device	Z No Qualifier
R Diaphragm, Right S Diaphragm, Left	0 Open 3 Percutaneous 4 Percutaneous Endoscopic	2 Monitoring Device M Diaphragmatic Pacemaker Lead	Z No Qualifier

Section	0	Medical and Surgical		
Body System	B	Respiratory System		
Operation	J	Inspection: Visually and/or manually exploring a body part		

Body Part (Character 4)	Approach (Character 5)	Device (Character 6)	Qualifier (Character 7)
0 Tracheobronchial Tree 1 Trachea K Lung, Right L Lung, Left Q Pleura T Diaphragm	0 Open 3 Percutaneous 4 Percutaneous Endoscopic 7 Via Natural or Artificial Opening 8 Via Natural or Artificial Opening Endoscopic X External	Z No Device	Z No Qualifier

Section	0	Medical and Surgical		
Body System	B	Respiratory System		
Operation	L	Occlusion: Completely closing an orifice or the lumen of a tubular body part		

Body Part (Character 4)	Approach (Character 5)	Device (Character 6)	Qualifier (Character 7)
1 Trachea 2 Carina 3 Main Bronchus, Right 4 Upper Lobe Bronchus, Right 5 Middle Lobe Bronchus, Right 6 Lower Lobe Bronchus, Right 7 Main Bronchus, Left 8 Upper Lobe Bronchus, Left 9 Lingula Bronchus B Lower Lobe Bronchus, Left	0 Open 3 Percutaneous 4 Percutaneous Endoscopic	C Extraluminal Device D Intraluminal Device Z No Device	Z No Qualifier
1 Trachea 2 Carina 3 Main Bronchus, Right 4 Upper Lobe Bronchus, Right 5 Middle Lobe Bronchus, Right 6 Lower Lobe Bronchus, Right 7 Main Bronchus, Left 8 Upper Lobe Bronchus, Left 9 Lingula Bronchus B Lower Lobe Bronchus, Left	7 Via Natural or Artificial Opening 8 Via Natural or Artificial Opening Endoscopic	D Intraluminal Device Z No Device	Z No Qualifier

Section	0	Medical and Surgical		
Body System	B	Respiratory System		
Operation	M	Reattachment Putting back in or on all or a portion of a separated body part to its normal location or other suitable location		

Body Part (Character 4)	Approach (Character 5)	Device (Character 6)	Qualifier (Character 7)
1 Trachea 2 Carina 3 Main Bronchus, Right 4 Upper Lobe Bronchus, Right 5 Middle Lobe Bronchus, Right 6 Lower Lobe Bronchus, Right 7 Main Bronchus, Left 8 Upper Lobe Bronchus, Left 9 Lingula Bronchus B Lower Lobe Bronchus, Left C Upper Lung Lobe, Right D Middle Lung Lobe, Right F Lower Lung Lobe, Right G Upper Lung Lobe, Left H Lung Lingula J Lower Lung Lobe, Left K Lung, Right L Lung, Left R Diaphragm, Right S Diaphragm, Left	0 Open	Z No Device	Z No Qualifier

Section	0	Medical and Surgical		
Body System	B	Respiratory System		
Operation	N	Release: Freeing a body part from an abnormal physical constraint by cutting or by the use of force		

Body Part (Character 4)	Approach (Character 5)	Device (Character 6)	Qualifier (Character 7)
1 Trachea 2 Carina 3 Main Bronchus, Right 4 Upper Lobe Bronchus, Right 5 Middle Lobe Bronchus, Right 6 Lower Lobe Bronchus, Right 7 Main Bronchus, Left 8 Upper Lobe Bronchus, Left 9 Lingula Bronchus B Lower Lobe Bronchus, Left C Upper Lung Lobe, Right D Middle Lung Lobe, Right F Lower Lung Lobe, Right G Upper Lung Lobe, Left H Lung Lingula J Lower Lung Lobe, Left K Lung, Right L Lung, Left M Lungs, Bilateral	0 Open 3 Percutaneous 4 Percutaneous Endoscopic 7 Via Natural or Artificial Opening 8 Via Natural or Artificial Opening Endoscopic	Z No Device	Z No Qualifier
N Pleura, Right P Pleura, Left R Diaphragm, Right S Diaphragm, Left	0 Open 3 Percutaneous 4 Percutaneous Endoscopic	Z No Device	Z No Qualifier

Section	0	Medical and Surgical		
Body System	B	Respiratory System		
Operation	P	Removal: Taking out or off a device from a body part		

Body Part (Character 4)	Approach (Character 5)	Device (Character 6)	Qualifier (Character 7)
0 Tracheobronchial Tree	0 Open 3 Percutaneous 4 Percutaneous Endoscopic 7 Via Natural or Artificial Opening 8 Via Natural or Artificial Opening Endoscopic	0 Drainage Device 1 Radioactive Element 2 Monitoring Device 3 Infusion Device 7 Autologous Tissue Substitute C Extraluminal Device D Intraluminal Device J Synthetic Substitute K Nonautologous Tissue Substitute	Z No Qualifier
0 Tracheobronchial Tree	X External	0 Drainage Device 1 Radioactive Element 2 Monitoring Device 3 Infusion Device D Intraluminal Device	Z No Qualifier
1 Trachea	0 Open 3 Percutaneous 4 Percutaneous Endoscopic 7 Via Natural or Artificial Opening 8 Via Natural or Artificial Opening Endoscopic	0 Drainage Device 2 Monitoring Device 7 Autologous Tissue Substitute C Extraluminal Device D Intraluminal Device F Tracheostomy Device J Synthetic Substitute K Nonautologous Tissue Substitute	Z No Qualifier
1 Trachea	X External	0 Drainage Device 2 Monitoring Device D Intraluminal Device F Tracheostomy Device	Z No Qualifier
K Lung, Right L Lung, Left	0 Open 3 Percutaneous 4 Percutaneous Endoscopic 7 Via Natural or Artificial Opening 8 Via Natural or Artificial Opening Endoscopic X External	0 Drainage Device 1 Radioactive Element 2 Monitoring Device 3 Infusion Device	Z No Qualifier

Section	0	Medical and Surgical		
Body System	B	Respiratory System		
Operation	P	Removal: Taking out or off a device from a body part		

Body Part (Character 4)	Approach (Character 5)	Device (Character 6)	Qualifier (Character 7)
Q Pleura	0 Open 3 Percutaneous 4 Percutaneous Endoscopic 7 Via Natural or Artificial Opening 8 Via Natural or Artificial Opening Endoscopic X External	0 Drainage Device 1 Radioactive Element 2 Monitoring Device	Z No Qualifier
T Diaphragm	0 Open 3 Percutaneous 4 Percutaneous Endoscopic 7 Via Natural or Artificial Opening 8 Via Natural or Artificial Opening Endoscopic	0 Drainage Device 2 Monitoring Device 7 Autologous Tissue Substitute J Synthetic Substitute K Nonautologous Tissue Substitute M Diaphragmatic Pacemaker Lead	Z No Qualifier
T Diaphragm	X External	0 Drainage Device 2 Monitoring Device M Diaphragmatic Pacemaker Lead	Z No Qualifier

Section	0	Medical and Surgical		
Body System	B	Respiratory System		
Operation	Q	Repair: Restoring, to the extent possible, a body part to its normal anatomic structure and function		

Body Part (Character 4)	Approach (Character 5)	Device (Character 6)	Qualifier (Character 7)
1 Trachea 2 Carina 3 Main Bronchus, Right 4 Upper Lobe Bronchus, Right 5 Middle Lobe Bronchus, Right 6 Lower Lobe Bronchus, Right 7 Main Bronchus, Left 8 Upper Lobe Bronchus, Left 9 Lingula Bronchus B Lower Lobe Bronchus, Left C Upper Lung Lobe, Right D Middle Lung Lobe, Right F Lower Lung Lobe, Right G Upper Lung Lobe, Left H Lung Lingula J Lower Lung Lobe, Left K Lung, Right L Lung, Left M Lungs, Bilateral	0 Open 3 Percutaneous 4 Percutaneous Endoscopic 7 Via Natural or Artificial Opening 8 Via Natural or Artificial Opening Endoscopic	Z No Device	Z No Qualifier
N Pleura, Right P Pleura, Left R Diaphragm, Right S Diaphragm, Left	0 Open 3 Percutaneous 4 Percutaneous Endoscopic	Z No Device	Z No Qualifier

Section	0	Medical and Surgical		
Body System	B	Respiratory System		
Operation	S	Reposition: Moving to its normal location, or other suitable location, all or a portion of a body part		

Body Part (Character 4)	Approach (Character 5)	Device (Character 6)	Qualifier (Character 7)
1 Trachea 2 Carina 3 Main Bronchus, Right 4 Upper Lobe Bronchus, Right 5 Middle Lobe Bronchus, Right 6 Lower Lobe Bronchus, Right 7 Main Bronchus, Left 8 Upper Lobe Bronchus, Left 9 Lingula Bronchus B Lower Lobe Bronchus, Left C Upper Lung Lobe, Right D Middle Lung Lobe, Right F Lower Lung Lobe, Right G Upper Lung Lobe, Left H Lung Lingula J Lower Lung Lobe, Left K Lung, Right L Lung, Left R Diaphragm, Right S Diaphragm, Left	0 Open	Z No Device	Z No Qualifier

Section	0	Medical and Surgical		
Body System	B	Respiratory System		
Operation	T	Resection: Cutting out or off, without replacement, all of a body part		

Body Part (Character 4)	Approach (Character 5)	Device (Character 6)	Qualifier (Character 7)
1 Trachea 2 Carina 3 Main Bronchus, Right 4 Upper Lobe Bronchus, Right 5 Middle Lobe Bronchus, Right 6 Lower Lobe Bronchus, Right 7 Main Bronchus, Left 8 Upper Lobe Bronchus, Left 9 Lingula Bronchus B Lower Lobe Bronchus, Left C Upper Lung Lobe, Right D Middle Lung Lobe, Right F Lower Lung Lobe, Right G Upper Lung Lobe, Left H Lung Lingula J Lower Lung Lobe, Left K Lung, Right L Lung, Left M Lungs, Bilateral R Diaphragm, Right S Diaphragm, Left	0 Open 4 Percutaneous Endoscopic	Z No Device	Z No Qualifier

Section	0	Medical and Surgical		
Body System	B	Respiratory System		
Operation	U	Supplement: Putting in or on biological or synthetic material that physically reinforces and/or augments the function of a portion of a body part		

Body Part (Character 4)	Approach (Character 5)	Device (Character 6)	Qualifier (Character 7)
1 Trachea 2 Carina 3 Main Bronchus, Right 4 Upper Lobe Bronchus, Right 5 Middle Lobe Bronchus, Right 6 Lower Lobe Bronchus, Right 7 Main Bronchus, Left 8 Upper Lobe Bronchus, Left 9 Lingula Bronchus B Lower Lobe Bronchus, Left R Diaphragm, Right S Diaphragm, Left	0 Open 4 Percutaneous Endoscopic	7 Autologous Tissue Substitute J Synthetic Substitute K Nonautologous Tissue Substitute	Z No Qualifier

Section	0	Medical and Surgical		
Body System	B	Respiratory System		
Operation	V	Restriction: Partially closing an orifice or the lumen of a tubular body part		
Body Part (Character 4)	**Approach (Character 5)**		**Device (Character 6)**	**Qualifier (Character 7)**
1 Trachea 2 Carina 3 Main Bronchus, Right 4 Upper Lobe Bronchus, Right 5 Middle Lobe Bronchus, Right 6 Lower Lobe Bronchus, Right 7 Main Bronchus, Left 8 Upper Lobe Bronchus, Left 9 Lingula Bronchus B Lower Lobe Bronchus, Left	0 Open 3 Percutaneous 4 Percutaneous Endoscopic		C Extraluminal Device D Intraluminal Device Z No Device	Z No Qualifier
1 Trachea 2 Carina 3 Main Bronchus, Right 4 Upper Lobe Bronchus, Right 5 Middle Lobe Bronchus, Right 6 Lower Lobe Bronchus, Right 7 Main Bronchus, Left 8 Upper Lobe Bronchus, Left 9 Lingula Bronchus B Lower Lobe Bronchus, Left	7 Via Natural or Artificial Opening 8 Via Natural or Artificial Opening Endoscopic		D Intraluminal Device Z No Device	Z No Qualifier

Section	0	Medical and Surgical		
Body System	B	Respiratory System		
Operation	W	Revision: Correcting, to the extent possible, a portion of a malfunctioning device or the position of a displaced device		
Body Part (Character 4)	**Approach (Character 5)**		**Device (Character 6)**	**Qualifier (Character 7)**
0 Tracheobronchial Tree	0 Open 3 Percutaneous 4 Percutaneous Endoscopic 7 Via Natural or Artificial Opening 8 Via Natural or Artificial Opening Endoscopic X External		0 Drainage Device 2 Monitoring Device 3 Infusion Device 7 Autologous Tissue Substitute C Extraluminal Device D Intraluminal Device J Synthetic Substitute K Nonautologous Tissue Substitute	Z No Qualifier
1 Trachea	0 Open 3 Percutaneous 4 Percutaneous Endoscopic 7 Via Natural or Artificial Opening 8 Via Natural or Artificial Opening Endoscopic X External		0 Drainage Device 2 Monitoring Device 7 Autologous Tissue Substitute C Extraluminal Device D Intraluminal Device F Tracheostomy Device J Synthetic Substitute K Nonautologous Tissue Substitute	Z No Qualifier
K Lung, Right L Lung, Left	0 Open 3 Percutaneous 4 Percutaneous Endoscopic 7 Via Natural or Artificial Opening 8 Via Natural or Artificial Opening Endoscopic X External		0 Drainage Device 2 Monitoring Device 3 Infusion Device	Z No Qualifier
Q Pleura	0 Open 3 Percutaneous 4 Percutaneous Endoscopic 7 Via Natural or Artificial Opening 8 Via Natural or Artificial Opening Endoscopic X External		0 Drainage Device 2 Monitoring Device	Z No Qualifier
T Diaphragm	0 Open 3 Percutaneous 4 Percutaneous Endoscopic 7 Via Natural or Artificial Opening 8 Via Natural or Artificial Opening Endoscopic X External		0 Drainage Device 2 Monitoring Device 7 Autologous Tissue Substitute J Synthetic Substitute K Nonautologous Tissue Substitute M Diaphragmatic Pacemaker Lead	Z No Qualifier

Section	0	Medical and Surgical			
Body System	B	Respiratory System			
Operation	Y	Transplantation: Putting in or on all or a portion of a living body part taken from another individual or animal to physically take the place and/or function of all or a portion of a similar body part			

Body Part (Character 4)	Approach (Character 5)	Device (Character 6)	Qualifier (Character 7)
C Upper Lung Lobe, Right	0 Open	Z No Device	0 Allogeneic
D Middle Lung Lobe, Right			1 Syngeneic
F Lower Lung Lobe, Right			2 Zooplastic
G Upper Lung Lobe, Left			
H Lung Lingula			
J Lower Lung Lobe, Left			
K Lung, Right			
L Lung, Left			
M Lungs, Bilateral			

Section	0	Medical and Surgical		
Body System	C	Mouth and Throat		
Operation	0	Alteration: Modifying the anatomic structure of a body part without affecting the function of the body part		

Body Part (Character 4)	Approach (Character 5)	Device (Character 6)	Qualifier (Character 7)
0 Upper Lip **1** Lower Lip	**X** External	**7** Autologous Tissue Substitute **J** Synthetic Substitute **K** Nonautologous Tissue Substitute **Z** No Device	**Z** No Qualifier

Section	0	Medical and Surgical		
Body System	C	Mouth and Throat		
Operation	2	Change: Taking out or off a device from a body part and putting back an identical or similar device in or on the same body part without cutting or puncturing the skin or a mucous membrane		

Body Part (Character 4)	Approach (Character 5)	Device (Character 6)	Qualifier (Character 7)
A Salivary Gland **S** Larynx **Y** Mouth and Throat	**X** External	**0** Drainage Device **Y** Other Device	**Z** No Qualifier

Section	0	Medical and Surgical		
Body System	C	Mouth and Throat		
Operation	5	Destruction: Physical eradication of all or a portion of a body part by the direct use of energy, force, or a destructive agent		

Body Part (Character 4)	Approach (Character 5)	Device (Character 6)	Qualifier (Character 7)
0 Upper Lip **1** Lower Lip **2** Hard Palate **3** Soft Palate **4** Buccal Mucosa **5** Upper Gingiva **6** Lower Gingiva **7** Tongue **N** Uvula **P** Tonsils **Q** Adenoids	**0** Open **3** Percutaneous **X** External	**Z** No Device	**Z** No Qualifier
8 Parotid Gland, Right **9** Parotid Gland, Left **B** Parotid Duct, Right **C** Parotid Duct, Left **D** Sublingual Gland, Right **F** Sublingual Gland, Left **G** Submaxillary Gland, Right **H** Submaxillary Gland, Left **J** Minor Salivary Gland	**0** Open **3** Percutaneous	**Z** No Device	**Z** No Qualifier
M Pharynx **R** Epiglottis **S** Larynx **T** Vocal Cord, Right **V** Vocal Cord, Left	**0** Open **3** Percutaneous **4** Percutaneous Endoscopic **7** Via Natural or Artificial Opening **8** Via Natural or Artificial Opening Endoscopic	**Z** No Device	**Z** No Qualifier
W Upper Tooth **X** Lower Tooth	**0** Open **X** External	**Z** No Device	**0** Single **1** Multiple **2** All

Section	0	Medical and Surgical		
Body System	C	Mouth and Throat		
Operation	7	Dilation: Expanding an orifice or the lumen of a tubular body part		

Body Part (Character 4)	Approach (Character 5)	Device (Character 6)	Qualifier (Character 7)
B Parotid Duct, Right **C** Parotid Duct, Left	**0** Open **3** Percutaneous **7** Via Natural or Artificial Opening	**D** Intraluminal Device **Z** No Device	**Z** No Qualifier
M Pharynx	**7** Via Natural or Artificial Opening **8** Via Natural or Artificial Opening Endoscopic	**D** Intraluminal Device **Z** No Device	**Z** No Qualifier
S Larynx	**0** Open **3** Percutaneous **4** Percutaneous Endoscopic **7** Via Natural or Artificial Opening **8** Via Natural or Artificial Opening Endoscopic	**D** Intraluminal Device **Z** No Device	**Z** No Qualifier

Section	0	Medical and Surgical		
Body System	C	Mouth and Throat		
Operation	9	Drainage: Taking or letting out fluids and/or gases from a body part		

Body Part (Character 4)	Approach (Character 5)	Device (Character 6)	Qualifier (Character 7)
0 Upper Lip 1 Lower Lip 2 Hard Palate 3 Soft Palate 4 Buccal Mucosa 5 Upper Gingiva 6 Lower Gingiva 7 Tongue N Uvula P Tonsils Q Adenoids	0 Open 3 Percutaneous X External	0 Drainage Device	Z No Qualifier
0 Upper Lip 1 Lower Lip 2 Hard Palate 3 Soft Palate 4 Buccal Mucosa 5 Upper Gingiva 6 Lower Gingiva 7 Tongue N Uvula P Tonsils Q Adenoids	0 Open 3 Percutaneous X External	Z No Device	X Diagnostic Z No Qualifier
8 Parotid Gland, Right 9 Parotid Gland, Left B Parotid Duct, Right C Parotid Duct, Left D Sublingual Gland, Right F Sublingual Gland, Left G Submaxillary Gland, Right H Submaxillary Gland, Left J Minor Salivary Gland	0 Open 3 Percutaneous	0 Drainage Device	Z No Qualifier

Section	0	Medical and Surgical		
Body System	C	Mouth and Throat		
Operation	9	Drainage: Taking or letting out fluids and/or gases from a body part		

Body Part (Character 4)	Approach (Character 5)	Device (Character 6)	Qualifier (Character 7)
8 Parotid Gland, Right 9 Parotid Gland, Left B Parotid Duct, Right C Parotid Duct, Left D Sublingual Gland, Right F Sublingual Gland, Left G Submaxillary Gland, Right H Submaxillary Gland, Left J Minor Salivary Gland	0 Open 3 Percutaneous	Z No Device	X Diagnostic Z No Qualifier
M Pharynx R Epiglottis S Larynx T Vocal Cord, Right V Vocal Cord, Left	0 Open 3 Percutaneous 4 Percutaneous Endoscopic 7 Via Natural or Artificial Opening 8 Via Natural or Artificial Opening Endoscopic	0 Drainage Device	Z No Qualifier
M Pharynx R Epiglottis S Larynx T Vocal Cord, Right V Vocal Cord, Left	0 Open 3 Percutaneous 4 Percutaneous Endoscopic 7 Via Natural or Artificial Opening 8 Via Natural or Artificial Opening Endoscopic	Z No Device	X Diagnostic Z No Qualifier
W Upper Tooth X Lower Tooth	0 Open X External	0 Drainage Device Z No Device	0 Single 1 Multiple 2 All

Section	0	Medical and Surgical		
Body System	C	Mouth and Throat		
Operation	B	Excision: Cutting out or off, without replacement, a portion of a body part		
Body Part (Character 4)		**Approach (Character 5)**	**Device (Character 6)**	**Qualifier (Character 7)**
0 Upper Lip 1 Lower Lip 2 Hard Palate 3 Soft Palate 4 Buccal Mucosa 5 Upper Gingiva 6 Lower Gingiva 7 Tongue N Uvula P Tonsils Q Adenoids		0 Open 3 Percutaneous X External	Z No Device	X Diagnostic Z No Qualifier
8 Parotid Gland, Right 9 Parotid Gland, Left B Parotid Duct, Right C Parotid Duct, Left D Sublingual Gland, Right F Sublingual Gland, Left G Submaxillary Gland, Right H Submaxillary Gland, Left J Minor Salivary Gland		0 Open 3 Percutaneous	Z No Device	X Diagnostic Z No Qualifier
M Pharynx R Epiglottis S Larynx T Vocal Cord, Right V Vocal Cord, Left		0 Open 3 Percutaneous 4 Percutaneous Endoscopic 7 Via Natural or Artificial Opening 8 Via Natural or Artificial Opening Endoscopic	Z No Device	X Diagnostic Z No Qualifier
W Upper Tooth X Lower Tooth		0 Open X External	Z No Device	0 Single 1 Multiple 2 All

Section	0	Medical and Surgical		
Body System	C	Mouth and Throat		
Operation	C	Extirpation: Taking or cutting out solid matter from a body part		
Body Part (Character 4)		**Approach (Character 5)**	**Device (Character 6)**	**Qualifier (Character 7)**
0 Upper Lip 1 Lower Lip 2 Hard Palate 3 Soft Palate 4 Buccal Mucosa 5 Upper Gingiva 6 Lower Gingiva 7 Tongue N Uvula P Tonsils Q Adenoids		0 Open 3 Percutaneous X External	Z No Device	Z No Qualifier
8 Parotid Gland, Right 9 Parotid Gland, Left B Parotid Duct, Right C Parotid Duct, Left D Sublingual Gland, Right F Sublingual Gland, Left G Submaxillary Gland, Right H Submaxillary Gland, Left J Minor Salivary Gland		0 Open 3 Percutaneous	Z No Device	Z No Qualifier
M Pharynx R Epiglottis S Larynx T Vocal Cord, Right V Vocal Cord, Left		0 Open 3 Percutaneous 4 Percutaneous Endoscopic 7 Via Natural or Artificial Opening 8 Via Natural or Artificial Opening Endoscopic	Z No Device	Z No Qualifier
W Upper Tooth X Lower Tooth		0 Open X External	Z No Device	0 Single 1 Multiple 2 All

Section	0	Medical and Surgical		
Body System	C	Mouth and Throat		
Operation	D	Extraction: Pulling or stripping out or off all or a portion of a body part by the use of force		
Body Part (Character 4)		Approach (Character 5)	Device (Character 6)	Qualifier (Character 7)
T Vocal Cord, Right V Vocal Cord, Left		0 Open 3 Percutaneous 4 Percutaneous Endoscopic 7 Via Natural or Artificial Opening 8 Via Natural or Artificial Opening Endoscopic	Z No Device	Z No Qualifier
W Upper Tooth X Lower Tooth		X External	Z No Device	0 Single 1 Multiple 2 All

Section	0	Medical and Surgical		
Body System	C	Mouth and Throat		
Operation	F	Fragmentation: Breaking solid matter in a body part into pieces		
Body Part (Character 4)		Approach (Character 5)	Device (Character 6)	Qualifier (Character 7)
B Parotid Duct, Right C Parotid Duct, Left		0 Open 3 Percutaneous 7 Via Natural or Artificial Opening X External	Z No Device	Z No Qualifier

Section	0	Medical and Surgical		
Body System	C	Mouth and Throat		
Operation	H	Insertion: Putting in a nonbiological appliance that monitors, assists, performs, or prevents a physiological function but does not physically take the place of a body part		
Body Part (Character 4)		Approach (Character 5)	Device (Character 6)	Qualifier (Character 7)
7 Tongue		0 Open 3 Percutaneous X External	1 Radioactive Element	Z No Qualifier
Y Mouth and Throat		7 Via Natural or Artificial Opening 8 Via Natural or Artificial Opening Endoscopic	B Intraluminal Device, Airway	Z No Qualifier

Section	0	Medical and Surgical		
Body System	C	Mouth and Throat		
Operation	J	Inspection: Visually and/or manually exploring a body part		
Body Part (Character 4)		Approach (Character 5)	Device (Character 6)	Qualifier (Character 7)
A Salivary Gland		0 Open 3 Percutaneous X External	Z No Device	Z No Qualifier
S Larynx Y Mouth and Throat		0 Open 3 Percutaneous 4 Percutaneous Endoscopic 7 Via Natural or Artificial Opening 8 Via Natural or Artificial Opening Endoscopic X External	Z No Device	Z No Qualifier

Section	0	Medical and Surgical		
Body System	C	Mouth and Throat		
Operation	L	Occlusion: Completely closing an orifice or the lumen of a tubular body part		
Body Part (Character 4)		Approach (Character 5)	Device (Character 6)	Qualifier (Character 7)
B Parotid Duct, Right C Parotid Duct, Left		0 Open 3 Percutaneous 4 Percutaneous Endoscopic	C Extraluminal Device D Intraluminal Device Z No Device	Z No Qualifier
B Parotid Duct, Right C Parotid Duct, Left		7 Via Natural or Artificial Opening 8 Via Natural or Artificial Opening Endoscopic	D Intraluminal Device Z No Device	Z No Qualifier

Section	0	Medical and Surgical		
Body System	C	Mouth and Throat		
Operation	M	Reattachment Putting back in or on all or a portion of a separated body part to its normal location or other suitable location		

Body Part (Character 4)	Approach (Character 5)	Device (Character 6)	Qualifier (Character 7)
0 Upper Lip 1 Lower Lip 3 Soft Palate 7 Tongue N Uvula	0 Open	Z No Device	Z No Qualifier
W Upper Tooth X Lower Tooth	0 Open X External	Z No Device	0 Single 1 Multiple 2 All

Section	0	Medical and Surgical		
Body System	C	Mouth and Throat		
Operation	N	Release: Freeing a body part from an abnormal physical constraint by cutting or by the use of force		

Body Part (Character 4)	Approach (Character 5)	Device (Character 6)	Qualifier (Character 7)
0 Upper Lip 1 Lower Lip 2 Hard Palate 3 Soft Palate 4 Buccal Mucosa 5 Upper Gingiva 6 Lower Gingiva 7 Tongue N Uvula P Tonsils Q Adenoids	0 Open 3 Percutaneous X External	Z No Device	Z No Qualifier
8 Parotid Gland, Right 9 Parotid Gland, Left B Parotid Duct, Right C Parotid Duct, Left D Sublingual Gland, Right F Sublingual Gland, Left G Submaxillary Gland, Right H Submaxillary Gland, Left J Minor Salivary Gland	0 Open 3 Percutaneous	Z No Device	Z No Qualifier
M Pharynx R Epiglottis S Larynx T Vocal Cord, Right V Vocal Cord, Left	0 Open 3 Percutaneous 4 Percutaneous Endoscopic 7 Via Natural or Artificial Opening 8 Via Natural or Artificial Opening Endoscopic	Z No Device	Z No Qualifier
W Upper Tooth X Lower Tooth	0 Open X External	Z No Device	0 Single 1 Multiple 2 All

Section	0	Medical and Surgical		
Body System	C	Mouth and Throat		
Operation	P	Removal: Taking out or off a device from a body part		

Body Part (Character 4)	Approach (Character 5)	Device (Character 6)	Qualifier (Character 7)
A Salivary Gland	0 Open 3 Percutaneous	0 Drainage Device C Extraluminal Device	Z No Qualifier
S Larynx	0 Open 3 Percutaneous 7 Via Natural or Artificial Opening 8 Via Natural or Artificial Opening Endoscopic X External	0 Drainage Device 7 Autologous Tissue Substitute D Intraluminal Device J Synthetic Substitute K Nonautologous Tissue Substitute	Z No Qualifier
Y Mouth and Throat	0 Open 3 Percutaneous 7 Via Natural or Artificial Opening 8 Via Natural or Artificial Opening Endoscopic X External	0 Drainage Device 1 Radioactive Element 7 Autologous Tissue Substitute D Intraluminal Device J Synthetic Substitute K Nonautologous Tissue Substitute	Z No Qualifier

Section	0	Medical and Surgical
Body System	C	Mouth and Throat
Operation	Q	Repair: Restoring, to the extent possible, a body part to its normal anatomic structure and function

Body Part (Character 4)	Approach (Character 5)	Device (Character 6)	Qualifier (Character 7)
0 Upper Lip 1 Lower Lip 2 Hard Palate 3 Soft Palate 4 Buccal Mucosa 5 Upper Gingiva 6 Lower Gingiva 7 Tongue N Uvula P Tonsils Q Adenoids	0 Open 3 Percutaneous X External	Z No Device	Z No Qualifier
8 Parotid Gland, Right 9 Parotid Gland, Left B Parotid Duct, Right C Parotid Duct, Left D Sublingual Gland, Right F Sublingual Gland, Left G Submaxillary Gland, Right H Submaxillary Gland, Left J Minor Salivary Gland	0 Open 3 Percutaneous	Z No Device	Z No Qualifier
M Pharynx R Epiglottis S Larynx T Vocal Cord, Right V Vocal Cord, Left	0 Open 3 Percutaneous 4 Percutaneous Endoscopic 7 Via Natural or Artificial Opening 8 Via Natural or Artificial Opening Endoscopic	Z No Device	Z No Qualifier
W Upper Tooth X Lower Tooth	0 Open X External	Z No Device	0 Single 1 Multiple 2 All

Section	0	Medical and Surgical
Body System	C	Mouth and Throat
Operation	R	Replacement: Putting in or on biological or synthetic material that physically takes the place and/or function of all or a portion of a body part

Body Part (Character 4)	Approach (Character 5)	Device (Character 6)	Qualifier (Character 7)
0 Upper Lip 1 Lower Lip 2 Hard Palate 3 Soft Palate 4 Buccal Mucosa 5 Upper Gingiva 6 Lower Gingiva 7 Tongue N Uvula	0 Open 3 Percutaneous X External	7 Autologous Tissue Substitute J Synthetic Substitute K Nonautologous Tissue Substitute	Z No Qualifier
B Parotid Duct, Right C Parotid Duct, Left	0 Open 3 Percutaneous	7 Autologous Tissue Substitute J Synthetic Substitute K Nonautologous Tissue Substitute	Z No Qualifier
M Pharynx R Epiglottis S Larynx T Vocal Cord, Right V Vocal Cord, Left	0 Open 7 Via Natural or Artificial Opening 8 Via Natural or Artificial Opening Endoscopic	7 Autologous Tissue Substitute J Synthetic Substitute K Nonautologous Tissue Substitute	Z No Qualifier
W Upper Tooth X Lower Tooth	0 Open X External	7 Autologous Tissue Substitute J Synthetic Substitute K Nonautologous Tissue Substitute	0 Single 1 Multiple 2 All

Section	0	Medical and Surgical
Body System	C	Mouth and Throat
Operation	S	Reposition: Moving to its normal location, or other suitable location, all or a portion of a body part

Body Part (Character 4)	Approach (Character 5)	Device (Character 6)	Qualifier (Character 7)
0 Upper Lip 1 Lower Lip 2 Hard Palate 3 Soft Palate 7 Tongue N Uvula	0 Open X External	Z No Device	Z No Qualifier
B Parotid Duct, Right C Parotid Duct, Left	0 Open 3 Percutaneous	Z No Device	Z No Qualifier
R Epiglottis T Vocal Cord, Right V Vocal Cord, Left	0 Open 7 Via Natural or Artificial Opening 8 Via Natural or Artificial Opening Endoscopic	Z No Device	Z No Qualifier
W Upper Tooth X Lower Tooth	0 Open X External	5 External Fixation Device Z No Device	0 Single 1 Multiple 2 All

Section	0	Medical and Surgical
Body System	C	Mouth and Throat
Operation	T	Resection: Cutting out or off, without replacement, all of a body part

Body Part (Character 4)	Approach (Character 5)	Device (Character 6)	Qualifier (Character 7)
0 Upper Lip 1 Lower Lip 2 Hard Palate 3 Soft Palate 7 Tongue N Uvula P Tonsils Q Adenoids	0 Open X External	Z No Device	Z No Qualifier
8 Parotid Gland, Right 9 Parotid Gland, Left B Parotid Duct, Right C Parotid Duct, Left D Sublingual Gland, Right F Sublingual Gland, Left G Submaxillary Gland, Right H Submaxillary Gland, Left J Minor Salivary Gland	0 Open	Z No Device	Z No Qualifier
M Pharynx R Epiglottis S Larynx T Vocal Cord, Right V Vocal Cord, Left	0 Open 4 Percutaneous Endoscopic 7 Via Natural or Artificial Opening 8 Via Natural or Artificial Opening Endoscopic	Z No Device	Z No Qualifier
W Upper Tooth X Lower Tooth	0 Open	Z No Device	0 Single 1 Multiple 2 All

Section	0	Medical and Surgical
Body System	C	Mouth and Throat
Operation	U	Supplement: Putting in or on biological or synthetic material that physically reinforces and/or augments the function of a portion of a body part

Body Part (Character 4)	Approach (Character 5)	Device (Character 6)	Qualifier (Character 7)
0 Upper Lip 1 Lower Lip 2 Hard Palate 3 Soft Palate 4 Buccal Mucosa 5 Upper Gingiva 6 Lower Gingiva 7 Tongue N Uvula	0 Open 3 Percutaneous X External	7 Autologous Tissue Substitute J Synthetic Substitute K Nonautologous Tissue Substitute	Z No Qualifier
M Pharynx R Epiglottis S Larynx T Vocal Cord, Right V Vocal Cord, Left	0 Open 7 Via Natural or Artificial Opening 8 Via Natural or Artificial Opening Endoscopic	7 Autologous Tissue Substitute J Synthetic Substitute K Nonautologous Tissue Substitute	Z No Qualifier

Section	0	Medical and Surgical		
Body System	C	Mouth and Throat		
Operation	V	Restriction: Partially closing an orifice or the lumen of a tubular body part		
Body Part (Character 4)		**Approach (Character 5)**	**Device (Character 6)**	**Qualifier (Character 7)**
B Parotid Duct, Right **C** Parotid Duct, Left		**0** Open **3** Percutaneous	**C** Extraluminal Device **D** Intraluminal Device **Z** No Device	**Z** No Qualifier
B Parotid Duct, Right **C** Parotid Duct, Left		**7** Via Natural or Artificial Opening **8** Via Natural or Artificial Opening Endoscopic	**D** Intraluminal Device **Z** No Device	**Z** No Qualifier

Section	0	Medical and Surgical		
Body System	C	Mouth and Throat		
Operation	W	Revision: Correcting, to the extent possible, a portion of a malfunctioning device or the position of a displaced device		
Body Part (Character 4)		**Approach (Character 5)**	**Device (Character 6)**	**Qualifier (Character 7)**
A Salivary Gland		**0** Open **3** Percutaneous **X** External	**0** Drainage Device **C** Extraluminal Device	**Z** No Qualifier
S Larynx		**0** Open **3** Percutaneous **7** Via Natural or Artificial Opening **8** Via Natural or Artificial Opening Endoscopic **X** External	**0** Drainage Device **7** Autologous Tissue Substitute **D** Intraluminal Device **J** Synthetic Substitute **K** Nonautologous Tissue Substitute	**Z** No Qualifier
Y Mouth and Throat		**0** Open **3** Percutaneous **7** Via Natural or Artificial Opening **8** Via Natural or Artificial Opening Endoscopic **X** External	**0** Drainage Device **1** Radioactive Element **7** Autologous Tissue Substitute **D** Intraluminal Device **J** Synthetic Substitute **K** Nonautologous Tissue Substitute	**Z** No Qualifier

Section	0	Medical and Surgical		
Body System	C	Mouth and Throat		
Operation	X	Transfer: Moving, without taking out, all or a portion of a body part to another location to take over the function of all or a portion of a body part		
Body Part (Character 4)		**Approach (Character 5)**	**Device (Character 6)**	**Qualifier (Character 7)**
0 Upper Lip **1** Lower Lip **3** Soft Palate **4** Buccal Mucosa **5** Upper Gingiva **6** Lower Gingiva **7** Tongue		**0** Open **X** External	**Z** No Device	**Z** No Qualifier

Section	0	Medical and Surgical
Body System	D	Gastrointestinal System
Operation	1	Bypass: Altering the route of passage of the contents of a tubular body part

Body Part (Character 4)	Approach (Character 5)	Device (Character 6)	Qualifier (Character 7)
1 Esophagus, Upper 2 Esophagus, Middle 3 Esophagus, Lower 5 Esophagus	0 Open 4 Percutaneous Endoscopic 8 Via Natural or Artificial Opening Endoscopic	7 Autologous Tissue Substitute J Synthetic Substitute K Nonautologous Tissue Substitute Z No Device	4 Cutaneous 6 Stomach 9 Duodenum A Jejunum B Ileum
1 Esophagus, Upper 2 Esophagus, Middle 3 Esophagus, Lower 5 Esophagus	3 Percutaneous	J Synthetic Substitute	4 Cutaneous
6 Stomach 9 Duodenum	0 Open 4 Percutaneous Endoscopic 8 Via Natural or Artificial Opening Endoscopic	7 Autologous Tissue Substitute J Synthetic Substitute K Nonautologous Tissue Substitute Z No Device	4 Cutaneous 9 Duodenum A Jejunum B Ileum L Transverse Colon
6 Stomach 9 Duodenum	3 Percutaneous	J Synthetic Substitute	4 Cutaneous
A Jejunum	0 Open 4 Percutaneous Endoscopic 8 Via Natural or Artificial Opening Endoscopic	7 Autologous Tissue Substitute J Synthetic Substitute K Nonautologous Tissue Substitute Z No Device	4 Cutaneous A Jejunum B Ileum H Cecum K Ascending Colon L Transverse Colon M Descending Colon N Sigmoid Colon P Rectum Q Anus
A Jejunum	3 Percutaneous	J Synthetic Substitute	4 Cutaneous
B Ileum	0 Open 4 Percutaneous Endoscopic 8 Via Natural or Artificial Opening Endoscopic	7 Autologous Tissue Substitute J Synthetic Substitute K Nonautologous Tissue Substitute Z No Device	4 Cutaneous B Ileum H Cecum K Ascending Colon L Transverse Colon M Descending Colon N Sigmoid Colon P Rectum Q Anus

Section	0	Medical and Surgical
Body System	D	Gastrointestinal System
Operation	1	Bypass: Altering the route of passage of the contents of a tubular body part

Body Part (Character 4)	Approach (Character 5)	Device (Character 6)	Qualifier (Character 7)
B Ileum	3 Percutaneous	J Synthetic Substitute	4 Cutaneous
H Cecum	0 Open 4 Percutaneous Endoscopic 8 Via Natural or Artificial Opening Endoscopic	7 Autologous Tissue Substitute J Synthetic Substitute K Nonautologous Tissue Substitute Z No Device	4 Cutaneous H Cecum K Ascending Colon L Transverse Colon M Descending Colon N Sigmoid Colon P Rectum
H Cecum	3 Percutaneous	J Synthetic Substitute	4 Cutaneous
K Ascending Colon	0 Open 4 Percutaneous Endoscopic 8 Via Natural or Artificial Opening Endoscopic	7 Autologous Tissue Substitute J Synthetic Substitute K Nonautologous Tissue Substitute Z No Device	4 Cutaneous K Ascending Colon L Transverse Colon M Descending Colon N Sigmoid Colon P Rectum
K Ascending Colon	3 Percutaneous	J Synthetic Substitute	4 Cutaneous
L Transverse Colon	0 Open 4 Percutaneous Endoscopic 8 Via Natural or Artificial Opening Endoscopic	7 Autologous Tissue Substitute J Synthetic Substitute K Nonautologous Tissue Substitute Z No Device	4 Cutaneous L Transverse Colon M Descending Colon N Sigmoid Colon P Rectum
L Transverse Colon	3 Percutaneous	J Synthetic Substitute	4 Cutaneous
M Descending Colon	0 Open 4 Percutaneous Endoscopic 8 Via Natural or Artificial Opening Endoscopic	7 Autologous Tissue Substitute J Synthetic Substitute K Nonautologous Tissue Substitute Z No Device	4 Cutaneous M Descending Colon N Sigmoid Colon P Rectum

Section	0	Medical and Surgical	
Body System	D	Gastrointestinal System	[continued]
Operation	1	Bypass: Altering the route of passage of the contents of a tubular body part	

Body Part (Character 4)	Body Part (Character 4)	Body Part (Character 4)	Body Part (Character 4)
M Descending Colon	3 Percutaneous	J Synthetic Substitute	4 Cutaneous
N Sigmoid Colon	0 Open 4 Percutaneous Endoscopic 8 Via Natural or Artificial Opening Endoscopic	7 Autologous Tissue Substitute J Synthetic Substitute K Nonautologous Tissue Substitute Z No Device	4 Cutaneous N Sigmoid Colon P Rectum
N Sigmoid Colon	3 Percutaneous	J Synthetic Substitute	4 Cutaneous

Section	0	Medical and Surgical
Body System	D	Gastrointestinal System
Operation	2	Change: Taking out or off a device from a body part and putting back an identical or similar device in or on the same body part without cutting or puncturing the skin or a mucous membrane

Body Part (Character 4)	Body Part (Character 4)	Body Part (Character 4)	Body Part (Character 4)
0 Upper Intestinal Tract D Lower Intestinal Tract	X External	0 Drainage Device U Feeding Device Y Other Device	Z No Qualifier
U Omentum V Mesentery W Peritoneum	X External	0 Drainage Device Y Other Device	Z No Qualifier

Section	0	Medical and Surgical
Body System	D	Gastrointestinal System
Operation	5	Destruction: Physical eradication of all or a portion of a body part by the direct use of energy, force, or a destructive agent

Body Part (Character 4)	Body Part (Character 4)	Body Part (Character 4)	Body Part (Character 4)
1 Esophagus, Upper 2 Esophagus, Middle 3 Esophagus, Lower 4 Esophagogastric Junction 5 Esophagus 6 Stomach 7 Stomach, Pylorus 8 Small Intestine 9 Duodenum A Jejunum B Ileum C Ileocecal Valve E Large Intestine F Large Intestine, Right G Large Intestine, Left H Cecum J Appendix K Ascending Colon L Transverse Colon M Descending Colon N Sigmoid Colon P Rectum	0 Open 3 Percutaneous 4 Percutaneous Endoscopic 7 Via Natural or Artificial Opening 8 Via Natural or Artificial Opening Endoscopic	Z No Device	Z No Qualifier
Q Anus	0 Open 3 Percutaneous 4 Percutaneous Endoscopic 7 Via Natural or Artificial Opening 8 Via Natural or Artificial Opening Endoscopic X External	Z No Device	Z No Qualifier
R Anal Sphincter S Greater Omentum T Lesser Omentum V Mesentery W Peritoneum	0 Open 3 Percutaneous 4 Percutaneous Endoscopic	Z No Device	Z No Qualifier

Section	0	Medical and Surgical		
Body System	D	Gastrointestinal System		
Operation	7	Dilation: Expanding an orifice or the lumen of a tubular body part		
Body Part (Character 4)		**Body Part (Character 4)**	**Body Part (Character 4)**	**Body Part (Character 4)**
1 Esophagus, Upper 2 Esophagus, Middle 3 Esophagus, Lower 4 Esophagogastric Junction 5 Esophagus 6 Stomach 7 Stomach, Pylorus 8 Small Intestine 9 Duodenum A Jejunum B Ileum C Ileocecal Valve E Large Intestine F Large Intestine, Right G Large Intestine, Left H Cecum K Ascending Colon L Transverse Colon M Descending Colon N Sigmoid Colon P Rectum Q Anus		0 Open 3 Percutaneous 4 Percutaneous Endoscopic 7 Via Natural or Artificial Opening 8 Via Natural or Artificial Opening Endoscopic	D Intraluminal Device Z No Device	Z No Qualifier

Section	0	Medical and Surgical		
Body System	D	Gastrointestinal System		
Operation	8	Division: Cutting into a body part, without draining fluids and/or gases from the body part, in order to separate or transect a body part		
Body Part (Character 4)		**Body Part (Character 4)**	**Body Part (Character 4)**	**Body Part (Character 4)**
4 Esophagogastric Junction 7 Stomach, Pylorus		0 Open 3 Percutaneous 4 Percutaneous Endoscopic 7 Via Natural or Artificial Opening 8 Via Natural or Artificial Opening Endoscopic	Z No Device	Z No Qualifier
R Anal Sphincter		0 Open 3 Percutaneous	Z No Device	Z No Qualifier

Section	0	Medical and Surgical		
Body System	D	Gastrointestinal System		
Operation	9	Drainage: Taking or letting out fluids and/or gases from a body part		
Body Part (Character 4)		**Body Part (Character 4)**	**Body Part (Character 4)**	**Body Part (Character 4)**
1 Esophagus, Upper 2 Esophagus, Middle 3 Esophagus, Lower 4 Esophagogastric Junction 5 Esophagus 6 Stomach 7 Stomach, Pylorus 8 Small Intestine 9 Duodenum A Jejunum B Ileum C Ileocecal Valve E Large Intestine F Large Intestine, Right G Large Intestine, Left H Cecum J Appendix K Ascending Colon L Transverse Colon M Descending Colon N Sigmoid Colon P Rectum		0 Open 3 Percutaneous 4 Percutaneous Endoscopic 7 Via Natural or Artificial Opening 8 Via Natural or Artificial Opening Endoscopic	0 Drainage Device	Z No Qualifier

Section	0	Medical and Surgical
Body System	D	Gastrointestinal System
Operation	9	Drainage: Taking or letting out fluids and/or gases from a body part

Body Part (Character 4)	Body Part (Character 4)	Body Part (Character 4)	Body Part (Character 4)
1 Esophagus, Upper **2** Esophagus, Middle **3** Esophagus, Lower **4** Esophagogastric Junction **5** Esophagus **6** Stomach **7** Stomach, Pylorus **8** Small Intestine **9** Duodenum **A** Jejunum **B** Ileum **C** Ileocecal Valve **E** Large Intestine **F** Large Intestine, Right **G** Large Intestine, Left **H** Cecum **J** Appendix **K** Ascending Colon **L** Transverse Colon **M** Descending Colon **N** Sigmoid Colon **P** Rectum	**0** Open **3** Percutaneous **4** Percutaneous Endoscopic **7** Via Natural or Artificial Opening **8** Via Natural or Artificial Opening Endoscopic	**Z** No Device	**X** Diagnostic **Z** No Qualifier
Q Anus	**0** Open **3** Percutaneous **4** Percutaneous Endoscopic **7** Via Natural or Artificial Opening **8** Via Natural or Artificial Opening Endoscopic **X** External	**0** Drainage Device	**Z** No Qualifier
Q Anus	**0** Open **3** Percutaneous **4** Percutaneous Endoscopic **7** Via Natural or Artificial Opening **8** Via Natural or Artificial Opening Endoscopic **X** External	**Z** No Device	**X** Diagnostic **Z** No Qualifier

Section	0	Medical and Surgical
Body System	D	Gastrointestinal System
Operation	9	Drainage: Taking or letting out fluids and/or gases from a body part

Body Part (Character 4)	Body Part (Character 4)	Body Part (Character 4)	Body Part (Character 4)
R Anal Sphincter **S** Greater Omentum **T** Lesser Omentum **V** Mesentery **W** Peritoneum	**0** Open **3** Percutaneous **4** Percutaneous Endoscopic	**0** Drainage Device	**Z** No Qualifier
R Anal Sphincter **S** Greater Omentum **T** Lesser Omentum **V** Mesentery **W** Peritoneum	**0** Open **3** Percutaneous **4** Percutaneous Endoscopic	**Z** No Device	**X** Diagnostic **Z** No Qualifier

Section	0	Medical and Surgical		
Body System	D	Gastrointestinal System		
Operation	B	Excision: Cutting out or off, without replacement, a portion of a body part		
Body Part (Character 4)	**Body Part (Character 4)**		**Body Part (Character 4)**	**Body Part (Character 4)**
1 Esophagus, Upper 2 Esophagus, Middle 3 Esophagus, Lower 4 Esophagogastric Junction 5 Esophagus 7 Stomach, Pylorus 8 Small Intestine 9 Duodenum A Jejunum B Ileum C Ileocecal Valve E Large Intestine F Large Intestine, Right G Large Intestine, Left H Cecum J Appendix K Ascending Colon L Transverse Colon M Descending Colon N Sigmoid Colon P Rectum	0 Open 3 Percutaneous 4 Percutaneous Endoscopic 7 Via Natural or Artificial Opening 8 Via Natural or Artificial Opening Endoscopic		Z No Device	X Diagnostic Z No Qualifier
6 Stomach	0 Open 3 Percutaneous 4 Percutaneous Endoscopic 7 Via Natural or Artificial Opening 8 Via Natural or Artificial Opening Endoscopic		Z No Device	3 Vertical X Diagnostic Z No Qualifier
Q Anus	0 Open 3 Percutaneous 4 Percutaneous Endoscopic 7 Via Natural or Artificial Opening 8 Via Natural or Artificial Opening Endoscopic X External		Z No Device	X Diagnostic Z No Qualifier

Section	0	Medical and Surgical		
Body System	D	Gastrointestinal System		
Operation	B	Excision: Cutting out or off, without replacement, a portion of a body part		
Body Part (Character 4)	**Body Part (Character 4)**		**Body Part (Character 4)**	**Body Part (Character 4)**
R Anal Sphincter S Greater Omentum T Lesser Omentum V Mesentery W Peritoneum	0 Open 3 Percutaneous 4 Percutaneous Endoscopic		Z No Device	X Diagnostic Z No Qualifier

Section	0	Medical and Surgical		
Body System	D	Gastrointestinal System		
Operation	C	Extirpation: Taking or cutting out solid matter from a body part		

Body Part (Character 4)	Body Part (Character 4)	Body Part (Character 4)	Body Part (Character 4)
1 Esophagus, Upper 2 Esophagus, Middle 3 Esophagus, Lower 4 Esophagogastric Junction 5 Esophagus 6 Stomach 7 Stomach, Pylorus 8 Small Intestine 9 Duodenum A Jejunum B Ileum C Ileocecal Valve E Large Intestine F Large Intestine, Right G Large Intestine, Left H Cecum J Appendix K Ascending Colon L Transverse Colon M Descending Colon N Sigmoid Colon P Rectum	0 Open 3 Percutaneous 4 Percutaneous Endoscopic 7 Via Natural or Artificial Opening 8 Via Natural or Artificial Opening Endoscopic	Z No Device	Z No Qualifier
Q Anus	0 Open 3 Percutaneous 4 Percutaneous Endoscopic 7 Via Natural or Artificial Opening 8 Via Natural or Artificial Opening Endoscopic X External	Z No Device	Z No Qualifier
R Anal Sphincter S Greater Omentum T Lesser Omentum V Mesentery W Peritoneum	0 Open 3 Percutaneous 4 Percutaneous Endoscopic	Z No Device	Z No Qualifier

Section	0	Medical and Surgical		
Body System	D	Gastrointestinal System		
Operation	F	Fragmentation: Breaking solid matter in a body part into pieces		

Body Part (Character 4)	Body Part (Character 4)	Body Part (Character 4)	Body Part (Character 4)
5 Esophagus 6 Stomach 8 Small Intestine 9 Duodenum A Jejunum B Ileum E Large Intestine F Large Intestine, Right G Large Intestine, Left H Cecum J Appendix K Ascending Colon L Transverse Colon M Descending Colon N Sigmoid Colon P Rectum Q Anus	0 Open 3 Percutaneous 4 Percutaneous Endoscopic 7 Via Natural or Artificial Opening 8 Via Natural or Artificial Opening Endoscopic X External	Z No Device	Z No Qualifier

Section	0	Medical and Surgical			
Body System	D	Gastrointestinal System			
Operation	H	Insertion: Putting in a nonbiological appliance that monitors, assists, performs, or prevents a physiological function but does not physically take the place of a body part			

Body Part (Character 4)	Approach (Character 5)	Device (Character 6)	Qualifier (Character 7)
5 Esophagus	0 Open 3 Percutaneous 4 Percutaneous Endoscopic	1 Radioactive Element 2 Monitoring Device 3 Infusion Device D Intraluminal Device U Feeding Device	Z No Qualifier
5 Esophagus	7 Via Natural or Artificial Opening 8 Via Natural or Artificial Opening Endoscopic	1 Radioactive Element 2 Monitoring Device 3 Infusion Device B Intraluminal Device, Airway D Intraluminal Device U Feeding Device	Z No Qualifier
6 Stomach	0 Open 3 Percutaneous 4 Percutaneous Endoscopic	2 Monitoring Device 3 Infusion Device D Intraluminal Device M Stimulator Lead U Feeding Device	Z No Qualifier
6 Stomach	7 Via Natural or Artificial Opening 8 Via Natural or Artificial Opening Endoscopic	2 Monitoring Device 3 Infusion Device D Intraluminal Device U Feeding Device	Z No Qualifier
8 Small Intestine 9 Duodenum A Jejunum B Ileum	0 Open 3 Percutaneous 4 Percutaneous Endoscopic 7 Via Natural or Artificial Opening 8 Via Natural or Artificial Opening Endoscopic	2 Monitoring Device 3 Infusion Device D Intraluminal Device U Feeding Device	Z No Qualifier
E Large Intestine	0 Open 3 Percutaneous 4 Percutaneous Endoscopic 7 Via Natural or Artificial Opening 8 Via Natural or Artificial Opening Endoscopic	D Intraluminal Device	Z No Qualifier
P Rectum	0 Open 3 Percutaneous 4 Percutaneous Endoscopic 7 Via Natural or Artificial Opening 8 Via Natural or Artificial Opening Endoscopic	1 Radioactive Element D Intraluminal Device	Z No Qualifier

Section	0	Medical and Surgical			
Body System	D	Gastrointestinal System			
Operation	H	Insertion: Putting in a nonbiological appliance that monitors, assists, performs, or prevents a physiological function but does not physically take the place of a body part			

Body Part (Character 4)	Approach (Character 5)	Device (Character 6)	Qualifier (Character 7)
Q Anus	0 Open 3 Percutaneous 4 Percutaneous Endoscopic	D Intraluminal Device L Artificial Sphincter	Z No Qualifier
Q Anus	7 Via Natural or Artificial Opening 8 Via Natural or Artificial Opening Endoscopic	D Intraluminal Device	Z No Qualifier
R Anal Sphincter	0 Open 3 Percutaneous 4 Percutaneous Endoscopic	M Stimulator Lead	Z No Qualifier

Section	0	Medical and Surgical		
Body System	D	Gastrointestinal System		
Operation	J	Inspection: Visually and/or manually exploring a body part		
Body Part (Character 4)		Body Part (Character 4)	Body Part (Character 4)	Body Part (Character 4)
0 Upper Intestinal Tract **6** Stomach **D** Lower Intestinal Tract		**0** Open **3** Percutaneous **4** Percutaneous Endoscopic **7** Via Natural or Artificial Opening **8** Via Natural or Artificial Opening Endoscopic **X** External	**Z** No Device	**Z** No Qualifier
U Omentum **V** Mesentery **W** Peritoneum		**0** Open **3** Percutaneous **4** Percutaneous Endoscopic **X** External	**Z** No Device	**Z** No Qualifier

Section	0	Medical and Surgical		
Body System	D	Gastrointestinal System		
Operation	L	Occlusion: Completely closing an orifice or the lumen of a tubular body part		
Body Part (Character 4)		Body Part (Character 4)	Body Part (Character 4)	Body Part (Character 4)
1 Esophagus, Upper **2** Esophagus, Middle **3** Esophagus, Lower **4** Esophagogastric Junction **5** Esophagus **6** Stomach **7** Stomach, Pylorus **8** Small Intestine **9** Duodenum **A** Jejunum **B** Ileum **C** Ileocecal Valve **E** Large Intestine **F** Large Intestine, Right **G** Large Intestine, Left **H** Cecum **K** Ascending Colon **L** Transverse Colon **M** Descending Colon **N** Sigmoid Colon **P** Rectum		**0** Open **3** Percutaneous **4** Percutaneous Endoscopic	**C** Extraluminal Device **D** Intraluminal Device **Z** No Device	**Z** No Qualifier

Section	0	Medical and Surgical		
Body System	D	Gastrointestinal System		
Operation	L	Occlusion: Completely closing an orifice or the lumen of a tubular body part		
Body Part (Character 4)		Body Part (Character 4)	Body Part (Character 4)	Body Part (Character 4)
1 Esophagus, Upper **2** Esophagus, Middle **3** Esophagus, Lower **4** Esophagogastric Junction **5** Esophagus **6** Stomach **7** Stomach, Pylorus **8** Small Intestine **9** Duodenum **A** Jejunum **B** Ileum **C** Ileocecal Valve **E** Large Intestine **F** Large Intestine, Right **G** Large Intestine, Left **H** Cecum **K** Ascending Colon **L** Transverse Colon **M** Descending Colon **N** Sigmoid Colon **P** Rectum		**7** Via Natural or Artificial Opening **8** Via Natural or Artificial Opening Endoscopic	**D** Intraluminal Device **Z** No Device	**Z** No Qualifier

Section	0	Medical and Surgical	
Body System	D	Gastrointestinal System	[continued]
Operation	L	Occlusion: Completely closing an orifice or the lumen of a tubular body part	

Body Part (Character 4)	Body Part (Character 4)	Body Part (Character 4)	Body Part (Character 4)
Q Anus	0 Open 3 Percutaneous 4 Percutaneous Endoscopic X External	C Extraluminal Device D Intraluminal Device Z No Device	Z No Qualifier
Q Anus	7 Via Natural or Artificial Opening 8 Via Natural or Artificial Opening Endoscopic	D Intraluminal Device Z No Device	Z No Qualifier

Section	0	Medical and Surgical	
Body System	D	Gastrointestinal System	
Operation	M	Reattachment Putting back in or on all or a portion of a separated body part to its normal location or other suitable location	

Body Part (Character 4)	Body Part (Character 4)	Body Part (Character 4)	Body Part (Character 4)
5 Esophagus 6 Stomach 8 Small Intestine 9 Duodenum A Jejunum B Ileum E Large Intestine F Large Intestine, Right G Large Intestine, Left H Cecum K Ascending Colon L Transverse Colon M Descending Colon N Sigmoid Colon P Rectum	0 Open 4 Percutaneous Endoscopic	Z No Device	Z No Qualifier

Section	0	Medical and Surgical	
Body System	D	Gastrointestinal System	
Operation	N	Release: Freeing a body part from an abnormal physical constraint by cutting or by the use of force	

Body Part (Character 4)	Body Part (Character 4)	Body Part (Character 4)	Body Part (Character 4)
1 Esophagus, Upper 2 Esophagus, Middle 3 Esophagus, Lower 4 Esophagogastric Junction 5 Esophagus 6 Stomach 7 Stomach, Pylorus 8 Small Intestine 9 Duodenum A Jejunum B Ileum C Ileocecal Valve E Large Intestine F Large Intestine, Right G Large Intestine, Left H Cecum J Appendix K Ascending Colon L Transverse Colon M Descending Colon N Sigmoid Colon P Rectum	0 Open 3 Percutaneous 4 Percutaneous Endoscopic 7 Via Natural or Artificial Opening 8 Via Natural or Artificial Opening Endoscopic	Z No Device	Z No Qualifier
Q Anus	0 Open 3 Percutaneous 4 Percutaneous Endoscopic 7 Via Natural or Artificial Opening 8 Via Natural or Artificial Opening Endoscopic X External	Z No Device	Z No Qualifier
R Anal Sphincter S Greater Omentum T Lesser Omentum V Mesentery W Peritoneum	0 Open 3 Percutaneous 4 Percutaneous Endoscopic	Z No Device	Z No Qualifier

Section	0	Medical and Surgical		
Body System	D	Gastrointestinal System		
Operation	P	Removal: Taking out or off a device from a body part		

Body Part (Character 4)	Body Part (Character 4)	Body Part (Character 4)	Body Part (Character 4)
0 Upper Intestinal Tract D Lower Intestinal Tract	0 Open 3 Percutaneous 4 Percutaneous Endoscopic 7 Via Natural or Artificial Opening 8 Via Natural or Artificial Opening Endoscopic	0 Drainage Device 2 Monitoring Device 3 Infusion Device 7 Autologous Tissue Substitute C Extraluminal Device D Intraluminal Device J Synthetic Substitute K Nonautologous Tissue Substitute U Feeding Device	Z No Qualifier
0 Upper Intestinal Tract D Lower Intestinal Tract	X External	0 Drainage Device 2 Monitoring Device 3 Infusion Device D Intraluminal Device U Feeding Device	Z No Qualifier
5 Esophagus	0 Open 3 Percutaneous 4 Percutaneous Endoscopic	1 Radioactive Element 2 Monitoring Device 3 Infusion Device U Feeding Device	Z No Qualifier
5 Esophagus	7 Via Natural or Artificial Opening 8 Via Natural or Artificial Opening Endoscopic	1 Radioactive Element D Intraluminal Device	Z No Qualifier
5 Esophagus	X External	1 Radioactive Element 2 Monitoring Device 3 Infusion Device D Intraluminal Device U Feeding Device	Z No Qualifier
6 Stomach	0 Open 3 Percutaneous 4 Percutaneous Endoscopic	0 Drainage Device 2 Monitoring Device 3 Infusion Device 7 Autologous Tissue Substitute C Extraluminal Device D Intraluminal Device J Synthetic Substitute K Nonautologous Tissue Substitute M Stimulator Lead U Feeding Device	Z No Qualifier

Section	0	Medical and Surgical		
Body System	D	Gastrointestinal System		
Operation	P	Removal: Taking out or off a device from a body part		

Body Part (Character 4)	Body Part (Character 4)	Body Part (Character 4)	Body Part (Character 4)
6 Stomach	7 Via Natural or Artificial Opening 8 Via Natural or Artificial Opening Endoscopic	0 Drainage Device 2 Monitoring Device 3 Infusion Device 7 Autologous Tissue Substitute C Extraluminal Device D Intraluminal Device J Synthetic Substitute K Nonautologous Tissue Substitute U Feeding Device	Z No Qualifier
6 Stomach	X External	0 Drainage Device 2 Monitoring Device 3 Infusion Device D Intraluminal Device U Feeding Device	Z No Qualifier
P Rectum	0 Open 3 Percutaneous 4 Percutaneous Endoscopic 7 Via Natural or Artificial Opening 8 Via Natural or Artificial Opening Endoscopic X External	1 Radioactive Element	Z No Qualifier

Section	0	Medical and Surgical		
Body System	D	Gastrointestinal System		[continued]
Operation	P	Removal: Taking out or off a device from a body part		
Body Part (Character 4)	**Body Part (Character 4)**		**Body Part (Character 4)**	**Body Part (Character 4)**
Q Anus	0 Open 3 Percutaneous 4 Percutaneous Endoscopic 7 Via Natural or Artificial Opening 8 Via Natural or Artificial Opening Endoscopic		L Artificial Sphincter	Z No Qualifier
R Anal Sphincter	0 Open 3 Percutaneous 4 Percutaneous Endoscopic		M Stimulator Lead	Z No Qualifier
U Omentum V Mesentery W Peritoneum	0 Open 3 Percutaneous 4 Percutaneous Endoscopic		0 Drainage Device 1 Radioactive Element 7 Autologous Tissue Substitute J Synthetic Substitute K Nonautologous Tissue Substitute	Z No Qualifier

Section	0	Medical and Surgical		
Body System	D	Gastrointestinal System		
Operation	Q	Repair: Restoring, to the extent possible, a body part to its normal anatomic structure and function		
Body Part (Character 4)	**Body Part (Character 4)**		**Body Part (Character 4)**	**Body Part (Character 4)**
1 Esophagus, Upper 2 Esophagus, Middle 3 Esophagus, Lower 4 Esophagogastric Junction 5 Esophagus 6 Stomach 7 Stomach, Pylorus 8 Small Intestine 9 Duodenum A Jejunum B Ileum C Ileocecal Valve E Large Intestine F Large Intestine, Right G Large Intestine, Left H Cecum J Appendix K Ascending Colon L Transverse Colon M Descending Colon N Sigmoid Colon P Rectum	0 Open 3 Percutaneous 4 Percutaneous Endoscopic 7 Via Natural or Artificial Opening 8 Via Natural or Artificial Opening Endoscopic		Z No Device	Z No Qualifier
Q Anus	0 Open 3 Percutaneous 4 Percutaneous Endoscopic 7 Via Natural or Artificial Opening 8 Via Natural or Artificial Opening Endoscopic X External		Z No Device	Z No Qualifier
R Anal Sphincter S Greater Omentum T Lesser Omentum V Mesentery W Peritoneum	0 Open 3 Percutaneous 4 Percutaneous Endoscopic		Z No Device	Z No Qualifier

Section	0	Medical and Surgical	
Body System	D	Gastrointestinal System	
Operation	R	Replacement: Putting in or on biological or synthetic material that physically takes the place and/or function of all or a portion of a body part	

Body Part (Character 4)	Body Part (Character 4)	Body Part (Character 4)	Body Part (Character 4)
5 Esophagus	0 Open 4 Percutaneous Endoscopic 7 Via Natural or Artificial Opening 8 Via Natural or Artificial Opening Endoscopic	7 Autologous Tissue Substitute J Synthetic Substitute K Nonautologous Tissue Substitute	Z No Qualifier
R Anal Sphincter S Greater Omentum T Lesser Omentum V Mesentery W Peritoneum	0 Open 4 Percutaneous Endoscopic	7 Autologous Tissue Substitute J Synthetic Substitute K Nonautologous Tissue Substitute	Z No Qualifier

Section	0	Medical and Surgical	
Body System	D	Gastrointestinal System	
Operation	S	Reposition: Moving to its normal location, or other suitable location, all or a portion of a body part	

Body Part (Character 4)	Body Part (Character 4)	Body Part (Character 4)	Body Part (Character 4)
5 Esophagus 6 Stomach 9 Duodenum A Jejunum B Ileum H Cecum K Ascending Colon L Transverse Colon M Descending Colon N Sigmoid Colon P Rectum Q Anus	0 Open 4 Percutaneous Endoscopic 7 Via Natural or Artificial Opening 8 Via Natural or Artificial Opening Endoscopic X External	Z No Device	Z No Qualifier

Section	0	Medical and Surgical	
Body System	D	Gastrointestinal System	
Operation	T	Resection: Cutting out or off, without replacement, all of a body part	

Body Part (Character 4)	Body Part (Character 4)	Body Part (Character 4)	Body Part (Character 4)
1 Esophagus, Upper 2 Esophagus, Middle 3 Esophagus, Lower 4 Esophagogastric Junction 5 Esophagus 6 Stomach 7 Stomach, Pylorus 8 Small Intestine 9 Duodenum A Jejunum B Ileum C Ileocecal Valve E Large Intestine F Large Intestine, Right G Large Intestine, Left H Cecum J Appendix K Ascending Colon L Transverse Colon M Descending Colon N Sigmoid Colon P Rectum Q Anus	0 Open 4 Percutaneous Endoscopic 7 Via Natural or Artificial Opening 8 Via Natural or Artificial Opening Endoscopic	Z No Device	Z No Qualifier
R Anal Sphincter S Greater Omentum T Lesser Omentum	0 Open 4 Percutaneous Endoscopic	Z No Device	Z No Qualifier

Section	0	Medical and Surgical		
Body System	D	Gastrointestinal System		
Operation	U	Supplement: Putting in or on biological or synthetic material that physically reinforces and/or augments the function of a portion of a body part		
Body Part (Character 4)	Body Part (Character 4)	Body Part (Character 4)	Body Part (Character 4)
---	---	---	---
1 Esophagus, Upper 2 Esophagus, Middle 3 Esophagus, Lower 4 Esophagogastric Junction 5 Esophagus 6 Stomach 7 Stomach, Pylorus 8 Small Intestine 9 Duodenum A Jejunum B Ileum C Ileocecal Valve E Large Intestine F Large Intestine, Right G Large Intestine, Left H Cecum K Ascending Colon L Transverse Colon M Descending Colon N Sigmoid Colon P Rectum	0 Open 4 Percutaneous Endoscopic 7 Via Natural or Artificial Opening 8 Via Natural or Artificial Opening Endoscopic	7 Autologous Tissue Substitute J Synthetic Substitute K Nonautologous Tissue Substitute	Z No Qualifier
Q Anus	0 Open 4 Percutaneous Endoscopic 7 Via Natural or Artificial Opening 8 Via Natural or Artificial Opening Endoscopic X External	7 Autologous Tissue Substitute J Synthetic Substitute K Nonautologous Tissue Substitute	Z No Qualifier
R Anal Sphincter S Greater Omentum T Lesser Omentum V Mesentery W Peritoneum	0 Open 4 Percutaneous Endoscopic	7 Autologous Tissue Substitute J Synthetic Substitute K Nonautologous Tissue Substitute	Z No Qualifier

Section	0	Medical and Surgical		
Body System	D	Gastrointestinal System		
Operation	V	Restriction: Partially closing an orifice or the lumen of a tubular body part		
Body Part (Character 4)	Body Part (Character 4)	Body Part (Character 4)	Body Part (Character 4)
---	---	---	---
1 Esophagus, Upper 2 Esophagus, Middle 3 Esophagus, Lower 4 Esophagogastric Junction 5 Esophagus 6 Stomach 7 Stomach, Pylorus 8 Small Intestine 9 Duodenum A Jejunum B Ileum C Ileocecal Valve E Large Intestine F Large Intestine, Right G Large Intestine, Left H Cecum K Ascending Colon L Transverse Colon M Descending Colon N Sigmoid Colon P Rectum	0 Open 3 Percutaneous 4 Percutaneous Endoscopic	C Extraluminal Device D Intraluminal Device Z No Device	Z No Qualifier

Section	0	Medical and Surgical			
Body System	D	Gastrointestinal System			
Operation	V	Restriction: Partially closing an orifice or the lumen of a tubular body part			
Body Part (Character 4)		**Body Part (Character 4)**	**Body Part (Character 4)**	**Body Part (Character 4)**
1 Esophagus, Upper 2 Esophagus, Middle 3 Esophagus, Lower 4 Esophagogastric Junction 5 Esophagus 6 Stomach 7 Stomach, Pylorus 8 Small Intestine 9 Duodenum A Jejunum B Ileum C Ileocecal Valve E Large Intestine F Large Intestine, Right G Large Intestine, Left H Cecum K Ascending Colon L Transverse Colon M Descending Colon N Sigmoid Colon P Rectum		7 Via Natural or Artificial Opening 8 Via Natural or Artificial Opening Endoscopic	D Intraluminal Device Z No Device	Z No Qualifier
Q Anus		0 Open 3 Percutaneous 4 Percutaneous Endoscopic X External	C Extraluminal Device D Intraluminal Device Z No Device	Z No Qualifier
Q Anus		7 Via Natural or Artificial Opening 8 Via Natural or Artificial Opening Endoscopic	D Intraluminal Device Z No Device	Z No Qualifier

Section	0	Medical and Surgical			
Body System	D	Gastrointestinal System			
Operation	W	Revision: Correcting, to the extent possible, a portion of a malfunctioning device or the position of a displaced device			
Body Part (Character 4)		**Body Part (Character 4)**	**Body Part (Character 4)**	**Body Part (Character 4)**
0 Upper Intestinal Tract D Lower Intestinal Tract		0 Open 3 Percutaneous 4 Percutaneous Endoscopic 7 Via Natural or Artificial Opening 8 Via Natural or Artificial Opening Endoscopic X External	0 Drainage Device 2 Monitoring Device 3 Infusion Device 7 Autologous Tissue Substitute C Extraluminal Device D Intraluminal Device J Synthetic Substitute K Nonautologous Tissue Substitute U Feeding Device	Z No Qualifier
5 Esophagus		7 Via Natural or Artificial Opening 8 Via Natural or Artificial Opening Endoscopic X External	D Intraluminal Device	Z No Qualifier
6 Stomach		0 Open 3 Percutaneous 4 Percutaneous Endoscopic	0 Drainage Device 2 Monitoring Device 3 Infusion Device 7 Autologous Tissue Substitute C Extraluminal Device D Intraluminal Device J Synthetic Substitute K Nonautologous Tissue Substitute M Stimulator Lead U Feeding Device	Z No Qualifier

Section	0	Medical and Surgical	
Body System	D	Gastrointestinal System	[continued]
Operation	W	Revision: Correcting, to the extent possible, a portion of a malfunctioning device or the position of a displaced device	

Body Part (Character 4)	Body Part (Character 4)	Body Part (Character 4)	Body Part (Character 4)
6 Stomach	7 Via Natural or Artificial Opening 8 Via Natural or Artificial Opening Endoscopic X External	0 Drainage Device 2 Monitoring Device 3 Infusion Device 7 Autologous Tissue Substitute C Extraluminal Device D Intraluminal Device J Synthetic Substitute K Nonautologous Tissue Substitute U Feeding Device	Z No Qualifier
8 Small Intestine E Large Intestine	0 Open 4 Percutaneous Endoscopic 7 Via Natural or Artificial Opening 8 Via Natural or Artificial Opening Endoscopic	7 Autologous Tissue Substitute J Synthetic Substitute K Nonautologous Tissue Substitute	Z No Qualifier
Q Anus	0 Open 3 Percutaneous 4 Percutaneous Endoscopic 7 Via Natural or Artificial Opening 8 Via Natural or Artificial Opening Endoscopic	L Artificial Sphincter	Z No Qualifier
R Anal Sphincter	0 Open 3 Percutaneous 4 Percutaneous Endoscopic	M Stimulator Lead	Z No Qualifier
U Omentum V Mesentery W Peritoneum	0 Open 3 Percutaneous 4 Percutaneous Endoscopic	0 Drainage Device 7 Autologous Tissue Substitute J Synthetic Substitute K Nonautologous Tissue Substitute	Z No Qualifier

Section	0	Medical and Surgical	
Body System	D	Gastrointestinal System	
Operation	X	Transfer: Moving, without taking out, all or a portion of a body part to another location to take over the function of all or a portion of a body part	

Body Part (Character 4)	Body Part (Character 4)	Body Part (Character 4)	Body Part (Character 4)
6 Stomach 8 Small Intestine E Large Intestine	0 Open 4 Percutaneous Endoscopic	Z No Device	5 Esophagus

Section	0	Medical and Surgical	
Body System	D	Gastrointestinal System	
Operation	Y	Transplantation: Putting in or on all or a portion of a living body part taken from another individual or animal to physically take the place and/or function of all or a portion of a similar body part	

Body Part (Character 4)	Body Part (Character 4)	Body Part (Character 4)	Body Part (Character 4)
5 Esophagus 6 Stomach 8 Small Intestine E Large Intestine	0 Open	Z No Device	0 Allogeneic 1 Syngeneic 2 Zooplastic

Section	0	Medical and Surgical		
Body System	F	Hepatobiliary System and Pancreas		
Operation	1	Bypass: Altering the route of passage of the contents of a tubular body part		
Body Part (Character 4)		Approach (Character 5)	Device (Character 6)	Qualifier (Character 7)
4 Gallbladder 5 Hepatic Duct, Right 6 Hepatic Duct, Left 8 Cystic Duct 9 Common Bile Duct		0 Open 4 Percutaneous Endoscopic	D Intraluminal Device Z No Device	3 Duodenum 4 Stomach 5 Hepatic Duct, Right 6 Hepatic Duct, Left 7 Hepatic Duct, Caudate 8 Cystic Duct 9 Common Bile Duct B Small Intestine
D Pancreatic Duct F Pancreatic Duct, Accessory G Pancreas		0 Open 4 Percutaneous Endoscopic	D Intraluminal Device Z No Device	3 Duodenum B Small Intestine C Large Intestine

Section	0	Medical and Surgical		
Body System	F	Hepatobiliary System and Pancreas		
Operation	2	Change: Taking out or off a device from a body part and putting back an identical or similar device in or on the same body part without cutting or puncturing the skin or a mucous membrane		
Body Part (Character 4)		Approach (Character 5)	Device (Character 6)	Qualifier (Character 7)
0 Liver 4 Gallbladder B Hepatobiliary Duct D Pancreatic Duct G Pancreas		X External	0 Drainage Device Y Other Device	Z No Qualifier

Section	0	Medical and Surgical		
Body System	F	Hepatobiliary System and Pancreas		
Operation	5	Destruction: Physical eradication of all or a portion of a body part by the direct use of energy, force, or a destructive agent		
Body Part (Character 4)		Approach (Character 5)	Device (Character 6)	Qualifier (Character 7)
0 Liver 1 Liver, Right Lobe 2 Liver, Left Lobe 4 Gallbladder G Pancreas		0 Open 3 Percutaneous 4 Percutaneous Endoscopic	Z No Device	Z No Qualifier
5 Hepatic Duct, Right 6 Hepatic Duct, Left 8 Cystic Duct 9 Common Bile Duct C Ampulla of Vater D Pancreatic Duct F Pancreatic Duct, Accessory		0 Open 3 Percutaneous 4 Percutaneous Endoscopic 7 Via Natural or Artificial Opening 8 Via Natural or Artificial Opening Endoscopic	Z No Device	Z No Qualifier

Section	0	Medical and Surgical		
Body System	F	Hepatobiliary System and Pancreas		
Operation	7	Dilation: Expanding an orifice or the lumen of a tubular body part		
Body Part (Character 4)		Approach (Character 5)	Device (Character 6)	Qualifier (Character 7)
5 Hepatic Duct, Right 6 Hepatic Duct, Left 8 Cystic Duct 9 Common Bile Duct C Ampulla of Vater D Pancreatic Duct F Pancreatic Duct, Accessory		0 Open 3 Percutaneous 4 Percutaneous Endoscopic 7 Via Natural or Artificial Opening 8 Via Natural or Artificial Opening Endoscopic	D Intraluminal Device Z No Device	Z No Qualifier

Section	0	Medical and Surgical		
Body System	F	Hepatobiliary System and Pancreas		
Operation	8	Division: Cutting into a body part, without draining fluids and/or gases from the body part, in order to separate or transect a body part		
Body Part (Character 4)		Approach (Character 5)	Device (Character 6)	Qualifier (Character 7)
G Pancreas		0 Open 3 Percutaneous 4 Percutaneous Endoscopic	Z No Device	Z No Qualifier

Section	0	Medical and Surgical		
Body System	F	Hepatobiliary System and Pancreas		
Operation	9	Drainage: Taking or letting out fluids and/or gases from a body part		
Body Part (Character 4)		**Approach (Character 5)**	**Device (Character 6)**	**Qualifier (Character 7)**
0 Liver 1 Liver, Right Lobe 2 Liver, Left Lobe 4 Gallbladder G Pancreas		0 Open 3 Percutaneous 4 Percutaneous Endoscopic	0 Drainage Device	Z No Qualifier
0 Liver 1 Liver, Right Lobe 2 Liver, Left Lobe 4 Gallbladder G Pancreas		0 Open 3 Percutaneous 4 Percutaneous Endoscopic	Z No Device	X Diagnostic Z No Qualifier
5 Hepatic Duct, Right 6 Hepatic Duct, Left 8 Cystic Duct 9 Common Bile Duct C Ampulla of Vater D Pancreatic Duct F Pancreatic Duct, Accessory		0 Open 3 Percutaneous 4 Percutaneous Endoscopic 7 Via Natural or Artificial Opening 8 Via Natural or Artificial Opening Endoscopic	0 Drainage Device	Z No Qualifier
5 Hepatic Duct, Right 6 Hepatic Duct, Left 8 Cystic Duct 9 Common Bile Duct C Ampulla of Vater D Pancreatic Duct F Pancreatic Duct, Accessory		0 Open 3 Percutaneous 4 Percutaneous Endoscopic 7 Via Natural or Artificial Opening 8 Via Natural or Artificial Opening Endoscopic	Z No Device	X Diagnostic Z No Qualifier

Section	0	Medical and Surgical		
Body System	F	Hepatobiliary System and Pancreas		
Operation	B	Excision: Cutting out or off, without replacement, a portion of a body part		
Body Part (Character 4)		**Approach (Character 5)**	**Device (Character 6)**	**Qualifier (Character 7)**
0 Liver 1 Liver, Right Lobe 2 Liver, Left Lobe 4 Gallbladder G Pancreas		0 Open 3 Percutaneous 4 Percutaneous Endoscopic	Z No Device	X Diagnostic Z No Qualifier
5 Hepatic Duct, Right 6 Hepatic Duct, Left 8 Cystic Duct 9 Common Bile Duct C Ampulla of Vater D Pancreatic Duct F Pancreatic Duct, Accessory		0 Open 3 Percutaneous 4 Percutaneous Endoscopic 7 Via Natural or Artificial Opening 8 Via Natural or Artificial Opening Endoscopic	Z No Device	X Diagnostic Z No Qualifier

Section	0	Medical and Surgical		
Body System	F	Hepatobiliary System and Pancreas		
Operation	C	Extirpation: Taking or cutting out solid matter from a body part		
Body Part (Character 4)		**Approach (Character 5)**	**Device (Character 6)**	**Qualifier (Character 7)**
0 Liver 1 Liver, Right Lobe 2 Liver, Left Lobe 4 Gallbladder G Pancreas		0 Open 3 Percutaneous 4 Percutaneous Endoscopic	Z No Device	Z No Qualifier
5 Hepatic Duct, Right 6 Hepatic Duct, Left 8 Cystic Duct 9 Common Bile Duct C Ampulla of Vater D Pancreatic Duct F Pancreatic Duct, Accessory		0 Open 3 Percutaneous 4 Percutaneous Endoscopic 7 Via Natural or Artificial Opening 8 Via Natural or Artificial Opening Endoscopic	Z No Device	Z No Qualifier

Section	0	Medical and Surgical		
Body System	F	Hepatobiliary System and Pancreas		
Operation	F	Fragmentation: Breaking solid matter in a body part into pieces		
Body Part (Character 4)		Approach (Character 5)	Device (Character 6)	Qualifier (Character 7)
4 Gallbladder 5 Hepatic Duct, Right 6 Hepatic Duct, Left 8 Cystic Duct 9 Common Bile Duct C Ampulla of Vater D Pancreatic Duct F Pancreatic Duct, Accessory		0 Open 3 Percutaneous 4 Percutaneous Endoscopic 7 Via Natural or Artificial Opening 8 Via Natural or Artificial Opening Endoscopic X External	Z No Device	Z No Qualifier

Section	0	Medical and Surgical		
Body System	F	Hepatobiliary System and Pancreas		
Operation	H	Insertion: Putting in a nonbiological appliance that monitors, assists, performs, or prevents a physiological function but does not physically take the place of a body part		
Body Part (Character 4)		Approach (Character 5)	Device (Character 6)	Qualifier (Character 7)
0 Liver 1 Liver, Right Lobe 2 Liver, Left Lobe 4 Gallbladder G Pancreas		0 Open 3 Percutaneous 4 Percutaneous Endoscopic	2 Monitoring Device 3 Infusion Device	Z No Qualifier
B Hepatobiliary Duct D Pancreatic Duct		0 Open 3 Percutaneous 4 Percutaneous Endoscopic 7 Via Natural or Artificial Opening 8 Via Natural or Artificial Opening Endoscopic	1 Radioactive Element 2 Monitoring Device 3 Infusion Device D Intraluminal Device	Z No Qualifier

Section	0	Medical and Surgical		
Body System	F	Hepatobiliary System and Pancreas		
Operation	J	Inspection: Visually and/or manually exploring a body part		
Body Part (Character 4)		Approach (Character 5)	Device (Character 6)	Qualifier (Character 7)
0 Liver 4 Gallbladder G Pancreas		0 Open 3 Percutaneous 4 Percutaneous Endoscopic X External	Z No Device	Z No Qualifier
B Hepatobiliary Duct D Pancreatic Duct		0 Open 3 Percutaneous 4 Percutaneous Endoscopic 7 Via Natural or Artificial Opening 8 Via Natural or Artificial Opening Endoscopic	Z No Device	Z No Qualifier

Section	0	Medical and Surgical		
Body System	F	Hepatobiliary System and Pancreas		
Operation	L	Occlusion: Completely closing an orifice or the lumen of a tubular body part		
Body Part (Character 4)		Approach (Character 5)	Device (Character 6)	Qualifier (Character 7)
5 Hepatic Duct, Right 6 Hepatic Duct, Left 8 Cystic Duct 9 Common Bile Duct C Ampulla of Vater D Pancreatic Duct F Pancreatic Duct, Accessory		0 Open 3 Percutaneous 4 Percutaneous Endoscopic	C Extraluminal Device D Intraluminal Device Z No Device	Z No Qualifier
5 Hepatic Duct, Right 6 Hepatic Duct, Left 8 Cystic Duct 9 Common Bile Duct C Ampulla of Vater D Pancreatic Duct F Pancreatic Duct, Accessory		7 Via Natural or Artificial Opening 8 Via Natural or Artificial Opening Endoscopic	D Intraluminal Device Z No Device	Z No Qualifier

Section	0	Medical and Surgical		
Body System	F	Hepatobiliary System and Pancreas		
Operation	M	Reattachment Putting back in or on all or a portion of a separated body part to its normal location or other suitable location		

Body Part (Character 4)	Approach (Character 5)	Device (Character 6)	Qualifier (Character 7)
0 Liver 1 Liver, Right Lobe 2 Liver, Left Lobe 4 Gallbladder 5 Hepatic Duct, Right 6 Hepatic Duct, Left 8 Cystic Duct 9 Common Bile Duct C Ampulla of Vater D Pancreatic Duct F Pancreatic Duct, Accessory G Pancreas	0 Open 4 Percutaneous Endoscopic	Z No Device	Z No Qualifier

Section	0	Medical and Surgical		
Body System	F	Hepatobiliary System and Pancreas		
Operation	N	Release: Freeing a body part from an abnormal physical constraint by cutting or by the use of force		

Body Part (Character 4)	Approach (Character 5)	Device (Character 6)	Qualifier (Character 7)
0 Liver 1 Liver, Right Lobe 2 Liver, Left Lobe 4 Gallbladder G Pancreas	0 Open 3 Percutaneous 4 Percutaneous Endoscopic	Z No Device	Z No Qualifier
5 Hepatic Duct, Right 6 Hepatic Duct, Left 8 Cystic Duct 9 Common Bile Duct C Ampulla of Vater D Pancreatic Duct F Pancreatic Duct, Accessory	0 Open 3 Percutaneous 4 Percutaneous Endoscopic 7 Via Natural or Artificial Opening 8 Via Natural or Artificial Opening Endoscopic	Z No Device	Z No Qualifier

Section	0	Medical and Surgical		
Body System	F	Hepatobiliary System and Pancreas		
Operation	P	Removal: Taking out or off a device from a body part		

Body Part (Character 4)	Approach (Character 5)	Device (Character 6)	Qualifier (Character 7)
0 Liver	0 Open 3 Percutaneous 4 Percutaneous Endoscopic X External	0 Drainage Device 2 Monitoring Device 3 Infusion Device	Z No Qualifier
4 Gallbladder G Pancreas	0 Open 3 Percutaneous 4 Percutaneous Endoscopic X External	0 Drainage Device 2 Monitoring Device 3 Infusion Device D Intraluminal Device	Z No Qualifier
B Hepatobiliary Duct D Pancreatic Duct	0 Open 3 Percutaneous 4 Percutaneous Endoscopic 7 Via Natural or Artificial Opening 8 Via Natural or Artificial Opening Endoscopic	0 Drainage Device 1 Radioactive Element 2 Monitoring Device 3 Infusion Device 7 Autologous Tissue Substitute C Extraluminal Device D Intraluminal Device J Synthetic Substitute K Nonautologous Tissue Substitute	Z No Qualifier
B Hepatobiliary Duct D Pancreatic Duct	X External	0 Drainage Device 1 Radioactive Element 2 Monitoring Device 3 Infusion Device D Intraluminal Device	Z No Qualifier

Section	0	Medical and Surgical		
Body System	F	Hepatobiliary System and Pancreas		
Operation	Q	Repair: Restoring, to the extent possible, a body part to its normal anatomic structure and function		
Body Part (Character 4)		Approach (Character 5)	Device (Character 6)	Qualifier (Character 7)
0 Liver 1 Liver, Right Lobe 2 Liver, Left Lobe 4 Gallbladder G Pancreas		0 Open 3 Percutaneous 4 Percutaneous Endoscopic	Z No Device	Z No Qualifier
5 Hepatic Duct, Right 6 Hepatic Duct, Left 8 Cystic Duct 9 Common Bile Duct C Ampulla of Vater D Pancreatic Duct F Pancreatic Duct, Accessory		0 Open 3 Percutaneous 4 Percutaneous Endoscopic 7 Via Natural or Artificial Opening 8 Via Natural or Artificial Opening Endoscopic	Z No Device	Z No Qualifier

Section	0	Medical and Surgical		
Body System	F	Hepatobiliary System and Pancreas		
Operation	R	Replacement: Putting in or on biological or synthetic material that physically takes the place and/or function of all or a portion of a body part		
Body Part (Character 4)		Approach (Character 5)	Device (Character 6)	Qualifier (Character 7)
5 Hepatic Duct, Right 6 Hepatic Duct, Left 8 Cystic Duct 9 Common Bile Duct C Ampulla of Vater D Pancreatic Duct F Pancreatic Duct, Accessory		0 Open 4 Percutaneous Endoscopic	7 Autologous Tissue Substitute J Synthetic Substitute K Nonautologous Tissue Substitute	Z No Qualifier

Section	0	Medical and Surgical		
Body System	F	Hepatobiliary System and Pancreas		
Operation	S	Reposition: Moving to its normal location, or other suitable location, all or a portion of a body part		
Body Part (Character 4)		Approach (Character 5)	Device (Character 6)	Qualifier (Character 7)
0 Liver 4 Gallbladder 5 Hepatic Duct, Right 6 Hepatic Duct, Left 8 Cystic Duct 9 Common Bile Duct C Ampulla of Vater D Pancreatic Duct F Pancreatic Duct, Accessory G Pancreas		0 Open 4 Percutaneous Endoscopic	Z No Device	Z No Qualifier

Section	0	Medical and Surgical		
Body System	F	Hepatobiliary System and Pancreas		
Operation	T	Resection: Cutting out or off, without replacement, all of a body part		
Body Part (Character 4)		Approach (Character 5)	Device (Character 6)	Qualifier (Character 7)
0 Liver 1 Liver, Right Lobe 2 Liver, Left Lobe 4 Gallbladder G Pancreas		0 Open 4 Percutaneous Endoscopic	Z No Device	Z No Qualifier
5 Hepatic Duct, Right 6 Hepatic Duct, Left 8 Cystic Duct 9 Common Bile Duct C Ampulla of Vater D Pancreatic Duct F Pancreatic Duct, Accessory		0 Open 4 Percutaneous Endoscopic 7 Via Natural or Artificial Opening 8 Via Natural or Artificial Opening Endoscopic	Z No Device	Z No Qualifier

Section	0	Medical and Surgical		
Body System	F	Hepatobiliary System and Pancreas		
Operation	U	Supplement: Putting in or on biological or synthetic material that physically reinforces and/or augments the function of a portion of a body part		
Body Part (Character 4)		**Approach (Character 5)**	**Device (Character 6)**	**Qualifier (Character 7)**
5 Hepatic Duct, Right 6 Hepatic Duct, Left 8 Cystic Duct 9 Common Bile Duct C Ampulla of Vater D Pancreatic Duct F Pancreatic Duct, Accessory		0 Open 3 Percutaneous 4 Percutaneous Endoscopic	7 Autologous Tissue Substitute J Synthetic Substitute K Nonautologous Tissue Substitute	Z No Qualifier

Section	0	Medical and Surgical		
Body System	F	Hepatobiliary System and Pancreas		
Operation	V	Restriction: Partially closing an orifice or the lumen of a tubular body part		
Body Part (Character 4)		**Approach (Character 5)**	**Device (Character 6)**	**Qualifier (Character 7)**
5 Hepatic Duct, Right 6 Hepatic Duct, Left 8 Cystic Duct 9 Common Bile Duct C Ampulla of Vater D Pancreatic Duct F Pancreatic Duct, Accessory		0 Open 3 Percutaneous 4 Percutaneous Endoscopic	C Extraluminal Device D Intraluminal Device Z No Device	Z No Qualifier
5 Hepatic Duct, Right 6 Hepatic Duct, Left 8 Cystic Duct 9 Common Bile Duct C Ampulla of Vater D Pancreatic Duct F Pancreatic Duct, Accessory		7 Via Natural or Artificial Opening 8 Via Natural or Artificial Opening Endoscopic	D Intraluminal Device Z No Device	Z No Qualifier

Section	0	Medical and Surgical		
Body System	F	Hepatobiliary System and Pancreas		
Operation	W	Revision: Correcting, to the extent possible, a portion of a malfunctioning device or the position of a displaced device		
Body Part (Character 4)		**Approach (Character 5)**	**Device (Character 6)**	**Qualifier (Character 7)**
0 Liver		0 Open 3 Percutaneous 4 Percutaneous Endoscopic X External	0 Drainage Device 2 Monitoring Device 3 Infusion Device	Z No Qualifier
4 Gallbladder G Pancreas		0 Open 3 Percutaneous 4 Percutaneous Endoscopic X External	0 Drainage Device 2 Monitoring Device 3 Infusion Device D Intraluminal Device	Z No Qualifier
B Hepatobiliary Duct D Pancreatic Duct		0 Open 3 Percutaneous 4 Percutaneous Endoscopic 7 Via Natural or Artificial Opening 8 Via Natural or Artificial Opening Endoscopic X External	0 Drainage Device 2 Monitoring Device 3 Infusion Device 7 Autologous Tissue Substitute C Extraluminal Device D Intraluminal Device J Synthetic Substitute K Nonautologous Tissue Substitute	Z No Qualifier

Section	0	Medical and Surgical		
Body System	F	Hepatobiliary System and Pancreas		
Operation	Y	Transplantation: Putting in or on all or a portion of a living body part taken from another individual or animal to physically take the place and/or function of all or a portion of a similar body part		
Body Part (Character 4)		**Approach (Character 5)**	**Device (Character 6)**	**Qualifier (Character 7)**
0 Liver G Pancreas		0 Open	Z No Device	0 Allogeneic 1 Syngeneic 2 Zooplastic

Section	0	Medical and Surgical		
Body System	G	Endocrine System		
Operation	2	Change: Taking out or off a device from a body part and putting back an identical or similar device in or on the same body part without cutting or puncturing the skin or a mucous membrane		
Body Part (Character 4)		Approach (Character 5)	Device (Character 6)	Qualifier (Character 7)
0 Pituitary Gland 1 Pineal Body 5 Adrenal Gland K Thyroid Gland R Parathyroid Gland S Endocrine Gland		X External	0 Drainage Device Y Other Device	Z No Qualifier

Section	0	Medical and Surgical		
Body System	G	Endocrine System		
Operation	5	Destruction: Physical eradication of all or a portion of a body part by the direct use of energy, force, or a destructive agent		
Body Part (Character 4)		Approach (Character 5)	Device (Character 6)	Qualifier (Character 7)
0 Pituitary Gland 1 Pineal Body 2 Adrenal Gland, Left 3 Adrenal Gland, Right 4 Adrenal Glands, Bilateral 6 Carotid Body, Left 7 Carotid Body, Right 8 Carotid Bodies, Bilateral 9 Para-aortic Body B Coccygeal Glomus C Glomus Jugulare D Aortic Body F Paraganglion Extremity G Thyroid Gland Lobe, Left H Thyroid Gland Lobe, Right K Thyroid Gland L Superior Parathyroid Gland, Right M Superior Parathyroid Gland, Left N Inferior Parathyroid Gland, Right P Inferior Parathyroid Gland, Left Q Parathyroid Glands, Multiple R Parathyroid Gland		0 Open 3 Percutaneous 4 Percutaneous Endoscopic	Z No Device	Z No Qualifier

Section	0	Medical and Surgical		
Body System	G	Endocrine System		
Operation	8	Division: Cutting into a body part, without draining fluids and/or gases from the body part, in order to separate or transect a body part		
Body Part (Character 4)		Approach (Character 5)	Device (Character 6)	Qualifier (Character 7)
0 Pituitary Gland J Thyroid Gland Isthmus		0 Open 3 Percutaneous 4 Percutaneous Endoscopic	Z No Device	Z No Qualifier

Section	0	Medical and Surgical		
Body System	G	Endocrine System		
Operation	9	Drainage: Taking or letting out fluids and/or gases from a body part		

Body Part (Character 4)	Approach (Character 5)	Device (Character 6)	Qualifier (Character 7)
0 Pituitary Gland **1** Pineal Body **2** Adrenal Gland, Left **3** Adrenal Gland, Right **4** Adrenal Glands, Bilateral **6** Carotid Body, Left **7** Carotid Body, Right **8** Carotid Bodies, Bilateral **9** Para-aortic Body **B** Coccygeal Glomus **C** Glomus Jugulare **D** Aortic Body **F** Paraganglion Extremity **G** Thyroid Gland Lobe, Left **H** Thyroid Gland Lobe, Right **K** Thyroid Gland **L** Superior Parathyroid Gland, Right **M** Superior Parathyroid Gland, Left **N** Inferior Parathyroid Gland, Right **P** Inferior Parathyroid Gland, Left **Q** Parathyroid Glands, Multiple **R** Parathyroid Gland	**0** Open **3** Percutaneous **4** Percutaneous Endoscopic	**0** Drainage Device	**Z** No Qualifier

Section	0	Medical and Surgical		
Body System	G	Endocrine System		
Operation	9	Drainage: Taking or letting out fluids and/or gases from a body part		

Body Part (Character 4)	Approach (Character 5)	Device (Character 6)	Qualifier (Character 7)
0 Pituitary Gland **1** Pineal Body **2** Adrenal Gland, Left **3** Adrenal Gland, Right **4** Adrenal Glands, Bilateral **6** Carotid Body, Left **7** Carotid Body, Right **8** Carotid Bodies, Bilateral **9** Para-aortic Body **B** Coccygeal Glomus **C** Glomus Jugulare **D** Aortic Body **F** Paraganglion Extremity **G** Thyroid Gland Lobe, Left **H** Thyroid Gland Lobe, Right **K** Thyroid Gland **L** Superior Parathyroid Gland, Right **M** Superior Parathyroid Gland, Left **N** Inferior Parathyroid Gland, Right **P** Inferior Parathyroid Gland, Left **Q** Parathyroid Glands, Multiple **R** Parathyroid Gland	**0** Open **3** Percutaneous **4** Percutaneous Endoscopic	**Z** No Device	**X** Diagnostic **Z** No Qualifier

Section	0	Medical and Surgical			
Body System	G	Endocrine System			
Operation	B	Excision: Cutting out or off, without replacement, a portion of a body part			
Body Part (Character 4)		**Approach (Character 5)**	**Device (Character 6)**	**Qualifier (Character 7)**	
0 Pituitary Gland **1** Pineal Body **2** Adrenal Gland, Left **3** Adrenal Gland, Right **4** Adrenal Glands, Bilateral **6** Carotid Body, Left **7** Carotid Body, Right **8** Carotid Bodies, Bilateral **9** Para-aortic Body **B** Coccygeal Glomus **C** Glomus Jugulare **D** Aortic Body **F** Paraganglion Extremity **G** Thyroid Gland Lobe, Left **H** Thyroid Gland Lobe, Right **L** Superior Parathyroid Gland, Right **M** Superior Parathyroid Gland, Left **N** Inferior Parathyroid Gland, Right **P** Inferior Parathyroid Gland, Left **Q** Parathyroid Glands, Multiple **R** Parathyroid Gland		**0** Open **3** Percutaneous **4** Percutaneous Endoscopic	**Z** No Device	**X** Diagnostic **Z** No Qualifier	

Section	0	Medical and Surgical			
Body System	G	Endocrine System			
Operation	C	Extirpation: Taking or cutting out solid matter from a body part			
Body Part (Character 4)		**Approach (Character 5)**	**Device (Character 6)**	**Qualifier (Character 7)**	
0 Pituitary Gland **1** Pineal Body **2** Adrenal Gland, Left **3** Adrenal Gland, Right **4** Adrenal Glands, Bilateral **6** Carotid Body, Left **7** Carotid Body, Right **8** Carotid Bodies, Bilateral **9** Para-aortic Body **B** Coccygeal Glomus **C** Glomus Jugulare **D** Aortic Body **F** Paraganglion Extremity **G** Thyroid Gland Lobe, Left **H** Thyroid Gland Lobe, Right **K** Thyroid Gland **L** Superior Parathyroid Gland, Right **M** Superior Parathyroid Gland, Left **N** Inferior Parathyroid Gland, Right **P** Inferior Parathyroid Gland, Left **Q** Parathyroid Glands, Multiple **R** Parathyroid Gland		**0** Open **3** Percutaneous **4** Percutaneous Endoscopic	**Z** No Device	**Z** No Qualifier	

Section	0	Medical and Surgical			
Body System	G	Endocrine System			
Operation	H	Insertion: Putting in a nonbiological appliance that monitors, assists, performs, or prevents a physiological function but does not physically take the place of a body part			
Body Part (Character 4)		**Approach (Character 5)**	**Device (Character 6)**	**Qualifier (Character 7)**	
S Endocrine Gland		**0** Open **3** Percutaneous **4** Percutaneous Endoscopic	**2** Monitoring Device **3** Infusion Device	**Z** No Qualifier	

Section	0	Medical and Surgical		
Body System	G	Endocrine System		
Operation	J	Inspection: Visually and/or manually exploring a body part		

Body Part (Character 4)	Approach (Character 5)	Device (Character 6)	Qualifier (Character 7)
0 Pituitary Gland **1** Pineal Body **5** Adrenal Gland **K** Thyroid Gland **R** Parathyroid Gland **S** Endocrine Gland	**0** Open **3** Percutaneous **4** Percutaneous Endoscopic	**Z** No Device	**Z** No Qualifier

Section	0	Medical and Surgical		
Body System	G	Endocrine System		
Operation	M	Reattachment Putting back in or on all or a portion of a separated body part to its normal location or other suitable location		

Body Part (Character 4)	Approach (Character 5)	Device (Character 6)	Qualifier (Character 7)
2 Adrenal Gland, Left **3** Adrenal Gland, Right **G** Thyroid Gland Lobe, Left **H** Thyroid Gland Lobe, Right **L** Superior Parathyroid Gland, Right **M** Superior Parathyroid Gland, Left **N** Inferior Parathyroid Gland, Right **P** Inferior Parathyroid Gland, Left **Q** Parathyroid Glands, Multiple **R** Parathyroid Gland	**0** Open **4** Percutaneous Endoscopic	**Z** No Device	**Z** No Qualifier

Section	0	Medical and Surgical		
Body System	G	Endocrine System		
Operation	N	Release: Freeing a body part from an abnormal physical constraint by cutting or by the use of force		

Body Part (Character 4)	Approach (Character 5)	Device (Character 6)	Qualifier (Character 7)
0 Pituitary Gland **1** Pineal Body **2** Adrenal Gland, Left **3** Adrenal Gland, Right **4** Adrenal Glands, Bilateral **6** Carotid Body, Left **7** Carotid Body, Right **8** Carotid Bodies, Bilateral **9** Para-aortic Body **B** Coccygeal Glomus **C** Glomus Jugulare **D** Aortic Body **F** Paraganglion Extremity **G** Thyroid Gland Lobe, Left **H** Thyroid Gland Lobe, Right **K** Thyroid Gland **L** Superior Parathyroid Gland, Right **M** Superior Parathyroid Gland, Left **N** Inferior Parathyroid Gland, Right **P** Inferior Parathyroid Gland, Left **Q** Parathyroid Glands, Multiple **R** Parathyroid Gland	**0** Open **3** Percutaneous **4** Percutaneous Endoscopic	**Z** No Device	**Z** No Qualifier

Section	0	Medical and Surgical		
Body System	G	Endocrine System		
Operation	P	Removal: Taking out or off a device from a body part		
Body Part (Character 4)		**Approach (Character 5)**	**Device (Character 6)**	**Qualifier (Character 7)**
0 Pituitary Gland 1 Pineal Body 5 Adrenal Gland K Thyroid Gland R Parathyroid Gland		0 Open 3 Percutaneous 4 Percutaneous Endoscopic X External	0 Drainage Device	Z No Qualifier
S Endocrine Gland		0 Open 3 Percutaneous 4 Percutaneous Endoscopic X External	0 Drainage Device 2 Monitoring Device 3 Infusion Device	Z No Qualifier

Section	0	Medical and Surgical		
Body System	G	Endocrine System		
Operation	Q	Repair: Restoring, to the extent possible, a body part to its normal anatomic structure and function		
Body Part (Character 4)		**Approach (Character 5)**	**Device (Character 6)**	**Qualifier (Character 7)**
0 Pituitary Gland 1 Pineal Body 2 Adrenal Gland, Left 3 Adrenal Gland, Right 4 Adrenal Glands, Bilateral 6 Carotid Body, Left 7 Carotid Body, Right 8 Carotid Bodies, Bilateral 9 Para-aortic Body B Coccygeal Glomus C Glomus Jugulare D Aortic Body F Paraganglion Extremity G Thyroid Gland Lobe, Left H Thyroid Gland Lobe, Right J Thyroid Gland Isthmus K Thyroid Gland L Superior Parathyroid Gland, Right M Superior Parathyroid Gland, Left N Inferior Parathyroid Gland, Right P Inferior Parathyroid Gland, Left Q Parathyroid Glands, Multiple R Parathyroid Gland		0 Open 3 Percutaneous 4 Percutaneous Endoscopic	Z No Device	Z No Qualifier

Section	0	Medical and Surgical		
Body System	G	Endocrine System		
Operation	S	Reposition: Moving to its normal location, or other suitable location, all or a portion of a body part		
Body Part (Character 4)		**Approach (Character 5)**	**Device (Character 6)**	**Qualifier (Character 7)**
2 Adrenal Gland, Left 3 Adrenal Gland, Right G Thyroid Gland Lobe, Left H Thyroid Gland Lobe, Right L Superior Parathyroid Gland, Right M Superior Parathyroid Gland, Left N Inferior Parathyroid Gland, Right P Inferior Parathyroid Gland, Left Q Parathyroid Glands, Multiple R Parathyroid Gland		0 Open 4 Percutaneous Endoscopic	Z No Device	Z No Qualifier

Section	0	Medical and Surgical		
Body System	G	Endocrine System		
Operation	T	Resection: Cutting out or off, without replacement, all of a body part		

Body Part (Character 4)	Approach (Character 5)	Device (Character 6)	Qualifier (Character 7)
0 Pituitary Gland **1** Pineal Body **2** Adrenal Gland, Left **3** Adrenal Gland, Right **4** Adrenal Glands, Bilateral **6** Carotid Body, Left **7** Carotid Body, Right **8** Carotid Bodies, Bilateral **9** Para-aortic Body **B** Coccygeal Glomus **C** Glomus Jugulare **D** Aortic Body **F** Paraganglion Extremity **G** Thyroid Gland Lobe, Left **H** Thyroid Gland Lobe, Right **K** Thyroid Gland **L** Superior Parathyroid Gland, Right **M** Superior Parathyroid Gland, Left **N** Inferior Parathyroid Gland, Right **P** Inferior Parathyroid Gland, Left **Q** Parathyroid Glands, Multiple **R** Parathyroid Gland	**0** Open **4** Percutaneous Endoscopic	**Z** No Device	**Z** No Qualifier

Section	0	Medical and Surgical		
Body System	G	Endocrine System		
Operation	W	Revision: Correcting, to the extent possible, a portion of a malfunctioning device or the position of a displaced device		

Body Part (Character 4)	Approach (Character 5)	Device (Character 6)	Qualifier (Character 7)
0 Pituitary Gland **1** Pineal Body **5** Adrenal Gland **K** Thyroid Gland **R** Parathyroid Gland	**0** Open **3** Percutaneous **4** Percutaneous Endoscopic **X** External	**0** Drainage Device	**Z** No Qualifier
S Endocrine Gland	**0** Open **3** Percutaneous **4** Percutaneous Endoscopic **X** External	**0** Drainage Device **2** Monitoring Device **3** Infusion Device	**Z** No Qualifier

Section	0	Medical and Surgical		
Body System	H	Skin and Breast		
Operation	0	Alteration: Modifying the anatomic structure of a body part without affecting the function of the body part		
Body Part (Character 4)		**Approach (Character 5)**	**Device (Character 6)**	**Qualifier (Character 7)**
T Breast, Right U Breast, Left V Breast, Bilateral		0 Open 3 Percutaneous X External	7 Autologous Tissue Substitute J Synthetic Substitute K Nonautologous Tissue Substitute Z No Device	Z No Qualifier

Section	0	Medical and Surgical		
Body System	H	Skin and Breast		
Operation	2	Change: Taking out or off a device from a body part and putting back an identical or similar device in or on the same body part without cutting or puncturing the skin or a mucous membrane		
Body Part (Character 4)		**Approach (Character 5)**	**Device (Character 6)**	**Qualifier (Character 7)**
P Skin T Breast, Right U Breast, Left		X External	0 Drainage Device Y Other Device	Z No Qualifier

Section	0	Medical and Surgical		
Body System	H	Skin and Breast		
Operation	5	Destruction: Physical eradication of all or a portion of a body part by the direct use of energy, force, or a destructive agent		
Body Part (Character 4)		**Approach (Character 5)**	**Device (Character 6)**	**Qualifier (Character 7)**
0 Skin, Scalp 1 Skin, Face 2 Skin, Right Ear 3 Skin, Left Ear 4 Skin, Neck 5 Skin, Chest 6 Skin, Back 7 Skin, Abdomen 8 Skin, Buttock 9 Skin, Perineum A Skin, Genitalia B Skin, Right Upper Arm C Skin, Left Upper Arm D Skin, Right Lower Arm E Skin, Left Lower Arm F Skin, Right Hand G Skin, Left Hand H Skin, Right Upper Leg J Skin, Left Upper Leg K Skin, Right Lower Leg L Skin, Left Lower Leg M Skin, Right Foot N Skin, Left Foot		X External	Z No Device	D Multiple Z No Qualifier
Q Finger Nail R Toe Nail		X External	Z No Device	Z No Qualifier
T Breast, Right U Breast, Left V Breast, Bilateral W Nipple, Right X Nipple, Left		0 Open 3 Percutaneous 7 Via Natural or Artificial Opening 8 Via Natural or Artificial Opening Endoscopic X External	Z No Device	Z No Qualifier

Section	0	Medical and Surgical			
Body System	H	Skin and Breast			
Operation	8	Division: Cutting into a body part, without draining fluids and/or gases from the body part, in order to separate or transect a body part			

Body Part (Character 4)	Approach (Character 5)	Device (Character 6)	Qualifier (Character 7)
0 Skin, Scalp	X External	Z No Device	Z No Qualifier
1 Skin, Face			
2 Skin, Right Ear			
3 Skin, Left Ear			
4 Skin, Neck			
5 Skin, Chest			
6 Skin, Back			
7 Skin, Abdomen			
8 Skin, Buttock			
9 Skin, Perineum			
A Skin, Genitalia			
B Skin, Right Upper Arm			
C Skin, Left Upper Arm			
D Skin, Right Lower Arm			
E Skin, Left Lower Arm			
F Skin, Right Hand			
G Skin, Left Hand			
H Skin, Right Upper Leg			
J Skin, Left Upper Leg			
K Skin, Right Lower Leg			
L Skin, Left Lower Leg			
M Skin, Right Foot			
N Skin, Left Foot			

Section	0	Medical and Surgical			
Body System	H	Skin and Breast			
Operation	9	Drainage: Taking or letting out fluids and/or gases from a body part			

Body Part (Character 4)	Approach (Character 5)	Device (Character 6)	Qualifier (Character 7)
0 Skin, Scalp	X External	0 Drainage Device	Z No Qualifier
1 Skin, Face			
2 Skin, Right Ear			
3 Skin, Left Ear			
4 Skin, Neck			
5 Skin, Chest			
6 Skin, Back			
7 Skin, Abdomen			
8 Skin, Buttock			
9 Skin, Perineum			
A Skin, Genitalia			
B Skin, Right Upper Arm			
C Skin, Left Upper Arm			
D Skin, Right Lower Arm			
E Skin, Left Lower Arm			
F Skin, Right Hand			
G Skin, Left Hand			
H Skin, Right Upper Leg			
J Skin, Left Upper Leg			
K Skin, Right Lower Leg			
L Skin, Left Lower Leg			
M Skin, Right Foot			
N Skin, Left Foot			
Q Finger Nail			
R Toe Nail			

Section	0	Medical and Surgical	
Body System	H	Skin and Breast	[continued]
Operation	9	Drainage: Taking or letting out fluids and/or gases from a body part	

Body Part (Character 4)	Approach (Character 5)	Device (Character 6)	Qualifier (Character 7)
0 Skin, Scalp **1** Skin, Face **2** Skin, Right Ear **3** Skin, Left Ear **4** Skin, Neck **5** Skin, Chest **6** Skin, Back **7** Skin, Abdomen **8** Skin, Buttock **9** Skin, Perineum **A** Skin, Genitalia **B** Skin, Right Upper Arm **C** Skin, Left Upper Arm **D** Skin, Right Lower Arm **E** Skin, Left Lower Arm **F** Skin, Right Hand **G** Skin, Left Hand **H** Skin, Right Upper Leg **J** Skin, Left Upper Leg **K** Skin, Right Lower Leg **L** Skin, Left Lower Leg **M** Skin, Right Foot **N** Skin, Left Foot **Q** Finger Nail **R** Toe Nail	**X** External	**Z** No Device	**X** Diagnostic **Z** No Qualifier
T Breast, Right **U** Breast, Left **V** Breast, Bilateral **W** Nipple, Right **X** Nipple, Left	**0** Open **3** Percutaneous **7** Via Natural or Artificial Opening **8** Via Natural or Artificial Opening Endoscopic **X** External	**0** Drainage Device	**Z** No Qualifier
T Breast, Right **U** Breast, Left **V** Breast, Bilateral **W** Nipple, Right **X** Nipple, Left	**0** Open **3** Percutaneous **7** Via Natural or Artificial Opening **8** Via Natural or Artificial Opening Endoscopic **X** External	**Z** No Device	**X** Diagnostic **Z** No Qualifier

Section	0	Medical and Surgical
Body System	H	Skin and Breast
Operation	B	Excision: Cutting out or off, without replacement, a portion of a body part

Body Part (Character 4)	Approach (Character 5)	Device (Character 6)	Qualifier (Character 7)
0 Skin, Scalp **1** Skin, Face **2** Skin, Right Ear **3** Skin, Left Ear **4** Skin, Neck **5** Skin, Chest **6** Skin, Back **7** Skin, Abdomen **8** Skin, Buttock **9** Skin, Perineum **A** Skin, Genitalia **B** Skin, Right Upper Arm **C** Skin, Left Upper Arm **D** Skin, Right Lower Arm **E** Skin, Left Lower Arm **F** Skin, Right Hand **G** Skin, Left Hand **H** Skin, Right Upper Leg **J** Skin, Left Upper Leg **K** Skin, Right Lower Leg **L** Skin, Left Lower Leg **M** Skin, Right Foot **N** Skin, Left Foot **Q** Finger Nail **R** Toe Nail	**X** External	**Z** No Device	**X** Diagnostic **Z** No Qualifier

Section	0	Medical and Surgical		
Body System	H	Skin and Breast		[continued]
Operation	B	Excision: Cutting out or off, without replacement, a portion of a body part		

Body Part (Character 4)	Body Part (Character 4)		
T Breast, Right **U** Breast, Left **V** Breast, Bilateral **W** Nipple, Right **X** Nipple, Left **Y** Supernumerary Breast	**0** Open **3** Percutaneous **7** Via Natural or Artificial Opening **8** Via Natural or Artificial Opening Endoscopic **X** External	**Z** No Device	**X** Diagnostic **Z** No Qualifier

Section	0	Medical and Surgical		
Body System	H	Skin and Breast		
Operation	C	Extirpation: Taking or cutting out solid matter from a body part		

Body Part (Character 4)	Approach (Character 5)	Device (Character 6)	Qualifier (Character 7)
0 Skin, Scalp **1** Skin, Face **2** Skin, Right Ear **3** Skin, Left Ear **4** Skin, Neck **5** Skin, Chest **6** Skin, Back **7** Skin, Abdomen **8** Skin, Buttock **9** Skin, Perineum **A** Skin, Genitalia **B** Skin, Right Upper Arm **C** Skin, Left Upper Arm **D** Skin, Right Lower Arm **E** Skin, Left Lower Arm **F** Skin, Right Hand **G** Skin, Left Hand **H** Skin, Right Upper Leg **J** Skin, Left Upper Leg **K** Skin, Right Lower Leg **L** Skin, Left Lower Leg **M** Skin, Right Foot **N** Skin, Left Foot **Q** Finger Nail **R** Toe Nail	**X** External	**Z** No Device	**Z** No Qualifier
T Breast, Right **U** Breast, Left **V** Breast, Bilateral **W** Nipple, Right **X** Nipple, Left	**0** Open **3** Percutaneous **7** Via Natural or Artificial Opening **8** Via Natural or Artificial Opening Endoscopic **X** External	**Z** No Device	**Z** No Qualifier

Section	0	Medical and Surgical		
Body System	**H**	**Skin and Breast**		
Operation	**D**	**Extraction: Pulling or stripping out or off all or a portion of a body part by the use of force**		
Body Part (Character 4)		**Approach (Character 5)**	**Device (Character 6)**	**Qualifier (Character 7)**
0 Skin, Scalp **1** Skin, Face **2** Skin, Right Ear **3** Skin, Left Ear **4** Skin, Neck **5** Skin, Chest **6** Skin, Back **7** Skin, Abdomen **8** Skin, Buttock **9** Skin, Perineum **A** Skin, Genitalia **B** Skin, Right Upper Arm **C** Skin, Left Upper Arm **D** Skin, Right Lower Arm **E** Skin, Left Lower Arm **F** Skin, Right Hand **G** Skin, Left Hand **H** Skin, Right Upper Leg **J** Skin, Left Upper Leg **K** Skin, Right Lower Leg **L** Skin, Left Lower Leg **M** Skin, Right Foot **N** Skin, Left Foot **Q** Finger Nail **R** Toe Nail **S** Hair		**X** External	**Z** No Device	**Z** No Qualifier

Section	0	Medical and Surgical		
Body System	**H**	**Skin and Breast**		
Operation	**H**	**Insertion: Putting in a nonbiological appliance that monitors, assists, performs, or prevents a physiological function but does not physically take the place of a body part**		
Body Part (Character 4)		**Approach (Character 5)**	**Device (Character 6)**	**Qualifier (Character 7)**
T Breast, Right **U** Breast, Left **V** Breast, Bilateral **W** Nipple, Right **X** Nipple, Left		**0** Open **3** Percutaneous **7** Via Natural or Artificial Opening **8** Via Natural or Artificial Opening Endoscopic	**1** Radioactive Element **N** Tissue Expander	**Z** No Qualifier
T Breast, Right **U** Breast, Left **V** Breast, Bilateral **W** Nipple, Right **X** Nipple, Left		**X** External	**1** Radioactive Element	**Z** No Qualifier

Section	0	Medical and Surgical		
Body System	**H**	**Skin and Breast**		
Operation	**J**	**Inspection: Visually and/or manually exploring a body part**		
Body Part (Character 4)		**Approach (Character 5)**	**Device (Character 6)**	**Qualifier (Character 7)**
P Skin **Q** Finger Nail **R** Toe Nail		**X** External	**Z** No Device	**Z** No Qualifier
T Breast, Right **U** Breast, Left		**0** Open **3** Percutaneous **7** Via Natural or Artificial Opening **8** Via Natural or Artificial Opening Endoscopic **X** External	**Z** No Device	**Z** No Qualifier

Section	0	Medical and Surgical		
Body System	H	Skin and Breast		
Operation	M	Reattachment Putting back in or on all or a portion of a separated body part to its normal location or other suitable location		

Body Part (Character 4)	Approach (Character 5)	Device (Character 6)	Qualifier (Character 7)
0 Skin, Scalp **1** Skin, Face **2** Skin, Right Ear **3** Skin, Left Ear **4** Skin, Neck **5** Skin, Chest **6** Skin, Back **7** Skin, Abdomen **8** Skin, Buttock **9** Skin, Perineum **A** Skin, Genitalia **B** Skin, Right Upper Arm **C** Skin, Left Upper Arm **D** Skin, Right Lower Arm **E** Skin, Left Lower Arm **F** Skin, Right Hand **G** Skin, Left Hand **H** Skin, Right Upper Leg **J** Skin, Left Upper Leg **K** Skin, Right Lower Leg **L** Skin, Left Lower Leg **M** Skin, Right Foot **N** Skin, Left Foot **T** Breast, Right **U** Breast, Left **V** Breast, Bilateral **W** Nipple, Right **X** Nipple, Left	**X** External	**Z** No Device	**Z** No Qualifier

Section	0	Medical and Surgical		
Body System	H	Skin and Breast		
Operation	N	Release: Freeing a body part from an abnormal physical constraint by cutting or by the use of force		

Body Part (Character 4)	Approach (Character 5)	Device (Character 6)	Qualifier (Character 7)
0 Skin, Scalp **1** Skin, Face **2** Skin, Right Ear **3** Skin, Left Ear **4** Skin, Neck **5** Skin, Chest **6** Skin, Back **7** Skin, Abdomen **8** Skin, Buttock **9** Skin, Perineum **A** Skin, Genitalia **B** Skin, Right Upper Arm **C** Skin, Left Upper Arm **D** Skin, Right Lower Arm **E** Skin, Left Lower Arm **F** Skin, Right Hand **G** Skin, Left Hand **H** Skin, Right Upper Leg **J** Skin, Left Upper Leg **K** Skin, Right Lower Leg **L** Skin, Left Lower Leg **M** Skin, Right Foot **N** Skin, Left Foot **Q** Finger Nail **R** Toe Nail	**X** External	**Z** No Device	**Z** No Qualifier
T Breast, Right **U** Breast, Left **V** Breast, Bilateral **W** Nipple, Right **X** Nipple, Left	**0** Open **3** Percutaneous **7** Via Natural or Artificial Opening **8** Via Natural or Artificial Opening Endoscopic **X** External	**Z** No Device	**Z** No Qualifier

Section	0	Medical and Surgical
Body System	H	Skin and Breast
Operation	P	Removal: Taking out or off a device from a body part

Body Part (Character 4)	Approach (Character 5)	Device (Character 6)	Qualifier (Character 7)
P Skin Q Finger Nail R Toe Nail	X External	0 Drainage Device 7 Autologous Tissue Substitute J Synthetic Substitute K Nonautologous Tissue Substitute	Z No Qualifier
S Hair	X External	7 Autologous Tissue Substitute J Synthetic Substitute K Nonautologous Tissue Substitute	Z No Qualifier
T Breast, Right U Breast, Left	0 Open 3 Percutaneous 7 Via Natural or Artificial Opening 8 Via Natural or Artificial Opening Endoscopic	0 Drainage Device 1 Radioactive Element 7 Autologous Tissue Substitute J Synthetic Substitute K Nonautologous Tissue Substitute N Tissue Expander	Z No Qualifier
T Breast, Right U Breast, Left	X External	0 Drainage Device 1 Radioactive Element 7 Autologous Tissue Substitute J Synthetic Substitute K Nonautologous Tissue Substitute	Z No Qualifier

Section	0	Medical and Surgical
Body System	H	Skin and Breast
Operation	Q	Repair: Restoring, to the extent possible, a body part to its normal anatomic structure and function

Body Part (Character 4)	Approach (Character 5)	Device (Character 6)	Qualifier (Character 7)
0 Skin, Scalp 1 Skin, Face 2 Skin, Right Ear 3 Skin, Left Ear 4 Skin, Neck 5 Skin, Chest 6 Skin, Back 7 Skin, Abdomen 8 Skin, Buttock 9 Skin, Perineum A Skin, Genitalia B Skin, Right Upper Arm C Skin, Left Upper Arm D Skin, Right Lower Arm E Skin, Left Lower Arm F Skin, Right Hand G Skin, Left Hand H Skin, Right Upper Leg J Skin, Left Upper Leg K Skin, Right Lower Leg L Skin, Left Lower Leg M Skin, Right Foot N Skin, Left Foot Q Finger Nail R Toe Nail	X External	Z No Device	Z No Qualifier
T Breast, Right U Breast, Left V Breast, Bilateral W Nipple, Right X Nipple, Left Y Supernumerary Breast	0 Open 3 Percutaneous 7 Via Natural or Artificial Opening 8 Via Natural or Artificial Opening Endoscopic X External	Z No Device	Z No Qualifier

Section	0	Medical and Surgical		
Body System	H	Skin and Breast		
Operation	R	Replacement: Putting in or on biological or synthetic material that physically takes the place and/or function of all or a portion of a body part		

Body Part (Character 4)	Approach (Character 5)	Device (Character 6)	Qualifier (Character 7)
0 Skin, Scalp 1 Skin, Face 2 Skin, Right Ear 3 Skin, Left Ear 4 Skin, Neck 5 Skin, Chest 6 Skin, Back 7 Skin, Abdomen 8 Skin, Buttock 9 Skin, Perineum A Skin, Genitalia B Skin, Right Upper Arm C Skin, Left Upper Arm D Skin, Right Lower Arm E Skin, Left Lower Arm F Skin, Right Hand G Skin, Left Hand H Skin, Right Upper Leg J Skin, Left Upper Leg K Skin, Right Lower Leg L Skin, Left Lower Leg M Skin, Right Foot N Skin, Left Foot	X External	7 Autologous Tissue Substitute K Nonautologous Tissue Substitute	3 Full Thickness 4 Partial Thickness

Section	0	Medical and Surgical		
Body System	H	Skin and Breast		
Operation	R	Replacement: Putting in or on biological or synthetic material that physically takes the place and/or function of all or a portion of a body part		

Body Part (Character 4)	Approach (Character 5)	Device (Character 6)	Qualifier (Character 7)
0 Skin, Scalp 1 Skin, Face 2 Skin, Right Ear 3 Skin, Left Ear 4 Skin, Neck 5 Skin, Chest 6 Skin, Back 7 Skin, Abdomen 8 Skin, Buttock 9 Skin, Perineum A Skin, Genitalia B Skin, Right Upper Arm C Skin, Left Upper Arm D Skin, Right Lower Arm E Skin, Left Lower Arm F Skin, Right Hand G Skin, Left Hand H Skin, Right Upper Leg J Skin, Left Upper Leg K Skin, Right Lower Leg L Skin, Left Lower Leg M Skin, Right Foot N Skin, Left Foot	X External	J Synthetic Substitute	3 Full Thickness 4 Partial Thickness Z No Qualifier
Q Finger Nail R Toe Nail S Hair	X External	7 Autologous Tissue Substitute J Synthetic Substitute K Nonautologous Tissue Substitute	Z No Qualifier
T Breast, Right U Breast, Left V Breast, Bilateral	0 Open	7 Autologous Tissue Substitute	5 Latissimus Dorsi Myocutaneous Flap 6 Transverse Rectus Abdominis Myocutaneous Flap 7 Deep Inferior Epigastric Artery Perforator Flap 8 Superficial Inferior Epigastric Artery Flap 9 Gluteal Artery Perforator Flap Z No Qualifier

Section	0	Medical and Surgical		
Body System	H	Skin and Breast		[continued]
Operation	R	Replacement: Putting in or on biological or synthetic material that physically takes the place and/or function of all or a portion of a body part		

Body Part (Character 4)	Body Part (Character 4)	Body Part (Character 4)	Body Part (Character 4)
T Breast, Right U Breast, Left V Breast, Bilateral	0 Open	J Synthetic Substitute K Nonautologous Tissue Substitute	Z No Qualifier

Section	0	Medical and Surgical		
Body System	H	Skin and Breast		
Operation	R	Replacement: Putting in or on biological or synthetic material that physically takes the place and/or function of all or a portion of a body part		

Body Part (Character 4)	Approach (Character 5)	Device (Character 6)	Qualifier (Character 7)
T Breast, Right U Breast, Left V Breast, Bilateral	3 Percutaneous X External	7 Autologous Tissue Substitute J Synthetic Substitute K Nonautologous Tissue Substitute	Z No Qualifier
W Nipple, Right X Nipple, Left	0 Open 3 Percutaneous X External	7 Autologous Tissue Substitute J Synthetic Substitute K Nonautologous Tissue Substitute	Z No Qualifier

Section	0	Medical and Surgical		
Body System	H	Skin and Breast		
Operation	S	Reposition: Moving to its normal location, or other suitable location, all or a portion of a body part		

Body Part (Character 4)	Approach (Character 5)	Device (Character 6)	Qualifier (Character 7)
S Hair W Nipple, Right X Nipple, Left	X External	Z No Device	Z No Qualifier
T Breast, Right U Breast, Left V Breast, Bilateral	0 Open	Z No Device	Z No Qualifier

Section	0	Medical and Surgical		
Body System	H	Skin and Breast		
Operation	T	Resection: Cutting out or off, without replacement, all of a body part		

Body Part (Character 4)	Approach (Character 5)	Device (Character 6)	Qualifier (Character 7)
Q Finger Nail R Toe Nail W Nipple, Right X Nipple, Left	X External	Z No Device	Z No Qualifier
T Breast, Right U Breast, Left V Breast, Bilateral Y Supernumerary Breast	0 Open	Z No Device	Z No Qualifier

Section	0	Medical and Surgical		
Body System	H	Skin and Breast		
Operation	U	Supplement: Putting in or on biological or synthetic material that physically reinforces and/or augments the function of a portion of a body part		

Body Part (Character 4)	Approach (Character 5)	Device (Character 6)	Qualifier (Character 7)
T Breast, Right U Breast, Left V Breast, Bilateral W Nipple, Right X Nipple, Left	0 Open 3 Percutaneous 7 Via Natural or Artificial Opening 8 Via Natural or Artificial Opening Endoscopic X External	7 Autologous Tissue Substitute J Synthetic Substitute K Nonautologous Tissue Substitute	Z No Qualifier

Section	0	Medical and Surgical		
Body System	H	Skin and Breast		
Operation	W	Revision: Correcting, to the extent possible, a portion of a malfunctioning device or the position of a displaced device		

Body Part (Character 4)	Approach (Character 5)	Device (Character 6)	Qualifier (Character 7)
P Skin Q Finger Nail R Toe Nail	X External	0 Drainage Device 7 Autologous Tissue Substitute J Synthetic Substitute K Nonautologous Tissue Substitute	Z No Qualifier
S Hair	X External	7 Autologous Tissue Substitute J Synthetic Substitute K Nonautologous Tissue Substitute	Z No Qualifier
T Breast, Right U Breast, Left	0 Open 3 Percutaneous 7 Via Natural or Artificial Opening 8 Via Natural or Artificial Opening Endoscopic	0 Drainage Device 7 Autologous Tissue Substitute J Synthetic Substitute K Nonautologous Tissue Substitute N Tissue Expander	Z No Qualifier
T Breast, Right U Breast, Left	X External	0 Drainage Device 7 Autologous Tissue Substitute J Synthetic Substitute K Nonautologous Tissue Substitute	Z No Qualifier

Section	0	Medical and Surgical		
Body System	H	Skin and Breast		
Operation	X	Transfer: Moving, without taking out, all or a portion of a body part to another location to take over the function of all or a portion of a body part		

Body Part (Character 4)	Approach (Character 5)	Device (Character 6)	Qualifier (Character 7)
0 Skin, Scalp 1 Skin, Face 2 Skin, Right Ear 3 Skin, Left Ear 4 Skin, Neck 5 Skin, Chest 6 Skin, Back 7 Skin, Abdomen 8 Skin, Buttock 9 Skin, Perineum A Skin, Genitalia B Skin, Right Upper Arm C Skin, Left Upper Arm D Skin, Right Lower Arm E Skin, Left Lower Arm F Skin, Right Hand G Skin, Left Hand H Skin, Right Upper Leg J Skin, Left Upper Leg K Skin, Right Lower Leg L Skin, Left Lower Leg M Skin, Right Foot N Skin, Left Foot	X External	Z No Device	Z No Qualifier

Section	0	Medical and Surgical
Body System	J	Subcutaneous Tissue and Fascia
Operation	0	Alteration: Modifying the anatomic structure of a body part without affecting the function of the body part

Body Part (Character 4)	Approach (Character 5)	Device (Character 6)	Qualifier (Character 7)
1 Subcutaneous Tissue and Fascia, Face 4 Subcutaneous Tissue and Fascia, Anterior Neck 5 Subcutaneous Tissue and Fascia, Posterior Neck 6 Subcutaneous Tissue and Fascia, Chest 7 Subcutaneous Tissue and Fascia, Back 8 Subcutaneous Tissue and Fascia, Abdomen 9 Subcutaneous Tissue and Fascia, Buttock D Subcutaneous Tissue and Fascia, Right Upper Arm F Subcutaneous Tissue and Fascia, Left Upper Arm G Subcutaneous Tissue and Fascia, Right Lower Arm H Subcutaneous Tissue and Fascia, Left Lower Arm L Subcutaneous Tissue and Fascia, Right Upper Leg M Subcutaneous Tissue and Fascia, Left Upper Leg N Subcutaneous Tissue and Fascia, Right Lower Leg P Subcutaneous Tissue and Fascia, Left Lower Leg	0 Open 3 Percutaneous	Z No Device	Z No Qualifier

Section	0	Medical and Surgical
Body System	J	Subcutaneous Tissue and Fascia
Operation	2	Change: Taking out or off a device from a body part and putting back an identical or similar device in or on the same body part without cutting or puncturing the skin or a mucous membrane

Body Part (Character 4)	Approach (Character 5)	Device (Character 6)	Qualifier (Character 7)
S Subcutaneous Tissue and Fascia, Head and Neck T Subcutaneous Tissue and Fascia, Trunk V Subcutaneous Tissue and Fascia, Upper Extremity W Subcutaneous Tissue and Fascia, Lower Extremity	X External	0 Drainage Device Y Other Device	Z No Qualifier

Section	0	Medical and Surgical
Body System	J	Subcutaneous Tissue and Fascia
Operation	5	Destruction: Physical eradication of all or a portion of a body part by the direct use of energy, force, or a destructive agent

Body Part (Character 4)	Approach (Character 5)	Device (Character 6)	Qualifier (Character 7)
0 Subcutaneous Tissue and Fascia, Scalp **1** Subcutaneous Tissue and Fascia, Face **4** Subcutaneous Tissue and Fascia, Anterior Neck **5** Subcutaneous Tissue and Fascia, Posterior Neck **6** Subcutaneous Tissue and Fascia, Chest **7** Subcutaneous Tissue and Fascia, Back **8** Subcutaneous Tissue and Fascia, Abdomen **9** Subcutaneous Tissue and Fascia, Buttock **B** Subcutaneous Tissue and Fascia, Perineum **C** Subcutaneous Tissue and Fascia, Pelvic Region **D** Subcutaneous Tissue and Fascia, Right Upper Arm **F** Subcutaneous Tissue and Fascia, Left Upper Arm **G** Subcutaneous Tissue and Fascia, Right Lower Arm **H** Subcutaneous Tissue and Fascia, Left Lower Arm **J** Subcutaneous Tissue and Fascia, Right Hand **K** Subcutaneous Tissue and Fascia, Left Hand **L** Subcutaneous Tissue and Fascia, Right Upper Leg **M** Subcutaneous Tissue and Fascia, Left Upper Leg **N** Subcutaneous Tissue and Fascia, Right Lower Leg **P** Subcutaneous Tissue and Fascia, Left Lower Leg **Q** Subcutaneous Tissue and Fascia, Right Foot **R** Subcutaneous Tissue and Fascia, Left Foot	**0** Open **3** Percutaneous	**Z** No Device	**Z** No Qualifier

Section	0	Medical and Surgical		
Body System	J	Subcutaneous Tissue and Fascia		
Operation	8	Division: Cutting into a body part, without draining fluids and/or gases from the body part, in order to separate or transect a body part		

Body Part (Character 4)	Approach (Character 5)	Device (Character 6)	Qualifier (Character 7)
0 Subcutaneous Tissue and Fascia, Scalp **1** Subcutaneous Tissue and Fascia, Face **4** Subcutaneous Tissue and Fascia, Anterior Neck **5** Subcutaneous Tissue and Fascia, Posterior Neck **6** Subcutaneous Tissue and Fascia, Chest **7** Subcutaneous Tissue and Fascia, Back **8** Subcutaneous Tissue and Fascia, Abdomen **9** Subcutaneous Tissue and Fascia, Buttock **B** Subcutaneous Tissue and Fascia, Perineum **C** Subcutaneous Tissue and Fascia, Pelvic Region **D** Subcutaneous Tissue and Fascia, Right Upper Arm **F** Subcutaneous Tissue and Fascia, Left Upper Arm **G** Subcutaneous Tissue and Fascia, Right Lower Arm **H** Subcutaneous Tissue and Fascia, Left Lower Arm **J** Subcutaneous Tissue and Fascia, Right Hand **K** Subcutaneous Tissue and Fascia, Left Hand **L** Subcutaneous Tissue and Fascia, Right Upper Leg **M** Subcutaneous Tissue and Fascia, Left Upper Leg **N** Subcutaneous Tissue and Fascia, Right Lower Leg **P** Subcutaneous Tissue and Fascia, Left Lower Leg **Q** Subcutaneous Tissue and Fascia, Right Foot **R** Subcutaneous Tissue and Fascia, Left Foot **S** Subcutaneous Tissue and Fascia, Head and Neck **T** Subcutaneous Tissue and Fascia, Trunk **V** Subcutaneous Tissue and Fascia, Upper Extremity **W** Subcutaneous Tissue and Fascia, Lower Extremity	**0** Open **3** Percutaneous	**Z** No Device	**Z** No Qualifier

Section	0	Medical and Surgical		
Body System	J	Subcutaneous Tissue and Fascia		
Operation	9	Drainage: Taking or letting out fluids and/or gases from a body part		

Body Part (Character 4)	Approach (Character 5)	Device (Character 6)	Qualifier (Character 7)
0 Subcutaneous Tissue and Fascia, Scalp **1** Subcutaneous Tissue and Fascia, Face **4** Subcutaneous Tissue and Fascia, Anterior Neck **5** Subcutaneous Tissue and Fascia, Posterior Neck **6** Subcutaneous Tissue and Fascia, Chest **7** Subcutaneous Tissue and Fascia, Back **8** Subcutaneous Tissue and Fascia, Abdomen **9** Subcutaneous Tissue and Fascia, Buttock **B** Subcutaneous Tissue and Fascia, Perineum **C** Subcutaneous Tissue and Fascia, Pelvic Region **D** Subcutaneous Tissue and Fascia, Right Upper Arm **F** Subcutaneous Tissue and Fascia, Left Upper Arm **G** Subcutaneous Tissue and Fascia, Right Lower Arm **H** Subcutaneous Tissue and Fascia, Left Lower Arm **J** Subcutaneous Tissue and Fascia, Right Hand **K** Subcutaneous Tissue and Fascia, Left Hand **L** Subcutaneous Tissue and Fascia, Right Upper Leg **M** Subcutaneous Tissue and Fascia, Left Upper Leg **N** Subcutaneous Tissue and Fascia, Right Lower Leg **P** Subcutaneous Tissue and Fascia, Left Lower Leg **Q** Subcutaneous Tissue and Fascia, Right Foot **R** Subcutaneous Tissue and Fascia, Left Foot	**0** Open **3** Percutaneous	**Z** No Device	**X** Diagnostic **Z** No Qualifier

Section	0	Medical and Surgical		
Body System	J	Subcutaneous Tissue and Fascia		
Operation	B	Excision: Cutting out or off, without replacement, a portion of a body part		

Body Part (Character 4)	Approach (Character 5)	Device (Character 6)	Qualifier (Character 7)
0 Subcutaneous Tissue and Fascia, Scalp **1** Subcutaneous Tissue and Fascia, Face **4** Subcutaneous Tissue and Fascia, Anterior Neck **5** Subcutaneous Tissue and Fascia, Posterior Neck **6** Subcutaneous Tissue and Fascia, Chest **7** Subcutaneous Tissue and Fascia, Back **8** Subcutaneous Tissue and Fascia, Abdomen **9** Subcutaneous Tissue and Fascia, Buttock **B** Subcutaneous Tissue and Fascia, Perineum **C** Subcutaneous Tissue and Fascia, Pelvic Region **D** Subcutaneous Tissue and Fascia, Right Upper Arm **F** Subcutaneous Tissue and Fascia, Left Upper Arm **G** Subcutaneous Tissue and Fascia, Right Lower Arm **H** Subcutaneous Tissue and Fascia, Left Lower Arm **J** Subcutaneous Tissue and Fascia, Right Hand **K** Subcutaneous Tissue and Fascia, Left Hand **L** Subcutaneous Tissue and Fascia, Right Upper Leg **M** Subcutaneous Tissue and Fascia, Left Upper Leg **N** Subcutaneous Tissue and Fascia, Right Lower Leg **P** Subcutaneous Tissue and Fascia, Left Lower Leg **Q** Subcutaneous Tissue and Fascia, Right Foot **R** Subcutaneous Tissue and Fascia, Left Foot	**0** Open **3** Percutaneous	**Z** No Device	**X** Diagnostic **Z** No Qualifier

Section	0	Medical and Surgical		
Body System	J	Subcutaneous Tissue and Fascia		
Operation	C	Extirpation: Taking or cutting out solid matter from a body part		

Body Part (Character 4)	Approach (Character 5)	Device (Character 6)	Qualifier (Character 7)
0 Subcutaneous Tissue and Fascia, Scalp 1 Subcutaneous Tissue and Fascia, Face 4 Subcutaneous Tissue and Fascia, Anterior Neck 5 Subcutaneous Tissue and Fascia, Posterior Neck 6 Subcutaneous Tissue and Fascia, Chest 7 Subcutaneous Tissue and Fascia, Back 8 Subcutaneous Tissue and Fascia, Abdomen 9 Subcutaneous Tissue and Fascia, Buttock B Subcutaneous Tissue and Fascia, Perineum C Subcutaneous Tissue and Fascia, Pelvic Region D Subcutaneous Tissue and Fascia, Right Upper Arm F Subcutaneous Tissue and Fascia, Left Upper Arm G Subcutaneous Tissue and Fascia, Right Lower Arm H Subcutaneous Tissue and Fascia, Left Lower Arm J Subcutaneous Tissue and Fascia, Right Hand K Subcutaneous Tissue and Fascia, Left Hand L Subcutaneous Tissue and Fascia, Right Upper Leg M Subcutaneous Tissue and Fascia, Left Upper Leg N Subcutaneous Tissue and Fascia, Right Lower Leg P Subcutaneous Tissue and Fascia, Left Lower Leg Q Subcutaneous Tissue and Fascia, Right Foot R Subcutaneous Tissue and Fascia, Left Foot	0 Open 3 Percutaneous	Z No Device	Z No Qualifier

Section	0	Medical and Surgical		
Body System	J	Subcutaneous Tissue and Fascia		
Operation	D	Extraction: Pulling or stripping out or off all or a portion of a body part by the use of force		

Body Part (Character 4)	Approach (Character 5)	Device (Character 6)	Qualifier (Character 7)
0 Subcutaneous Tissue and Fascia, Scalp **1** Subcutaneous Tissue and Fascia, Face **4** Subcutaneous Tissue and Fascia, Anterior Neck **5** Subcutaneous Tissue and Fascia, Posterior Neck **6** Subcutaneous Tissue and Fascia, Chest **7** Subcutaneous Tissue and Fascia, Back **8** Subcutaneous Tissue and Fascia, Abdomen **9** Subcutaneous Tissue and Fascia, Buttock **B** Subcutaneous Tissue and Fascia, Perineum **C** Subcutaneous Tissue and Fascia, Pelvic Region **D** Subcutaneous Tissue and Fascia, Right Upper Arm **F** Subcutaneous Tissue and Fascia, Left Upper Arm **G** Subcutaneous Tissue and Fascia, Right Lower Arm **H** Subcutaneous Tissue and Fascia, Left Lower Arm **J** Subcutaneous Tissue and Fascia, Right Hand **K** Subcutaneous Tissue and Fascia, Left Hand **L** Subcutaneous Tissue and Fascia, Right Upper Leg **M** Subcutaneous Tissue and Fascia, Left Upper Leg **N** Subcutaneous Tissue and Fascia, Right Lower Leg **P** Subcutaneous Tissue and Fascia, Left Lower Leg **Q** Subcutaneous Tissue and Fascia, Right Foot **R** Subcutaneous Tissue and Fascia, Left Foot	**0** Open **3** Percutaneous	**Z** No Device	**Z** No Qualifier

Section	0	Medical and Surgical
Body System	J	Subcutaneous Tissue and Fascia
Operation	H	Insertion: Putting in a nonbiological appliance that monitors, assists, performs, or prevents a physiological function but does not physically take the place of a body part

Body Part (Character 4)	Approach (Character 5)	Device (Character 6)	Qualifier (Character 7)
0 Subcutaneous Tissue and Fascia, Scalp **1** Subcutaneous Tissue and Fascia, Face **4** Subcutaneous Tissue and Fascia, Anterior Neck **5** Subcutaneous Tissue and Fascia, Posterior Neck **9** Subcutaneous Tissue and Fascia, Buttock **B** Subcutaneous Tissue and Fascia, Perineum **C** Subcutaneous Tissue and Fascia, Pelvic Region **J** Subcutaneous Tissue and Fascia, Right Hand **K** Subcutaneous Tissue and Fascia, Left Hand **Q** Subcutaneous Tissue and Fascia, Right Foot **R** Subcutaneous Tissue and Fascia, Left Foot	**0** Open **3** Percutaneous	**N** Tissue Expander **0** Monitoring Device, Hemodynamic **2** Monitoring Device **4** Pacemaker, Single Chamber **5** Pacemaker, Single Chamber Rate Responsive **6** Pacemaker, Dual Chamber **7** Cardiac Resynchronization Pacemaker Pulse Generator **8** Defibrillator Generator **9** Cardiac Resynchronization Defibrillator Pulse Generator	**Z** No Qualifier
6 Subcutaneous Tissue and Fascia, Chest **8** Subcutaneous Tissue and Fascia, Abdomen	**0** Open **3** Percutaneous	**A** Contractility Modulation Device **B** Stimulator Generator, Single Array **C** Stimulator Generator, Single Array Rechargeable **D** Stimulator Generator, Multiple Array **E** Stimulator Generator, Multiple Array Rechargeable **H** Contraceptive Device **M** Stimulator Generator **N** Tissue Expander **P** Cardiac Rhythm Related Device **V** Infusion Device, Pump **W** Vascular Access Device, Reservoir **X** Vascular Access Device	**Z** No Qualifier

Section	0	Medical and Surgical		
Body System	J	Subcutaneous Tissue and Fascia		
Operation	H	Insertion: Putting in a nonbiological appliance that monitors, assists, performs, or prevents a physiological function but does not physically take the place of a body part		

Body Part (Character 4)	Approach (Character 5)	Device (Character 6)	Qualifier (Character 7)
7 Subcutaneous Tissue and Fascia, Back	0 Open 3 Percutaneous	B Stimulator Generator, Single Array C Stimulator Generator, Single Array Rechargeable D Stimulator Generator, Multiple Array E Stimulator Generator, Multiple Array Rechargeable M Stimulator Generator N Tissue Expander V Infusion Device, Pump	Z No Qualifier
D Subcutaneous Tissue and Fascia, Right Upper Arm F Subcutaneous Tissue and Fascia, Left Upper Arm G Subcutaneous Tissue and Fascia, Right Lower Arm H Subcutaneous Tissue and Fascia, Left Lower Arm L Subcutaneous Tissue and Fascia, Right Upper Leg M Subcutaneous Tissue and Fascia, Left Upper Leg N Subcutaneous Tissue and Fascia, Right Lower Leg P Subcutaneous Tissue and Fascia, Left Lower Leg	0 Open 3 Percutaneous	H Contraceptive Device N Tissue Expander V Infusion Device, Pump W Vascular Access Device, Reservoir X Vascular Access Device	Z No Qualifier
S Subcutaneous Tissue and Fascia, Head and Neck V Subcutaneous Tissue and Fascia, Upper Extremity W Subcutaneous Tissue and Fascia, Lower Extremity	0 Open 3 Percutaneous	1 Radioactive Element 3 Infusion Device	Z No Qualifier
T Subcutaneous Tissue and Fascia, Trunk	0 Open 3 Percutaneous	1 Radioactive Element 3 Infusion Device V Infusion Device, Pump	Z No Qualifier

Section	0	Medical and Surgical		
Body System	J	Subcutaneous Tissue and Fascia		
Operation	J	Inspection: Visually and/or manually exploring a body part		

Body Part (Character 4)	Approach (Character 5)	Device (Character 6)	Qualifier (Character 7)
S Subcutaneous Tissue and Fascia, Head and Neck T Subcutaneous Tissue and Fascia, Trunk V Subcutaneous Tissue and Fascia, Upper Extremity W Subcutaneous Tissue and Fascia, Lower Extremity	0 Open 3 Percutaneous X External	Z No Device	Z No Qualifier

Section	0	Medical and Surgical			
Body System	J	Subcutaneous Tissue and Fascia			
Operation	N	Release: Freeing a body part from an abnormal physical constraint by cutting or by the use of force			

Body Part (Character 4)	Approach (Character 5)	Device (Character 6)	Qualifier (Character 7)
0 Subcutaneous Tissue and Fascia, Scalp 1 Subcutaneous Tissue and Fascia, Face 4 Subcutaneous Tissue and Fascia, Anterior Neck 5 Subcutaneous Tissue and Fascia, Posterior Neck 6 Subcutaneous Tissue and Fascia, Chest 7 Subcutaneous Tissue and Fascia, Back 8 Subcutaneous Tissue and Fascia, Abdomen 9 Subcutaneous Tissue and Fascia, Buttock B Subcutaneous Tissue and Fascia, Perineum C Subcutaneous Tissue and Fascia, Pelvic Region D Subcutaneous Tissue and Fascia, Right Upper Arm F Subcutaneous Tissue and Fascia, Left Upper Arm G Subcutaneous Tissue and Fascia, Right Lower Arm H Subcutaneous Tissue and Fascia, Left Lower Arm J Subcutaneous Tissue and Fascia, Right Hand K Subcutaneous Tissue and Fascia, Left Hand L Subcutaneous Tissue and Fascia, Right Upper Leg M Subcutaneous Tissue and Fascia, Left Upper Leg N Subcutaneous Tissue and Fascia, Right Lower Leg P Subcutaneous Tissue and Fascia, Left Lower Leg Q Subcutaneous Tissue and Fascia, Right Foot R Subcutaneous Tissue and Fascia, Left Foot	0 Open 3 Percutaneous X External	Z No Device	Z No Qualifier

Section	0	Medical and Surgical		
Body System	J	Subcutaneous Tissue and Fascia		
Operation	P	Removal: Taking out or off a device from a body part		

Body Part (Character 4)	Approach (Character 5)	Device (Character 6)	Qualifier (Character 7)
S Subcutaneous Tissue and Fascia, Head and Neck	**0** Open **3** Percutaneous	**0** Drainage Device **1** Radioactive Element **3** Infusion Device **7** Autologous Tissue Substitute **J** Synthetic Substitute **K** Nonautologous Tissue Substitute **N** Tissue Expander	**Z** No Qualifier
S Subcutaneous Tissue and Fascia, Head and Neck	**X** External	**0** Drainage Device **1** Radioactive Element **3** Infusion Device	**Z** No Qualifier
T Subcutaneous Tissue and Fascia, Trunk	**0** Open **3** Percutaneous	**0** Drainage Device **1** Radioactive Element **2** Monitoring Device **3** Infusion Device **7** Autologous Tissue Substitute **H** Contraceptive Device **J** Synthetic Substitute **K** Nonautologous Tissue Substitute **M** Stimulator Generator **N** Tissue Expander **P** Cardiac Rhythm Related Device **V** Infusion Device, Pump **W** Vascular Access Device, Reservoir **X** Vascular Access Device	**Z** No Qualifier
T Subcutaneous Tissue and Fascia, Trunk	**X** External	**0** Drainage Device **1** Radioactive Element **2** Monitoring Device **3** Infusion Device **H** Contraceptive Device **V** Infusion Device, Pump **X** Vascular Access Device	**Z** No Qualifier

Section	0	Medical and Surgical		
Body System	J	Subcutaneous Tissue and Fascia		
Operation	P	Removal: Taking out or off a device from a body part		

Body Part (Character 4)	Approach (Character 5)	Device (Character 6)	Qualifier (Character 7)
V Subcutaneous Tissue and Fascia, Upper Extremity **W** Subcutaneous Tissue and Fascia, Lower Extremity	**0** Open **3** Percutaneous	**0** Drainage Device **1** Radioactive Element **3** Infusion Device **7** Autologous Tissue Substitute **H** Contraceptive Device **J** Synthetic Substitute **K** Nonautologous Tissue Substitute **N** Tissue Expander **V** Infusion Device, Pump **W** Vascular Access Device, Reservoir **X** Vascular Access Device	**Z** No Qualifier
V Subcutaneous Tissue and Fascia, Upper Extremity **W** Subcutaneous Tissue and Fascia, Lower Extremity	**X** External	**0** Drainage Device **1** Radioactive Element **3** Infusion Device **H** Contraceptive Device **V** Infusion Device, Pump **X** Vascular Access Device	**Z** No Qualifier

Section	0	Medical and Surgical
Body System	J	Subcutaneous Tissue and Fascia
Operation	Q	Repair: Restoring, to the extent possible, a body part to its normal anatomic structure and function

Body Part (Character 4)	Approach (Character 5)	Device (Character 6)	Qualifier (Character 7)
0 Subcutaneous Tissue and Fascia, Scalp **1** Subcutaneous Tissue and Fascia, Face **4** Subcutaneous Tissue and Fascia, Anterior Neck **5** Subcutaneous Tissue and Fascia, Posterior Neck **6** Subcutaneous Tissue and Fascia, Chest **7** Subcutaneous Tissue and Fascia, Back **8** Subcutaneous Tissue and Fascia, Abdomen **9** Subcutaneous Tissue and Fascia, Buttock **B** Subcutaneous Tissue and Fascia, Perineum **C** Subcutaneous Tissue and Fascia, Pelvic Region **D** Subcutaneous Tissue and Fascia, Right Upper Arm **F** Subcutaneous Tissue and Fascia, Left Upper Arm **G** Subcutaneous Tissue and Fascia, Right Lower Arm **H** Subcutaneous Tissue and Fascia, Left Lower Arm **J** Subcutaneous Tissue and Fascia, Right Hand **K** Subcutaneous Tissue and Fascia, Left Hand **L** Subcutaneous Tissue and Fascia, Right Upper Leg **M** Subcutaneous Tissue and Fascia, Left Upper Leg **N** Subcutaneous Tissue and Fascia, Right Lower Leg **P** Subcutaneous Tissue and Fascia, Left Lower Leg **Q** Subcutaneous Tissue and Fascia, Right Foot **R** Subcutaneous Tissue and Fascia, Left Foot	**0** Open **3** Percutaneous	**Z** No Device	**Z** No Qualifier

Section	0	Medical and Surgical
Body System	J	Subcutaneous Tissue and Fascia
Operation	W	Revision: Correcting, to the extent possible, a portion of a malfunctioning device or the position of a displaced device

Body Part (Character 4)	Approach (Character 5)	Device (Character 6)	Qualifier (Character 7)
S Subcutaneous Tissue and Fascia, Head and Neck	**0** Open **3** Percutaneous **X** External	**0** Drainage Device **3** Infusion Device **7** Autologous Tissue Substitute **J** Synthetic Substitute **K** Nonautologous Tissue Substitute **N** Tissue Expander	**Z** No Qualifier
T Subcutaneous Tissue and Fascia, Trunk	**0** Open **3** Percutaneous **X** External	**0** Drainage Device **2** Monitoring Device **3** Infusion Device **7** Autologous Tissue Substitute **H** Contraceptive Device **J** Synthetic Substitute **K** Nonautologous Tissue Substitute **M** Stimulator Generator **N** Tissue Expander **P** Cardiac Rhythm Related Device **V** Infusion Device, Pump **W** Vascular Access Device, Reservoir **X** Vascular Access Device	**Z** No Qualifier
V Subcutaneous Tissue and Fascia, Upper Extremity **W** Subcutaneous Tissue and Fascia, Lower Extremity	**0** Open **3** Percutaneous **X** External	**0** Drainage Device **3** Infusion Device **7** Autologous Tissue Substitute **H** Contraceptive Device **J** Synthetic Substitute **K** Nonautologous Tissue Substitute **N** Tissue Expander **V** Infusion Device, Pump **W** Vascular Access Device, Reservoir **X** Vascular Access Device	**Z** No Qualifier

Section	0	Medical and Surgical		
Body System	J	Subcutaneous Tissue and Fascia		
Operation	X	Transfer: Moving, without taking out, all or a portion of a body part to another location to take over the function of all or a portion of a body part		

Body Part (Character 4)	Approach (Character 5)	Device (Character 6)	Qualifier (Character 7)
0 Subcutaneous Tissue and Fascia, Scalp **1** Subcutaneous Tissue and Fascia, Face **4** Subcutaneous Tissue and Fascia, Anterior Neck **5** Subcutaneous Tissue and Fascia, Posterior Neck **6** Subcutaneous Tissue and Fascia, Chest **7** Subcutaneous Tissue and Fascia, Back **8** Subcutaneous Tissue and Fascia, Abdomen **9** Subcutaneous Tissue and Fascia, Buttock **B** Subcutaneous Tissue and Fascia, Perineum **C** Subcutaneous Tissue and Fascia, Pelvic Region **D** Subcutaneous Tissue and Fascia, Right Upper Arm **F** Subcutaneous Tissue and Fascia, Left Upper Arm **G** Subcutaneous Tissue and Fascia, Right Lower Arm **H** Subcutaneous Tissue and Fascia, Left Lower Arm **J** Subcutaneous Tissue and Fascia, Right Hand **K** Subcutaneous Tissue and Fascia, Left Hand **L** Subcutaneous Tissue and Fascia, Right Upper Leg **M** Subcutaneous Tissue and Fascia, Left Upper Leg **N** Subcutaneous Tissue and Fascia, Right Lower Leg **P** Subcutaneous Tissue and Fascia, Left Lower Leg **Q** Subcutaneous Tissue and Fascia, Right Foot **R** Subcutaneous Tissue and Fascia, Left Foot	**0** Open **3** Percutaneous	**Z** No Device	**B** Skin and Subcutaneous Tissue **C** Skin, Subcutaneous Tissue and Fascia **Z** No Qualifier

Section	0	Medical and Surgical		
Body System	K	Muscles		
Operation	2	Change: Taking out or off a device from a body part and putting back an identical or similar device in or on the same body part without cutting or puncturing the skin or a mucous membrane		
Body Part (Character 4)		**Approach (Character 5)**	**Device (Character 6)**	**Qualifier (Character 7)**
X Upper Muscle		X External	0 Drainage Device	Z No Qualifier
Y Lower Muscle			Y Other Device	

Section	0	Medical and Surgical		
Body System	K	Muscles		
Operation	5	Destruction: Physical eradication of all or a portion of a body part by the direct use of energy, force, or a destructive agent		
Body Part (Character 4)		**Approach (Character 5)**	**Device (Character 6)**	**Qualifier (Character 7)**
0 Head Muscle		0 Open	Z No Device	Z No Qualifier
1 Facial Muscle		3 Percutaneous		
2 Neck Muscle, Right		4 Percutaneous Endoscopic		
3 Neck Muscle, Left				
4 Tongue, Palate, Pharynx Muscle				
5 Shoulder Muscle, Right				
6 Shoulder Muscle, Left				
7 Upper Arm Muscle, Right				
8 Upper Arm Muscle, Left				
9 Lower Arm and Wrist Muscle, Right				
B Lower Arm and Wrist Muscle, Left				
C Hand Muscle, Right				
D Hand Muscle, Left				
F Trunk Muscle, Right				
G Trunk Muscle, Left				
H Thorax Muscle, Right				
J Thorax Muscle, Left				
K Abdomen Muscle, Right				
L Abdomen Muscle, Left				
M Perineum Muscle				
N Hip Muscle, Right				
P Hip Muscle, Left				
Q Upper Leg Muscle, Right				
R Upper Leg Muscle, Left				
S Lower Leg Muscle, Right				
T Lower Leg Muscle, Left				
V Foot Muscle, Right				
W Foot Muscle, Left				

Section	0	Medical and Surgical		
Body System	K	Muscles		
Operation	8	Division: Cutting into a body part, without draining fluids and/or gases from the body part, in order to separate or transect a body part		

Body Part (Character 4)	Approach (Character 5)	Device (Character 6)	Qualifier (Character 7)
0 Head Muscle 1 Facial Muscle 2 Neck Muscle, Right 3 Neck Muscle, Left 4 Tongue, Palate, Pharynx Muscle 5 Shoulder Muscle, Right 6 Shoulder Muscle, Left 7 Upper Arm Muscle, Right 8 Upper Arm Muscle, Left 9 Lower Arm and Wrist Muscle, Right B Lower Arm and Wrist Muscle, Left C Hand Muscle, Right D Hand Muscle, Left F Trunk Muscle, Right G Trunk Muscle, Left H Thorax Muscle, Right J Thorax Muscle, Left K Abdomen Muscle, Right L Abdomen Muscle, Left M Perineum Muscle N Hip Muscle, Right P Hip Muscle, Left Q Upper Leg Muscle, Right R Upper Leg Muscle, Left S Lower Leg Muscle, Right T Lower Leg Muscle, Left V Foot Muscle, Right W Foot Muscle, Left	0 Open 3 Percutaneous 4 Percutaneous Endoscopic	Z No Device	Z No Qualifier

Section	0	Medical and Surgical				
Body System	K	Muscles				
Operation	9	Drainage: Taking or letting out fluids and/or gases from a body part				

Body Part (Character 4)	Approach (Character 5)	Device (Character 6)	Qualifier (Character 7)
0 Head Muscle	**0** Open	**0** Drainage Device	**Z** No Qualifier
1 Facial Muscle	**3** Percutaneous		
2 Neck Muscle, Right	**4** Percutaneous Endoscopic		
3 Neck Muscle, Left			
4 Tongue, Palate, Pharynx Muscle			
5 Shoulder Muscle, Right			
6 Shoulder Muscle, Left			
7 Upper Arm Muscle, Right			
8 Upper Arm Muscle, Left			
9 Lower Arm and Wrist Muscle, Right			
B Lower Arm and Wrist Muscle, Left			
C Hand Muscle, Right			
D Hand Muscle, Left			
F Trunk Muscle, Right			
G Trunk Muscle, Left			
H Thorax Muscle, Right			
J Thorax Muscle, Left			
K Abdomen Muscle, Right			
L Abdomen Muscle, Left			
M Perineum Muscle			
N Hip Muscle, Right			
P Hip Muscle, Left			
Q Upper Leg Muscle, Right			
R Upper Leg Muscle, Left			
S Lower Leg Muscle, Right			
T Lower Leg Muscle, Left			
V Foot Muscle, Right			
W Foot Muscle, Left			

Section	0	Medical and Surgical				
Body System	K	Muscles				
Operation	9	Drainage: Taking or letting out fluids and/or gases from a body part				

Body Part (Character 4)	Approach (Character 5)	Device (Character 6)	Qualifier (Character 7)
0 Head Muscle	**0** Open	**Z** No Device	**X** Diagnostic
1 Facial Muscle	**3** Percutaneous		**Z** No Qualifier
2 Neck Muscle, Right	**4** Percutaneous Endoscopic		
3 Neck Muscle, Left			
4 Tongue, Palate, Pharynx Muscle			
5 Shoulder Muscle, Right			
6 Shoulder Muscle, Left			
7 Upper Arm Muscle, Right			
8 Upper Arm Muscle, Left			
9 Lower Arm and Wrist Muscle, Right			
B Lower Arm and Wrist Muscle, Left			
C Hand Muscle, Right			
D Hand Muscle, Left			
F Trunk Muscle, Right			
G Trunk Muscle, Left			
H Thorax Muscle, Right			
J Thorax Muscle, Left			
K Abdomen Muscle, Right			
L Abdomen Muscle, Left			
M Perineum Muscle			
N Hip Muscle, Right			
P Hip Muscle, Left			
Q Upper Leg Muscle, Right			
R Upper Leg Muscle, Left			
S Lower Leg Muscle, Right			
T Lower Leg Muscle, Left			
V Foot Muscle, Right			
W Foot Muscle, Left			

Section	0	Medical and Surgical		
Body System	K	Muscles		
Operation	B	Excision: Cutting out or off, without replacement, a portion of a body part		

Body Part (Character 4)	Approach (Character 5)	Device (Character 6)	Qualifier (Character 7)
0 Head Muscle 1 Facial Muscle 2 Neck Muscle, Right 3 Neck Muscle, Left 4 Tongue, Palate, Pharynx Muscle 5 Shoulder Muscle, Right 6 Shoulder Muscle, Left 7 Upper Arm Muscle, Right 8 Upper Arm Muscle, Left 9 Lower Arm and Wrist Muscle, Right B Lower Arm and Wrist Muscle, Left C Hand Muscle, Right D Hand Muscle, Left F Trunk Muscle, Right G Trunk Muscle, Left H Thorax Muscle, Right J Thorax Muscle, Left K Abdomen Muscle, Right L Abdomen Muscle, Left M Perineum Muscle N Hip Muscle, Right P Hip Muscle, Left Q Upper Leg Muscle, Right R Upper Leg Muscle, Left S Lower Leg Muscle, Right T Lower Leg Muscle, Left V Foot Muscle, Right W Foot Muscle, Left	0 Open 3 Percutaneous 4 Percutaneous Endoscopic	Z No Device	X Diagnostic Z No Qualifier

Section	0	Medical and Surgical		
Body System	K	Muscles		
Operation	C	Extirpation: Taking or cutting out solid matter from a body part		

Body Part (Character 4)	Approach (Character 5)	Device (Character 6)	Qualifier (Character 7)
0 Head Muscle 1 Facial Muscle 2 Neck Muscle, Right 3 Neck Muscle, Left 4 Tongue, Palate, Pharynx Muscle 5 Shoulder Muscle, Right 6 Shoulder Muscle, Left 7 Upper Arm Muscle, Right 8 Upper Arm Muscle, Left 9 Lower Arm and Wrist Muscle, Right B Lower Arm and Wrist Muscle, Left C Hand Muscle, Right D Hand Muscle, Left F Trunk Muscle, Right G Trunk Muscle, Left H Thorax Muscle, Right J Thorax Muscle, Left K Abdomen Muscle, Right L Abdomen Muscle, Left M Perineum Muscle N Hip Muscle, Right P Hip Muscle, Left Q Upper Leg Muscle, Right R Upper Leg Muscle, Left S Lower Leg Muscle, Right T Lower Leg Muscle, Left V Foot Muscle, Right W Foot Muscle, Left	0 Open 3 Percutaneous 4 Percutaneous Endoscopic	Z No Device	Z No Qualifier

Section	0	Medical and Surgical		
Body System	K	Muscles		
Operation	H	Insertion: Putting in a nonbiological appliance that monitors, assists, performs, or prevents a physiological function but does not physically take the place of a body part		
Body Part (Character 4)		**Approach (Character 5)**	**Device (Character 6)**	**Qualifier (Character 7)**
X Upper Muscle Y Lower Muscle		0 Open 3 Percutaneous 4 Percutaneous Endoscopic	M Stimulator Lead	Z No Qualifier

Section	0	Medical and Surgical		
Body System	K	Muscles		
Operation	J	Inspection: Visually and/or manually exploring a body part		
Body Part (Character 4)		**Approach (Character 5)**	**Device (Character 6)**	**Qualifier (Character 7)**
X Upper Muscle Y Lower Muscle		0 Open 3 Percutaneous 4 Percutaneous Endoscopic X External	Z No Device	Z No Qualifier

Section	0	Medical and Surgical		
Body System	K	Muscles		
Operation	M	Reattachment Putting back in or on all or a portion of a separated body part to its normal location or other suitable location		
Body Part (Character 4)		**Approach (Character 5)**	**Device (Character 6)**	**Qualifier (Character 7)**
0 Head Muscle 1 Facial Muscle 2 Neck Muscle, Right 3 Neck Muscle, Left 4 Tongue, Palate, Pharynx Muscle 5 Shoulder Muscle, Right 6 Shoulder Muscle, Left 7 Upper Arm Muscle, Right 8 Upper Arm Muscle, Left 9 Lower Arm and Wrist Muscle, Right B Lower Arm and Wrist Muscle, Left C Hand Muscle, Right D Hand Muscle, Left F Trunk Muscle, Right G Trunk Muscle, Left H Thorax Muscle, Right J Thorax Muscle, Left K Abdomen Muscle, Right L Abdomen Muscle, Left M Perineum Muscle N Hip Muscle, Right P Hip Muscle, Left Q Upper Leg Muscle, Right R Upper Leg Muscle, Left S Lower Leg Muscle, Right T Lower Leg Muscle, Left V Foot Muscle, Right W Foot Muscle, Left		0 Open 4 Percutaneous Endoscopic	Z No Device	Z No Qualifier

Section	0	Medical and Surgical		
Body System	K	Muscles		
Operation	N	Release: Freeing a body part from an abnormal physical constraint by cutting or by the use of force		

Body Part (Character 4)	Approach (Character 5)	Device (Character 6)	Qualifier (Character 7)
0 Head Muscle 1 Facial Muscle 2 Neck Muscle, Right 3 Neck Muscle, Left 4 Tongue, Palate, Pharynx Muscle 5 Shoulder Muscle, Right 6 Shoulder Muscle, Left 7 Upper Arm Muscle, Right 8 Upper Arm Muscle, Left 9 Lower Arm and Wrist Muscle, Right B Lower Arm and Wrist Muscle, Left C Hand Muscle, Right D Hand Muscle, Left F Trunk Muscle, Right G Trunk Muscle, Left H Thorax Muscle, Right J Thorax Muscle, Left K Abdomen Muscle, Right L Abdomen Muscle, Left M Perineum Muscle N Hip Muscle, Right P Hip Muscle, Left Q Upper Leg Muscle, Right R Upper Leg Muscle, Left S Lower Leg Muscle, Right T Lower Leg Muscle, Left V Foot Muscle, Right W Foot Muscle, Left	0 Open 3 Percutaneous 4 Percutaneous Endoscopic X External	Z No Device	Z No Qualifier

Section	0	Medical and Surgical		
Body System	K	Muscles		
Operation	P	Removal: Taking out or off a device from a body part		

Body Part (Character 4)	Approach (Character 5)	Device (Character 6)	Qualifier (Character 7)
X Upper Muscle Y Lower Muscle	0 Open 3 Percutaneous 4 Percutaneous Endoscopic	0 Drainage Device 7 Autologous Tissue Substitute J Synthetic Substitute K Nonautologous Tissue Substitute M Stimulator Lead	Z No Qualifier
X Upper Muscle Y Lower Muscle	X External	0 Drainage Device M Stimulator Lead	Z No Qualifier

Section	0	Medical and Surgical			
Body System	K	Muscles			
Operation	Q	Repair: Restoring, to the extent possible, a body part to its normal anatomic structure and function			

Body Part (Character 4)	Approach (Character 5)	Device (Character 6)	Qualifier (Character 7)
0 Head Muscle **1** Facial Muscle **2** Neck Muscle, Right **3** Neck Muscle, Left **4** Tongue, Palate, Pharynx Muscle **5** Shoulder Muscle, Right **6** Shoulder Muscle, Left **7** Upper Arm Muscle, Right **8** Upper Arm Muscle, Left **9** Lower Arm and Wrist Muscle, Right **B** Lower Arm and Wrist Muscle, Left **C** Hand Muscle, Right **D** Hand Muscle, Left **F** Trunk Muscle, Right **G** Trunk Muscle, Left **H** Thorax Muscle, Right **J** Thorax Muscle, Left **K** Abdomen Muscle, Right **L** Abdomen Muscle, Left **M** Perineum Muscle **N** Hip Muscle, Right **P** Hip Muscle, Left **Q** Upper Leg Muscle, Right **R** Upper Leg Muscle, Left **S** Lower Leg Muscle, Right **T** Lower Leg Muscle, Left **V** Foot Muscle, Right **W** Foot Muscle, Left	**0** Open **3** Percutaneous **4** Percutaneous Endoscopic	**Z** No Device	**Z** No Qualifier

Section	0	Medical and Surgical			
Body System	K	Muscles			
Operation	S	Reposition: Moving to its normal location, or other suitable location, all or a portion of a body part			

Body Part (Character 4)	Approach (Character 5)	Device (Character 6)	Qualifier (Character 7)
0 Head Muscle **1** Facial Muscle **2** Neck Muscle, Right **3** Neck Muscle, Left **4** Tongue, Palate, Pharynx Muscle **5** Shoulder Muscle, Right **6** Shoulder Muscle, Left **7** Upper Arm Muscle, Right **8** Upper Arm Muscle, Left **9** Lower Arm and Wrist Muscle, Right **B** Lower Arm and Wrist Muscle, Left **C** Hand Muscle, Right **D** Hand Muscle, Left **F** Trunk Muscle, Right **G** Trunk Muscle, Left **H** Thorax Muscle, Right **J** Thorax Muscle, Left **K** Abdomen Muscle, Right **L** Abdomen Muscle, Left **M** Perineum Muscle **N** Hip Muscle, Right **P** Hip Muscle, Left **Q** Upper Leg Muscle, Right **R** Upper Leg Muscle, Left **S** Lower Leg Muscle, Right **T** Lower Leg Muscle, Left **V** Foot Muscle, Right **W** Foot Muscle, Left	**0** Open **4** Percutaneous Endoscopic	**Z** No Device	**Z** No Qualifier

Section	0	Medical and Surgical			
Body System	K	Muscles			
Operation	T	Resection: Cutting out or off, without replacement, all of a body part			

Body Part (Character 4)	Approach (Character 5)	Device (Character 6)	Qualifier (Character 7)
0 Head Muscle 1 Facial Muscle 2 Neck Muscle, Right 3 Neck Muscle, Left 4 Tongue, Palate, Pharynx Muscle 5 Shoulder Muscle, Right 6 Shoulder Muscle, Left 7 Upper Arm Muscle, Right 8 Upper Arm Muscle, Left 9 Lower Arm and Wrist Muscle, Right B Lower Arm and Wrist Muscle, Left C Hand Muscle, Right D Hand Muscle, Left F Trunk Muscle, Right G Trunk Muscle, Left H Thorax Muscle, Right J Thorax Muscle, Left K Abdomen Muscle, Right L Abdomen Muscle, Left M Perineum Muscle N Hip Muscle, Right P Hip Muscle, Left Q Upper Leg Muscle, Right R Upper Leg Muscle, Left S Lower Leg Muscle, Right T Lower Leg Muscle, Left V Foot Muscle, Right W Foot Muscle, Left	0 Open 4 Percutaneous Endoscopic	Z No Device	Z No Qualifier

Section	0	Medical and Surgical			
Body System	K	Muscles			
Operation	U	Supplement: Putting in or on biological or synthetic material that physically reinforces and/or augments the function of a portion of a body part			

Body Part (Character 4)	Approach (Character 5)	Device (Character 6)	Qualifier (Character 7)
0 Head Muscle 1 Facial Muscle 2 Neck Muscle, Right 3 Neck Muscle, Left 4 Tongue, Palate, Pharynx Muscle 5 Shoulder Muscle, Right 6 Shoulder Muscle, Left 7 Upper Arm Muscle, Right 8 Upper Arm Muscle, Left 9 Lower Arm and Wrist Muscle, Right B Lower Arm and Wrist Muscle, Left C Hand Muscle, Right D Hand Muscle, Left F Trunk Muscle, Right G Trunk Muscle, Left H Thorax Muscle, Right J Thorax Muscle, Left K Abdomen Muscle, Right L Abdomen Muscle, Left M Perineum Muscle N Hip Muscle, Right P Hip Muscle, Left Q Upper Leg Muscle, Right R Upper Leg Muscle, Left S Lower Leg Muscle, Right T Lower Leg Muscle, Left V Foot Muscle, Right W Foot Muscle, Left	0 Open 4 Percutaneous Endoscopic	7 Autologous Tissue Substitute J Synthetic Substitute K Nonautologous Tissue Substitute	Z No Qualifier

Section	0	Medical and Surgical		
Body System	K	Muscles		
Operation	W	Revision: Correcting, to the extent possible, a portion of a malfunctioning device or the position of a displaced device		

Body Part (Character 4)	Approach (Character 5)	Device (Character 6)	Qualifier (Character 7)
X Upper Muscle **Y** Lower Muscle	**0** Open **3** Percutaneous **4** Percutaneous Endoscopic **X** External	**0** Drainage Device **7** Autologous Tissue Substitute **J** Synthetic Substitute **K** Nonautologous Tissue Substitute **M** Stimulator Lead	**Z** No Qualifier

Section	0	Medical and Surgical		
Body System	K	Muscles		
Operation	X	Transfer: Moving, without taking out, all or a portion of a body part to another location to take over the function of all or a portion of a body part		

Body Part (Character 4)	Approach (Character 5)	Device (Character 6)	Qualifier (Character 7)
0 Head Muscle **1** Facial Muscle **2** Neck Muscle, Right **3** Neck Muscle, Left **4** Tongue, Palate, Pharynx Muscle **5** Shoulder Muscle, Right **6** Shoulder Muscle, Left **7** Upper Arm Muscle, Right **8** Upper Arm Muscle, Left **9** Lower Arm and Wrist Muscle, Right **B** Lower Arm and Wrist Muscle, Left **C** Hand Muscle, Right **D** Hand Muscle, Left **F** Trunk Muscle, Right **G** Trunk Muscle, Left **H** Thorax Muscle, Right **J** Thorax Muscle, Left **M** Perineum Muscle **N** Hip Muscle, Right **P** Hip Muscle, Left **Q** Upper Leg Muscle, Right **R** Upper Leg Muscle, Left **S** Lower Leg Muscle, Right **T** Lower Leg Muscle, Left **V** Foot Muscle, Right **W** Foot Muscle, Left	**0** Open **4** Percutaneous Endoscopic	**Z** No Device	**0** Skin **1** Subcutaneous Tissue **2** Skin and Subcutaneous Tissue **Z** No Qualifier
K Abdomen Muscle, Right **L** Abdomen Muscle, Left	**0** Open **4** Percutaneous Endoscopic	**Z** No Device	**0** Skin **1** Subcutaneous Tissue **2** Skin and Subcutaneous Tissue **6** Transverse Rectus Abdominis Myocutaneous Flap **Z** No Qualifier

Section	0	Medical and Surgical		
Body System	L	Tendons		
Operation	2	Change: Taking out or off a device from a body part and putting back an identical or similar device in or on the same body part without cutting or puncturing the skin or a mucous membrane		

Body Part (Character 4)	Approach (Character 5)	Device (Character 6)	Qualifier (Character 7)
X Upper Tendon Y Lower Tendon	X External	0 Drainage Device Y Other Device	Z No Qualifier

Section	0	Medical and Surgical		
Body System	L	Tendons		
Operation	5	Destruction: Physical eradication of all or a portion of a body part by the direct use of energy, force, or a destructive agent		

Body Part (Character 4)	Approach (Character 5)	Device (Character 6)	Qualifier (Character 7)
0 Head and Neck Tendon 1 Shoulder Tendon, Right 2 Shoulder Tendon, Left 3 Upper Arm Tendon, Right 4 Upper Arm Tendon, Left 5 Lower Arm and Wrist Tendon, Right 6 Lower Arm and Wrist Tendon, Left 7 Hand Tendon, Right 8 Hand Tendon, Left 9 Trunk Tendon, Right B Trunk Tendon, Left C Thorax Tendon, Right D Thorax Tendon, Left F Abdomen Tendon, Right G Abdomen Tendon, Left H Perineum Tendon J Hip Tendon, Right K Hip Tendon, Left L Upper Leg Tendon, Right M Upper Leg Tendon, Left N Lower Leg Tendon, Right P Lower Leg Tendon, Left Q Knee Tendon, Right R Knee Tendon, Left S Ankle Tendon, Right T Ankle Tendon, Left V Foot Tendon, Right W Foot Tendon, Left	0 Open 3 Percutaneous 4 Percutaneous Endoscopic	Z No Device	Z No Qualifier

Section	0	Medical and Surgical		
Body System	L	Tendons		
Operation	8	Division: Cutting into a body part, without draining fluids and/or gases from the body part, in order to separate or transect a body part		

Body Part (Character 4)	Approach (Character 5)	Device (Character 6)	Qualifier (Character 7)
0 Head and Neck Tendon **1** Shoulder Tendon, Right **2** Shoulder Tendon, Left **3** Upper Arm Tendon, Right **4** Upper Arm Tendon, Left **5** Lower Arm and Wrist Tendon, Right **6** Lower Arm and Wrist Tendon, Left **7** Hand Tendon, Right **8** Hand Tendon, Left **9** Trunk Tendon, Right **B** Trunk Tendon, Left **C** Thorax Tendon, Right **D** Thorax Tendon, Left **F** Abdomen Tendon, Right **G** Abdomen Tendon, Left **H** Perineum Tendon **J** Hip Tendon, Right **K** Hip Tendon, Left **L** Upper Leg Tendon, Right **M** Upper Leg Tendon, Left **N** Lower Leg Tendon, Right **P** Lower Leg Tendon, Left **Q** Knee Tendon, Right **R** Knee Tendon, Left **S** Ankle Tendon, Right **T** Ankle Tendon, Left **V** Foot Tendon, Right **W** Foot Tendon, Left	**0** Open **3** Percutaneous **4** Percutaneous Endoscopic	**Z** No Device	**Z** No Qualifier

Section	0	Medical and Surgical		
Body System	L	Tendons		
Operation	9	Drainage: Taking or letting out fluids and/or gases from a body part		

Body Part (Character 4)	Approach (Character 5)	Device (Character 6)	Qualifier (Character 7)
0 Head and Neck Tendon **1** Shoulder Tendon, Right **2** Shoulder Tendon, Left **3** Upper Arm Tendon, Right **4** Upper Arm Tendon, Left **5** Lower Arm and Wrist Tendon, Right **6** Lower Arm and Wrist Tendon, Left **7** Hand Tendon, Right **8** Hand Tendon, Left **9** Trunk Tendon, Right **B** Trunk Tendon, Left **C** Thorax Tendon, Right **D** Thorax Tendon, Left **F** Abdomen Tendon, Right **G** Abdomen Tendon, Left **H** Perineum Tendon **J** Hip Tendon, Right **K** Hip Tendon, Left **L** Upper Leg Tendon, Right **M** Upper Leg Tendon, Left **N** Lower Leg Tendon, Right **P** Lower Leg Tendon, Left **Q** Knee Tendon, Right **R** Knee Tendon, Left **S** Ankle Tendon, Right **T** Ankle Tendon, Left **V** Foot Tendon, Right **W** Foot Tendon, Left	**0** Open **3** Percutaneous **4** Percutaneous Endoscopic	**0** Drainage Device	**Z** No Qualifier

Section	0	Medical and Surgical			
Body System	L	Tendons			
Operation	9	Drainage: Taking or letting out fluids and/or gases from a body part			

Body Part (Character 4)	Approach (Character 5)	Device (Character 6)	Qualifier (Character 7)
0 Head and Neck Tendon **1** Shoulder Tendon, Right **2** Shoulder Tendon, Left **3** Upper Arm Tendon, Right **4** Upper Arm Tendon, Left **5** Lower Arm and Wrist Tendon, Right **6** Lower Arm and Wrist Tendon, Left **7** Hand Tendon, Right **8** Hand Tendon, Left **9** Trunk Tendon, Right **B** Trunk Tendon, Left **C** Thorax Tendon, Right **D** Thorax Tendon, Left **F** Abdomen Tendon, Right **G** Abdomen Tendon, Left **H** Perineum Tendon **J** Hip Tendon, Right **K** Hip Tendon, Left **L** Upper Leg Tendon, Right **M** Upper Leg Tendon, Left **N** Lower Leg Tendon, Right **P** Lower Leg Tendon, Left **Q** Knee Tendon, Right **R** Knee Tendon, Left **S** Ankle Tendon, Right **T** Ankle Tendon, Left **V** Foot Tendon, Right **W** Foot Tendon, Left	**0** Open **3** Percutaneous **4** Percutaneous Endoscopic	**Z** No Device	**X** Diagnostic **Z** No Qualifier

Section	0	Medical and Surgical			
Body System	L	Tendons			
Operation	B	Excision: Cutting out or off, without replacement, a portion of a body part			

Body Part (Character 4)	Approach (Character 5)	Device (Character 6)	Qualifier (Character 7)
0 Head and Neck Tendon **1** Shoulder Tendon, Right **2** Shoulder Tendon, Left **3** Upper Arm Tendon, Right **4** Upper Arm Tendon, Left **5** Lower Arm and Wrist Tendon, Right **6** Lower Arm and Wrist Tendon, Left **7** Hand Tendon, Right **8** Hand Tendon, Left **9** Trunk Tendon, Right **B** Trunk Tendon, Left **C** Thorax Tendon, Right **D** Thorax Tendon, Left **F** Abdomen Tendon, Right **G** Abdomen Tendon, Left **H** Perineum Tendon **J** Hip Tendon, Right **K** Hip Tendon, Left **L** Upper Leg Tendon, Right **M** Upper Leg Tendon, Left **N** Lower Leg Tendon, Right **P** Lower Leg Tendon, Left **Q** Knee Tendon, Right **R** Knee Tendon, Left **S** Ankle Tendon, Right **T** Ankle Tendon, Left **V** Foot Tendon, Right **W** Foot Tendon, Left	**0** Open **3** Percutaneous **4** Percutaneous Endoscopic	**Z** No Device	**X** Diagnostic **Z** No Qualifier

Section	0	Medical and Surgical		
Body System	L	Tendons		
Operation	C	Extirpation: Taking or cutting out solid matter from a body part		

Body Part (Character 4)	Approach (Character 5)	Device (Character 6)	Qualifier (Character 7)
0 Head and Neck Tendon **1** Shoulder Tendon, Right **2** Shoulder Tendon, Left **3** Upper Arm Tendon, Right **4** Upper Arm Tendon, Left **5** Lower Arm and Wrist Tendon, Right **6** Lower Arm and Wrist Tendon, Left **7** Hand Tendon, Right **8** Hand Tendon, Left **9** Trunk Tendon, Right **B** Trunk Tendon, Left **C** Thorax Tendon, Right **D** Thorax Tendon, Left **F** Abdomen Tendon, Right **G** Abdomen Tendon, Left **H** Perineum Tendon **J** Hip Tendon, Right **K** Hip Tendon, Left **L** Upper Leg Tendon, Right **M** Upper Leg Tendon, Left **N** Lower Leg Tendon, Right **P** Lower Leg Tendon, Left **Q** Knee Tendon, Right **R** Knee Tendon, Left **S** Ankle Tendon, Right **T** Ankle Tendon, Left **V** Foot Tendon, Right **W** Foot Tendon, Left	**0** Open **3** Percutaneous **4** Percutaneous Endoscopic	**Z** No Device	**Z** No Qualifier

Section	0	Medical and Surgical		
Body System	L	Tendons		
Operation	J	Inspection: Visually and/or manually exploring a body part		

Body Part (Character 4)	Approach (Character 5)	Device (Character 6)	Qualifier (Character 7)
X Upper Tendon **Y** Lower Tendon	**0** Open **3** Percutaneous **4** Percutaneous Endoscopic **X** External	**Z** No Device	**Z** No Qualifier

Section	0	Medical and Surgical		
Body System	L	Tendons		
Operation	M	Reattachment Putting back in or on all or a portion of a separated body part to its normal location or other suitable location		

Body Part (Character 4)	Approach (Character 5)	Device (Character 6)	Qualifier (Character 7)
0 Head and Neck Tendon 1 Shoulder Tendon, Right 2 Shoulder Tendon, Left 3 Upper Arm Tendon, Right 4 Upper Arm Tendon, Left 5 Lower Arm and Wrist Tendon, Right 6 Lower Arm and Wrist Tendon, Left 7 Hand Tendon, Right 8 Hand Tendon, Left 9 Trunk Tendon, Right B Trunk Tendon, Left C Thorax Tendon, Right D Thorax Tendon, Left F Abdomen Tendon, Right G Abdomen Tendon, Left H Perineum Tendon J Hip Tendon, Right K Hip Tendon, Left L Upper Leg Tendon, Right M Upper Leg Tendon, Left N Lower Leg Tendon, Right P Lower Leg Tendon, Left Q Knee Tendon, Right R Knee Tendon, Left S Ankle Tendon, Right T Ankle Tendon, Left V Foot Tendon, Right W Foot Tendon, Left	0 Open 4 Percutaneous Endoscopic	Z No Device	Z No Qualifier

Section	0	Medical and Surgical		
Body System	L	Tendons		
Operation	N	Release: Freeing a body part from an abnormal physical constraint by cutting or by the use of force		

Body Part (Character 4)	Approach (Character 5)	Device (Character 6)	Qualifier (Character 7)
0 Head and Neck Tendon 1 Shoulder Tendon, Right 2 Shoulder Tendon, Left 3 Upper Arm Tendon, Right 4 Upper Arm Tendon, Left 5 Lower Arm and Wrist Tendon, Right 6 Lower Arm and Wrist Tendon, Left 7 Hand Tendon, Right 8 Hand Tendon, Left 9 Trunk Tendon, Right B Trunk Tendon, Left C Thorax Tendon, Right D Thorax Tendon, Left F Abdomen Tendon, Right G Abdomen Tendon, Left H Perineum Tendon J Hip Tendon, Right K Hip Tendon, Left L Upper Leg Tendon, Right M Upper Leg Tendon, Left N Lower Leg Tendon, Right P Lower Leg Tendon, Left Q Knee Tendon, Right R Knee Tendon, Left S Ankle Tendon, Right T Ankle Tendon, Left V Foot Tendon, Right W Foot Tendon, Left	0 Open 3 Percutaneous 4 Percutaneous Endoscopic X External	Z No Device	Z No Qualifier

Section	0	Medical and Surgical		
Body System	L	Tendons		
Operation	P	Removal: Taking out or off a device from a body part		

Body Part (Character 4)	Approach (Character 5)	Device (Character 6)	Qualifier (Character 7)
X Upper Tendon Y Lower Tendon	0 Open 3 Percutaneous 4 Percutaneous Endoscopic	0 Drainage Device 7 Autologous Tissue Substitute J Synthetic Substitute K Nonautologous Tissue Substitute	Z No Qualifier
X Upper Tendon Y Lower Tendon	X External	0 Drainage Device	Z No Qualifier

Section	0	Medical and Surgical		
Body System	L	Tendons		
Operation	Q	Repair: Restoring, to the extent possible, a body part to its normal anatomic structure and function		

Body Part (Character 4)	Approach (Character 5)	Device (Character 6)	Qualifier (Character 7)
0 Head and Neck Tendon 1 Shoulder Tendon, Right 2 Shoulder Tendon, Left 3 Upper Arm Tendon, Right 4 Upper Arm Tendon, Left 5 Lower Arm and Wrist Tendon, Right 6 Lower Arm and Wrist Tendon, Left 7 Hand Tendon, Right 8 Hand Tendon, Left 9 Trunk Tendon, Right B Trunk Tendon, Left C Thorax Tendon, Right D Thorax Tendon, Left F Abdomen Tendon, Right G Abdomen Tendon, Left H Perineum Tendon J Hip Tendon, Right K Hip Tendon, Left L Upper Leg Tendon, Right M Upper Leg Tendon, Left N Lower Leg Tendon, Right P Lower Leg Tendon, Left Q Knee Tendon, Right R Knee Tendon, Left S Ankle Tendon, Right T Ankle Tendon, Left V Foot Tendon, Right W Foot Tendon, Left	0 Open 3 Percutaneous 4 Percutaneous Endoscopic	Z No Device	Z No Qualifier

Section	0	Medical and Surgical		
Body System	L	Tendons		
Operation	R	Replacement: Putting in or on biological or synthetic material that physically takes the place and/or function of all or a portion of a body part		

Body Part (Character 4)	Approach (Character 5)	Device (Character 6)	Qualifier (Character 7)
0 Head and Neck Tendon **1** Shoulder Tendon, Right **2** Shoulder Tendon, Left **3** Upper Arm Tendon, Right **4** Upper Arm Tendon, Left **5** Lower Arm and Wrist Tendon, Right **6** Lower Arm and Wrist Tendon, Left **7** Hand Tendon, Right **8** Hand Tendon, Left **9** Trunk Tendon, Right **B** Trunk Tendon, Left **C** Thorax Tendon, Right **D** Thorax Tendon, Left **F** Abdomen Tendon, Right **G** Abdomen Tendon, Left **H** Perineum Tendon **J** Hip Tendon, Right **K** Hip Tendon, Left **L** Upper Leg Tendon, Right **M** Upper Leg Tendon, Left **N** Lower Leg Tendon, Right **P** Lower Leg Tendon, Left **Q** Knee Tendon, Right **R** Knee Tendon, Left **S** Ankle Tendon, Right **T** Ankle Tendon, Left **V** Foot Tendon, Right **W** Foot Tendon, Left	**0** Open **4** Percutaneous Endoscopic	**7** Autologous Tissue Substitute **J** Synthetic Substitute **K** Nonautologous Tissue Substitute	**Z** No Qualifier

Section	0	Medical and Surgical		
Body System	L	Tendons		
Operation	S	Reposition: Moving to its normal location, or other suitable location, all or a portion of a body part		

Body Part (Character 4)	Approach (Character 5)	Device (Character 6)	Qualifier (Character 7)
0 Head and Neck Tendon **1** Shoulder Tendon, Right **2** Shoulder Tendon, Left **3** Upper Arm Tendon, Right **4** Upper Arm Tendon, Left **5** Lower Arm and Wrist Tendon, Right **6** Lower Arm and Wrist Tendon, Left **7** Hand Tendon, Right **8** Hand Tendon, Left **9** Trunk Tendon, Right **B** Trunk Tendon, Left **C** Thorax Tendon, Right **D** Thorax Tendon, Left **F** Abdomen Tendon, Right **G** Abdomen Tendon, Left **H** Perineum Tendon **J** Hip Tendon, Right **K** Hip Tendon, Left **L** Upper Leg Tendon, Right **M** Upper Leg Tendon, Left **N** Lower Leg Tendon, Right **P** Lower Leg Tendon, Left **Q** Knee Tendon, Right **R** Knee Tendon, Left **S** Ankle Tendon, Right **T** Ankle Tendon, Left **V** Foot Tendon, Right **W** Foot Tendon, Left	**0** Open **4** Percutaneous Endoscopic	**Z** No Device	**Z** No Qualifier

Section	0	Medical and Surgical
Body System	L	Tendons
Operation	T	Resection: Cutting out or off, without replacement, all of a body part

Body Part (Character 4)	Approach (Character 5)	Device (Character 6)	Qualifier (Character 7)
0 Head and Neck Tendon 1 Shoulder Tendon, Right 2 Shoulder Tendon, Left 3 Upper Arm Tendon, Right 4 Upper Arm Tendon, Left 5 Lower Arm and Wrist Tendon, Right 6 Lower Arm and Wrist Tendon, Left 7 Hand Tendon, Right 8 Hand Tendon, Left 9 Trunk Tendon, Right B Trunk Tendon, Left C Thorax Tendon, Right D Thorax Tendon, Left F Abdomen Tendon, Right G Abdomen Tendon, Left H Perineum Tendon J Hip Tendon, Right K Hip Tendon, Left L Upper Leg Tendon, Right M Upper Leg Tendon, Left N Lower Leg Tendon, Right P Lower Leg Tendon, Left Q Knee Tendon, Right R Knee Tendon, Left S Ankle Tendon, Right T Ankle Tendon, Left V Foot Tendon, Right W Foot Tendon, Left	0 Open 4 Percutaneous Endoscopic	Z No Device	Z No Qualifier

Section	0	Medical and Surgical
Body System	L	Tendons
Operation	U	Supplement: Putting in or on biological or synthetic material that physically reinforces and/or augments the function of a portion of a body part

Body Part (Character 4)	Approach (Character 5)	Device (Character 6)	Qualifier (Character 7)
0 Head and Neck Tendon 1 Shoulder Tendon, Right 2 Shoulder Tendon, Left 3 Upper Arm Tendon, Right 4 Upper Arm Tendon, Left 5 Lower Arm and Wrist Tendon, Right 6 Lower Arm and Wrist Tendon, Left 7 Hand Tendon, Right 8 Hand Tendon, Left 9 Trunk Tendon, Right B Trunk Tendon, Left C Thorax Tendon, Right D Thorax Tendon, Left F Abdomen Tendon, Right G Abdomen Tendon, Left H Perineum Tendon J Hip Tendon, Right K Hip Tendon, Left L Upper Leg Tendon, Right M Upper Leg Tendon, Left N Lower Leg Tendon, Right P Lower Leg Tendon, Left Q Knee Tendon, Right R Knee Tendon, Left S Ankle Tendon, Right T Ankle Tendon, Left V Foot Tendon, Right W Foot Tendon, Left	0 Open 4 Percutaneous Endoscopic	7 Autologous Tissue Substitute J Synthetic Substitute K Nonautologous Tissue Substitute	Z No Qualifier

Section	0	Medical and Surgical		
Body System	L	Tendons		
Operation	W	Revision: Correcting, to the extent possible, a portion of a malfunctioning device or the position of a displaced device		

Body Part (Character 4)	Approach (Character 5)	Device (Character 6)	Qualifier (Character 7)
X Upper Tendon Y Lower Tendon	0 Open 3 Percutaneous 4 Percutaneous Endoscopic X External	0 Drainage Device 7 Autologous Tissue Substitute J Synthetic Substitute K Nonautologous Tissue Substitute	Z No Qualifier

Section	0	Medical and Surgical		
Body System	L	Tendons		
Operation	X	Transfer: Moving, without taking out, all or a portion of a body part to another location to take over the function of all or a portion of a body part		

Body Part (Character 4)	Approach (Character 5)	Device (Character 6)	Qualifier (Character 7)
0 Head and Neck Tendon 1 Shoulder Tendon, Right 2 Shoulder Tendon, Left 3 Upper Arm Tendon, Right 4 Upper Arm Tendon, Left 5 Lower Arm and Wrist Tendon, Right 6 Lower Arm and Wrist Tendon, Left 7 Hand Tendon, Right 8 Hand Tendon, Left 9 Trunk Tendon, Right B Trunk Tendon, Left C Thorax Tendon, Right D Thorax Tendon, Left F Abdomen Tendon, Right G Abdomen Tendon, Left H Perineum Tendon J Hip Tendon, Right K Hip Tendon, Left L Upper Leg Tendon, Right M Upper Leg Tendon, Left N Lower Leg Tendon, Right P Lower Leg Tendon, Left Q Knee Tendon, Right R Knee Tendon, Left S Ankle Tendon, Right T Ankle Tendon, Left V Foot Tendon, Right W Foot Tendon, Left	0 Open 4 Percutaneous Endoscopic	Z No Device	Z No Qualifier

Section	0	Medical and Surgical			
Body System	M	Bursae and Ligaments			
Operation	2	Change: Taking out or off a device from a body part and putting back an identical or similar device in or on the same body part without cutting or puncturing the skin or a mucous membrane			

Body Part (Character 4)	Approach (Character 5)	Device (Character 6)	Qualifier (Character 7)
X Upper Bursa and Ligament	X External	0 Drainage Device	Z No Qualifier
Y Lower Bursa and Ligament		Y Other Device	

Section	0	Medical and Surgical			
Body System	M	Bursae and Ligaments			
Operation	5	Destruction: Physical eradication of all or a portion of a body part by the direct use of energy, force, or a destructive agent			

Body Part (Character 4)	Approach (Character 5)	Device (Character 6)	Qualifier (Character 7)
0 Head and Neck Bursa and Ligament	0 Open	Z No Device	Z No Qualifier
1 Shoulder Bursa and Ligament, Right	3 Percutaneous		
2 Shoulder Bursa and Ligament, Left	4 Percutaneous Endoscopic		
3 Elbow Bursa and Ligament, Right			
4 Elbow Bursa and Ligament, Left			
5 Wrist Bursa and Ligament, Right			
6 Wrist Bursa and Ligament, Left			
7 Hand Bursa and Ligament, Right			
8 Hand Bursa and Ligament, Left			
9 Upper Extremity Bursa and Ligament, Right			
B Upper Extremity Bursa and Ligament, Left			
C Trunk Bursa and Ligament, Right			
D Trunk Bursa and Ligament, Left			
F Thorax Bursa and Ligament, Right			
G Thorax Bursa and Ligament, Left			
H Abdomen Bursa and Ligament, Right			
J Abdomen Bursa and Ligament, Left			
K Perineum Bursa and Ligament			
L Hip Bursa and Ligament, Right			
M Hip Bursa and Ligament, Left			
N Knee Bursa and Ligament, Right			
P Knee Bursa and Ligament, Left			
Q Ankle Bursa and Ligament, Right			
R Ankle Bursa and Ligament, Left			
S Foot Bursa and Ligament, Right			
T Foot Bursa and Ligament, Left			
V Lower Extremity Bursa and Ligament, Right			
W Lower Extremity Bursa and Ligament, Left			

Section	0	Medical and Surgical		
Body System	M	Bursae and Ligaments		
Operation	8	Division: Cutting into a body part, without draining fluids and/or gases from the body part, in order to separate or transect a body part		

Body Part (Character 4)	Approach (Character 5)	Device (Character 6)	Qualifier (Character 7)
0 Head and Neck Bursa and Ligament **1** Shoulder Bursa and Ligament, Right **2** Shoulder Bursa and Ligament, Left **3** Elbow Bursa and Ligament, Right **4** Elbow Bursa and Ligament, Left **5** Wrist Bursa and Ligament, Right **6** Wrist Bursa and Ligament, Left **7** Hand Bursa and Ligament, Right **8** Hand Bursa and Ligament, Left **9** Upper Extremity Bursa and Ligament, Right **B** Upper Extremity Bursa and Ligament, Left **C** Trunk Bursa and Ligament, Right **D** Trunk Bursa and Ligament, Left **F** Thorax Bursa and Ligament, Right **G** Thorax Bursa and Ligament, Left **H** Abdomen Bursa and Ligament, Right **J** Abdomen Bursa and Ligament, Left **K** Perineum Bursa and Ligament **L** Hip Bursa and Ligament, Right **M** Hip Bursa and Ligament, Left **N** Knee Bursa and Ligament, Right **P** Knee Bursa and Ligament, Left **Q** Ankle Bursa and Ligament, Right **R** Ankle Bursa and Ligament, Left **S** Foot Bursa and Ligament, Right **T** Foot Bursa and Ligament, Left **V** Lower Extremity Bursa and Ligament, Right **W** Lower Extremity Bursa and Ligament, Left	**0** Open **3** Percutaneous **4** Percutaneous Endoscopic	**Z** No Device	**Z** No Qualifier

Section	0	Medical and Surgical				
Body System	M	Bursae and Ligaments				
Operation	9	Drainage: Taking or letting out fluids and/or gases from a body part				

Body Part (Character 4)	Approach (Character 5)	Device (Character 6)	Qualifier (Character 7)
0 Head and Neck Bursa and Ligament **1** Shoulder Bursa and Ligament, Right **2** Shoulder Bursa and Ligament, Left **3** Elbow Bursa and Ligament, Right **4** Elbow Bursa and Ligament, Left **5** Wrist Bursa and Ligament, Right **6** Wrist Bursa and Ligament, Left **7** Hand Bursa and Ligament, Right **8** Hand Bursa and Ligament, Left **9** Upper Extremity Bursa and Ligament, Right **B** Upper Extremity Bursa and Ligament, Left **C** Trunk Bursa and Ligament, Right **D** Trunk Bursa and Ligament, Left **F** Thorax Bursa and Ligament, Right **G** Thorax Bursa and Ligament, Left **H** Abdomen Bursa and Ligament, Right **J** Abdomen Bursa and Ligament, Left **K** Perineum Bursa and Ligament **L** Hip Bursa and Ligament, Right **M** Hip Bursa and Ligament, Left **N** Knee Bursa and Ligament, Right **P** Knee Bursa and Ligament, Left **Q** Ankle Bursa and Ligament, Right **R** Ankle Bursa and Ligament, Left **S** Foot Bursa and Ligament, Right **T** Foot Bursa and Ligament, Left **V** Lower Extremity Bursa and Ligament, Right **W** Lower Extremity Bursa and Ligament, Left	**0** Open **3** Percutaneous **4** Percutaneous Endoscopic	**0** Drainage Device	**Z** No Qualifier

Section	0	Medical and Surgical		
Body System	M	Bursae and Ligaments		
Operation	9	Drainage: Taking or letting out fluids and/or gases from a body part		

Body Part (Character 4)	Approach (Character 5)	Device (Character 6)	Qualifier (Character 7)
0 Head and Neck Bursa and Ligament **1** Shoulder Bursa and Ligament, Right **2** Shoulder Bursa and Ligament, Left **3** Elbow Bursa and Ligament, Right **4** Elbow Bursa and Ligament, Left **5** Wrist Bursa and Ligament, Right **6** Wrist Bursa and Ligament, Left **7** Hand Bursa and Ligament, Right **8** Hand Bursa and Ligament, Left **9** Upper Extremity Bursa and Ligament, Right **B** Upper Extremity Bursa and Ligament, Left **C** Trunk Bursa and Ligament, Right **D** Trunk Bursa and Ligament, Left **F** Thorax Bursa and Ligament, Right **G** Thorax Bursa and Ligament, Left **H** Abdomen Bursa and Ligament, Right **J** Abdomen Bursa and Ligament, Left **K** Perineum Bursa and Ligament **L** Hip Bursa and Ligament, Right **M** Hip Bursa and Ligament, Left **N** Knee Bursa and Ligament, Right **P** Knee Bursa and Ligament, Left **Q** Ankle Bursa and Ligament, Right **R** Ankle Bursa and Ligament, Left **S** Foot Bursa and Ligament, Right **T** Foot Bursa and Ligament, Left **V** Lower Extremity Bursa and Ligament, Right **W** Lower Extremity Bursa and Ligament, Left	**0** Open **3** Percutaneous **4** Percutaneous Endoscopic	**Z** No Device	**X** Diagnostic **Z** No Qualifier

Section	0	Medical and Surgical		
Body System	M	Bursae and Ligaments		
Operation	B	Excision: Cutting out or off, without replacement, a portion of a body part		

Body Part (Character 4)	Approach (Character 5)	Device (Character 6)	Qualifier (Character 7)
0 Head and Neck Bursa and Ligament **1** Shoulder Bursa and Ligament, Right **2** Shoulder Bursa and Ligament, Left **3** Elbow Bursa and Ligament, Right **4** Elbow Bursa and Ligament, Left **5** Wrist Bursa and Ligament, Right **6** Wrist Bursa and Ligament, Left **7** Hand Bursa and Ligament, Right **8** Hand Bursa and Ligament, Left **9** Upper Extremity Bursa and Ligament, Right **B** Upper Extremity Bursa and Ligament, Left **C** Trunk Bursa and Ligament, Right **D** Trunk Bursa and Ligament, Left **F** Thorax Bursa and Ligament, Right **G** Thorax Bursa and Ligament, Left **H** Abdomen Bursa and Ligament, Right **J** Abdomen Bursa and Ligament, Left **K** Perineum Bursa and Ligament **L** Hip Bursa and Ligament, Right **M** Hip Bursa and Ligament, Left **N** Knee Bursa and Ligament, Right **P** Knee Bursa and Ligament, Left **Q** Ankle Bursa and Ligament, Right **R** Ankle Bursa and Ligament, Left **S** Foot Bursa and Ligament, Right **T** Foot Bursa and Ligament, Left **V** Lower Extremity Bursa and Ligament, Right **W** Lower Extremity Bursa and Ligament, Left	**0** Open **3** Percutaneous **4** Percutaneous Endoscopic	**Z** No Device	**X** Diagnostic **Z** No Qualifier

Section	0	Medical and Surgical		
Body System	M	Bursae and Ligaments		
Operation	C	Extirpation: Taking or cutting out solid matter from a body part		

Body Part (Character 4)	Approach (Character 5)	Device (Character 6)	Qualifier (Character 7)
0 Head and Neck Bursa and Ligament **1** Shoulder Bursa and Ligament, Right **2** Shoulder Bursa and Ligament, Left **3** Elbow Bursa and Ligament, Right **4** Elbow Bursa and Ligament, Left **5** Wrist Bursa and Ligament, Right **6** Wrist Bursa and Ligament, Left **7** Hand Bursa and Ligament, Right **8** Hand Bursa and Ligament, Left **9** Upper Extremity Bursa and Ligament, Right **B** Upper Extremity Bursa and Ligament, Left **C** Trunk Bursa and Ligament, Right **D** Trunk Bursa and Ligament, Left **F** Thorax Bursa and Ligament, Right **G** Thorax Bursa and Ligament, Left **H** Abdomen Bursa and Ligament, Right **J** Abdomen Bursa and Ligament, Left **K** Perineum Bursa and Ligament **L** Hip Bursa and Ligament, Right **M** Hip Bursa and Ligament, Left **N** Knee Bursa and Ligament, Right **P** Knee Bursa and Ligament, Left **Q** Ankle Bursa and Ligament, Right **R** Ankle Bursa and Ligament, Left **S** Foot Bursa and Ligament, Right **T** Foot Bursa and Ligament, Left **V** Lower Extremity Bursa and Ligament, Right **W** Lower Extremity Bursa and Ligament, Left	**0** Open **3** Percutaneous **4** Percutaneous Endoscopic	**Z** No Device	**Z** No Qualifier

Section	0	Medical and Surgical		
Body System	M	Bursae and Ligaments		
Operation	D	Extraction: Pulling or stripping out or off all or a portion of a body part by the use of force		

Body Part (Character 4)	Approach (Character 5)	Device (Character 6)	Qualifier (Character 7)
0 Head and Neck Bursa and Ligament 1 Shoulder Bursa and Ligament, Right 2 Shoulder Bursa and Ligament, Left 3 Elbow Bursa and Ligament, Right 4 Elbow Bursa and Ligament, Left 5 Wrist Bursa and Ligament, Right 6 Wrist Bursa and Ligament, Left 7 Hand Bursa and Ligament, Right 8 Hand Bursa and Ligament, Left 9 Upper Extremity Bursa and Ligament, Right B Upper Extremity Bursa and Ligament, Left C Trunk Bursa and Ligament, Right D Trunk Bursa and Ligament, Left F Thorax Bursa and Ligament, Right G Thorax Bursa and Ligament, Left H Abdomen Bursa and Ligament, Right J Abdomen Bursa and Ligament, Left K Perineum Bursa and Ligament L Hip Bursa and Ligament, Right M Hip Bursa and Ligament, Left N Knee Bursa and Ligament, Right P Knee Bursa and Ligament, Left Q Ankle Bursa and Ligament, Right R Ankle Bursa and Ligament, Left S Foot Bursa and Ligament, Right T Foot Bursa and Ligament, Left V Lower Extremity Bursa and Ligament, Right W Lower Extremity Bursa and Ligament, Left	0 Open 3 Percutaneous 4 Percutaneous Endoscopic	Z No Device	Z No Qualifier

Section	0	Medical and Surgical		
Body System	M	Bursae and Ligaments		
Operation	J	Inspection: Visually and/or manually exploring a body part		

Body Part (Character 4)	Approach (Character 5)	Device (Character 6)	Qualifier (Character 7)
X Upper Bursa and Ligament Y Lower Bursa and Ligament	0 Open 3 Percutaneous 4 Percutaneous Endoscopic X External	Z No Device	Z No Qualifier

Section	0	Medical and Surgical				
Body System	M	Bursae and Ligaments				
Operation	M	Reattachment Putting back in or on all or a portion of a separated body part to its normal location or other suitable location				

Body Part (Character 4)	Approach (Character 5)	Device (Character 6)	Qualifier (Character 7)
0 Head and Neck Bursa and Ligament **1** Shoulder Bursa and Ligament, Right **2** Shoulder Bursa and Ligament, Left **3** Elbow Bursa and Ligament, Right **4** Elbow Bursa and Ligament, Left **5** Wrist Bursa and Ligament, Right **6** Wrist Bursa and Ligament, Left **7** Hand Bursa and Ligament, Right **8** Hand Bursa and Ligament, Left **9** Upper Extremity Bursa and Ligament, Right **B** Upper Extremity Bursa and Ligament, Left **C** Trunk Bursa and Ligament, Right **D** Trunk Bursa and Ligament, Left **F** Thorax Bursa and Ligament, Right **G** Thorax Bursa and Ligament, Left **H** Abdomen Bursa and Ligament, Right **J** Abdomen Bursa and Ligament, Left **K** Perineum Bursa and Ligament **L** Hip Bursa and Ligament, Right **M** Hip Bursa and Ligament, Left **N** Knee Bursa and Ligament, Right **P** Knee Bursa and Ligament, Left **Q** Ankle Bursa and Ligament, Right **R** Ankle Bursa and Ligament, Left **S** Foot Bursa and Ligament, Right **T** Foot Bursa and Ligament, Left **V** Lower Extremity Bursa and Ligament, Right **W** Lower Extremity Bursa and Ligament, Left	**0** Open **4** Percutaneous Endoscopic	**Z** No Device	**Z** No Qualifier

Section	0	Medical and Surgical		
Body System	M	Bursae and Ligaments		
Operation	N	Release: Freeing a body part from an abnormal physical constraint by cutting or by the use of force		

Body Part (Character 4)	Approach (Character 5)	Device (Character 6)	Qualifier (Character 7)
0 Head and Neck Bursa and Ligament **1** Shoulder Bursa and Ligament, Right **2** Shoulder Bursa and Ligament, Left **3** Elbow Bursa and Ligament, Right **4** Elbow Bursa and Ligament, Left **5** Wrist Bursa and Ligament, Right **6** Wrist Bursa and Ligament, Left **7** Hand Bursa and Ligament, Right **8** Hand Bursa and Ligament, Left **9** Upper Extremity Bursa and Ligament, Right **B** Upper Extremity Bursa and Ligament, Left **C** Trunk Bursa and Ligament, Right **D** Trunk Bursa and Ligament, Left **F** Thorax Bursa and Ligament, Right **G** Thorax Bursa and Ligament, Left **H** Abdomen Bursa and Ligament, Right **J** Abdomen Bursa and Ligament, Left **K** Perineum Bursa and Ligament **L** Hip Bursa and Ligament, Right **M** Hip Bursa and Ligament, Left **N** Knee Bursa and Ligament, Right **P** Knee Bursa and Ligament, Left **Q** Ankle Bursa and Ligament, Right **R** Ankle Bursa and Ligament, Left **S** Foot Bursa and Ligament, Right **T** Foot Bursa and Ligament, Left **V** Lower Extremity Bursa and Ligament, Right **W** Lower Extremity Bursa and Ligament, Left	**0** Open **3** Percutaneous **4** Percutaneous Endoscopic **X** External	**Z** No Device	**Z** No Qualifier

Section	0	Medical and Surgical		
Body System	M	Bursae and Ligaments		
Operation	P	Removal: Taking out or off a device from a body part		

Body Part (Character 4)	Approach (Character 5)	Device (Character 6)	Qualifier (Character 7)
X Upper Bursa and Ligament **Y** Lower Bursa and Ligament	**0** Open **3** Percutaneous **4** Percutaneous Endoscopic	**0** Drainage Device **7** Autologous Tissue Substitute **J** Synthetic Substitute **K** Nonautologous Tissue Substitute	**Z** No Qualifier
X Upper Bursa and Ligament **Y** Lower Bursa and Ligament	**X** External	**0** Drainage Device	**Z** No Qualifier

Section	0	Medical and Surgical		
Body System	M	Bursae and Ligaments		
Operation	Q	Repair: Restoring, to the extent possible, a body part to its normal anatomic structure and function		

Body Part (Character 4)	Approach (Character 5)	Device (Character 6)	Qualifier (Character 7)
0 Head and Neck Bursa and Ligament 1 Shoulder Bursa and Ligament, Right 2 Shoulder Bursa and Ligament, Left 3 Elbow Bursa and Ligament, Right 4 Elbow Bursa and Ligament, Left 5 Wrist Bursa and Ligament, Right 6 Wrist Bursa and Ligament, Left 7 Hand Bursa and Ligament, Right 8 Hand Bursa and Ligament, Left 9 Upper Extremity Bursa and Ligament, Right B Upper Extremity Bursa and Ligament, Left C Trunk Bursa and Ligament, Right D Trunk Bursa and Ligament, Left F Thorax Bursa and Ligament, Right G Thorax Bursa and Ligament, Left H Abdomen Bursa and Ligament, Right J Abdomen Bursa and Ligament, Left K Perineum Bursa and Ligament L Hip Bursa and Ligament, Right M Hip Bursa and Ligament, Left N Knee Bursa and Ligament, Right P Knee Bursa and Ligament, Left Q Ankle Bursa and Ligament, Right R Ankle Bursa and Ligament, Left S Foot Bursa and Ligament, Right T Foot Bursa and Ligament, Left V Lower Extremity Bursa and Ligament, Right W Lower Extremity Bursa and Ligament, Left	0 Open 3 Percutaneous 4 Percutaneous Endoscopic	Z No Device	Z No Qualifier

Section	0	**Medical and Surgical**		
Body System	M	**Bursae and Ligaments**		
Operation	S	**Reposition: Moving to its normal location, or other suitable location, all or a portion of a body part**		

Body Part (Character 4)	Approach (Character 5)	Device (Character 6)	Qualifier (Character 7)
0 Head and Neck Bursa and Ligament **1** Shoulder Bursa and Ligament, Right **2** Shoulder Bursa and Ligament, Left **3** Elbow Bursa and Ligament, Right **4** Elbow Bursa and Ligament, Left **5** Wrist Bursa and Ligament, Right **6** Wrist Bursa and Ligament, Left **7** Hand Bursa and Ligament, Right **8** Hand Bursa and Ligament, Left **9** Upper Extremity Bursa and Ligament, Right **B** Upper Extremity Bursa and Ligament, Left **C** Trunk Bursa and Ligament, Right **D** Trunk Bursa and Ligament, Left **F** Thorax Bursa and Ligament, Right **G** Thorax Bursa and Ligament, Left **H** Abdomen Bursa and Ligament, Right **J** Abdomen Bursa and Ligament, Left **K** Perineum Bursa and Ligament **L** Hip Bursa and Ligament, Right **M** Hip Bursa and Ligament, Left **N** Knee Bursa and Ligament, Right **P** Knee Bursa and Ligament, Left **Q** Ankle Bursa and Ligament, Right **R** Ankle Bursa and Ligament, Left **S** Foot Bursa and Ligament, Right **T** Foot Bursa and Ligament, Left **V** Lower Extremity Bursa and Ligament, Right **W** Lower Extremity Bursa and Ligament, Left	**0** Open **4** Percutaneous Endoscopic	**Z** No Device	**Z** No Qualifier

Section	0	Medical and Surgical		
Body System	M	Bursae and Ligaments		
Operation	T	Resection: Cutting out or off, without replacement, all of a body part		

Body Part (Character 4)	Approach (Character 5)	Device (Character 6)	Qualifier (Character 7)
0 Head and Neck Bursa and Ligament 1 Shoulder Bursa and Ligament, Right 2 Shoulder Bursa and Ligament, Left 3 Elbow Bursa and Ligament, Right 4 Elbow Bursa and Ligament, Left 5 Wrist Bursa and Ligament, Right 6 Wrist Bursa and Ligament, Left 7 Hand Bursa and Ligament, Right 8 Hand Bursa and Ligament, Left 9 Upper Extremity Bursa and Ligament, Right B Upper Extremity Bursa and Ligament, Left C Trunk Bursa and Ligament, Right D Trunk Bursa and Ligament, Left F Thorax Bursa and Ligament, Right G Thorax Bursa and Ligament, Left H Abdomen Bursa and Ligament, Right J Abdomen Bursa and Ligament, Left K Perineum Bursa and Ligament L Hip Bursa and Ligament, Right M Hip Bursa and Ligament, Left N Knee Bursa and Ligament, Right P Knee Bursa and Ligament, Left Q Ankle Bursa and Ligament, Right R Ankle Bursa and Ligament, Left S Foot Bursa and Ligament, Right T Foot Bursa and Ligament, Left V Lower Extremity Bursa and Ligament, Right W Lower Extremity Bursa and Ligament, Left	0 Open 4 Percutaneous Endoscopic	Z No Device	Z No Qualifier

Section	0	Medical and Surgical		
Body System	M	Bursae and Ligaments		
Operation	U	Supplement: Putting in or on biological or synthetic material that physically reinforces and/or augments the function of a portion of a body part		

Body Part (Character 4)	Approach (Character 5)	Device (Character 6)	Qualifier (Character 7)
0 Head and Neck Bursa and Ligament **1** Shoulder Bursa and Ligament, Right **2** Shoulder Bursa and Ligament, Left **3** Elbow Bursa and Ligament, Right **4** Elbow Bursa and Ligament, Left **5** Wrist Bursa and Ligament, Right **6** Wrist Bursa and Ligament, Left **7** Hand Bursa and Ligament, Right **8** Hand Bursa and Ligament, Left **9** Upper Extremity Bursa and Ligament, Right **B** Upper Extremity Bursa and Ligament, Left **C** Trunk Bursa and Ligament, Right **D** Trunk Bursa and Ligament, Left **F** Thorax Bursa and Ligament, Right **G** Thorax Bursa and Ligament, Left **H** Abdomen Bursa and Ligament, Right **J** Abdomen Bursa and Ligament, Left **K** Perineum Bursa and Ligament **L** Hip Bursa and Ligament, Right **M** Hip Bursa and Ligament, Left **N** Knee Bursa and Ligament, Right **P** Knee Bursa and Ligament, Left **Q** Ankle Bursa and Ligament, Right **R** Ankle Bursa and Ligament, Left **S** Foot Bursa and Ligament, Right **T** Foot Bursa and Ligament, Left **V** Lower Extremity Bursa and Ligament, Right **W** Lower Extremity Bursa and Ligament, Left	**0** Open **4** Percutaneous Endoscopic	**7** Autologous Tissue Substitute **J** Synthetic Substitute **K** Nonautologous Tissue Substitute	**Z** No Qualifier

Section	0	Medical and Surgical		
Body System	M	Bursae and Ligaments		
Operation	W	Revision: Correcting, to the extent possible, a portion of a malfunctioning device or the position of a displaced device		

Body Part (Character 4)	Approach (Character 5)	Device (Character 6)	Qualifier (Character 7)
X Upper Bursa and Ligament **Y** Lower Bursa and Ligament	**0** Open **3** Percutaneous **4** Percutaneous Endoscopic **X** External	**0** Drainage Device **7** Autologous Tissue Substitute **J** Synthetic Substitute **K** Nonautologous Tissue Substitute	**Z** No Qualifier

Section	0	Medical and Surgical
Body System	M	Bursae and Ligaments
Operation	X	Transfer: Moving, without taking out, all or a portion of a body part to another location to take over the function of all or a portion of a body part

Body Part (Character 4)	Approach (Character 5)	Device (Character 6)	Qualifier (Character 7)
0 Head and Neck Bursa and Ligament **1** Shoulder Bursa and Ligament, Right **2** Shoulder Bursa and Ligament, Left **3** Elbow Bursa and Ligament, Right **4** Elbow Bursa and Ligament, Left **5** Wrist Bursa and Ligament, Right **6** Wrist Bursa and Ligament, Left **7** Hand Bursa and Ligament, Right **8** Hand Bursa and Ligament, Left **9** Upper Extremity Bursa and Ligament, Right **B** Upper Extremity Bursa and Ligament, Left **C** Trunk Bursa and Ligament, Right **D** Trunk Bursa and Ligament, Left **F** Thorax Bursa and Ligament, Right **G** Thorax Bursa and Ligament, Left **H** Abdomen Bursa and Ligament, Right **J** Abdomen Bursa and Ligament, Left **K** Perineum Bursa and Ligament **L** Hip Bursa and Ligament, Right **M** Hip Bursa and Ligament, Left **N** Knee Bursa and Ligament, Right **P** Knee Bursa and Ligament, Left **Q** Ankle Bursa and Ligament, Right **R** Ankle Bursa and Ligament, Left **S** Foot Bursa and Ligament, Right **T** Foot Bursa and Ligament, Left **V** Lower Extremity Bursa and Ligament, Right **W** Lower Extremity Bursa and Ligament, Left	**0** Open **4** Percutaneous Endoscopic	**Z** No Device	**Z** No Qualifier

Section	0	Medical and Surgical			
Body System	N	Head and Facial Bones			
Operation	2	Change: Taking out or off a device from a body part and putting back an identical or similar device in or on the same body part without cutting or puncturing the skin or a mucous membrane			

Body Part (Character 4)	Approach (Character 5)	Device (Character 6)	Qualifier (Character 7)
0 Skull B Nasal Bone W Facial Bone	X External	0 Drainage Device Y Other Device	Z No Qualifier

Section	0	Medical and Surgical			
Body System	N	Head and Facial Bones			
Operation	5	Destruction: Physical eradication of all or a portion of a body part by the direct use of energy, force, or a destructive agent			

Body Part (Character 4)	Approach (Character 5)	Device (Character 6)	Qualifier (Character 7)
0 Skull 1 Frontal Bone, Right 2 Frontal Bone, Left 3 Parietal Bone, Right 4 Parietal Bone, Left 5 Temporal Bone, Right 6 Temporal Bone, Left 7 Occipital Bone, Right 8 Occipital Bone, Left B Nasal Bone C Sphenoid Bone, Right D Sphenoid Bone, Left F Ethmoid Bone, Right G Ethmoid Bone, Left H Lacrimal Bone, Right J Lacrimal Bone, Left K Palatine Bone, Right L Palatine Bone, Left M Zygomatic Bone, Right N Zygomatic Bone, Left P Orbit, Right Q Orbit, Left R Maxilla, Right S Maxilla, Left T Mandible, Right V Mandible, Left X Hyoid Bone	0 Open 3 Percutaneous 4 Percutaneous Endoscopic	Z No Device	Z No Qualifier

Section	0	Medical and Surgical		
Body System	N	Head and Facial Bones		
Operation	8	Division: Cutting into a body part, without draining fluids and/or gases from the body part, in order to separate or transect a body part		

Body Part (Character 4)	Approach (Character 5)	Device (Character 6)	Qualifier (Character 7)
0 Skull 1 Frontal Bone, Right 2 Frontal Bone, Left 3 Parietal Bone, Right 4 Parietal Bone, Left 5 Temporal Bone, Right 6 Temporal Bone, Left 7 Occipital Bone, Right 8 Occipital Bone, Left B Nasal Bone C Sphenoid Bone, Right D Sphenoid Bone, Left F Ethmoid Bone, Right G Ethmoid Bone, Left H Lacrimal Bone, Right J Lacrimal Bone, Left K Palatine Bone, Right L Palatine Bone, Left M Zygomatic Bone, Right N Zygomatic Bone, Left P Orbit, Right Q Orbit, Left R Maxilla, Right S Maxilla, Left T Mandible, Right V Mandible, Left X Hyoid Bone	0 Open 3 Percutaneous 4 Percutaneous Endoscopic	Z No Device	Z No Qualifier

Section	0	Medical and Surgical		
Body System	N	Head and Facial Bones		
Operation	9	Drainage: Taking or letting out fluids and/or gases from a body part		

Body Part (Character 4)	Approach (Character 5)	Device (Character 6)	Qualifier (Character 7)
0 Skull 1 Frontal Bone, Right 2 Frontal Bone, Left 3 Parietal Bone, Right 4 Parietal Bone, Left 5 Temporal Bone, Right 6 Temporal Bone, Left 7 Occipital Bone, Right 8 Occipital Bone, Left B Nasal Bone C Sphenoid Bone, Right D Sphenoid Bone, Left F Ethmoid Bone, Right G Ethmoid Bone, Left H Lacrimal Bone, Right J Lacrimal Bone, Left K Palatine Bone, Right L Palatine Bone, Left M Zygomatic Bone, Right N Zygomatic Bone, Left P Orbit, Right Q Orbit, Left R Maxilla, Right S Maxilla, Left T Mandible, Right V Mandible, Left X Hyoid Bone	0 Open 3 Percutaneous 4 Percutaneous Endoscopic	0 Drainage Device	Z No Qualifier

Section	0	Medical and Surgical		
Body System	N	Head and Facial Bones		
Operation	9	Drainage: Taking or letting out fluids and/or gases from a body part		

Body Part (Character 4)	Approach (Character 5)	Device (Character 6)	Qualifier (Character 7)
0 Skull	0 Open	Z No Device	X Diagnostic
1 Frontal Bone, Right	3 Percutaneous		Z No Qualifier
2 Frontal Bone, Left	4 Percutaneous Endoscopic		
3 Parietal Bone, Right			
4 Parietal Bone, Left			
5 Temporal Bone, Right			
6 Temporal Bone, Left			
7 Occipital Bone, Right			
8 Occipital Bone, Left			
B Nasal Bone			
C Sphenoid Bone, Right			
D Sphenoid Bone, Left			
F Ethmoid Bone, Right			
G Ethmoid Bone, Left			
H Lacrimal Bone, Right			
J Lacrimal Bone, Left			
K Palatine Bone, Right			
L Palatine Bone, Left			
M Zygomatic Bone, Right			
N Zygomatic Bone, Left			
P Orbit, Right			
Q Orbit, Left			
R Maxilla, Right			
S Maxilla, Left			
T Mandible, Right			
V Mandible, Left			
X Hyoid Bone			

Section	0	Medical and Surgical		
Body System	N	Head and Facial Bones		
Operation	B	Excision: Cutting out or off, without replacement, a portion of a body part		

Body Part (Character 4)	Approach (Character 5)	Device (Character 6)	Qualifier (Character 7)
0 Skull	0 Open	Z No Device	X Diagnostic
1 Frontal Bone, Right	3 Percutaneous		Z No Qualifier
2 Frontal Bone, Left	4 Percutaneous Endoscopic		
3 Parietal Bone, Right			
4 Parietal Bone, Left			
5 Temporal Bone, Right			
6 Temporal Bone, Left			
7 Occipital Bone, Right			
8 Occipital Bone, Left			
B Nasal Bone			
C Sphenoid Bone, Right			
D Sphenoid Bone, Left			
F Ethmoid Bone, Right			
G Ethmoid Bone, Left			
H Lacrimal Bone, Right			
J Lacrimal Bone, Left			
K Palatine Bone, Right			
L Palatine Bone, Left			
M Zygomatic Bone, Right			
N Zygomatic Bone, Left			
P Orbit, Right			
Q Orbit, Left			
R Maxilla, Right			
S Maxilla, Left			
T Mandible, Right			
V Mandible, Left			
X Hyoid Bone			

Section	0	Medical and Surgical		
Body System	N	Head and Facial Bones		
Operation	C	Extirpation: Taking or cutting out solid matter from a body part		

Body Part (Character 4)	Approach (Character 5)	Device (Character 6)	Qualifier (Character 7)
1 Frontal Bone, Right 2 Frontal Bone, Left 3 Parietal Bone, Right 4 Parietal Bone, Left 5 Temporal Bone, Right 6 Temporal Bone, Left 7 Occipital Bone, Right 8 Occipital Bone, Left B Nasal Bone C Sphenoid Bone, Right D Sphenoid Bone, Left F Ethmoid Bone, Right G Ethmoid Bone, Left H Lacrimal Bone, Right J Lacrimal Bone, Left K Palatine Bone, Right L Palatine Bone, Left M Zygomatic Bone, Right N Zygomatic Bone, Left P Orbit, Right Q Orbit, Left R Maxilla, Right S Maxilla, Left T Mandible, Right V Mandible, Left X Hyoid Bone	0 Open 3 Percutaneous 4 Percutaneous Endoscopic	Z No Device	Z No Qualifier

Section	0	Medical and Surgical		
Body System	N	Head and Facial Bones		
Operation	H	Insertion: Putting in a nonbiological appliance that monitors, assists, performs, or prevents a physiological function but does not physically take the place of a body part		

Body Part (Character 4)	Approach (Character 5)	Device (Character 6)	Qualifier (Character 7)
0 Skull	0 Open	4 Internal Fixation Device 5 External Fixation Device M Bone Growth Stimulator N Neurostimulator Generator	Z No Qualifier
0 Skull	3 Percutaneous 4 Percutaneous Endoscopic	4 Internal Fixation Device 5 External Fixation Device M Bone Growth Stimulator	Z No Qualifier
1 Frontal Bone, Right 2 Frontal Bone, Left 3 Parietal Bone, Right 4 Parietal Bone, Left 7 Occipital Bone, Right 8 Occipital Bone, Left C Sphenoid Bone, Right D Sphenoid Bone, Left F Ethmoid Bone, Right G Ethmoid Bone, Left H Lacrimal Bone, Right J Lacrimal Bone, Left K Palatine Bone, Right L Palatine Bone, Left M Zygomatic Bone, Right N Zygomatic Bone, Left P Orbit, Right Q Orbit, Left X Hyoid Bone	0 Open 3 Percutaneous 4 Percutaneous Endoscopic	4 Internal Fixation Device	Z No Qualifier
5 Temporal Bone, Right 6 Temporal Bone, Left	0 Open 3 Percutaneous 4 Percutaneous Endoscopic	4 Internal Fixation Device 5 Hearing Device	Z No Qualifier
B Nasal Bone	0 Open 3 Percutaneous 4 Percutaneous Endoscopic	4 Internal Fixation Device M Bone Growth Stimulator	Z No Qualifier
R Maxilla, Right S Maxilla, Left T Mandible, Right V Mandible, Left	0 Open 3 Percutaneous 4 Percutaneous Endoscopic	4 Internal Fixation Device 5 External Fixation Device	Z No Qualifier

Section	0	Medical and Surgical		
Body System	N	Head and Facial Bones		
Operation	H	Insertion: Putting in a nonbiological appliance that monitors, assists, performs, or prevents a physiological function but does not physically take the place of a body part		

Body Part (Character 4)	Approach (Character 5)	Device (Character 6)	Qualifier (Character 7)
W Facial Bone	0 Open 3 Percutaneous 4 Percutaneous Endoscopic	M Bone Growth Stimulator	Z No Qualifier

Section	0	Medical and Surgical		
Body System	N	Head and Facial Bones		
Operation	J	Inspection: Visually and/or manually exploring a body part		

Body Part (Character 4)	Approach (Character 5)	Device (Character 6)	Qualifier (Character 7)
0 Skull B Nasal Bone W Facial Bone	0 Open 3 Percutaneous 4 Percutaneous Endoscopic X External	Z No Device	Z No Qualifier

Section	0	Medical and Surgical		
Body System	N	Head and Facial Bones		
Operation	N	Release: Freeing a body part from an abnormal physical constraint by cutting or by the use of force		

Body Part (Character 4)	Approach (Character 5)	Device (Character 6)	Qualifier (Character 7)
1 Frontal Bone, Right 2 Frontal Bone, Left 3 Parietal Bone, Right 4 Parietal Bone, Left 5 Temporal Bone, Right 6 Temporal Bone, Left 7 Occipital Bone, Right 8 Occipital Bone, Left B Nasal Bone C Sphenoid Bone, Right D Sphenoid Bone, Left F Ethmoid Bone, Right G Ethmoid Bone, Left H Lacrimal Bone, Right J Lacrimal Bone, Left K Palatine Bone, Right L Palatine Bone, Left M Zygomatic Bone, Right N Zygomatic Bone, Left P Orbit, Right Q Orbit, Left R Maxilla, Right S Maxilla, Left T Mandible, Right V Mandible, Left X Hyoid Bone	0 Open 3 Percutaneous 4 Percutaneous Endoscopic	Z No Device	Z No Qualifier

Section	0	Medical and Surgical		
Body System	N	Head and Facial Bones		
Operation	P	Removal: Taking out or off a device from a body part		

Body Part (Character 4)	Approach (Character 5)	Device (Character 6)	Qualifier (Character 7)
0 Skull	0 Open	0 Drainage Device 4 Internal Fixation Device 5 External Fixation Device 7 Autologous Tissue Substitute J Synthetic Substitute K Nonautologous Tissue Substitute M Bone Growth Stimulator N Neurostimulator Generator S Hearing Device	Z No Qualifier
0 Skull	3 Percutaneous 4 Percutaneous Endoscopic	0 Drainage Device 4 Internal Fixation Device 5 External Fixation Device 7 Autologous Tissue Substitute J Synthetic Substitute K Nonautologous Tissue Substitute M Bone Growth Stimulator S Hearing Device	Z No Qualifier

Section	0	Medical and Surgical			
Body System	N	Head and Facial Bones			
Operation	P	Removal: Taking out or off a device from a body part			

Body Part (Character 4)	Approach (Character 5)	Device (Character 6)	Qualifier (Character 7)
0 Skull	**X** External	**0** Drainage Device **4** Internal Fixation Device **5** External Fixation Device **M** Bone Growth Stimulator **S** Hearing Device	**Z** No Qualifier
B Nasal Bone **W** Facial Bone	**0** Open **3** Percutaneous **4** Percutaneous Endoscopic	**0** Drainage Device **4** Internal Fixation Device **7** Autologous Tissue Substitute **J** Synthetic Substitute **K** Nonautologous Tissue Substitute **M** Bone Growth Stimulator	**Z** No Qualifier
B Nasal Bone **W** Facial Bone	**X** External	**0** Drainage Device **4** Internal Fixation Device **M** Bone Growth Stimulator	**Z** No Qualifier

Section	0	Medical and Surgical			
Body System	N	Head and Facial Bones			
Operation	Q	Repair: Restoring, to the extent possible, a body part to its normal anatomic structure and function			

Body Part (Character 4)	Approach (Character 5)	Device (Character 6)	Qualifier (Character 7)
0 Skull **1** Frontal Bone, Right **2** Frontal Bone, Left **3** Parietal Bone, Right **4** Parietal Bone, Left **5** Temporal Bone, Right **6** Temporal Bone, Left **7** Occipital Bone, Right **8** Occipital Bone, Left **B** Nasal Bone **C** Sphenoid Bone, Right **D** Sphenoid Bone, Left **F** Ethmoid Bone, Right **G** Ethmoid Bone, Left **H** Lacrimal Bone, Right **J** Lacrimal Bone, Left **K** Palatine Bone, Right **L** Palatine Bone, Left **M** Zygomatic Bone, Right **N** Zygomatic Bone, Left **P** Orbit, Right **Q** Orbit, Left **R** Maxilla, Right **S** Maxilla, Left **T** Mandible, Right **V** Mandible, Left **X** Hyoid Bone	**0** Open **3** Percutaneous **4** Percutaneous Endoscopic **X** External	**Z** No Device	**Z** No Qualifier

Section	0	Medical and Surgical
Body System	N	Head and Facial Bones
Operation	R	Replacement: Putting in or on biological or synthetic material that physically takes the place and/or function of all or a portion of a body part

Body Part (Character 4)	Approach (Character 5)	Device (Character 6)	Qualifier (Character 7)
0 Skull 1 Frontal Bone, Right 2 Frontal Bone, Left 3 Parietal Bone, Right 4 Parietal Bone, Left 5 Temporal Bone, Right 6 Temporal Bone, Left 7 Occipital Bone, Right 8 Occipital Bone, Left B Nasal Bone C Sphenoid Bone, Right D Sphenoid Bone, Left F Ethmoid Bone, Right G Ethmoid Bone, Left H Lacrimal Bone, Right J Lacrimal Bone, Left K Palatine Bone, Right L Palatine Bone, Left M Zygomatic Bone, Right N Zygomatic Bone, Left P Orbit, Right Q Orbit, Left R Maxilla, Right S Maxilla, Left T Mandible, Right V Mandible, Left X Hyoid Bone	0 Open 3 Percutaneous 4 Percutaneous Endoscopic	7 Autologous Tissue Substitute J Synthetic Substitute K Nonautologous Tissue Substitute	Z No Qualifier

Section	0	Medical and Surgical
Body System	N	Head and Facial Bones
Operation	S	Reposition: Moving to its normal location, or other suitable location, all or a portion of a body part

Body Part (Character 4)	Approach (Character 5)	Device (Character 6)	Qualifier (Character 7)
0 Skull R Maxilla, Right S Maxilla, Left T Mandible, Right V Mandible, Left	0 Open 3 Percutaneous 4 Percutaneous Endoscopic	4 Internal Fixation Device 5 External Fixation Device Z No Device	Z No Qualifier
0 Skull R Maxilla, Right S Maxilla, Left T Mandible, Right V Mandible, Left	X External	Z No Device	Z No Qualifier
1 Frontal Bone, Right 2 Frontal Bone, Left 3 Parietal Bone, Right 4 Parietal Bone, Left 5 Temporal Bone, Right 6 Temporal Bone, Left 7 Occipital Bone, Right 8 Occipital Bone, Left B Nasal Bone C Sphenoid Bone, Right D Sphenoid Bone, Left F Ethmoid Bone, Right G Ethmoid Bone, Left H Lacrimal Bone, Right J Lacrimal Bone, Left K Palatine Bone, Right L Palatine Bone, Left M Zygomatic Bone, Right N Zygomatic Bone, Left P Orbit, Right Q Orbit, Left X Hyoid Bone	0 Open 3 Percutaneous 4 Percutaneous Endoscopic	4 Internal Fixation Device Z No Device	Z No Qualifier

Section	0	Medical and Surgical		
Body System	N	Head and Facial Bones		
Operation	S	Reposition: Moving to its normal location, or other suitable location, all or a portion of a body part		

Body Part (Character 4)	Approach (Character 5)	Device (Character 6)	Qualifier (Character 7)
1 Frontal Bone, Right	X External	Z No Device	Z No Qualifier
2 Frontal Bone, Left			
3 Parietal Bone, Right			
4 Parietal Bone, Left			
5 Temporal Bone, Right			
6 Temporal Bone, Left			
7 Occipital Bone, Right			
8 Occipital Bone, Left			
B Nasal Bone			
C Sphenoid Bone, Right			
D Sphenoid Bone, Left			
F Ethmoid Bone, Right			
G Ethmoid Bone, Left			
H Lacrimal Bone, Right			
J Lacrimal Bone, Left			
K Palatine Bone, Right			
L Palatine Bone, Left			
M Zygomatic Bone, Right			
N Zygomatic Bone, Left			
P Orbit, Right			
Q Orbit, Left			
X Hyoid Bone			

Section	0	Medical and Surgical		
Body System	N	Head and Facial Bones		
Operation	T	Resection: Cutting out or off, without replacement, all of a body part		

Body Part (Character 4)	Approach (Character 5)	Device (Character 6)	Qualifier (Character 7)
1 Frontal Bone, Right	0 Open	Z No Device	Z No Qualifier
2 Frontal Bone, Left			
3 Parietal Bone, Right			
4 Parietal Bone, Left			
5 Temporal Bone, Right			
6 Temporal Bone, Left			
7 Occipital Bone, Right			
8 Occipital Bone, Left			
B Nasal Bone			
C Sphenoid Bone, Right			
D Sphenoid Bone, Left			
F Ethmoid Bone, Right			
G Ethmoid Bone, Left			
H Lacrimal Bone, Right			
J Lacrimal Bone, Left			
K Palatine Bone, Right			
L Palatine Bone, Left			
M Zygomatic Bone, Right			
N Zygomatic Bone, Left			
P Orbit, Right			
Q Orbit, Left			
R Maxilla, Right			
S Maxilla, Left			
T Mandible, Right			
V Mandible, Left			
X Hyoid Bone			

Section	0	Medical and Surgical		
Body System	N	Head and Facial Bones		
Operation	U	Supplement: Putting in or on biological or synthetic material that physically reinforces and/or augments the function of a portion of a body part		

Body Part (Character 4)	Approach (Character 5)	Device (Character 6)	Qualifier (Character 7)
0 Skull 1 Frontal Bone, Right 2 Frontal Bone, Left 3 Parietal Bone, Right 4 Parietal Bone, Left 5 Temporal Bone, Right 6 Temporal Bone, Left 7 Occipital Bone, Right 8 Occipital Bone, Left B Nasal Bone C Sphenoid Bone, Right D Sphenoid Bone, Left F Ethmoid Bone, Right G Ethmoid Bone, Left H Lacrimal Bone, Right J Lacrimal Bone, Left K Palatine Bone, Right L Palatine Bone, Left M Zygomatic Bone, Right N Zygomatic Bone, Left P Orbit, Right Q Orbit, Left R Maxilla, Right S Maxilla, Left T Mandible, Right V Mandible, Left X Hyoid Bone	0 Open 3 Percutaneous 4 Percutaneous Endoscopic	7 Autologous Tissue Substitute J Synthetic Substitute K Nonautologous Tissue Substitute	Z No Qualifier

Section	0	Medical and Surgical		
Body System	N	Head and Facial Bones		
Operation	W	Revision: Correcting, to the extent possible, a portion of a malfunctioning device or the position of a displaced device		

Body Part (Character 4)	Approach (Character 5)	Device (Character 6)	Qualifier (Character 7)
0 Skull	0 Open	0 Drainage Device 4 Internal Fixation Device 5 External Fixation Device 7 Autologous Tissue Substitute J Synthetic Substitute K Nonautologous Tissue Substitute M Bone Growth Stimulator N Neurostimulator Generator S Hearing Device	Z No Qualifier
0 Skull	3 Percutaneous 4 Percutaneous Endoscopic X External	0 Drainage Device 4 Internal Fixation Device 5 External Fixation Device 7 Autologous Tissue Substitute J Synthetic Substitute K Nonautologous Tissue Substitute M Bone Growth Stimulator S Hearing Device	Z No Qualifier
B Nasal Bone W Facial Bone	0 Open 3 Percutaneous 4 Percutaneous Endoscopic X External	0 Drainage Device 4 Internal Fixation Device 7 Autologous Tissue Substitute J Synthetic Substitute K Nonautologous Tissue Substitute M Bone Growth Stimulator	Z No Qualifier

Section	0	Medical and Surgical			
Body System	P	Upper Bones			
Operation	2	Change: Taking out or off a device from a body part and putting back an identical or similar device in or on the same body part without cutting or puncturing the skin or a mucous membrane			
Body Part (Character 4)		Approach (Character 5)	Device (Character 6)		Qualifier (Character 7)
Y Upper Bone		X External	0 Drainage Device Y Other Device		Z No Qualifier

Section	0	Medical and Surgical		
Body System	P	Upper Bones		
Operation	5	Destruction: Physical eradication of all or a portion of a body part by the direct use of energy, force, or a destructive agent		
Body Part (Character 4)	Approach (Character 5)	Device (Character 6)	Qualifier (Character 7)
0 Sternum 1 Rib, Right 2 Rib, Left 3 Cervical Vertebra 4 Thoracic Vertebra 5 Scapula, Right 6 Scapula, Left 7 Glenoid Cavity, Right 8 Glenoid Cavity, Left 9 Clavicle, Right B Clavicle, Left C Humeral Head, Right D Humeral Head, Left F Humeral Shaft, Right G Humeral Shaft, Left H Radius, Right J Radius, Left K Ulna, Right L Ulna, Left M Carpal, Right N Carpal, Left P Metacarpal, Right Q Metacarpal, Left R Thumb Phalanx, Right S Thumb Phalanx, Left T Finger Phalanx, Right V Finger Phalanx, Left	0 Open 3 Percutaneous 4 Percutaneous Endoscopic	Z No Device	Z No Qualifier

Section	0	Medical and Surgical		
Body System	P	Upper Bones		
Operation	8	Division: Cutting into a body part, without draining fluids and/or gases from the body part, in order to separate or transect a body part		
Body Part (Character 4)	Approach (Character 5)	Device (Character 6)	Qualifier (Character 7)
0 Sternum 1 Rib, Right 2 Rib, Left 3 Cervical Vertebra 4 Thoracic Vertebra 5 Scapula, Right 6 Scapula, Left 7 Glenoid Cavity, Right 8 Glenoid Cavity, Left 9 Clavicle, Right B Clavicle, Left C Humeral Head, Right D Humeral Head, Left F Humeral Shaft, Right G Humeral Shaft, Left H Radius, Right J Radius, Left K Ulna, Right L Ulna, Left M Carpal, Right N Carpal, Left P Metacarpal, Right Q Metacarpal, Left R Thumb Phalanx, Right S Thumb Phalanx, Left T Finger Phalanx, Right V Finger Phalanx, Left	0 Open 3 Percutaneous 4 Percutaneous Endoscopic	Z No Device	Z No Qualifier

Section	0	Medical and Surgical		
Body System	P	Upper Bones		
Operation	9	Drainage: Taking or letting out fluids and/or gases from a body part		

Body Part (Character 4)	Approach (Character 5)	Device (Character 6)	Qualifier (Character 7)
0 Sternum	**0** Open	**0** Drainage Device	**Z** No Qualifier
1 Rib, Right	**3** Percutaneous		
2 Rib, Left	**4** Percutaneous Endoscopic		
3 Cervical Vertebra			
4 Thoracic Vertebra			
5 Scapula, Right			
6 Scapula, Left			
7 Glenoid Cavity, Right			
8 Glenoid Cavity, Left			
9 Clavicle, Right			
B Clavicle, Left			
C Humeral Head, Right			
D Humeral Head, Left			
F Humeral Shaft, Right			
G Humeral Shaft, Left			
H Radius, Right			
J Radius, Left			
K Ulna, Right			
L Ulna, Left			
M Carpal, Right			
N Carpal, Left			
P Metacarpal, Right			
Q Metacarpal, Left			
R Thumb Phalanx, Right			
S Thumb Phalanx, Left			
T Finger Phalanx, Right			
V Finger Phalanx, Left			

Section	0	Medical and Surgical		
Body System	P	Upper Bones		
Operation	9	Drainage: Taking or letting out fluids and/or gases from a body part		

Body Part (Character 4)	Approach (Character 5)	Device (Character 6)	Qualifier (Character 7)
0 Sternum	**0** Open	**Z** No Device	**X** Diagnostic
1 Rib, Right	**3** Percutaneous		**Z** No Qualifier
2 Rib, Left	**4** Percutaneous Endoscopic		
3 Cervical Vertebra			
4 Thoracic Vertebra			
5 Scapula, Right			
6 Scapula, Left			
7 Glenoid Cavity, Right			
8 Glenoid Cavity, Left			
9 Clavicle, Right			
B Clavicle, Left			
C Humeral Head, Right			
D Humeral Head, Left			
F Humeral Shaft, Right			
G Humeral Shaft, Left			
H Radius, Right			
J Radius, Left			
K Ulna, Right			
L Ulna, Left			
M Carpal, Right			
N Carpal, Left			
P Metacarpal, Right			
Q Metacarpal, Left			
R Thumb Phalanx, Right			
S Thumb Phalanx, Left			
T Finger Phalanx, Right			
V Finger Phalanx, Left			

Section	0	Medical and Surgical		
Body System	P	Upper Bones		
Operation	B	Excision: Cutting out or off, without replacement, a portion of a body part		

Body Part (Character 4)	Approach (Character 5)	Device (Character 6)	Qualifier (Character 7)
0 Sternum 1 Rib, Right 2 Rib, Left 3 Cervical Vertebra 4 Thoracic Vertebra 5 Scapula, Right 6 Scapula, Left 7 Glenoid Cavity, Right 8 Glenoid Cavity, Left 9 Clavicle, Right B Clavicle, Left C Humeral Head, Right D Humeral Head, Left F Humeral Shaft, Right G Humeral Shaft, Left H Radius, Right J Radius, Left K Ulna, Right L Ulna, Left M Carpal, Right N Carpal, Left P Metacarpal, Right Q Metacarpal, Left R Thumb Phalanx, Right S Thumb Phalanx, Left T Finger Phalanx, Right V Finger Phalanx, Left	0 Open 3 Percutaneous 4 Percutaneous Endoscopic	Z No Device	X Diagnostic Z No Qualifier

Section	0	Medical and Surgical		
Body System	P	Upper Bones		
Operation	C	Extirpation: Taking or cutting out solid matter from a body part		

Body Part (Character 4)	Approach (Character 5)	Device (Character 6)	Qualifier (Character 7)
0 Sternum 1 Rib, Right 2 Rib, Left 3 Cervical Vertebra 4 Thoracic Vertebra 5 Scapula, Right 6 Scapula, Left 7 Glenoid Cavity, Right 8 Glenoid Cavity, Left 9 Clavicle, Right B Clavicle, Left C Humeral Head, Right D Humeral Head, Left F Humeral Shaft, Right G Humeral Shaft, Left H Radius, Right J Radius, Left K Ulna, Right L Ulna, Left M Carpal, Right N Carpal, Left P Metacarpal, Right Q Metacarpal, Left R Thumb Phalanx, Right S Thumb Phalanx, Left T Finger Phalanx, Right V Finger Phalanx, Left	0 Open 3 Percutaneous 4 Percutaneous Endoscopic	Z No Device	Z No Qualifier

Section	0	Medical and Surgical		
Body System	P	Upper Bones		
Operation	H	Insertion: Putting in a nonbiological appliance that monitors, assists, performs, or prevents a physiological function but does not physically take the place of a body part		
Body Part (Character 4)		**Approach (Character 5)**	**Device (Character 6)**	**Qualifier (Character 7)**
0 Sternum		0 Open 3 Percutaneous 4 Percutaneous Endoscopic	0 Internal Fixation Device, Rigid Plate 4 Internal Fixation Device	Z No Qualifier
1 Rib, Right 2 Rib, Left 3 Cervical Vertebra 4 Thoracic Vertebra 5 Scapula, Right 6 Scapula, Left 7 Glenoid Cavity, Right 8 Glenoid Cavity, Left 9 Clavicle, Right B Clavicle, Left		0 Open 3 Percutaneous 4 Percutaneous Endoscopic	4 Internal Fixation Device	Z No Qualifier
C Humeral Head, Right D Humeral Head, Left F Humeral Shaft, Right G Humeral Shaft, Left H Radius, Right J Radius, Left K Ulna, Right L Ulna, Left		0 Open 3 Percutaneous 4 Percutaneous Endoscopic	4 Internal Fixation Device 5 External Fixation Device 6 Internal Fixation Device, Intramedullary 8 External Fixation Device, Limb Lengthening B External Fixation Device, Monoplanar C External Fixation Device, Ring D External Fixation Device, Hybrid	Z No Qualifier
M Carpal, Right N Carpal, Left P Metacarpal, Right Q Metacarpal, Left R Thumb Phalanx, Right S Thumb Phalanx, Left T Finger Phalanx, Right V Finger Phalanx, Left		0 Open 3 Percutaneous 4 Percutaneous Endoscopic	4 Internal Fixation Device 5 External Fixation Device	Z No Qualifier
Y Upper Bone		0 Open 3 Percutaneous 4 Percutaneous Endoscopic	M Bone Growth Stimulator	Z No Qualifier

Section	0	Medical and Surgical		
Body System	P	Upper Bones		
Operation	J	Inspection: Visually and/or manually exploring a body part		
Body Part (Character 4)		**Approach (Character 5)**	**Device (Character 6)**	**Qualifier (Character 7)**
Y Upper Bone		0 Open 3 Percutaneous 4 Percutaneous Endoscopic X External	Z No Device	Z No Qualifier

Section	0	Medical and Surgical
Body System	P	Upper Bones
Operation	N	Release: Freeing a body part from an abnormal physical constraint by cutting or by the use of force

Body Part (Character 4)	Approach (Character 5)	Device (Character 6)	Qualifier (Character 7)
0 Sternum **1** Rib, Right **2** Rib, Left **3** Cervical Vertebra **4** Thoracic Vertebra **5** Scapula, Right **6** Scapula, Left **7** Glenoid Cavity, Right **8** Glenoid Cavity, Left **9** Clavicle, Right **B** Clavicle, Left **C** Humeral Head, Right **D** Humeral Head, Left **F** Humeral Shaft, Right **G** Humeral Shaft, Left **H** Radius, Right **J** Radius, Left **K** Ulna, Right **L** Ulna, Left **M** Carpal, Right **N** Carpal, Left **P** Metacarpal, Right **Q** Metacarpal, Left **R** Thumb Phalanx, Right **S** Thumb Phalanx, Left **T** Finger Phalanx, Right **V** Finger Phalanx, Left	**0** Open **3** Percutaneous **4** Percutaneous Endoscopic	**Z** No Device	**Z** No Qualifier

Section	0	Medical and Surgical
Body System	P	Upper Bones
Operation	P	Removal: Taking out or off a device from a body part

Body Part (Character 4)	Approach (Character 5)	Device (Character 6)	Qualifier (Character 7)
0 Sternum **1** Rib, Right **2** Rib, Left **3** Cervical Vertebra **4** Thoracic Vertebra **5** Scapula, Right **6** Scapula, Left **7** Glenoid Cavity, Right **8** Glenoid Cavity, Left **9** Clavicle, Right **B** Clavicle, Left	**0** Open **3** Percutaneous **4** Percutaneous Endoscopic	**4** Internal Fixation Device **7** Autologous Tissue Substitute **J** Synthetic Substitute **K** Nonautologous Tissue Substitute	**Z** No Qualifier
0 Sternum **1** Rib, Right **2** Rib, Left **3** Cervical Vertebra **4** Thoracic Vertebra **5** Scapula, Right **6** Scapula, Left **7** Glenoid Cavity, Right **8** Glenoid Cavity, Left **9** Clavicle, Right **B** Clavicle, Left	**X** External	**4** Internal Fixation Device	**Z** No Qualifier

Section	0	Medical and Surgical		
Body System	P	Upper Bones		
Operation	P	Removal: Taking out or off a device from a body part		

Body Part (Character 4)	Approach (Character 5)	Device (Character 6)	Qualifier (Character 7)
C Humeral Head, Right D Humeral Head, Left F Humeral Shaft, Right G Humeral Shaft, Left H Radius, Right J Radius, Left K Ulna, Right L Ulna, Left M Carpal, Right N Carpal, Left P Metacarpal, Right Q Metacarpal, Left R Thumb Phalanx, Right S Thumb Phalanx, Left T Finger Phalanx, Right V Finger Phalanx, Left	0 Open 3 Percutaneous 4 Percutaneous Endoscopic	4 Internal Fixation Device 5 External Fixation Device 7 Autologous Tissue Substitute J Synthetic Substitute K Nonautologous Tissue Substitute	Z No Qualifier
C Humeral Head, Right D Humeral Head, Left F Humeral Shaft, Right G Humeral Shaft, Left H Radius, Right J Radius, Left K Ulna, Right L Ulna, Left M Carpal, Right N Carpal, Left P Metacarpal, Right Q Metacarpal, Left R Thumb Phalanx, Right S Thumb Phalanx, Left T Finger Phalanx, Right V Finger Phalanx, Left	X External	4 Internal Fixation Device 5 External Fixation Device	Z No Qualifier
Y Upper Bone	0 Open 3 Percutaneous 4 Percutaneous Endoscopic X External	0 Drainage Device M Bone Growth Stimulator	Z No Qualifier

Section	0	Medical and Surgical		
Body System	P	Upper Bones		
Operation	Q	Repair: Restoring, to the extent possible, a body part to its normal anatomic structure and function		

Body Part (Character 4)	Approach (Character 5)	Device (Character 6)	Qualifier (Character 7)
0 Sternum 1 Rib, Right 2 Rib, Left 3 Cervical Vertebra 4 Thoracic Vertebra 5 Scapula, Right 6 Scapula, Left 7 Glenoid Cavity, Right 8 Glenoid Cavity, Left 9 Clavicle, Right B Clavicle, Left C Humeral Head, Right D Humeral Head, Left F Humeral Shaft, Right G Humeral Shaft, Left H Radius, Right J Radius, Left K Ulna, Right L Ulna, Left M Carpal, Right N Carpal, Left P Metacarpal, Right Q Metacarpal, Left R Thumb Phalanx, Right S Thumb Phalanx, Left T Finger Phalanx, Right V Finger Phalanx, Left	0 Open 3 Percutaneous 4 Percutaneous Endoscopic X External	Z No Device	Z No Qualifier

Section	0	Medical and Surgical					
Body System	P	Upper Bones					
Operation	R	Replacement: Putting in or on biological or synthetic material that physically takes the place and/or function of all or a portion of a body part					

Body Part (Character 4)	Approach (Character 5)	Device (Character 6)	Qualifier (Character 7)
0 Sternum 1 Rib, Right 2 Rib, Left 3 Cervical Vertebra 4 Thoracic Vertebra 5 Scapula, Right 6 Scapula, Left 7 Glenoid Cavity, Right 8 Glenoid Cavity, Left 9 Clavicle, Right B Clavicle, Left C Humeral Head, Right D Humeral Head, Left F Humeral Shaft, Right G Humeral Shaft, Left H Radius, Right J Radius, Left K Ulna, Right L Ulna, Left M Carpal, Right N Carpal, Left P Metacarpal, Right Q Metacarpal, Left R Thumb Phalanx, Right S Thumb Phalanx, Left T Finger Phalanx, Right V Finger Phalanx, Left	0 Open 3 Percutaneous 4 Percutaneous Endoscopic	7 Autologous Tissue Substitute J Synthetic Substitute K Nonautologous Tissue Substitute	Z No Qualifier

Section	0	Medical and Surgical					
Body System	P	Upper Bones					
Operation	S	Reposition: Moving to its normal location, or other suitable location, all or a portion of a body part					

Body Part (Character 4)	Approach (Character 5)	Device (Character 6)	Qualifier (Character 7)
0 Sternum	0 Open 3 Percutaneous 4 Percutaneous Endoscopic	0 Internal Fixation Device, Rigid Plate 4 Internal Fixation Device Z No Device	Z No Qualifier
0 Sternum	X External	Z No Device	Z No Qualifier
1 Rib, Right 2 Rib, Left 3 Cervical Vertebra 4 Thoracic Vertebra 5 Scapula, Right 6 Scapula, Left 7 Glenoid Cavity, Right 8 Glenoid Cavity, Left 9 Clavicle, Right B Clavicle, Left	0 Open 3 Percutaneous 4 Percutaneous Endoscopic	4 Internal Fixation Device Z No Device	Z No Qualifier
1 Rib, Right 2 Rib, Left 3 Cervical Vertebra 4 Thoracic Vertebra 5 Scapula, Right 6 Scapula, Left 7 Glenoid Cavity, Right 8 Glenoid Cavity, Left 9 Clavicle, Right B Clavicle, Left	X External	Z No Device	Z No Qualifier
C Humeral Head, Right D Humeral Head, Left F Humeral Shaft, Right G Humeral Shaft, Left H Radius, Right J Radius, Left K Ulna, Right L Ulna, Left	0 Open 3 Percutaneous 4 Percutaneous Endoscopic	4 Internal Fixation Device 5 External Fixation Device 6 Internal Fixation Device, Intramedullary B External Fixation Device, Monoplanar C External Fixation Device, Ring D External Fixation Device, Hybrid Z No Device	Z No Qualifier

Section	0	Medical and Surgical
Body System	P	Upper Bones
Operation	S	Reposition: Moving to its normal location, or other suitable location, all or a portion of a body part

Body Part (Character 4)	Approach (Character 5)	Device (Character 6)	Qualifier (Character 7)
C Humeral Head, Right D Humeral Head, Left F Humeral Shaft, Right G Humeral Shaft, Left H Radius, Right J Radius, Left K Ulna, Right L Ulna, Left	X External	Z No Device	Z No Qualifier
M Carpal, Right N Carpal, Left P Metacarpal, Right Q Metacarpal, Left R Thumb Phalanx, Right S Thumb Phalanx, Left T Finger Phalanx, Right V Finger Phalanx, Left	0 Open 3 Percutaneous 4 Percutaneous Endoscopic	4 Internal Fixation Device 5 External Fixation Device Z No Device	Z No Qualifier
M Carpal, Right N Carpal, Left P Metacarpal, Right Q Metacarpal, Left R Thumb Phalanx, Right S Thumb Phalanx, Left T Finger Phalanx, Right V Finger Phalanx, Left	X External	Z No Device	Z No Qualifier

Section	0	Medical and Surgical
Body System	P	Upper Bones
Operation	T	Resection: Cutting out or off, without replacement, all of a body part

Body Part (Character 4)	Approach (Character 5)	Device (Character 6)	Qualifier (Character 7)
0 Sternum 1 Rib, Right 2 Rib, Left 5 Scapula, Right 6 Scapula, Left 7 Glenoid Cavity, Right 8 Glenoid Cavity, Left 9 Clavicle, Right B Clavicle, Left C Humeral Head, Right D Humeral Head, Left F Humeral Shaft, Right G Humeral Shaft, Left H Radius, Right J Radius, Left K Ulna, Right L Ulna, Left M Carpal, Right N Carpal, Left P Metacarpal, Right Q Metacarpal, Left R Thumb Phalanx, Right S Thumb Phalanx, Left T Finger Phalanx, Right V Finger Phalanx, Left	0 Open	Z No Device	Z No Qualifier

Section	0	Medical and Surgical		
Body System	P	Upper Bones		
Operation	U	Supplement: Putting in or on biological or synthetic material that physically reinforces and/or augments the function of a portion of a body part		

Body Part (Character 4)	Approach (Character 5)	Device (Character 6)	Qualifier (Character 7)
0 Sternum **1** Rib, Right **2** Rib, Left **3** Cervical Vertebra **4** Thoracic Vertebra **5** Scapula, Right **6** Scapula, Left **7** Glenoid Cavity, Right **8** Glenoid Cavity, Left **9** Clavicle, Right **B** Clavicle, Left **C** Humeral Head, Right **D** Humeral Head, Left **F** Humeral Shaft, Right **G** Humeral Shaft, Left **H** Radius, Right **J** Radius, Left **K** Ulna, Right **L** Ulna, Left **M** Carpal, Right **N** Carpal, Left **P** Metacarpal, Right **Q** Metacarpal, Left **R** Thumb Phalanx, Right **S** Thumb Phalanx, Left **T** Finger Phalanx, Right **V** Finger Phalanx, Left	**0** Open **3** Percutaneous **4** Percutaneous Endoscopic	**7** Autologous Tissue Substitute **J** Synthetic Substitute **K** Nonautologous Tissue Substitute	**Z** No Qualifier

Section	0	Medical and Surgical		
Body System	P	Upper Bones		
Operation	W	Revision: Correcting, to the extent possible, a portion of a malfunctioning device or the position of a displaced device		

Body Part (Character 4)	Approach (Character 5)	Device (Character 6)	Qualifier (Character 7)
0 Sternum **1** Rib, Right **2** Rib, Left **3** Cervical Vertebra **4** Thoracic Vertebra **5** Scapula, Right **6** Scapula, Left **7** Glenoid Cavity, Right **8** Glenoid Cavity, Left **9** Clavicle, Right **B** Clavicle, Left	**0** Open **3** Percutaneous **4** Percutaneous Endoscopic **X** External	**4** Internal Fixation Device **7** Autologous Tissue Substitute **J** Synthetic Substitute **K** Nonautologous Tissue Substitute	**Z** No Qualifier
C Humeral Head, Right **D** Humeral Head, Left **F** Humeral Shaft, Right **G** Humeral Shaft, Left **H** Radius, Right **J** Radius, Left **K** Ulna, Right **L** Ulna, Left **M** Carpal, Right **N** Carpal, Left **P** Metacarpal, Right **Q** Metacarpal, Left **R** Thumb Phalanx, Right **S** Thumb Phalanx, Left **T** Finger Phalanx, Right **V** Finger Phalanx, Left	**0** Open **3** Percutaneous **4** Percutaneous Endoscopic **X** External	**4** Internal Fixation Device **5** External Fixation Device **7** Autologous Tissue Substitute **J** Synthetic Substitute **K** Nonautologous Tissue Substitute	**Z** No Qualifier
Y Upper Bone	**0** Open **3** Percutaneous **4** Percutaneous Endoscopic **X** External	**0** Drainage Device **M** Bone Growth Stimulator	**Z** No Qualifier

Section	0	Medical and Surgical		
Body System	Q	Lower Bones		
Operation	2	Change: Taking out or off a device from a body part and putting back an identical or similar device in or on the same body part without cutting or puncturing the skin or a mucous membrane		

Body Part (Character 4)	Approach (Character 5)	Device (Character 6)	Qualifier (Character 7)
Y Lower Bone	X External	0 Drainage Device Y Other Device	Z No Qualifier

Section	0	Medical and Surgical		
Body System	Q	Lower Bones		
Operation	5	Destruction: Physical eradication of all or a portion of a body part by the direct use of energy, force, or a destructive agent		

Body Part (Character 4)	Approach (Character 5)	Device (Character 6)	Qualifier (Character 7)
0 Lumbar Vertebra 1 Sacrum 2 Pelvic Bone, Right 3 Pelvic Bone, Left 4 Acetabulum, Right 5 Acetabulum, Left 6 Upper Femur, Right 7 Upper Femur, Left 8 Femoral Shaft, Right 9 Femoral Shaft, Left B Lower Femur, Right C Lower Femur, Left D Patella, Right F Patella, Left G Tibia, Right H Tibia, Left J Fibula, Right K Fibula, Left L Tarsal, Right M Tarsal, Left N Metatarsal, Right P Metatarsal, Left Q Toe Phalanx, Right R Toe Phalanx, Left S Coccyx	0 Open 3 Percutaneous 4 Percutaneous Endoscopic	Z No Device	Z No Qualifier

Section	0	Medical and Surgical		
Body System	Q	Lower Bones		
Operation	8	Division: Cutting into a body part, without draining fluids and/or gases from the body part, in order to separate or transect a body part		

Body Part (Character 4)	Approach (Character 5)	Device (Character 6)	Qualifier (Character 7)
0 Lumbar Vertebra 1 Sacrum 2 Pelvic Bone, Right 3 Pelvic Bone, Left 4 Acetabulum, Right 5 Acetabulum, Left 6 Upper Femur, Right 7 Upper Femur, Left 8 Femoral Shaft, Right 9 Femoral Shaft, Left B Lower Femur, Right C Lower Femur, Left D Patella, Right F Patella, Left G Tibia, Right H Tibia, Left J Fibula, Right K Fibula, Left L Tarsal, Right M Tarsal, Left N Metatarsal, Right P Metatarsal, Left Q Toe Phalanx, Right R Toe Phalanx, Left S Coccyx	0 Open 3 Percutaneous 4 Percutaneous Endoscopic	Z No Device	Z No Qualifier

Section	0	Medical and Surgical		
Body System	Q	Lower Bones		
Operation	9	Drainage: Taking or letting out fluids and/or gases from a body part		
Body Part (Character 4)		**Approach (Character 5)**	**Device (Character 6)**	**Qualifier (Character 7)**
0 Lumbar Vertebra		**0** Open	**0** Drainage Device	**Z** No Qualifier
1 Sacrum		**3** Percutaneous		
2 Pelvic Bone, Right		**4** Percutaneous Endoscopic		
3 Pelvic Bone, Left				
4 Acetabulum, Right				
5 Acetabulum, Left				
6 Upper Femur, Right				
7 Upper Femur, Left				
8 Femoral Shaft, Right				
9 Femoral Shaft, Left				
B Lower Femur, Right				
C Lower Femur, Left				
D Patella, Right				
F Patella, Left				
G Tibia, Right				
H Tibia, Left				
J Fibula, Right				
K Fibula, Left				
L Tarsal, Right				
M Tarsal, Left				
N Metatarsal, Right				
P Metatarsal, Left				
Q Toe Phalanx, Right				
R Toe Phalanx, Left				
S Coccyx				

Section	0	Medical and Surgical		
Body System	Q	Lower Bones		
Operation	9	Drainage: Taking or letting out fluids and/or gases from a body part		
Body Part (Character 4)		**Approach (Character 5)**	**Device (Character 6)**	**Qualifier (Character 7)**
0 Lumbar Vertebra		**0** Open	**Z** No Device	**X** Diagnostic
1 Sacrum		**3** Percutaneous		**Z** No Qualifier
2 Pelvic Bone, Right		**4** Percutaneous Endoscopic		
3 Pelvic Bone, Left				
4 Acetabulum, Right				
5 Acetabulum, Left				
6 Upper Femur, Right				
7 Upper Femur, Left				
8 Femoral Shaft, Right				
9 Femoral Shaft, Left				
B Lower Femur, Right				
C Lower Femur, Left				
D Patella, Right				
F Patella, Left				
G Tibia, Right				
H Tibia, Left				
J Fibula, Right				
K Fibula, Left				
L Tarsal, Right				
M Tarsal, Left				
N Metatarsal, Right				
P Metatarsal, Left				
Q Toe Phalanx, Right				
R Toe Phalanx, Left				
S Coccyx				

Section	0	Medical and Surgical			
Body System	Q	Lower Bones			
Operation	B	Excision: Cutting out or off, without replacement, a portion of a body part			

Body Part (Character 4)	Approach (Character 5)	Device (Character 6)	Qualifier (Character 7)
0 Lumbar Vertebra **1** Sacrum **2** Pelvic Bone, Right **3** Pelvic Bone, Left **4** Acetabulum, Right **5** Acetabulum, Left **6** Upper Femur, Right **7** Upper Femur, Left **8** Femoral Shaft, Right **9** Femoral Shaft, Left **B** Lower Femur, Right **C** Lower Femur, Left **D** Patella, Right **F** Patella, Left **G** Tibia, Right **H** Tibia, Left **J** Fibula, Right **K** Fibula, Left **L** Tarsal, Right **M** Tarsal, Left **N** Metatarsal, Right **P** Metatarsal, Left **Q** Toe Phalanx, Right **R** Toe Phalanx, Left **S** Coccyx	**0** Open **3** Percutaneous **4** Percutaneous Endoscopic	**Z** No Device	**X** Diagnostic **Z** No Qualifier

Section	0	Medical and Surgical			
Body System	Q	Lower Bones			
Operation	C	Extirpation: Taking or cutting out solid matter from a body part			

Body Part (Character 4)	Approach (Character 5)	Device (Character 6)	Qualifier (Character 7)
0 Lumbar Vertebra **1** Sacrum **2** Pelvic Bone, Right **3** Pelvic Bone, Left **4** Acetabulum, Right **5** Acetabulum, Left **6** Upper Femur, Right **7** Upper Femur, Left **8** Femoral Shaft, Right **9** Femoral Shaft, Left **B** Lower Femur, Right **C** Lower Femur, Left **D** Patella, Right **F** Patella, Left **G** Tibia, Right **H** Tibia, Left **J** Fibula, Right **K** Fibula, Left **L** Tarsal, Right **M** Tarsal, Left **N** Metatarsal, Right **P** Metatarsal, Left **Q** Toe Phalanx, Right **R** Toe Phalanx, Left **S** Coccyx	**0** Open **3** Percutaneous **4** Percutaneous Endoscopic	**Z** No Device	**Z** No Qualifier

Section	0	Medical and Surgical		
Body System	Q	Lower Bones		
Operation	H	Insertion: Putting in a nonbiological appliance that monitors, assists, performs, or prevents a physiological function but does not physically take the place of a body part		

Body Part (Character 4)	Approach (Character 5)	Device (Character 6)	Qualifier (Character 7)
0 Lumbar Vertebra **1** Sacrum **2** Pelvic Bone, Right **3** Pelvic Bone, Left **4** Acetabulum, Right **5** Acetabulum, Left **D** Patella, Right **F** Patella, Left **L** Tarsal, Right **M** Tarsal, Left **N** Metatarsal, Right **P** Metatarsal, Left **Q** Toe Phalanx, Right **R** Toe Phalanx, Left **S** Coccyx	**0** Open **3** Percutaneous **4** Percutaneous Endoscopic	**4** Internal Fixation Device **5** External Fixation Device	**Z** No Qualifier
6 Upper Femur, Right **7** Upper Femur, Left **8** Femoral Shaft, Right **9** Femoral Shaft, Left **B** Lower Femur, Right **C** Lower Femur, Left **G** Tibia, Right **H** Tibia, Left **J** Fibula, Right **K** Fibula, Left	**0** Open **3** Percutaneous **4** Percutaneous Endoscopic	**4** Internal Fixation Device **5** External Fixation Device **6** Internal Fixation Device, Intramedullary **8** External Fixation Device, Limb Lengthening **B** External Fixation Device, Monoplanar **C** External Fixation Device, Ring **D** External Fixation Device, Hybrid	**Z** No Qualifier
Y Lower Bone	**0** Open **3** Percutaneous **4** Percutaneous Endoscopic	**M** Bone Growth Stimulator	**Z** No Qualifier

Section	0	Medical and Surgical		
Body System	Q	Lower Bones		
Operation	J	Inspection: Visually and/or manually exploring a body part		

Body Part (Character 4)	Approach (Character 5)	Device (Character 6)	Qualifier (Character 7)
Y Lower Bone	**0** Open **3** Percutaneous **4** Percutaneous Endoscopic **X** External	**Z** No Device	**Z** No Qualifier

Section	0	Medical and Surgical		
Body System	Q	Lower Bones		
Operation	N	Release: Freeing a body part from an abnormal physical constraint by cutting or by the use of force		

Body Part (Character 4)	Approach (Character 5)	Device (Character 6)	Qualifier (Character 7)
0 Lumbar Vertebra	0 Open	Z No Device	Z No Qualifier
1 Sacrum	3 Percutaneous		
2 Pelvic Bone, Right	4 Percutaneous Endoscopic		
3 Pelvic Bone, Left			
4 Acetabulum, Right			
5 Acetabulum, Left			
6 Upper Femur, Right			
7 Upper Femur, Left			
8 Femoral Shaft, Right			
9 Femoral Shaft, Left			
B Lower Femur, Right			
C Lower Femur, Left			
D Patella, Right			
F Patella, Left			
G Tibia, Right			
H Tibia, Left			
J Fibula, Right			
K Fibula, Left			
L Tarsal, Right			
M Tarsal, Left			
N Metatarsal, Right			
P Metatarsal, Left			
Q Toe Phalanx, Right			
R Toe Phalanx, Left			
S Coccyx			

Section	0	Medical and Surgical		
Body System	Q	Lower Bones		
Operation	P	Removal: Taking out or off a device from a body part		

Body Part (Character 4)	Approach (Character 5)	Device (Character 6)	Qualifier (Character 7)
0 Lumbar Vertebra	0 Open	4 Internal Fixation Device	Z No Qualifier
1 Sacrum	3 Percutaneous	7 Autologous Tissue Substitute	
4 Acetabulum, Right	4 Percutaneous Endoscopic	J Synthetic Substitute	
5 Acetabulum, Left		K Nonautologous Tissue Substitute	
S Coccyx			
0 Lumbar Vertebra	X External	4 Internal Fixation Device	Z No Qualifier
1 Sacrum			
4 Acetabulum, Right			
5 Acetabulum, Left			
S Coccyx			
2 Pelvic Bone, Right	0 Open	4 Internal Fixation Device	Z No Qualifier
3 Pelvic Bone, Left	3 Percutaneous	5 External Fixation Device	
6 Upper Femur, Right	4 Percutaneous Endoscopic	7 Autologous Tissue Substitute	
7 Upper Femur, Left		J Synthetic Substitute	
8 Femoral Shaft, Right		K Nonautologous Tissue Substitute	
9 Femoral Shaft, Left			
B Lower Femur, Right			
C Lower Femur, Left			
D Patella, Right			
F Patella, Left			
G Tibia, Right			
H Tibia, Left			
J Fibula, Right			
K Fibula, Left			
L Tarsal, Right			
M Tarsal, Left			
N Metatarsal, Right			
P Metatarsal, Left			
Q Toe Phalanx, Right			
R Toe Phalanx, Left			

Section	0	Medical and Surgical			
Body System	Q	Lower Bones			
Operation	P	Removal: Taking out or off a device from a body part			

Body Part (Character 4)	Approach (Character 5)	Device (Character 6)	Qualifier (Character 7)
2 Pelvic Bone, Right 3 Pelvic Bone, Left 6 Upper Femur, Right 7 Upper Femur, Left 8 Femoral Shaft, Right 9 Femoral Shaft, Left B Lower Femur, Right C Lower Femur, Left D Patella, Right F Patella, Left G Tibia, Right H Tibia, Left J Fibula, Right K Fibula, Left L Tarsal, Right M Tarsal, Left N Metatarsal, Right P Metatarsal, Left Q Toe Phalanx, Right R Toe Phalanx, Left	X External	4 Internal Fixation Device 5 External Fixation Device	Z No Qualifier
Y Lower Bone	0 Open 3 Percutaneous 4 Percutaneous Endoscopic X External	0 Drainage Device M Bone Growth Stimulator	Z No Qualifier

Section	0	Medical and Surgical			
Body System	Q	Lower Bones			
Operation	Q	Repair: Restoring, to the extent possible, a body part to its normal anatomic structure and function			

Body Part (Character 4)	Approach (Character 5)	Device (Character 6)	Qualifier (Character 7)
0 Lumbar Vertebra 1 Sacrum 2 Pelvic Bone, Right 3 Pelvic Bone, Left 4 Acetabulum, Right 5 Acetabulum, Left 6 Upper Femur, Right 7 Upper Femur, Left 8 Femoral Shaft, Right 9 Femoral Shaft, Left B Lower Femur, Right C Lower Femur, Left D Patella, Right F Patella, Left G Tibia, Right H Tibia, Left J Fibula, Right K Fibula, Left L Tarsal, Right M Tarsal, Left N Metatarsal, Right P Metatarsal, Left Q Toe Phalanx, Right R Toe Phalanx, Left S Coccyx	0 Open 3 Percutaneous 4 Percutaneous Endoscopic X External	Z No Device	Z No Qualifier

Section	0	Medical and Surgical
Body System	Q	Lower Bones
Operation	R	Replacement: Putting in or on biological or synthetic material that physically takes the place and/or function of all or a portion of a body part

Body Part (Character 4)	Approach (Character 5)	Device (Character 6)	Qualifier (Character 7)
0 Lumbar Vertebra 1 Sacrum 2 Pelvic Bone, Right 3 Pelvic Bone, Left 4 Acetabulum, Right 5 Acetabulum, Left 6 Upper Femur, Right 7 Upper Femur, Left 8 Femoral Shaft, Right 9 Femoral Shaft, Left B Lower Femur, Right C Lower Femur, Left D Patella, Right F Patella, Left G Tibia, Right H Tibia, Left J Fibula, Right K Fibula, Left L Tarsal, Right M Tarsal, Left N Metatarsal, Right P Metatarsal, Left Q Toe Phalanx, Right R Toe Phalanx, Left S Coccyx	0 Open 3 Percutaneous 4 Percutaneous Endoscopic	7 Autologous Tissue Substitute J Synthetic Substitute K Nonautologous Tissue Substitute	Z No Qualifier

Section	0	Medical and Surgical
Body System	Q	Lower Bones
Operation	S	Reposition: Moving to its normal location, or other suitable location, all or a portion of a body part

Body Part (Character 4)	Approach (Character 5)	Device (Character 6)	Qualifier (Character 7)
0 Lumbar Vertebra 1 Sacrum 4 Acetabulum, Right 5 Acetabulum, Left S Coccyx	0 Open 3 Percutaneous 4 Percutaneous Endoscopic	4 Internal Fixation Device Z No Device	Z No Qualifier
0 Lumbar Vertebra 1 Sacrum 4 Acetabulum, Right 5 Acetabulum, Left S Coccyx	X External	Z No Device	Z No Qualifier
2 Pelvic Bone, Right 3 Pelvic Bone, Left D Patella, Right F Patella, Left L Tarsal, Right M Tarsal, Left N Metatarsal, Right P Metatarsal, Left Q Toe Phalanx, Right R Toe Phalanx, Left	0 Open 3 Percutaneous 4 Percutaneous Endoscopic	4 Internal Fixation Device 5 External Fixation Device Z No Device	Z No Qualifier
2 Pelvic Bone, Right 3 Pelvic Bone, Left D Patella, Right F Patella, Left L Tarsal, Right M Tarsal, Left N Metatarsal, Right P Metatarsal, Left Q Toe Phalanx, Right R Toe Phalanx, Left	X External	Z No Device	Z No Qualifier

Section	0	Medical and Surgical		
Body System	Q	Lower Bones		
Operation	S	Reposition: Moving to its normal location, or other suitable location, all or a portion of a body part		

Body Part (Character 4)	Approach (Character 5)	Device (Character 6)	Qualifier (Character 7)
6 Upper Femur, Right 7 Upper Femur, Left 8 Femoral Shaft, Right 9 Femoral Shaft, Left B Lower Femur, Right C Lower Femur, Left G Tibia, Right H Tibia, Left J Fibula, Right K Fibula, Left	0 Open 3 Percutaneous 4 Percutaneous Endoscopic	4 Internal Fixation Device 5 External Fixation Device 6 Internal Fixation Device, Intramedullary B External Fixation Device, Monoplanar C External Fixation Device, Ring D External Fixation Device, Hybrid Z No Device	Z No Qualifier
6 Upper Femur, Right 7 Upper Femur, Left 8 Femoral Shaft, Right 9 Femoral Shaft, Left B Lower Femur, Right C Lower Femur, Left G Tibia, Right H Tibia, Left J Fibula, Right K Fibula, Left	X External	Z No Device	Z No Qualifier

Section	0	Medical and Surgical		
Body System	Q	Lower Bones		
Operation	T	Resection: Cutting out or off, without replacement, all of a body part		

Body Part (Character 4)	Approach (Character 5)	Device (Character 6)	Qualifier (Character 7)
2 Pelvic Bone, Right 3 Pelvic Bone, Left 4 Acetabulum, Right 5 Acetabulum, Left 6 Upper Femur, Right 7 Upper Femur, Left 8 Femoral Shaft, Right 9 Femoral Shaft, Left B Lower Femur, Right C Lower Femur, Left D Patella, Right F Patella, Left G Tibia, Right H Tibia, Left J Fibula, Right K Fibula, Left L Tarsal, Right M Tarsal, Left N Metatarsal, Right P Metatarsal, Left Q Toe Phalanx, Right R Toe Phalanx, Left S Coccyx	0 Open	Z No Device	Z No Qualifier

Section	0	Medical and Surgical
Body System	Q	Lower Bones
Operation	U	Supplement: Putting in or on biological or synthetic material that physically reinforces and/or augments the function of a portion of a body part

Body Part (Character 4)	Approach (Character 5)	Device (Character 6)	Qualifier (Character 7)
0 Lumbar Vertebra 1 Sacrum 2 Pelvic Bone, Right 3 Pelvic Bone, Left 4 Acetabulum, Right 5 Acetabulum, Left 6 Upper Femur, Right 7 Upper Femur, Left 8 Femoral Shaft, Right 9 Femoral Shaft, Left B Lower Femur, Right C Lower Femur, Left D Patella, Right F Patella, Left G Tibia, Right H Tibia, Left J Fibula, Right K Fibula, Left L Tarsal, Right M Tarsal, Left N Metatarsal, Right P Metatarsal, Left Q Toe Phalanx, Right R Toe Phalanx, Left S Coccyx	0 Open 3 Percutaneous 4 Percutaneous Endoscopic	7 Autologous Tissue Substitute J Synthetic Substitute K Nonautologous Tissue Substitute	Z No Qualifier

Section	0	Medical and Surgical
Body System	Q	Lower Bones
Operation	W	Revision: Correcting, to the extent possible, a portion of a malfunctioning device or the position of a displaced device

Body Part (Character 4)	Approach (Character 5)	Device (Character 6)	Qualifier (Character 7)
0 Lumbar Vertebra 1 Sacrum 4 Acetabulum, Right 5 Acetabulum, Left S Coccyx	0 Open 3 Percutaneous 4 Percutaneous Endoscopic X External	4 Internal Fixation Device 7 Autologous Tissue Substitute J Synthetic Substitute K Nonautologous Tissue Substitute	Z No Qualifier
2 Pelvic Bone, Right 3 Pelvic Bone, Left 6 Upper Femur, Right 7 Upper Femur, Left 8 Femoral Shaft, Right 9 Femoral Shaft, Left B Lower Femur, Right C Lower Femur, Left D Patella, Right F Patella, Left G Tibia, Right H Tibia, Left J Fibula, Right K Fibula, Left L Tarsal, Right M Tarsal, Left N Metatarsal, Right P Metatarsal, Left Q Toe Phalanx, Right R Toe Phalanx, Left	0 Open 3 Percutaneous 4 Percutaneous Endoscopic X External	4 Internal Fixation Device 5 External Fixation Device 7 Autologous Tissue Substitute J Synthetic Substitute K Nonautologous Tissue Substitute	Z No Qualifier
Y Lower Bone	0 Open 3 Percutaneous 4 Percutaneous Endoscopic X External	0 Drainage Device M Bone Growth Stimulator	Z No Qualifier

Section	0	Medical and Surgical			
Body System	R	Upper Joints			
Operation	2	Change: Taking out or off a device from a body part and putting back an identical or similar device in or on the same body part without cutting or puncturing the skin or a mucous membrane			

Body Part (Character 4)	Approach (Character 5)	Device (Character 6)	Qualifier (Character 7)
Y Upper Joint	X External	0 Drainage Device Y Other Device	Z No Qualifier

Section	0	Medical and Surgical			
Body System	R	Upper Joints			
Operation	5	Destruction: Physical eradication of all or a portion of a body part by the direct use of energy, force, or a destructive agent			

Body Part (Character 4)	Approach (Character 5)	Device (Character 6)	Qualifier (Character 7)
0 Occipital-cervical Joint	0 Open	Z No Device	Z No Qualifier
1 Cervical Vertebral Joint	3 Percutaneous		
3 Cervical Vertebral Disc	4 Percutaneous Endoscopic		
4 Cervicothoracic Vertebral Joint			
5 Cervicothoracic Vertebral Disc			
6 Thoracic Vertebral Joint			
9 Thoracic Vertebral Disc			
A Thoracolumbar Vertebral Joint			
B Thoracolumbar Vertebral Disc			
C Temporomandibular Joint, Right			
D Temporomandibular Joint, Left			
E Sternoclavicular Joint, Right			
F Sternoclavicular Joint, Left			
G Acromioclavicular Joint, Right			
H Acromioclavicular Joint, Left			
J Shoulder Joint, Right			
K Shoulder Joint, Left			
L Elbow Joint, Right			
M Elbow Joint, Left			
N Wrist Joint, Right			
P Wrist Joint, Left			
Q Carpal Joint, Right			
R Carpal Joint, Left			
S Metacarpocarpal Joint, Right			
T Metacarpocarpal Joint, Left			
U Metacarpophalangeal Joint, Right			
V Metacarpophalangeal Joint, Left			
W Finger Phalangeal Joint, Right			
X Finger Phalangeal Joint, Left			

Section	0	Medical and Surgical		
Body System	R	Upper Joints		
Operation	9	Drainage: Taking or letting out fluids and/or gases from a body part		

Body Part (Character 4)	Approach (Character 5)	Device (Character 6)	Qualifier (Character 7)
0 Occipital-cervical Joint 1 Cervical Vertebral Joint 3 Cervical Vertebral Disc 4 Cervicothoracic Vertebral Joint 5 Cervicothoracic Vertebral Disc 6 Thoracic Vertebral Joint 9 Thoracic Vertebral Disc A Thoracolumbar Vertebral Joint B Thoracolumbar Vertebral Disc C Temporomandibular Joint, Right D Temporomandibular Joint, Left E Sternoclavicular Joint, Right F Sternoclavicular Joint, Left G Acromioclavicular Joint, Right H Acromioclavicular Joint, Left J Shoulder Joint, Right K Shoulder Joint, Left L Elbow Joint, Right M Elbow Joint, Left N Wrist Joint, Right P Wrist Joint, Left Q Carpal Joint, Right R Carpal Joint, Left S Metacarpocarpal Joint, Right T Metacarpocarpal Joint, Left U Metacarpophalangeal Joint, Right V Metacarpophalangeal Joint, Left W Finger Phalangeal Joint, Right X Finger Phalangeal Joint, Left	0 Open 3 Percutaneous 4 Percutaneous Endoscopic	0 Drainage Device	Z No Qualifier

Section	0	Medical and Surgical		
Body System	R	Upper Joints		
Operation	9	Drainage: Taking or letting out fluids and/or gases from a body part		

Body Part (Character 4)	Approach (Character 5)	Device (Character 6)	Qualifier (Character 7)
0 Occipital-cervical Joint 1 Cervical Vertebral Joint 3 Cervical Vertebral Disc 4 Cervicothoracic Vertebral Joint 5 Cervicothoracic Vertebral Disc 6 Thoracic Vertebral Joint 9 Thoracic Vertebral Disc A Thoracolumbar Vertebral Joint B Thoracolumbar Vertebral Disc C Temporomandibular Joint, Right D Temporomandibular Joint, Left E Sternoclavicular Joint, Right F Sternoclavicular Joint, Left G Acromioclavicular Joint, Right H Acromioclavicular Joint, Left J Shoulder Joint, Right K Shoulder Joint, Left L Elbow Joint, Right M Elbow Joint, Left N Wrist Joint, Right P Wrist Joint, Left Q Carpal Joint, Right R Carpal Joint, Left S Metacarpocarpal Joint, Right T Metacarpocarpal Joint, Left U Metacarpophalangeal Joint, Right V Metacarpophalangeal Joint, Left W Finger Phalangeal Joint, Right X Finger Phalangeal Joint, Left	0 Open 3 Percutaneous 4 Percutaneous Endoscopic	Z No Device	X Diagnostic Z No Qualifier

Section	0	Medical and Surgical		
Body System	R	Upper Joints		
Operation	B	Excision: Cutting out or off, without replacement, a portion of a body part		
Body Part (Character 4)		**Approach (Character 5)**	**Device (Character 6)**	**Qualifier (Character 7)**
0 Occipital-cervical Joint		0 Open	Z No Device	X Diagnostic
1 Cervical Vertebral Joint		3 Percutaneous		Z No Qualifier
3 Cervical Vertebral Disc		4 Percutaneous Endoscopic		
4 Cervicothoracic Vertebral Joint				
5 Cervicothoracic Vertebral Disc				
6 Thoracic Vertebral Joint				
9 Thoracic Vertebral Disc				
A Thoracolumbar Vertebral Joint				
B Thoracolumbar Vertebral Disc				
C Temporomandibular Joint, Right				
D Temporomandibular Joint, Left				
E Sternoclavicular Joint, Right				
F Sternoclavicular Joint, Left				
G Acromioclavicular Joint, Right				
H Acromioclavicular Joint, Left				
J Shoulder Joint, Right				
K Shoulder Joint, Left				
L Elbow Joint, Right				
M Elbow Joint, Left				
N Wrist Joint, Right				
P Wrist Joint, Left				
Q Carpal Joint, Right				
R Carpal Joint, Left				
S Metacarpocarpal Joint, Right				
T Metacarpocarpal Joint, Left				
U Metacarpophalangeal Joint, Right				
V Metacarpophalangeal Joint, Left				
W Finger Phalangeal Joint, Right				
X Finger Phalangeal Joint, Left				

Section	0	Medical and Surgical		
Body System	R	Upper Joints		
Operation	C	Extirpation: Taking or cutting out solid matter from a body part		
Body Part (Character 4)		**Approach (Character 5)**	**Device (Character 6)**	**Qualifier (Character 7)**
0 Occipital-cervical Joint		0 Open	Z No Device	Z No Qualifier
1 Cervical Vertebral Joint		3 Percutaneous		
3 Cervical Vertebral Disc		4 Percutaneous Endoscopic		
4 Cervicothoracic Vertebral Joint				
5 Cervicothoracic Vertebral Disc				
6 Thoracic Vertebral Joint				
9 Thoracic Vertebral Disc				
A Thoracolumbar Vertebral Joint				
B Thoracolumbar Vertebral Disc				
C Temporomandibular Joint, Right				
D Temporomandibular Joint, Left				
E Sternoclavicular Joint, Right				
F Sternoclavicular Joint, Left				
G Acromioclavicular Joint, Right				
H Acromioclavicular Joint, Left				
J Shoulder Joint, Right				
K Shoulder Joint, Left				
L Elbow Joint, Right				
M Elbow Joint, Left				
N Wrist Joint, Right				
P Wrist Joint, Left				
Q Carpal Joint, Right				
R Carpal Joint, Left				
S Metacarpocarpal Joint, Right				
T Metacarpocarpal Joint, Left				
U Metacarpophalangeal Joint, Right				
V Metacarpophalangeal Joint, Left				
W Finger Phalangeal Joint, Right				
X Finger Phalangeal Joint, Left				

Section	0	Medical and Surgical		
Body System	R	Upper Joints		
Operation	G	Fusion: Joining together portions of an articular body part rendering the articular body part immobile		

Body Part (Character 4)	Approach (Character 5)	Device (Character 6)	Qualifier (Character 7)
0 Occipital-cervical Joint **1** Cervical Vertebral Joint **2** Cervical Vertebral Joints, 2 or more **4** Cervicothoracic Vertebral Joint **6** Thoracic Vertebral Joint **7** Thoracic Vertebral Joints, 2-7 **8** Thoracic Vertebral Joints, 8 or more **A** Thoracolumbar Vertebral Joint	**0** Open **3** Percutaneous **4** Percutaneous Endoscopic	**7** Autologous Tissue Substitute **A** Interbody Fusion Device **J** Synthetic Substitute **K** Nonautologous Tissue Substitute **Z** No Device	**0** Anterior Approach, Anterior Column **1** Posterior Approach, Posterior Column **J** Posterior Approach, Anterior Column
C Temporomandibular Joint, Right **D** Temporomandibular Joint, Left **E** Sternoclavicular Joint, Right **F** Sternoclavicular Joint, Left **G** Acromioclavicular Joint, Right **H** Acromioclavicular Joint, Left **J** Shoulder Joint, Right **K** Shoulder Joint, Left	**0** Open **3** Percutaneous **4** Percutaneous Endoscopic	**4** Internal Fixation Device **7** Autologous Tissue Substitute **J** Synthetic Substitute **K** Nonautologous Tissue Substitute **Z** No Device	**Z** No Qualifier
L Elbow Joint, Right **M** Elbow Joint, Left **N** Wrist Joint, Right **P** Wrist Joint, Left **Q** Carpal Joint, Right **R** Carpal Joint, Left **S** Metacarpocarpal Joint, Right **T** Metacarpocarpal Joint, Left **U** Metacarpophalangeal Joint, Right **V** Metacarpophalangeal Joint, Left **W** Finger Phalangeal Joint, Right **X** Finger Phalangeal Joint, Left	**0** Open **3** Percutaneous **4** Percutaneous Endoscopic	**4** Internal Fixation Device **5** External Fixation Device **7** Autologous Tissue Substitute **J** Synthetic Substitute **K** Nonautologous Tissue Substitute **Z** No Device	**Z** No Qualifier

Section	0	Medical and Surgical		
Body System	R	Upper Joints		
Operation	H	Insertion: Putting in a nonbiological appliance that monitors, assists, performs, or prevents a physiological function but does not physically take the place of a body part		

Body Part (Character 4)	Approach (Character 5)	Device (Character 6)	Qualifier (Character 7)
0 Occipital-cervical Joint **1** Cervical Vertebral Joint **4** Cervicothoracic Vertebral Joint **6** Thoracic Vertebral Joint **A** Thoracolumbar Vertebral Joint	**0** Open **3** Percutaneous **4** Percutaneous Endoscopic	**3** Infusion Device **4** Internal Fixation Device **8** Spacer **B** Spinal Stabilization Device, Interspinous Process **C** Spinal Stabilization Device, Pedicle-Based **D** Spinal Stabilization Device, Facet Replacement	**Z** No Qualifier
3 Cervical Vertebral Disc **5** Cervicothoracic Vertebral Disc **9** Thoracic Vertebral Disc **B** Thoracolumbar Vertebral Disc	**0** Open **3** Percutaneous **4** Percutaneous Endoscopic	**3** Infusion Device	**Z** No Qualifier
C Temporomandibular Joint, Right **D** Temporomandibular Joint, Left **E** Sternoclavicular Joint, Right **F** Sternoclavicular Joint, Left **G** Acromioclavicular Joint, Right **H** Acromioclavicular Joint, Left **J** Shoulder Joint, Right **K** Shoulder Joint, Left	**0** Open **3** Percutaneous **4** Percutaneous Endoscopic	**3** Infusion Device **4** Internal Fixation Device **8** Spacer	**Z** No Qualifier
L Elbow Joint, Right **M** Elbow Joint, Left **N** Wrist Joint, Right **P** Wrist Joint, Left **Q** Carpal Joint, Right **R** Carpal Joint, Left **S** Metacarpocarpal Joint, Right **T** Metacarpocarpal Joint, Left **U** Metacarpophalangeal Joint, Right **V** Metacarpophalangeal Joint, Left **W** Finger Phalangeal Joint, Right **X** Finger Phalangeal Joint, Left	**0** Open **3** Percutaneous **4** Percutaneous Endoscopic	**3** Infusion Device **4** Internal Fixation Device **5** External Fixation Device **8** Spacer	**Z** No Qualifier

Section	0	Medical and Surgical		
Body System	R	Upper Joints		
Operation	J	Inspection: Visually and/or manually exploring a body part		

Body Part (Character 4)	Approach (Character 5)	Device (Character 6)	Qualifier (Character 7)
0 Occipital-cervical Joint 1 Cervical Vertebral Joint 3 Cervical Vertebral Disc 4 Cervicothoracic Vertebral Joint 5 Cervicothoracic Vertebral Disc 6 Thoracic Vertebral Joint 9 Thoracic Vertebral Disc A Thoracolumbar Vertebral Joint B Thoracolumbar Vertebral Disc C Temporomandibular Joint, Right D Temporomandibular Joint, Left E Sternoclavicular Joint, Right F Sternoclavicular Joint, Left G Acromioclavicular Joint, Right H Acromioclavicular Joint, Left J Shoulder Joint, Right K Shoulder Joint, Left L Elbow Joint, Right M Elbow Joint, Left N Wrist Joint, Right P Wrist Joint, Left Q Carpal Joint, Right R Carpal Joint, Left S Metacarpocarpal Joint, Right T Metacarpocarpal Joint, Left U Metacarpophalangeal Joint, Right V Metacarpophalangeal Joint, Left W Finger Phalangeal Joint, Right X Finger Phalangeal Joint, Left	0 Open 3 Percutaneous 4 Percutaneous Endoscopic X External	Z No Device	Z No Qualifier

Section	0	Medical and Surgical		
Body System	R	Upper Joints		
Operation	N	Release: Freeing a body part from an abnormal physical constraint by cutting or by the use of force		

Body Part (Character 4)	Approach (Character 5)	Device (Character 6)	Qualifier (Character 7)
0 Occipital-cervical Joint 1 Cervical Vertebral Joint 3 Cervical Vertebral Disc 4 Cervicothoracic Vertebral Joint 5 Cervicothoracic Vertebral Disc 6 Thoracic Vertebral Joint 9 Thoracic Vertebral Disc A Thoracolumbar Vertebral Joint B Thoracolumbar Vertebral Disc C Temporomandibular Joint, Right D Temporomandibular Joint, Left E Sternoclavicular Joint, Right F Sternoclavicular Joint, Left G Acromioclavicular Joint, Right H Acromioclavicular Joint, Left J Shoulder Joint, Right K Shoulder Joint, Left L Elbow Joint, Right M Elbow Joint, Left N Wrist Joint, Right P Wrist Joint, Left Q Carpal Joint, Right R Carpal Joint, Left S Metacarpocarpal Joint, Right T Metacarpocarpal Joint, Left U Metacarpophalangeal Joint, Right V Metacarpophalangeal Joint, Left W Finger Phalangeal Joint, Right X Finger Phalangeal Joint, Left	0 Open 3 Percutaneous 4 Percutaneous Endoscopic X External	Z No Device	Z No Qualifier

Section	0	Medical and Surgical		
Body System	R	Upper Joints		
Operation	P	Removal: Taking out or off a device from a body part		

Body Part (Character 4)	Approach (Character 5)	Device (Character 6)	Qualifier (Character 7)
0 Occipital-cervical Joint 1 Cervical Vertebral Joint 4 Cervicothoracic Vertebral Joint 6 Thoracic Vertebral Joint A Thoracolumbar Vertebral Joint	0 Open 3 Percutaneous 4 Percutaneous Endoscopic	0 Drainage Device 3 Infusion Device 4 Internal Fixation Device 7 Autologous Tissue Substitute 8 Spacer A Interbody Fusion Device J Synthetic Substitute K Nonautologous Tissue Substitute	Z No Qualifier
0 Occipital-cervical Joint 1 Cervical Vertebral Joint 4 Cervicothoracic Vertebral Joint 6 Thoracic Vertebral Joint A Thoracolumbar Vertebral Joint	X External	0 Drainage Device 3 Infusion Device 4 Internal Fixation Device	Z No Qualifier
3 Cervical Vertebral Disc 5 Cervicothoracic Vertebral Disc 9 Thoracic Vertebral Disc B Thoracolumbar Vertebral Disc	0 Open 3 Percutaneous 4 Percutaneous Endoscopic	0 Drainage Device 3 Infusion Device 7 Autologous Tissue Substitute J Synthetic Substitute K Nonautologous Tissue Substitute	Z No Qualifier
3 Cervical Vertebral Disc 5 Cervicothoracic Vertebral Disc 9 Thoracic Vertebral Disc B Thoracolumbar Vertebral Disc	X External	0 Drainage Device 3 Infusion Device	Z No Qualifier
C Temporomandibular Joint, Right D Temporomandibular Joint, Left E Sternoclavicular Joint, Right F Sternoclavicular Joint, Left G Acromioclavicular Joint, Right H Acromioclavicular Joint, Left J Shoulder Joint, Right K Shoulder Joint, Left	0 Open 3 Percutaneous 4 Percutaneous Endoscopic	0 Drainage Device 3 Infusion Device 4 Internal Fixation Device 7 Autologous Tissue Substitute 8 Spacer J Synthetic Substitute K Nonautologous Tissue Substitute	Z No Qualifier

Section	0	Medical and Surgical		
Body System	R	Upper Joints		
Operation	P	Removal: Taking out or off a device from a body part		

Body Part (Character 4)	Approach (Character 5)	Device (Character 6)	Qualifier (Character 7)
C Temporomandibular Joint, Right D Temporomandibular Joint, Left E Sternoclavicular Joint, Right F Sternoclavicular Joint, Left G Acromioclavicular Joint, Right H Acromioclavicular Joint, Left J Shoulder Joint, Right K Shoulder Joint, Left	X External	0 Drainage Device 3 Infusion Device 4 Internal Fixation Device	Z No Qualifier
L Elbow Joint, Right M Elbow Joint, Left N Wrist Joint, Right P Wrist Joint, Left Q Carpal Joint, Right R Carpal Joint, Left S Metacarpocarpal Joint, Right T Metacarpocarpal Joint, Left U Metacarpophalangeal Joint, Right V Metacarpophalangeal Joint, Left W Finger Phalangeal Joint, Right X Finger Phalangeal Joint, Left	0 Open 3 Percutaneous 4 Percutaneous Endoscopic	0 Drainage Device 3 Infusion Device 4 Internal Fixation Device 5 External Fixation Device 7 Autologous Tissue Substitute 8 Spacer J Synthetic Substitute K Nonautologous Tissue Substitute	Z No Qualifier
L Elbow Joint, Right M Elbow Joint, Left N Wrist Joint, Right P Wrist Joint, Left Q Carpal Joint, Right R Carpal Joint, Left S Metacarpocarpal Joint, Right T Metacarpocarpal Joint, Left U Metacarpophalangeal Joint, Right V Metacarpophalangeal Joint, Left W Finger Phalangeal Joint, Right X Finger Phalangeal Joint, Left	X External	0 Drainage Device 3 Infusion Device 4 Internal Fixation Device 5 External Fixation Device	Z No Qualifier

Section	0	Medical and Surgical		
Body System	R	Upper Joints		
Operation	Q	Repair: Restoring, to the extent possible, a body part to its normal anatomic structure and function		

Body Part (Character 4)	Approach (Character 5)	Device (Character 6)	Qualifier (Character 7)
0 Occipital-cervical Joint 1 Cervical Vertebral Joint 3 Cervical Vertebral Disc 4 Cervicothoracic Vertebral Joint 5 Cervicothoracic Vertebral Disc 6 Thoracic Vertebral Joint 9 Thoracic Vertebral Disc A Thoracolumbar Vertebral Joint B Thoracolumbar Vertebral Disc C Temporomandibular Joint, Right D Temporomandibular Joint, Left E Sternoclavicular Joint, Right F Sternoclavicular Joint, Left G Acromioclavicular Joint, Right H Acromioclavicular Joint, Left J Shoulder Joint, Right K Shoulder Joint, Left L Elbow Joint, Right M Elbow Joint, Left N Wrist Joint, Right P Wrist Joint, Left Q Carpal Joint, Right R Carpal Joint, Left S Metacarpocarpal Joint, Right T Metacarpocarpal Joint, Left U Metacarpophalangeal Joint, Right V Metacarpophalangeal Joint, Left W Finger Phalangeal Joint, Right X Finger Phalangeal Joint, Left	0 Open 3 Percutaneous 4 Percutaneous Endoscopic X External	Z No Device	Z No Qualifier

Section	0	Medical and Surgical		
Body System	R	Upper Joints		
Operation	R	Replacement: Putting in or on biological or synthetic material that physically takes the place and/or function of all or a portion of a body part		

Body Part (Character 4)	Approach (Character 5)	Device (Character 6)	Qualifier (Character 7)
0 Occipital-cervical Joint 1 Cervical Vertebral Joint 3 Cervical Vertebral Disc 4 Cervicothoracic Vertebral Joint 5 Cervicothoracic Vertebral Disc 6 Thoracic Vertebral Joint 9 Thoracic Vertebral Disc A Thoracolumbar Vertebral Joint B Thoracolumbar Vertebral Disc C Temporomandibular Joint, Right D Temporomandibular Joint, Left E Sternoclavicular Joint, Right F Sternoclavicular Joint, Left G Acromioclavicular Joint, Right H Acromioclavicular Joint, Left L Elbow Joint, Right M Elbow Joint, Left N Wrist Joint, Right P Wrist Joint, Left Q Carpal Joint, Right R Carpal Joint, Left S Metacarpocarpal Joint, Right T Metacarpocarpal Joint, Left U Metacarpophalangeal Joint, Right V Metacarpophalangeal Joint, Left W Finger Phalangeal Joint, Right X Finger Phalangeal Joint, Left	0 Open	7 Autologous Tissue Substitute J Synthetic Substitute K Nonautologous Tissue Substitute	Z No Qualifier
J Shoulder Joint, Right K Shoulder Joint, Left	0 Open	0 Synthetic Substitute, Reverse Ball and Socket 7 Autologous Tissue Substitute K Nonautologous Tissue Substitute	Z No Qualifier
J Shoulder Joint, Right K Shoulder Joint, Left	0 Open	J Synthetic Substitute	6 Humeral Surface 7 Glenoid Surface Z No Qualifier

Section	0	Medical and Surgical		
Body System	R	Upper Joints		
Operation	S	Reposition: Moving to its normal location, or other suitable location, all or a portion of a body part		

Body Part (Character 4)	Approach (Character 5)	Device (Character 6)	Qualifier (Character 7)
0 Occipital-cervical Joint **1** Cervical Vertebral Joint **4** Cervicothoracic Vertebral Joint **6** Thoracic Vertebral Joint **A** Thoracolumbar Vertebral Joint **C** Temporomandibular Joint, Right **D** Temporomandibular Joint, Left **E** Sternoclavicular Joint, Right **F** Sternoclavicular Joint, Left **G** Acromioclavicular Joint, Right **H** Acromioclavicular Joint, Left **J** Shoulder Joint, Right **K** Shoulder Joint, Left	**0** Open **3** Percutaneous **4** Percutaneous Endoscopic **X** External	**4** Internal Fixation Device **Z** No Device	**Z** No Qualifier
L Elbow Joint, Right **M** Elbow Joint, Left **N** Wrist Joint, Right **P** Wrist Joint, Left **Q** Carpal Joint, Right **R** Carpal Joint, Left **S** Metacarpocarpal Joint, Right **T** Metacarpocarpal Joint, Left **U** Metacarpophalangeal Joint, Right **V** Metacarpophalangeal Joint, Left **W** Finger Phalangeal Joint, Right **X** Finger Phalangeal Joint, Left	**0** Open **3** Percutaneous **4** Percutaneous Endoscopic **X** External	**4** Internal Fixation Device **5** External Fixation Device **Z** No Device	**Z** No Qualifier

Section	0	Medical and Surgical		
Body System	R	Upper Joints		
Operation	T	Resection: Cutting out or off, without replacement, all of a body part		

Body Part (Character 4)	Approach (Character 5)	Device (Character 6)	Qualifier (Character 7)
3 Cervical Vertebral Disc **4** Cervicothoracic Vertebral Joint **5** Cervicothoracic Vertebral Disc **9** Thoracic Vertebral Disc **B** Thoracolumbar Vertebral Disc **C** Temporomandibular Joint, Right **D** Temporomandibular Joint, Left **E** Sternoclavicular Joint, Right **F** Sternoclavicular Joint, Left **G** Acromioclavicular Joint, Right **H** Acromioclavicular Joint, Left **J** Shoulder Joint, Right **K** Shoulder Joint, Left **L** Elbow Joint, Right **M** Elbow Joint, Left **N** Wrist Joint, Right **P** Wrist Joint, Left **Q** Carpal Joint, Right **R** Carpal Joint, Left **S** Metacarpocarpal Joint, Right **T** Metacarpocarpal Joint, Left **U** Metacarpophalangeal Joint, Right **V** Metacarpophalangeal Joint, Left **W** Finger Phalangeal Joint, Right **X** Finger Phalangeal Joint, Left	**0** Open	**Z** No Device	**Z** No Qualifier

Section	0	Medical and Surgical			
Body System	R	Upper Joints			
Operation	U	Supplement: Putting in or on biological or synthetic material that physically reinforces and/or augments the function of a portion of a body part			

Body Part (Character 4)	Approach (Character 5)	Device (Character 6)	Qualifier (Character 7)
0 Occipital-cervical Joint **1** Cervical Vertebral Joint **3** Cervical Vertebral Disc **4** Cervicothoracic Vertebral Joint **5** Cervicothoracic Vertebral Disc **6** Thoracic Vertebral Joint **9** Thoracic Vertebral Disc **A** Thoracolumbar Vertebral Joint **B** Thoracolumbar Vertebral Disc **C** Temporomandibular Joint, Right **D** Temporomandibular Joint, Left **E** Sternoclavicular Joint, Right **F** Sternoclavicular Joint, Left **G** Acromioclavicular Joint, Right **H** Acromioclavicular Joint, Left **J** Shoulder Joint, Right **K** Shoulder Joint, Left **L** Elbow Joint, Right **M** Elbow Joint, Left **N** Wrist Joint, Right **P** Wrist Joint, Left **Q** Carpal Joint, Right **R** Carpal Joint, Left **S** Metacarpocarpal Joint, Right **T** Metacarpocarpal Joint, Left **U** Metacarpophalangeal Joint, Right **V** Metacarpophalangeal Joint, Left **W** Finger Phalangeal Joint, Right **X** Finger Phalangeal Joint, Left	**0** Open **3** Percutaneous **4** Percutaneous Endoscopic	**7** Autologous Tissue Substitute **J** Synthetic Substitute **K** Nonautologous Tissue Substitute	**Z** No Qualifier

Section	0	Medical and Surgical			
Body System	R	Upper Joints			
Operation	W	Revision: Correcting, to the extent possible, a portion of a malfunctioning device or the position of a displaced device			

Body Part (Character 4)	Approach (Character 5)	Device (Character 6)	Qualifier (Character 7)
0 Occipital-cervical Joint **1** Cervical Vertebral Joint **4** Cervicothoracic Vertebral Joint **6** Thoracic Vertebral Joint **A** Thoracolumbar Vertebral Joint	**0** Open **3** Percutaneous **4** Percutaneous Endoscopic **X** External	**0** Drainage Device **3** Infusion Device **4** Internal Fixation Device **7** Autologous Tissue Substitute **8** Spacer **A** Interbody Fusion Device **J** Synthetic Substitute **K** Nonautologous Tissue Substitute	**Z** No Qualifier
3 Cervical Vertebral Disc **5** Cervicothoracic Vertebral Disc **9** Thoracic Vertebral Disc **B** Thoracolumbar Vertebral Disc	**0** Open **3** Percutaneous **4** Percutaneous Endoscopic **X** External	**0** Drainage Device **3** Infusion Device **7** Autologous Tissue Substitute **J** Synthetic Substitute **K** Nonautologous Tissue Substitute	**Z** No Qualifier
C Temporomandibular Joint, Right **D** Temporomandibular Joint, Left **E** Sternoclavicular Joint, Right **F** Sternoclavicular Joint, Left **G** Acromioclavicular Joint, Right **H** Acromioclavicular Joint, Left **J** Shoulder Joint, Right **K** Shoulder Joint, Left	**0** Open **3** Percutaneous **4** Percutaneous Endoscopic **X** External	**0** Drainage Device **3** Infusion Device **4** Internal Fixation Device **7** Autologous Tissue Substitute **8** Spacer **J** Synthetic Substitute **K** Nonautologous Tissue Substitute	**Z** No Qualifier
L Elbow Joint, Right **M** Elbow Joint, Left **N** Wrist Joint, Right **P** Wrist Joint, Left **Q** Carpal Joint, Right **R** Carpal Joint, Left **S** Metacarpocarpal Joint, Right **T** Metacarpocarpal Joint, Left **U** Metacarpophalangeal Joint, Right **V** Metacarpophalangeal Joint, Left **W** Finger Phalangeal Joint, Right **X** Finger Phalangeal Joint, Left	**0** Open **3** Percutaneous **4** Percutaneous Endoscopic **X** External	**0** Drainage Device **3** Infusion Device **4** Internal Fixation Device **5** External Fixation Device **7** Autologous Tissue Substitute **8** Spacer **J** Synthetic Substitute **K** Nonautologous Tissue Substitute	**Z** No Qualifier

Section	0	Medical and Surgical		
Body System	S	Lower Joints		
Operation	2	Change: Taking out or off a device from a body part and putting back an identical or similar device in or on the same body part without cutting or puncturing the skin or a mucous membrane		
Body Part (Character 4)		**Approach (Character 5)**	**Device (Character 6)**	**Qualifier (Character 7)**
Y Lower Joint		**X** External	**0** Drainage Device **Y** Other Device	**Z** No Qualifier

Section	0	Medical and Surgical		
Body System	S	Lower Joints		
Operation	5	Destruction: Physical eradication of all or a portion of a body part by the direct use of energy, force, or a destructive agent		
Body Part (Character 4)		**Approach (Character 5)**	**Device (Character 6)**	**Qualifier (Character 7)**
0 Lumbar Vertebral Joint **2** Lumbar Vertebral Disc **3** Lumbosacral Joint **4** Lumbosacral Disc **5** Sacrococcygeal Joint **6** Coccygeal Joint **7** Sacroiliac Joint, Right **8** Sacroiliac Joint, Left **9** Hip Joint, Right **B** Hip Joint, Left **C** Knee Joint, Right **D** Knee Joint, Left **F** Ankle Joint, Right **G** Ankle Joint, Left **H** Tarsal Joint, Right **J** Tarsal Joint, Left **K** Metatarsal-Tarsal Joint, Right **L** Metatarsal-Tarsal Joint, Left **M** Metatarsal-Phalangeal Joint, Right **N** Metatarsal-Phalangeal Joint, Left **P** Toe Phalangeal Joint, Right **Q** Toe Phalangeal Joint, Left		**0** Open **3** Percutaneous **4** Percutaneous Endoscopic	**Z** No Device	**Z** No Qualifier

Section	0	Medical and Surgical		
Body System	S	Lower Joints		
Operation	9	Drainage: Taking or letting out fluids and/or gases from a body part		
Body Part (Character 4)		**Approach (Character 5)**	**Device (Character 6)**	**Qualifier (Character 7)**
0 Lumbar Vertebral Joint **2** Lumbar Vertebral Disc **3** Lumbosacral Joint **4** Lumbosacral Disc **5** Sacrococcygeal Joint **6** Coccygeal Joint **7** Sacroiliac Joint, Right **8** Sacroiliac Joint, Left **9** Hip Joint, Right **B** Hip Joint, Left **C** Knee Joint, Right **D** Knee Joint, Left **F** Ankle Joint, Right **G** Ankle Joint, Left **H** Tarsal Joint, Right **J** Tarsal Joint, Left **K** Metatarsal-Tarsal Joint, Right **L** Metatarsal-Tarsal Joint, Left **M** Metatarsal-Phalangeal Joint, Right **N** Metatarsal-Phalangeal Joint, Left **P** Toe Phalangeal Joint, Right **Q** Toe Phalangeal Joint, Left		**0** Open **3** Percutaneous **4** Percutaneous Endoscopic	**0** Drainage Device	**Z** No Qualifier

Section	0	Medical and Surgical			
Body System	S	Lower Joints			
Operation	9	Drainage: Taking or letting out fluids and/or gases from a body part			

Body Part (Character 4)	Approach (Character 5)	Device (Character 6)	Qualifier (Character 7)
0 Lumbar Vertebral Joint	0 Open	Z No Device	X Diagnostic
2 Lumbar Vertebral Disc	3 Percutaneous		Z No Qualifier
3 Lumbosacral Joint	4 Percutaneous Endoscopic		
4 Lumbosacral Disc			
5 Sacrococcygeal Joint			
6 Coccygeal Joint			
7 Sacroiliac Joint, Right			
8 Sacroiliac Joint, Left			
9 Hip Joint, Right			
B Hip Joint, Left			
C Knee Joint, Right			
D Knee Joint, Left			
F Ankle Joint, Right			
G Ankle Joint, Left			
H Tarsal Joint, Right			
J Tarsal Joint, Left			
K Metatarsal-Tarsal Joint, Right			
L Metatarsal-Tarsal Joint, Left			
M Metatarsal-Phalangeal Joint, Right			
N Metatarsal-Phalangeal Joint, Left			
P Toe Phalangeal Joint, Right			
Q Toe Phalangeal Joint, Left			

Section	0	Medical and Surgical			
Body System	S	Lower Joints			
Operation	B	Excision: Cutting out or off, without replacement, a portion of a body part			

Body Part (Character 4)	Approach (Character 5)	Device (Character 6)	Qualifier (Character 7)
0 Lumbar Vertebral Joint	0 Open	Z No Device	X Diagnostic
2 Lumbar Vertebral Disc	3 Percutaneous		Z No Qualifier
3 Lumbosacral Joint	4 Percutaneous Endoscopic		
4 Lumbosacral Disc			
5 Sacrococcygeal Joint			
6 Coccygeal Joint			
7 Sacroiliac Joint, Right			
8 Sacroiliac Joint, Left			
9 Hip Joint, Right			
B Hip Joint, Left			
C Knee Joint, Right			
D Knee Joint, Left			
F Ankle Joint, Right			
G Ankle Joint, Left			
H Tarsal Joint, Right			
J Tarsal Joint, Left			
K Metatarsal-Tarsal Joint, Right			
L Metatarsal-Tarsal Joint, Left			
M Metatarsal-Phalangeal Joint, Right			
N Metatarsal-Phalangeal Joint, Left			
P Toe Phalangeal Joint, Right			
Q Toe Phalangeal Joint, Left			

Section	0	Medical and Surgical		
Body System	S	Lower Joints		
Operation	C	Extirpation: Taking or cutting out solid matter from a body part		

Body Part (Character 4)	Approach (Character 5)	Device (Character 6)	Qualifier (Character 7)
0 Lumbar Vertebral Joint **2** Lumbar Vertebral Disc **3** Lumbosacral Joint **4** Lumbosacral Disc **5** Sacrococcygeal Joint **6** Coccygeal Joint **7** Sacroiliac Joint, Right **8** Sacroiliac Joint, Left **9** Hip Joint, Right **B** Hip Joint, Left **C** Knee Joint, Right **D** Knee Joint, Left **F** Ankle Joint, Right **G** Ankle Joint, Left **H** Tarsal Joint, Right **J** Tarsal Joint, Left **K** Metatarsal-Tarsal Joint, Right **L** Metatarsal-Tarsal Joint, Left **M** Metatarsal-Phalangeal Joint, Right **N** Metatarsal-Phalangeal Joint, Left **P** Toe Phalangeal Joint, Right **Q** Toe Phalangeal Joint, Left	**0** Open **3** Percutaneous **4** Percutaneous Endoscopic	**Z** No Device	**Z** No Qualifier

Section	0	Medical and Surgical		
Body System	S	Lower Joints		
Operation	G	Fusion: Joining together portions of an articular body part rendering the articular body part immobile		

Body Part (Character 4)	Approach (Character 5)	Device (Character 6)	Qualifier (Character 7)
0 Lumbar Vertebral Joint **1** Lumbar Vertebral Joints, **2** or more **3** Lumbosacral Joint	**0** Open **3** Percutaneous **4** Percutaneous Endoscopic	**7** Autologous Tissue Substitute **A** Interbody Fusion Device **J** Synthetic Substitute **K** Nonautologous Tissue Substitute **Z** No Device	**0** Anterior **Approach** **Character 5**, Anterior Column **1** Posterior **Approach** **Character 5**, Posterior Column **J** Posterior **Approach** **Character 5**, Anterior Column
5 Sacrococcygeal Joint **6** Coccygeal Joint **7** Sacroiliac Joint, Right **8** Sacroiliac Joint, Left	**0** Open **3** Percutaneous **4** Percutaneous Endoscopic	**4** Internal Fixation Device **7** Autologous Tissue Substitute **J** Synthetic Substitute **K** Nonautologous Tissue Substitute **Z** No Device	**Z** No Qualifier
9 Hip Joint, Right **B** Hip Joint, Left **C** Knee Joint, Right **D** Knee Joint, Left **F** Ankle Joint, Right **G** Ankle Joint, Left **H** Tarsal Joint, Right **J** Tarsal Joint, Left **K** Metatarsal-Tarsal Joint, Right **L** Metatarsal-Tarsal Joint, Left **M** Metatarsal-Phalangeal Joint, Right **N** Metatarsal-Phalangeal Joint, Left **P** Toe Phalangeal Joint, Right **Q** Toe Phalangeal Joint, Left	**0** Open **3** Percutaneous **4** Percutaneous Endoscopic	**4** Internal Fixation Device **5** External Fixation Device **7** Autologous Tissue Substitute **J** Synthetic Substitute **K** Nonautologous Tissue Substitute **Z** No Device	**Z** No Qualifier

Section	0	Medical and Surgical		
Body System	S	Lower Joints		
Operation	H	Insertion: Putting in a nonbiological appliance that monitors, assists, performs, or prevents a physiological function but does not physically take the place of a body part		

Body Part (Character 4)	Approach (Character 5)	Device (Character 6)	Qualifier (Character 7)
0 Lumbar Vertebral Joint **3** Lumbosacral Joint	**0** Open **3** Percutaneous **4** Percutaneous Endoscopic	**3** Infusion Device **4** Internal Fixation Device **8** Spacer **B** Spinal Stabilization Device, Interspinous Process **C** Spinal Stabilization Device, Pedicle-Based **D** Spinal Stabilization Device, Facet Replacement	**Z** No Qualifier
2 Lumbar Vertebral Disc **4** Lumbosacral Disc	**0** Open **3** Percutaneous **4** Percutaneous Endoscopic	**3** Infusion Device **8** Spacer	**Z** No Qualifier
5 Sacrococcygeal Joint **6** Coccygeal Joint **7** Sacroiliac Joint, Right **8** Sacroiliac Joint, Left	**0** Open **3** Percutaneous **4** Percutaneous Endoscopic	**3** Infusion Device **4** Internal Fixation Device **8** Spacer	**Z** No Qualifier
9 Hip Joint, Right **B** Hip Joint, Left **C** Knee Joint, Right **D** Knee Joint, Left **F** Ankle Joint, Right **G** Ankle Joint, Left **H** Tarsal Joint, Right **J** Tarsal Joint, Left **K** Metatarsal-Tarsal Joint, Right **L** Metatarsal-Tarsal Joint, Left **M** Metatarsal-Phalangeal Joint, Right **N** Metatarsal-Phalangeal Joint, Left **P** Toe Phalangeal Joint, Right **Q** Toe Phalangeal Joint, Left	**0** Open **3** Percutaneous **4** Percutaneous Endoscopic	**3** Infusion Device **4** Internal Fixation Device **5** External Fixation Device **8** Spacer	**Z** No Qualifier

Section	0	Medical and Surgical		
Body System	S	Lower Joints		
Operation	J	Inspection: Visually and/or manually exploring a body part		

Body Part (Character 4)	Approach (Character 5)	Device (Character 6)	Qualifier (Character 7)
0 Lumbar Vertebral Joint **2** Lumbar Vertebral Disc **3** Lumbosacral Joint **4** Lumbosacral Disc **5** Sacrococcygeal Joint **6** Coccygeal Joint **7** Sacroiliac Joint, Right **8** Sacroiliac Joint, Left **9** Hip Joint, Right **B** Hip Joint, Left **C** Knee Joint, Right **D** Knee Joint, Left **F** Ankle Joint, Right **G** Ankle Joint, Left **H** Tarsal Joint, Right **J** Tarsal Joint, Left **K** Metatarsal-Tarsal Joint, Right **L** Metatarsal-Tarsal Joint, Left **M** Metatarsal-Phalangeal Joint, Right **N** Metatarsal-Phalangeal Joint, Left **P** Toe Phalangeal Joint, Right **Q** Toe Phalangeal Joint, Left	**0** Open **3** Percutaneous **4** Percutaneous Endoscopic **X** External	**Z** No Device	**Z** No Qualifier

Section	0	Medical and Surgical		
Body System	S	**Lower Joints**		
Operation	N	Release: Freeing a body part from an abnormal physical constraint by cutting or by the use of force		
Body Part (Character 4)		**Approach (Character 5)**	**Device (Character 6)**	**Qualifier (Character 7)**
0 Lumbar Vertebral Joint		**0** Open	**Z** No Device	**Z** No Qualifier
2 Lumbar Vertebral Disc		**3** Percutaneous		
3 Lumbosacral Joint		**4** Percutaneous Endoscopic		
4 Lumbosacral Disc		**X** External		
5 Sacrococcygeal Joint				
6 Coccygeal Joint				
7 Sacroiliac Joint, Right				
8 Sacroiliac Joint, Left				
9 Hip Joint, Right				
B Hip Joint, Left				
C Knee Joint, Right				
D Knee Joint, Left				
F Ankle Joint, Right				
G Ankle Joint, Left				
H Tarsal Joint, Right				
J Tarsal Joint, Left				
K Metatarsal-Tarsal Joint, Right				
L Metatarsal-Tarsal Joint, Left				
M Metatarsal-Phalangeal Joint, Right				
N Metatarsal-Phalangeal Joint, Left				
P Toe Phalangeal Joint, Right				
Q Toe Phalangeal Joint, Left				

Section	0	**Medical and Surgical**		
Body System	S	**Lower Joints**		
Operation	P	**Removal: Taking out or off a device from a body part**		
Body Part (Character 4)		**Approach (Character 5)**	**Device (Character 6)**	**Qualifier (Character 7)**
0 Lumbar Vertebral Joint **3** Lumbosacral Joint		**0** Open **3** Percutaneous **4** Percutaneous Endoscopic	**0** Drainage Device **3** Infusion Device **4** Internal Fixation Device **7** Autologous Tissue Substitute **8** Spacer **A** Interbody Fusion Device **J** Synthetic Substitute **K** Nonautologous Tissue Substitute	**Z** No Qualifier
0 Lumbar Vertebral Joint **3** Lumbosacral Joint		**X** External	**0** Drainage Device **3** Infusion Device **4** Internal Fixation Device	**Z** No Qualifier
2 Lumbar Vertebral Disc **4** Lumbosacral Disc		**0** Open **3** Percutaneous **4** Percutaneous Endoscopic	**0** Drainage Device **3** Infusion Device **7** Autologous Tissue Substitute **J** Synthetic Substitute **K** Nonautologous Tissue Substitute	**Z** No Qualifier
2 Lumbar Vertebral Disc **4** Lumbosacral Disc		**X** External	**0** Drainage Device **3** Infusion Device	**Z** No Qualifier
5 Sacrococcygeal Joint **6** Coccygeal Joint **7** Sacroiliac Joint, Right **8** Sacroiliac Joint, Left		**0** Open **3** Percutaneous **4** Percutaneous Endoscopic	**0** Drainage Device **3** Infusion Device **4** Internal Fixation Device **7** Autologous Tissue Substitute **8** Spacer **J** Synthetic Substitute **K** Nonautologous Tissue Substitute	**Z** No Qualifier
5 Sacrococcygeal Joint **6** Coccygeal Joint **7** Sacroiliac Joint, Right **8** Sacroiliac Joint, Left		**X** External	**0** Drainage Device **3** Infusion Device **4** Internal Fixation Device	**Z** No Qualifier

Section	0	Medical and Surgical		
Body System	S	Lower Joints		
Operation	P	Removal: Taking out or off a device from a body part		

Body Part (Character 4)	Approach (Character 5)	Device (Character 6)	Qualifier (Character 7)
9 Hip Joint, Right **B** Hip Joint, Left	**0** Open	**0** Drainage Device **3** Infusion Device **4** Internal Fixation Device **5** External Fixation Device **7** Autologous Tissue Substitute **8** Spacer **9** Liner **B** Resurfacing Device **J** Synthetic Substitute **K** Nonautologous Tissue Substitute	**Z** No Qualifier
9 Hip Joint, Right **B** Hip Joint, Left	**3** Percutaneous **4** Percutaneous Endoscopic	**0** Drainage Device **3** Infusion Device **4** Internal Fixation Device **5** External Fixation Device **7** Autologous Tissue Substitute **8** Spacer **J** Synthetic Substitute **K** Nonautologous Tissue Substitute	**Z** No Qualifier
9 Hip Joint, Right **B** Hip Joint, Left	**X** External	**0** Drainage Device **3** Infusion Device **4** Internal Fixation Device **5** External Fixation Device	**Z** No Qualifier
C Knee Joint, Right **D** Knee Joint, Left	**0** Open	**0** Drainage Device **3** Infusion Device **4** Internal Fixation Device **5** External Fixation Device **7** Autologous Tissue Substitute **8** Spacer **9** Liner **J** Synthetic Substitute **K** Nonautologous Tissue Substitute	**Z** No Qualifier

Section	0	Medical and Surgical		
Body System	S	Lower Joints		
Operation	P	Removal: Taking out or off a device from a body part		

Body Part (Character 4)	Approach (Character 5)	Device (Character 6)	Qualifier (Character 7)
C Knee Joint, Right **D** Knee Joint, Left	**3** Percutaneous **4** Percutaneous Endoscopic	**0** Drainage Device **3** Infusion Device **4** Internal Fixation Device **5** External Fixation Device **7** Autologous Tissue Substitute **8** Spacer **J** Synthetic Substitute **K** Nonautologous Tissue Substitute	**Z** No Qualifier
C Knee Joint, Right **D** Knee Joint, Left	**X** External	**0** Drainage Device **3** Infusion Device **4** Internal Fixation Device **5** External Fixation Device	**Z** No Qualifier
F Ankle Joint, Right **G** Ankle Joint, Left **H** Tarsal Joint, Right **J** Tarsal Joint, Left **K** Metatarsal-Tarsal Joint, Right **L** Metatarsal-Tarsal Joint, Left **M** Metatarsal-Phalangeal Joint, Right **N** Metatarsal-Phalangeal Joint, Left **P** Toe Phalangeal Joint, Right **Q** Toe Phalangeal Joint, Left	**0** Open **3** Percutaneous **4** Percutaneous Endoscopic	**0** Drainage Device **3** Infusion Device **4** Internal Fixation Device **5** External Fixation Device **7** Autologous Tissue Substitute **8** Spacer **J** Synthetic Substitute **K** Nonautologous Tissue Substitute	**Z** No Qualifier
F Ankle Joint, Right **G** Ankle Joint, Left **H** Tarsal Joint, Right **J** Tarsal Joint, Left **K** Metatarsal-Tarsal Joint, Right **L** Metatarsal-Tarsal Joint, Left **M** Metatarsal-Phalangeal Joint, Right **N** Metatarsal-Phalangeal Joint, Left **P** Toe Phalangeal Joint, Right **Q** Toe Phalangeal Joint, Left	**X** External	**0** Drainage Device **3** Infusion Device **4** Internal Fixation Device **5** External Fixation Device	**Z** No Qualifier

Section	0	Medical and Surgical		
Body System	S	Lower Joints		
Operation	Q	Repair: Restoring, to the extent possible, a body part to its normal anatomic structure and function		
Body Part (Character 4)		**Approach (Character 5)**	**Device (Character 6)**	**Qualifier (Character 7)**
0 Lumbar Vertebral Joint 2 Lumbar Vertebral Disc 3 Lumbosacral Joint 4 Lumbosacral Disc 5 Sacrococcygeal Joint 6 Coccygeal Joint 7 Sacroiliac Joint, Right 8 Sacroiliac Joint, Left 9 Hip Joint, Right B Hip Joint, Left C Knee Joint, Right D Knee Joint, Left F Ankle Joint, Right G Ankle Joint, Left H Tarsal Joint, Right J Tarsal Joint, Left K Metatarsal-Tarsal Joint, Right L Metatarsal-Tarsal Joint, Left M Metatarsal-Phalangeal Joint, Right N Metatarsal-Phalangeal Joint, Left P Toe Phalangeal Joint, Right Q Toe Phalangeal Joint, Left		0 Open 3 Percutaneous 4 Percutaneous Endoscopic X External	Z No Device	Z No Qualifier

Section	0	Medical and Surgical		
Body System	S	Lower Joints		
Operation	R	Replacement: Putting in or on biological or synthetic material that physically takes the place and/or function of all or a portion of a body part		
Body Part (Character 4)		**Approach (Character 5)**	**Device (Character 6)**	**Qualifier (Character 7)**
0 Lumbar Vertebral Joint 2 Lumbar Vertebral Disc 3 Lumbosacral Joint 4 Lumbosacral Disc 5 Sacrococcygeal Joint 6 Coccygeal Joint 7 Sacroiliac Joint, Right 8 Sacroiliac Joint, Left H Tarsal Joint, Right J Tarsal Joint, Left K Metatarsal-Tarsal Joint, Right L Metatarsal-Tarsal Joint, Left M Metatarsal-Phalangeal Joint, Right N Metatarsal-Phalangeal Joint, Left P Toe Phalangeal Joint, Right Q Toe Phalangeal Joint, Left		0 Open	7 Autologous Tissue Substitute J Synthetic Substitute K Nonautologous Tissue Substitute	Z No Qualifier
9 Hip Joint, Right B Hip Joint, Left		0 Open	1 Synthetic Substitute, Metal 2 Synthetic Substitute, Metal on Polyethylene 3 Synthetic Substitute, Ceramic 4 Synthetic Substitute, Ceramic on Polyethylene J Synthetic Substitute	9 Cemented A Uncemented Z No Qualifier
9 Hip Joint, Right B Hip Joint, Left		0 Open	7 Autologous Tissue Substitute K Nonautologous Tissue Substitute	Z No Qualifier
A Hip Joint, Acetabular Surface, Right E Hip Joint, Acetabular Surface, Left		0 Open	0 Synthetic Substitute, Polyethylene 1 Synthetic Substitute, Metal 3 Synthetic Substitute, Ceramic J Synthetic Substitute	9 Cemented A Uncemented Z No Qualifier
A Hip Joint, Acetabular Surface, Right E Hip Joint, Acetabular Surface, Left		0 Open	7 Autologous Tissue Substitute K Nonautologous Tissue Substitute	Z No Qualifier

Section	0	Medical and Surgical
Body System	S	Lower Joints
Operation	R	Replacement: Putting in or on biological or synthetic material that physically takes the place and/or function of all or a portion of a body part

Body Part (Character 4)	Approach (Character 5)	Device (Character 6)	Qualifier (Character 7)
C Knee Joint, Right D Knee Joint, Left F Ankle Joint, Right G Ankle Joint, Left T Knee Joint, Femoral Surface, Right U Knee Joint, Femoral Surface, Left V Knee Joint, Tibial Surface, Right W Knee Joint, Tibial Surface, Left	0 Open	7 Autologous Tissue Substitute K Nonautologous Tissue Substitute	Z No Qualifier
C Knee Joint, Right D Knee Joint, Left F Ankle Joint, Right G Ankle Joint, Left T Knee Joint, Femoral Surface, Right U Knee Joint, Femoral Surface, Left V Knee Joint, Tibial Surface, Right W Knee Joint, Tibial Surface, Left	0 Open	J Synthetic Substitute	9 Cemented A Uncemented Z No Qualifier
R Hip Joint, Femoral Surface, Right S Hip Joint, Femoral Surface, Left	0 Open	1 Synthetic Substitute, Metal 3 Synthetic Substitute, Ceramic J Synthetic Substitute	9 Cemented A Uncemented Z No Qualifier
R Hip Joint, Femoral Surface, Right S Hip Joint, Femoral Surface, Left	0 Open	7 Autologous Tissue Substitute K Nonautologous Tissue Substitute	Z No Qualifier

Section	0	Medical and Surgical
Body System	S	Lower Joints
Operation	S	Reposition: Moving to its normal location, or other suitable location, all or a portion of a body part

Body Part (Character 4)	Approach (Character 5)	Device (Character 6)	Qualifier (Character 7)
0 Lumbar Vertebral Joint 3 Lumbosacral Joint 5 Sacrococcygeal Joint 6 Coccygeal Joint 7 Sacroiliac Joint, Right 8 Sacroiliac Joint, Left	0 Open 3 Percutaneous 4 Percutaneous Endoscopic X External	4 Internal Fixation Device Z No Device	Z No Qualifier
9 Hip Joint, Right B Hip Joint, Left C Knee Joint, Right D Knee Joint, Left F Ankle Joint, Right G Ankle Joint, Left H Tarsal Joint, Right J Tarsal Joint, Left K Metatarsal-Tarsal Joint, Right L Metatarsal-Tarsal Joint, Left M Metatarsal-Phalangeal Joint, Right N Metatarsal-Phalangeal Joint, Left P Toe Phalangeal Joint, Right Q Toe Phalangeal Joint, Left	0 Open 3 Percutaneous 4 Percutaneous Endoscopic X External	4 Internal Fixation Device 5 External Fixation Device Z No Device	Z No Qualifier

Section	0	Medical and Surgical		
Body System	S	Lower Joints		
Operation	T	Resection: Cutting out or off, without replacement, all of a body part		
Body Part **Character 4**		**Approach** **Character 5**	Device	Qualifier
2 Lumbar Vertebral Disc 4 Lumbosacral Disc 5 Sacrococcygeal Joint 6 Coccygeal Joint 7 Sacroiliac Joint, Right 8 Sacroiliac Joint, Left 9 Hip Joint, Right B Hip Joint, Left C Knee Joint, Right D Knee Joint, Left F Ankle Joint, Right G Ankle Joint, Left H Tarsal Joint, Right J Tarsal Joint, Left K Metatarsal-Tarsal Joint, Right L Metatarsal-Tarsal Joint, Left M Metatarsal-Phalangeal Joint, Right N Metatarsal-Phalangeal Joint, Left P Toe Phalangeal Joint, Right Q Toe Phalangeal Joint, Left		0 Open	Z No Device	Z No Qualifier

Section	0	Medical and Surgical		
Body System	S	Lower Joints		
Operation	U	Supplement: Putting in or on biological or synthetic material that physically reinforces and/or augments the function of a portion of a body part		
Body Part (Character 4)		**Approach (Character 5)**	**Device (Character 6)**	**Qualifier (Character 7)**
0 Lumbar Vertebral Joint 2 Lumbar Vertebral Disc 3 Lumbosacral Joint 4 Lumbosacral Disc 5 Sacrococcygeal Joint 6 Coccygeal Joint 7 Sacroiliac Joint, Right 8 Sacroiliac Joint, Left F Ankle Joint, Right G Ankle Joint, Left H Tarsal Joint, Right J Tarsal Joint, Left K Metatarsal-Tarsal Joint, Right L Metatarsal-Tarsal Joint, Left M Metatarsal-Phalangeal Joint, Right N Metatarsal-Phalangeal Joint, Left P Toe Phalangeal Joint, Right Q Toe Phalangeal Joint, Left		0 Open 3 Percutaneous 4 Percutaneous Endoscopic	7 Autologous Tissue Substitute J Synthetic Substitute K Nonautologous Tissue Substitute	Z No Qualifier
9 Hip Joint, Right B Hip Joint, Left		0 Open	7 Autologous Tissue Substitute 9 Liner B Resurfacing Device J Synthetic Substitute K Nonautologous Tissue Substitute	Z No Qualifier
9 Hip Joint, Right B Hip Joint, Left		3 Percutaneous 4 Percutaneous Endoscopic	7 Autologous Tissue Substitute J Synthetic Substitute K Nonautologous Tissue Substitute	Z No Qualifier
A Hip Joint, Acetabular Surface, Right E Hip Joint, Acetabular Surface, Left R Hip Joint, Femoral Surface, Right S Hip Joint, Femoral Surface, Left		0 Open	9 Liner B Resurfacing Device	Z No Qualifier
C Knee Joint, Right D Knee Joint, Left		0 Open	7 Autologous Tissue Substitute J Synthetic Substitute K Nonautologous Tissue Substitute	Z No Qualifier
C Knee Joint, Right D Knee Joint, Left		0 Open	9 Liner	C Patellar Surface Z No Qualifier

Section	0	Medical and Surgical		
Body System	S	Lower Joints		
Operation	U	Supplement: Putting in or on biological or synthetic material that physically reinforces and/or augments the function of a portion of a body part		

Body Part (Character 4)	Approach (Character 5)	Device (Character 6)	Qualifier (Character 7)
C Knee Joint, Right D Knee Joint, Left	3 Percutaneous 4 Percutaneous Endoscopic	7 Autologous Tissue Substitute J Synthetic Substitute K Nonautologous Tissue Substitute	Z No Qualifier
T Knee Joint, Femoral Surface, Right U Knee Joint, Femoral Surface, Left V Knee Joint, Tibial Surface, Right W Knee Joint, Tibial Surface, Left	0 Open	9 Liner	Z No Qualifier

Section	0	Medical and Surgical		
Body System	S	Lower Joints		
Operation	W	Revision: Correcting, to the extent possible, a portion of a malfunctioning device or the position of a displaced device		

Body Part (Character 4)	Approach (Character 5)	Device (Character 6)	Qualifier (Character 7)
0 Lumbar Vertebral Joint 3 Lumbosacral Joint	0 Open 3 Percutaneous 4 Percutaneous Endoscopic X External	0 Drainage Device 3 Infusion Device 4 Internal Fixation Device 7 Autologous Tissue Substitute 8 Spacer A Interbody Fusion Device J Synthetic Substitute K Nonautologous Tissue Substitute	Z No Qualifier
2 Lumbar Vertebral Disc 4 Lumbosacral Disc	0 Open 3 Percutaneous 4 Percutaneous Endoscopic X External	0 Drainage Device 3 Infusion Device 7 Autologous Tissue Substitute J Synthetic Substitute K Nonautologous Tissue Substitute	Z No Qualifier
5 Sacrococcygeal Joint 6 Coccygeal Joint 7 Sacroiliac Joint, Right 8 Sacroiliac Joint, Left	0 Open 3 Percutaneous 4 Percutaneous Endoscopic X External	0 Drainage Device 3 Infusion Device 4 Internal Fixation Device 7 Autologous Tissue Substitute 8 Spacer J Synthetic Substitute K Nonautologous Tissue Substitute	Z No Qualifier
9 Hip Joint, Right B Hip Joint, Left	0 Open	0 Drainage Device 3 Infusion Device 4 Internal Fixation Device 5 External Fixation Device 7 Autologous Tissue Substitute 8 Spacer 9 Liner B Resurfacing Device J Synthetic Substitute K Nonautologous Tissue Substitute	Z No Qualifier

Section	0	Medical and Surgical		
Body System	S	Lower Joints		
Operation	W	Revision: Correcting, to the extent possible, a portion of a malfunctioning device or the position of a displaced device		

Body Part (Character 4)	Approach (Character 5)	Device (Character 6)	Qualifier (Character 7)
9 Hip Joint, Right B Hip Joint, Left	3 Percutaneous 4 Percutaneous Endoscopic X External	0 Drainage Device 3 Infusion Device 4 Internal Fixation Device 5 External Fixation Device 7 Autologous Tissue Substitute 8 Spacer J Synthetic Substitute K Nonautologous Tissue Substitute	Z No Qualifier
C Knee Joint, Right D Knee Joint, Left	0 Open	0 Drainage Device 3 Infusion Device 4 Internal Fixation Device 5 External Fixation Device 7 Autologous Tissue Substitute 8 Spacer 9 Liner J Synthetic Substitute K Nonautologous Tissue Substitute	Z No Qualifier
C Knee Joint, Right D Knee Joint, Left	3 Percutaneous 4 Percutaneous Endoscopic X External	0 Drainage Device 3 Infusion Device 4 Internal Fixation Device 5 External Fixation Device 7 Autologous Tissue Substitute 8 Spacer J Synthetic Substitute K Nonautologous Tissue Substitute	Z No Qualifier
F Ankle Joint, Right G Ankle Joint, Left H Tarsal Joint, Right J Tarsal Joint, Left K Metatarsal-Tarsal Joint, Right L Metatarsal-Tarsal Joint, Left M Metatarsal-Phalangeal Joint, Right N Metatarsal-Phalangeal Joint, Left P Toe Phalangeal Joint, Right Q Toe Phalangeal Joint, Left	0 Open 3 Percutaneous 4 Percutaneous Endoscopic X External	0 Drainage Device 3 Infusion Device 4 Internal Fixation Device 5 External Fixation Device 7 Autologous Tissue Substitute 8 Spacer J Synthetic Substitute K Nonautologous Tissue Substitute	Z No Qualifier

Section	0	Medical and Surgical	
Body System	T	Urinary System	
Operation	1	Bypass: Altering the route of passage of the contents of a tubular body part	
Body Part (Character 4)	**Approach (Character 5)**	**Device (Character 6)**	**Qualifier (Character 7)**
3 Kidney Pelvis, Right 4 Kidney Pelvis, Left	0 Open 4 Percutaneous Endoscopic	7 Autologous Tissue Substitute J Synthetic Substitute K Nonautologous Tissue Substitute Z No Device	3 Kidney Pelvis, Right 4 Kidney Pelvis, Left 6 Ureter, Right 7 Ureter, Left 8 Colon 9 Colocutaneous A Ileum B Bladder C Ileocutaneous D Cutaneous
3 Kidney Pelvis, Right 4 Kidney Pelvis, Left	3 Percutaneous	J Synthetic Substitute	D Cutaneous
6 Ureter, Right 7 Ureter, Left 8 Ureters, Bilateral	0 Open 4 Percutaneous Endoscopic	7 Autologous Tissue Substitute J Synthetic Substitute K Nonautologous Tissue Substitute Z No Device	6 Ureter, Right 7 Ureter, Left 8 Colon 9 Colocutaneous A Ileum B Bladder C Ileocutaneous D Cutaneous
6 Ureter, Right 7 Ureter, Left 8 Ureters, Bilateral	3 Percutaneous	J Synthetic Substitute	D Cutaneous
B Bladder	0 Open 4 Percutaneous Endoscopic	7 Autologous Tissue Substitute J Synthetic Substitute K Nonautologous Tissue Substitute Z No Device	9 Colocutaneous C Ileocutaneous D Cutaneous
B Bladder	3 Percutaneous	J Synthetic Substitute	D Cutaneous

Section	0	Medical and Surgical	
Body System	T	Urinary System	
Operation	2	Change: Taking out or off a device from a body part and putting back an identical or similar device in or on the same body part without cutting or puncturing the skin or a mucous membrane	
Body Part (Character 4)	**Approach (Character 5)**	**Device (Character 6)**	**Qualifier (Character 7)**
5 Kidney 9 Ureter B Bladder D Urethra	X External	0 Drainage Device Y Other Device	Z No Qualifier

Section	0	Medical and Surgical	
Body System	T	Urinary System	
Operation	5	Destruction: Physical eradication of all or a portion of a body part by the direct use of energy, force, or a destructive agent	
Body Part Character 4	**Approach Character 5**	**Device**	**Qualifier**
0 Kidney, Right 1 Kidney, Left 3 Kidney Pelvis, Right 4 Kidney Pelvis, Left 6 Ureter, Right 7 Ureter, Left B Bladder C Bladder Neck	0 Open 3 Percutaneous 4 Percutaneous Endoscopic 7 Via Natural or Artificial Opening 8 Via Natural or Artificial Opening Endoscopic	Z No Device	Z No Qualifier
D Urethra	0 Open 3 Percutaneous 4 Percutaneous Endoscopic 7 Via Natural or Artificial Opening 8 Via Natural or Artificial Opening Endoscopic X External	Z No Device	Z No Qualifier

Section	0	Medical and Surgical		
Body System	T	Urinary System		
Operation	7	Dilation: Expanding an orifice or the lumen of a tubular body part		

Body Part (Character 4)	Approach (Character 5)	Device (Character 6)	Qualifier (Character 7)
3 Kidney Pelvis, Right 4 Kidney Pelvis, Left 6 Ureter, Right 7 Ureter, Left 8 Ureters, Bilateral B Bladder C Bladder Neck D Urethra	0 Open 3 Percutaneous 4 Percutaneous Endoscopic 7 Via Natural or Artificial Opening 8 Via Natural or Artificial Opening Endoscopic	D Intraluminal Device Z No Device	Z No Qualifier

Section	0	Medical and Surgical		
Body System	T	Urinary System		
Operation	8	Division: Cutting into a body part, without draining fluids and/or gases from the body part, in order to separate or transect a body part		

Body Part (Character 4)	Approach (Character 5)	Device (Character 6)	Qualifier (Character 7)
2 Kidneys, Bilateral C Bladder Neck	0 Open 3 Percutaneous 4 Percutaneous Endoscopic	Z No Device	Z No Qualifier

Section	0	Medical and Surgical		
Body System	T	Urinary System		
Operation	9	Drainage: Taking or letting out fluids and/or gases from a body part		

Body Part (Character 4)	Approach (Character 5)	Device (Character 6)	Qualifier (Character 7)
0 Kidney, Right 1 Kidney, Left 3 Kidney Pelvis, Right 4 Kidney Pelvis, Left 6 Ureter, Right 7 Ureter, Left 8 Ureters, Bilateral B Bladder C Bladder Neck	0 Open 3 Percutaneous 4 Percutaneous Endoscopic 7 Via Natural or Artificial Opening 8 Via Natural or Artificial Opening Endoscopic	0 Drainage Device	Z No Qualifier
0 Kidney, Right 1 Kidney, Left 3 Kidney Pelvis, Right 4 Kidney Pelvis, Left 6 Ureter, Right 7 Ureter, Left 8 Ureters, Bilateral B Bladder C Bladder Neck	0 Open 3 Percutaneous 4 Percutaneous Endoscopic 7 Via Natural or Artificial Opening 8 Via Natural or Artificial Opening Endoscopic	Z No Device	X Diagnostic Z No Qualifier
D Urethra	0 Open 3 Percutaneous 4 Percutaneous Endoscopic 7 Via Natural or Artificial Opening 8 Via Natural or Artificial Opening Endoscopic X External	0 Drainage Device	Z No Qualifier
D Urethra	0 Open 3 Percutaneous 4 Percutaneous Endoscopic 7 Via Natural or Artificial Opening 8 Via Natural or Artificial Opening Endoscopic X External	Z No Device	X Diagnostic Z No Qualifier

Section	0	Medical and Surgical
Body System	T	Urinary System
Operation	B	Excision: Cutting out or off, without replacement, a portion of a body part

Body Part (Character 4)	Approach (Character 5)	Device (Character 6)	Qualifier (Character 7)
0 Kidney, Right 1 Kidney, Left 3 Kidney Pelvis, Right 4 Kidney Pelvis, Left 6 Ureter, Right 7 Ureter, Left B Bladder C Bladder Neck	0 Open 3 Percutaneous 4 Percutaneous Endoscopic 7 Via Natural or Artificial Opening 8 Via Natural or Artificial Opening Endoscopic	Z No Device	X Diagnostic Z No Qualifier
D Urethra	0 Open 3 Percutaneous 4 Percutaneous Endoscopic 7 Via Natural or Artificial Opening 8 Via Natural or Artificial Opening Endoscopic X External	Z No Device	X Diagnostic Z No Qualifier

Section	0	Medical and Surgical
Body System	T	Urinary System
Operation	C	Extirpation: Taking or cutting out solid matter from a body part

Body Part (Character 4)	Approach (Character 5)	Device (Character 6)	Qualifier (Character 7)
0 Kidney, Right 1 Kidney, Left 3 Kidney Pelvis, Right 4 Kidney Pelvis, Left 6 Ureter, Right 7 Ureter, Left B Bladder C Bladder Neck	0 Open 3 Percutaneous 4 Percutaneous Endoscopic 7 Via Natural or Artificial Opening 8 Via Natural or Artificial Opening Endoscopic	Z No Device	Z No Qualifier
D Urethra	0 Open 3 Percutaneous 4 Percutaneous Endoscopic 7 Via Natural or Artificial Opening 8 Via Natural or Artificial Opening Endoscopic X External	Z No Device	Z No Qualifier

Section	0	Medical and Surgical
Body System	T	Urinary System
Operation	D	Extraction: Pulling or stripping out or off all or a portion of a body part by the use of force

Body Part (Character 4)	Approach (Character 5)	Device (Character 6)	Qualifier (Character 7)
0 Kidney, Right 1 Kidney, Left	0 Open 3 Percutaneous 4 Percutaneous Endoscopic	Z No Device	Z No Qualifier

Section	0	Medical and Surgical
Body System	T	Urinary System
Operation	F	Fragmentation: Breaking solid matter in a body part into pieces

Body Part (Character 4)	Approach (Character 5)	Device (Character 6)	Qualifier (Character 7)
3 Kidney Pelvis, Right 4 Kidney Pelvis, Left 6 Ureter, Right 7 Ureter, Left B Bladder C Bladder Neck D Urethra	0 Open 3 Percutaneous 4 Percutaneous Endoscopic 7 Via Natural or Artificial Opening 8 Via Natural or Artificial Opening Endoscopic X External	Z No Device	Z No Qualifier

Section	0	Medical and Surgical		
Body System	T	Urinary System		
Operation	H	Insertion: Putting in a nonbiological appliance that monitors, assists, performs, or prevents a physiological function but does not physically take the place of a body part		

Body Part (Character 4)	Approach (Character 5)	Device (Character 6)	Qualifier (Character 7)
5 Kidney	0 Open 3 Percutaneous 4 Percutaneous Endoscopic 7 Via Natural or Artificial Opening 8 Via Natural or Artificial Opening Endoscopic	2 Monitoring Device 3 Infusion Device	Z No Qualifier
9 Ureter	0 Open 3 Percutaneous 4 Percutaneous Endoscopic 7 Via Natural or Artificial Opening 8 Via Natural or Artificial Opening Endoscopic	2 Monitoring Device 3 Infusion Device M Stimulator Lead	Z No Qualifier
B Bladder	0 Open 3 Percutaneous 4 Percutaneous Endoscopic 7 Via Natural or Artificial Opening 8 Via Natural or Artificial Opening Endoscopic	2 Monitoring Device 3 Infusion Device L Artificial Sphincter M Stimulator Lead	Z No Qualifier
C Bladder Neck	0 Open 3 Percutaneous 4 Percutaneous Endoscopic 7 Via Natural or Artificial Opening 8 Via Natural or Artificial Opening Endoscopic	L Artificial Sphincter	Z No Qualifier
D Urethra	0 Open 3 Percutaneous 4 Percutaneous Endoscopic 7 Via Natural or Artificial Opening 8 Via Natural or Artificial Opening Endoscopic X External	2 Monitoring Device 3 Infusion Device L Artificial Sphincter	Z No Qualifier

Section	0	Medical and Surgical		
Body System	T	Urinary System		
Operation	J	Inspection: Visually and/or manually exploring a body part		

Body Part (Character 4)	Approach (Character 5)	Device (Character 6)	Qualifier (Character 7)
5 Kidney 9 Ureter B Bladder D Urethra	0 Open 3 Percutaneous 4 Percutaneous Endoscopic 7 Via Natural or Artificial Opening 8 Via Natural or Artificial Opening Endoscopic X External	Z No Device	Z No Qualifier

Section	0	Medical and Surgical		
Body System	T	Urinary System		
Operation	L	Occlusion: Completely closing an orifice or the lumen of a tubular body part		
Body Part (Character 4)		**Approach (Character 5)**	**Device (Character 6)**	**Qualifier (Character 7)**
3 Kidney Pelvis, Right 4 Kidney Pelvis, Left 6 Ureter, Right 7 Ureter, Left B Bladder C Bladder Neck		0 Open 3 Percutaneous 4 Percutaneous Endoscopic	C Extraluminal Device D Intraluminal Device Z No Device	Z No Qualifier
3 Kidney Pelvis, Right 4 Kidney Pelvis, Left 6 Ureter, Right 7 Ureter, Left B Bladder C Bladder Neck		7 Via Natural or Artificial Opening 8 Via Natural or Artificial Opening Endoscopic	D Intraluminal Device Z No Device	Z No Qualifier
D Urethra		0 Open 3 Percutaneous 4 Percutaneous Endoscopic X External	C Extraluminal Device D Intraluminal Device Z No Device	Z No Qualifier
D Urethra		7 Via Natural or Artificial Opening 8 Via Natural or Artificial Opening Endoscopic	D Intraluminal Device Z No Device	Z No Qualifier

Section	0	Medical and Surgical		
Body System	T	Urinary System		
Operation	M	Reattachment Putting back in or on all or a portion of a separated body part to its normal location or other suitable location		
Body Part (Character 4)		**Approach (Character 5)**	**Device (Character 6)**	**Qualifier (Character 7)**
0 Kidney, Right 1 Kidney, Left 2 Kidneys, Bilateral 3 Kidney Pelvis, Right 4 Kidney Pelvis, Left 6 Ureter, Right 7 Ureter, Left 8 Ureters, Bilateral B Bladder C Bladder Neck D Urethra		0 Open 4 Percutaneous Endoscopic	Z No Device	Z No Qualifier

Section	0	Medical and Surgical		
Body System	T	Urinary System		
Operation	N	Release: Freeing a body part from an abnormal physical constraint by cutting or by the use of force		
Body Part (Character 4)		**Approach (Character 5)**	**Device (Character 6)**	**Qualifier (Character 7)**
0 Kidney, Right 1 Kidney, Left 3 Kidney Pelvis, Right 4 Kidney Pelvis, Left 6 Ureter, Right 7 Ureter, Left B Bladder C Bladder Neck		0 Open 3 Percutaneous 4 Percutaneous Endoscopic 7 Via Natural or Artificial Opening 8 Via Natural or Artificial Opening Endoscopic	Z No Device	Z No Qualifier
D Urethra		0 Open 3 Percutaneous 4 Percutaneous Endoscopic 7 Via Natural or Artificial Opening 8 Via Natural or Artificial Opening Endoscopic X External	Z No Device	Z No Qualifier

Section	0	Medical and Surgical
Body System	T	Urinary System
Operation	P	Removal: Taking out or off a device from a body part

Body Part (Character 4)	Approach (Character 5)	Device (Character 6)	Qualifier (Character 7)
5 Kidney	**0** Open **3** Percutaneous **4** Percutaneous Endoscopic **7** Via Natural or Artificial Opening **8** Via Natural or Artificial Opening Endoscopic	**0** Drainage Device **2** Monitoring Device **3** Infusion Device **7** Autologous Tissue Substitute **C** Extraluminal Device **D** Intraluminal Device **J** Synthetic Substitute **K** Nonautologous Tissue Substitute	**Z** No Qualifier
5 Kidney	**X** External	**0** Drainage Device **2** Monitoring Device **3** Infusion Device **D** Intraluminal Device	**Z** No Qualifier
9 Ureter	**0** Open **3** Percutaneous **4** Percutaneous Endoscopic **7** Via Natural or Artificial Opening **8** Via Natural or Artificial Opening Endoscopic	**0** Drainage Device **2** Monitoring Device **3** Infusion Device **7** Autologous Tissue Substitute **C** Extraluminal Device **D** Intraluminal Device **J** Synthetic Substitute **K** Nonautologous Tissue Substitute **M** Stimulator Lead	**Z** No Qualifier
9 Ureter	**X** External	**0** Drainage Device **2** Monitoring Device **3** Infusion Device **D** Intraluminal Device **M** Stimulator Lead	**Z** No Qualifier
B Bladder	**0** Open **3** Percutaneous **4** Percutaneous Endoscopic **7** Via Natural or Artificial Opening **8** Via Natural or Artificial Opening Endoscopic	**0** Drainage Device **2** Monitoring Device **3** Infusion Device **7** Autologous Tissue Substitute **C** Extraluminal Device **D** Intraluminal Device **J** Synthetic Substitute **K** Nonautologous Tissue Substitute **L** Artificial Sphincter **M** Stimulator Lead	**Z** No Qualifier

Section	0	Medical and Surgical
Body System	T	Urinary System
Operation	P	Removal: Taking out or off a device from a body part

Body Part (Character 4)	Approach (Character 5)	Device (Character 6)	Qualifier (Character 7)
B Bladder	**X** External	**0** Drainage Device **2** Monitoring Device **3** Infusion Device **D** Intraluminal Device **L** Artificial Sphincter **M** Stimulator Lead	**Z** No Qualifier
D Urethra	**0** Open **3** Percutaneous **4** Percutaneous Endoscopic **7** Via Natural or Artificial Opening **8** Via Natural or Artificial Opening Endoscopic	**0** Drainage Device **2** Monitoring Device **3** Infusion Device **7** Autologous Tissue Substitute **C** Extraluminal Device **D** Intraluminal Device **J** Synthetic Substitute **K** Nonautologous Tissue Substitute **L** Artificial Sphincter	**Z** No Qualifier
D Urethra	**X** External	**0** Drainage Device **2** Monitoring Device **3** Infusion Device **D** Intraluminal Device **L** Artificial Sphincter	**Z** No Qualifier

Section	0	Medical and Surgical		
Body System	T	Urinary System		
Operation	Q	Repair: Restoring, to the extent possible, a body part to its normal anatomic structure and function		

Body Part (Character 4)	Approach (Character 5)	Device (Character 6)	Qualifier (Character 7)
0 Kidney, Right 1 Kidney, Left 3 Kidney Pelvis, Right 4 Kidney Pelvis, Left 6 Ureter, Right 7 Ureter, Left B Bladder C Bladder Neck	0 Open 3 Percutaneous 4 Percutaneous Endoscopic 7 Via Natural or Artificial Opening 8 Via Natural or Artificial Opening Endoscopic	Z No Device	Z No Qualifier
D Urethra	0 Open 3 Percutaneous 4 Percutaneous Endoscopic 7 Via Natural or Artificial Opening 8 Via Natural or Artificial Opening Endoscopic X External	Z No Device	Z No Qualifier

Section	0	Medical and Surgical		
Body System	T	Urinary System		
Operation	R	Replacement: Putting in or on biological or synthetic material that physically takes the place and/or function of all or a portion of a body part		

Body Part (Character 4)	Approach (Character 5)	Device (Character 6)	Qualifier (Character 7)
3 Kidney Pelvis, Right 4 Kidney Pelvis, Left 6 Ureter, Right 7 Ureter, Left B Bladder C Bladder Neck	0 Open 4 Percutaneous Endoscopic 7 Via Natural or Artificial Opening 8 Via Natural or Artificial Opening Endoscopic	7 Autologous Tissue Substitute J Synthetic Substitute K Nonautologous Tissue Substitute	Z No Qualifier
D Urethra	0 Open 4 Percutaneous Endoscopic 7 Via Natural or Artificial Opening 8 Via Natural or Artificial Opening Endoscopic X External	7 Autologous Tissue Substitute J Synthetic Substitute K Nonautologous Tissue Substitute	Z No Qualifier

Section	0	Medical and Surgical		
Body System	T	Urinary System		
Operation	S	Reposition: Moving to its normal location, or other suitable location, all or a portion of a body part		

Body Part (Character 4)	Approach (Character 5)	Device (Character 6)	Qualifier (Character 7)
0 Kidney, Right 1 Kidney, Left 2 Kidneys, Bilateral 3 Kidney Pelvis, Right 4 Kidney Pelvis, Left 6 Ureter, Right 7 Ureter, Left 8 Ureters, Bilateral B Bladder C Bladder Neck D Urethra	0 Open 4 Percutaneous Endoscopic	Z No Device	Z No Qualifier

Section	0	Medical and Surgical		
Body System	T	Urinary System		
Operation	T	Resection: Cutting out or off, without replacement, all of a body part		

Body Part (Character 4)	Approach (Character 5)	Device (Character 6)	Qualifier (Character 7)
0 Kidney, Right 1 Kidney, Left 2 Kidneys, Bilateral	0 Open 4 Percutaneous Endoscopic	Z No Device	Z No Qualifier
3 Kidney Pelvis, Right 4 Kidney Pelvis, Left 6 Ureter, Right 7 Ureter, Left B Bladder C Bladder Neck D Urethra	0 Open 4 Percutaneous Endoscopic 7 Via Natural or Artificial Opening 8 Via Natural or Artificial Opening Endoscopic	Z No Device	Z No Qualifier

Section	0	Medical and Surgical		
Body System	T	Urinary System		
Operation	U	Supplement: Putting in or on biological or synthetic material that physically reinforces and/or augments the function of a portion of a body part		

Body Part (Character 4)	Approach (Character 5)	Device (Character 6)	Qualifier (Character 7)
3 Kidney Pelvis, Right 4 Kidney Pelvis, Left 6 Ureter, Right 7 Ureter, Left B Bladder C Bladder Neck	0 Open 4 Percutaneous Endoscopic 7 Via Natural or Artificial Opening 8 Via Natural or Artificial Opening Endoscopic	7 Autologous Tissue Substitute J Synthetic Substitute K Nonautologous Tissue Substitute	Z No Qualifier
D Urethra	0 Open 4 Percutaneous Endoscopic 7 Via Natural or Artificial Opening 8 Via Natural or Artificial Opening Endoscopic X External	7 Autologous Tissue Substitute J Synthetic Substitute K Nonautologous Tissue Substitute	Z No Qualifier

Section	0	Medical and Surgical		
Body System	T	Urinary System		
Operation	V	Restriction: Partially closing an orifice or the lumen of a tubular body part		

Body Part (Character 4)	Approach (Character 5)	Device (Character 6)	Qualifier (Character 7)
3 Kidney Pelvis, Right 4 Kidney Pelvis, Left 6 Ureter, Right 7 Ureter, Left B Bladder C Bladder Neck	0 Open 3 Percutaneous 4 Percutaneous Endoscopic	C Extraluminal Device D Intraluminal Device Z No Device	Z No Qualifier
3 Kidney Pelvis, Right 4 Kidney Pelvis, Left 6 Ureter, Right 7 Ureter, Left B Bladder C Bladder Neck	7 Via Natural or Artificial Opening 8 Via Natural or Artificial Opening Endoscopic	D Intraluminal Device Z No Device	Z No Qualifier
D Urethra	0 Open 3 Percutaneous 4 Percutaneous Endoscopic	C Extraluminal Device D Intraluminal Device Z No Device	Z No Qualifier
D Urethra	7 Via Natural or Artificial Opening 8 Via Natural or Artificial Opening Endoscopic	D Intraluminal Device Z No Device	Z No Qualifier
D Urethra	X External	Z No Device	Z No Qualifier

Section	0	Medical and Surgical		
Body System	T	Urinary System		
Operation	W	Revision: Correcting, to the extent possible, a portion of a malfunctioning device or the position of a displaced device		

Body Part (Character 4)	Approach (Character 5)	Device (Character 6)	Qualifier (Character 7)
5 Kidney	0 Open 3 Percutaneous 4 Percutaneous Endoscopic 7 Via Natural or Artificial Opening 8 Via Natural or Artificial Opening Endoscopic X External	0 Drainage Device 2 Monitoring Device 3 Infusion Device 7 Autologous Tissue Substitute C Extraluminal Device D Intraluminal Device J Synthetic Substitute K Nonautologous Tissue Substitute	Z No Qualifier
9 Ureter	0 Open 3 Percutaneous 4 Percutaneous Endoscopic 7 Via Natural or Artificial Opening 8 Via Natural or Artificial Opening Endoscopic X External	0 Drainage Device 2 Monitoring Device 3 Infusion Device 7 Autologous Tissue Substitute C Extraluminal Device D Intraluminal Device J Synthetic Substitute K Nonautologous Tissue Substitute M Stimulator Lead	Z No Qualifier
B Bladder	0 Open 3 Percutaneous 4 Percutaneous Endoscopic 7 Via Natural or Artificial Opening 8 Via Natural or Artificial Opening Endoscopic X External	0 Drainage Device 2 Monitoring Device 3 Infusion Device 7 Autologous Tissue Substitute C Extraluminal Device D Intraluminal Device J Synthetic Substitute K Nonautologous Tissue Substitute L Artificial Sphincter M Stimulator Lead	Z No Qualifier
D Urethra	0 Open 3 Percutaneous 4 Percutaneous Endoscopic 7 Via Natural or Artificial Opening 8 Via Natural or Artificial Opening Endoscopic X External	0 Drainage Device 2 Monitoring Device 3 Infusion Device 7 Autologous Tissue Substitute C Extraluminal Device D Intraluminal Device J Synthetic Substitute K Nonautologous Tissue Substitute L Artificial Sphincter	Z No Qualifier

Section	0	Medical and Surgical		
Body System	T	Urinary System		
Operation	Y	Transplantation: Putting in or on all or a portion of a living body part taken from another individual or animal to physically take the place and/or function of all or a portion of a similar body part		

Body Part (Character 4)	Approach (Character 5)	Device (Character 6)	Qualifier (Character 7)
0 Kidney, Right 1 Kidney, Left	0 Open	Z No Device	0 Allogeneic 1 Syngeneic 2 Zooplastic

Section	0	Medical and Surgical		
Body System	U	Female Reproductive System		
Operation	1	Bypass: Altering the route of passage of the contents of a tubular body part		
Body Part (Character 4)		Approach (Character 5)	Device (Character 6)	Qualifier (Character 7)
5 Fallopian Tube, Right 6 Fallopian Tube, Left		0 Open 4 Percutaneous Endoscopic	7 Autologous Tissue Substitute J Synthetic Substitute K Nonautologous Tissue Substitute Z No Device	5 Fallopian Tube, Right 6 Fallopian Tube, Left 9 Uterus

Section	0	Medical and Surgical		
Body System	U	Female Reproductive System		
Operation	2	Change: Taking out or off a device from a body part and putting back an identical or similar device in or on the same body part without cutting or puncturing the skin or a mucous membrane		
Body Part (Character 4)		Approach (Character 5)	Device (Character 6)	Qualifier (Character 7)
3 Ovary 8 Fallopian Tube M Vulva		X External	0 Drainage Device Y Other Device	Z No Qualifier
D Uterus and Cervix		X External	0 Drainage Device H Contraceptive Device Y Other Device	Z No Qualifier
H Vagina and Cul-de-sac		X External	0 Drainage Device G Intraluminal Device, Pessary Y Other Device	Z No Qualifier

Section	0	Medical and Surgical		
Body System	U	Female Reproductive System		
Operation	5	Destruction: Physical eradication of all or a portion of a body part by the direct use of energy, force, or a destructive agent		
Body Part (Character 4)		Approach (Character 5)	Device (Character 6)	Qualifier (Character 7)
0 Ovary, Right 1 Ovary, Left 2 Ovaries, Bilateral 4 Uterine Supporting Structure		0 Open 3 Percutaneous 4 Percutaneous Endoscopic	Z No Device	Z No Qualifier
5 Fallopian Tube, Right 6 Fallopian Tube, Left 7 Fallopian Tubes, Bilateral 9 Uterus B Endometrium C Cervix F Cul-de-sac		0 Open 3 Percutaneous 4 Percutaneous Endoscopic 7 Via Natural or Artificial Opening 8 Via Natural or Artificial Opening Endoscopic	Z No Device	Z No Qualifier
G Vagina K Hymen		0 Open 3 Percutaneous 4 Percutaneous Endoscopic 7 Via Natural or Artificial Opening 8 Via Natural or Artificial Opening Endoscopic X External	Z No Device	Z No Qualifier
J Clitoris L Vestibular Gland M Vulva		0 Open X External	Z No Device	Z No Qualifier

Section	0	Medical and Surgical		
Body System	U	Female Reproductive System		
Operation	7	Dilation: Expanding an orifice or the lumen of a tubular body part		
Body Part (Character 4)		Approach (Character 5)	Device (Character 6)	Qualifier (Character 7)
5 Fallopian Tube, Right 6 Fallopian Tube, Left 7 Fallopian Tubes, Bilateral 9 Uterus C Cervix G Vagina		0 Open 3 Percutaneous 4 Percutaneous Endoscopic 7 Via Natural or Artificial Opening 8 Via Natural or Artificial Opening Endoscopic	D Intraluminal Device Z No Device	Z No Qualifier
K Hymen		0 Open 3 Percutaneous 4 Percutaneous Endoscopic 7 Via Natural or Artificial Opening 8 Via Natural or Artificial Opening Endoscopic X External	D Intraluminal Device Z No Device	Z No Qualifier

Section	0	Medical and Surgical
Body System	U	Female Reproductive System
Operation	8	Division: Cutting into a body part, without draining fluids and/or gases from the body part, in order to separate or transect a body part

Body Part (Character 4)	Approach (Character 5)	Device (Character 6)	Qualifier (Character 7)
0 Ovary, Right **1** Ovary, Left **2** Ovaries, Bilateral **4** Uterine Supporting Structure	**0** Open **3** Percutaneous **4** Percutaneous Endoscopic	**Z** No Device	**Z** No Qualifier
K Hymen	**7** Via Natural or Artificial Opening **8** Via Natural or Artificial Opening Endoscopic **X** External	**Z** No Device	**Z** No Qualifier

Section	0	Medical and Surgical
Body System	U	Female Reproductive System
Operation	9	Drainage: Taking or letting out fluids and/or gases from a body part

Body Part Character 4	Approach Character 5	Device	Qualifier
0 Ovary, Right **1** Ovary, Left **2** Ovaries, Bilateral	**0** Open **3** Percutaneous **4** Percutaneous Endoscopic	**0** Drainage Device	**Z** No Qualifier
0 Ovary, Right **1** Ovary, Left **2** Ovaries, Bilateral	**0** Open **3** Percutaneous **4** Percutaneous Endoscopic	**Z** No Device	**X** Diagnostic **Z** No Qualifier
0 Ovary, Right **1** Ovary, Left **2** Ovaries, Bilateral	**X** External	**Z** No Device	**Z** No Qualifier
4 Uterine Supporting Structure	**0** Open **3** Percutaneous **4** Percutaneous Endoscopic	**0** Drainage Device	**Z** No Qualifier
4 Uterine Supporting Structure	**0** Open **3** Percutaneous **4** Percutaneous Endoscopic	**Z** No Device	**X** Diagnostic **Z** No Qualifier
5 Fallopian Tube, Right **6** Fallopian Tube, Left **7** Fallopian Tubes, Bilateral **9** Uterus **C** Cervix **F** Cul-de-sac	**0** Open **3** Percutaneous **4** Percutaneous Endoscopic **7** Via Natural or Artificial Opening **8** Via Natural or Artificial Opening Endoscopic	**0** Drainage Device	**Z** No Qualifier
5 Fallopian Tube, Right **6** Fallopian Tube, Left **7** Fallopian Tubes, Bilateral **9** Uterus **C** Cervix **F** Cul-de-sac	**0** Open **3** Percutaneous **4** Percutaneous Endoscopic **7** Via Natural or Artificial Opening **8** Via Natural or Artificial Opening Endoscopic	**Z** No Device	**X** Diagnostic **Z** No Qualifier
G Vagina **K** Hymen	**0** Open **3** Percutaneous **4** Percutaneous Endoscopic **7** Via Natural or Artificial Opening **8** Via Natural or Artificial Opening Endoscopic **X** External	**0** Drainage Device	**Z** No Qualifier

Section	0	Medical and Surgical
Body System	U	Female Reproductive System
Operation	9	Drainage: Taking or letting out fluids and/or gases from a body part

Body Part (Character 4)	Approach (Character 5)	Device (Character 6)	Qualifier (Character 7)
G Vagina **K** Hymen	**0** Open **3** Percutaneous **4** Percutaneous Endoscopic **7** Via Natural or Artificial Opening **8** Via Natural or Artificial Opening Endoscopic **X** External	**Z** No Device	**X** Diagnostic **Z** No Qualifier
J Clitoris **L** Vestibular Gland **M** Vulva	**0** Open **X** External	**0** Drainage Device	**Z** No Qualifier
J Clitoris **L** Vestibular Gland **M** Vulva	**0** Open **X** External	**Z** No Device	**X** Diagnostic **Z** No Qualifier

Section	0	Medical and Surgical

Body System	U	Female Reproductive System			
Operation	B	Excision: Cutting out or off, without replacement, a portion of a body part			
Body Part (Character 4)		Approach (Character 5)	Device (Character 6)	Qualifier (Character 7)	
0 Ovary, Right 1 Ovary, Left 2 Ovaries, Bilateral 4 Uterine Supporting Structure 5 Fallopian Tube, Right 6 Fallopian Tube, Left 7 Fallopian Tubes, Bilateral 9 Uterus C Cervix F Cul-de-sac		0 Open 3 Percutaneous 4 Percutaneous Endoscopic 7 Via Natural or Artificial Opening 8 Via Natural or Artificial Opening Endoscopic	Z No Device	X Diagnostic Z No Qualifier	
G Vagina K Hymen		0 Open 3 Percutaneous 4 Percutaneous Endoscopic 7 Via Natural or Artificial Opening 8 Via Natural or Artificial Opening Endoscopic X External	Z No Device	X Diagnostic Z No Qualifier	
J Clitoris L Vestibular Gland M Vulva		0 Open X External	Z No Device	X Diagnostic Z No Qualifier	

Section	0	Medical and Surgical			
Body System	U	Female Reproductive System			
Operation	C	Extirpation: Taking or cutting out solid matter from a body part			
Body Part (Character 4)		Approach (Character 5)	Device (Character 6)	Qualifier (Character 7)	
0 Ovary, Right 1 Ovary, Left 2 Ovaries, Bilateral 4 Uterine Supporting Structure		0 Open 3 Percutaneous 4 Percutaneous Endoscopic	Z No Device	Z No Qualifier	
5 Fallopian Tube, Right 6 Fallopian Tube, Left 7 Fallopian Tubes, Bilateral 9 Uterus B Endometrium C Cervix F Cul-de-sac		0 Open 3 Percutaneous 4 Percutaneous Endoscopic 7 Via Natural or Artificial Opening 8 Via Natural or Artificial Opening Endoscopic	Z No Device	Z No Qualifier	
G Vagina K Hymen		0 Open 3 Percutaneous 4 Percutaneous Endoscopic 7 Via Natural or Artificial Opening 8 Via Natural or Artificial Opening Endoscopic X External	Z No Device	Z No Qualifier	
J Clitoris L Vestibular Gland M Vulva		0 Open X External	Z No Device	Z No Qualifier	

Section	0	Medical and Surgical			
Body System	U	Female Reproductive System			
Operation	D	Extraction: Pulling or stripping out or off all or a portion of a body part by the use of force			
Body Part (Character 4)		Approach (Character 5)	Device (Character 6)	Qualifier (Character 7)	
B Endometrium		7 Via Natural or Artificial Opening 8 Via Natural or Artificial Opening Endoscopic	Z No Device	X Diagnostic Z No Qualifier	
N Ova		0 Open 3 Percutaneous 4 Percutaneous Endoscopic	Z No Device	Z No Qualifier	

Section	0	Medical and Surgical		
Body System	U	Female Reproductive System		
Operation	F	Fragmentation: Breaking solid matter in a body part into pieces		

Body Part (Character 4)	Approach (Character 5)	Device (Character 6)	Qualifier (Character 7)
5 Fallopian Tube, Right 6 Fallopian Tube, Left 7 Fallopian Tubes, Bilateral 9 Uterus	0 Open 3 Percutaneous 4 Percutaneous Endoscopic 7 Via Natural or Artificial Opening 8 Via Natural or Artificial Opening Endoscopic X External	Z No Device	Z No Qualifier

Section	0	Medical and Surgical		
Body System	U	Female Reproductive System		
Operation	H	Insertion: Putting in a nonbiological appliance that monitors, assists, performs, or prevents a physiological function but does not physically take the place of a body part		

Body Part (Character 4)	Approach (Character 5)	Device (Character 6)	Qualifier (Character 7)
3 Ovary	0 Open 3 Percutaneous 4 Percutaneous Endoscopic	3 Infusion Device	Z No Qualifier
8 Fallopian Tube D Uterus and Cervix H Vagina and Cul-de-sac	0 Open 3 Percutaneous 4 Percutaneous Endoscopic 7 Via Natural or Artificial Opening 8 Via Natural or Artificial Opening Endoscopic	3 Infusion Device	Z No Qualifier
9 Uterus	7 Via Natural or Artificial Opening 8 Via Natural or Artificial Opening Endoscopic	H Contraceptive Device	Z No Qualifier
C Cervix	0 Open 3 Percutaneous 4 Percutaneous Endoscopic	1 Radioactive Element	Z No Qualifier
C Cervix	7 Via Natural or Artificial Opening 8 Via Natural or Artificial Opening Endoscopic	1 Radioactive Element H Contraceptive Device	Z No Qualifier
F Cul-de-sac	7 Via Natural or Artificial Opening 8 Via Natural or Artificial Opening Endoscopic	G Intraluminal Device, Pessary	Z No Qualifier
G Vagina	0 Open 3 Percutaneous 4 Percutaneous Endoscopic X External	1 Radioactive Element	Z No Qualifier
G Vagina	7 Via Natural or Artificial Opening 8 Via Natural or Artificial Opening Endoscopic	1 Radioactive Element G Intraluminal Device, Pessary	Z No Qualifier

Section	0	Medical and Surgical		
Body System	U	Female Reproductive System		
Operation	J	Inspection: Visually and/or manually exploring a body part		

Body Part (Character 4)	Approach (Character 5)	Device (Character 6)	Qualifier (Character 7)
3 Ovary	0 Open 3 Percutaneous 4 Percutaneous Endoscopic X External	Z No Device	Z No Qualifier
8 Fallopian Tube D Uterus and Cervix H Vagina and Cul-de-sac	0 Open 3 Percutaneous 4 Percutaneous Endoscopic 7 Via Natural or Artificial Opening 8 Via Natural or Artificial Opening Endoscopic X External	Z No Device	Z No Qualifier
M Vulva	0 Open X External	Z No Device	Z No Qualifier

Section	0	Medical and Surgical		
Body System	U	Female Reproductive System		
Operation	L	Occlusion: Completely closing an orifice or the lumen of a tubular body part		

Body Part (Character 4)	Approach (Character 5)	Device (Character 6)	Qualifier (Character 7)
5 Fallopian Tube, Right 6 Fallopian Tube, Left 7 Fallopian Tubes, Bilateral	0 Open 3 Percutaneous 4 Percutaneous Endoscopic	C Extraluminal Device D Intraluminal Device Z No Device	Z No Qualifier
5 Fallopian Tube, Right 6 Fallopian Tube, Left 7 Fallopian Tubes, Bilateral	7 Via Natural or Artificial Opening 8 Via Natural or Artificial Opening Endoscopic	D Intraluminal Device Z No Device	Z No Qualifier
F Cul-de-sac G Vagina	7 Via Natural or Artificial Opening 8 Via Natural or Artificial Opening Endoscopic	D Intraluminal Device Z No Device	Z No Qualifier

Section	0	Medical and Surgical		
Body System	U	Female Reproductive System		
Operation	M	Reattachment Putting back in or on all or a portion of a separated body part to its normal location or other suitable location		

Body Part (Character 4)	Approach (Character 5)	Device (Character 6)	Qualifier (Character 7)
0 Ovary, Right 1 Ovary, Left 2 Ovaries, Bilateral 4 Uterine Supporting Structure 5 Fallopian Tube, Right 6 Fallopian Tube, Left 7 Fallopian Tubes, Bilateral 9 Uterus C Cervix F Cul-de-sac G Vagina	0 Open 4 Percutaneous Endoscopic	Z No Device	Z No Qualifier
J Clitoris M Vulva	X External	Z No Device	Z No Qualifier
K Hymen	0 Open 4 Percutaneous Endoscopic X External	Z No Device	Z No Qualifier

Section	0	Medical and Surgical		
Body System	U	Female Reproductive System		
Operation	N	Release: Freeing a body part from an abnormal physical constraint by cutting or by the use of force		

Body Part (Character 4)	Approach (Character 5)	Device (Character 6)	Qualifier (Character 7)
0 Ovary, Right 1 Ovary, Left 2 Ovaries, Bilateral 4 Uterine Supporting Structure	0 Open 3 Percutaneous 4 Percutaneous Endoscopic	Z No Device	Z No Qualifier
5 Fallopian Tube, Right 6 Fallopian Tube, Left 7 Fallopian Tubes, Bilateral 9 Uterus C Cervix F Cul-de-sac	0 Open 3 Percutaneous 4 Percutaneous Endoscopic 7 Via Natural or Artificial Opening 8 Via Natural or Artificial Opening Endoscopic	Z No Device	Z No Qualifier
G Vagina K Hymen	0 Open 3 Percutaneous 4 Percutaneous Endoscopic 7 Via Natural or Artificial Opening 8 Via Natural or Artificial Opening Endoscopic X External	Z No Device	Z No Qualifier
J Clitoris L Vestibular Gland M Vulva	0 Open X External	Z No Device	Z No Qualifier

Section	0	Medical and Surgical		
Body System	U	Female Reproductive System		
Operation	P	Removal: Taking out or off a device from a body part		

Body Part (Character 4)	Approach (Character 5)	Device (Character 6)	Qualifier (Character 7)
3 Ovary	0 Open 3 Percutaneous 4 Percutaneous Endoscopic X External	0 Drainage Device 3 Infusion Device	Z No Qualifier
8 Fallopian Tube	0 Open 3 Percutaneous 4 Percutaneous Endoscopic 7 Via Natural or Artificial Opening 8 Via Natural or Artificial Opening Endoscopic	0 Drainage Device 3 Infusion Device 7 Autologous Tissue Substitute C Extraluminal Device D Intraluminal Device J Synthetic Substitute K Nonautologous Tissue Substitute	Z No Qualifier
8 Fallopian Tube	X External	0 Drainage Device 3 Infusion Device D Intraluminal Device	Z No Qualifier
D Uterus and Cervix	0 Open 3 Percutaneous 4 Percutaneous Endoscopic 7 Via Natural or Artificial Opening 8 Via Natural or Artificial Opening Endoscopic	0 Drainage Device 1 Radioactive Element 3 Infusion Device 7 Autologous Tissue Substitute C Extraluminal Device D Intraluminal Device H Contraceptive Device J Synthetic Substitute K Nonautologous Tissue Substitute	Z No Qualifier
D Uterus and Cervix	X External	0 Drainage Device 3 Infusion Device D Intraluminal Device H Contraceptive Device	Z No Qualifier
H Vagina and Cul-de-sac	0 Open 3 Percutaneous 4 Percutaneous Endoscopic 7 Via Natural or Artificial Opening 8 Via Natural or Artificial Opening Endoscopic	0 Drainage Device 1 Radioactive Element 3 Infusion Device 7 Autologous Tissue Substitute D Intraluminal Device J Synthetic Substitute K Nonautologous Tissue Substitute	Z No Qualifier

Section	0	Medical and Surgical		
Body System	U	Female Reproductive System		
Operation	P	Removal: Taking out or off a device from a body part		

Body Part (Character 4)	Approach (Character 5)	Device (Character 6)	Qualifier (Character 7)
H Vagina and Cul-de-sac	X External	0 Drainage Device 1 Radioactive Element 3 Infusion Device D Intraluminal Device	Z No Qualifier
M Vulva	0 Open	0 Drainage Device 7 Autologous Tissue Substitute J Synthetic Substitute K Nonautologous Tissue Substitute	Z No Qualifier
M Vulva	X External	0 Drainage Device	Z No Qualifier

Section	0	Medical and Surgical
Body System	U	Female Reproductive System
Operation	Q	Repair: Restoring, to the extent possible, a body part to its normal anatomic structure and function

Body Part (Character 4)	Approach (Character 5)	Device (Character 6)	Qualifier (Character 7)
0 Ovary, Right 1 Ovary, Left 2 Ovaries, Bilateral 4 Uterine Supporting Structure	0 Open 3 Percutaneous 4 Percutaneous Endoscopic	Z No Device	Z No Qualifier
5 Fallopian Tube, Right 6 Fallopian Tube, Left 7 Fallopian Tubes, Bilateral 9 Uterus C Cervix F Cul-de-sac	0 Open 3 Percutaneous 4 Percutaneous Endoscopic 7 Via Natural or Artificial Opening 8 Via Natural or Artificial Opening Endoscopic	Z No Device	Z No Qualifier
G Vagina K Hymen	0 Open 3 Percutaneous 4 Percutaneous Endoscopic 7 Via Natural or Artificial Opening 8 Via Natural or Artificial Opening Endoscopic X External	Z No Device	Z No Qualifier
J Clitoris L Vestibular Gland M Vulva	0 Open X External	Z No Device	Z No Qualifier

Section	0	Medical and Surgical
Body System	U	Female Reproductive System
Operation	S	Reposition: Moving to its normal location, or other suitable location, all or a portion of a body part

Body Part (Character 4)	Approach (Character 5)	Device (Character 6)	Qualifier (Character 7)
0 Ovary, Right 1 Ovary, Left 2 Ovaries, Bilateral 4 Uterine Supporting Structure 5 Fallopian Tube, Right 6 Fallopian Tube, Left 7 Fallopian Tubes, Bilateral C Cervix F Cul-de-sac	0 Open 4 Percutaneous Endoscopic	Z No Device	Z No Qualifier
9 Uterus G Vagina	0 Open 4 Percutaneous Endoscopic X External	Z No Device	Z No Qualifier

Section	0	Medical and Surgical
Body System	U	Female Reproductive System
Operation	T	Resection: Cutting out or off, without replacement, all of a body part

Body Part (Character 4)	Approach (Character 5)	Device (Character 6)	Qualifier (Character 7)
0 Ovary, Right 1 Ovary, Left 2 Ovaries, Bilateral 5 Fallopian Tube, Right 6 Fallopian Tube, Left 7 Fallopian Tubes, Bilateral 9 Uterus	0 Open 4 Percutaneous Endoscopic 7 Via Natural or Artificial Opening 8 Via Natural or Artificial Opening Endoscopic F Via Natural or Artificial Opening With Percutaneous Endoscopic Assistance	Z No Device	Z No Qualifier
4 Uterine Supporting Structure C Cervix F Cul-de-sac G Vagina	0 Open 4 Percutaneous Endoscopic 7 Via Natural or Artificial Opening 8 Via Natural or Artificial Opening Endoscopic	Z No Device	Z No Qualifier
J Clitoris L Vestibular Gland M Vulva	0 Open X External	Z No Device	Z No Qualifier
K Hymen	0 Open 4 Percutaneous Endoscopic 7 Via Natural or Artificial Opening 8 Via Natural or Artificial Opening Endoscopic X External	Z No Device	Z No Qualifier

Section	0	Medical and Surgical		
Body System	U	Female Reproductive System		
Operation	U	Supplement: Putting in or on biological or synthetic material that physically reinforces and/or augments the function of a portion of a body part		

Body Part (Character 4)	Approach (Character 5)	Device (Character 6)	Qualifier (Character 7)
4 Uterine Supporting Structure	0 Open 4 Percutaneous Endoscopic	7 Autologous Tissue Substitute J Synthetic Substitute K Nonautologous Tissue Substitute	Z No Qualifier
5 Fallopian Tube, Right 6 Fallopian Tube, Left 7 Fallopian Tubes, Bilateral F Cul-de-sac	0 Open 4 Percutaneous Endoscopic 7 Via Natural or Artificial Opening 8 Via Natural or Artificial Opening Endoscopic	7 Autologous Tissue Substitute J Synthetic Substitute K Nonautologous Tissue Substitute	Z No Qualifier
G Vagina K Hymen	0 Open 4 Percutaneous Endoscopic 7 Via Natural or Artificial Opening 8 Via Natural or Artificial Opening Endoscopic X External	7 Autologous Tissue Substitute J Synthetic Substitute K Nonautologous Tissue Substitute	Z No Qualifier
J Clitoris M Vulva	0 Open X External	7 Autologous Tissue Substitute J Synthetic Substitute K Nonautologous Tissue Substitute	Z No Qualifier

Section	0	Medical and Surgical		
Body System	U	Female Reproductive System		
Operation	V	Restriction: Partially closing an orifice or the lumen of a tubular body part		

Body Part (Character 4)	Approach (Character 5)	Device (Character 6)	Qualifier (Character 7)
C Cervix	0 Open 3 Percutaneous 4 Percutaneous Endoscopic	C Extraluminal Device D Intraluminal Device Z No Device	Z No Qualifier
C Cervix	7 Via Natural or Artificial Opening 8 Via Natural or Artificial Opening Endoscopic	D Intraluminal Device Z No Device	Z No Qualifier

Section	0	Medical and Surgical
Body System	U	Female Reproductive System
Operation	W	Revision: Correcting, to the extent possible, a portion of a malfunctioning device or the position of a displaced device

Body Part (Character 4)	Approach (Character 5)	Device (Character 6)	Qualifier (Character 7)
3 Ovary	0 Open 3 Percutaneous 4 Percutaneous Endoscopic X External	0 Drainage Device 3 Infusion Device	Z No Qualifier
8 Fallopian Tube	0 Open 3 Percutaneous 4 Percutaneous Endoscopic 7 Via Natural or Artificial Opening 8 Via Natural or Artificial Opening Endoscopic X External	0 Drainage Device 3 Infusion Device 7 Autologous Tissue Substitute C Extraluminal Device D Intraluminal Device J Synthetic Substitute K Nonautologous Tissue Substitute	Z No Qualifier
D Uterus and Cervix	0 Open 3 Percutaneous 4 Percutaneous Endoscopic 7 Via Natural or Artificial Opening 8 Via Natural or Artificial Opening Endoscopic	0 Drainage Device 1 Radioactive Element 3 Infusion Device 7 Autologous Tissue Substitute C Extraluminal Device D Intraluminal Device H Contraceptive Device J Synthetic Substitute K Nonautologous Tissue Substitute	Z No Qualifier
D Uterus and Cervix	X External	0 Drainage Device 3 Infusion Device 7 Autologous Tissue Substitute C Extraluminal Device D Intraluminal Device H Contraceptive Device J Synthetic Substitute K Nonautologous Tissue Substitute	Z No Qualifier
H Vagina and Cul-de-sac	0 Open 3 Percutaneous 4 Percutaneous Endoscopic 7 Via Natural or Artificial Opening 8 Via Natural or Artificial Opening Endoscopic	0 Drainage Device 1 Radioactive Element 3 Infusion Device 7 Autologous Tissue Substitute D Intraluminal Device J Synthetic Substitute K Nonautologous Tissue Substitute	Z No Qualifier

Section	0	Medical and Surgical
Body System	U	Female Reproductive System
Operation	W	Revision: Correcting, to the extent possible, a portion of a malfunctioning device or the position of a displaced device

Body Part (Character 4)	Approach (Character 5)	Device (Character 6)	Qualifier (Character 7)
H Vagina and Cul-de-sac	X External	0 Drainage Device 3 Infusion Device 7 Autologous Tissue Substitute D Intraluminal Device J Synthetic Substitute K Nonautologous Tissue Substitute	Z No Qualifier
M Vulva	0 Open X External	0 Drainage Device 7 Autologous Tissue Substitute J Synthetic Substitute K Nonautologous Tissue Substitute	Z No Qualifier

Section	0	Medical and Surgical
Body System	U	Female Reproductive System
Operation	Y	Transplantation: Putting in or on all or a portion of a living body part taken from another individual or animal to physically take the place and/or function of all or a portion of a similar body part

Body Part (Character 4)	Approach (Character 5)	Device (Character 6)	Qualifier (Character 7)
0 Ovary, Right 1 Ovary, Left	0 Open	Z No Device	0 Allogeneic 1 Syngeneic 2 Zooplastic

Section	0	Medical and Surgical		
Body System	V	Male Reproductive System		
Operation	1	Bypass: Altering the route of passage of the contents of a tubular body part		
Body Part (Character 4)		**Approach (Character 5)**	**Device (Character 6)**	**Qualifier (Character 7)**
N Vas Deferens, Right P Vas Deferens, Left Q Vas Deferens, Bilateral		0 Open 4 Percutaneous Endoscopic	7 Autologous Tissue Substitute J Synthetic Substitute K Nonautologous Tissue Substitute Z No Device	J Epididymis, Right K Epididymis, Left N Vas Deferens, Right P Vas Deferens, Left

Section	0	Medical and Surgical		
Body System	V	Male Reproductive System		
Operation	2	Change: Taking out or off a device from a body part and putting back an identical or similar device in or on the same body part without cutting or puncturing the skin or a mucous membrane		
Body Part (Character 4)		**Approach (Character 5)**	**Device (Character 6)**	**Qualifier (Character 7)**
4 Prostate and Seminal Vesicles 8 Scrotum and Tunica Vaginalis D Testis M Epididymis and Spermatic Cord R Vas Deferens 5 Penis		X External	0 Drainage Device Y Other Device	Z No Qualifier

Section	0	Medical and Surgical		
Body System	V	Male Reproductive System		
Operation	5	Destruction: Physical eradication of all or a portion of a body part by the direct use of energy, force, or a destructive agent		
Body Part (Character 4)		**Approach (Character 5)**	**Device (Character 6)**	**Qualifier (Character 7)**
0 Prostate		0 Open 3 Percutaneous 4 Percutaneous Endoscopic 7 Via Natural or Artificial Opening 8 Via Natural or Artificial Opening Endoscopic	Z No Device	Z No Qualifier
1 Seminal Vesicle, Right 2 Seminal Vesicle, Left 3 Seminal Vesicles, Bilateral 6 Tunica Vaginalis, Right 7 Tunica Vaginalis, Left 9 Testis, Right B Testis, Left C Testes, Bilateral F Spermatic Cord, Right G Spermatic Cord, Left H Spermatic Cords, Bilateral J Epididymis, Right K Epididymis, Left L Epididymis, Bilateral N Vas Deferens, Right P Vas Deferens, Left Q Vas Deferens, Bilateral		0 Open 3 Percutaneous 4 Percutaneous Endoscopic	Z No Device	Z No Qualifier
5 Scrotum S Penis T Prepuce		0 Open 3 Percutaneous 4 Percutaneous Endoscopic X External	Z No Device	Z No Qualifier

Section	0	Medical and Surgical		
Body System	V	Male Reproductive System		
Operation	7	Dilation: Expanding an orifice or the lumen of a tubular body part		
Body Part (Character 4)		**Approach (Character 5)**	**Device (Character 6)**	**Qualifier (Character 7)**
N Vas Deferens, Right P Vas Deferens, Left Q Vas Deferens, Bilateral		0 Open 3 Percutaneous 4 Percutaneous Endoscopic	D Intraluminal Device Z No Device	Z No Qualifier

Section	0	Medical and Surgical		
Body System	V	Male Reproductive System		
Operation	9	Drainage: Taking or letting out fluids and/or gases from a body part		

Body Part (Character 4)	Approach (Character 5)	Device (Character 6)	Qualifier (Character 7)
0 Prostate	**0** Open **3** Percutaneous **4** Percutaneous Endoscopic **7** Via Natural or Artificial Opening **8** Via Natural or Artificial Opening Endoscopic	**0** Drainage Device	**Z** No Qualifier
0 Prostate	**0** Open **3** Percutaneous **4** Percutaneous Endoscopic **7** Via Natural or Artificial Opening **8** Via Natural or Artificial Opening Endoscopic	**Z** No Device	**X** Diagnostic **Z** No Qualifier
1 Seminal Vesicle, Right **2** Seminal Vesicle, Left **3** Seminal Vesicles, Bilateral **6** Tunica Vaginalis, Right **7** Tunica Vaginalis, Left **9** Testis, Right **B** Testis, Left **C** Testes, Bilateral **F** Spermatic Cord, Right **G** Spermatic Cord, Left **H** Spermatic Cords, Bilateral **J** Epididymis, Right **K** Epididymis, Left **L** Epididymis, Bilateral **N** Vas Deferens, Right **P** Vas Deferens, Left **Q** Vas Deferens, Bilateral	**0** Open **3** Percutaneous **4** Percutaneous Endoscopic	**0** Drainage Device	**Z** No Qualifier

Section	0	Medical and Surgical		
Body System	V	Male Reproductive System		
Operation	9	Drainage: Taking or letting out fluids and/or gases from a body part		

Body Part (Character 4)	Approach (Character 5)	Device (Character 6)	Qualifier (Character 7)
1 Seminal Vesicle, Right **2** Seminal Vesicle, Left **3** Seminal Vesicles, Bilateral **6** Tunica Vaginalis, Right **7** Tunica Vaginalis, Left **9** Testis, Right **B** Testis, Left **C** Testes, Bilateral **F** Spermatic Cord, Right **G** Spermatic Cord, Left **H** Spermatic Cords, Bilateral **J** Epididymis, Right **K** Epididymis, Left **L** Epididymis, Bilateral **N** Vas Deferens, Right **P** Vas Deferens, Left **Q** Vas Deferens, Bilateral	**0** Open **3** Percutaneous **4** Percutaneous Endoscopic	**Z** No Device	**X** Diagnostic **Z** No Qualifier
5 Scrotum **S** Penis **T** Prepuce	**0** Open **3** Percutaneous **4** Percutaneous Endoscopic **X** External	**0** Drainage Device	**Z** No Qualifier
5 Scrotum **S** Penis **T** Prepuce	**0** Open **3** Percutaneous **4** Percutaneous Endoscopic **X** External	**Z** No Device	**X** Diagnostic **Z** No Qualifier

Section	0	Medical and Surgical		
Body System	V	Male Reproductive System		
Operation	B	Excision: Cutting out or off, without replacement, a portion of a body part		

Body Part (Character 4)	Approach (Character 5)	Device (Character 6)	Qualifier (Character 7)
0 Prostate	**0** Open **3** Percutaneous **4** Percutaneous Endoscopic **7** Via Natural or Artificial Opening **8** Via Natural or Artificial Opening Endoscopic	**Z** No Device	**X** Diagnostic **Z** No Qualifier
1 Seminal Vesicle, Right **2** Seminal Vesicle, Left **3** Seminal Vesicles, Bilateral **6** Tunica Vaginalis, Right **7** Tunica Vaginalis, Left **9** Testis, Right **B** Testis, Left **C** Testes, Bilateral **F** Spermatic Cord, Right **G** Spermatic Cord, Left **H** Spermatic Cords, Bilateral **J** Epididymis, Right **K** Epididymis, Left **L** Epididymis, Bilateral **N** Vas Deferens, Right **P** Vas Deferens, Left **Q** Vas Deferens, Bilateral	**0** Open **3** Percutaneous **4** Percutaneous Endoscopic	**Z** No Device	**X** Diagnostic **Z** No Qualifier
5 Scrotum **S** Penis **T** Prepuce	**0** Open **3** Percutaneous **4** Percutaneous Endoscopic **X** External	**Z** No Device	**X** Diagnostic **Z** No Qualifier

Section	0	Medical and Surgical		
Body System	V	Male Reproductive System		
Operation	C	Extirpation: Taking or cutting out solid matter from a body part		

Body Part (Character 4)	Approach (Character 5)	Device (Character 6)	Qualifier (Character 7)
0 Prostate	**0** Open **3** Percutaneous **4** Percutaneous Endoscopic **7** Via Natural or Artificial Opening **8** Via Natural or Artificial Opening Endoscopic	**Z** No Device	**Z** No Qualifier
1 Seminal Vesicle, Right **2** Seminal Vesicle, Left **3** Seminal Vesicles, Bilateral **6** Tunica Vaginalis, Right **7** Tunica Vaginalis, Left **9** Testis, Right **B** Testis, Left **C** Testes, Bilateral **F** Spermatic Cord, Right **G** Spermatic Cord, Left **H** Spermatic Cords, Bilateral **J** Epididymis, Right **K** Epididymis, Left **L** Epididymis, Bilateral **N** Vas Deferens, Right **P** Vas Deferens, Left **Q** Vas Deferens, Bilateral	**0** Open **3** Percutaneous **4** Percutaneous Endoscopic	**Z** No Device	**Z** No Qualifier
5 Scrotum **S** Penis **T** Prepuce	**0** Open **3** Percutaneous **4** Percutaneous Endoscopic **X** External	**Z** No Device	**Z** No Qualifier

Section	0	Medical and Surgical		
Body System	V	Male Reproductive System		
Operation	H	Insertion: Putting in a nonbiological appliance that monitors, assists, performs, or prevents a physiological function but does not physically take the place of a body part		

Body Part (Character 4)	Approach (Character 5)	Device (Character 6)	Qualifier (Character 7)
0 Prostate	**0** Open **3** Percutaneous **4** Percutaneous Endoscopic **7** Via Natural or Artificial Opening **8** Via Natural or Artificial Opening Endoscopic	**1** Radioactive Element	**Z** No Qualifier
4 Prostate and Seminal Vesicles **8** Scrotum and Tunica Vaginalis **D** Testis **M** Epididymis and Spermatic Cord **R** Vas Deferens	**0** Open **3** Percutaneous **4** Percutaneous Endoscopic **7** Via Natural or Artificial Opening **8** Via Natural or Artificial Opening Endoscopic	**3** Infusion Device	**Z** No Qualifier
S Penis	**0** Open **3** Percutaneous **4** Percutaneous Endoscopic **X** External	**3** Infusion Device	**Z** No Qualifier

Section	0	Medical and Surgical		
Body System	V	Male Reproductive System		
Operation	J	Inspection: Visually and/or manually exploring a body part		

Body Part (Character 4)	Approach (Character 5)	Device (Character 6)	Qualifier (Character 7)
4 Prostate and Seminal Vesicles **8** Scrotum and Tunica Vaginalis **D** Testis **M** Epididymis and Spermatic Cord **R** Vas Deferens **5** Penis	**0** Open **3** Percutaneous **4** Percutaneous Endoscopic **X** External	**Z** No Device	**Z** No Qualifier

Section	0	Medical and Surgical		
Body System	V	Male Reproductive System		
Operation	L	Occlusion: Completely closing an orifice or the lumen of a tubular body part		

Body Part (Character 4)	Approach (Character 5)	Device (Character 6)	Qualifier (Character 7)
F Spermatic Cord, Right **G** Spermatic Cord, Left **H** Spermatic Cords, Bilateral **N** Vas Deferens, Right **P** Vas Deferens, Left **Q** Vas Deferens, Bilateral	**0** Open **3** Percutaneous **4** Percutaneous Endoscopic	**C** Extraluminal Device **D** Intraluminal Device **Z** No Device	**Z** No Qualifier

Section	0	Medical and Surgical		
Body System	V	Male Reproductive System		
Operation	M	Reattachment Putting back in or on all or a portion of a separated body part to its normal location or other suitable location		

Body Part (Character 4)	Approach (Character 5)	Device (Character 6)	Qualifier (Character 7)
5 Scrotum **S** Penis	**X** External	**Z** No Device	**Z** No Qualifier
6 Tunica Vaginalis, Right **7** Tunica Vaginalis, Left **9** Testis, Right **B** Testis, Left **C** Testes, Bilateral **F** Spermatic Cord, Right **G** Spermatic Cord, Left **H** Spermatic Cords, Bilateral	**0** Open **4** Percutaneous Endoscopic	**Z** No Device	**Z** No Qualifier

Section	0	Medical and Surgical			
Body System	V	Male Reproductive System			
Operation	N	Release: Freeing a body part from an abnormal physical constraint by cutting or by the use of force			

Body Part (Character 4)	Approach (Character 5)	Device (Character 6)	Qualifier (Character 7)
0 Prostate	**0** Open **3** Percutaneous **4** Percutaneous Endoscopic **7** Via Natural or Artificial Opening **8** Via Natural or Artificial Opening Endoscopic	**Z** No Device	**Z** No Qualifier
1 Seminal Vesicle, Right **2** Seminal Vesicle, Left **3** Seminal Vesicles, Bilateral **6** Tunica Vaginalis, Right **7** Tunica Vaginalis, Left **9** Testis, Right **B** Testis, Left **C** Testes, Bilateral **F** Spermatic Cord, Right **G** Spermatic Cord, Left **H** Spermatic Cords, Bilateral **J** Epididymis, Right **K** Epididymis, Left **L** Epididymis, Bilateral **N** Vas Deferens, Right **P** Vas Deferens, Left **Q** Vas Deferens, Bilateral	**0** Open **3** Percutaneous **4** Percutaneous Endoscopic	**Z** No Device	**Z** No Qualifier
5 Scrotum **S** Penis **T** Prepuce	**0** Open **3** Percutaneous **4** Percutaneous Endoscopic **X** External	**Z** No Device	**Z** No Qualifier

Section	0	Medical and Surgical		
Body System	V	Male Reproductive System		
Operation	P	Removal: Taking out or off a device from a body part		

Body Part (Character 4)	Approach (Character 5)	Device (Character 6)	Qualifier (Character 7)
4 Prostate and Seminal Vesicles	**0** Open **3** Percutaneous **4** Percutaneous Endoscopic **7** Via Natural or Artificial Opening **8** Via Natural or Artificial Opening Endoscopic	**0** Drainage Device **1** Radioactive Element **3** Infusion Device **7** Autologous Tissue Substitute **J** Synthetic Substitute **K** Nonautologous Tissue Substitute	**Z** No Qualifier
4 Prostate and Seminal Vesicles	**X** External	**0** Drainage Device **1** Radioactive Element **3** Infusion Device	**Z** No Qualifier
8 Scrotum and Tunica Vaginalis **D** Testis **S** Penis	**0** Open **3** Percutaneous **4** Percutaneous Endoscopic **7** Via Natural or Artificial Opening **8** Via Natural or Artificial Opening Endoscopic	**0** Drainage Device **3** Infusion Device **7** Autologous Tissue Substitute **J** Synthetic Substitute **K** Nonautologous Tissue Substitute	**Z** No Qualifier
8 Scrotum and Tunica Vaginalis **D** Testis **S** Penis	**X** External	**0** Drainage Device **3** Infusion Device	**Z** No Qualifier
M Epididymis and Spermatic Cord	**0** Open **3** Percutaneous **4** Percutaneous Endoscopic **7** Via Natural or Artificial Opening **8** Via Natural or Artificial Opening Endoscopic	**0** Drainage Device **3** Infusion Device **7** Autologous Tissue Substitute **C** Extraluminal Device **J** Synthetic Substitute **K** Nonautologous Tissue Substitute	**Z** No Qualifier
M Epididymis and Spermatic Cord	**X** External	**0** Drainage Device **3** Infusion Device	**Z** No Qualifier
R Vas Deferens	**0** Open **3** Percutaneous **4** Percutaneous Endoscopic **7** Via Natural or Artificial Opening **8** Via Natural or Artificial Opening Endoscopic	**0** Drainage Device **3** Infusion Device **7** Autologous Tissue Substitute **C** Extraluminal Device **D** Intraluminal Device **J** Synthetic Substitute **K** Nonautologous Tissue Substitute	**Z** No Qualifier
R Vas Deferens	**X** External	**0** Drainage Device **3** Infusion Device **D** Intraluminal Device	**Z** No Qualifier

Section	0	Medical and Surgical		
Body System	V	Male Reproductive System		
Operation	Q	Repair: Restoring, to the extent possible, a body part to its normal anatomic structure and function		

Body Part (Character 4)	Approach (Character 5)	Device (Character 6)	Qualifier (Character 7)
0 Prostate	0 Open 3 Percutaneous 4 Percutaneous Endoscopic 7 Via Natural or Artificial Opening 8 Via Natural or Artificial Opening Endoscopic	Z No Device	Z No Qualifier
1 Seminal Vesicle, Right 2 Seminal Vesicle, Left 3 Seminal Vesicles, Bilateral 6 Tunica Vaginalis, Right 7 Tunica Vaginalis, Left 9 Testis, Right B Testis, Left C Testes, Bilateral F Spermatic Cord, Right G Spermatic Cord, Left H Spermatic Cords, Bilateral J Epididymis, Right K Epididymis, Left L Epididymis, Bilateral N Vas Deferens, Right P Vas Deferens, Left Q Vas Deferens, Bilateral	0 Open 3 Percutaneous 4 Percutaneous Endoscopic	Z No Device	Z No Qualifier
5 Scrotum S Penis T Prepuce	0 Open 3 Percutaneous 4 Percutaneous Endoscopic X External	Z No Device	Z No Qualifier

Section	0	Medical and Surgical		
Body System	V	Male Reproductive System		
Operation	R	Replacement: Putting in or on biological or synthetic material that physically takes the place and/or function of all or a portion of a body part		

Body Part (Character 4)	Approach (Character 5)	Device (Character 6)	Qualifier (Character 7)
9 Testis, Right B Testis, Left C Testes, Bilateral	0 Open	J Synthetic Substitute	Z No Qualifier

Section	0	Medical and Surgical		
Body System	V	Male Reproductive System		
Operation	S	Reposition: Moving to its normal location, or other suitable location, all or a portion of a body part		

Body Part (Character 4)	Approach (Character 5)	Device (Character 6)	Qualifier (Character 7)
9 Testis, Right B Testis, Left C Testes, Bilateral F Spermatic Cord, Right G Spermatic Cord, Left H Spermatic Cords, Bilateral	0 Open 3 Percutaneous 4 Percutaneous Endoscopic	Z No Device	Z No Qualifier

Section	0	Medical and Surgical
Body System	V	Male Reproductive System
Operation	T	Resection: Cutting out or off, without replacement, all of a body part

Body Part (Character 4)	Approach (Character 5)	Device (Character 6)	Qualifier (Character 7)
0 Prostate	**0** Open **4** Percutaneous Endoscopic **7** Via Natural or Artificial Opening **8** Via Natural or Artificial Opening Endoscopic	**Z** No Device	**Z** No Qualifier
1 Seminal Vesicle, Right **2** Seminal Vesicle, Left **3** Seminal Vesicles, Bilateral **6** Tunica Vaginalis, Right **7** Tunica Vaginalis, Left **9** Testis, Right **B** Testis, Left **C** Testes, Bilateral **F** Spermatic Cord, Right **G** Spermatic Cord, Left **H** Spermatic Cords, Bilateral **J** Epididymis, Right **K** Epididymis, Left **L** Epididymis, Bilateral **N** Vas Deferens, Right **P** Vas Deferens, Left **Q** Vas Deferens, Bilateral	**0** Open **4** Percutaneous Endoscopic	**Z** No Device	**Z** No Qualifier
5 Scrotum **S** Penis **T** Prepuce	**0** Open **4** Percutaneous Endoscopic **X** External	**Z** No Device	**Z** No Qualifier

Section	0	Medical and Surgical
Body System	V	Male Reproductive System
Operation	U	Supplement: Putting in or on biological or synthetic material that physically reinforces and/or augments the function of a portion of a body part

Body Part (Character 4)	Approach (Character 5)	Device (Character 6)	Qualifier (Character 7)
1 Seminal Vesicle, Right **2** Seminal Vesicle, Left **3** Seminal Vesicles, Bilateral **6** Tunica Vaginalis, Right **7** Tunica Vaginalis, Left **F** Spermatic Cord, Right **G** Spermatic Cord, Left **H** Spermatic Cords, Bilateral **J** Epididymis, Right **K** Epididymis, Left **L** Epididymis, Bilateral **N** Vas Deferens, Right **P** Vas Deferens, Left **Q** Vas Deferens, Bilateral	**0** Open **4** Percutaneous Endoscopic	**7** Autologous Tissue Substitute **J** Synthetic Substitute **K** Nonautologous Tissue Substitute	**Z** No Qualifier
5 Scrotum **S** Penis **T** Prepuce	**0** Open **4** Percutaneous Endoscopic **X** External	**7** Autologous Tissue Substitute **J** Synthetic Substitute **K** Nonautologous Tissue Substitute	**Z** No Qualifier
9 Testis, Right **B** Testis, Left **C** Testes, Bilateral	**0** Open	**7** Autologous Tissue Substitute **J** Synthetic Substitute **K** Nonautologous Tissue Substitute	**Z** No Qualifier

Section	0	Medical and Surgical		
Body System	V	Male Reproductive System		
Operation	W	Revision: Correcting, to the extent possible, a portion of a malfunctioning device or the position of a displaced device		

Body Part (Character 4)	Approach (Character 5)	Device (Character 6)	Qualifier (Character 7)
4 Prostate and Seminal Vesicles **8** Scrotum and Tunica Vaginalis **D** Testis **5** Penis	**0** Open **3** Percutaneous **4** Percutaneous Endoscopic **7** Via Natural or Artificial Opening **8** Via Natural or Artificial Opening Endoscopic **X** External	**0** Drainage Device **3** Infusion Device **7** Autologous Tissue Substitute **J** Synthetic Substitute **K** Nonautologous Tissue Substitute	**Z** No Qualifier
M Epididymis and Spermatic Cord	**0** Open **3** Percutaneous **4** Percutaneous Endoscopic **7** Via Natural or Artificial Opening **8** Via Natural or Artificial Opening Endoscopic **X** External	**0** Drainage Device **3** Infusion Device **7** Autologous Tissue Substitute **C** Extraluminal Device **J** Synthetic Substitute **K** Nonautologous Tissue Substitute	**Z** No Qualifier
R Vas Deferens	**0** Open **3** Percutaneous **4** Percutaneous Endoscopic **7** Via Natural or Artificial Opening **8** Via Natural or Artificial Opening Endoscopic **X** External	**0** Drainage Device **3** Infusion Device **7** Autologous Tissue Substitute **C** Extraluminal Device **D** Intraluminal Device **J** Synthetic Substitute **K** Nonautologous Tissue Substitute	**Z** No Qualifier

Section	0	Medical and Surgical		
Body System	W	Anatomical Regions, General		
Operation	0	Alteration: Modifying the anatomic structure of a body part without affecting the function of the body part		

Body Part (Character 4)	Approach (Character 5)	Device (Character 6)	Qualifier (Character 7)
0 Head 2 Face 4 Upper Jaw 5 Lower Jaw 6 Neck 8 Chest Wall F Abdominal Wall K Upper Back L Lower Back M Perineum, Male N Perineum, Female	0 Open 3 Percutaneous 4 Percutaneous Endoscopic	7 Autologous Tissue Substitute J Synthetic Substitute K Nonautologous Tissue Substitute Z No Device	Z No Qualifier

Section	0	Medical and Surgical		
Body System	W	Anatomical Regions, General		
Operation	1	Bypass: Altering the route of passage of the contents of a tubular body part		

Body Part (Character 4)	Approach (Character 5)	Device (Character 6)	Qualifier (Character 7)
1 Cranial Cavity	0 Open	J Synthetic Substitute	9 Pleural Cavity, Right B Pleural Cavity, Left G Peritoneal Cavity J Pelvic Cavity
9 Pleural Cavity, Right B Pleural Cavity, Left G Peritoneal Cavity J Pelvic Cavity	0 Open 4 Percutaneous Endoscopic	J Synthetic Substitute	4 Cutaneous 9 Pleural Cavity, Right B Pleural Cavity, Left G Peritoneal Cavity J Pelvic Cavity Y Lower Vein
9 Pleural Cavity, Right B Pleural Cavity, Left G Peritoneal Cavity J Pelvic Cavity	3 Percutaneous	J Synthetic Substitute	4 Cutaneous

Section	0	Medical and Surgical		
Body System	W	Anatomical Regions, General		
Operation	2	Change: Taking out or off a device from a body part and putting back an identical or similar device in or on the same body part without cutting or puncturing the skin or a mucous membrane		

Body Part (Character 4)	Approach (Character 5)	Device (Character 6)	Qualifier (Character 7)
0 Head 1 Cranial Cavity 2 Face 4 Upper Jaw 5 Lower Jaw 6 Neck 8 Chest Wall 9 Pleural Cavity, Right B Pleural Cavity, Left C Mediastinum D Pericardial Cavity F Abdominal Wall G Peritoneal Cavity H Retroperitoneum J Pelvic Cavity K Upper Back L Lower Back M Perineum, Male N Perineum, Female	X External	0 Drainage Device Y Other Device	Z No Qualifier

Section	0	Medical and Surgical		
Body System	W	Anatomical Regions, General		
Operation	3	Control: Stopping, or attempting to stop, postprocedural bleeding		
Body Part (Character 4)		Approach (Character 5)	Device (Character 6)	Qualifier (Character 7)
0 Head 1 Cranial Cavity 2 Face 4 Upper Jaw 5 Lower Jaw 6 Neck 8 Chest Wall 9 Pleural Cavity, Right B Pleural Cavity, Left C Mediastinum D Pericardial Cavity F Abdominal Wall G Peritoneal Cavity H Retroperitoneum J Pelvic Cavity K Upper Back L Lower Back M Perineum, Male N Perineum, Female		0 Open 3 Percutaneous 4 Percutaneous Endoscopic	Z No Device	Z No Qualifier
3 Oral Cavity and Throat		0 Open 3 Percutaneous 4 Percutaneous Endoscopic 7 Via Natural or Artificial Opening 8 Via Natural or Artificial Opening Endoscopic X External	Z No Device	Z No Qualifier
P Gastrointestinal Tract Q Respiratory Tract R Genitourinary Tract		0 Open 3 Percutaneous 4 Percutaneous Endoscopic 7 Via Natural or Artificial Opening 8 Via Natural or Artificial Opening Endoscopic	Z No Device	Z No Qualifier

Section	0	Medical and Surgical		
Body System	W	Anatomical Regions, General		
Operation	4	Creation: Making a new genital structure that does not take over the function of a body part		
Body Part (Character 4)		Approach (Character 5)	Device (Character 6)	Qualifier (Character 7)
M Perineum, Male		0 Open	7 Autologous Tissue Substitute J Synthetic Substitute K Nonautologous Tissue Substitute Z No Device	0 Vagina
N Perineum, Female		0 Open	7 Autologous Tissue Substitute J Synthetic Substitute K Nonautologous Tissue Substitute Z No Device	1 Penis

Section	0	Medical and Surgical		
Body System	W	Anatomical Regions, General		
Operation	8	Division: Cutting into a body part, without draining fluids and/or gases from the body part, in order to separate or transect a body part		
Body Part (Character 4)		Approach (Character 5)	Device (Character 6)	Qualifier (Character 7)
N Perineum, Female		X External	Z No Device	Z No Qualifier

Section	0	Medical and Surgical		
Body System	W	Anatomical Regions, General		
Operation	9	Drainage: Taking or letting out fluids and/or gases from a body part		
Body Part (Character 4)		Approach (Character 5)	Device (Character 6)	Qualifier (Character 7)
0 Head 1 Cranial Cavity 2 Face 3 Oral Cavity and Throat 4 Upper Jaw 5 Lower Jaw 6 Neck 8 Chest Wall 9 Pleural Cavity, Right B Pleural Cavity, Left C Mediastinum D Pericardial Cavity F Abdominal Wall G Peritoneal Cavity H Retroperitoneum J Pelvic Cavity K Upper Back L Lower Back M Perineum, Male N Perineum, Female		0 Open 3 Percutaneous 4 Percutaneous Endoscopic	0 Drainage Device	Z No Qualifier

Section	0	Medical and Surgical		
Body System	W	Anatomical Regions, General		
Operation	9	Drainage: Taking or letting out fluids and/or gases from a body part		
Body Part (Character 4)		Approach (Character 5)	Device (Character 6)	Qualifier (Character 7)
0 Head 1 Cranial Cavity 2 Face 3 Oral Cavity and Throat 4 Upper Jaw 5 Lower Jaw 6 Neck 8 Chest Wall 9 Pleural Cavity, Right B Pleural Cavity, Left C Mediastinum D Pericardial Cavity F Abdominal Wall G Peritoneal Cavity H Retroperitoneum J Pelvic Cavity K Upper Back L Lower Back M Perineum, Male N Perineum, Female		0 Open 3 Percutaneous 4 Percutaneous Endoscopic	Z No Device	X Diagnostic Z No Qualifier

Section	0	Medical and Surgical		
Body System	W	Anatomical Regions, General		
Operation	B	Excision: Cutting out or off, without replacement, a portion of a body part		
Body Part (Character 4)		Approach (Character 5)	Device (Character 6)	Qualifier (Character 7)
0 Head 2 Face 4 Upper Jaw 5 Lower Jaw 8 Chest Wall K Upper Back L Lower Back M Perineum, Male N Perineum, Female		0 Open 3 Percutaneous 4 Percutaneous Endoscopic X External	Z No Device	X Diagnostic Z No Qualifier
6 Neck F Abdominal Wall		0 Open 3 Percutaneous 4 Percutaneous Endoscopic	Z No Device	X Diagnostic Z No Qualifier
6 Neck F Abdominal Wall		X External	Z No Device	2 Stoma X Diagnostic Z No Qualifier
C Mediastinum H Retroperitoneum		0 Open 3 Percutaneous 4 Percutaneous Endoscopic	Z No Device	X Diagnostic Z No Qualifier

Section	0	Medical and Surgical		
Body System	W	Anatomical Regions, General		
Operation	C	Extirpation: Taking or cutting out solid matter from a body part		

Body Part (Character 4)	Approach (Character 5)	Device (Character 6)	Qualifier (Character 7)
1 Cranial Cavity **3** Oral Cavity and Throat **9** Pleural Cavity, Right **B** Pleural Cavity, Left **C** Mediastinum **D** Pericardial Cavity **G** Peritoneal Cavity **J** Pelvic Cavity	**0** Open **3** Percutaneous **4** Percutaneous Endoscopic **X** External	**Z** No Device	**Z** No Qualifier
P Gastrointestinal Tract **Q** Respiratory Tract **R** Genitourinary Tract	**0** Open **3** Percutaneous **4** Percutaneous Endoscopic **7** Via Natural or Artificial Opening **8** Via Natural or Artificial Opening Endoscopic **X** External	**Z** No Device	**Z** No Qualifier

Section	0	Medical and Surgical		
Body System	W	Anatomical Regions, General		
Operation	F	Fragmentation: Breaking solid matter in a body part into pieces		

Body Part (Character 4)	Approach (Character 5)	Device (Character 6)	Qualifier (Character 7)
1 Cranial Cavity **3** Oral Cavity and Throat **9** Pleural Cavity, Right **B** Pleural Cavity, Left **C** Mediastinum **D** Pericardial Cavity **G** Peritoneal Cavity **J** Pelvic Cavity	**0** Open **3** Percutaneous **4** Percutaneous Endoscopic **X** External	**Z** No Device	**Z** No Qualifier
P Gastrointestinal Tract **Q** Respiratory Tract **R** Genitourinary Tract	**0** Open **3** Percutaneous **4** Percutaneous Endoscopic **7** Via Natural or Artificial Opening **8** Via Natural or Artificial Opening Endoscopic **X** External	**Z** No Device	**Z** No Qualifier

Section	0	Medical and Surgical		
Body System	W	Anatomical Regions, General		
Operation	H	Insertion: Putting in a nonbiological appliance that monitors, assists, performs, or prevents a physiological function but does not physically take the place of a body part		

Body Part (Character 4)	Approach (Character 5)	Device (Character 6)	Qualifier (Character 7)
0 Head **1** Cranial Cavity **2** Face **3** Oral Cavity and Throat **4** Upper Jaw **5** Lower Jaw **6** Neck **8** Chest Wall **9** Pleural Cavity, Right **B** Pleural Cavity, Left **C** Mediastinum **D** Pericardial Cavity **F** Abdominal Wall **G** Peritoneal Cavity **H** Retroperitoneum **J** Pelvic Cavity **K** Upper Back **L** Lower Back **M** Perineum, Male **N** Perineum, Female	**0** Open **3** Percutaneous **4** Percutaneous Endoscopic	**1** Radioactive Element **3** Infusion Device **Y** Other Device	**Z** No Qualifier
P Gastrointestinal Tract **Q** Respiratory Tract **R** Genitourinary Tract	**0** Open **3** Percutaneous **4** Percutaneous Endoscopic **7** Via Natural or Artificial Opening **8** Via Natural or Artificial Opening Endoscopic	**1** Radioactive Element **3** Infusion Device **Y** Other Device	**Z** No Qualifier

Section	0	Medical and Surgical		
Body System	W	Anatomical Regions, General		
Operation	J	Inspection: Visually and/or manually exploring a body part		
Body Part (Character 4)		Approach (Character 5)	Device (Character 6)	Qualifier (Character 7)
0 Head 2 Face 3 Oral Cavity and Throat 4 Upper Jaw 5 Lower Jaw 6 Neck 8 Chest Wall F Abdominal Wall K Upper Back L Lower Back M Perineum, Male N Perineum, Female		0 Open 3 Percutaneous 4 Percutaneous Endoscopic X External	Z No Device	Z No Qualifier
1 Cranial Cavity 9 Pleural Cavity, Right B Pleural Cavity, Left C Mediastinum D Pericardial Cavity G Peritoneal Cavity H Retroperitoneum J Pelvic Cavity		0 Open 3 Percutaneous 4 Percutaneous Endoscopic	Z No Device	Z No Qualifier
P Gastrointestinal Tract Q Respiratory Tract R Genitourinary Tract		0 Open 3 Percutaneous 4 Percutaneous Endoscopic 7 Via Natural or Artificial Opening 8 Via Natural or Artificial Opening Endoscopic	Z No Device	Z No Qualifier

Section	0	Medical and Surgical		
Body System	W	Anatomical Regions, General		
Operation	M	Reattachment Putting back in or on all or a portion of a separated body part to its normal location or other suitable location		
Body Part (Character 4)		Approach (Character 5)	Device (Character 6)	Qualifier (Character 7)
2 Face 4 Upper Jaw 5 Lower Jaw 6 Neck 8 Chest Wall F Abdominal Wall K Upper Back L Lower Back M Perineum, Male N Perineum, Female		0 Open	Z No Device	Z No Qualifier

Section	0	Medical and Surgical		
Body System	W	Anatomical Regions, General		
Operation	P	Removal: Taking out or off a device from a body part		

Body Part (Character 4)	Approach (Character 5)	Device (Character 6)	Qualifier (Character 7)
0 Head 2 Face 4 Upper Jaw 5 Lower Jaw 6 Neck 8 Chest Wall C Mediastinum F Abdominal Wall K Upper Back L Lower Back M Perineum, Male N Perineum, Female	0 Open 3 Percutaneous 4 Percutaneous Endoscopic X External	0 Drainage Device 1 Radioactive Element 3 Infusion Device 7 Autologous Tissue Substitute J Synthetic Substitute K Nonautologous Tissue Substitute Y Other Device	Z No Qualifier
1 Cranial Cavity 9 Pleural Cavity, Right B Pleural Cavity, Left G Peritoneal Cavity J Pelvic Cavity	0 Open 3 Percutaneous 4 Percutaneous Endoscopic	0 Drainage Device 1 Radioactive Element 3 Infusion Device J Synthetic Substitute Y Other Device	Z No Qualifier
1 Cranial Cavity 9 Pleural Cavity, Right B Pleural Cavity, Left G Peritoneal Cavity J Pelvic Cavity	X External	0 Drainage Device 1 Radioactive Element 3 Infusion Device	Z No Qualifier
D Pericardial Cavity H Retroperitoneum	0 Open 3 Percutaneous 4 Percutaneous Endoscopic	0 Drainage Device 1 Radioactive Element 3 Infusion Device Y Other Device	Z No Qualifier
D Pericardial Cavity H Retroperitoneum	X External	0 Drainage Device 1 Radioactive Element 3 Infusion Device	Z No Qualifier

P Gastrointestinal Tract
Q Respiratory Tract
R Genitourinary Tract
	0 Open
	3 Percutaneous
	4 Percutaneous Endoscopic
	7 Via Natural or Artificial
	  Opening
	8 Via Natural or Artificial
	  Opening Endoscopic
	X External
		1 Radioactive Element
		3 Infusion Device
		Y Other Device
			Z No Qualifier

Section	0	Medical and Surgical		
Body System	W	Anatomical Regions, General		
Operation	Q	Repair: Restoring, to the extent possible, a body part to its normal anatomic structure and function		

Body Part (Character 4)	Approach (Character 5)	Device (Character 6)	Qualifier (Character 7)
0 Head 2 Face 4 Upper Jaw 5 Lower Jaw 8 Chest Wall K Upper Back L Lower Back M Perineum, Male N Perineum, Female	0 Open 3 Percutaneous 4 Percutaneous Endoscopic X External	Z No Device	Z No Qualifier
6 Neck F Abdominal Wall	0 Open 3 Percutaneous 4 Percutaneous Endoscopic	Z No Device	Z No Qualifier
6 Neck F Abdominal Wall	X External	Z No Device	2 Stoma Z No Qualifier
C Mediastinum	0 Open 3 Percutaneous 4 Percutaneous Endoscopic	Z No Device	Z No Qualifier

Section	0	Medical and Surgical		
Body System	W	Anatomical Regions, General		
Operation	U	Supplement: Putting in or on biological or synthetic material that physically reinforces and/or augments the function of a portion of a body part		

Body Part (Character 4)	Approach (Character 5)	Device (Character 6)	Qualifier (Character 7)
0 Head 2 Face 4 Upper Jaw 5 Lower Jaw 6 Neck 8 Chest Wall C Mediastinum F Abdominal Wall K Upper Back L Lower Back M Perineum, Male N Perineum, Female	0 Open 4 Percutaneous Endoscopic	7 Autologous Tissue Substitute J Synthetic Substitute K Nonautologous Tissue Substitute	Z No Qualifier

Section	0	Medical and Surgical		
Body System	W	Anatomical Regions, General		
Operation	W	Revision: Correcting, to the extent possible, a portion of a malfunctioning device or the position of a displaced device		

Body Part (Character 4)	Approach (Character 5)	Device (Character 6)	Qualifier (Character 7)
0 Head 2 Face 4 Upper Jaw 5 Lower Jaw 6 Neck 8 Chest Wall C Mediastinum F Abdominal Wall K Upper Back L Lower Back M Perineum, Male N Perineum, Female	0 Open 3 Percutaneous 4 Percutaneous Endoscopic X External	0 Drainage Device 1 Radioactive Element 3 Infusion Device 7 Autologous Tissue Substitute J Synthetic Substitute K Nonautologous Tissue Substitute Y Other Device	Z No Qualifier
1 Cranial Cavity 9 Pleural Cavity, Right B Pleural Cavity, Left G Peritoneal Cavity J Pelvic Cavity	0 Open 3 Percutaneous 4 Percutaneous Endoscopic X External	0 Drainage Device 1 Radioactive Element 3 Infusion Device J Synthetic Substitute Y Other Device	Z No Qualifier
D Pericardial Cavity H Retroperitoneum	0 Open 3 Percutaneous 4 Percutaneous Endoscopic X External	0 Drainage Device 1 Radioactive Element 3 Infusion Device Y Other Device	Z No Qualifier
P Gastrointestinal Tract Q Respiratory Tract R Genitourinary Tract	0 Open 3 Percutaneous 4 Percutaneous Endoscopic 7 Via Natural or Artificial Opening 8 Via Natural or Artificial Opening Endoscopic X External	1 Radioactive Element 3 Infusion Device Y Other Device	Z No Qualifier

Section	0	Medical and Surgical		
Body System	X	Anatomical Regions, Upper Extremities		
Operation	0	Alteration: Modifying the anatomic structure of a body part without affecting the function of the body part		

Body Part (Character 4)	Approach (Character 5)	Device (Character 6)	Qualifier (Character 7)
2 Shoulder Region, Right	0 Open	7 Autologous Tissue Substitute	Z No Qualifier
3 Shoulder Region, Left	3 Percutaneous	J Synthetic Substitute	
4 Axilla, Right	4 Percutaneous Endoscopic	K Nonautologous Tissue	
5 Axilla, Left		Substitute	
6 Upper Extremity, Right		Z No Device	
7 Upper Extremity, Left			
8 Upper Arm, Right			
9 Upper Arm, Left			
B Elbow Region, Right			
C Elbow Region, Left			
D Lower Arm, Right			
F Lower Arm, Left			
G Wrist Region, Right			
H Wrist Region, Left			

Section	0	Medical and Surgical		
Body System	X	Anatomical Regions, Upper Extremities		
Operation	2	Change: Taking out or off a device from a body part and putting back an identical or similar device in or on the same body part without cutting or puncturing the skin or a mucous membrane		

Body Part (Character 4)	Approach (Character 5)	Device (Character 6)	Qualifier (Character 7)
6 Upper Extremity, Right	X External	0 Drainage Device	Z No Qualifier
7 Upper Extremity, Left		Y Other Device	

Section	0	Medical and Surgical		
Body System	X	Anatomical Regions, Upper Extremities		
Operation	3	Control: Stopping, or attempting to stop, postprocedural bleeding		

Body Part (Character 4)	Approach (Character 5)	Device (Character 6)	Qualifier (Character 7)
2 Shoulder Region, Right	0 Open	Z No Device	Z No Qualifier
3 Shoulder Region, Left	3 Percutaneous		
4 Axilla, Right	4 Percutaneous Endoscopic		
5 Axilla, Left			
6 Upper Extremity, Right			
7 Upper Extremity, Left			
8 Upper Arm, Right			
9 Upper Arm, Left			
B Elbow Region, Right			
C Elbow Region, Left			
D Lower Arm, Right			
F Lower Arm, Left			
G Wrist Region, Right			
H Wrist Region, Left			
J Hand, Right			
K Hand, Left			

Section	0	Medical and Surgical		
Body System	X	Anatomical Regions, Upper Extremities		
Operation	6	Detachment: Cutting off all or a portion of the upper or lower extremities		

Body Part (Character 4)	Approach (Character 5)	Device (Character 6)	Qualifier (Character 7)
0 Forequarter, Right 1 Forequarter, Left 2 Shoulder Region, Right 3 Shoulder Region, Left B Elbow Region, Right C Elbow Region, Left	0 Open	Z No Device	Z No Qualifier
8 Upper Arm, Right 9 Upper Arm, Left D Lower Arm, Right F Lower Arm, Left	0 Open	Z No Device	1 High 2 Mid 3 Low
J Hand, Right K Hand, Left	0 Open	Z No Device	0 Complete 4 Complete 1st Ray 5 Complete 2nd Ray 6 Complete 3rd Ray 7 Complete 4th Ray 8 Complete 5th Ray 9 Partial 1st Ray B Partial 2nd Ray C Partial 3rd Ray D Partial 4th Ray F Partial 5th Ray
L Thumb, Right M Thumb, Left N Index Finger, Right P Index Finger, Left Q Middle Finger, Right R Middle Finger, Left S Ring Finger, Right T Ring Finger, Left V Little Finger, Right W Little Finger, Left	0 Open	Z No Device	0 Complete 1 High 2 Mid 3 Low

Section	0	Medical and Surgical		
Body System	X	Anatomical Regions, Upper Extremities		
Operation	9	Drainage: Taking or letting out fluids and/or gases from a body part		

Body Part (Character 4)	Approach (Character 5)	Device (Character 6)	Qualifier (Character 7)
2 Shoulder Region, Right 3 Shoulder Region, Left 4 Axilla, Right 5 Axilla, Left 6 Upper Extremity, Right 7 Upper Extremity, Left 8 Upper Arm, Right 9 Upper Arm, Left B Elbow Region, Right C Elbow Region, Left D Lower Arm, Right F Lower Arm, Left G Wrist Region, Right H Wrist Region, Left J Hand, Right K Hand, Left	0 Open 3 Percutaneous 4 Percutaneous Endoscopic	0 Drainage Device	Z No Qualifier
2 Shoulder Region, Right 3 Shoulder Region, Left 4 Axilla, Right 5 Axilla, Left 6 Upper Extremity, Right 7 Upper Extremity, Left 8 Upper Arm, Right 9 Upper Arm, Left B Elbow Region, Right C Elbow Region, Left D Lower Arm, Right F Lower Arm, Left G Wrist Region, Right H Wrist Region, Left J Hand, Right K Hand, Left	0 Open 3 Percutaneous 4 Percutaneous Endoscopic	Z No Device	X Diagnostic Z No Qualifier

Section	0	Medical and Surgical		
Body System	X	Anatomical Regions, Upper Extremities		
Operation	B	Excision: Cutting out or off, without replacement, a portion of a body part		

Body Part (Character 4)	Approach (Character 5)	Device (Character 6)	Qualifier (Character 7)
2 Shoulder Region, Right 3 Shoulder Region, Left 4 Axilla, Right 5 Axilla, Left 6 Upper Extremity, Right 7 Upper Extremity, Left 8 Upper Arm, Right 9 Upper Arm, Left B Elbow Region, Right C Elbow Region, Left D Lower Arm, Right F Lower Arm, Left G Wrist Region, Right H Wrist Region, Left J Hand, Right K Hand, Left	0 Open 3 Percutaneous 4 Percutaneous Endoscopic	Z No Device	X Diagnostic Z No Qualifier

Section	0	Medical and Surgical		
Body System	X	Anatomical Regions, Upper Extremities		
Operation	H	Insertion: Putting in a nonbiological appliance that monitors, assists, performs, or prevents a physiological function but does not physically take the place of a body part		

Body Part (Character 4)	Approach (Character 5)	Device (Character 6)	Qualifier (Character 7)
2 Shoulder Region, Right 3 Shoulder Region, Left 4 Axilla, Right 5 Axilla, Left 6 Upper Extremity, Right 7 Upper Extremity, Left 8 Upper Arm, Right 9 Upper Arm, Left B Elbow Region, Right C Elbow Region, Left D Lower Arm, Right F Lower Arm, Left G Wrist Region, Right H Wrist Region, Left J Hand, Right K Hand, Left	0 Open 3 Percutaneous 4 Percutaneous Endoscopic	1 Radioactive Element 3 Infusion Device Y Other Device	Z No Qualifier

Section	0	Medical and Surgical		
Body System	X	Anatomical Regions, Upper Extremities		
Operation	J	Inspection: Visually and/or manually exploring a body part		

Body Part (Character 4)	Approach (Character 5)	Device (Character 6)	Qualifier (Character 7)
2 Shoulder Region, Right 3 Shoulder Region, Left 4 Axilla, Right 5 Axilla, Left 6 Upper Extremity, Right 7 Upper Extremity, Left 8 Upper Arm, Right 9 Upper Arm, Left B Elbow Region, Right C Elbow Region, Left D Lower Arm, Right F Lower Arm, Left G Wrist Region, Right H Wrist Region, Left J Hand, Right K Hand, Left	0 Open 3 Percutaneous 4 Percutaneous Endoscopic X External	Z No Device	Z No Qualifier

Section	0	Medical and Surgical		
Body System	X	Anatomical Regions, Upper Extremities		
Operation	M	Reattachment Putting back in or on all or a portion of a separated body part to its normal location or other suitable location		

Body Part (Character 4)	Approach (Character 5)	Device (Character 6)	Qualifier (Character 7)
0 Forequarter, Right 1 Forequarter, Left 2 Shoulder Region, Right 3 Shoulder Region, Left 4 Axilla, Right 5 Axilla, Left 6 Upper Extremity, Right 7 Upper Extremity, Left 8 Upper Arm, Right 9 Upper Arm, Left B Elbow Region, Right C Elbow Region, Left D Lower Arm, Right F Lower Arm, Left G Wrist Region, Right H Wrist Region, Left J Hand, Right K Hand, Left L Thumb, Right M Thumb, Left N Index Finger, Right P Index Finger, Left Q Middle Finger, Right R Middle Finger, Left S Ring Finger, Right T Ring Finger, Left V Little Finger, Right W Little Finger, Left	0 Open	Z No Device	Z No Qualifier

Section	0	Medical and Surgical		
Body System	X	Anatomical Regions, Upper Extremities		
Operation	P	Removal: Taking out or off a device from a body part		

Body Part (Character 4)	Approach (Character 5)	Device (Character 6)	Qualifier (Character 7)
6 Upper Extremity, Right 7 Upper Extremity, Left	0 Open 3 Percutaneous 4 Percutaneous Endoscopic X External	0 Drainage Device 1 Radioactive Element 3 Infusion Device 7 Autologous Tissue Substitute J Synthetic Substitute K Nonautologous Tissue Substitute Y Other Device	Z No Qualifier

Section	0	Medical and Surgical		
Body System	X	Anatomical Regions, Upper Extremities		
Operation	Q	Repair: Restoring, to the extent possible, a body part to its normal anatomic structure and function		

Body Part (Character 4)	Approach (Character 5)	Device (Character 6)	Qualifier (Character 7)
2 Shoulder Region, Right 3 Shoulder Region, Left 4 Axilla, Right 5 Axilla, Left 6 Upper Extremity, Right 7 Upper Extremity, Left 8 Upper Arm, Right 9 Upper Arm, Left B Elbow Region, Right C Elbow Region, Left D Lower Arm, Right F Lower Arm, Left G Wrist Region, Right H Wrist Region, Left J Hand, Right K Hand, Left L Thumb, Right M Thumb, Left N Index Finger, Right P Index Finger, Left Q Middle Finger, Right R Middle Finger, Left S Ring Finger, Right T Ring Finger, Left V Little Finger, Right W Little Finger, Left	0 Open 3 Percutaneous 4 Percutaneous Endoscopic X External	Z No Device	Z No Qualifier

Section	0	Medical and Surgical		
Body System	X	Anatomical Regions, Upper Extremities		
Operation	R	Replacement: Putting in or on biological or synthetic material that physically takes the place and/or function of all or a portion of a body part		

Body Part (Character 4)	Approach (Character 5)	Device (Character 6)	Qualifier (Character 7)
L Thumb, Right M Thumb, Left		0 Open 4 Percutaneous Endoscopic	7 Autologous Tissue Substitute

Section	0	Medical and Surgical		
Body System	X	Anatomical Regions, Upper Extremities		
Operation	U	Supplement: Putting in or on biological or synthetic material that physically reinforces and/or augments the function of a portion of a body part		

Body Part (Character 4)	Approach (Character 5)	Device (Character 6)	Qualifier (Character 7)
2 Shoulder Region, Right 3 Shoulder Region, Left 4 Axilla, Right 5 Axilla, Left 6 Upper Extremity, Right 7 Upper Extremity, Left 8 Upper Arm, Right 9 Upper Arm, Left B Elbow Region, Right C Elbow Region, Left D Lower Arm, Right F Lower Arm, Left G Wrist Region, Right H Wrist Region, Left J Hand, Right K Hand, Left L Thumb, Right M Thumb, Left N Index Finger, Right P Index Finger, Left Q Middle Finger, Right R Middle Finger, Left S Ring Finger, Right T Ring Finger, Left V Little Finger, Right W Little Finger, Left	0 Open 4 Percutaneous Endoscopic	7 Autologous Tissue Substitute J Synthetic Substitute K Nonautologous Tissue Substitute	Z No Qualifier

Section	0	Medical and Surgical		
Body System	X	Anatomical Regions, Upper Extremities		
Operation	W	Revision: Correcting, to the extent possible, a portion of a malfunctioning device or the position of a displaced device		

Body Part (Character 4)	Approach (Character 5)	Device (Character 6)	Qualifier (Character 7)
6 Upper Extremity, Right 7 Upper Extremity, Left	0 Open 3 Percutaneous 4 Percutaneous Endoscopic X External	0 Drainage Device 3 Infusion Device 7 Autologous Tissue Substitute J Synthetic Substitute K Nonautologous Tissue Substitute Y Other Device	Z No Qualifier

Section	0	Medical and Surgical		
Body System	X	Anatomical Regions, Upper Extremities		
Operation	X	Transfer: Moving, without taking out, all or a portion of a body part to another location to take over the function of all or a portion of a body part		

Body Part (Character 4)	Approach (Character 5)	Device (Character 6)	Qualifier (Character 7)
N Index Finger, Right	0 Open	Z No Device	L Thumb, Right
P Index Finger, Left	0 Open	Z No Device	M Thumb, Left

Section	0	Medical and Surgical		
Body System	Y	Anatomical Regions, Lower Extremities		
Operation	0	Alteration: Modifying the anatomic structure of a body part without affecting the function of the body part		
Body Part (Character 4)		**Approach (Character 5)**	**Device (Character 6)**	**Qualifier (Character 7)**
0 Buttock, Right 1 Buttock, Left 9 Lower Extremity, Right B Lower Extremity, Left C Upper Leg, Right D Upper Leg, Left F Knee Region, Right G Knee Region, Left H Lower Leg, Right J Lower Leg, Left K Ankle Region, Right L Ankle Region, Left		0 Open 3 Percutaneous 4 Percutaneous Endoscopic	7 Autologous Tissue Substitute J Synthetic Substitute K Nonautologous Tissue Substitute Z No Device	Z No Qualifier

Section	0	Medical and Surgical		
Body System	Y	Anatomical Regions, Lower Extremities		
Operation	2	Change: Taking out or off a device from a body part and putting back an identical or similar device in or on the same body part without cutting or puncturing the skin or a mucous membrane		
Body Part (Character 4)		**Approach (Character 5)**	**Device (Character 6)**	**Qualifier (Character 7)**
9 Lower Extremity, Right B Lower Extremity, Left		X External	0 Drainage Device Y Other Device	Z No Qualifier

Section	0	Medical and Surgical		
Body System	Y	Anatomical Regions, Lower Extremities		
Operation	3	Control: Stopping, or attempting to stop, postprocedural bleeding		
Body Part (Character 4)		**Approach (Character 5)**	**Device (Character 6)**	**Qualifier (Character 7)**
0 Buttock, Right 1 Buttock, Left 5 Inguinal Region, Right 6 Inguinal Region, Left 7 Femoral Region, Right 8 Femoral Region, Left 9 Lower Extremity, Right B Lower Extremity, Left C Upper Leg, Right D Upper Leg, Left F Knee Region, Right G Knee Region, Left H Lower Leg, Right J Lower Leg, Left K Ankle Region, Right L Ankle Region, Left M Foot, Right N Foot, Left		0 Open 3 Percutaneous 4 Percutaneous Endoscopic	Z No Device	Z No Qualifier

Section	0	Medical and Surgical	
Body System	Y	Anatomical Regions, Lower Extremities	
Operation	6	Detachment: Cutting off all or a portion of the upper or lower extremities	

Body Part (Character 4)	Approach (Character 5)	Device (Character 6)	Qualifier (Character 7)
2 Hindquarter, Right 3 Hindquarter, Left 4 Hindquarter, Bilateral 7 Femoral Region, Right 8 Femoral Region, Left F Knee Region, Right G Knee Region, Left	0 Open	Z No Device	Z No Qualifier
C Upper Leg, Right D Upper Leg, Left H Lower Leg, Right J Lower Leg, Left	0 Open	Z No Device	1 High 2 Mid 3 Low
M Foot, Right N Foot, Left	0 Open	Z No Device	0 Complete 4 Complete 1st Ray 5 Complete 2nd Ray 6 Complete 3rd Ray 7 Complete 4th Ray 8 Complete 5th Ray 9 Partial 1st Ray B Partial 2nd Ray C Partial 3rd Ray D Partial 4th Ray F Partial 5th Ray
P 1st Toe, Right Q 1st Toe, Left R 2nd Toe, Right S 2nd Toe, Left T 3rd Toe, Right U 3rd Toe, Left V 4th Toe, Right W 4th Toe, Left X 5th Toe, Right Y 5th Toe, Left	0 Open	Z No Device	0 Complete 1 High 2 Mid 3 Low

Section	0	Medical and Surgical		
Body System	Y	Anatomical Regions, Lower Extremities		
Operation	9	Drainage: Taking or letting out fluids and/or gases from a body part		

Body Part (Character 4)	Approach (Character 5)	Device (Character 6)	Qualifier (Character 7)
0 Buttock, Right 1 Buttock, Left 5 Inguinal Region, Right 6 Inguinal Region, Left 7 Femoral Region, Right 8 Femoral Region, Left 9 Lower Extremity, Right B Lower Extremity, Left C Upper Leg, Right D Upper Leg, Left F Knee Region, Right G Knee Region, Left H Lower Leg, Right J Lower Leg, Left K Ankle Region, Right L Ankle Region, Left M Foot, Right N Foot, Left	0 Open 3 Percutaneous 4 Percutaneous Endoscopic	0 Drainage Device	Z No Qualifier
0 Buttock, Right 1 Buttock, Left 5 Inguinal Region, Right 6 Inguinal Region, Left 7 Femoral Region, Right 8 Femoral Region, Left 9 Lower Extremity, Right B Lower Extremity, Left C Upper Leg, Right D Upper Leg, Left F Knee Region, Right G Knee Region, Left H Lower Leg, Right J Lower Leg, Left K Ankle Region, Right L Ankle Region, Left M Foot, Right N Foot, Left	0 Open 3 Percutaneous 4 Percutaneous Endoscopic	Z No Device	X Diagnostic Z No Qualifier

Section	0	Medical and Surgical		
Body System	Y	Anatomical Regions, Lower Extremities		
Operation	B	Excision: Cutting out or off, without replacement, a portion of a body part		

Body Part (Character 4)	Approach (Character 5)	Device (Character 6)	Qualifier (Character 7)
0 Buttock, Right 1 Buttock, Left 5 Inguinal Region, Right 6 Inguinal Region, Left 7 Femoral Region, Right 8 Femoral Region, Left 9 Lower Extremity, Right B Lower Extremity, Left C Upper Leg, Right D Upper Leg, Left F Knee Region, Right G Knee Region, Left H Lower Leg, Right J Lower Leg, Left K Ankle Region, Right L Ankle Region, Left M Foot, Right N Foot, Left	0 Open 3 Percutaneous 4 Percutaneous Endoscopic	Z No Device	X Diagnostic Z No Qualifier

Section	0	Medical and Surgical		
Body System	Y	Anatomical Regions, Lower Extremities		
Operation	H	Insertion: Putting in a nonbiological appliance that monitors, assists, performs, or prevents a physiological function but does not physically take the place of a body part		

Body Part (Character 4)	Approach (Character 5)	Device (Character 6)	Qualifier (Character 7)
0 Buttock, Right	0 Open	1 Radioactive Element	Z No Qualifier
1 Buttock, Left	3 Percutaneous	3 Infusion Device	
5 Inguinal Region, Right	4 Percutaneous Endoscopic	Y Other Device	
6 Inguinal Region, Left			
7 Femoral Region, Right			
8 Femoral Region, Left			
9 Lower Extremity, Right			
B Lower Extremity, Left			
C Upper Leg, Right			
D Upper Leg, Left			
F Knee Region, Right			
G Knee Region, Left			
H Lower Leg, Right			
J Lower Leg, Left			
K Ankle Region, Right			
L Ankle Region, Left			
M Foot, Right			
N Foot, Left			

Section	0	Medical and Surgical		
Body System	Y	Anatomical Regions, Lower Extremities		
Operation	J	Inspection: Visually and/or manually exploring a body part		

Body Part (Character 4)	Approach (Character 5)	Device (Character 6)	Qualifier (Character 7)
0 Buttock, Right	0 Open	Z No Device	Z No Qualifier
1 Buttock, Left	3 Percutaneous		
5 Inguinal Region, Right	4 Percutaneous Endoscopic		
6 Inguinal Region, Left	X External		
7 Femoral Region, Right			
8 Femoral Region, Left			
9 Lower Extremity, Right			
A Inguinal Region, Bilateral			
B Lower Extremity, Left			
C Upper Leg, Right			
D Upper Leg, Left			
E Femoral Region, Bilateral			
F Knee Region, Right			
G Knee Region, Left			
H Lower Leg, Right			
J Lower Leg, Left			
K Ankle Region, Right			
L Ankle Region, Left			
M Foot, Right			
N Foot, Left			

Section	0	Medical and Surgical				
Body System	Y	Anatomical Regions, Lower Extremities				
Operation	M	Reattachment Putting back in or on all or a portion of a separated body part to its normal location or other suitable location				

Body Part (Character 4)	Approach (Character 5)	Device (Character 6)	Qualifier (Character 7)
0 Buttock, Right 1 Buttock, Left 2 Hindquarter, Right 3 Hindquarter, Left 4 Hindquarter, Bilateral 5 Inguinal Region, Right 6 Inguinal Region, Left 7 Femoral Region, Right 8 Femoral Region, Left 9 Lower Extremity, Right B Lower Extremity, Left C Upper Leg, Right D Upper Leg, Left F Knee Region, Right G Knee Region, Left H Lower Leg, Right J Lower Leg, Left K Ankle Region, Right L Ankle Region, Left M Foot, Right N Foot, Left P 1st Toe, Right Q 1st Toe, Left R 2nd Toe, Right S 2nd Toe, Left T 3rd Toe, Right U 3rd Toe, Left V 4th Toe, Right W 4th Toe, Left X 5th Toe, Right Y 5th Toe, Left	0 Open	Z No Device	Z No Qualifier

Section	0	Medical and Surgical				
Body System	Y	Anatomical Regions, Lower Extremities				
Operation	P	Removal: Taking out or off a device from a body part				

Body Part (Character 4)	Approach (Character 5)	Device (Character 6)	Qualifier (Character 7)
9 Lower Extremity, Right B Lower Extremity, Left	0 Open 3 Percutaneous 4 Percutaneous Endoscopic X External	0 Drainage Device 1 Radioactive Element 3 Infusion Device 7 Autologous Tissue Substitute J Synthetic Substitute K Nonautologous Tissue Substitute Y Other Device	Z No Qualifier

Section	0	Medical and Surgical		
Body System	Y	Anatomical Regions, Lower Extremities		
Operation	Q	Repair: Restoring, to the extent possible, a body part to its normal anatomic structure and function		

Body Part (Character 4)	Approach (Character 5)	Device (Character 6)	Qualifier (Character 7)
0 Buttock, Right 1 Buttock, Left 5 Inguinal Region, Right 6 Inguinal Region, Left 7 Femoral Region, Right 8 Femoral Region, Left 9 Lower Extremity, Right A Inguinal Region, Bilateral B Lower Extremity, Left C Upper Leg, Right D Upper Leg, Left E Femoral Region, Bilateral F Knee Region, Right G Knee Region, Left H Lower Leg, Right J Lower Leg, Left K Ankle Region, Right L Ankle Region, Left M Foot, Right N Foot, Left P 1st Toe, Right Q 1st Toe, Left R 2nd Toe, Right S 2nd Toe, Left T 3rd Toe, Right U 3rd Toe, Left V 4th Toe, Right W 4th Toe, Left X 5th Toe, Right Y 5th Toe, Left	0 Open 3 Percutaneous 4 Percutaneous Endoscopic X External	Z No Device	Z No Qualifier

Section	0	Medical and Surgical		
Body System	Y	Anatomical Regions, Lower Extremities		
Operation	U	Supplement: Putting in or on biological or synthetic material that physically reinforces and/or augments the function of a portion of a body part		

Body Part (Character 4)	Approach (Character 5)	Device (Character 6)	Qualifier (Character 7)
0 Buttock, Right 1 Buttock, Left 5 Inguinal Region, Right 6 Inguinal Region, Left 7 Femoral Region, Right 8 Femoral Region, Left 9 Lower Extremity, Right A Inguinal Region, Bilateral B Lower Extremity, Left C Upper Leg, Right D Upper Leg, Left E Femoral Region, Bilateral F Knee Region, Right G Knee Region, Left H Lower Leg, Right J Lower Leg, Left K Ankle Region, Right L Ankle Region, Left M Foot, Right N Foot, Left P 1st Toe, Right Q 1st Toe, Left R 2nd Toe, Right S 2nd Toe, Left T 3rd Toe, Right U 3rd Toe, Left V 4th Toe, Right W 4th Toe, Left X 5th Toe, Right Y 5th Toe, Left	0 Open 4 Percutaneous Endoscopic	7 Autologous Tissue Substitute J Synthetic Substitute K Nonautologous Tissue Substitute	Z No Qualifier

Section	0	Medical and Surgical		
Body System	Y	Anatomical Regions, Lower Extremities		
Operation	W	Revision: Correcting, to the extent possible, a portion of a malfunctioning device or the position of a displaced device		

Body Part (Character 4)	Approach (Character 5)	Device (Character 6)	Qualifier (Character 7)
9 Lower Extremity, Right B Lower Extremity, Left	0 Open 3 Percutaneous 4 Percutaneous Endoscopic X External	0 Drainage Device 3 Infusion Device 7 Autologous Tissue Substitute J Synthetic Substitute K Nonautologous Tissue Substitute Y Other Device	Z No Qualifier

Section	1	Obstetrics
Body System	0	Pregnancy
Operation	2	Change: Taking out or off a device from a body part and putting back an identical or similar device in or on the same body part without cutting or puncturing the skin or a mucous membrane

Body Part (Character 4)	Approach (Character 5)	Device (Character 6)	Qualifier (Character 7)
0 Products of Conception	7 Via Natural or Artificial Opening	3 Monitoring Electrode Y Other Device	Z No Qualifier

Section	1	Obstetrics
Body System	0	Pregnancy
Operation	9	Drainage: Taking or letting out fluids and/or gases from a body part

Body Part (Character 4)	Approach (Character 5)	Device (Character 6)	Qualifier (Character 7)
0 Products of Conception	0 Open 3 Percutaneous 4 Percutaneous Endoscopic 7 Via Natural or Artificial Opening 8 Via Natural or Artificial Opening Endoscopic	Z No Device	9 Fetal Blood A Fetal Cerebrospinal Fluid B Fetal Fluid, Other C Amniotic Fluid, Therapeutic D Fluid, Other U Amniotic Fluid, Diagnostic

Section	1	Obstetrics
Body System	0	Pregnancy
Operation	A	Abortion: Artificially terminating a pregnancy

Body Part (Character 4)	Approach (Character 5)	Device (Character 6)	Qualifier (Character 7)
0 Products of Conception	0 Open 3 Percutaneous 4 Percutaneous Endoscopic 8 Via Natural or Artificial Opening Endoscopic	Z No Device	Z No Qualifier
0 Products of Conception	7 Via Natural or Artificial Opening	Z No Device	6 Vacuum W Laminaria X Abortifacient Z No Qualifier

Section	1	Obstetrics
Body System	0	Pregnancy
Operation	D	Extraction: Pulling or stripping out or off all or a portion of a body part by the use of force

Body Part (Character 4)	Approach (Character 5)	Device (Character 6)	Qualifier (Character 7)
0 Products of Conception	0 Open	Z No Device	0 Classical 1 Low Cervical 2 Extraperitoneal
0 Products of Conception	7 Via Natural or Artificial Opening	Z No Device	3 Low Forceps 4 Mid Forceps 5 High Forceps 6 Vacuum 7 Internal Version 8 Other
1 Products of Conception, Retained 2 Products of Conception, Ectopic	7 Via Natural or Artificial Opening 8 Via Natural or Artificial Opening Endoscopic	Z No Device	Z No Qualifier

Section	1	Obstetrics
Body System	0	Pregnancy
Operation	E	Delivery: Assisting the passage of the products of conception from the genital canal

Body Part (Character 4)	Approach (Character 5)	Device (Character 6)	Qualifier (Character 7)
0 Products of Conception	X External	Z No Device	Z No Qualifier

Section	1	Obstetrics
Body System	0	Pregnancy
Operation	H	Insertion: Putting in a nonbiological appliance that monitors, assists, performs, or prevents a physiological function but does not physically take the place of a body part

Body Part (Character 4)	Approach (Character 5)	Device (Character 6)	Qualifier (Character 7)
0 Products of Conception	0 Open 7 Via Natural or Artificial Opening	3 Monitoring Electrode Y Other Device	Z No Qualifier

Section	1	Obstetrics		
Body System	0	Pregnancy		
Operation	J	Inspection: Visually and/or manually exploring a body part		
Body Part (Character 4)	Approach (Character 5)		Device (Character 6)	Qualifier (Character 7)
0 Products of Conception 1 Products of Conception, Retained 2 Products of Conception, Ectopic	0 Open 3 Percutaneous 4 Percutaneous Endoscopic 7 Via Natural or Artificial Opening 8 Via Natural or Artificial Opening Endoscopic X External		Z No Device	Z No Qualifier

Section	1	Obstetrics		
Body System	0	Pregnancy		
Operation	P	Removal: Taking out or off a device from a body part, region or orifice		
Body Part (Character 4)	Approach (Character 5)		Device (Character 6)	Qualifier (Character 7)
0 Products of Conception	0 Open 7 Via Natural or Artificial Opening		3 Monitoring Electrode Y Other Device	Z No Qualifier

Section	1	Obstetrics		
Body System	0	Pregnancy		
Operation	Q	Repair: Restoring, to the extent possible, a body part to its normal anatomic structure and function		
Body Part (Character 4)	Approach (Character 5)		Device (Character 6)	Qualifier (Character 7)
0 Products of Conception	0 Open 3 Percutaneous 4 Percutaneous Endoscopic 7 Via Natural or Artificial Opening 8 Via Natural or Artificial Opening Endoscopic		Y Other Device Z No Device	E Nervous System F Cardiovascular System G Lymphatics and Hemic H Eye J Ear, Nose and Sinus K Respiratory System L Mouth and Throat M Gastrointestinal System N Hepatobiliary and Pancreas P Endocrine System Q Skin R Musculoskeletal System S Urinary System T Female Reproductive System V Male Reproductive System Y Other Body System

Section	1	Obstetrics		
Body System	0	Pregnancy		
Operation	S	Reposition: Moving to its normal location, or other suitable location, all or a portion of a body part		
Body Part (Character 4)	Approach (Character 5)		Device (Character 6)	Qualifier (Character 7)
0 Products of Conception	7 Via Natural or Artificial Opening X External		Z No Device	Z No Qualifier
2 Products of Conception, Ectopic	0 Open 3 Percutaneous 4 Percutaneous Endoscopic 7 Via Natural or Artificial Opening 8 Via Natural or Artificial Opening Endoscopic		Z No Device	Z No Qualifier

Section	1	Obstetrics		
Body System	0	Pregnancy		
Operation	T	Resection: Cutting out or off, without replacement, all of a body part		
Body Part (Character 4)	Approach (Character 5)		Device (Character 6)	Qualifier (Character 7)
2 Products of Conception, Ectopic	0 Open 3 Percutaneous 4 Percutaneous Endoscopic 7 Via Natural or Artificial Opening 8 Via Natural or Artificial Opening Endoscopic		Z No Device	Z No Qualifier

Section	1	Obstetrics
Body System	0	Pregnancy
Operation	Y	Transplantation: Putting in or on all or a portion of a living body part taken from another individual or animal to physically take the place and/or function of all or a portion of a similar body part

Body Part (Character 4)	Approach (Character 5)	Device (Character 6)	Qualifier (Character 7)
0 Products of Conception	**3** Percutaneous **4** Percutaneous Endoscopic **7** Via Natural or Artificial Opening	**Z** No Device	**E** Nervous System **F** Cardiovascular System **G** Lymphatics and Hemic **H** Eye **J** Ear, Nose and Sinus **K** Respiratory System **L** Mouth and Throat **M** Gastrointestinal System **N** Hepatobiliary and Pancreas **P** Endocrine System **Q** Skin **R** Musculoskeletal System **S** Urinary System **T** Female Reproductive System **V** Male Reproductive System **Y** Other Body System

Section	2	Placement			
Body System	W	Anatomical Regions			
Operation	0	Change: Taking out or off a device from a body part and putting back an identical or similar device in or on the same body part without cutting or puncturing the skin or a mucous membrane			

Body Region (Character 4)	Approach (Character 5)	Device (Character 6)	Qualifier (Character 7)
0 Head	X External	0 Traction Apparatus	Z No Qualifier
2 Neck		1 Splint	
3 Abdominal Wall		2 Cast	
4 Chest Wall		3 Brace	
5 Back		4 Bandage	
6 Inguinal Region, Right		5 Packing Material	
7 Inguinal Region, Left		6 Pressure Dressing	
8 Upper Extremity, Right		7 Intermittent Pressure Device	
9 Upper Extremity, Left		Y Other Device	
A Upper Arm, Right			
B Upper Arm, Left			
C Lower Arm, Right			
D Lower Arm, Left			
E Hand, Right			
F Hand, Left			
G Thumb, Right			
H Thumb, Left			
J Finger, Right			
K Finger, Left			
L Lower Extremity, Right			
M Lower Extremity, Left			
N Upper Leg, Right			
P Upper Leg, Left			
Q Lower Leg, Right			
R Lower Leg, Left			
S Foot, Right			
T Foot, Left			
U Toe, Right			
V Toe, Left			

Section	2	Placement			
Body System	W	Anatomical Regions			
Operation	0	Change: Taking out or off a device from a body part and putting back an identical or similar device in or on the same body part without cutting or puncturing the skin or a mucous membrane			

Body Region (Character 4)	Approach (Character 5)	Device (Character 6)	Qualifier (Character 7)
1 Face	X External	0 Traction Apparatus	Z No Qualifier
		1 Splint	
		2 Cast	
		3 Brace	
		4 Bandage	
		5 Packing Material	
		6 Pressure Dressing	
		7 Intermittent Pressure Device	
		9 Wire	
		Y Other Device	

Section	2	Placement			
Body System	W	Anatomical Regions			
Operation	1	Compression: Putting pressure on a body region			

Body Region (Character 4)	Approach (Character 5)	Device (Character 6)	Qualifier (Character 7)
0 Head 1 Face 2 Neck 3 Abdominal Wall 4 Chest Wall 5 Back 6 Inguinal Region, Right 7 Inguinal Region, Left 8 Upper Extremity, Right 9 Upper Extremity, Left A Upper Arm, Right B Upper Arm, Left C Lower Arm, Right D Lower Arm, Left E Hand, Right F Hand, Left G Thumb, Right H Thumb, Left J Finger, Right K Finger, Left L Lower Extremity, Right M Lower Extremity, Left N Upper Leg, Right P Upper Leg, Left Q Lower Leg, Right R Lower Leg, Left S Foot, Right T Foot, Left U Toe, Right V Toe, Left	X External	6 Pressure Dressing 7 Intermittent Pressure Device	Z No Qualifier

Section	2	Placement			
Body System	W	Anatomical Regions			
Operation	2	Dressing: Putting material on a body region for protection			

Body Region (Character 4)	Approach (Character 5)	Device (Character 6)	Qualifier (Character 7)
0 Head 1 Face 2 Neck 3 Abdominal Wall 4 Chest Wall 5 Back 6 Inguinal Region, Right 7 Inguinal Region, Left 8 Upper Extremity, Right 9 Upper Extremity, Left A Upper Arm, Right B Upper Arm, Left C Lower Arm, Right D Lower Arm, Left E Hand, Right F Hand, Left G Thumb, Right H Thumb, Left J Finger, Right K Finger, Left L Lower Extremity, Right M Lower Extremity, Left N Upper Leg, Right P Upper Leg, Left Q Lower Leg, Right R Lower Leg, Left S Foot, Right T Foot, Left U Toe, Right V Toe, Left	X External	4 Bandage	Z No Qualifier

Section	2	Placement			
Body System	W	Anatomical Regions			
Operation	3	Immobilization: Limiting or preventing motion of a body region			

Body Region (Character 4)	Approach (Character 5)	Device (Character 6)	Qualifier (Character 7)
0 Head 2 Neck 3 Abdominal Wall 4 Chest Wall 5 Back 6 Inguinal Region, Right 7 Inguinal Region, Left 8 Upper Extremity, Right 9 Upper Extremity, Left A Upper Arm, Right B Upper Arm, Left C Lower Arm, Right D Lower Arm, Left E Hand, Right F Hand, Left G Thumb, Right H Thumb, Left J Finger, Right K Finger, Left L Lower Extremity, Right M Lower Extremity, Left N Upper Leg, Right P Upper Leg, Left Q Lower Leg, Right R Lower Leg, Left S Foot, Right T Foot, Left U Toe, Right V Toe, Left	X External	1 Splint 2 Cast 3 Brace Y Other Device	Z No Qualifier
1 Face	X External	1 Splint 2 Cast 3 Brace 9 Wire Y Other Device	Z No Qualifier

Section	2	Placement			
Body System	W	Anatomical Regions			
Operation	4	Packing: Putting material in a body region or orifice			

Body Region (Character 4)	Approach (Character 5)	Device (Character 6)	Qualifier (Character 7)
0 Head 1 Face 2 Neck 3 Abdominal Wall 4 Chest Wall 5 Back 6 Inguinal Region, Right 7 Inguinal Region, Left 8 Upper Extremity, Right 9 Upper Extremity, Left A Upper Arm, Right B Upper Arm, Left C Lower Arm, Right D Lower Arm, Left E Hand, Right F Hand, Left G Thumb, Right H Thumb, Left J Finger, Right K Finger, Left L Lower Extremity, Right M Lower Extremity, Left N Upper Leg, Right P Upper Leg, Left Q Lower Leg, Right R Lower Leg, Left S Foot, Right T Foot, Left U Toe, Right V Toe, Left	X External	5 Packing Material	Z No Qualifier

Section	2	Placement			
Body System	W	Anatomical Regions			
Operation	5	Removal: Taking out or off a device from a body part			

Body Region (Character 4)	Approach (Character 5)	Device (Character 6)	Qualifier (Character 7)
0 Head	X External	0 Traction Apparatus	Z No Qualifier
2 Neck		1 Splint	
3 Abdominal Wall		2 Cast	
4 Chest Wall		3 Brace	
5 Back		4 Bandage	
6 Inguinal Region, Right		5 Packing Material	
7 Inguinal Region, Left		6 Pressure Dressing	
8 Upper Extremity, Right		7 Intermittent Pressure Device	
9 Upper Extremity, Left		Y Other Device	
A Upper Arm, Right			
B Upper Arm, Left			
C Lower Arm, Right			
D Lower Arm, Left			
E Hand, Right			
F Hand, Left			
G Thumb, Right			
H Thumb, Left			
J Finger, Right			
K Finger, Left			
L Lower Extremity, Right			
M Lower Extremity, Left			
N Upper Leg, Right			
P Upper Leg, Left			
Q Lower Leg, Right			
R Lower Leg, Left			
S Foot, Right			
T Foot, Left			
U Toe, Right			
V Toe, Left			

Section	2	Placement			
Body System	W	Anatomical Regions			
Operation	5	Removal: Taking out or off a device from a body part			

Body Region (Character 4)	Approach (Character 5)	Device (Character 6)	Qualifier (Character 7)
1 Face	X External	0 Traction Apparatus	Z No Qualifier
		1 Splint	
		2 Cast	
		3 Brace	
		4 Bandage	
		5 Packing Material	
		6 Pressure Dressing	
		7 Intermittent Pressure Device	
		9 Wire	
		Y Other Device	

Section	2	Placement			
Body System	W	Anatomical Regions			
Operation	6	Traction: Exerting a pulling force on a body region in a distal direction			

Body Region (Character 4)	Approach (Character 5)	Device (Character 6)	Qualifier (Character 7)
0 Head	X External	0 Traction Apparatus	Z No Qualifier
1 Face		Z No Device	
2 Neck			
3 Abdominal Wall			
4 Chest Wall			
5 Back			
6 Inguinal Region, Right			
7 Inguinal Region, Left			
8 Upper Extremity, Right			
9 Upper Extremity, Left			
A Upper Arm, Right			
B Upper Arm, Left			
C Lower Arm, Right			
D Lower Arm, Left			
E Hand, Right			
F Hand, Left			
G Thumb, Right			
H Thumb, Left			
J Finger, Right			
K Finger, Left			
L Lower Extremity, Right			
M Lower Extremity, Left			
N Upper Leg, Right			
P Upper Leg, Left			
Q Lower Leg, Right			
R Lower Leg, Left			
S Foot, Right			
T Foot, Left			
U Toe, Right			
V Toe, Left			

Section	2	Placement			
Body System	Y	Anatomical Orifices			
Operation	0	Change: Taking out or off a device from a body part and putting back an identical or similar device in or on the same body part without cutting or puncturing the skin or a mucous membrane			

Body Region (Character 4)	Approach (Character 5)	Device (Character 6)	Qualifier (Character 7)
0 Mouth and Pharynx	X External	5 Packing Material	Z No Qualifier
1 Nasal			
2 Ear			
3 Anorectal			
4 Female Genital Tract			
5 Urethra			

Section	2	Placement			
Body System	Y	Anatomical Orifices			
Operation	4	Packing: Putting material in a body region or orifice			

Body Region (Character 4)	Approach (Character 5)	Device (Character 6)	Qualifier (Character 7)
0 Mouth and Pharynx	X External	5 Packing Material	Z No Qualifier
1 Nasal			
2 Ear			
3 Anorectal			
4 Female Genital Tract			
5 Urethra			

Section	2	Placement			
Body System	Y	Anatomical Orifices			
Operation	5	Removal: Taking out or off a device from a body part			

Body Region (Character 4)	Approach (Character 5)	Device (Character 6)	Qualifier (Character 7)
0 Mouth and Pharynx	X External	5 Packing Material	Z No Qualifier
1 Nasal			
2 Ear			
3 Anorectal			
4 Female Genital Tract			
5 Urethra			

Section	3	Administration
Body System	0	Circulatory
Operation	2	Transfusion: Putting in blood or blood products

Body System/Region (Character 4)	Approach (Character 5)	Substance (Character 6)	Qualifier (Character 7)
3 Peripheral Vein 4 Central Vein	0 Open 3 Percutaneous	A Stem Cells, Embryonic	Z No Qualifier
3 Peripheral Vein 4 Central Vein	0 Open 3 Percutaneous	G Bone Marrow H Whole Blood J Serum Albumin K Frozen Plasma L Fresh Plasma M Plasma Cryoprecipitate N Red Blood Cells P Frozen Red Cells Q White Cells R Platelets S Globulin T Fibrinogen V Antihemophilic Factors W Factor IX X Stem Cells, Cord Blood Y Stem Cells, Hematopoietic	0 Autologous 1 Nonautologous
5 Peripheral Artery 6 Central Artery	0 Open 3 Percutaneous	G Bone Marrow H Whole Blood J Serum Albumin K Frozen Plasma L Fresh Plasma M Plasma Cryoprecipitate N Red Blood Cells P Frozen Red Cells Q White Cells R Platelets S Globulin T Fibrinogen V Antihemophilic Factors W Factor IX X Stem Cells, Cord Blood Y Stem Cells, Hematopoietic	0 Autologous 1 Nonautologous

Section	3	Administration
Body System	0	Circulatory
Operation	2	Transfusion: Putting in blood or blood products

Body System/Region (Character 4)	Approach (Character 5)	Substance (Character 6)	Qualifier (Character 7)
7 Products of Conception, Circulatory	3 Percutaneous 7 Via Natural or Artificial Opening	H Whole Blood J Serum Albumin K Frozen Plasma L Fresh Plasma M Plasma Cryoprecipitate N Red Blood Cells P Frozen Red Cells Q White Cells R Platelets S Globulin T Fibrinogen V Antihemophilic Factors W Factor IX	1 Nonautologous

Section	3	Administration
Body System	C	Indwelling Device
Operation	1	Irrigation: Putting in or on a cleansing substance

Body System/Region (Character 4)	Approach (Character 5)	Substance (Character 6)	Qualifier (Character 7)
Z None	X External	8 Irrigating Substance	Z No Qualifier

Section	3	Administration
Body System	E	Physiological Systems and Anatomical Regions
Operation	0	Introduction: Putting in or on a therapeutic, diagnostic, nutritional, physiological, or prophylactic substance except blood or blood products

Body System/Region (Character 4)	Approach (Character 5)	Substance (Character 6)	Qualifier (Character 7)
0 Skin and Mucous Membranes	X External	0 Antineoplastic	5 Other Antineoplastic M Monoclonal Antibody
0 Skin and Mucous Membranes	X External	2 Anti-infective	8 Oxazolidinones 9 Other Anti-infective
0 Skin and Mucous Membranes	X External	3 Anti-inflammatory 4 Serum, Toxoid and Vaccine B Local Anesthetic K Other Diagnostic Substance M Pigment N Analgesics, Hypnotics, Sedatives T Destructive Agent	Z No Qualifier
0 Skin and Mucous Membranes	X External	G Other Therapeutic Substance	C Other Substance
1 Subcutaneous Tissue	0 Open	2 Anti-infective	A Anti-Infective Envelope
1 Subcutaneous Tissue	3 Percutaneous	0 Antineoplastic	5 Other Antineoplastic M Monoclonal Antibody
1 Subcutaneous Tissue	3 Percutaneous	2 Anti-infective	8 Oxazolidinones 9 Other Anti-infective A Anti-Infective Envelope
1 Subcutaneous Tissue	3 Percutaneous	3 Anti-inflammatory 4 Serum, Toxoid and Vaccine 6 Nutritional Substance 7 Electrolytic and Water Balance Substance B Local Anesthetic H Radioactive Substance K Other Diagnostic Substance N Analgesics, Hypnotics, Sedatives T Destructive Agent	Z No Qualifier
1 Subcutaneous Tissue	3 Percutaneous	G Other Therapeutic Substance	C Other Substance
1 Subcutaneous Tissue	3 Percutaneous	V Hormone	G Insulin J Other Hormone
2 Muscle	3 Percutaneous	0 Antineoplastic	5 Other Antineoplastic M Monoclonal Antibody
2 Muscle	3 Percutaneous	2 Anti-infective	8 Oxazolidinones 9 Other Anti-infective

Section	3	Administration
Body System	E	Physiological Systems and Anatomical Regions
Operation	0	Introduction: Putting in or on a therapeutic, diagnostic, nutritional, physiological, or prophylactic substance except blood or blood products

Body System/Region (Character 4)	Approach (Character 5)	Substance (Character 6)	Qualifier (Character 7)
2 Muscle	3 Percutaneous	3 Anti-inflammatory 4 Serum, Toxoid and Vaccine 6 Nutritional Substance 7 Electrolytic and Water Balance Substance B Local Anesthetic H Radioactive Substance K Other Diagnostic Substance N Analgesics, Hypnotics, Sedatives T Destructive Agent	Z No Qualifier
2 Muscle	3 Percutaneous	G Other Therapeutic Substance	C Other Substance
3 Peripheral Vein	0 Open	0 Antineoplastic	2 High-dose Interleukin-2 3 Low-dose Interleukin-2 5 Other Antineoplastic M Monoclonal Antibody P Clofarabine
3 Peripheral Vein	0 Open	1 Thrombolytic	6 Recombinant Human-activated Protein C 7 Other Thrombolytic
3 Peripheral Vein	0 Open	2 Anti-infective	8 Oxazolidinones 9 Other Anti-infective
3 Peripheral Vein	0 Open	3 Anti-inflammatory 4 Serum, Toxoid and Vaccine 6 Nutritional Substance 7 Electrolytic and Water Balance Substance F Intracirculatory Anesthetic H Radioactive Substance K Other Diagnostic Substance N Analgesics, Hypnotics, Sedatives P Platelet Inhibitor R Antiarrhythmic T Destructive Agent X Vasopressor	Z No Qualifier
3 Peripheral Vein	0 Open	G Other Therapeutic Substance	C Other Substance N Blood Brain Barrier Disruption
3 Peripheral Vein	0 Open	U Pancreatic Islet Cells	0 Autologous 1 Nonautologous

Section	3	Administration
Body System	E	Physiological Systems and Anatomical Regions
Operation	0	Introduction: Putting in or on a therapeutic, diagnostic, nutritional, physiological, or prophylactic substance except blood or blood products

Body System/Region (Character 4)	Approach (Character 5)	Substance (Character 6)	Qualifier (Character 7)
3 Peripheral Vein	0 Open	V Hormone	G Insulin H Human B-Type Natriuretic Peptide J Other Hormone
3 Peripheral Vein	0 Open	W Immunotherapeutic	K Immunostimulator L Immunosuppressive
3 Peripheral Vein	3 Percutaneous	0 Antineoplastic	2 High-dose Interleukin-2 3 Low-dose Interleukin-2 5 Other Antineoplastic M Monoclonal Antibody P Clofarabine
3 Peripheral Vein	3 Percutaneous	1 Thrombolytic	6 Recombinant Human-activated Protein C 7 Other Thrombolytic
3 Peripheral Vein	3 Percutaneous	2 Anti-infective	8 Oxazolidinones 9 Other Anti-infective
3 Peripheral Vein	3 Percutaneous	3 Anti-inflammatory 4 Serum, Toxoid and Vaccine 6 Nutritional Substance 7 Electrolytic and Water Balance Substance F Intracirculatory Anesthetic H Radioactive Substance K Other Diagnostic Substance N Analgesics, Hypnotics, Sedatives P Platelet Inhibitor R Antiarrhythmic T Destructive Agent X Vasopressor	Z No Qualifier
3 Peripheral Vein	3 Percutaneous	G Other Therapeutic Substance	C Other Substance N Blood Brain Barrier Disruption Q Glucarpidase
3 Peripheral Vein	3 Percutaneous	U Pancreatic Islet Cells	0 Autologous 1 Nonautologous
3 Peripheral Vein	3 Percutaneous	V Hormone	G Insulin H Human B-Type Natriuretic Peptide J Other Hormone
3 Peripheral Vein	3 Percutaneous	W Immunotherapeutic	K Immunostimulator L Immunosuppressive

Section	3	Administration		
Body System	E	Physiological Systems and Anatomical Regions		
Operation	0	Introduction: Putting in or on a therapeutic, diagnostic, nutritional, physiological, or prophylactic substance except blood or blood products		

Body System/Region (Character 4)	Approach (Character 5)	Substance (Character 6)	Qualifier (Character 7)
4 Central Vein	0 Open	0 Antineoplastic	2 High-dose Interleukin-2 3 Low-dose Interleukin-2 5 Other Antineoplastic M Monoclonal Antibody P Clofarabine
4 Central Vein	0 Open	1 Thrombolytic	6 Recombinant Human-activated Protein C 7 Other Thrombolytic
4 Central Vein	0 Open	2 Anti-infective	8 Oxazolidinones 9 Other Anti-infective
4 Central Vein	0 Open	3 Anti-inflammatory 4 Serum, Toxoid and Vaccine 6 Nutritional Substance 7 Electrolytic and Water Balance Substance F Intracirculatory Anesthetic H Radioactive Substance K Other Diagnostic Substance N Analgesics, Hypnotics, Sedatives P Platelet Inhibitor R Antiarrhythmic T Destructive Agent X Vasopressor	Z No Qualifier
4 Central Vein	0 Open	G Other Therapeutic Substance	C Other Substance N Blood Brain Barrier Disruption
4 Central Vein	0 Open	V Hormone	G Insulin H Human B-Type Natriuretic Peptide J Other Hormone
4 Central Vein	0 Open	W Immunotherapeutic	K Immunostimulator L Immunosuppressive
4 Central Vein	3 Percutaneous	0 Antineoplastic	2 High-dose Interleukin-2 3 Low-dose Interleukin-2 5 Other Antineoplastic M Monoclonal Antibody P Clofarabine
4 Central Vein	3 Percutaneous	1 Thrombolytic	6 Recombinant Human-activated Protein C 7 Other Thrombolytic

Section	3	Administration
Body System	E	Physiological Systems and Anatomical Regions
Operation	0	Introduction: Putting in or on a therapeutic, diagnostic, nutritional, physiological, or prophylactic substance except blood or blood products

Body System/Region (Character 4)	Approach (Character 5)	Substance (Character 6)	Qualifier (Character 7)
4 Central Vein	3 Percutaneous	2 Anti-infective	8 Oxazolidinones 9 Other Anti-infective
4 Central Vein	3 Percutaneous	3 Anti-inflammatory 4 Serum, Toxoid and Vaccine 6 Nutritional Substance 7 Electrolytic and Water Balance Substance F Intracirculatory Anesthetic H Radioactive Substance K Other Diagnostic Substance N Analgesics, Hypnotics, Sedatives P Platelet Inhibitor R Antiarrhythmic T Destructive Agent X Vasopressor	Z No Qualifier
4 Central Vein	3 Percutaneous	G Other Therapeutic Substance	C Other Substance N Blood Brain Barrier Disruption Q Glucarpidase
4 Central Vein	3 Percutaneous	V Hormone	G Insulin H Human B-Type Natriuretic Peptide J Other Hormone
4 Central Vein	3 Percutaneous	W Immunotherapeutic	K Immunostimulator L Immunosuppressive
5 Peripheral Artery 6 Central Artery	0 Open 3 Percutaneous	0 Antineoplastic	2 High-dose Interleukin-2 3 Low-dose Interleukin-2 5 Other Antineoplastic M Monoclonal Antibody P Clofarabine
5 Peripheral Artery 6 Central Artery	0 Open 3 Percutaneous	1 Thrombolytic	6 Recombinant Human-activated Protein C 7 Other Thrombolytic
5 Peripheral Artery 6 Central Artery	0 Open 3 Percutaneous	2 Anti-infective	8 Oxazolidinones 9 Other Anti-infective

Section	3	Administration
Body System	E	Physiological Systems and Anatomical Regions
Operation	0	Introduction: Putting in or on a therapeutic, diagnostic, nutritional, physiological, or prophylactic substance except blood or blood products

Body System/Region (Character 4)	Approach (Character 5)	Substance (Character 6)	Qualifier (Character 7)
5 Peripheral Artery 6 Central Artery	0 Open 3 Percutaneous	3 Anti-inflammatory 4 Serum, Toxoid and Vaccine 6 Nutritional Substance 7 Electrolytic and Water Balance Substance F Intracirculatory Anesthetic H Radioactive Substance K Other Diagnostic Substance N Analgesics, Hypnotics, Sedatives P Platelet Inhibitor R Antiarrhythmic T Destructive Agent X Vasopressor	Z No Qualifier
5 Peripheral Artery 6 Central Artery	0 Open 3 Percutaneous	G Other Therapeutic Substance	C Other Substance N Blood Brain Barrier Disruption
5 Peripheral Artery 6 Central Artery	0 Open 3 Percutaneous	V Hormone	G Insulin H Human B-Type Natriuretic Peptide J Other Hormone
5 Peripheral Artery 6 Central Artery	0 Open 3 Percutaneous	W Immunotherapeutic	K Immunostimulator L Immunosuppressive
7 Coronary Artery 8 Heart	0 Open 3 Percutaneous	1 Thrombolytic	6 Recombinant Human-activated Protein C 7 Other Thrombolytic
7 Coronary Artery 8 Heart	0 Open 3 Percutaneous	G Other Therapeutic Substance	C Other Substance
7 Coronary Artery 8 Heart	0 Open 3 Percutaneous	K Other Diagnostic Substance P Platelet Inhibitor	Z No Qualifier
9 Nose	3 Percutaneous 7 Via Natural or Artificial Opening X External	0 Antineoplastic	5 Other Antineoplastic M Monoclonal Antibody
9 Nose	3 Percutaneous 7 Via Natural or Artificial Opening X External	2 Anti-infective	8 Oxazolidinones 9 Other Anti-infective

Section	3	Administration		
Body System	E	Physiological Systems and Anatomical Regions		
Operation	0	Introduction: Putting in or on a therapeutic, diagnostic, nutritional, physiological, or prophylactic substance except blood or blood products		

Body System/Region (Character 4)	Approach (Character 5)	Substance (Character 6)	Qualifier (Character 7)
9 Nose	3 Percutaneous 7 Via Natural or Artificial Opening X External	3 Anti-inflammatory 4 Serum, Toxoid and Vaccine B Local Anesthetic H Radioactive Substance K Other Diagnostic Substance N Analgesics, Hypnotics, Sedatives T Destructive Agent	Z No Qualifier
9 Nose	3 Percutaneous 7 Via Natural or Artificial Opening X External	G Other Therapeutic Substance	C Other Substance
A Bone Marrow	3 Percutaneous	0 Antineoplastic	5 Other Antineoplastic M Monoclonal Antibody
A Bone Marrow	3 Percutaneous	G Other Therapeutic Substance	C Other Substance
B Ear	3 Percutaneous 7 Via Natural or Artificial Opening X External	0 Antineoplastic	4 Liquid Brachytherapy Radioisotope 5 Other Antineoplastic M Monoclonal Antibody
B Ear	3 Percutaneous 7 Via Natural or Artificial Opening X External	2 Anti-infective	8 Oxazolidinones 9 Other Anti-infective
B Ear	3 Percutaneous 7 Via Natural or Artificial Opening X External	3 Anti-inflammatory B Local Anesthetic H Radioactive Substance K Other Diagnostic Substance N Analgesics, Hypnotics, Sedatives T Destructive Agent	Z No Qualifier
B Ear	3 Percutaneous 7 Via Natural or Artificial Opening X External	G Other Therapeutic Substance	C Other Substance
C Eye	3 Percutaneous 7 Via Natural or Artificial Opening X External	0 Antineoplastic	4 Liquid Brachytherapy Radioisotope 5 Other Antineoplastic M Monoclonal Antibody
C Eye	3 Percutaneous 7 Via Natural or Artificial Opening X External	2 Anti-infective	8 Oxazolidinones 9 Other Anti-infective

Section	3	Administration
Body System	E	Physiological Systems and Anatomical Regions
Operation	0	Introduction: Putting in or on a therapeutic, diagnostic, nutritional, physiological, or prophylactic substance except blood or blood products

Body System/Region (Character 4)	Approach (Character 5)	Substance (Character 6)	Qualifier (Character 7)
C Eye	3 Percutaneous 7 Via Natural or Artificial Opening X External	3 Anti-inflammatory B Local Anesthetic H Radioactive Substance K Other Diagnostic Substance M Pigment N Analgesics, Hypnotics, Sedatives T Destructive Agent	Z No Qualifier
C Eye	3 Percutaneous 7 Via Natural or Artificial Opening X External	G Other Therapeutic Substance	C Other Substance
C Eye	3 Percutaneous 7 Via Natural or Artificial Opening X External	S Gas	F Other Gas
D Mouth and Pharynx	3 Percutaneous 7 Via Natural or Artificial Opening X External	0 Antineoplastic	4 Liquid Brachytherapy Radioisotope 5 Other Antineoplastic M Monoclonal Antibody
D Mouth and Pharynx	3 Percutaneous 7 Via Natural or Artificial Opening X External	2 Anti-infective	8 Oxazolidinones 9 Other Anti-infective
D Mouth and Pharynx	3 Percutaneous 7 Via Natural or Artificial Opening X External	3 Anti-inflammatory 4 Serum, Toxoid and Vaccine 6 Nutritional Substance 7 Electrolytic and Water Balance Substance B Local Anesthetic H Radioactive Substance K Other Diagnostic Substance N Analgesics, Hypnotics, Sedatives R Antiarrhythmic T Destructive Agent	Z No Qualifier
D Mouth and Pharynx	3 Percutaneous 7 Via Natural or Artificial Opening X External	G Other Therapeutic Substance	C Other Substance

Section	3	Administration
Body System	E	Physiological Systems and Anatomical Regions
Operation	0	Introduction: Putting in or on a therapeutic, diagnostic, nutritional, physiological, or prophylactic substance except blood or blood products

Body System/Region (Character 4)	Approach (Character 5)	Substance (Character 6)	Qualifier (Character 7)
E Products of Conception G Upper GI H Lower GI K Genitourinary Tract N Male Reproductive	3 Percutaneous 7 Via Natural or Artificial Opening 8 Via Natural or Artificial Opening Endoscopic	0 Antineoplastic	4 Liquid Brachytherapy Radioisotope 5 Other Antineoplastic M Monoclonal Antibody
E Products of Conception G Upper GI H Lower GI K Genitourinary Tract N Male Reproductive	3 Percutaneous 7 Via Natural or Artificial Opening 8 Via Natural or Artificial Opening Endoscopic	2 Anti-infective	8 Oxazolidinones 9 Other Anti-infective
E Products of Conception G Upper GI H Lower GI K Genitourinary Tract N Male Reproductive	3 Percutaneous 7 Via Natural or Artificial Opening 8 Via Natural or Artificial Opening Endoscopic	3 Anti-inflammatory 6 Nutritional Substance 7 Electrolytic and Water Balance Substance B Local Anesthetic H Radioactive Substance K Other Diagnostic Substance N Analgesics, Hypnotics, Sedatives T Destructive Agent	Z No Qualifier
E Products of Conception G Upper GI H Lower GI K Genitourinary Tract N Male Reproductive	3 Percutaneous 7 Via Natural or Artificial Opening 8 Via Natural or Artificial Opening Endoscopic	G Other Therapeutic Substance	C Other Substance
E Products of Conception G Upper GI H Lower GI K Genitourinary Tract N Male Reproductive	3 Percutaneous 7 Via Natural or Artificial Opening 8 Via Natural or Artificial Opening Endoscopic	S Gas	F Other Gas
F Respiratory Tract	3 Percutaneous	0 Antineoplastic	4 Liquid Brachytherapy Radioisotope 5 Other Antineoplastic M Monoclonal Antibody
F Respiratory Tract	3 Percutaneous	2 Anti-infective	8 Oxazolidinones 9 Other Anti-infective

Section	3	Administration
Body System	E	Physiological Systems and Anatomical Regions
Operation	0	Introduction: Putting in or on a therapeutic, diagnostic, nutritional, physiological, or prophylactic substance except blood or blood products

Body System/Region (Character 4)	Approach (Character 5)	Substance (Character 6)	Qualifier (Character 7)
F Respiratory Tract	3 Percutaneous	3 Anti-inflammatory 6 Nutritional Substance 7 Electrolytic and Water Balance Substance B Local Anesthetic H Radioactive Substance K Other Diagnostic Substance N Analgesics, Hypnotics, Sedatives T Destructive Agent	Z No Qualifier
F Respiratory Tract	3 Percutaneous	G Other Therapeutic Substance	C Other Substance
F Respiratory Tract	3 Percutaneous	S Gas	D Nitric Oxide F Other Gas
F Respiratory Tract	7 Via Natural or Artificial Opening 8 Via Natural or Artificial Opening Endoscopic	0 Antineoplastic	4 Liquid Brachytherapy Radioisotope 5 Other Antineoplastic M Monoclonal Antibody
F Respiratory Tract	7 Via Natural or Artificial Opening 8 Via Natural or Artificial Opening Endoscopic	2 Anti-infective	8 Oxazolidinones 9 Other Anti-infective
F Respiratory Tract	7 Via Natural or Artificial Opening 8 Via Natural or Artificial Opening Endoscopic	3 Anti-inflammatory 6 Nutritional Substance 7 Electrolytic and Water Balance Substance B Local Anesthetic D Inhalation Anesthetic H Radioactive Substance K Other Diagnostic Substance N Analgesics, Hypnotics, Sedatives T Destructive Agent	Z No Qualifier
F Respiratory Tract	7 Via Natural or Artificial Opening 8 Via Natural or Artificial Opening Endoscopic	G Other Therapeutic Substance	C Other Substance
F Respiratory Tract	7 Via Natural or Artificial Opening 8 Via Natural or Artificial Opening Endoscopic	S Gas	D Nitric Oxide F Other Gas
J Biliary and Pancreatic Tract	3 Percutaneous 7 Via Natural or Artificial Opening 8 Via Natural or Artificial Opening Endoscopic	0 Antineoplastic	4 Liquid Brachytherapy Radioisotope 5 Other Antineoplastic M Monoclonal Antibody
J Biliary and Pancreatic Tract	3 Percutaneous 7 Via Natural or Artificial Opening 8 Via Natural or Artificial Opening Endoscopic	2 Anti-infective	8 Oxazolidinones 9 Other Anti-infective

Section	3	Administration
Body System	E	Physiological Systems and Anatomical Regions
Operation	0	Introduction: Putting in or on a therapeutic, diagnostic, nutritional, physiological, or prophylactic substance except blood or blood products

Body System/Region (Character 4)	Approach (Character 5)	Substance (Character 6)	Qualifier (Character 7)
J Biliary and Pancreatic Tract	3 Percutaneous 7 Via Natural or Artificial Opening 8 Via Natural or Artificial Opening Endoscopic	3 Anti-inflammatory 6 Nutritional Substance 7 Electrolytic and Water Balance Substance B Local Anesthetic H Radioactive Substance K Other Diagnostic Substance N Analgesics, Hypnotics, Sedatives T Destructive Agent	Z No Qualifier
J Biliary and Pancreatic Tract	3 Percutaneous 7 Via Natural or Artificial Opening 8 Via Natural or Artificial Opening Endoscopic	G Other Therapeutic Substance	C Other Substance
J Biliary and Pancreatic Tract	3 Percutaneous 7 Via Natural or Artificial Opening 8 Via Natural or Artificial Opening Endoscopic	S Gas	F Other Gas
J Biliary and Pancreatic Tract	3 Percutaneous 7 Via Natural or Artificial Opening 8 Via Natural or Artificial Opening Endoscopic	U Pancreatic Islet Cells	0 Autologous 1 Nonautologous
L Pleural Cavity M Peritoneal Cavity	0 Open	5 Adhesion Barrier	Z No Qualifier
L Pleural Cavity M Peritoneal Cavity	3 Percutaneous	0 Antineoplastic	4 Liquid Brachytherapy Radioisotope 5 Other Antineoplastic M Monoclonal Antibody
L Pleural Cavity M Peritoneal Cavity	3 Percutaneous	2 Anti-infective	8 Oxazolidinones 9 Other Anti-infective
L Pleural Cavity M Peritoneal Cavity	3 Percutaneous	3 Anti-inflammatory 6 Nutritional Substance 7 Electrolytic and Water Balance Substance B Local Anesthetic H Radioactive Substance K Other Diagnostic Substance N Analgesics, Hypnotics, Sedatives T Destructive Agent	Z No Qualifier
L Pleural Cavity M Peritoneal Cavity	3 Percutaneous	G Other Therapeutic Substance	C Other Substance
L Pleural Cavity M Peritoneal Cavity	3 Percutaneous	S Gas	F Other Gas

Section	3	Administration
Body System	E	Physiological Systems and Anatomical Regions
Operation	0	Introduction: Putting in or on a therapeutic, diagnostic, nutritional, physiological, or prophylactic substance except blood or blood products

Body System/Region (Character 4)	Approach (Character 5)	Substance (Character 6)	Qualifier (Character 7)
L Pleural Cavity M Peritoneal Cavity	7 Via Natural or Artificial Opening	0 Antineoplastic	4 Liquid Brachytherapy Radioisotope 5 Other Antineoplastic M Monoclonal Antibody
L Pleural Cavity M Peritoneal Cavity	7 Via Natural or Artificial Opening	S Gas	F Other Gas
P Female Reproductive	0 Open	5 Adhesion Barrier	Z No Qualifier
P Female Reproductive	3 Percutaneous 7 Via Natural or Artificial Opening	0 Antineoplastic	4 Liquid Brachytherapy Radioisotope 5 Other Antineoplastic M Monoclonal Antibody
P Female Reproductive	3 Percutaneous 7 Via Natural or Artificial Opening	2 Anti-infective	8 Oxazolidinones 9 Other Anti-infective
P Female Reproductive	3 Percutaneous 7 Via Natural or Artificial Opening	3 Anti-inflammatory 6 Nutritional Substance 7 Electrolytic and Water Balance Substance B Local Anesthetic H Radioactive Substance K Other Diagnostic Substance L Sperm N Analgesics, Hypnotics, Sedatives T Destructive Agent	Z No Qualifier
P Female Reproductive	3 Percutaneous 7 Via Natural or Artificial Opening	G Other Therapeutic Substance	C Other Substance
P Female Reproductive	3 Percutaneous 7 Via Natural or Artificial Opening	Q Fertilized Ovum	0 Autologous 1 Nonautologous
P Female Reproductive	3 Percutaneous 7 Via Natural or Artificial Opening	S Gas	F Other Gas
P Female Reproductive	8 Via Natural or Artificial Opening Endoscopic	0 Antineoplastic	4 Liquid Brachytherapy Radioisotope 5 Other Antineoplastic M Monoclonal Antibody
P Female Reproductive	8 Via Natural or Artificial Opening Endoscopic	2 Anti-infective	8 Oxazolidinones 9 Other Anti-infective

Section	3	Administration		
Body System	E	Physiological Systems and Anatomical Regions		
Operation	0	Introduction: Putting in or on a therapeutic, diagnostic, nutritional, physiological, or prophylactic substance except blood or blood products		

Body System/Region (Character 4)	Approach (Character 5)	Substance (Character 6)	Qualifier (Character 7)
P Female Reproductive	8 Via Natural or Artificial Opening Endoscopic	3 Anti-inflammatory 6 Nutritional Substance 7 Electrolytic and Water Balance Substance B Local Anesthetic H Radioactive Substance K Other Diagnostic Substance N Analgesics, Hypnotics, Sedatives T Destructive Agent	Z No Qualifier
P Female Reproductive	8 Via Natural or Artificial Opening Endoscopic	G Other Therapeutic Substance	C Other Substance
P Female Reproductive	8 Via Natural or Artificial Opening Endoscopic	S Gas	F Other Gas
Q Cranial Cavity and Brain	0 Open	A Stem Cells, Embryonic	Z No Qualifier
Q Cranial Cavity and Brain	0 Open	E Stem Cells, Somatic	0 Autologous 1 Nonautologous
Q Cranial Cavity and Brain	3 Percutaneous	0 Antineoplastic	4 Liquid Brachytherapy Radioisotope 5 Other Antineoplastic M Monoclonal Antibody
Q Cranial Cavity and Brain	3 Percutaneous	2 Anti-infective	8 Oxazolidinones 9 Other Anti-infective
Q Cranial Cavity and Brain	3 Percutaneous	3 Anti-inflammatory 6 Nutritional Substance 7 Electrolytic and Water Balance Substance A Stem Cells, Embryonic B Local Anesthetic H Radioactive Substance K Other Diagnostic Substance N Analgesics, Hypnotics, Sedatives T Destructive Agent	Z No Qualifier
Q Cranial Cavity and Brain	3 Percutaneous	E Stem Cells, Somatic	0 Autologous 1 Nonautologous
Q Cranial Cavity and Brain	3 Percutaneous	G Other Therapeutic Substance	C Other Substance
Q Cranial Cavity and Brain	3 Percutaneous	S Gas	F Other Gas
Q Cranial Cavity and Brain	7 Via Natural or Artificial Opening	0 Antineoplastic	4 Liquid Brachytherapy Radioisotope 5 Other Antineoplastic M Monoclonal Antibody
Q Cranial Cavity and Brain	7 Via Natural or Artificial Opening	S Gas	F Other Gas
R Spinal Canal	0 Open	A Stem Cells, Embryonic	Z No Qualifier

Section	3	Administration		
Body System	E	Physiological Systems and Anatomical Regions		
Operation	0	Introduction: Putting in or on a therapeutic, diagnostic, nutritional, physiological, or prophylactic substance except blood or blood products		

Body System/Region (Character 4)	Approach (Character 5)	Substance (Character 6)	Qualifier (Character 7)
R Spinal Canal	0 Open	E Stem Cells, Somatic	0 Autologous 1 Nonautologous
R Spinal Canal	3 Percutaneous	0 Antineoplastic	2 High-dose Interleukin-2 3 Low-dose Interleukin-2 4 Liquid Brachytherapy Radioisotope 5 Other Antineoplastic M Monoclonal Antibody
R Spinal Canal	3 Percutaneous	2 Anti-infective	8 Oxazolidinones 9 Other Anti-infective
R Spinal Canal	3 Percutaneous	3 Anti-inflammatory 6 Nutritional Substance 7 Electrolytic and Water Balance Substance A Stem Cells, Embryonic B Local Anesthetic C Regional Anesthetic H Radioactive Substance K Other Diagnostic Substance N Analgesics, Hypnotics, Sedatives T Destructive Agent	Z No Qualifier
R Spinal Canal	3 Percutaneous	E Stem Cells, Somatic	0 Autologous 1 Nonautologous
R Spinal Canal	3 Percutaneous	G Other Therapeutic Substance	C Other Substance
R Spinal Canal	3 Percutaneous	S Gas	F Other Gas
R Spinal Canal	7 Via Natural or Artificial Opening	S Gas	F Other Gas
S Epidural Space	3 Percutaneous	0 Antineoplastic	2 High-dose Interleukin-2 3 Low-dose Interleukin-2 4 Liquid Brachytherapy Radioisotope 5 Other Antineoplastic M Monoclonal Antibody
S Epidural Space	3 Percutaneous	2 Anti-infective	8 Oxazolidinones 9 Other Anti-infective

Section	3	Administration
Body System	E	Physiological Systems and Anatomical Regions
Operation	0	Introduction: Putting in or on a therapeutic, diagnostic, nutritional, physiological, or prophylactic substance except blood or blood products

Body System/Region (Character 4)	Approach (Character 5)	Substance (Character 6)	Qualifier (Character 7)
S Epidural Space	3 Percutaneous	3 Anti-inflammatory 6 Nutritional Substance 7 Electrolytic and Water Balance Substance B Local Anesthetic C Regional Anesthetic H Radioactive Substance K Other Diagnostic Substance N Analgesics, Hypnotics, Sedatives T Destructive Agent	Z No Qualifier
S Epidural Space	3 Percutaneous	G Other Therapeutic Substance	C Other Substance
S Epidural Space	3 Percutaneous	S Gas	F Other Gas
S Epidural Space	7 Via Natural or Artificial Opening	S Gas	F Other Gas
T Peripheral Nerves and Plexi X Cranial Nerves	3 Percutaneous	3 Anti-inflammatory B Local Anesthetic C Regional Anesthetic T Destructive Agent	Z No Qualifier
T Peripheral Nerves and Plexi X Cranial Nerves	3 Percutaneous	G Other Therapeutic Substance	C Other Substance
U Joints	0 Open	2 Anti-infective	8 Oxazolidinones 9 Other Anti-infective
U Joints	0 Open	G Other Therapeutic Substance	B Recombinant Bone Morphogenetic Protein
U Joints	3 Percutaneous	0 Antineoplastic	4 Liquid Brachytherapy Radioisotope 5 Other Antineoplastic M Monoclonal Antibody
U Joints	3 Percutaneous	2 Anti-infective	8 Oxazolidinones 9 Other Anti-infective
U Joints	3 Percutaneous	3 Anti-inflammatory 6 Nutritional Substance 7 Electrolytic and Water Balance Substance B Local Anesthetic H Radioactive Substance K Other Diagnostic Substance N Analgesics, Hypnotics, Sedatives T Destructive Agent	Z No Qualifier
U Joints	3 Percutaneous	G Other Therapeutic Substance	B Recombinant Bone Morphogenetic Protein C Other Substance

Section	3	Administration
Body System	E	Physiological Systems and Anatomical Regions
Operation	0	Introduction: Putting in or on a therapeutic, diagnostic, nutritional, physiological, or prophylactic substance except blood or blood products

Body System/Region (Character 4)	Approach (Character 5)	Substance (Character 6)	Qualifier (Character 7)
U Joints	**3** Percutaneous	**S** Gas	**F** Other Gas
V Bones	**0** Open	**G** Other Therapeutic Substance	**B** Recombinant Bone Morphogenetic Protein
V Bones	**3** Percutaneous	**0** Antineoplastic	**5** Other Antineoplastic **M** Monoclonal Antibody
V Bones	**3** Percutaneous	**2** Anti-infective	**8** Oxazolidinones **9** Other Anti-infective
V Bones	**3** Percutaneous	**3** Anti-inflammatory **6** Nutritional Substance **7** Electrolytic and Water Balance Substance **B** Local Anesthetic **H** Radioactive Substance **K** Other Diagnostic Substance **N** Analgesics, Hypnotics, Sedatives **T** Destructive Agent	**Z** No Qualifier
V Bones	**3** Percutaneous	**G** Other Therapeutic Substance	**B** Recombinant Bone Morphogenetic Protein **C** Other Substance
W Lymphatics	**3** Percutaneous	**0** Antineoplastic	**5** Other Antineoplastic **M** Monoclonal Antibody
W Lymphatics	**3** Percutaneous	**2** Anti-infective	**8** Oxazolidinones **9** Other Anti-infective
W Lymphatics	**3** Percutaneous	**3** Anti-inflammatory **6** Nutritional Substance **7** Electrolytic and Water Balance Substance **B** Local Anesthetic **H** Radioactive Substance **K** Other Diagnostic Substance **N** Analgesics, Hypnotics, Sedatives **T** Destructive Agent	**Z** No Qualifier
W Lymphatics	**3** Percutaneous	**G** Other Therapeutic Substance	**C** Other Substance
Y Pericardial Cavity	**3** Percutaneous	**0** Antineoplastic	**4** Liquid Brachytherapy Radioisotope **5** Other Antineoplastic **M** Monoclonal Antibody
Y Pericardial Cavity	**3** Percutaneous	**2** Anti-infective	**8** Oxazolidinones **9** Other Anti-infective

Section	3	Administration
Body System	E	Physiological Systems and Anatomical Regions
Operation	0	Introduction: Putting in or on a therapeutic, diagnostic, nutritional, physiological, or prophylactic substance except blood or blood products

Body System/Region (Character 4)	Approach (Character 5)	Substance (Character 6)	Qualifier (Character 7)
Y Pericardial Cavity	3 Percutaneous	3 Anti-inflammatory 6 Nutritional Substance 7 Electrolytic and Water Balance Substance B Local Anesthetic H Radioactive Substance K Other Diagnostic Substance N Analgesics, Hypnotics, Sedatives T Destructive Agent	Z No Qualifier
Y Pericardial Cavity	3 Percutaneous	G Other Therapeutic Substance	C Other Substance
Y Pericardial Cavity	3 Percutaneous	S Gas	F Other Gas
Y Pericardial Cavity	7 Via Natural or Artificial Opening	0 Antineoplastic	4 Liquid Brachytherapy Radioisotope 5 Other Antineoplastic M Monoclonal Antibody
Y Pericardial Cavity	7 Via Natural or Artificial Opening	S Gas	F Other Gas

Section	3	Administration
Body System	E	Physiological Systems and Anatomical Regions
Operation	1	Irrigation: Putting in or on a cleansing substance

Body System/Region (Character 4)	Approach (Character 5)	Substance (Character 6)	Qualifier (Character 7)
0 Skin and Mucous Membranes C Eye	3 Percutaneous X External	8 Irrigating Substance	X Diagnostic Z No Qualifier
9 Nose B Ear F Respiratory Tract G Upper GI H Lower GI J Biliary and Pancreatic Tract K Genitourinary Tract N Male Reproductive P Female Reproductive	3 Percutaneous 7 Via Natural or Artificial Opening 8 Via Natural or Artificial Opening Endoscopic	8 Irrigating Substance	X Diagnostic Z No Qualifier
L Pleural Cavity Q Cranial Cavity and Brain R Spinal Canal S Epidural Space U Joints Y Pericardial Cavity	3 Percutaneous	8 Irrigating Substance	X Diagnostic Z No Qualifier
M Peritoneal Cavity	3 Percutaneous	8 Irrigating Substance	X Diagnostic Z No Qualifier
M Peritoneal Cavity	3 Percutaneous	9 Dialysate	Z No Qualifier

Section	4	Measurement and Monitoring
Body System	A	Physiological Systems
Operation	0	Measurement: Determining the level of a physiological or physical function at a point in time

Body System (Character 4)	Approach (Character 5)	Function/Device (Character 6)	Qualifier (Character 7)
0 Central Nervous	**0** Open	**2** Conductivity **4** Electrical Activity **B** Pressure	**Z** No Qualifier
0 Central Nervous	**3** Percutaneous	**4** Electrical Activity	**Z** No Qualifier
0 Central Nervous	**3** Percutaneous	**B** Pressure **K** Temperature **R** Saturation	**D** Intracranial
0 Central Nervous	**7** Via Natural or Artificial Opening	**B** Pressure **K** Temperature **R** Saturation	**D** Intracranial
0 Central Nervous	**X** External	**2** Conductivity **4** Electrical Activity	**Z** No Qualifier
1 Peripheral Nervous	**0** Open **3** Percutaneous **X** External	**2** Conductivity	**9** Sensory **B** Motor
1 Peripheral Nervous	**0** Open **3** Percutaneous **X** External	**4** Electrical Activity	**Z** No Qualifier
2 Cardiac	**0** Open **3** Percutaneous	**4** Electrical Activity **9** Output **C** Rate **F** Rhythm **H** Sound **P** Action Currents	**Z** No Qualifier
2 Cardiac	**0** Open **3** Percutaneous	**N** Sampling and Pressure	**6** Right Heart **7** Left Heart **8** Bilateral
2 Cardiac	**X** External	**4** Electrical Activity	**A** Guidance **Z** No Qualifier
2 Cardiac	**X** External	**9** Output **C** Rate **F** Rhythm **H** Sound **P** Action Currents	**Z** No Qualifier
2 Cardiac	**X** External	**M** Total Activity	**4** Stress
3 Arterial	**0** Open **3** Percutaneous	**5** Flow **J** Pulse	**1** Peripheral **3** Pulmonary **C** Coronary
3 Arterial	**0** Open **3** Percutaneous	**B** Pressure	**1** Peripheral **3** Pulmonary **C** Coronary **F** Other Thoracic
3 Arterial	**0** Open **3** Percutaneous	**H** Sound **R** Saturation	**1** Peripheral
3 Arterial	**X** External	**5** Flow **B** Pressure **H** Sound **J** Pulse **R** Saturation	**1** Peripheral
4 Venous	**0** Open **3** Percutaneous	**5** Flow **B** Pressure **J** Pulse	**0** Central **1** Peripheral **2** Portal **3** Pulmonary
4 Venous	**0** Open **3** Percutaneous	**R** Saturation	**1** Peripheral
4 Venous	**X** External	**5** Flow **B** Pressure **J** Pulse **R** Saturation	**1** Peripheral
5 Circulatory	**X** External	**L** Volume	**Z** No Qualifier
6 Lymphatic	**0** Open **3** Percutaneous	**5** Flow **B** Pressure	**Z** No Qualifier
7 Visual	**X** External	**0** Acuity **7** Mobility **B** Pressure	**Z** No Qualifier
8 Olfactory	**X** External	**0** Acuity	**Z** No Qualifier

Section	4	Measurement and Monitoring	
Body System	A	Physiological Systems	[continued]
Operation	0	Measurement: Determining the level of a physiological or physical function at a point in time	

Body System (Character 4)	Approach (Character 5)	Function/Device (Character 6)	Qualifier (Character 7)
9 Respiratory	7 Via Natural or Artificial Opening 8 Via Natural or Artificial Opening Endoscopic X External	1 Capacity 5 Flow C Rate D Resistance L Volume M Total Activity	Z No Qualifier
B Gastrointestinal	7 Via Natural or Artificial Opening 8 Via Natural or Artificial Opening Endoscopic	8 Motility B Pressure G Secretion	Z No Qualifier
C Biliary	3 Percutaneous 4 Percutaneous Endoscopic 7 Via Natural or Artificial Opening 8 Via Natural or Artificial Opening Endoscopic	5 Flow B Pressure	Z No Qualifier
D Urinary	7 Via Natural or Artificial Opening	3 Contractility 5 Flow B Pressure D Resistance L Volume	Z No Qualifier
F Musculoskeletal	3 Percutaneous X External	3 Contractility	Z No Qualifier
H Products of Conception, Cardiac	7 Via Natural or Artificial Opening 8 Via Natural or Artificial Opening Endoscopic X External	4 Electrical Activity C Rate F Rhythm H Sound	Z No Qualifier
J Products of Conception, Nervous	7 Via Natural or Artificial Opening 8 Via Natural or Artificial Opening Endoscopic X External	2 Conductivity 4 Electrical Activity B Pressure	Z No Qualifier
Z None	7 Via Natural or Artificial Opening	6 Metabolism K Temperature	Z No Qualifier
Z None	X External	6 Metabolism K Temperature Q Sleep	Z No Qualifier

Section	4	Measurement and Monitoring
Body System	A	Physiological Systems
Operation	1	Monitoring Determining the level of a physiological or physical function repetitively over a period of time

Body System (Character 4)	Approach (Character 5)	Function/Device (Character 6)	Qualifier (Character 7)
0 Central Nervous	0 Open	2 Conductivity B Pressure	Z No Qualifier
0 Central Nervous	0 Open	4 Electrical Activity	G Intraoperative Z No Qualifier
0 Central Nervous	3 Percutaneous	4 Electrical Activity	G Intraoperative Z No Qualifier
0 Central Nervous	3 Percutaneous	B Pressure K Temperature R Saturation	D Intracranial
0 Central Nervous	7 Via Natural or Artificial Opening	B Pressure K Temperature R Saturation	D Intracranial
0 Central Nervous	X External	2 Conductivity	Z No Qualifier
0 Central Nervous	X External	4 Electrical Activity	G Intraoperative Z No Qualifier
1 Peripheral Nervous	0 Open 3 Percutaneous X External	2 Conductivity	9 Sensory B Motor
1 Peripheral Nervous	0 Open 3 Percutaneous X External	4 Electrical Activity	G Intraoperative Z No Qualifier
2 Cardiac	0 Open 3 Percutaneous	4 Electrical Activity 9 Output C Rate F Rhythm H Sound	Z No Qualifier
2 Cardiac	X External	4 Electrical Activity	5 Ambulatory Z No Qualifier
2 Cardiac	X External	9 Output C Rate F Rhythm H Sound	Z No Qualifier
2 Cardiac	X External	M Total Activity	4 Stress
3 Arterial	0 Open 3 Percutaneous	5 Flow B Pressure J Pulse	1 Peripheral 3 Pulmonary C Coronary
3 Arterial	0 Open 3 Percutaneous	H Sound R Saturation	1 Peripheral
3 Arterial	X External	5 Flow B Pressure H Sound J Pulse R Saturation	1 Peripheral
4 Venous	0 Open 3 Percutaneous	5 Flow B Pressure J Pulse	0 Central 1 Peripheral 2 Portal 3 Pulmonary
4 Venous	0 Open 3 Percutaneous	R Saturation	0 Central 2 Portal 3 Pulmonary
4 Venous	X External	5 Flow B Pressure J Pulse	1 Peripheral
6 Lymphatic	0 Open 3 Percutaneous	5 Flow B Pressure	Z No Qualifier
9 Respiratory	7 Via Natural or Artificial Opening X External	1 Capacity 5 Flow C Rate D Resistance L Volume	Z No Qualifier
B Gastrointestinal	7 Via Natural or Artificial Opening 8 Via Natural or Artificial Opening Endoscopic	8 Motility B Pressure G Secretion	Z No Qualifier
D Urinary	7 Via Natural or Artificial Opening	3 Contractility 5 Flow B Pressure D Resistance L Volume	Z No Qualifier

Section	4	Measurement and Monitoring		
Body System	A	Physiological Systems		continued]
Operation	1	Monitoring Determining the level of a physiological or physical function repetitively over a period of time		

Body System (Character 4)	Approach (Character 5)	Function/Device (Character 6)	Qualifier (Character 7)
H Products of Conception, Cardiac	7 Via Natural or Artificial Opening 8 Via Natural or Artificial Opening Endoscopic X External	4 Electrical Activity C Rate F Rhythm H Sound	Z No Qualifier
J Products of Conception, Nervous	7 Via Natural or Artificial Opening 8 Via Natural or Artificial Opening Endoscopic X External	2 Conductivity 4 Electrical Activity B Pressure	Z No Qualifier
Z None	7 Via Natural or Artificial Opening	K Temperature	Z No Qualifier
Z None	X External	K Temperature Q Sleep	Z No Qualifier

Section	4	Measurement and Monitoring		
Body System	B	Physiological Devices		
Operation	0	Measurement: Determining the level of a physiological or physical function at a point in time		

Body System (Character 4)	Approach (Character 5)	Function/Device (Character 6)	Qualifier (Character 7)
0 Central Nervous 1 Peripheral Nervous F Musculoskeletal	X External	V Stimulator	Z No Qualifier
2 Cardiac	X External	S Pacemaker T Defibrillator	Z No Qualifier
9 Respiratory	X External	S Pacemaker	Z No Qualifier

Section	5	Extracorporeal Assistance and Performance		
Body System	A	Physiological Systems		
Operation	0	Assistance: Taking over a portion of a physiological function by extracorporeal means		

Body System (Character 4)	Duration (Character 5)	Function (Character 6)	Qualifier (Character 7)
2 Cardiac	1 Intermittent 2 Continuous	1 Output	0 Balloon Pump 5 Pulsatile Compression 6 Other Pump D Impeller Pump
5 Circulatory	1 Intermittent 2 Continuous	2 Oxygenation	1 Hyperbaric C Supersaturated
9 Respiratory	3 Less than 24 Consecutive Hours 4 24-96 Consecutive Hours 5 Greater than 96 Consecutive Hours	5 Ventilation	7 Continuous Positive Airway Pressure 8 Intermittent Positive Airway Pressure 9 Continuous Negative Airway Pressure B Intermittent Negative Airway Pressure Z No Qualifier

Section	5	Extracorporeal Assistance and Performance	
Body System	A	Physiological Systems	
Operation	1	Performance: Completely taking over a physiological function by extracorporeal means	

Body System (Character 4)	Duration (Character 5)	Function (Character 6)	Qualifier (Character 7)
2 Cardiac	0 Single	1 Output	2 Manual
2 Cardiac	1 Intermittent	3 Pacing	Z No Qualifier
2 Cardiac	2 Continuous	1 Output 3 Pacing	Z No Qualifier
5 Circulatory	2 Continuous	2 Oxygenation	3 Membrane
9 Respiratory	0 Single	5 Ventilation	4 Nonmechanical
9 Respiratory	3 Less than 24 Consecutive Hours 4 24-96 Consecutive Hours 5 Greater than 96 Consecutive Hours	5 Ventilation	Z No Qualifier
C Biliary D Urinary	0 Single 6 Multiple	0 Filtration	Z No Qualifier

Section	5	Extracorporeal Assistance and Performance	
Body System	A	Physiological Systems	
Operation	2	Restoration: Returning, or attempting to return, a physiological function to its original state by extracorporeal means	

Body System (Character 4)	Duration (Character 5)	Function (Character 6)	Qualifier (Character 7)
2 Cardiac	0 Single	4 Rhythm	Z No Qualifier

Section	6	Extracorporeal Therapies		
Body System	A	Physiological Systems		
Operation	0	Atmospheric Control: Extracorporeal control of atmospheric pressure and composition		
Body System (Character 4)		**Duration (Character 5)**	**Qualifier (Character 6)**	**Qualifier (Character 7)**
Z None		0 Single 1 Multiple	Z No Qualifier	Z No Qualifier

Section	6	Extracorporeal Therapies		
Body System	A	Physiological Systems		
Operation	1	Decompression: Extracorporeal elimination of undissolved gas from body fluids		
Body System (Character 4)		**Duration (Character 5)**	**Qualifier (Character 6)**	**Qualifier (Character 7)**
5 Circulatory		0 Single 1 Multiple	Z No Qualifier	Z No Qualifier

Section	6	Extracorporeal Therapies		
Body System	A	Physiological Systems		
Operation	2	Electromagnetic Therapy: Extracorporeal treatment by electromagnetic rays		
Body System (Character 4)		**Duration (Character 5)**	**Qualifier (Character 6)**	**Qualifier (Character 7)**
1 Urinary 2 Central Nervous		0 Single 1 Multiple	Z No Qualifier	Z No Qualifier

Section	6	Extracorporeal Therapies		
Body System	A	Physiological Systems		
Operation	3	Hyperthermia: Extracorporeal raising of body temperature		
Body System (Character 4)		**Duration (Character 5)**	**Qualifier (Character 6)**	**Qualifier (Character 7)**
Z None		0 Single 1 Multiple	Z No Qualifier	Z No Qualifier

Section	6	Extracorporeal Therapies		
Body System	A	Physiological Systems		
Operation	4	Extracorporeal Therapies Physiological Systems Hypothermia: Extracorporeal lowering of body temperature		
Body System (Character 4)		**Duration (Character 5)**	**Qualifier (Character 6)**	**Qualifier (Character 7)**
Z None		0 Single 1 Multiple	Z No Qualifier	Z No Qualifier

Section	6	Extracorporeal Therapies		
Body System	A	Physiological Systems		
Operation	5	Pheresis: Extracorporeal separation of blood products		
Body System (Character 4)		**Duration (Character 5)**	**Qualifier (Character 6)**	**Qualifier (Character 7)**
5 Circulatory		0 Single 1 Multiple	Z No Qualifier	0 Erythrocytes 1 Leukocytes 2 Platelets 3 Plasma T Stem Cells, Cord Blood V Stem Cells, Hematopoietic

Section	6	Extracorporeal Therapies		
Body System	A	Physiological Systems		
Operation	6	Phototherapy: Extracorporeal treatment by light rays		
Body System (Character 4)		**Duration (Character 5)**	**Qualifier (Character 6)**	**Qualifier (Character 7)**
0 Skin 5 Circulatory		0 Single 1 Multiple	Z No Qualifier	Z No Qualifier

Section	6	Extracorporeal Therapies		
Body System	A	Physiological Systems		
Operation	7	Ultrasound Therapy: Extracorporeal treatment by ultrasound		
Body System (Character 4)		**Duration (Character 5)**	**Qualifier (Character 6)**	**Qualifier (Character 7)**
5 Circulatory		0 Single 1 Multiple	Z No Qualifier	4 Head and Neck Vessels 5 Heart 6 Peripheral Vessels 7 Other Vessels Z No Qualifier

Section	6	Extracorporeal Therapies		
Body System	A	Physiological Systems		
Operation	8	Ultraviolet Light Therapy: Extracorporeal treatment by ultraviolet light		
Body System (Character 4)		**Duration (Character 5)**	**Qualifier (Character 6)**	**Qualifier (Character 7)**
0 Skin		0 Single 1 Multiple	Z No Qualifier	Z No Qualifier

Section	6 Extracorporeal Therapies		
Body System	A Physiological Systems		
Operation	9 Shock Wave Therapy: Extracorporeal treatment by shock waves		
Body System (Character 4)	**Duration (Character 5)**	**Qualifier (Character 6)**	**Qualifier (Character 7)**
3 Musculoskeletal	0 Single 1 Multiple	Z No Qualifier	Z No Qualifier

Section	7	Osteopathic			
Body System	W	Anatomical Regions			
Operation	0	Treatment: Manual treatment to eliminate or alleviate somatic dysfunction and related disorders			

Body Region (Character 4)	Approach (Character 5)	Method (Character 6)	Qualifier (Character 7)
0 Head	X External	0 Articulatory-Raising	Z None
1 Cervical		1 Fascial Release	
2 Thoracic		2 General Mobilization	
3 Lumbar		3 High Velocity-Low Amplitude	
4 Sacrum		4 Indirect	
5 Pelvis		5 Low Velocity-High Amplitude	
6 Lower Extremities		6 Lymphatic Pump	
7 Upper Extremities		7 Muscle Energy-Isometric	
8 Rib Cage		8 Muscle Energy-Isotonic	
9 Abdomen		9 Other Method	

Section	8	Other Procedures			
Body System	C	Indwelling Device			
Operation	0	Other Procedures: Methodologies which attempt to remediate or cure a disorder or disease			

Body Region (Character 4)	Approach (Character 5)	Method (Character 6)	Qualifier (Character 7)
1 Nervous System	X External	6 Collection	J Cerebrospinal Fluid L Other Fluid
2 Circulatory System	X External	6 Collection	K Blood L Other Fluid

Section	8	Other Procedures			
Body System	E	Physiological Systems and Anatomical Regions			
Operation	0	Other Procedures: Methodologies which attempt to remediate or cure a disorder or disease			

Body Region (Character 4)	Approach (Character 5)	Method (Character 6)	Qualifier (Character 7)
1 Nervous System U Female Reproductive System	X External	Y Other Method	7 Examination
2 Circulatory System	3 Percutaneous	D Near Infrared Spectroscopy	Z No Qualifier
9 Head and Neck Region W Trunk Region	0 Open 3 Percutaneous 4 Percutaneous Endoscopic 7 Via Natural or Artificial Opening 8 Via Natural or Artificial Opening Endoscopic	C Robotic Assisted Procedure	Z No Qualifier
9 Head and Neck Region W Trunk Region	X External	B Computer Assisted Procedure	F With Fluoroscopy G With Computerized Tomography H With Magnetic Resonance Imaging Z No Qualifier
9 Head and Neck Region W Trunk Region	X External	C Robotic Assisted Procedure	Z No Qualifier
9 Head and Neck Region W Trunk Region	X External	Y Other Method	8 Suture Removal
H Integumentary System and Breast	3 Percutaneous	0 Acupuncture	0 Anesthesia Z No Qualifier
H Integumentary System and Breast	X External	6 Collection	2 Breast Milk
H Integumentary System and Breast	X External	Y Other Method	9 Piercing
K Musculoskeletal System	X External	1 Therapeutic Massage	Z No Qualifier
K Musculoskeletal System	X External	Y Other Method	7 Examination
V Male Reproductive System	X External	1 Therapeutic Massage	C Prostate D Rectum
V Male Reproductive System	X External	6 Collection	3 Sperm
X Upper Extremity Y Lower Extremity	0 Open 3 Percutaneous 4 Percutaneous Endoscopic	C Robotic Assisted Procedure	Z No Qualifier
X Upper Extremity Y Lower Extremity	X External	B Computer Assisted Procedure	F With Fluoroscopy G With Computerized Tomography H With Magnetic Resonance Imaging Z No Qualifier
X Upper Extremity Y Lower Extremity	X External	C Robotic Assisted Procedure	Z No Qualifier
X Upper Extremity Y Lower Extremity	X External	Y Other Method	8 Suture Removal
Z None	X External	Y Other Method	1 In Vitro Fertilization 4 Yoga Therapy 5 Meditation 6 Isolation

Section	9	Chiropractic			
Body System	W	Anatomical Regions			
Operation	B	Manipulation: Manual procedure that involves a directed thrust to move a joint past the physiological range of motion, without exceeding the anatomical limit			

Body Region (Character 4)	Approach (Character 5)	Method (Character 6)	Qualifier (Character 7)
0 Head	X External	B Non-Manual	Z None
1 Cervical		C Indirect Visceral	
2 Thoracic		D Extra-Articular	
3 Lumbar		F Direct Visceral	
4 Sacrum		G Long Lever Specific Contact	
5 Pelvis		H Short Lever Specific Contact	
6 Lower Extremities		J Long and Short Lever	
7 Upper Extremities		Specific Contact	
8 Rib Cage		K Mechanically Assisted	
9 Abdomen		L Other Method	

Section	B	Imaging		
Body System	0	Central Nervous System		
Type	0	Plain Radiography: Planar display of an image developed from the capture of external ionizing radiation on photographic or photoconductive plate		
Body Part (Character 4)		**Contrast (Character 5)**	**Qualifier (Character 6)**	**Qualifier (Character 7)**
B Spinal Cord		0 High Osmolar 1 Low Osmolar Y Other Contrast Z None	Z None	Z None

Section	B	Imaging		
Body System	0	Central Nervous System		
Type	1	Fluoroscopy: Single plane or bi-plane real time display of an image developed from the capture of external ionizing radiation on a fluorescent screen. The image may also be stored by either digital or analog means		
Body Part (Character 4)		**Contrast (Character 5)**	**Qualifier (Character 6)**	**Qualifier (Character 7)**
B Spinal Cord		0 High Osmolar 1 Low Osmolar Y Other Contrast Z None	Z None	Z None

Section	B	Imaging		
Body System	0	Central Nervous System		
Type	2	Computerized Tomography (CT Scan): Computer reformatted digital display of multiplanar images developed from the capture of multiple exposures of external ionizing radiation		
Body Part (Character 4)		**Contrast (Character 5)**	**Qualifier (Character 6)**	**Qualifier (Character 7)**
0 Brain 7 Cisterna 8 Cerebral Ventricle(s) 9 Sella Turcica/Pituitary Gland B Spinal Cord		0 High Osmolar 1 Low Osmolar Y Other Contrast	0 Unenhanced and Enhanced Z None	Z None
0 Brain 7 Cisterna 8 Cerebral Ventricle(s) 9 Sella Turcica/Pituitary Gland B Spinal Cord		Z None	Z None	Z None

Section	B	Imaging		
Body System	0	Central Nervous System		
Type	3	Magnetic Resonance Imaging (MRI): Computer reformatted digital display of multiplanar images developed from the capture of radiofrequency signals emitted by nuclei in a body site excited within a magnetic field		
Body Part (Character 4)		**Contrast (Character 5)**	**Qualifier (Character 6)**	**Qualifier (Character 7)**
0 Brain 9 Sella Turcica/Pituitary Gland B Spinal Cord C Acoustic Nerves		Y Other Contrast	0 Unenhanced and Enhanced Z None	Z None
0 Brain 9 Sella Turcica/Pituitary Gland B Spinal Cord C Acoustic Nerves		Z None	Z None	Z None

Section	B	Imaging		
Body System	0	Central Nervous System		
Type	4	Ultrasonography: Real time display of images of anatomy or flow information developed from the capture of reflected and attenuated high frequency sound waves		
Body Part (Character 4)		**Contrast (Character 5)**	**Qualifier (Character 6)**	**Qualifier (Character 7)**
0 Brain B Spinal Cord		Z None	Z None	Z None

Section	B	Imaging
Body System	2	Heart
Type	0	Plain Radiography: Planar display of an image developed from the capture of external ionizing radiation on photographic or photoconductive plate

Body Part (Character 4)	Contrast (Character 5)	Qualifier (Character 6)	Qualifier (Character 7)
0 Coronary Artery, Single **1** Coronary Arteries, Multiple **2** Coronary Artery Bypass Graft, Single **3** Coronary Artery Bypass Grafts, Multiple **4** Heart, Right **5** Heart, Left **6** Heart, Right and Left **7** Internal Mammary Bypass Graft, Right **8** Internal Mammary Bypass Graft, Left **F** Bypass Graft, Other	**0** High Osmolar **1** Low Osmolar **Y** Other Contrast	**Z** None	**Z** None

Section	B	Imaging
Body System	2	Heart
Type	1	Fluoroscopy: Single plane or bi-plane real time display of an image developed from the capture of external ionizing radiation on a fluorescent screen. The image may also be stored by either digital or analog means

Body Part (Character 4)	Contrast (Character 5)	Qualifier (Character 6)	Qualifier (Character 7)
0 Coronary Artery, Single **1** Coronary Arteries, Multiple **2** Coronary Artery Bypass Graft, Single **3** Coronary Artery Bypass Grafts, Multiple	**0** High Osmolar **1** Low Osmolar **Y** Other Contrast	**1** Laser	**0** Intraoperative
0 Coronary Artery, Single **1** Coronary Arteries, Multiple **2** Coronary Artery Bypass Graft, Single **3** Coronary Artery Bypass Grafts, Multiple	**0** High Osmolar **1** Low Osmolar **Y** Other Contrast	**Z** None	**Z** None
4 Heart, Right **5** Heart, Left **6** Heart, Right and Left **7** Internal Mammary Bypass Graft, Right **8** Internal Mammary Bypass Graft, Left **F** Bypass Graft, Other	**0** High Osmolar **1** Low Osmolar **Y** Other Contrast	**Z** None	**Z** None

Section	B	Imaging
Body System	2	Heart
Type	2	Computerized Tomography (CT Scan): Computer reformatted digital display of multiplanar images developed from the capture of multiple exposures of external ionizing radiation

Body Part (Character 4)	Contrast (Character 5)	Qualifier (Character 6)	Qualifier (Character 7)
1 Coronary Arteries, Multiple **3** Coronary Artery Bypass Grafts, Multiple **6** Heart, Right and Left	**0** High Osmolar **1** Low Osmolar **Y** Other Contrast	**0** Unenhanced and Enhanced **Z** None	**Z** None
1 Coronary Arteries, Multiple **3** Coronary Artery Bypass Grafts, Multiple **6** Heart, Right and Left	**Z** None	**2** Intravascular Optical Coherence **Z** None	**Z** None

Section	B	Imaging
Body System	2	Heart
Type	3	Magnetic Resonance Imaging (MRI): Computer reformatted digital display of multiplanar images developed from the capture of radiofrequency signals emitted by nuclei in a body site excited within a magnetic field

Body Part (Character 4)	Contrast (Character 5)	Qualifier (Character 6)	Qualifier (Character 7)
1 Coronary Arteries, Multiple **3** Coronary Artery Bypass Grafts, Multiple **6** Heart, Right and Left	**Y** Other Contrast	**0** Unenhanced and Enhanced **Z** None	**Z** None
1 Coronary Arteries, Multiple **3** Coronary Artery Bypass Grafts, Multiple **6** Heart, Right and Left	**Z** None	**Z** None	**Z** None

Section	B	Imaging		
Body System	2	Heart		
Type	4	Ultrasonography: Real time display of images of anatomy or flow information developed from the capture of reflected and attenuated high frequency sound waves		

Body Part (Character 4)	Contrast (Character 5)	Qualifier (Character 6)	Qualifier (Character 7)
0 Coronary Artery, Single **1** Coronary Arteries, Multiple **4** Heart, Right **5** Heart, Left **6** Heart, Right and Left **B** Heart with Aorta **C** Pericardium **D** Pediatric Heart	**Y** Other Contrast	**Z** None	**Z** None
0 Coronary Artery, Single **1** Coronary Arteries, Multiple **4** Heart, Right **5** Heart, Left **6** Heart, Right and Left **B** Heart with Aorta **C** Pericardium **D** Pediatric Heart	**Z** None	**Z** None	**3** Intravascular **4** Transesophageal **Z** None

Section	B	Imaging		
Body System	3	Upper Arteries		
Type	0	Plain Radiography: Planar display of an image developed from the capture of external ionizing radiation on photographic or photoconductive plate		

Body Part (Character 4)	Contrast (Character 5)	Qualifier (Character 6)	Qualifier (Character 7)
0 Thoracic Aorta **1** Brachiocephalic-Subclavian Artery, Right **2** Subclavian Artery, Left **3** Common Carotid Artery, Right **4** Common Carotid Artery, Left **5** Common Carotid Arteries, Bilateral **6** Internal Carotid Artery, Right **7** Internal Carotid Artery, Left **8** Internal Carotid Arteries, Bilateral **9** External Carotid Artery, Right **B** External Carotid Artery, Left **C** External Carotid Arteries, Bilateral **D** Vertebral Artery, Right **F** Vertebral Artery, Left **G** Vertebral Arteries, Bilateral **H** Upper Extremity Arteries, Right **J** Upper Extremity Arteries, Left **K** Upper Extremity Arteries, Bilateral **L** Intercostal and Bronchial Arteries **M** Spinal Arteries **N** Upper Arteries, Other **P** Thoraco-Abdominal Aorta **Q** Cervico-Cerebral Arch **R** Intracranial Arteries **S** Pulmonary Artery, Right **T** Pulmonary Artery, Left	**0** High Osmolar **1** Low Osmolar **Y** Other Contrast **Z** None	**Z** None	**Z** None

Section	B	Imaging
Body System	3	Upper Arteries
Type	1	Fluoroscopy: Single plane or bi-plane real time display of an image developed from the capture of external ionizing radiation on a fluorescent screen. The image may also be stored by either digital or analog means

Body Part (Character 4)	Contrast (Character 5)	Qualifier (Character 6)	Qualifier (Character 7)
0 Thoracic Aorta **1** Brachiocephalic-Subclavian Artery, Right **2** Subclavian Artery, Left **3** Common Carotid Artery, Right **4** Common Carotid Artery, Left **5** Common Carotid Arteries, Bilateral **6** Internal Carotid Artery, Right **7** Internal Carotid Artery, Left **8** Internal Carotid Arteries, Bilateral **9** External Carotid Artery, Right **B** External Carotid Artery, Left **C** External Carotid Arteries, Bilateral **D** Vertebral Artery, Right **F** Vertebral Artery, Left **G** Vertebral Arteries, Bilateral **H** Upper Extremity Arteries, Right **J** Upper Extremity Arteries, Left **K** Upper Extremity Arteries, Bilateral **L** Intercostal and Bronchial Arteries **M** Spinal Arteries **N** Upper Arteries, Other **P** Thoraco-Abdominal Aorta **Q** Cervico-Cerebral Arch **R** Intracranial Arteries **S** Pulmonary Artery, Right **T** Pulmonary Artery, Left	**0** High Osmolar **1** Low Osmolar **Y** Other Contrast	**1** Laser	**0** Intraoperative

Section	B	Imaging
Body System	3	Upper Arteries
Type	1	Fluoroscopy: Single plane or bi-plane real time display of an image developed from the capture of external ionizing radiation on a fluorescent screen. The image may also be stored by either digital or analog means

Body Part (Character 4)	Contrast (Character 5)	Qualifier (Character 6)	Qualifier (Character 7)
0 Thoracic Aorta **1** Brachiocephalic-Subclavian Artery, Right **2** Subclavian Artery, Left **3** Common Carotid Artery, Right **4** Common Carotid Artery, Left **5** Common Carotid Arteries, Bilateral **6** Internal Carotid Artery, Right **7** Internal Carotid Artery, Left **8** Internal Carotid Arteries, Bilateral **9** External Carotid Artery, Right **B** External Carotid Artery, Left **C** External Carotid Arteries, Bilateral **D** Vertebral Artery, Right **F** Vertebral Artery, Left **G** Vertebral Arteries, Bilateral **H** Upper Extremity Arteries, Right **J** Upper Extremity Arteries, Left **K** Upper Extremity Arteries, Bilateral **L** Intercostal and Bronchial Arteries **M** Spinal Arteries **N** Upper Arteries, Other **P** Thoraco-Abdominal Aorta **Q** Cervico-Cerebral Arch **R** Intracranial Arteries **S** Pulmonary Artery, Right **T** Pulmonary Artery, Left	**0** High Osmolar **1** Low Osmolar **Y** Other Contrast	**Z** None	**Z** None

Section	B	Imaging		
Body System	3	Upper Arteries		
Type	1	Fluoroscopy: Single plane or bi-plane real time display of an image developed from the capture of external ionizing radiation on a fluorescent screen. The image may also be stored by either digital or analog means		

Body Part (Character 4)	Contrast (Character 5)	Qualifier (Character 6)	Qualifier (Character 7)
0 Thoracic Aorta **1** Brachiocephalic-Subclavian Artery, Right **2** Subclavian Artery, Left **3** Common Carotid Artery, Right **4** Common Carotid Artery, Left **5** Common Carotid Arteries, Bilateral **6** Internal Carotid Artery, Right **7** Internal Carotid Artery, Left **8** Internal Carotid Arteries, Bilateral **9** External Carotid Artery, Right **B** External Carotid Artery, Left **C** External Carotid Arteries, Bilateral **D** Vertebral Artery, Right **F** Vertebral Artery, Left **G** Vertebral Arteries, Bilateral **H** Upper Extremity Arteries, Right **J** Upper Extremity Arteries, Left **K** Upper Extremity Arteries, Bilateral **L** Intercostal and Bronchial Arteries **M** Spinal Arteries **N** Upper Arteries, Other **P** Thoraco-Abdominal Aorta **Q** Cervico-Cerebral Arch **R** Intracranial Arteries **S** Pulmonary Artery, Right **T** Pulmonary Artery, Left	**Z** None	**Z** None	**Z** None

Section	B	Imaging		
Body System	3	Upper Arteries		
Type	2	Computerized Tomography (CT Scan): Computer reformatted digital display of multiplanar images developed from the capture of multiple exposures of external ionizing radiation		

Body Part (Character 4)	Contrast (Character 5)	Qualifier (Character 6)	Qualifier (Character 7)
0 Thoracic Aorta **5** Common Carotid Arteries, Bilateral **8** Internal Carotid Arteries, Bilateral **G** Vertebral Arteries, Bilateral **R** Intracranial Arteries **S** Pulmonary Artery, Right **T** Pulmonary Artery, Left	**0** High Osmolar **1** Low Osmolar **Y** Other Contrast	**Z** None	**Z** None
0 Thoracic Aorta **5** Common Carotid Arteries, Bilateral **8** Internal Carotid Arteries, Bilateral **G** Vertebral Arteries, Bilateral **R** Intracranial Arteries **S** Pulmonary Artery, Right **T** Pulmonary Artery, Left	**Z** None	**2** Intravascular Optical Coherence **Z** None	**Z** None

Section	B	Imaging		
Body System	3	Upper Arteries		
Type	3	Magnetic Resonance Imaging (MRI): Computer reformatted digital display of multiplanar images developed from the capture of radiofrequency signals emitted by nuclei in a body site excited within a magnetic field		

Body Part (Character 4)	Contrast (Character 5)	Qualifier (Character 6)	Qualifier (Character 7)
0 Thoracic Aorta **5** Common Carotid Arteries, Bilateral **8** Internal Carotid Arteries, Bilateral **G** Vertebral Arteries, Bilateral **H** Upper Extremity Arteries, Right **J** Upper Extremity Arteries, Left **K** Upper Extremity Arteries, Bilateral **M** Spinal Arteries **Q** Cervico-Cerebral Arch **R** Intracranial Arteries	**Y** Other Contrast	**0** Unenhanced and Enhanced **Z** None	**Z** None
0 Thoracic Aorta **5** Common Carotid Arteries, Bilateral **8** Internal Carotid Arteries, Bilateral **G** Vertebral Arteries, Bilateral **H** Upper Extremity Arteries, Right **J** Upper Extremity Arteries, Left **K** Upper Extremity Arteries, Bilateral **M** Spinal Arteries **Q** Cervico-Cerebral Arch **R** Intracranial Arteries	**Z** None	**Z** None	**Z** None

Section	B	Imaging		
Body System	3	Upper Arteries		
Type	4	Ultrasonography: Real time display of images of anatomy or flow information developed from the capture of reflected and attenuated high frequency sound waves		

Body Part (Character 4)	Contrast (Character 5)	Qualifier (Character 6)	Qualifier (Character 7)
0 Thoracic Aorta **1** Brachiocephalic-Subclavian Artery, Right **2** Subclavian Artery, Left **3** Common Carotid Artery, Right **4** Common Carotid Artery, Left **5** Common Carotid Arteries, Bilateral **6** Internal Carotid Artery, Right **7** Internal Carotid Artery, Left **8** Internal Carotid Arteries, Bilateral **H** Upper Extremity Arteries, Right **J** Upper Extremity Arteries, Left **K** Upper Extremity Arteries, Bilateral **R** Intracranial Arteries **S** Pulmonary Artery, Right **T** Pulmonary Artery, Left **V** Ophthalmic Arteries	**Z** None	**Z** None	**3** Intravascular **Z** None

Section	B	Imaging		
Body System	4	Lower Arteries		
Type	0	Plain Radiography: Planar display of an image developed from the capture of external ionizing radiation on photographic or photoconductive plate		

Body Part (Character 4)	Contrast (Character 5)	Qualifier (Character 6)	Qualifier (Character 7)
0 Abdominal Aorta **2** Hepatic Artery **3** Splenic Arteries **4** Superior Mesenteric Artery **5** Inferior Mesenteric Artery **6** Renal Artery, Right **7** Renal Artery, Left **8** Renal Arteries, Bilateral **9** Lumbar Arteries **B** Intra-Abdominal Arteries, Other **C** Pelvic Arteries **D** Aorta and Bilateral Lower Extremity Arteries **F** Lower Extremity Arteries, Right **G** Lower Extremity Arteries, Left **J** Lower Arteries, Other **M** Renal Artery Transplant	**0** High Osmolar **1** Low Osmolar **Y** Other Contrast	**Z** None	**Z** None

Section	B	Imaging		
Body System	4	Lower Arteries		
Type	1	Fluoroscopy: Single plane or bi-plane real time display of an image developed from the capture of external ionizing radiation on a fluorescent screen. The image may also be stored by either digital or analog means		

Body Part (Character 4)	Contrast (Character 5)	Qualifier (Character 6)	Qualifier (Character 7)
0 Abdominal Aorta **2** Hepatic Artery **3** Splenic Arteries **4** Superior Mesenteric Artery **5** Inferior Mesenteric Artery **6** Renal Artery, Right **7** Renal Artery, Left **8** Renal Arteries, Bilateral **9** Lumbar Arteries **B** Intra-Abdominal Arteries, Other **C** Pelvic Arteries **D** Aorta and Bilateral Lower Extremity Arteries **F** Lower Extremity Arteries, Right **G** Lower Extremity Arteries, Left **J** Lower Arteries, Other	**0** High Osmolar **1** Low Osmolar **Y** Other Contrast	**1** Laser	**0** Intraoperative
0 Abdominal Aorta **2** Hepatic Artery **3** Splenic Arteries **4** Superior Mesenteric Artery **5** Inferior Mesenteric Artery **6** Renal Artery, Right **7** Renal Artery, Left **8** Renal Arteries, Bilateral **9** Lumbar Arteries **B** Intra-Abdominal Arteries, Other **C** Pelvic Arteries **D** Aorta and Bilateral Lower Extremity Arteries **F** Lower Extremity Arteries, Right **G** Lower Extremity Arteries, Left **J** Lower Arteries, Other	**0** High Osmolar **1** Low Osmolar **Y** Other Contrast	**Z** None	**Z** None

Section	B	Imaging
Body System	4	Lower Arteries
Type	1	Fluoroscopy: Single plane or bi-plane real time display of an image developed from the capture of external ionizing radiation on a fluorescent screen. The image may also be stored by either digital or analog means

Body Part (Character 4)	Contrast (Character 5)	Qualifier (Character 6)	Qualifier (Character 7)
0 Abdominal Aorta 2 Hepatic Artery 3 Splenic Arteries 4 Superior Mesenteric Artery 5 Inferior Mesenteric Artery 6 Renal Artery, Right 7 Renal Artery, Left 8 Renal Arteries, Bilateral 9 Lumbar Arteries B Intra-Abdominal Arteries, Other C Pelvic Arteries D Aorta and Bilateral Lower Extremity Arteries F Lower Extremity Arteries, Right G Lower Extremity Arteries, Left J Lower Arteries, Other	Z None	Z None	Z None

Section	B	Imaging
Body System	4	Lower Arteries
Type	2	Computerized Tomography (CT Scan): Computer reformatted digital display of multiplanar images developed from the capture of multiple exposures of external ionizing radiation

Body Part (Character 4)	Contrast (Character 5)	Qualifier (Character 6)	Qualifier (Character 7)
0 Abdominal Aorta 1 Celiac Artery 4 Superior Mesenteric Artery 8 Renal Arteries, Bilateral C Pelvic Arteries F Lower Extremity Arteries, Right G Lower Extremity Arteries, Left H Lower Extremity Arteries, Bilateral M Renal Artery Transplant	0 High Osmolar 1 Low Osmolar Y Other Contrast	Z None	Z None
0 Abdominal Aorta 1 Celiac Artery 4 Superior Mesenteric Artery 8 Renal Arteries, Bilateral C Pelvic Arteries F Lower Extremity Arteries, Right G Lower Extremity Arteries, Left H Lower Extremity Arteries, Bilateral M Renal Artery Transplant	Z None	2 Intravascular Optical Coherence Z None	Z None

Section	B	Imaging
Body System	4	Lower Arteries
Type	3	Magnetic Resonance Imaging (MRI): Computer reformatted digital display of multiplanar images developed from the capture of radiofrequency signals emitted by nuclei in a body site excited within a magnetic field

Body Part (Character 4)	Contrast (Character 5)	Qualifier (Character 6)	Qualifier (Character 7)
0 Abdominal Aorta 1 Celiac Artery 4 Superior Mesenteric Artery 8 Renal Arteries, Bilateral C Pelvic Arteries F Lower Extremity Arteries, Right G Lower Extremity Arteries, Left H Lower Extremity Arteries, Bilateral	Y Other Contrast	0 Unenhanced and Enhanced Z None	Z None
0 Abdominal Aorta 1 Celiac Artery 4 Superior Mesenteric Artery 8 Renal Arteries, Bilateral C Pelvic Arteries F Lower Extremity Arteries, Right G Lower Extremity Arteries, Left H Lower Extremity Arteries, Bilateral	Z None	Z None	Z None

Section	B	Imaging		
Body System	4	Lower Arteries		
Type	4	Ultrasonography: Real time display of images of anatomy or flow information developed from the capture of reflected and attenuated high frequency sound waves		

Body Part (Character 4)	Contrast (Character 5)	Qualifier (Character 6)	Qualifier (Character 7)
0 Abdominal Aorta **4** Superior Mesenteric Artery **5** Inferior Mesenteric Artery **6** Renal Artery, Right **7** Renal Artery, Left **8** Renal Arteries, Bilateral **B** Intra-Abdominal Arteries, Other **F** Lower Extremity Arteries, Right **G** Lower Extremity Arteries, Left **H** Lower Extremity Arteries, Bilateral **K** Celiac and Mesenteric Arteries **L** Femoral Artery **N** Penile Arteries	**Z** None	**Z** None	**3** Intravascular **Z** None

Section	B	Imaging		
Body System	5	Veins		
Type	0	Plain Radiography: Planar display of an image developed from the capture of external ionizing radiation on photographic or photoconductive plate		

Body Part (Character 4)	Contrast (Character 5)	Qualifier (Character 6)	Qualifier (Character 7)
0 Epidural Veins **1** Cerebral and Cerebellar Veins **2** Intracranial Sinuses **3** Jugular Veins, Right **4** Jugular Veins, Left **5** Jugular Veins, Bilateral **6** Subclavian Vein, Right **7** Subclavian Vein, Left **8** Superior Vena Cava **9** Inferior Vena Cava **B** Lower Extremity Veins, Right **C** Lower Extremity Veins, Left **D** Lower Extremity Veins, Bilateral **F** Pelvic (Iliac) Veins, Right **G** Pelvic (Iliac) Veins, Left **H** Pelvic (Iliac) Veins, Bilateral **J** Renal Vein, Right **K** Renal Vein, Left **L** Renal Veins, Bilateral **M** Upper Extremity Veins, Right **N** Upper Extremity Veins, Left **P** Upper Extremity Veins, Bilateral **Q** Pulmonary Vein, Right **R** Pulmonary Vein, Left **S** Pulmonary Veins, Bilateral **T** Portal and Splanchnic Veins **V** Veins, Other **W** Dialysis Shunt/Fistula	**0** High Osmolar **1** Low Osmolar **Y** Other Contrast	**Z** None	**Z** None

Section	B	Imaging		
Body System	5	Veins		
Type	1	Fluoroscopy: Single plane or bi-plane real time display of an image developed from the capture of external ionizing radiation on a fluorescent screen. The image may also be stored by either digital or analog means		

Body Part (Character 4)	Contrast (Character 5)	Qualifier (Character 6)	Qualifier (Character 7)
0 Epidural Veins	0 High Osmolar	Z None	A Guidance
1 Cerebral and Cerebellar Veins	1 Low Osmolar		Z None
2 Intracranial Sinuses	Y Other Contrast		
3 Jugular Veins, Right	Z None		
4 Jugular Veins, Left			
5 Jugular Veins, Bilateral			
6 Subclavian Vein, Right			
7 Subclavian Vein, Left			
8 Superior Vena Cava			
9 Inferior Vena Cava			
B Lower Extremity Veins, Right			
C Lower Extremity Veins, Left			
D Lower Extremity Veins, Bilateral			
F Pelvic (Iliac) Veins, Right			
G Pelvic (Iliac) Veins, Left			
H Pelvic (Iliac) Veins, Bilateral			
J Renal Vein, Right			
K Renal Vein, Left			
L Renal Veins, Bilateral			
M Upper Extremity Veins, Right			
N Upper Extremity Veins, Left			
P Upper Extremity Veins, Bilateral			
Q Pulmonary Vein, Right			
R Pulmonary Vein, Left			
S Pulmonary Veins, Bilateral			
T Portal and Splanchnic Veins			
V Veins, Other			
W Dialysis Shunt/Fistula			

Section	B	Imaging		
Body System	5	Veins		
Type	2	Computerized Tomography (CT Scan): Computer reformatted digital display of multiplanar images developed from the capture of multiple exposures of external ionizing radiation		

Body Part (Character 4)	Contrast (Character 5)	Qualifier (Character 6)	Qualifier (Character 7)
2 Intracranial Sinuses	0 High Osmolar	0 Unenhanced and Enhanced	Z None
8 Superior Vena Cava	1 Low Osmolar	Z None	
9 Inferior Vena Cava	Y Other Contrast		
F Pelvic (Iliac) Veins, Right			
G Pelvic (Iliac) Veins, Left			
H Pelvic (Iliac) Veins, Bilateral			
J Renal Vein, Right			
K Renal Vein, Left			
L Renal Veins, Bilateral			
Q Pulmonary Vein, Right			
R Pulmonary Vein, Left			
S Pulmonary Veins, Bilateral			
T Portal and Splanchnic Veins			
2 Intracranial Sinuses	Z None	2 Intravascular Optical Coherence	Z None
8 Superior Vena Cava		Z None	
9 Inferior Vena Cava			
F Pelvic (Iliac) Veins, Right			
G Pelvic (Iliac) Veins, Left			
H Pelvic (Iliac) Veins, Bilateral			
J Renal Vein, Right			
K Renal Vein, Left			
L Renal Veins, Bilateral			
Q Pulmonary Vein, Right			
R Pulmonary Vein, Left			
S Pulmonary Veins, Bilateral			
T Portal and Splanchnic Veins			

Section	B	Imaging		
Body System	5	Veins		
Type	3	Magnetic Resonance Imaging (MRI): Computer reformatted digital display of multiplanar images developed from the capture of radiofrequency signals emitted by nuclei in a body site excited within a magnetic field		

Body Part (Character 4)	Contrast (Character 5)	Qualifier (Character 6)	Qualifier (Character 7)
1 Cerebral and Cerebellar Veins **2** Intracranial Sinuses **5** Jugular Veins, Bilateral **8** Superior Vena Cava **9** Inferior Vena Cava **B** Lower Extremity Veins, Right **C** Lower Extremity Veins, Left **D** Lower Extremity Veins, Bilateral **H** Pelvic (Iliac) Veins, Bilateral **L** Renal Veins, Bilateral **M** Upper Extremity Veins, Right **N** Upper Extremity Veins, Left **P** Upper Extremity Veins, Bilateral **S** Pulmonary Veins, Bilateral **T** Portal and Splanchnic Veins **V** Veins, Other	**Y** Other Contrast	**0** Unenhanced and Enhanced **Z** None	**Z** None
1 Cerebral and Cerebellar Veins **2** Intracranial Sinuses **5** Jugular Veins, Bilateral **8** Superior Vena Cava **9** Inferior Vena Cava **B** Lower Extremity Veins, Right **C** Lower Extremity Veins, Left **D** Lower Extremity Veins, Bilateral **H** Pelvic (Iliac) Veins, Bilateral **L** Renal Veins, Bilateral **M** Upper Extremity Veins, Right **N** Upper Extremity Veins, Left **P** Upper Extremity Veins, Bilateral **S** Pulmonary Veins, Bilateral **T** Portal and Splanchnic Veins **V** Veins, Other	**Z** None	**Z** None	**Z** None

Section	B	Imaging		
Body System	5	Veins		
Type	4	Ultrasonography: Real time display of images of anatomy or flow information developed from the capture of reflected and attenuated high frequency sound waves		

Body Part (Character 4)	Contrast (Character 5)	Qualifier (Character 6)	Qualifier (Character 7)
3 Jugular Veins, Right **4** Jugular Veins, Left **6** Subclavian Vein, Right **7** Subclavian Vein, Left **8** Superior Vena Cava **9** Inferior Vena Cava **B** Lower Extremity Veins, Right **C** Lower Extremity Veins, Left **D** Lower Extremity Veins, Bilateral **J** Renal Vein, Right **K** Renal Vein, Left **L** Renal Veins, Bilateral **M** Upper Extremity Veins, Right **N** Upper Extremity Veins, Left **P** Upper Extremity Veins, Bilateral **T** Portal and Splanchnic Veins	**Z** None	**Z** None	**3** Intravascular **A** Guidance **Z** None

Section	B	Imaging		
Body System	7	Lymphatic System		
Type	0	Plain Radiography: Planar display of an image developed from the capture of external ionizing radiation on photographic or photoconductive plate		
Body Part (Character 4)		Contrast (Character 5)	Qualifier (Character 6)	Qualifier (Character 7)
0 Abdominal/Retroperitoneal Lymphatics, Unilateral 1 Abdominal/Retroperitoneal Lymphatics, Bilateral 4 Lymphatics, Head and Neck 5 Upper Extremity Lymphatics, Right 6 Upper Extremity Lymphatics, Left 7 Upper Extremity Lymphatics, Bilateral 8 Lower Extremity Lymphatics, Right 9 Lower Extremity Lymphatics, Left B Lower Extremity Lymphatics, Bilateral C Lymphatics, Pelvic		0 High Osmolar 1 Low Osmolar Y Other Contrast	Z None	Z None

Section	B	Imaging		
Body System	8	Eye		
Type	0	Plain Radiography: Planar display of an image developed from the capture of external ionizing radiation on photographic or photoconductive plate		
Body Part (Character 4)		Contrast (Character 5)	Qualifier (Character 6)	Qualifier (Character 7)
0 Lacrimal Duct, Right 1 Lacrimal Duct, Left 2 Lacrimal Ducts, Bilateral		0 High Osmolar 1 Low Osmolar Y Other Contrast	Z None	Z None
3 Optic Foramina, Right 4 Optic Foramina, Left 5 Eye, Right 6 Eye, Left 7 Eyes, Bilateral		Z None	Z None	Z None

Section	B	Imaging		
Body System	8	Eye		
Type	2	Computerized Tomography (CT Scan): Computer reformatted digital display of multiplanar images developed from the capture of multiple exposures of external ionizing radiation		
Body Part (Character 4)		Contrast (Character 5)	Qualifier (Character 6)	Qualifier (Character 7)
5 Eye, Right 6 Eye, Left 7 Eyes, Bilateral		0 High Osmolar 1 Low Osmolar Y Other Contrast	0 Unenhanced and Enhanced Z None	Z None
5 Eye, Right 6 Eye, Left 7 Eyes, Bilateral		Z None	Z None	Z None

Section	B	Imaging		
Body System	8	Eye		
Type	3	Magnetic Resonance Imaging (MRI): Computer reformatted digital display of multiplanar images developed from the capture of radiofrequency signals emitted by nuclei in a body site excited within a magnetic field		
Body Part (Character 4)		Contrast (Character 5)	Qualifier (Character 6)	Qualifier (Character 7)
5 Eye, Right 6 Eye, Left 7 Eyes, Bilateral		Y Other Contrast	0 Unenhanced and Enhanced Z None	Z None
5 Eye, Right 6 Eye, Left 7 Eyes, Bilateral		Z None	Z None	Z None

Section	B	Imaging		
Body System	8	Eye		
Type	4	Ultrasonography: Real time display of images of anatomy or flow information developed from the capture of reflected and attenuated high frequency sound waves		
Body Part (Character 4)		Contrast (Character 5)	Qualifier (Character 6)	Qualifier (Character 7)
5 Eye, Right 6 Eye, Left 7 Eyes, Bilateral			Z None	Z None

Section	B	Imaging		
Body System	9	Ear, Nose, Mouth and Throat		
Type	0	Plain Radiography: Planar display of an image developed from the capture of external ionizing radiation on photographic or photoconductive plate		
Body Part (Character 4)		Contrast (Character 5)	Qualifier (Character 6)	Qualifier (Character 7)
2 Paranasal Sinuses **F** Nasopharynx/Oropharynx **H** Mastoids		**Z** None	**Z** None	**Z** None
4 Parotid Gland, Right **5** Parotid Gland, Left **6** Parotid Glands, Bilateral **7** Submandibular Gland, Right **8** Submandibular Gland, Left **9** Submandibular Glands, Bilateral **B** Salivary Gland, Right **C** Salivary Gland, Left **D** Salivary Glands, Bilateral		**0** High Osmolar **1** Low Osmolar **Y** Other Contrast	**Z** None	**Z** None

Section	B	Imaging		
Body System	9	Ear, Nose, Mouth and Throat		
Type	1	Fluoroscopy: Single plane or bi-plane real time display of an image developed from the capture of external ionizing radiation on a fluorescent screen. The image may also be stored by either digital or analog means		
Body Part Character 4		Contrast	Qualifier	Qualifier
G Pharynx and Epiglottis **J** Larynx		**Y** Other Contrast **Z** None	**Z** None	**Z** None

Section	B	Imaging		
Body System	9	Ear, Nose, Mouth and Throat		
Type	2	Computerized Tomography (CT Scan): Computer reformatted digital display of multiplanar images developed from the capture of multiple exposures of external ionizing radiation		
Body Part (Character 4)		Contrast (Character 5)	Qualifier (Character 6)	Qualifier (Character 7)
0 Ear **2** Paranasal Sinuses **6** Parotid Glands, Bilateral **9** Submandibular Glands, Bilateral **D** Salivary Glands, Bilateral **F** Nasopharynx/Oropharynx **J** Larynx		**0** High Osmolar **1** Low Osmolar **Y** Other Contrast	**0** Unenhanced and Enhanced **Z** None	**Z** None
0 Ear **2** Paranasal Sinuses **6** Parotid Glands, Bilateral **9** Submandibular Glands, Bilateral **D** Salivary Glands, Bilateral **F** Nasopharynx/Oropharynx **J** Larynx		**Z** None	**Z** None	**Z** None

Section	B	Imaging		
Body System	9	Ear, Nose, Mouth and Throat		
Type	3	Magnetic Resonance Imaging (MRI): Computer reformatted digital display of multiplanar images developed from the capture of radiofrequency signals emitted by nuclei in a body site excited within a magnetic field		
Body Part (Character 4)		Contrast (Character 5)	Qualifier (Character 6)	Qualifier (Character 7)
0 Ear **2** Paranasal Sinuses **6** Parotid Glands, Bilateral **9** Submandibular Glands, Bilateral **D** Salivary Glands, Bilateral **F** Nasopharynx/Oropharynx **J** Larynx		**Y** Other Contrast	**0** Unenhanced and Enhanced **Z** None	**Z** None
0 Ear **2** Paranasal Sinuses **6** Parotid Glands, Bilateral **9** Submandibular Glands, Bilateral **D** Salivary Glands, Bilateral **F** Nasopharynx/Oropharynx **J** Larynx		**Z** None	**Z** None	**Z** None

Section	B	Imaging			
Body System	B	Respiratory System			
Type	0	Plain Radiography: Planar display of an image developed from the capture of external ionizing radiation on photographic or photoconductive plate			
Body Part (Character 4)		**Contrast (Character 5)**	**Qualifier (Character 6)**	**Qualifier (Character 7)**	
7 Tracheobronchial Tree, Right 8 Tracheobronchial Tree, Left 9 Tracheobronchial Trees, Bilateral		Y Other Contrast	Z None	Z None	
D Upper Airways		Z None	Z None	Z None	

Section	B	Imaging			
Body System	B	Respiratory System			
Type	1	Fluoroscopy: Single plane or bi-plane real time display of an image developed from the capture of external ionizing radiation on a fluorescent screen. The image may also be stored by either digital or analog means			
Body Part (Character 4)		**Contrast (Character 5)**	**Qualifier (Character 6)**	**Qualifier (Character 7)**	
2 Lung, Right 3 Lung, Left 4 Lungs, Bilateral 6 Diaphragm C Mediastinum D Upper Airways		Z None	Z None	Z None	
7 Tracheobronchial Tree, Right 8 Tracheobronchial Tree, Left 9 Tracheobronchial Trees, Bilateral		Y Other Contrast	Z None	Z None	

Section	B	Imaging			
Body System	B	Respiratory System			
Type	2	Computerized Tomography (CT Scan): Computer reformatted digital display of multiplanar images developed from the capture of multiple exposures of external ionizing radiation			
Body Part (Character 4)		**Contrast (Character 5)**	**Qualifier (Character 6)**	**Qualifier (Character 7)**	
4 Lungs, Bilateral 7 Tracheobronchial Tree, Right 8 Tracheobronchial Tree, Left 9 Tracheobronchial Trees, Bilateral F Trachea/Airways		0 High Osmolar 1 Low Osmolar Y Other Contrast	0 Unenhanced and Enhanced Z None	Z None	
4 Lungs, Bilateral 7 Tracheobronchial Tree, Right 8 Tracheobronchial Tree, Left 9 Tracheobronchial Trees, Bilateral F Trachea/Airways		Z None	Z None	Z None	

Section	B	Imaging			
Body System	B	Respiratory System			
Type	3	Magnetic Resonance Imaging (MRI): Computer reformatted digital display of multiplanar images developed from the capture of radiofrequency signals emitted by nuclei in a body site excited within a magnetic field			
Body Part (Character 4)		**Contrast (Character 5)**	**Qualifier (Character 6)**	**Qualifier (Character 7)**	
G Lung Apices		Y Other Contrast	0 Unenhanced and Enhanced Z None	Z None	
G Lung Apices		Z None	Z None	Z None	

Section	B	Imaging			
Body System	B	Respiratory System			
Type	4	Ultrasonography: Real time display of images of anatomy or flow information developed from the capture of reflected and attenuated high frequency sound waves			
Body Part (Character 4)		**Contrast (Character 5)**	**Qualifier (Character 6)**	**Qualifier (Character 7)**	
B Pleura C Mediastinum		Z None	Z None	Z None	

Section	B	Imaging			
Body System	D	Gastrointestinal System			
Type	1	Fluoroscopy: Single plane or bi-plane real time display of an image developed from the capture of external ionizing radiation on a fluorescent screen. The image may also be stored by either digital or analog means			
Body Part (Character 4)		**Contrast (Character 5)**	**Qualifier (Character 6)**	**Qualifier (Character 7)**	
1 Esophagus 2 Stomach 3 Small Bowel 4 Colon 5 Upper GI 6 Upper GI and Small Bowel 9 Duodenum B Mouth/Oropharynx		Y Other Contrast Z None	Z None	Z None	

Section	B	Imaging		
Body System	D	Gastrointestinal System		
Type	2	Computerized Tomography (CT Scan): Computer reformatted digital display of multiplanar images developed from the capture of multiple exposures of external ionizing radiation		
Body Part (Character 4)	Contrast (Character 5)	Qualifier (Character 6)	Qualifier (Character 7)
4 Colon	0 High Osmolar 1 Low Osmolar Y Other Contrast	0 Unenhanced and Enhanced Z None	Z None
4 Colon	Z None	Z None	Z None

Section	B	Imaging		
Body System	D	Gastrointestinal System		
Type	4	Ultrasonography: Real time display of images of anatomy or flow information developed from the capture of reflected and attenuated high frequency sound waves		
Body Part (Character 4)	Contrast (Character 5)	Qualifier (Character 6)	Qualifier (Character 7)
1 Esophagus 2 Stomach 7 Gastrointestinal Tract 8 Appendix 9 Duodenum C Rectum	Z None	Z None	Z None

Section	B	Imaging		
Body System	F	Hepatobiliary System and Pancreas		
Type	0	Plain Radiography: Planar display of an image developed from the capture of external ionizing radiation on photographic or photoconductive plate		
Body Part (Character 4)	Contrast (Character 5)	Qualifier (Character 6)	Qualifier (Character 7)
0 Bile Ducts 3 Gallbladder and Bile Ducts C Hepatobiliary System, All	0 High Osmolar 1 Low Osmolar Y Other Contrast	Z None	Z None

Section	B	Imaging		
Body System	F	Hepatobiliary System and Pancreas		
Type	1	Fluoroscopy: Single plane or bi-plane real time display of an image developed from the capture of external ionizing radiation on a fluorescent screen. The image may also be stored by either digital or analog means		
Body Part (Character 4)	Contrast (Character 5)	Qualifier (Character 6)	Qualifier (Character 7)
0 Bile Ducts 1 Biliary and Pancreatic Ducts 2 Gallbladder 3 Gallbladder and Bile Ducts 4 Gallbladder, Bile Ducts and Pancreatic Ducts 8 Pancreatic Ducts	0 High Osmolar 1 Low Osmolar Y Other Contrast	Z None	Z None

Section	B	Imaging		
Body System	F	Hepatobiliary System and Pancreas		
Type	2	Computerized Tomography (CT Scan): Computer reformatted digital display of multiplanar images developed from the capture of multiple exposures of external ionizing radiation		
Body Part (Character 4)	Contrast (Character 5)	Qualifier (Character 6)	Qualifier (Character 7)
5 Liver 6 Liver and Spleen 7 Pancreas C Hepatobiliary System, All	0 High Osmolar 1 Low Osmolar Y Other Contrast	0 Unenhanced and Enhanced Z None	Z None
5 Liver 6 Liver and Spleen 7 Pancreas C Hepatobiliary System, All	Z None	Z None	Z None

Section	B	Imaging		
Body System	F	Hepatobiliary System and Pancreas		
Type	3	Magnetic Resonance Imaging (MRI): Computer reformatted digital display of multiplanar images developed from the capture of radiofrequency signals emitted by nuclei in a body site excited within a magnetic field		
Body Part (Character 4)	Contrast (Character 5)	Qualifier (Character 6)	Qualifier (Character 7)
5 Liver 6 Liver and Spleen 7 Pancreas	Y Other Contrast	0 Unenhanced and Enhanced Z None	Z None
5 Liver 6 Liver and Spleen 7 Pancreas	Z None	Z None	Z None

Section	B	Imaging		
Body System	F	Hepatobiliary System and Pancreas		
Type	4	Ultrasonography: Real time display of images of anatomy or flow information developed from the capture of reflected and attenuated high frequency sound waves		
Body Part (Character 4)	Contrast (Character 5)	Qualifier (Character 6)	Qualifier (Character 7)
0 Bile Ducts 2 Gallbladder 3 Gallbladder and Bile Ducts 5 Liver 6 Liver and Spleen 7 Pancreas C Hepatobiliary System, All	Z None	Z None	Z None

Section	B	Imaging		
Body System	G	Endocrine System		
Type	2	Computerized Tomography (CT Scan): Computer reformatted digital display of multiplanar images developed from the capture of multiple exposures of external ionizing radiation		
Body Part (Character 4)	Contrast (Character 5)	Qualifier (Character 6)	Qualifier (Character 7)
2 Adrenal Glands, Bilateral 3 Parathyroid Glands 4 Thyroid Gland	0 High Osmolar 1 Low Osmolar Y Other Contrast	0 Unenhanced and Enhanced Z None	Z None
2 Adrenal Glands, Bilateral 3 Parathyroid Glands 4 Thyroid Gland	Z None	Z None	Z None

Section	B	Imaging		
Body System	G	Endocrine System		
Type	3	Magnetic Resonance Imaging (MRI): Computer reformatted digital display of multiplanar images developed from the capture of radiofrequency signals emitted by nuclei in a body site excited within a magnetic field		
Body Part (Character 4)	Contrast (Character 5)	Qualifier (Character 6)	Qualifier (Character 7)
2 Adrenal Glands, Bilateral 3 Parathyroid Glands 4 Thyroid Gland	Y Other Contrast	0 Unenhanced and Enhanced Z None	Z None
2 Adrenal Glands, Bilateral 3 Parathyroid Glands 4 Thyroid Gland	Z None	Z None	Z None

Section	B	Imaging		
Body System	G	Endocrine System		
Type	4	Ultrasonography: Real time display of images of anatomy or flow information developed from the capture of reflected and attenuated high frequency sound waves		
Body Part (Character 4)	Contrast (Character 5)	Qualifier (Character 6)	Qualifier (Character 7)
0 Adrenal Gland, Right 1 Adrenal Gland, Left 2 Adrenal Glands, Bilateral 3 Parathyroid Glands 4 Thyroid Gland	Z None	Z None	Z None

Section	B	Imaging		
Body System	H	Skin, Subcutaneous Tissue and Breast		
Type	0	Plain Radiography: Planar display of an image developed from the capture of external ionizing radiation on photographic or photoconductive plate		
Body Part (Character 4)	Contrast (Character 5)	Qualifier (Character 6)	Qualifier (Character 7)
0 Breast, Right 1 Breast, Left 2 Breasts, Bilateral	Z None	Z None	Z None
3 Single Mammary Duct, Right 4 Single Mammary Duct, Left 5 Multiple Mammary Ducts, Right 6 Multiple Mammary Ducts, Left	0 High Osmolar 1 Low Osmolar Y Other Contrast Z None	Z None	Z None

Section	B	Imaging
Body System	H	Skin, Subcutaneous Tissue and Breast
Type	3	Magnetic Resonance Imaging (MRI): Computer reformatted digital display of multiplanar images developed from the capture of radiofrequency signals emitted by nuclei in a body site excited within a magnetic field

Body Part (Character 4)	Contrast (Character 5)	Qualifier (Character 6)	Qualifier (Character 7)
0 Breast, Right 1 Breast, Left 2 Breasts, Bilateral D Subcutaneous Tissue, Head/Neck F Subcutaneous Tissue, Upper Extremity G Subcutaneous Tissue, Thorax H Subcutaneous Tissue, Abdomen and Pelvis J Subcutaneous Tissue, Lower Extremity	Y Other Contrast	0 Unenhanced and Enhanced Z None	Z None
0 Breast, Right 1 Breast, Left 2 Breasts, Bilateral D Subcutaneous Tissue, Head/Neck F Subcutaneous Tissue, Upper Extremity G Subcutaneous Tissue, Thorax H Subcutaneous Tissue, Abdomen and Pelvis J Subcutaneous Tissue, Lower Extremity	Z None	Z None	Z None

Section	B	Imaging
Body System	H	Skin, Subcutaneous Tissue and Breast
Type	4	Ultrasonography: Real time display of images of anatomy or flow information developed from the capture of reflected and attenuated high frequency sound waves

Body Part (Character 4)	Contrast (Character 5)	Qualifier (Character 6)	Qualifier (Character 7)
0 Breast, Right 1 Breast, Left 2 Breasts, Bilateral 7 Extremity, Upper 8 Extremity, Lower 9 Abdominal Wall B Chest Wall C Head and Neck	Z None	Z None	Z None

Section	B	Imaging
Body System	L	Connective Tissue
Type	3	Magnetic Resonance Imaging (MRI): Computer reformatted digital display of multiplanar images developed from the capture of radiofrequency signals emitted by nuclei in a body site excited within a magnetic field

Body Part (Character 4)	Contrast (Character 5)	Qualifier (Character 6)	Qualifier (Character 7)
0 Connective Tissue, Upper Extremity 1 Connective Tissue, Lower Extremity 2 Tendons, Upper Extremity 3 Tendons, Lower Extremity	Y Other Contrast	0 Unenhanced and Enhanced Z None	Z None
0 Connective Tissue, Upper Extremity 1 Connective Tissue, Lower Extremity 2 Tendons, Upper Extremity 3 Tendons, Lower Extremity	Z None	Z None	Z None

Section	B	Imaging
Body System	L	Connective Tissue
Type	4	Ultrasonography: Real time display of images of anatomy or flow information developed from the capture of reflected and attenuated high frequency sound waves

Body Part (Character 4)	Contrast (Character 5)	Qualifier (Character 6)	Qualifier (Character 7)
0 Connective Tissue, Upper Extremity 1 Connective Tissue, Lower Extremity 2 Tendons, Upper Extremity 3 Tendons, Lower Extremity	Z None	Z None	Z None

Section	B	Imaging		
Body System	N	Skull and Facial Bones		
Type	0	Plain Radiography: Planar display of an image developed from the capture of external ionizing radiation on photographic or photoconductive plate		
Body Part (Character 4)		**Contrast (Character 5)**	**Qualifier (Character 6)**	**Qualifier (Character 7)**
0 Skull 1 Orbit, Right 2 Orbit, Left 3 Orbits, Bilateral 4 Nasal Bones 5 Facial Bones 6 Mandible B Zygomatic Arch, Right C Zygomatic Arch, Left D Zygomatic Arches, Bilateral G Tooth, Single H Teeth, Multiple J Teeth, All		Z None	Z None	Z None
7 Temporomandibular Joint, Right 8 Temporomandibular Joint, Left 9 Temporomandibular Joints, Bilateral		0 High Osmolar 1 Low Osmolar Y Other Contrast Z None	Z None	Z None

Section	B	Imaging		
Body System	N	Skull and Facial Bones		
Type	1	Fluoroscopy: Single plane or bi-plane real time display of an image developed from the capture of external ionizing radiation on a fluorescent screen. The image may also be stored by either digital or analog means		
Body Part (Character 4)		**Contrast (Character 5)**	**Qualifier (Character 6)**	**Qualifier (Character 7)**
7 Temporomandibular Joint, Right 8 Temporomandibular Joint, Left 9 Temporomandibular Joints, Bilateral		0 High Osmolar 1 Low Osmolar Y Other Contrast Z None	Z None	Z None

Section	B	Imaging		
Body System	N	Skull and Facial Bones		
Type	2	Computerized Tomography (CT Scan): Computer reformatted digital display of multiplanar images developed from the capture of multiple exposures of external ionizing radiation		
Body Part (Character 4)		**Contrast (Character 5)**	**Qualifier (Character 6)**	**Qualifier (Character 7)**
0 Skull 3 Orbits, Bilateral 5 Facial Bones 6 Mandible 9 Temporomandibular Joints, Bilateral F Temporal Bones		0 High Osmolar 1 Low Osmolar Y Other Contrast Z None	Z None	Z None

Section	B	Imaging		
Body System	N	Skull and Facial Bones		
Type	3	Magnetic Resonance Imaging (MRI): Computer reformatted digital display of multiplanar images developed from the capture of radiofrequency signals emitted by nuclei in a body site excited within a magnetic field		
Body Part (Character 4)		**Contrast (Character 5)**	**Qualifier (Character 6)**	**Qualifier (Character 7)**
9 Temporomandibular Joints, Bilateral		Y Other Contrast Z None	Z None	Z None

Section	B	Imaging
Body System	P	Non-Axial Upper Bones
Type	0	Plain Radiography: Planar display of an image developed from the capture of external ionizing radiation on photographic or photoconductive plate

Body Part (Character 4)	Contrast (Character 5)	Qualifier (Character 6)	Qualifier (Character 7)
0 Sternoclavicular Joint, Right 1 Sternoclavicular Joint, Left 2 Sternoclavicular Joints, Bilateral 3 Acromioclavicular Joints, Bilateral 4 Clavicle, Right 5 Clavicle, Left 6 Scapula, Right 7 Scapula, Left A Humerus, Right B Humerus, Left E Upper Arm, Right F Upper Arm, Left J Forearm, Right K Forearm, Left N Hand, Right P Hand, Left R Finger(s), Right S Finger(s), Left X Ribs, Right Y Ribs, Left	Z None	Z None	Z None
8 Shoulder, Right 9 Shoulder, Left C Hand/Finger Joint, Right D Hand/Finger Joint, Left G Elbow, Right H Elbow, Left L Wrist, Right M Wrist, Left	0 High Osmolar 1 Low Osmolar Y Other Contrast Z None	Z None	Z None

Section	B	Imaging
Body System	P	Non-Axial Upper Bones
Type	1	Fluoroscopy: Single plane or bi-plane real time display of an image developed from the capture of external ionizing radiation on a fluorescent screen. The image may also be stored by either digital or analog means

Body Part (Character 4)	Contrast (Character 5)	Qualifier (Character 6)	Qualifier (Character 7)
0 Sternoclavicular Joint, Right 1 Sternoclavicular Joint, Left 2 Sternoclavicular Joints, Bilateral 3 Acromioclavicular Joints, Bilateral 4 Clavicle, Right 5 Clavicle, Left 6 Scapula, Right 7 Scapula, Left A Humerus, Right B Humerus, Left E Upper Arm, Right F Upper Arm, Left J Forearm, Right K Forearm, Left N Hand, Right P Hand, Left R Finger(s), Right S Finger(s), Left X Ribs, Right Y Ribs, Left	Z None	Z None	Z None
8 Shoulder, Right 9 Shoulder, Left L Wrist, Right M Wrist, Left	0 High Osmolar 1 Low Osmolar Y Other Contrast Z None	Z None	Z None
C Hand/Finger Joint, Right D Hand/Finger Joint, Left G Elbow, Right H Elbow, Left	0 High Osmolar 1 Low Osmolar Y Other Contrast	Z None	Z None

Section	B	Imaging		
Body System	P	Non-Axial Upper Bones		
Type	2	Computerized Tomography (CT Scan): Computer reformatted digital display of multiplanar images developed from the capture of multiple exposures of external ionizing radiation		

Body Part (Character 4)	Contrast (Character 5)	Qualifier (Character 6)	Qualifier (Character 7)
0 Sternoclavicular Joint, Right 1 Sternoclavicular Joint, Left W Thorax	0 High Osmolar 1 Low Osmolar Y Other Contrast	Z None	Z None
2 Sternoclavicular Joints, Bilateral 3 Acromioclavicular Joints, Bilateral 4 Clavicle, Right 5 Clavicle, Left 6 Scapula, Right 7 Scapula, Left 8 Shoulder, Right 9 Shoulder, Left A Humerus, Right B Humerus, Left E Upper Arm, Right F Upper Arm, Left G Elbow, Right H Elbow, Left J Forearm, Right K Forearm, Left L Wrist, Right M Wrist, Left N Hand, Right P Hand, Left Q Hands and Wrists, Bilateral R Finger(s), Right S Finger(s), Left T Upper Extremity, Right U Upper Extremity, Left V Upper Extremities, Bilateral X Ribs, Right Y Ribs, Left	0 High Osmolar 1 Low Osmolar Y Other Contrast Z None	Z None	Z None
C Hand/Finger Joint, Right D Hand/Finger Joint, Left	Z None	Z None	Z None

Section	B	Imaging		
Body System	P	Non-Axial Upper Bones		
Type	3	Magnetic Resonance Imaging (MRI): Computer reformatted digital display of multiplanar images developed from the capture of radiofrequency signals emitted by nuclei in a body site excited within a magnetic field		

Body Part (Character 4)	Contrast (Character 5)	Qualifier (Character 6)	Qualifier (Character 7)
8 Shoulder, Right 9 Shoulder, Left C Hand/Finger Joint, Right D Hand/Finger Joint, Left E Upper Arm, Right F Upper Arm, Left G Elbow, Right H Elbow, Left J Forearm, Right K Forearm, Left L Wrist, Right M Wrist, Left	Y Other Contrast	0 Unenhanced and Enhanced Z None	Z None
8 Shoulder, Right 9 Shoulder, Left C Hand/Finger Joint, Right D Hand/Finger Joint, Left E Upper Arm, Right F Upper Arm, Left G Elbow, Right H Elbow, Left J Forearm, Right K Forearm, Left L Wrist, Right M Wrist, Left	Z None	Z None	Z None

Section	B	Imaging
Body System	P	Non-Axial Upper Bones
Type	4	Ultrasonography: Real time display of images of anatomy or flow information developed from the capture of reflected and attenuated high frequency sound waves

Body Part (Character 4)	Contrast (Character 5)	Qualifier (Character 6)	Qualifier (Character 7)
8 Shoulder, Right 9 Shoulder, Left G Elbow, Right H Elbow, Left L Wrist, Right M Wrist, Left N Hand, Right P Hand, Left	Z None	Z None	1 Densitometry Z None

Section	B	Imaging
Body System	Q	Non-Axial Lower Bones
Type	0	Plain Radiography: Planar display of an image developed from the capture of external ionizing radiation on photographic or photoconductive plate

Body Part (Character 4)	Contrast (Character 5)	Qualifier (Character 6)	Qualifier (Character 7)
0 Hip, Right 1 Hip, Left	0 High Osmolar 1 Low Osmolar Y Other Contrast	Z None	Z None
0 Hip, Right 1 Hip, Left	Z None	Z None	1 Densitometry Z None
3 Femur, Right 4 Femur, Left	Z None	Z None	1 Densitometry Z None
7 Knee, Right 8 Knee, Left G Ankle, Right H Ankle, Left	0 High Osmolar 1 Low Osmolar Y Other Contrast Z None	Z None	Z None
D Lower Leg, Right F Lower Leg, Left J Calcaneus, Right K Calcaneus, Left L Foot, Right M Foot, Left P Toe(s), Right Q Toe(s), Left V Patella, Right W Patella, Left	Z None	Z None	Z None
X Foot/Toe Joint, Right Y Foot/Toe Joint, Left	0 High Osmolar 1 Low Osmolar Y Other Contrast	Z None	Z None

Section	B	Imaging
Body System	Q	Non-Axial Lower Bones
Type	1	Fluoroscopy: Single plane or bi-plane real time display of an image developed from the capture of external ionizing radiation on a fluorescent screen. The image may also be stored by either digital or analog means

Body Part (Character 4)	Contrast (Character 5)	Qualifier (Character 6)	Qualifier (Character 7)
0 Hip, Right 1 Hip, Left 7 Knee, Right 8 Knee, Left G Ankle, Right H Ankle, Left X Foot/Toe Joint, Right Y Foot/Toe Joint, Left	0 High Osmolar 1 Low Osmolar Y Other Contrast Z None	Z None	Z None
3 Femur, Right 4 Femur, Left D Lower Leg, Right F Lower Leg, Left J Calcaneus, Right K Calcaneus, Left L Foot, Right M Foot, Left P Toe(s), Right Q Toe(s), Left V Patella, Right W Patella, Left	Z None	Z None	Z None

Section	B	Imaging		
Body System	Q	Non-Axial Lower Bones		
Type	2	Computerized Tomography (CT Scan): Computer reformatted digital display of multiplanar images developed from the capture of multiple exposures of external ionizing radiation		

Body Part (Character 4)	Contrast (Character 5)	Qualifier (Character 6)	Qualifier (Character 7)
0 Hip, Right 1 Hip, Left 3 Femur, Right 4 Femur, Left 7 Knee, Right 8 Knee, Left D Lower Leg, Right F Lower Leg, Left G Ankle, Right H Ankle, Left J Calcaneus, Right K Calcaneus, Left L Foot, Right M Foot, Left P Toe(s), Right Q Toe(s), Left R Lower Extremity, Right S Lower Extremity, Left V Patella, Right W Patella, Left X Foot/Toe Joint, Right Y Foot/Toe Joint, Left	0 High Osmolar 1 Low Osmolar Y Other Contrast Z None	Z None	Z None
B Tibia/Fibula, Right C Tibia/Fibula, Left	0 High Osmolar 1 Low Osmolar Y Other Contrast	Z None	Z None

Section	B	Imaging		
Body System	Q	Non-Axial Lower Bones		
Type	3	Magnetic Resonance Imaging (MRI): Computer reformatted digital display of multiplanar images developed from the capture of radiofrequency signals emitted by nuclei in a body site excited within a magnetic field		

Body Part (Character 4)	Contrast (Character 5)	Qualifier (Character 6)	Qualifier (Character 7)
0 Hip, Right 1 Hip, Left 3 Femur, Right 4 Femur, Left 7 Knee, Right 8 Knee, Left D Lower Leg, Right F Lower Leg, Left G Ankle, Right H Ankle, Left J Calcaneus, Right K Calcaneus, Left L Foot, Right M Foot, Left P Toe(s), Right Q Toe(s), Left V Patella, Right W Patella, Left	Y Other Contrast	0 Unenhanced and Enhanced Z None	Z None
0 Hip, Right 1 Hip, Left 3 Femur, Right 4 Femur, Left 7 Knee, Right 8 Knee, Left D Lower Leg, Right F Lower Leg, Left G Ankle, Right H Ankle, Left J Calcaneus, Right K Calcaneus, Left L Foot, Right M Foot, Left P Toe(s), Right Q Toe(s), Left V Patella, Right W Patella, Left	Z None	Z None	Z None

Section	B	Imaging			
Body System	Q	Non-Axial Lower Bones			
Type	4	Ultrasonography: Real time display of images of anatomy or flow information developed from the capture of reflected and attenuated high frequency sound waves			
Body Part (Character 4)		**Contrast (Character 5)**	**Qualifier (Character 6)**		**Qualifier (Character 7)**
0 Hip, Right 1 Hip, Left 2 Hips, Bilateral 7 Knee, Right 8 Knee, Left 9 Knees, Bilateral		Z None	Z None		Z None

Section	B	Imaging			
Body System	R	Axial Skeleton, Except Skull and Facial Bones			
Type	0	Plain Radiography: Planar display of an image developed from the capture of external ionizing radiation on photographic or photoconductive plate			
Body Part (Character 4)		**Contrast (Character 5)**	**Qualifier (Character 6)**		**Qualifier (Character 7)**
0 Cervical Spine 7 Thoracic Spine 9 Lumbar Spine G Whole Spine		Z None	Z None		1 Densitometry Z None
1 Cervical Disc(s) 2 Thoracic Disc(s) 3 Lumbar Disc(s) 4 Cervical Facet Joint(s) 5 Thoracic Facet Joint(s) 6 Lumbar Facet Joint(s) D Sacroiliac Joints		0 High Osmolar 1 Low Osmolar Y Other Contrast Z None	Z None		Z None
8 Thoracolumbar Joint B Lumbosacral Joint C Pelvis F Sacrum and Coccyx H Sternum		Z None	Z None		Z None

Section	B	Imaging			
Body System	R	Axial Skeleton, Except Skull and Facial Bones			
Type	1	Fluoroscopy: Single plane or bi-plane real time display of an image developed from the capture of external ionizing radiation on a fluorescent screen. The image may also be stored by either digital or analog means			
Body Part (Character 4)		**Contrast (Character 5)**	**Qualifier (Character 6)**		**Qualifier (Character 7)**
0 Cervical Spine 1 Cervical Disc(s) 2 Thoracic Disc(s) 3 Lumbar Disc(s) 4 Cervical Facet Joint(s) 5 Thoracic Facet Joint(s) 6 Lumbar Facet Joint(s) 7 Thoracic Spine 8 Thoracolumbar Joint 9 Lumbar Spine B Lumbosacral Joint C Pelvis D Sacroiliac Joints F Sacrum and Coccyx G Whole Spine H Sternum		0 High Osmolar 1 Low Osmolar Y Other Contrast Z None	Z None		Z None

Section	B	Imaging			
Body System	R	Axial Skeleton, Except Skull and Facial Bones			
Type	2	Computerized Tomography (CT Scan): Computer reformatted digital display of multiplanar images developed from the capture of multiple exposures of external ionizing radiation			
Body Part (Character 4)		**Contrast (Character 5)**	**Qualifier (Character 6)**		**Qualifier (Character 7)**
0 Cervical Spine 7 Thoracic Spine 9 Lumbar Spine C Pelvis D Sacroiliac Joints F Sacrum and Coccyx		0 High Osmolar 1 Low Osmolar Y Other Contrast Z None	Z None		Z None

Section	B	Imaging		
Body System	R	Axial Skeleton, Except Skull and Facial Bones		
Type	3	Magnetic Resonance Imaging (MRI): Computer reformatted digital display of multiplanar images developed from the capture of radiofrequency signals emitted by nuclei in a body site excited within a magnetic field		

Body Part (Character 4)	Contrast (Character 5)	Qualifier (Character 6)	Qualifier (Character 7)
0 Cervical Spine 1 Cervical Disc(s) 2 Thoracic Disc(s) 3 Lumbar Disc(s) 7 Thoracic Spine 9 Lumbar Spine C Pelvis F Sacrum and Coccyx	Y Other Contrast	0 Unenhanced and Enhanced Z None	Z None
0 Cervical Spine 1 Cervical Disc(s) 2 Thoracic Disc(s) 3 Lumbar Disc(s) 7 Thoracic Spine 9 Lumbar Spine C Pelvis F Sacrum and Coccyx	Z None	Z None	Z None

Section	B	Imaging		
Body System	R	Axial Skeleton, Except Skull and Facial Bones		
Type	4	Ultrasonography: Real time display of images of anatomy or flow information developed from the capture of reflected and attenuated high frequency sound waves		

Body Part (Character 4)	Contrast (Character 5)	Qualifier (Character 6)	Qualifier (Character 7)
0 Cervical Spine 7 Thoracic Spine 9 Lumbar Spine F Sacrum and Coccyx	Z None	Z None	Z None

Section	B	Imaging		
Body System	T	Urinary System		
Type	0	Plain Radiography: Planar display of an image developed from the capture of external ionizing radiation on photographic or photoconductive plate		

Body Part (Character 4)	Contrast (Character 5)	Qualifier (Character 6)	Qualifier (Character 7)
0 Bladder 1 Kidney, Right 2 Kidney, Left 3 Kidneys, Bilateral 4 Kidneys, Ureters and Bladder 5 Urethra 6 Ureter, Right 7 Ureter, Left 8 Ureters, Bilateral B Bladder and Urethra C Ileal Diversion Loop	0 High Osmolar 1 Low Osmolar Y Other Contrast Z None	Z None	Z None

Section	B	Imaging		
Body System	T	Urinary System		
Type	1	Fluoroscopy: Single plane or bi-plane real time display of an image developed from the capture of external ionizing radiation on a fluorescent screen. The image may also be stored by either digital or analog means		

Body Part (Character 4)	Contrast (Character 5)	Qualifier (Character 6)	Qualifier (Character 7)
0 Bladder 1 Kidney, Right 2 Kidney, Left 3 Kidneys, Bilateral 4 Kidneys, Ureters and Bladder 5 Urethra 6 Ureter, Right 7 Ureter, Left B Bladder and Urethra C Ileal Diversion Loop D Kidney, Ureter and Bladder, Right F Kidney, Ureter and Bladder, Left G Ileal Loop, Ureters and Kidneys	0 High Osmolar 1 Low Osmolar Y Other Contrast Z None	Z None	Z None

Section	B	Imaging
Body System	T	Urinary System
Type	2	Computerized Tomography (CT Scan): Computer reformatted digital display of multiplanar images developed from the capture of multiple exposures of external ionizing radiation

Body Part (Character 4)	Contrast (Character 5)	Qualifier (Character 6)	Qualifier (Character 7)
0 Bladder 1 Kidney, Right 2 Kidney, Left 3 Kidneys, Bilateral 9 Kidney Transplant	0 High Osmolar 1 Low Osmolar Y Other Contrast	0 Unenhanced and Enhanced Z None	Z None
0 Bladder 1 Kidney, Right 2 Kidney, Left 3 Kidneys, Bilateral 9 Kidney Transplant	Z None	Z None	Z None

Section	B	Imaging
Body System	T	Urinary System
Type	3	Magnetic Resonance Imaging (MRI): Computer reformatted digital display of multiplanar images developed from the capture of radiofrequency signals emitted by nuclei in a body site excited within a magnetic field

Body Part (Character 4)	Contrast (Character 5)	Qualifier (Character 6)	Qualifier (Character 7)
0 Bladder 1 Kidney, Right 2 Kidney, Left 3 Kidneys, Bilateral 9 Kidney Transplant	Y Other Contrast	0 Unenhanced and Enhanced Z None	Z None
0 Bladder 1 Kidney, Right 2 Kidney, Left 3 Kidneys, Bilateral 9 Kidney Transplant	Z None	Z None	Z None

Section	B	Imaging
Body System	T	Urinary System
Type	4	Ultrasonography: Real time display of images of anatomy or flow information developed from the capture of reflected and attenuated high frequency sound waves

Body Part (Character 4)	Contrast (Character 5)	Qualifier (Character 6)	Qualifier (Character 7)
0 Bladder 1 Kidney, Right 2 Kidney, Left 3 Kidneys, Bilateral 5 Urethra 6 Ureter, Right 7 Ureter, Left 8 Ureters, Bilateral 9 Kidney Transplant J Kidneys and Bladder	Z None	Z None	Z None

Section	B	Imaging
Body System	U	Female Reproductive System
Type	0	Plain Radiography: Planar display of an image developed from the capture of external ionizing radiation on photographic or photoconductive plate

Body Part (Character 4)	Contrast (Character 5)	Qualifier (Character 6)	Qualifier (Character 7)
0 Fallopian Tube, Right 1 Fallopian Tube, Left 2 Fallopian Tubes, Bilateral 6 Uterus 8 Uterus and Fallopian Tubes 9 Vagina	0 High Osmolar 1 Low Osmolar Y Other Contrast	Z None	Z None

Section	B	Imaging
Body System	U	Female Reproductive System
Type	1	Fluoroscopy: Single plane or bi-plane real time display of an image developed from the capture of external ionizing radiation on a fluorescent screen. The image may also be stored by either digital or analog means

Body Part (Character 4)	Contrast (Character 5)	Qualifier (Character 6)	Qualifier (Character 7)
0 Fallopian Tube, Right 1 Fallopian Tube, Left 2 Fallopian Tubes, Bilateral 6 Uterus 8 Uterus and Fallopian Tubes 9 Vagina	0 High Osmolar 1 Low Osmolar Y Other Contrast Z None	Z None	Z None

Section	B	Imaging
Body System	U	Female Reproductive System
Type	3	Magnetic Resonance Imaging (MRI): Computer reformatted digital display of multiplanar images developed from the capture of radiofrequency signals emitted by nuclei in a body site excited within a magnetic field

Body Part (Character 4)	Contrast (Character 5)	Qualifier (Character 6)	Qualifier (Character 7)
3 Ovary, Right 4 Ovary, Left 5 Ovaries, Bilateral 6 Uterus 9 Vagina B Pregnant Uterus C Uterus and Ovaries	Y Other Contrast	0 Unenhanced and Enhanced Z None	Z None
3 Ovary, Right 4 Ovary, Left 5 Ovaries, Bilateral 6 Uterus 9 Vagina B Pregnant Uterus C Uterus and Ovaries	Z None	Z None	Z None

Section	B	Imaging
Body System	U	Female Reproductive System
Type	4	Ultrasonography: Real time display of images of anatomy or flow information developed from the capture of reflected and attenuated high frequency sound waves

Body Part (Character 4)	Contrast (Character 5)	Qualifier (Character 6)	Qualifier (Character 7)
0 Fallopian Tube, Right 1 Fallopian Tube, Left 2 Fallopian Tubes, Bilateral 3 Ovary, Right 4 Ovary, Left 5 Ovaries, Bilateral 6 Uterus C Uterus and Ovaries	Y Other Contrast Z None	Z None	Z None

Section	B	Imaging
Body System	V	Male Reproductive System
Type	0	Plain Radiography: Planar display of an image developed from the capture of external ionizing radiation on photographic or photoconductive plate

Body Part (Character 4)	Contrast (Character 5)	Qualifier (Character 6)	Qualifier (Character 7)
0 Corpora Cavernosa 1 Epididymis, Right 2 Epididymis, Left 3 Prostate 5 Testicle, Right 6 Testicle, Left 8 Vasa Vasorum	0 High Osmolar 1 Low Osmolar Y Other Contrast	Z None	Z None

Section	B	Imaging
Body System	V	Male Reproductive System
Type	1	Fluoroscopy: Single plane or bi-plane real time display of an image developed from the capture of external ionizing radiation on a fluorescent screen. The image may also be stored by either digital or analog means

Body Part (Character 4)	Contrast (Character 5)	Qualifier (Character 6)	Qualifier (Character 7)
0 Corpora Cavernosa 8 Vasa Vasorum	0 High Osmolar 1 Low Osmolar Y Other Contrast Z None	Z None	Z None

Section	B	Imaging
Body System	V	Male Reproductive System
Type	2	Computerized Tomography (CT Scan): Computer reformatted digital display of multiplanar images developed from the capture of multiple exposures of external ionizing radiation

Body Part (Character 4)	Contrast (Character 5)	Qualifier (Character 6)	Qualifier (Character 7)
3 Prostate	0 High Osmolar 1 Low Osmolar Y Other Contrast	0 Unenhanced and Enhanced Z None	Z None
3 Prostate	Z None	Z None	Z None

Section	B	Imaging			
Body System	V	Male Reproductive System			
Type	3	Magnetic Resonance Imaging (MRI): Computer reformatted digital display of multiplanar images developed from the capture of radiofrequency signals emitted by nuclei in a body site excited within a magnetic field			

Body Part (Character 4)	Contrast (Character 5)	Qualifier (Character 6)	Qualifier (Character 7)
0 Corpora Cavernosa 3 Prostate 4 Scrotum 5 Testicle, Right 6 Testicle, Left 7 Testicles, Bilateral	Y Other Contrast	0 Unenhanced and Enhanced Z None	Z None
0 Corpora Cavernosa 3 Prostate 4 Scrotum 5 Testicle, Right 6 Testicle, Left 7 Testicles, Bilateral	Z None	Z None	Z None

Section	B	Imaging			
Body System	V	Male Reproductive System			
Type	4	Ultrasonography: Real time display of images of anatomy or flow information developed from the capture of reflected and attenuated high frequency sound waves			

Body Part (Character 4)	Contrast (Character 5)	Qualifier (Character 6)	Qualifier (Character 7)
4 Scrotum 9 Prostate and Seminal Vesicles B Penis	Z None	Z None	Z None

Section	B	Imaging			
Body System	W	Anatomical Regions			
Type	0	Plain Radiography: Planar display of an image developed from the capture of external ionizing radiation on photographic or photoconductive plate			

Body Part (Character 4)	Contrast (Character 5)	Qualifier (Character 6)	Qualifier (Character 7)
0 Abdomen 1 Abdomen and Pelvis 3 Chest B Long Bones, All C Lower Extremity J Upper Extremity K Whole Body L Whole Skeleton M Whole Body, Infant	Z None	Z None	Z None

Section	B	Imaging			
Body System	W	Anatomical Regions			
Type	1	Fluoroscopy: Single plane or bi-plane real time display of an image developed from the capture of external ionizing radiation on a fluorescent screen. The image may also be stored by either digital or analog means			

Body Part (Character 4)	Contrast (Character 5)	Qualifier (Character 6)	Qualifier (Character 7)
1 Abdomen and Pelvis 9 Head and Neck C Lower Extremity J Upper Extremity	0 High Osmolar 1 Low Osmolar Y Other Contrast Z None	Z None	Z None

Section	B	Imaging			
Body System	W	Anatomical Regions			
Type	2	Computerized Tomography (CT Scan): Computer reformatted digital display of multiplanar images developed from the capture of multiple exposures of external ionizing radiation			

Body Part (Character 4)	Contrast (Character 5)	Qualifier (Character 6)	Qualifier (Character 7)
0 Abdomen 1 Abdomen and Pelvis 4 Chest and Abdomen 5 Chest, Abdomen and Pelvis 8 Head 9 Head and Neck F Neck G Pelvic Region	0 High Osmolar 1 Low Osmolar Y Other Contrast	0 Unenhanced and Enhanced Z None	Z None
0 Abdomen 1 Abdomen and Pelvis 4 Chest and Abdomen 5 Chest, Abdomen and Pelvis 8 Head 9 Head and Neck F Neck G Pelvic Region	Z None	Z None	Z None

Section	B	Imaging		
Body System	W	Anatomical Regions		
Type	3	Magnetic Resonance Imaging (MRI): Computer reformatted digital display of multiplanar images developed from the capture of radiofrequency signals emitted by nuclei in a body site excited within a magnetic field		

Body Part (Character 4)	Contrast (Character 5)	Qualifier (Character 6)	Qualifier (Character 7)
0 Abdomen 8 Head F Neck G Pelvic Region H Retroperitoneum P Brachial Plexus	Y Other Contrast	0 Unenhanced and Enhanced Z None	Z None
0 Abdomen 8 Head F Neck G Pelvic Region H Retroperitoneum P Brachial Plexus	Z None	Z None	Z None
3 Chest	Y Other Contrast	0 Unenhanced and Enhanced Z None	Z None

Section	B	Imaging		
Body System	W	Anatomical Regions		
Type	4	Ultrasonography: Real time display of images of anatomy or flow information developed from the capture of reflected and attenuated high frequency sound waves		

Body Part (Character 4)	Contrast (Character 5)	Qualifier (Character 6)	Qualifier (Character 7)
0 Abdomen 1 Abdomen and Pelvis F Neck G Pelvic Region	Z None	Z None	Z None

Section	B	Imaging		
Body System	Y	Fetus and Obstetrical		
Type	3	Magnetic Resonance Imaging (MRI): Computer reformatted digital display of multiplanar images developed from the capture of radiofrequency signals emitted by nuclei in a body site excited within a magnetic field		

Body Part (Character 4)	Contrast (Character 5)	Qualifier (Character 6)	Qualifier (Character 7)
0 Fetal Head 1 Fetal Heart 2 Fetal Thorax 3 Fetal Abdomen 4 Fetal Spine 5 Fetal Extremities 6 Whole Fetus	Y Other Contrast	0 Unenhanced and Enhanced Z None	Z None
0 Fetal Head 1 Fetal Heart 2 Fetal Thorax 3 Fetal Abdomen 4 Fetal Spine 5 Fetal Extremities 6 Whole Fetus	Z None	Z None	Z None

Section	B	Imaging		
Body System	Y	Fetus and Obstetrical		
Type	4	Ultrasonography: Real time display of images of anatomy or flow information developed from the capture of reflected and attenuated high frequency sound waves		

Body Part (Character 4)	Contrast (Character 5)	Qualifier (Character 6)	Qualifier (Character 7)
7 Fetal Umbilical Cord 8 Placenta 9 First Trimester, Single Fetus B First Trimester, Multiple Gestation C Second Trimester, Single Fetus D Second Trimester, Multiple Gestation F Third Trimester, Single Fetus G Third Trimester, Multiple Gestation	Z None	Z None	Z None

Section	C	Nuclear Medicine
Body System	0	Central Nervous System
Type	1	Planar Nuclear Medicine Imaging: Introduction of radioactive materials into the body for single plane display of images developed from the capture of radioactive emissions

Body Part (Character 4)	Radionuclide (Character 5)	Qualifier (Character 6)	Qualifier (Character 7)
0 Brain	1 Technetium 99m (Tc-99m) Y Other Radionuclide	Z None	Z None
5 Cerebrospinal Fluid	D Indium 111 (In-111) Y Other Radionuclide	Z None	Z None
Y Central Nervous System	Y Other Radionuclide	Z None	Z None

Section	C	Nuclear Medicine
Body System	0	Central Nervous System
Type	2	Tomographic (Tomo) Nuclear Medicine Imaging: Introduction of radioactive materials into the body for three dimensional display of images developed from the capture of radioactive emissions

Body Part (Character 4)	Radionuclide (Character 5)	Qualifier (Character 6)	Qualifier (Character 7)
0 Brain	1 Technetium 99m (Tc-99m) F Iodine 123 (I-123) S Thallium 201 (Tl-201) Y Other Radionuclide	Z None	Z None
5 Cerebrospinal Fluid	D Indium 111 (In-111) Y Other Radionuclide	Z None	Z None
Y Central Nervous System	Y Other Radionuclide	Z None	Z None

Section	C	Nuclear Medicine
Body System	0	Central Nervous System
Type	3	Positron Emission Tomographic (PET) Imaging: Introduction of radioactive materials into the body for three dimensional display of images developed from the simultaneous capture, 180 degrees apart, of radioactive emissions

Body Part (Character 4)	Radionuclide (Character 5)	Qualifier (Character 6)	Qualifier (Character 7)
0 Brain	B Carbon 11 (C-11) K Fluorine 18 (F-18) M Oxygen 15 (O-15) Y Other Radionuclide	Z None	Z None
Y Central Nervous System	Y Other Radionuclide	Z None	Z None

Section	C	Nuclear Medicine
Body System	0	Central Nervous System
Type	5	Nonimaging Nuclear Medicine Probe: Introduction of radioactive materials into the body for the study of distribution and fate of certain substances by the detection of radioactive emissions; or, alternatively, measurement of absorption of radioactive emissions from an external source

Body Part (Character 4)	Radionuclide (Character 5)	Qualifier (Character 6)	Qualifier (Character 7)
0 Brain	V Xenon 133 (Xe-133) Y Other Radionuclide	Z None	Z None
Y Central Nervous System	Y Other Radionuclide	Z None	Z None

Section	C	Nuclear Medicine
Body System	2	Heart
Type	1	Planar Nuclear Medicine Imaging: Introduction of radioactive materials into the body for single plane display of images developed from the capture of radioactive emissions

Body Part (Character 4)	Radionuclide (Character 5)	Qualifier (Character 6)	Qualifier (Character 7)
6 Heart, Right and Left	1 Technetium 99m (Tc-99m) Y Other Radionuclide	Z None	Z None
G Myocardium	1 Technetium 99m (Tc-99m) D Indium 111 (In-111) S Thallium 201 (Tl-201) Y Other Radionuclide Z None	Z None	Z None
Y Heart	Y Other Radionuclide	Z None	Z None

Section	C	Nuclear Medicine		
Body System	2	Heart		
Type	2	Tomographic (Tomo) Nuclear Medicine Imaging: Introduction of radioactive materials into the body for three dimensional display of images developed from the capture of radioactive emissions		
Body Part (Character 4)	Radionuclide (Character 5)		Qualifier (Character 6)	Qualifier (Character 7)
6 Heart, Right and Left	1 Technetium 99m (Tc-99m) Y Other Radionuclide		Z None	Z None
G Myocardium	1 Technetium 99m (Tc-99m) D Indium 111 (In-111) K Fluorine 18 (F-18) S Thallium 201 (Tl-201) Y Other Radionuclide Z None		Z None	Z None
Y Heart	Y Other Radionuclide		Z None	Z None

Section	C	Nuclear Medicine		
Body System	2	Heart		
Type	3	Positron Emission Tomographic (PET) Imaging: Introduction of radioactive materials into the body for three dimensional display of images developed from the simultaneous capture, 180 degrees apart, of radioactive emissions		
Body Part (Character 4)	Radionuclide (Character 5)		Qualifier (Character 6)	Qualifier (Character 7)
G Myocardium	K Fluorine 18 (F-18) M Oxygen 15 (O-15) Q Rubidium 82 (Rb-82) R Nitrogen 13 (N-13) Y Other Radionuclide		Z None	Z None
Y Heart	Y Other Radionuclide		Z None	Z None

Section	C	Nuclear Medicine		
Body System	2	Heart		
Type	5	Nonimaging Nuclear Medicine Probe: Introduction of radioactive materials into the body for the study of distribution and fate of certain substances by the detection of radioactive emissions; or, alternatively, measurement of absorption of radioactive emissions from an external source		
Body Part (Character 4)	Radionuclide (Character 5)		Qualifier (Character 6)	Qualifier (Character 7)
6 Heart, Right and Left	1 Technetium 99m (Tc-99m) Y Other Radionuclide		Z None	Z None
Y Heart	Y Other Radionuclide		Z None	Z None

Section	C	Nuclear Medicine		
Body System	5	Veins		
Type	1	Planar Nuclear Medicine Imaging: Introduction of radioactive materials into the body for single plane display of images developed from the capture of radioactive emissions		
Body Part (Character 4)	Radionuclide (Character 5)		Qualifier (Character 6)	Qualifier (Character 7)
B Lower Extremity Veins, Right C Lower Extremity Veins, Left D Lower Extremity Veins, Bilateral N Upper Extremity Veins, Right P Upper Extremity Veins, Left Q Upper Extremity Veins, Bilateral R Central Veins	1 Technetium 99m (Tc-99m) Y Other Radionuclide		Z None	Z None
Y Veins	Y Other Radionuclide		Z None	Z None

Section	C	Nuclear Medicine		
Body System	7	Lymphatic and Hematologic System		
Type	1	Planar Nuclear Medicine Imaging: Introduction of radioactive materials into the body for single plane display of images developed from the capture of radioactive emissions		
Body Part (Character 4)	Radionuclide (Character 5)		Qualifier (Character 6)	Qualifier (Character 7)
0 Bone Marrow	1 Technetium 99m (Tc-99m) D Indium 111 (In-111) Y Other Radionuclide		Z None	Z None
2 Spleen 5 Lymphatics, Head and Neck D Lymphatics, Pelvic J Lymphatics, Head K Lymphatics, Neck L Lymphatics, Upper Chest M Lymphatics, Trunk N Lymphatics, Upper Extremity P Lymphatics, Lower Extremity	1 Technetium 99m (Tc-99m) Y Other Radionuclide		Z None	Z None
3 Blood	D Indium 111 (In-111) Y Other Radionuclide		Z None	Z None
Y Lymphatic and Hematologic System	Y Other Radionuclide		Z None	Z None

Section	C	Nuclear Medicine		
Body System	7	Lymphatic and Hematologic System		
Type	2	Tomographic (Tomo) Nuclear Medicine Imaging: Introduction of radioactive materials into the body for three dimensional display of images developed from the capture of radioactive emissions		
Body Part (Character 4)		**Radionuclide (Character 5)**	**Qualifier (Character 6)**	**Qualifier (Character 7)**
2 Spleen		1 Technetium 99m (Tc-99m) Y **O**ther Radionuclide	Z None	Z None
Y Lymphatic and Hematologic System		Y Other Radionuclide	Z None	Z None

Section	C	Nuclear Medicine		
Body System	7	Lymphatic and Hematologic System		
Type	5	Nonimaging Nuclear Medicine Probe: Introduction of radioactive materials into the body for the study of distribution and fate of certain substances by the detection of radioactive emissions; or, alternatively, measurement of absorption of radioactive emissions from an external source		
Body Part (Character 4)		**Radionuclide (Character 5)**	**Qualifier (Character 6)**	**Qualifier (Character 7)**
5 Lymphatics, Head and Neck D Lymphatics, Pelvic J Lymphatics, Head K Lymphatics, Neck L Lymphatics, Upper Chest M Lymphatics, Trunk N Lymphatics, Upper Extremity P Lymphatics, Lower Extremity		1 Technetium 99m (Tc-99m) Y **O**ther Radionuclide	Z None	Z None
Y Lymphatic and Hematologic System		Y Other Radionuclide	Z None	Z None

Section	C	Nuclear Medicine		
Body System	7	Lymphatic and Hematologic System		
Type	6	Nonimaging Nuclear Medicine Assay: Introduction of radioactive materials into the body for the study of body fluids and blood elements, by the detection of radioactive emissions		
Body Part (Character 4)		**Radionuclide (Character 5)**	**Qualifier (Character 6)**	**Qualifier (Character 7)**
3 Blood		1 Technetium 99m (Tc-99m) 7 Cobalt 58 (Co-58) C Cobalt 57 (Co-57) D Indium 111 (In-111) H Iodine 125 (I-125) W Chromium (Cr-51) Y **O**ther Radionuclide	Z None	Z None
Y Lymphatic and Hematologic System		Y Other Radionuclide	Z None	Z None

Section	C	Nuclear Medicine		
Body System	8	Eye		
Type	1	Planar Nuclear Medicine Imaging: Introduction of radioactive materials into the body for single plane display of images developed from the capture of radioactive emissions		
Body Part (Character 4)		**Radionuclide (Character 5)**	**Qualifier (Character 6)**	**Qualifier (Character 7)**
9 Lacrimal Ducts, Bilateral		1 Technetium 99m (Tc-99m) Y **O**ther Radionuclide	Z None	Z None
Y Eye		Y Other Radionuclide	Z None	Z None

Section	C	Nuclear Medicine		
Body System	9	Ear, Nose, Mouth and Throat		
Type	1	Planar Nuclear Medicine Imaging: Introduction of radioactive materials into the body for single plane display of images developed from the capture of radioactive emissions		
Body Part Character 4		Radionuclide	Qualifier	Qualifier
B Salivary Glands, Bilateral		1 Technetium 99m (Tc-99m) Y **O**ther Radionuclide	Z None	Z None
Y Ear, Nose, Mouth and Throat		Y Other Radionuclide	Z None	Z None

Section	C	Nuclear Medicine		
Body System	B	Respiratory System		
Type	1	Planar Nuclear Medicine Imaging: Introduction of radioactive materials into the body for single plane display of images developed from the capture of radioactive emissions		
Body Part (Character 4)		**Radionuclide (Character 5)**	**Qualifier (Character 6)**	**Qualifier (Character 7)**
2 Lungs and Bronchi		1 Technetium 99m (Tc-99m) 9 Krypton (Kr-81m) T Xenon 127 (Xe-127) V Xenon 133 (Xe-133) Y **O**ther Radionuclide	Z None	Z None
Y Respiratory System		Y Other Radionuclide	Z None	Z None

Section	C	Nuclear Medicine		
Body System	B	Respiratory System		
Type	2	Tomographic (Tomo) Nuclear Medicine Imaging: Introduction of radioactive materials into the body for three dimensional display of images developed from the capture of radioactive emissions		
Body Part (Character 4)		**Radionuclide (Character 5)**	**Qualifier (Character 6)**	**Qualifier (Character 7)**
2 Lungs and Bronchi		1 Technetium 99m (Tc-99m) 9 Krypton (Kr-81m) Y Other Radionuclide	Z None	Z None
Y Respiratory System		Y Other Radionuclide	Z None	Z None

Section	C	Nuclear Medicine		
Body System	B	Respiratory System		
Type	3	Positron Emission Tomographic (PET) Imaging: Introduction of radioactive materials into the body for three dimensional display of images developed from the simultaneous capture, 180 degrees apart, of radioactive emissions		
Body Part (Character 4)		**Radionuclide (Character 5)**	**Qualifier (Character 6)**	**Qualifier (Character 7)**
2 Lungs and Bronchi		K Fluorine 18 (F-18) Y Other Radionuclide	Z None	Z None
Y Respiratory System		Y Other Radionuclide	Z None	Z None

Section	C	Nuclear Medicine		
Body System	D	Gastrointestinal System		
Type	1	Planar Nuclear Medicine Imaging: Introduction of radioactive materials into the body for single plane display of images developed from the capture of radioactive emissions		
Body Part (Character 4)		**Radionuclide (Character 5)**	**Qualifier (Character 6)**	**Qualifier (Character 7)**
5 Upper Gastrointestinal Tract 7 Gastrointestinal Tract		1 Technetium 99m (Tc-99m) D Indium 111 (In-111) Y Other Radionuclide	Z None	Z None
Y Digestive System		Y Other Radionuclide	Z None	Z None

Section	C	Nuclear Medicine		
Body System	D	Gastrointestinal System		
Type	2	Tomographic (Tomo) Nuclear Medicine Imaging: Introduction of radioactive materials into the body for three dimensional display of images developed from the capture of radioactive emissions		
Body Part (Character 4)		**Radionuclide (Character 5)**	**Qualifier (Character 6)**	**Qualifier (Character 7)**
7 Gastrointestinal Tract		1 Technetium 99m (Tc-99m) D Indium 111 (In-111) Y Other Radionuclide	Z None	Z None
Y Digestive System		Y Other Radionuclide	Z None	Z None

Section	C	Nuclear Medicine		
Body System	F	Hepatobiliary System and Pancreas		
Type	1	Planar Nuclear Medicine Imaging: Introduction of radioactive materials into the body for single plane display of images developed from the capture of radioactive emissions		
Body Part (Character 4)		**Radionuclide (Character 5)**	**Qualifier (Character 6)**	**Qualifier (Character 7)**
4 Gallbladder 5 Liver 6 Liver and Spleen C Hepatobiliary System, All		1 Technetium 99m (Tc-99m) Y Other Radionuclide	Z None	Z None
Y Hepatobiliary System and Pancreas		Y Other Radionuclide	Z None	Z None

Section	C	Nuclear Medicine		
Body System	F	Hepatobiliary System and Pancreas		
Type	2	Tomographic (Tomo) Nuclear Medicine Imaging: Introduction of radioactive materials into the body for three dimensional display of images developed from the capture of radioactive emissions		
Body Part (Character 4)		**Radionuclide (Character 5)**	**Qualifier (Character 6)**	**Qualifier (Character 7)**
4 Gallbladder 5 Liver 6 Liver and Spleen		1 Technetium 99m (Tc-99m) Y Other Radionuclide	Z None	Z None
Y Hepatobiliary System and Pancreas		Y Other Radionuclide	Z None	Z None

Section	C	Nuclear Medicine		
Body System	G	Endocrine System		
Type	1	Planar Nuclear Medicine Imaging: Introduction of radioactive materials into the body for single plane display of images developed from the capture of radioactive emissions		
Body Part (Character 4)	**Radionuclide (Character 5)**	**Qualifier (Character 6)**	**Qualifier (Character 7)**
1 Parathyroid Glands	1 Technetium 99m (Tc-99m) S Thallium 201 (Tl-201) Y Other Radionuclide	Z None	Z None
2 Thyroid Gland	1 Technetium 99m (Tc-99m) F Iodine 123 (I-123) G Iodine 131 (I-131) Y Other Radionuclide	Z None	Z None
4 Adrenal Glands, Bilateral	G Iodine 131 (I-131) Y Other Radionuclide	Z None	Z None
Y Endocrine System	Y Other Radionuclide	Z None	Z None

Section	C	Nuclear Medicine		
Body System	G	Endocrine System		
Type	2	Tomographic (Tomo) Nuclear Medicine Imaging: Introduction of radioactive materials into the body for three dimensional display of images developed from the capture of radioactive emissions		
Body Part (Character 4)	**Radionuclide (Character 5)**	**Qualifier (Character 6)**	**Qualifier (Character 7)**
1 Parathyroid Glands	1 Technetium 99m (Tc-99m) S Thallium 201 (Tl-201) Y Other Radionuclide	Z None	Z None
Y Endocrine System	Y Other Radionuclide	Z None	Z None

Section	C	Nuclear Medicine		
Body System	G	Endocrine System		
Type	4	Nonimaging Nuclear Medicine Uptake: Introduction of radioactive materials into the body for measurements of organ function, from the detection of radioactive emissions		
Body Part (Character 4)	**Radionuclide (Character 5)**	**Qualifier (Character 6)**	**Qualifier (Character 7)**
2 Thyroid Gland	1 Technetium 99m (Tc-99m) F Iodine 123 (I-123) G Iodine 131 (I-131) Y Other Radionuclide	Z None	Z None
Y Endocrine System	Y Other Radionuclide	Z None	Z None

Section	C	Nuclear Medicine		
Body System	H	Skin, Subcutaneous Tissue and Breast		
Type	1	Planar Nuclear Medicine Imaging: Introduction of radioactive materials into the body for single plane display of images developed from the capture of radioactive emissions		
Body Part (Character 4)	**Radionuclide (Character 5)**	**Qualifier (Character 6)**	**Qualifier (Character 7)**
0 Breast, Right 1 Breast, Left 2 Breasts, Bilateral	1 Technetium 99m (Tc-99m) S Thallium 201 (Tl-201) Y Other Radionuclide	Z None	Z None
Y Skin, Subcutaneous Tissue and Breast	Y Other Radionuclide	Z None	Z None

Section	C	Nuclear Medicine		
Body System	H	Skin, Subcutaneous Tissue and Breast		
Type	2	Tomographic (Tomo) Nuclear Medicine Imaging: Introduction of radioactive materials into the body for three dimensional display of images developed from the capture of radioactive emissions		
Body Part (Character 4)	**Radionuclide (Character 5)**	**Qualifier (Character 6)**	**Qualifier (Character 7)**
0 Breast, Right 1 Breast, Left 2 Breasts, Bilateral	1 Technetium 99m (Tc-99m) S Thallium 201 (Tl-201) Y Other Radionuclide	Z None	Z None
Y Skin, Subcutaneous Tissue and Breast	Y Other Radionuclide	Z None	Z None

Section	C	Nuclear Medicine		
Body System	P	Musculoskeletal System		
Type	1	Planar Nuclear Medicine Imaging: Introduction of radioactive materials into the body for single plane display of images developed from the capture of radioactive emissions		

Body Part (Character 4)	Radionuclide (Character 5)	Qualifier (Character 6)	Qualifier (Character 7)
1 Skull 4 Thorax 5 Spine 6 Pelvis 7 Spine and Pelvis 8 Upper Extremity, Right 9 Upper Extremity, Left B Upper Extremities, Bilateral C Lower Extremity, Right D Lower Extremity, Left F Lower Extremities, Bilateral Z Musculoskeletal System, All	1 Technetium 99m (Tc-99m) Y Other Radionuclide	Z None	Z None
Y Musculoskeletal System, Other	Y Other Radionuclide	Z None	Z None

Section	C	Nuclear Medicine		
Body System	P	Musculoskeletal System		
Type	2	Tomographic (Tomo) Nuclear Medicine Imaging: Introduction of radioactive materials into the body for three dimensional display of images developed from the capture of radioactive emissions		

Body Part (Character 4)	Radionuclide (Character 5)	Qualifier (Character 6)	Qualifier (Character 7)
1 Skull 2 Cervical Spine 3 Skull and Cervical Spine 4 Thorax 6 Pelvis 7 Spine and Pelvis 8 Upper Extremity, Right 9 Upper Extremity, Left B Upper Extremities, Bilateral C Lower Extremity, Right D Lower Extremity, Left F Lower Extremities, Bilateral G Thoracic Spine H Lumbar Spine J Thoracolumbar Spine	1 Technetium 99m (Tc-99m) Y Other Radionuclide	Z None	Z None
Y Musculoskeletal System, Other	Y Other Radionuclide	Z None	Z None

Section	C	Nuclear Medicine		
Body System	P	Musculoskeletal System		
Type	5	Nonimaging Nuclear Medicine Probe: Introduction of radioactive materials into the body for the study of distribution and fate of certain substances by the detection of radioactive emissions; or, alternatively, measurement of absorption of radioactive emissions from an external source		

Body Part (Character 4)	Radionuclide (Character 5)	Qualifier (Character 6)	Qualifier (Character 7)
5 Spine N Upper Extremities P Lower Extremities	Z None	Z None	Z None
Y Musculoskeletal System, Other	Y Other Radionuclide	Z None	Z None

Section	C	Nuclear Medicine		
Body System	T	Urinary System		
Type	1	Planar Nuclear Medicine Imaging: Introduction of radioactive materials into the body for single plane display of images developed from the capture of radioactive emissions		

Body Part (Character 4)	Radionuclide (Character 5)	Qualifier (Character 6)	Qualifier (Character 7)
3 Kidneys, Ureters and Bladder	1 Technetium 99m (Tc-99m) F Iodine 123 (I-123) G Iodine 131 (I-131) Y Other Radionuclide	Z None	Z None
H Bladder and Ureters	1 Technetium 99m (Tc-99m) Y Other Radionuclide	Z None	Z None
Y Urinary System	Y Other Radionuclide	Z None	Z None

Section	C	Nuclear Medicine		
Body System	T	Urinary System		
Type	2	Tomographic (Tomo) Nuclear Medicine Imaging: Introduction of radioactive materials into the body for three dimensional display of images developed from the capture of radioactive emissions		

Body Part (Character 4)	Radionuclide (Character 5)	Qualifier (Character 6)	Qualifier (Character 7)
3 Kidneys, Ureters and Bladder	1 Technetium 99m (Tc-99m) Y Other Radionuclide	Z None	Z None
Y Urinary System	Y Other Radionuclide	Z None	Z None

Section	C	Nuclear Medicine
Body System	T	Urinary System
Type	6	Nonimaging Nuclear Medicine Assay: Introduction of radioactive materials into the body for the study of body fluids and blood elements, by the detection of radioactive emissions

Body Part (Character 4)	Radionuclide (Character 5)	Qualifier (Character 6)	Qualifier (Character 7)
3 Kidneys, Ureters and Bladder	1 Technetium 99m (Tc-99m) F Iodine 123 (I-123) G Iodine 131 (I-131) H Iodine 125 (I-125) Y Other Radionuclide	Z None	Z None
Y Urinary System	Y Other Radionuclide	Z None	Z None

Section	C	Nuclear Medicine
Body System	V	Male Reproductive System
Type	1	Planar Nuclear Medicine Imaging: Introduction of radioactive materials into the body for single plane display of images developed from the capture of radioactive emissions

Body Part (Character 4)	Radionuclide (Character 5)	Qualifier (Character 6)	Qualifier (Character 7)
9 Testicles, Bilateral	1 Technetium 99m (Tc-99m) Y Other Radionuclide	Z None	Z None
Y Male Reproductive System	Y Other Radionuclide	Z None	Z None

Section	C	Nuclear Medicine
Body System	W	Anatomical Regions
Type	1	Planar Nuclear Medicine Imaging: Introduction of radioactive materials into the body for single plane display of images developed from the capture of radioactive emissions

Body Part (Character 4)	Radionuclide (Character 5)	Qualifier (Character 6)	Qualifier (Character 7)
0 Abdomen 1 Abdomen and Pelvis 4 Chest and Abdomen 6 Chest and Neck B Head and Neck D Lower Extremity J Pelvic Region M Upper Extremity N Whole Body	1 Technetium 99m (Tc-99m) D Indium 111 (In-111) F Iodine 123 (I-123) G Iodine 131 (I-131) L Gallium 67 (Ga-67) S Thallium 201 (Tl-201) Y Other Radionuclide	Z None	Z None
3 Chest	1 Technetium 99m (Tc-99m) D Indium 111 (In-111) F Iodine 123 (I-123) G Iodine 131 (I-131) K Fluorine 18 (F-18) L Gallium 67 (Ga-67) S Thallium 201 (Tl-201) Y Other Radionuclide	Z None	Z None
Y Anatomical Regions, Multiple	Y Other Radionuclide	Z None	Z None
Z Anatomical Region, Other	Z None	Z None	Z None

Section	C	Nuclear Medicine
Body System	W	Anatomical Regions
Type	2	Tomographic (Tomo) Nuclear Medicine Imaging: Introduction of radioactive materials into the body for three dimensional display of images developed from the capture of radioactive emissions

Body Part (Character 4)	Radionuclide (Character 5)	Qualifier (Character 6)	Qualifier (Character 7)
0 Abdomen 1 Abdomen and Pelvis 3 Chest 4 Chest and Abdomen 6 Chest and Neck B Head and Neck D Lower Extremity J Pelvic Region M Upper Extremity	1 Technetium 99m (Tc-99m) D Indium 111 (In-111) F Iodine 123 (I-123) G Iodine 131 (I-131) K Fluorine 18 (F-18) L Gallium 67 (Ga-67) S Thallium 201 (Tl-201) Y Other Radionuclide	Z None	Z None
Y Anatomical Regions, Multiple	Y Other Radionuclide	Z None	Z None

Section	C	Nuclear Medicine
Body System	W	Anatomical Regions
Type	3	Positron Emission Tomographic (PET) Imaging: Introduction of radioactive materials into the body for three dimensional display of images developed from the simultaneous capture, 180 degrees apart, of radioactive emissions

Body Part (Character 4)	Radionuclide (Character 5)	Qualifier (Character 6)	Qualifier (Character 7)
N Whole Body	Y Other Radionuclide	Z None	Z None

Section	C	Nuclear Medicine		
Body System	W	Anatomical Regions		
Type	5	Nonimaging Nuclear Medicine Probe: Introduction of radioactive materials into the body for the study of distribution and fate of certain substances by the detection of radioactive emissions; or, alternatively, measurement of absorption of radioactive emissions from an external source		

Body Part (Character 4)	Radionuclide (Character 5)	Qualifier (Character 6)	Qualifier (Character 7)
0 Abdomen 1 Abdomen and Pelvis 3 Chest 4 Chest and Abdomen 6 Chest and Neck B Head and Neck D Lower Extremity J Pelvic Region M Upper Extremity	1 Technetium 99m (Tc-99m) D Indium 111 (In-111) Y Other Radionuclide	Z None	Z None

Section	C	Nuclear Medicine		
Body System	W	Anatomical Regions		
Type	7	Systemic Nuclear Medicine Therapy: Introduction of unsealed radioactive materials into the body for treatment		

Body Part (Character 4)	Radionuclide (Character 5)	Qualifier (Character 6)	Qualifier (Character 7)
0 Abdomen 3 Chest	N Phosphorus 32 (P-32) Y Other Radionuclide	Z None	Z None
G Thyroid	G Iodine 131 (I-131) Y Other Radionuclide	Z None	Z None
N Whole Body	8 Samarium 153 (Sm-153) G Iodine 131 (I-131) N Phosphorus 32 (P-32) P Strontium 89 (Sr-89) Y Other Radionuclide	Z None	Z None
Y Anatomical Regions, Multiple	Y Other Radionuclide	Z None	Z None

Section	D	Radiation Oncology		
Body System	0	Central and Peripheral Nervous System		
Modality	0	Beam Radiation		
Treatment Site (Character 4)		**Modality Qualifier (Character 5)**	**Isotope (Character 6)**	**Qualifier (Character 7)**
0 Brain **1** Brain Stem **6** Spinal Cord **7** Peripheral Nerve		**0** Photons <1 MeV **1** Photons **1** - 10 MeV **2** Photons >10 MeV **4** Heavy Particles (Protons, Ions) **5** Neutrons **6** Neutron Capture	**Z** None	**Z** None
0 Brain **1** Brain Stem **6** Spinal Cord **7** Peripheral Nerve		**3** Electrons	**Z** None	**0** Intraoperative **Z** None

Section	D	Radiation Oncology		
Body System	0	Central and Peripheral Nervous System		
Modality	1	Brachytherapy		
Treatment Site (Character 4)		**Modality Qualifier (Character 5)**	**Isotope (Character 6)**	**Qualifier (Character 7)**
0 Brain **1** Brain Stem **6** Spinal Cord **7** Peripheral Nerve		**9** High Dose Rate (HDR) **B** Low Dose Rate (LDR)	**7** Cesium 137 (Cs-137) **8** Iridium 192 (Ir-192) **9** Iodine 125 (I-125) **B** Palladium 103 (Pd-103) **C** Californium 252 (Cf-252) **Y** Other Isotope	**Z** None

Section	D	Radiation Oncology		
Body System	0	Central and Peripheral Nervous System		
Modality	2	Stereotactic Radiosurgery		
Treatment Site (Character 4)		**Modality Qualifier (Character 5)**	**Isotope (Character 6)**	**Qualifier (Character 7)**
0 Brain **1** Brain Stem **6** Spinal Cord **7** Peripheral Nerve		**D** Stereotactic Other Photon Radiosurgery **H** Stereotactic Particulate Radiosurgery **J** Stereotactic Gamma Beam Radiosurgery	**Z** None	**Z** None

Section	D	Radiation Oncology		
Body System	0	Central and Peripheral Nervous System		
Modality	Y	Other Radiation		
Treatment Site (Character 4)		**Modality Qualifier (Character 5)**	**Isotope (Character 6)**	**Qualifier (Character 7)**
0 Brain **1** Brain Stem **6** Spinal Cord **7** Peripheral Nerve		**7** Contact Radiation **8** Hyperthermia **F** Plaque Radiation **K** Laser Interstitial Thermal Therapy	**Z** None	**Z** None

Section	D	Radiation Oncology		
Body System	7	Lymphatic and Hematologic System		
Modality	0	Beam Radiation		
Treatment Site (Character 4)		**Modality Qualifier (Character 5)**	**Isotope (Character 6)**	**Qualifier (Character 7)**
0 Bone Marrow **1** Thymus **2** Spleen **3** Lymphatics, Neck **4** Lymphatics, Axillary **5** Lymphatics, Thorax **6** Lymphatics, Abdomen **7** Lymphatics, Pelvis **8** Lymphatics, Inguinal		**0** Photons <1 MeV **1** Photons **1** - 10 MeV **2** Photons >10 MeV **4** Heavy Particles (Protons, Ions) **5** Neutrons **6** Neutron Capture	**Z** None	**Z** None
0 Bone Marrow **1** Thymus **2** Spleen **3** Lymphatics, Neck **4** Lymphatics, Axillary **5** Lymphatics, Thorax **6** Lymphatics, Abdomen **7** Lymphatics, Pelvis **8** Lymphatics, Inguinal		**3** Electrons	**Z** None	**0** Intraoperative **Z** None

Section	D	Radiation Oncology		
Body System	7	Lymphatic and Hematologic System		
Modality	1	Brachytherapy		
Treatment Site (Character 4)	Modality Qualifier (Character 5)	Isotope (Character 6)	Qualifier (Character 7)
0 Bone Marrow 1 Thymus 2 Spleen 3 Lymphatics, Neck 4 Lymphatics, Axillary 5 Lymphatics, Thorax 6 Lymphatics, Abdomen 7 Lymphatics, Pelvis 8 Lymphatics, Inguinal	9 High Dose Rate (HDR) B Low Dose Rate (LDR)	7 Cesium 137 (Cs-137) 8 Iridium 192 (Ir-192) 9 Iodine 125 (I-125) B Palladium 103 (Pd-103) C Californium 252 (Cf-252) Y Other Isotope	Z None

Section	D	Radiation Oncology		
Body System	7	Lymphatic and Hematologic System		
Modality	2	Stereotactic Radiosurgery		
Treatment Site (Character 4)	Modality Qualifier (Character 5)	Isotope (Character 6)	Qualifier (Character 7)
0 Bone Marrow 1 Thymus 2 Spleen 3 Lymphatics, Neck 4 Lymphatics, Axillary 5 Lymphatics, Thorax 6 Lymphatics, Abdomen 7 Lymphatics, Pelvis 8 Lymphatics, Inguinal	D Stereotactic Other Photon Radiosurgery H Stereotactic Particulate Radiosurgery J Stereotactic Gamma Beam Radiosurgery	Z None	Z None

Section	D	Radiation Oncology		
Body System	7	Lymphatic and Hematologic System		
Modality	Y	Other Radiation		
Treatment Site (Character 4)	Modality Qualifier (Character 5)	Isotope (Character 6)	Qualifier (Character 7)
0 Bone Marrow 1 Thymus 2 Spleen 3 Lymphatics, Neck 4 Lymphatics, Axillary 5 Lymphatics, Thorax 6 Lymphatics, Abdomen 7 Lymphatics, Pelvis 8 Lymphatics, Inguinal	8 Hyperthermia F Plaque Radiation	Z None	Z None

Section	D	Radiation Oncology		
Body System	8	Eye		
Modality	0	Beam Radiation		
Treatment Site (Character 4)	Modality Qualifier (Character 5)	Isotope (Character 6)	Qualifier (Character 7)
0 Eye	0 Photons <1 MeV 1 Photons 1 - 10 MeV 2 Photons >10 MeV 4 Heavy Particles (Protons, Ions) 5 Neutrons 6 Neutron Capture	Z None	Z None
0 Eye	3 Electrons	Z None	0 Intraoperative Z None

Section	D	Radiation Oncology		
Body System	8	Eye		
Modality	1	Brachytherapy		
Treatment Site (Character 4)	Modality Qualifier (Character 5)	Isotope (Character 6)	Qualifier (Character 7)
0 Eye	9 High Dose Rate (HDR) B Low Dose Rate (LDR)	7 Cesium 137 (Cs-137) 8 Iridium 192 (Ir-192) 9 Iodine 125 (I-125) B Palladium 103 (Pd-103) C Californium 252 (Cf-252) Y Other Isotope	Z None

Section	D	Radiation Oncology		
Body System	8	Eye		
Modality	2	Stereotactic Radiosurgery		
Treatment Site (Character 4)	Modality Qualifier (Character 5)		Isotope (Character 6)	Qualifier (Character 7)
0 Eye	**D** Stereotactic Other Photon Radiosurgery **H** Stereotactic Particulate Radiosurgery **J** Stereotactic Gamma Beam Radiosurgery		**Z** None	**Z** None

Section	D	Radiation Oncology		
Body System	8	Eye		
Modality	Y	Other Radiation		
Treatment Site (Character 4)	Modality Qualifier (Character 5)		Isotope (Character 6)	Qualifier (Character 7)
0 Eye	**7** Contact Radiation **8** Hyperthermia **F** Plaque Radiation		**Z** None	**Z** None

Section	D	Radiation Oncology		
Body System	9	Ear, Nose, Mouth and Throat		
Modality	0	Beam Radiation		
Treatment Site (Character 4)	Modality Qualifier (Character 5)		Isotope (Character 6)	Qualifier (Character 7)
0 Ear 1 Nose 3 Hypopharynx 4 Mouth 5 Tongue 6 Salivary Glands 7 Sinuses 8 Hard Palate 9 Soft Palate B Larynx D Nasopharynx F Oropharynx	**0** Photons <1 MeV **1** Photons **1** - 10 MeV **2** Photons >10 MeV **4** Heavy Particles (Protons, Ions) **5** Neutrons **6** Neutron Capture		**Z** None	**Z** None
0 Ear 1 Nose 3 Hypopharynx 4 Mouth 5 Tongue 6 Salivary Glands 7 Sinuses 8 Hard Palate 9 Soft Palate B Larynx D Nasopharynx F Oropharynx	**3** Electrons		**Z** None	**0** Intraoperative **Z** None

Section	D	Radiation Oncology		
Body System	9	Ear, Nose, Mouth and Throat		
Modality	1	Brachytherapy		
Treatment Site (Character 4)	Modality Qualifier (Character 5)	Isotope (Character 6)	Qualifier (Character 7)
0 Ear 1 Nose 3 Hypopharynx 4 Mouth 5 Tongue 6 Salivary Glands 7 Sinuses 8 Hard Palate 9 Soft Palate B Larynx D Nasopharynx F Oropharynx	**9** High Dose Rate (HDR) **B** Low Dose Rate (LDR)	**7** Cesium 137 (Cs-137) **8** Iridium 192 (Ir-192) **9** Iodine 125 (I-125) **B** Palladium 103 (Pd-103) **C** Californium 252 (Cf-252) **Y** Other Isotope	**Z** None

Section	D	Radiation Oncology			
Body System	9	Ear, Nose, Mouth and Throat			
Modality	2	Stereotactic Radiosurgery			

Treatment Site (Character 4)	Modality Qualifier (Character 5)	Isotope (Character 6)	Qualifier (Character 7)
0 Ear **1** Nose **4** Mouth **5** Tongue **6** Salivary Glands **7** Sinuses **8** Hard Palate **9** Soft Palate **B** Larynx **C** Pharynx **D** Nasopharynx	**D** Stereotactic Other Photon Radiosurgery **H** Stereotactic Particulate Radiosurgery **J** Stereotactic Gamma Beam Radiosurgery	**Z** None	**Z** None

Section	D	Radiation Oncology			
Body System	9	Ear, Nose, Mouth and Throat			
Modality	Y	Other Radiation			

Treatment Site (Character 4)	Modality Qualifier (Character 5)	Isotope (Character 6)	Qualifier (Character 7)
0 Ear **1** Nose **5** Tongue **6** Salivary Glands **7** Sinuses **8** Hard Palate **9** Soft Palate	**7** Contact Radiation **8** Hyperthermia **F** Plaque Radiation	**Z** None	**Z** None
3 Hypopharynx **F** Oropharynx	**7** Contact Radiation **8** Hyperthermia	**Z** None	**Z** None
4 Mouth **B** Larynx **D** Nasopharynx	**7** Contact Radiation **8** Hyperthermia **C** Intraoperative Radiation Therapy (IORT) **F** Plaque Radiation	**Z** None	**Z** None
C Pharynx	**C** Intraoperative Radiation Therapy (IORT) **F** Plaque Radiation	**Z** None	**Z** None

Section	D	Radiation Oncology			
Body System	B	Respiratory System			
Modality	0	Beam Radiation			

Treatment Site (Character 4)	Modality Qualifier (Character 5)	Isotope (Character 6)	Qualifier (Character 7)
0 Trachea **1** Bronchus **2** Lung **5** Pleura **6** Mediastinum **7** Chest Wall **8** Diaphragm	**0** Photons <1 MeV **1** Photons **1** - 10 MeV **2** Photons >10 MeV **4** Heavy Particles (Protons, Ions) **5** Neutrons **6** Neutron Capture	**Z** None	**Z** None
0 Trachea **1** Bronchus **2** Lung **5** Pleura **6** Mediastinum **7** Chest Wall **8** Diaphragm	**3** Electrons	**Z** None	**0** Intraoperative **Z** None

Section	D	Radiation Oncology			
Body System	B	Respiratory System			
Modality	1	Brachytherapy			

Treatment Site (Character 4)	Modality Qualifier (Character 5)	Isotope (Character 6)	Qualifier (Character 7)
0 Trachea **1** Bronchus **2** Lung **5** Pleura **6** Mediastinum **7** Chest Wall **8** Diaphragm	**9** High Dose Rate (HDR) **B** Low Dose Rate (LDR)	**7** Cesium 137 (Cs-137) **8** Iridium 192 (Ir-192) **9** Iodine 125 (I-125) **B** Palladium 103 (Pd-103) **C** Californium 252 (Cf-252) **Y** Other Isotope	**Z** None

Section	D	Radiation Oncology		
Body System	B	Respiratory System		
Modality	2	Stereotactic Radiosurgery		
Treatment Site (Character 4)	Modality Qualifier (Character 5)	Isotope (Character 6)	Qualifier (Character 7)
0 Trachea 1 Bronchus 2 Lung 5 Pleura 6 Mediastinum 7 Chest Wall 8 Diaphragm	D Stereotactic Other Photon Radiosurgery H Stereotactic Particulate Radiosurgery J Stereotactic Gamma Beam Radiosurgery	Z None	Z None

Section	D	Radiation Oncology		
Body System	B	Respiratory System		
Modality	Y	Other Radiation		
Treatment Site (Character 4)	Modality Qualifier (Character 5)	Isotope (Character 6)	Qualifier (Character 7)
0 Trachea 1 Bronchus 2 Lung 5 Pleura 6 Mediastinum 7 Chest Wall 8 Diaphragm	7 Contact Radiation 8 Hyperthermia F Plaque Radiation K Laser Interstitial Thermal Therapy	Z None	Z None

Section	D	Radiation Oncology		
Body System	D	Gastrointestinal System		
Modality	0	Beam Radiation		
Treatment Site (Character 4)	Modality Qualifier (Character 5)	Isotope (Character 6)	Qualifier (Character 7)
0 Esophagus 1 Stomach 2 Duodenum 3 Jejunum 4 Ileum 5 Colon 7 Rectum	0 Photons <1 MeV 1 Photons 1 - 10 MeV 2 Photons >10 MeV 4 Heavy Particles (Protons, Ions) 5 Neutrons 6 Neutron Capture	Z None	Z None
0 Esophagus 1 Stomach 2 Duodenum 3 Jejunum 4 Ileum 5 Colon 7 Rectum	3 Electrons	Z None	0 Intraoperative Z None

Section	D	Radiation Oncology		
Body System	D	Gastrointestinal System		
Modality	1	Brachytherapy		
Treatment Site (Character 4)	Modality Qualifier (Character 5)	Isotope (Character 6)	Qualifier (Character 7)
0 Esophagus 1 Stomach 2 Duodenum 3 Jejunum 4 Ileum 5 Colon 7 Rectum	9 High Dose Rate (HDR) B Low Dose Rate (LDR)	7 Cesium 137 (Cs-137) 8 Iridium 192 (Ir-192) 9 Iodine 125 (I-125) B Palladium 103 (Pd-103) C Californium 252 (Cf-252) Y Other Isotope	Z None

Section	D	Radiation Oncology		
Body System	D	Gastrointestinal System		
Modality	2	Stereotactic Radiosurgery		
Treatment Site (Character 4)	Modality Qualifier (Character 5)	Isotope (Character 6)	Qualifier (Character 7)
0 Esophagus 1 Stomach 2 Duodenum 3 Jejunum 4 Ileum 5 Colon 7 Rectum	D Stereotactic Other Photon Radiosurgery H Stereotactic Particulate Radiosurgery J Stereotactic Gamma Beam Radiosurgery	Z None	Z None

Section	D	Radiation Oncology			
Body System	D	Gastrointestinal System			
Modality	Y	Other Radiation			
Treatment Site (Character 4)		**Modality Qualifier (Character 5)**	**Isotope (Character 6)**	**Qualifier (Character 7)**	
0 Esophagus		7 Contact Radiation 8 Hyperthermia F Plaque Radiation K Laser Interstitial Thermal Therapy	Z None	Z None	
1 Stomach 2 Duodenum 3 Jejunum 4 Ileum 5 Colon 7 Rectum		7 Contact Radiation 8 Hyperthermia C Intraoperative Radiation Therapy (IORT) F Plaque Radiation K Laser Interstitial Thermal Therapy	Z None	Z None	
8 Anus		C Intraoperative Radiation Therapy (IORT) F Plaque Radiation K Laser Interstitial Thermal Therapy	Z None	Z None	

Section	D	Radiation Oncology			
Body System	F	Hepatobiliary System and Pancreas			
Modality	0	Beam Radiation			
Treatment Site (Character 4)		**Modality Qualifier (Character 5)**	**Isotope (Character 6)**	**Qualifier (Character 7)**	
0 Liver 1 Gallbladder 2 Bile Ducts 3 Pancreas		0 Photons <1 MeV 1 Photons 1 - 10 MeV 2 Photons >10 MeV 4 Heavy Particles (Protons, Ions) 5 Neutrons 6 Neutron Capture	Z None	Z None	
0 Liver 1 Gallbladder 2 Bile Ducts 3 Pancreas		3 Electrons	Z None	0 Intraoperative Z None	

Section	D	Radiation Oncology			
Body System	F	Hepatobiliary System and Pancreas			
Modality	1	Brachytherapy			
Treatment Site (Character 4)		**Modality Qualifier (Character 5)**	**Isotope (Character 6)**	**Qualifier (Character 7)**	
0 Liver 1 Gallbladder 2 Bile Ducts 3 Pancreas		9 High Dose Rate (HDR) B Low Dose Rate (LDR)	7 Cesium 137 (Cs-137) 8 Iridium 192 (Ir-192) 9 Iodine 125 (I-125) B Palladium 103 (Pd-103) C Californium 252 (Cf-252) Y Other Isotope	Z None	

Section	D	Radiation Oncology			
Body System	F	Hepatobiliary System and Pancreas			
Modality	2	Stereotactic Radiosurgery			
Treatment Site (Character 4)		**Modality Qualifier (Character 5)**	**Isotope (Character 6)**	**Qualifier (Character 7)**	
0 Liver 1 Gallbladder 2 Bile Ducts 3 Pancreas		D Stereotactic Other Photon Radiosurgery H Stereotactic Particulate Radiosurgery J Stereotactic Gamma Beam Radiosurgery	Z None	Z None	

Section	D	Radiation Oncology			
Body System	F	Hepatobiliary System and Pancreas			
Modality	Y	Other Radiation			
Treatment Site (Character 4)		**Modality Qualifier (Character 5)**	**Isotope (Character 6)**	**Qualifier (Character 7)**	
0 Liver 1 Gallbladder 2 Bile Ducts 3 Pancreas		7 Contact Radiation 8 Hyperthermia C Intraoperative Radiation Therapy (IORT) F Plaque Radiation K Laser Interstitial Thermal Therapy	Z None	Z None	

Section	D	Radiation Oncology			
Body System	G	Endocrine System			
Modality	0	Beam Radiation			
Treatment Site (Character 4)		**Modality Qualifier (Character 5)**	**Isotope (Character 6)**	**Qualifier (Character 7)**	
0 Pituitary Gland 1 Pineal Body 2 Adrenal Glands 4 Parathyroid Glands 5 Thyroid		0 Photons <1 MeV 1 Photons 1 - 10 MeV 2 Photons >10 MeV 5 Neutrons 6 Neutron Capture	Z None	Z None	
0 Pituitary Gland 1 Pineal Body 2 Adrenal Glands 4 Parathyroid Glands 5 Thyroid		3 Electrons	Z None	0 Intraoperative Z None	

Section	D	Radiation Oncology			
Body System	G	Endocrine System			
Modality	1	Brachytherapy			
Treatment Site (Character 4)		**Modality Qualifier (Character 5)**	**Isotope (Character 6)**	**Qualifier (Character 7)**	
0 Pituitary Gland 1 Pineal Body 2 Adrenal Glands 4 Parathyroid Glands 5 Thyroid		9 High Dose Rate (HDR) B Low Dose Rate (LDR)	7 Cesium 137 (Cs-137) 8 Iridium 192 (Ir-192) 9 Iodine 125 (I-125) B Palladium 103 (Pd-103) C Californium 252 (Cf-252) Y Other Isotope	Z None	

Section	D	Radiation Oncology			
Body System	G	Endocrine System			
Modality	2	Stereotactic Radiosurgery			
Treatment Site (Character 4)		**Modality Qualifier (Character 5)**	**Isotope (Character 6)**	**Qualifier (Character 7)**	
0 Pituitary Gland 1 Pineal Body 2 Adrenal Glands 4 Parathyroid Glands 5 Thyroid		D Stereotactic Other Photon Radiosurgery H Stereotactic Particulate Radiosurgery J Stereotactic Gamma Beam Radiosurgery	Z None	Z None	

Section	D	Radiation Oncology			
Body System	G	Endocrine System			
Modality	Y	Other Radiation			
Treatment Site (Character 4)		**Modality Qualifier (Character 5)**	**Isotope (Character 6)**	**Qualifier (Character 7)**	
0 Pituitary Gland 1 Pineal Body 2 Adrenal Glands 4 Parathyroid Glands 5 Thyroid		7 Contact Radiation 8 Hyperthermia F Plaque Radiation K Laser Interstitial Thermal Therapy	Z None	Z None	

Section	D	Radiation Oncology			
Body System	H	Skin			
Modality	0	Beam Radiation			
Treatment Site (Character 4)		**Modality Qualifier (Character 5)**	**Isotope (Character 6)**	**Qualifier (Character 7)**	
2 Skin, Face 3 Skin, Neck 4 Skin, Arm 6 Skin, Chest 7 Skin, Back 8 Skin, Abdomen 9 Skin, Buttock B Skin, Leg		0 Photons <1 MeV 1 Photons 1 - 10 MeV 2 Photons >10 MeV 4 Heavy Particles (Protons, Ions) 5 Neutrons 6 Neutron Capture	Z None	Z None	
2 Skin, Face 3 Skin, Neck 4 Skin, Arm 6 Skin, Chest 7 Skin, Back 8 Skin, Abdomen 9 Skin, Buttock B Skin, Leg		3 Electrons	Z None	0 Intraoperative Z None	

Section	D	Radiation Oncology		
Body System	H	Skin		
Modality	Y	Other Radiation		
Treatment Site (Character 4)	**Modality Qualifier (Character 5)**		**Isotope (Character 6)**	**Qualifier (Character 7)**
2 Skin, Face 3 Skin, Neck 4 Skin, Arm 6 Skin, Chest 7 Skin, Back 8 Skin, Abdomen 9 Skin, Buttock B Skin, Leg	7 Contact Radiation 8 Hyperthermia F Plaque Radiation		Z None	Z None
5 Skin, Hand C Skin, Foot	F Plaque Radiation		Z None	Z None

Section	D	Radiation Oncology		
Body System	M	Breast		
Modality	0	Beam Radiation		
Treatment Site (Character 4)	**Modality Qualifier (Character 5)**		**Isotope (Character 6)**	**Qualifier (Character 7)**
0 Breast, Left 1 Breast, Right	0 Photons <1 MeV 1 Photons 1 - 10 MeV 2 Photons >10 MeV 4 Heavy Particles (Protons, Ions) 5 Neutrons 6 Neutron Capture		Z None	Z None
0 Breast, Left 1 Breast, Right	3 Electrons		Z None	0 Intraoperative Z None

Section	D	Radiation Oncology		
Body System	M	Breast		
Modality	1	Brachytherapy		
Treatment Site (Character 4)	**Modality Qualifier (Character 5)**		**Isotope (Character 6)**	**Qualifier (Character 7)**
0 Breast, Left 1 Breast, Right	9 High Dose Rate (HDR) B Low Dose Rate (LDR)		7 Cesium 137 (Cs-137) 8 Iridium 192 (Ir-192) 9 Iodine 125 (I-125) B Palladium 103 (Pd-103) C Californium 252 (Cf-252) Y Other Isotope	Z None

Section	D	Radiation Oncology		
Body System	M	Breast		
Modality	2	Stereotactic Radiosurgery		
Treatment Site (Character 4)	**Modality Qualifier (Character 5)**		**Isotope (Character 6)**	**Qualifier (Character 7)**
0 Breast, Left 1 Breast, Right	D Stereotactic Other Photon Radiosurgery H Stereotactic Particulate Radiosurgery J Stereotactic Gamma Beam Radiosurgery		Z None	Z None

Section	D	Radiation Oncology		
Body System	M	Breast		
Modality	Y	Other Radiation		
Treatment Site (Character 4)	**Modality Qualifier (Character 5)**		**Isotope (Character 6)**	**Qualifier (Character 7)**
0 Breast, Left 1 Breast, Right	7 Contact Radiation 8 Hyperthermia F Plaque Radiation K Laser Interstitial Thermal Therapy		Z None	Z None

Section	D	Radiation Oncology		
Body System	P	Musculoskeletal System		
Modality	0	Beam Radiation		

Treatment Site (Character 4)	Modality Qualifier (Character 5)	Isotope (Character 6)	Qualifier (Character 7)
0 Skull 2 Maxilla 3 Mandible 4 Sternum 5 Rib(s) 6 Humerus 7 Radius/Ulna 8 Pelvic Bones 9 Femur B Tibia/Fibula C Other Bone	0 Photons <1 MeV 1 Photons 1 - 10 MeV 2 Photons >10 MeV 4 Heavy Particles (Protons, Ions) 5 Neutrons 6 Neutron Capture	Z None	Z None
0 Skull 2 Maxilla 3 Mandible 4 Sternum 5 Rib(s) 6 Humerus 7 Radius/Ulna 8 Pelvic Bones 9 Femur B Tibia/Fibula C Other Bone	3 Electrons	Z None	0 Intraoperative Z None

Section	D	Radiation Oncology		
Body System	P	Musculoskeletal System		
Modality	Y	Other Radiation		

Treatment Site (Character 4)	Modality Qualifier (Character 5)	Isotope (Character 6)	Qualifier (Character 7)
0 Skull 2 Maxilla 3 Mandible 4 Sternum 5 Rib(s) 6 Humerus 7 Radius/Ulna 8 Pelvic Bones 9 Femur B Tibia/Fibula C Other Bone	7 Contact Radiation 8 Hyperthermia F Plaque Radiation	Z None	Z None

Section	D	Radiation Oncology		
Body System	T	Urinary System		
Modality	0	Beam Radiation		

Treatment Site (Character 4)	Modality Qualifier (Character 5)	Isotope (Character 6)	Qualifier (Character 7)
0 Kidney 1 Ureter 2 Bladder 3 Urethra	0 Photons <1 MeV 1 Photons 1 - 10 MeV 2 Photons >10 MeV 4 Heavy Particles (Protons, Ions) 5 Neutrons 6 Neutron Capture	Z None	Z None
0 Kidney 1 Ureter 2 Bladder 3 Urethra	3 Electrons	Z None	0 Intraoperative Z None

Section	D	Radiation Oncology		
Body System	T	Urinary System		
Modality	1	Brachytherapy		

Treatment Site (Character 4)	Modality Qualifier (Character 5)	Isotope (Character 6)	Qualifier (Character 7)
0 Kidney 1 Ureter 2 Bladder 3 Urethra	9 High Dose Rate (HDR) B Low Dose Rate (LDR)	7 Cesium 137 (Cs-137) 8 Iridium 192 (Ir-192) 9 Iodine 125 (I-125) B Palladium 103 (Pd-103) C Californium 252 (Cf-252) Y Other Isotope	Z None

Section	D	Radiation Oncology			
Body System	T	Urinary System			
Modality	2	Stereotactic Radiosurgery			
Treatment Site (Character 4)		Modality Qualifier (Character 5)	Isotope (Character 6)	Qualifier (Character 7)	
0 Kidney 1 Ureter 2 Bladder 3 Urethra		D Stereotactic Other Photon Radiosurgery H Stereotactic Particulate Radiosurgery J Stereotactic Gamma Beam Radiosurgery	Z None	Z None	

Section	D	Radiation Oncology		
Body System	T	Urinary System		
Modality	Y	Other Radiation		
Treatment Site (Character 4)	Modality Qualifier (Character 5)	Isotope (Character 6)	Qualifier (Character 7)	
0 Kidney	7 Contact Radiation			
1 Ureter	8 Hyperthermia	Z None	Z None	
2 Bladder	C Intraoperative Radiation Therapy (IORT)			
3 Urethra	F Plaque Radiation			

Section	D	Radiation Oncology		
Body System	U	Female Reproductive System		
Modality	0	Beam Radiation		
Treatment Site (Character 4)	Modality Qualifier (Character 5)	Isotope (Character 6)	Qualifier (Character 7)	
0 Ovary 1 Cervix 2 Uterus	0 Photons <1 MeV 1 Photons 1 - 10 MeV 2 Photons >10 MeV 4 Heavy Particles (Protons, Ions) 5 Neutrons 6 Neutron Capture	Z None	Z None	
0 Ovary 1 Cervix 2 Uterus	3 Electrons	Z None	0 Intraoperative Z None	

Section	D	Radiation Oncology		
Body System	U	Female Reproductive System		
Modality	1	Brachytherapy		
Treatment Site (Character 4)	Modality Qualifier (Character 5)	Isotope (Character 6)	Qualifier (Character 7)	
0 Ovary 1 Cervix 2 Uterus	9 High Dose Rate (HDR) B Low Dose Rate (LDR)	7 Cesium 137 (Cs-137) 8 Iridium 192 (Ir-192) 9 Iodine 125 (I-125) B Palladium 103 (Pd-103) C Californium 252 (Cf-252) Y Other Isotope	Z None	

Section	D	Radiation Oncology			
Body System	U	Female Reproductive System			
Modality	2	Stereotactic Radiosurgery			
Treatment Site (Character 4)		Modality Qualifier (Character 5)	Isotope (Character 6)	Qualifier (Character 7)	
0 Ovary 1 Cervix 2 Uterus		D Stereotactic Other Photon Radiosurgery H Stereotactic Particulate Radiosurgery J Stereotactic Gamma Beam Radiosurgery	Z None	Z None	

Section	D	Radiation Oncology		
Body System	U	Female Reproductive System		
Modality	Y	Other Radiation		
Treatment Site (Character 4)	Modality Qualifier (Character 5)	Isotope (Character 6)	Qualifier (Character 7)	
0 Ovary 1 Cervix 2 Uterus	7 Contact Radiation 8 Hyperthermia C Intraoperative Radiation Therapy (IORT) F Plaque Radiation	Z None	Z None	

Section	D	Radiation Oncology		
Body System	V	Male Reproductive System		
Modality	0	Male Reproductive System 0 Beam Radiation		
Treatment Site (Character 4)	Modality Qualifier (Character 5)		Isotope (Character 6)	Qualifier (Character 7)
0 Prostate 1 Testis	0 Photons <1 MeV 1 Photons 1 - 10 MeV 2 Photons >10 MeV 4 Heavy Particles (Protons, Ions) 5 Neutrons 6 Neutron Capture		Z None	Z None
0 Prostate 1 Testis	3 Electrons		Z None	0 Intraoperative Z None

Section	D	Radiation Oncology		
Body System	V	Male Reproductive System		
Modality	1	Brachytherapy		
Treatment Site (Character 4)	Modality Qualifier (Character 5)		Isotope (Character 6)	Qualifier (Character 7)
0 Prostate 1 Testis	9 High Dose Rate (HDR) B Low Dose Rate (LDR)		7 Cesium 137 (Cs-137) 8 Iridium 192 (Ir-192) 9 Iodine 125 (I-125) B Palladium 103 (Pd-103) C Californium 252 (Cf-252) Y Other Isotope	Z None

Section	D	Radiation Oncology		
Body System	V	Male Reproductive System		
Modality	2	Stereotactic Radiosurgery		
Treatment Site (Character 4)	Modality Qualifier (Character 5)		Isotope (Character 6)	Qualifier (Character 7)
0 Prostate 1 Testis	D Stereotactic Other Photon Radiosurgery H Stereotactic Particulate Radiosurgery J Stereotactic Gamma Beam Radiosurgery		Z None	Z None

Section	D	Radiation Oncology		
Body System	V	Male Reproductive System		
Modality	Y	Other Radiation		
Treatment Site (Character 4)	Modality Qualifier (Character 5)		Isotope (Character 6)	Qualifier (Character 7)
0 Prostate	7 Contact Radiation 8 Hyperthermia C Intraoperative Radiation Therapy (IORT) F Plaque Radiation K Laser Interstitial Thermal Therapy		Z None	Z None
1 Testis	7 Contact Radiation 8 Hyperthermia F Plaque Radiation		Z None	Z None

Section	D	Radiation Oncology		
Body System	W	Anatomical Regions		
Modality	0	Beam Radiation		
Treatment Site (Character 4)	Modality Qualifier (Character 5)		Isotope (Character 6)	Qualifier (Character 7)
1 Head and Neck 2 Chest 3 Abdomen 4 Hemibody 5 Whole Body 6 Pelvic Region	0 Photons <1 MeV 1 Photons 1 - 10 MeV 2 Photons >10 MeV 4 Heavy Particles (Protons, Ions) 5 Neutrons 6 Neutron Capture		Z None	Z None
1 Head and Neck 2 Chest 3 Abdomen 4 Hemibody 5 Whole Body 6 Pelvic Region	3 Electrons		Z None	0 Intraoperative Z None

Section	D	Radiation Oncology			
Body System	W	Anatomical Regions			
Modality	1	Brachytherapy			
Treatment Site (Character 4)		**Modality Qualifier (Character 5)**	**Isotope (Character 6)**	**Qualifier (Character 7)**	
1 Head and Neck		9 High Dose Rate (HDR)	7 Cesium 137 (Cs-137)	Z None	
2 Chest		B Low Dose Rate (LDR)	8 Iridium 192 (Ir-192)		
3 Abdomen			9 Iodine 125 (I-125)		
6 Pelvic Region			B Palladium 103 (Pd-103)		
			C Californium 252 (Cf-252)		
			Y Other Isotope		

Section	D	Radiation Oncology			
Body System	W	Anatomical Regions			
Modality	2	Stereotactic Radiosurgery			
Treatment Site (Character 4)		**Modality Qualifier (Character 5)**	**Isotope (Character 6)**	**Qualifier (Character 7)**	
1 Head and Neck		D Stereotactic Other Photon Radiosurgery	Z None	Z None	
2 Chest		H Stereotactic Particulate Radiosurgery			
3 Abdomen		J Stereotactic Gamma Beam Radiosurgery			
6 Pelvic Region					

Section	D	Radiation Oncology			
Body System	W	Anatomical Regions			
Modality	Y	Other Radiation			
Treatment Site (Character 4)		**Modality Qualifier (Character 5)**	**Isotope (Character 6)**	**Qualifier (Character 7)**	
1 Head and Neck		7 Contact Radiation	Z None	Z None	
2 Chest		8 Hyperthermia			
3 Abdomen		F Plaque Radiation			
4 Hemibody					
6 Pelvic Region					
5 Whole Body		7 Contact Radiation	Z None	Z None	
		8 Hyperthermia			
		F Plaque Radiation			
5 Whole Body		G Isotope Administration	D Iodine 131 (I-131)	Z None	
			F Phosphorus 32 (P-32)		
			G Strontium 89 (Sr-89)		
			H Strontium 90 (Sr-90)		
			Y Other Isotope		

Section	F	Physical Rehabilitation and Diagnostic Audiology	
Section Qualifier	0	Rehabilitation	
Type	0	Speech Assessment: Measurement of speech and related functions	

Body System/Region (Character 4)	Type Qualifier (Character 5)	Equipment (Character 6)	Qualifier (Character 7)
3 Neurological System - Whole Body	G Communicative/Cognitive Integration Skills	K Audiovisual M Augmentative / Alternative Communication P Computer Y Other Equipment Z None	Z None
Z None	0 Filtered Speech 3 Staggered Spondaic Word Q Performance Intensity Phonetically Balanced Speech Discrimination R Brief Tone Stimuli S Distorted Speech T Dichotic Stimuli V Temporal Ordering of Stimuli W Masking Patterns	1 Audiometer 2 Sound Field / Booth K Audiovisual Z None	Z None
Z None	1 Speech Threshold 2 Speech/Word Recognition	1 Audiometer 2 Sound Field / Booth 9 Cochlear Implant K Audiovisual Z None	Z None
Z None	4 Sensorineural Acuity Level	1 Audiometer 2 Sound Field / Booth Z None	Z None
Z None	5 Synthetic Sentence Identification	1 Audiometer 2 Sound Field / Booth 9 Cochlear Implant K Audiovisual	Z None
Z None	6 Speech and/or Language Screening 7 Nonspoken Language 8 Receptive/Expressive Language C Aphasia G Communicative/Cognitive Integration Skills L Augmentative/Alternative Communication System	K Audiovisual M Augmentative / Alternative Communication P Computer Y Other Equipment Z None	Z None
Z None	9 Articulation/Phonology	K Audiovisual P Computer Q Speech Analysis Y Other Equipment Z None	Z None

Section	F	Physical Rehabilitation and Diagnostic Audiology		
Section Qualifier	0	Rehabilitation		
Type	0	Speech Assessment: Measurement of speech and related functions		
Body System/Region (Character 4)	Type Qualifier (Character 5)		Equipment (Character 6)	Qualifier (Character 7)
Z None	B Motor Speech		K Audiovisual N Biosensory Feedback P Computer Q Speech Analysis T Aerodynamic Function Y Other Equipment Z None	Z None
Z None	D Fluency		K Audiovisual N Biosensory Feedback P Computer Q Speech Analysis S Voice Analysis T Aerodynamic Function Y Other Equipment Z None	Z None
Z None	F Voice		K Audiovisual N Biosensory Feedback P Computer S Voice Analysis T Aerodynamic Function Y Other Equipment Z None	Z None
Z None	H Bedside Swallowing and Oral Function P Oral Peripheral Mechanism		Y Other Equipment Z None	Z None
Z None	J Instrumental Swallowing and Oral Function		T Aerodynamic Function W Swallowing Y Other Equipment	Z None
Z None	K Orofacial Myofunctional		K Audiovisual P Computer Y Other Equipment Z None	Z None

Section	F	Physical Rehabilitation and Diagnostic Audiology		
Section Qualifier	0	Rehabilitation		
Type	0	Speech Assessment: Measurement of speech and related functions		
Body System/Region (Character 4)	Type Qualifier (Character 5)		Equipment (Character 6)	Qualifier (Character 7)
Z None	M Voice Prosthetic		K Audiovisual P Computer S Voice Analysis V Speech Prosthesis Y Other Equipment Z None	Z None
Z None	N Non-invasive Instrumental Status		N Biosensory Feedback P Computer Q Speech Analysis S Voice Analysis T Aerodynamic Function Y Other Equipment	Z None
Z None	X Other Specified Central Auditory Processing		Z None	Z None

Section	F	Physical Rehabilitation and Diagnostic Audiology		
Section Qualifier	0	Rehabilitation		
Type	1	Motor and/or Nerve Function Assessment: Measurement of motor, nerve, and related functions		

Body System/Region (Character 4)	Type Qualifier (Character 5)	Equipment (Character 6)	Qualifier (Character 7)
0 Neurological System - Head and Neck **1** Neurological System - Upper Back / Upper Extremity **2** Neurological System - Lower Back / Lower Extremity **3** Neurological System - Whole Body	**0** Muscle Performance	**E** Orthosis **F** Assistive, Adaptive, Supportive or Protective **U** Prosthesis **Y** Other Equipment **Z** None	**Z** None
0 Neurological System - Head and Neck **1** Neurological System - Upper Back / Upper Extremity **2** Neurological System - Lower Back / Lower Extremity **3** Neurological System - Whole Body	**1** Integumentary Integrity **3** Coordination/Dexterity **4** Motor Function **G** Reflex Integrity	**Z** None	**Z** None
0 Neurological System - Head and Neck **1** Neurological System - Upper Back / Upper Extremity **2** Neurological System - Lower Back / Lower Extremity **3** Neurological System - Whole Body	**5** Range of Motion and Joint Integrity **6** Sensory Awareness/Processing/ Integrity	**Y** Other Equipment **Z** None	**Z** None
D Integumentary System - Head and Neck **F** Integumentary System - Upper Back / Upper Extremity **G** Integumentary System - Lower Back / Lower Extremity **H** Integumentary System - Whole Body **J** Musculoskeletal System - Head and Neck **K** Musculoskeletal System - Upper Back / Upper Extremity **L** Musculoskeletal System - Lower Back / Lower Extremity **M** Musculoskeletal System - Whole Body	**0** Muscle Performance	**E** Orthosis **F** Assistive, Adaptive, Supportive or Protective **U** Prosthesis **Y** Other Equipment **Z** None	**Z** None
D Integumentary System - Head and Neck **F** Integumentary System - Upper Back / Upper Extremity **G** Integumentary System - Lower Back / Lower Extremity **H** Integumentary System - Whole Body **J** Musculoskeletal System - Head and Neck **K** Musculoskeletal System - Upper Back / Upper Extremity **L** Musculoskeletal System - Lower Back / Lower Extremity **M** Musculoskeletal System - Whole Body	**1** Integumentary Integrity	**Z** None	**Z** None

Section	F	Physical Rehabilitation and Diagnostic Audiology	
Section Qualifier	0	Rehabilitation	
Type	1	Motor and/or Nerve Function Assessment: Measurement of motor, nerve, and related functions	

Body System/Region (Character 4)	Type Qualifier (Character 5)	Equipment (Character 6)	Qualifier (Character 7)
D Integumentary System - Head and Neck **F** Integumentary System - Upper Back / Upper Extremity **G** Integumentary System - Lower Back / Lower Extremity **H** Integumentary System - Whole Body **J** Musculoskeletal System - Head and Neck **K** Musculoskeletal System - Upper Back / Upper Extremity **L** Musculoskeletal System - Lower Back / Lower Extremity **M** Musculoskeletal System - Whole Body	**5** Range of Motion and Joint Integrity **6** Sensory Awareness/Processing/ Integrity	**Y** Other Equipment **Z** None	**Z** None
N Genitourinary System	**0** Muscle Performance	**E** Orthosis **F** Assistive, Adaptive, Supportive or Protective **U** Prosthesis **Y** Other Equipment **Z** None	**Z** None
Z None	**2** Visual Motor Integration	**K** Audiovisual **M** Augmentative / Alternative Communication **N** Biosensory Feedback **P** Computer **Q** Speech Analysis **S** Voice Analysis **Y** Other Equipment **Z** None	**Z** None
Z None	**7** Facial Nerve Function	**7** Electrophysiologic	**Z** None
Z None	**9** Somatosensory Evoked Potentials	**J** Somatosensory	**Z** None
Z None	**B** Bed Mobility **C** Transfer **F** Wheelchair Mobility	**E** Orthosis **F** Assistive, Adaptive, Supportive or Protective **U** Prosthesis **Z** None	**Z** None
Z None	**D** Gait and/or Balance	**E** Orthosis **F** Assistive, Adaptive, Supportive or Protective **U** Prosthesis **Y** Other Equipment **Z** None	**Z** None

Section	F	Physical Rehabilitation and Diagnostic Audiology
Section Qualifier	0	Rehabilitation
Type	2	Activities of Daily Living Assessment: Measurement of functional level for activities of daily living

Body System/Region (Character 4)	Type Qualifier (Character 5)	Equipment (Character 6)	Qualifier (Character 7)
0 Neurological System - Head and Neck	9 Cranial Nerve Integrity D Neuromotor Development	Y Other Equipment Z None	Z None
1 Neurological System - Upper Back / Upper Extremity 2 Neurological System - Lower Back / Lower Extremity 3 Neurological System - Whole Body	D Neuromotor Development	Y Other Equipment Z None	Z None
4 Circulatory System - Head and Neck 5 Circulatory System - Upper Back / Upper Extremity 6 Circulatory System - Lower Back / Lower Extremity 8 Respiratory System - Head and Neck 9 Respiratory System - Upper Back / Upper Extremity B Respiratory System - Lower Back / Lower Extremity	G Ventilation, Respiration and Circulation	C Mechanical G Aerobic Endurance and Conditioning Y Other Equipment Z None	Z None
7 Circulatory System - Whole Body C Respiratory System - Whole Body	7 Aerobic Capacity and Endurance	E Orthosis G Aerobic Endurance and Conditioning U Prosthesis Y Other Equipment Z None	Z None
7 Circulatory System - Whole Body C Respiratory System - Whole Body	G Ventilation, Respiration and Circulation	C Mechanical G Aerobic Endurance and Conditioning Y Other Equipment Z None	Z None
Z None	0 Bathing/Showering 1 Dressing 3 Grooming/Personal Hygiene 4 Home Management	E Orthosis F Assistive, Adaptive, Supportive or Protective U Prosthesis Z None	Z None
Z None	2 Feeding/Eating 8 Anthropometric Characteristics F Pain	Y Other Equipment Z None	Z None
Z None	5 Perceptual Processing	K Audiovisual M Augmentative / Alternative Communication N Biosensory Feedback P Computer Q Speech Analysis S Voice Analysis Y Other Equipment Z None	Z None
Z None	6 Psychosocial Skills	Z None	Z None

Section	F	Physical Rehabilitation and Diagnostic Audiology
Section Qualifier	0	Rehabilitation
Type	2	Activities of Daily Living Assessment: Measurement of functional level for activities of daily living

Body System/Region (Character 4)	Type Qualifier (Character 5)	Equipment (Character 6)	Qualifier (Character 7)
Z None	B Environmental, Home and Work Barriers C Ergonomics and Body Mechanics	E Orthosis F Assistive, Adaptive, Supportive or Protective U Prosthesis Y Other Equipment Z None	Z None
Z None	H Vocational Activities and Functional Community or Work Reintegration Skills	E Orthosis F Assistive, Adaptive, Supportive or Protective G Aerobic Endurance and Conditioning U Prosthesis Y Other Equipment Z None	Z None

Section	F		Physical Rehabilitation and Diagnostic Audiology		
Section Qualifier	0		Rehabilitation		
Type	6		Speech Treatment: Application of techniques to improve, augment, or compensate for speech and related functional impairment		

Body System/Region (Character 4)	Type Qualifier (Character 5)	Equipment (Character 6)	Qualifier (Character 7)
3 Neurological System - Whole Body	6 Communicative/Cognitive Integration Skills	K Audiovisual M Augmentative / Alternative Communication P Computer Y Other Equipment Z None	Z None
Z None	0 Nonspoken Language 3 Aphasia 6 Communicative/Cognitive Integration Skills	K Audiovisual M Augmentative / Alternative Communication P Computer Y Other Equipment Z None	Z None
Z None	1 Speech-Language Pathology and Related Disorders Counseling 2 Speech-Language Pathology and Related Disorders Prevention	K Audiovisual Z None	Z None
Z None	4 Articulation/Phonology	K Audiovisual P Computer Q Speech Analysis T Aerodynamic Function Y Other Equipment Z None	Z None
Z None	5 Aural Rehabilitation	K Audiovisual L Assistive Listening M Augmentative / Alternative Communication N Biosensory Feedback P Computer Q Speech Analysis S Voice Analysis Y Other Equipment Z None	Z None
Z None	7 Fluency	4 Electroacoustic Immittance / Acoustic Reflex K Audiovisual N Biosensory Feedback Q Speech Analysis 5 Voice Analysis T Aerodynamic Function Y Other Equipment Z None	Z None

Section	F	Physical Rehabilitation and Diagnostic Audiology		
Section Qualifier	0	Rehabilitation		
Type	6	Speech Treatment: Application of techniques to improve, augment, or compensate for speech and related functional impairment		

Body System/Region (Character 4)	Type Qualifier (Character 5)	Equipment (Character 6)	Qualifier (Character 7)
Z None	8 Motor Speech	K Audiovisual N Biosensory Feedback P Computer Q Speech Analysis S Voice Analysis T Aerodynamic Function Y Other Equipment Z None	Z None
Z None	9 Orofacial Myofunctional	K Audiovisual P Computer Y Other Equipment Z None	Z None
Z None	B Receptive/Expressive Language	K Audiovisual L Assistive Listening M Augmentative / Alternative Communication P Computer Y Other Equipment Z None	Z None
Z None	C Voice	K Audiovisual N Biosensory Feedback P Computer S Voice Analysis T Aerodynamic Function V Speech Prosthesis Y Other Equipment Z None	Z None
Z None	D Swallowing Dysfunction	M Augmentative / Alternative Communication T Aerodynamic Function V Speech Prosthesis Y Other Equipment Z None	Z None

Section	F	Physical Rehabilitation and Diagnostic Audiology		
Section Qualifier	0	Rehabilitation		
Type	7	Motor Treatment: Exercise or activities to increase or facilitate motor function		

Body System/Region (Character 4)	Type Qualifier (Character 5)	Equipment (Character 6)	Qualifier (Character 7)
0 Neurological System - Head and Neck 1 Neurological System - Upper Back / Upper Extremity 2 Neurological System - Lower Back / Lower Extremity 3 Neurological System - Whole Body D Integumentary System - Head and Neck F Integumentary System - Upper Back / Upper Extremity G Integumentary System - Lower Back / Lower Extremity H Integumentary System - Whole Body J Musculoskeletal System - Head and Neck K Musculoskeletal System - Upper Back / Upper Extremity L Musculoskeletal System - Lower Back / Lower Extremity M Musculoskeletal System - Whole Body	0 Range of Motion and Joint Mobility 1 Muscle Performance 2 Coordination/Dexterity 3 Motor Function	E Orthosis F Assistive, Adaptive, Supportive or Protective U Prosthesis Y Other Equipment Z None	Z None

Section		F	Physical Rehabilitation and Diagnostic Audiology		
Section Qualifier		0	Rehabilitation		[continued]
Type		7	Motor Treatment: Exercise or activities to increase or facilitate motor function		

Body System/Region (Character 4)	Type Qualifier (Character 5)	Equipment (Character 6)	Qualifier (Character 7)
0 Neurological System - Head and Neck **1** Neurological System - Upper Back / Upper Extremity **2** Neurological System - Lower Back / Lower Extremity **3** Neurological System - Whole Body **D** Integumentary System - Head and Neck **F** Integumentary System - Upper Back / Upper Extremity **G** Integumentary System - Lower Back / Lower Extremity **H** Integumentary System - Whole Body **J** Musculoskeletal System - Head and Neck **K** Musculoskeletal System - Upper Back / Upper Extremity **L** Musculoskeletal System - Lower Back / Lower Extremity **M** Musculoskeletal System - Whole Body	**6** Therapeutic Exercise	**B** Physical Agents **C** Mechanical **D** Electrotherapeutic **E** Orthosis **F** Assistive, Adaptive, Supportive or Protective **G** Aerobic Endurance and Conditioning **H** Mechanical or Electromechanical **U** Prosthesis **Y** Other Equipment **Z** None	**Z** None
4 Circulatory System - Head and Neck **5** Circulatory System - Upper Back / Upper Extremity **6** Circulatory System - Lower Back / Lower Extremity **7** Circulatory System - Whole Body **8** Respiratory System - Head and Neck **9** Respiratory System - Upper Back / Upper Extremity **B** Respiratory System - Lower Back / Lower Extremity **C** Respiratory System - Whole Body	**6** Therapeutic Exercise	**B** Physical Agents **C** Mechanical **D** Electrotherapeutic **E** Orthosis **F** Assistive, Adaptive, Supportive or Protective **G** Aerobic Endurance and Conditioning **H** Mechanical or Electromechanical **U** Prosthesis **Y** Other Equipment **Z** None	**Z** None
N Genitourinary System	**1** Muscle Performance	**E** Orthosis **F** Assistive, Adaptive, Supportive or Protective **U** Prosthesis **Y** Other Equipment **Z** None	**Z** None
N Genitourinary System	**6** Therapeutic Exercise	**B** Physical Agents **C** Mechanical **D** Electrotherapeutic **E** Orthosis **F** Assistive, Adaptive, Supportive or Protective **G** Aerobic Endurance and Conditioning **H** Mechanical or Electromechanical **U** Prosthesis **Y** Other Equipment **Z** None	**Z** None
Z None	**4** Wheelchair Mobility	**D** Electrotherapeutic **E** Orthosis **F** Assistive, Adaptive, Supportive or Protective **U** Prosthesis **Y** Other Equipment **Z** None	**Z** None

Section	F	Physical Rehabilitation and Diagnostic Audiology		
Section Qualifier	0	Rehabilitation		
Type	7	Motor Treatment: Exercise or activities to increase or facilitate motor function		

Body System/Region (Character 4)	Type Qualifier (Character 5)	Equipment (Character 6)	Qualifier (Character 7)
Z None	5 Bed Mobility	C Mechanical E Orthosis F Assistive, Adaptive, Supportive or Protective U Prosthesis Y Other Equipment Z None	Z None
Z None	8 Transfer Training	C Mechanical D Electrotherapeutic E Orthosis F Assistive, Adaptive, Supportive or Protective U Prosthesis Y Other Equipment Z None	Z None
Z None	9 Gait Training/Functional Ambulation	C Mechanical D Electrotherapeutic E Orthosis F Assistive, Adaptive, Supportive or Protective G Aerobic Endurance and Conditioning U Prosthesis Y Other Equipment Z None	Z None

Section	F	Physical Rehabilitation and Diagnostic Audiology		
Section Qualifier	0	Rehabilitation		
Type	8	Activities of Daily Living Treatment: Exercise or activities to facilitate functional competence for activities of daily living		

Body System/Region (Character 4)	Type Qualifier (Character 5)	Equipment (Character 6)	Qualifier (Character 7)
D Integumentary System - Head and Neck F Integumentary System - Upper Back / Upper Extremity G Integumentary System - Lower Back / Lower Extremity H Integumentary System - Whole Body J Musculoskeletal System - Head and Neck K Musculoskeletal System - Upper Back / Upper Extremity L Musculoskeletal System - Lower Back / Lower Extremity M Musculoskeletal System - Whole Body	5 Wound Management	B Physical Agents C Mechanical D Electrotherapeutic E Orthosis F Assistive, Adaptive, Supportive or Protective U Prosthesis Y Other Equipment Z None	Z None
Z None	0 Bathing/Showering Techniques 1 Dressing Techniques 2 Grooming/Personal Hygiene	E Orthosis F Assistive, Adaptive, Supportive or Protective U Prosthesis Y Other Equipment Z None	Z None
Z None	3 Feeding/Eating	C Mechanical D Electrotherapeutic E Orthosis F Assistive, Adaptive, Supportive or Protective U Prosthesis Y Other Equipment Z None	Z None
Z None	4 Home Management	D Electrotherapeutic E Orthosis F Assistive, Adaptive, Supportive or Protective U Prosthesis Y Other Equipment Z None	Z None

Section	F	Physical Rehabilitation and Diagnostic Audiology		
Section Qualifier	0	Rehabilitation		[continued]
Type	8	Activities of Daily Living Treatment: Exercise or activities to facilitate functional competence for activities of daily living		

Body System/Region (Character 4)	Type Qualifier (Character 5)	Equipment (Character 6)	Qualifier (Character 7)
Z None	6 Psychosocial Skills	Z None	Z None
Z None	7 Vocational Activities and Functional Community or Work Reintegration Skills	B Physical Agents C Mechanical D Electrotherapeutic E Orthosis F Assistive, Adaptive, Supportive or Protective G Aerobic Endurance and Conditioning U Prosthesis Y Other Equipment Z None	Z None

Section	F	Physical Rehabilitation and Diagnostic Audiology		
Section Qualifier	0	Rehabilitation		
Type	9	Hearing Treatment: Application of techniques to improve, augment, or compensate for hearing and related functional impairment		

Body System/Region (Character 4)	Type Qualifier (Character 5)	Equipment (Character 6)	Qualifier (Character 7)
Z None	0 Hearing and Related Disorders Counseling 1 Hearing and Related Disorders Prevention	K Audiovisual Z None	Z None
Z None	2 Auditory Processing	K Audiovisual L Assistive Listening P Computer Y Other Equipment Z None	Z None
Z None	3 Cerumen Management	X Cerumen Management Z None	Z None

Section	F	Physical Rehabilitation and Diagnostic Audiology		
Section Qualifier	0	Rehabilitation		
Type	B	Cochlear Implant Treatment: Application of techniques to improve the communication abilities of individuals with cochlear implant		

Body System/Region (Character 4)	Type Qualifier (Character 5)	Equipment (Character 6)	Qualifier (Character 7)
Z None	0 Cochlear Implant Rehabilitation	1 Audiometer 2 Sound Field / Booth 9 Cochlear Implant K Audiovisual P Computer Y Other Equipment	Z None

Section	F	Physical Rehabilitation and Diagnostic Audiology		
Section Qualifier	0	Rehabilitation		
Type	C	Vestibular Treatment: Application of techniques to improve, augment, or compensate for vestibular and related functional impairment		

Body System/Region (Character 4)	Type Qualifier (Character 5)	Equipment (Character 6)	Qualifier (Character 7)
3 Neurological System - Whole Body H Integumentary System - Whole Body M Musculoskeletal System - Whole Body	3 Postural Control	E Orthosis F Assistive, Adaptive, Supportive or Protective U Prosthesis Y Other Equipment Z None	Z None
Z None	0 Vestibular	8 Vestibular / Balance Z None	Z None
Z None	1 Perceptual Processing 2 Visual Motor Integration	K Audiovisual L Assistive Listening N Biosensory Feedback P Computer Q Speech Analysis S Voice Analysis T Aerodynamic Function Y Other Equipment Z None	Z None

Section	F	Physical Rehabilitation and Diagnostic Audiology		
Section Qualifier	0	Rehabilitation		
Type	D	Device Fitting: Fitting of a device designed to facilitate or support achievement of a higher level of function		

Body System/Region (Character 4)	Type Qualifier (Character 5)	Equipment (Character 6)	Qualifier (Character 7)
Z None	0 Tinnitus Masker	5 Hearing Aid Selection / Fitting / Test Z None	Z None
Z None	1 Monaural Hearing Aid 2 Binaural Hearing Aid 5 Assistive Listening Device	1 Audiometer 2 Sound Field / Booth 5 Hearing Aid Selection / Fitting / Test K Audiovisual L Assistive Listening Z None	Z None
Z None	3 Augmentative/Alternative Communication System	M Augmentative / Alternative Communication	Z None
Z None	4 Voice Prosthetic	S Voice Analysis V Speech Prosthesis	Z None
Z None	6 Dynamic Orthosis 7 Static Orthosis 8 Prosthesis 9 Assistive, Adaptive, Supportive or Protective Devices	E Orthosis F Assistive, Adaptive, Supportive or Protective U Prosthesis Z None	Z None

Section	F	Physical Rehabilitation and Diagnostic Audiology		
Section Qualifier	0	Rehabilitation		
Type	F	Caregiver Training: Training in activities to support patient's optimal level of function		

Body System/Region (Character 4)	Type Qualifier (Character 5)	Equipment (Character 6)	Qualifier (Character 7)
Z None	0 Bathing/Showering Technique 1 Dressing 2 Feeding and Eating 3 Grooming/Personal Hygiene 4 Bed Mobility 5 Transfer 6 Wheelchair Mobility 7 Therapeutic Exercise 8 Airway Clearance Techniques 9 Wound Management B Vocational Activities and Functional Community or Work Reintegration Skills C Gait Training/Functional Ambulation D Application, Proper Use and Care of Devices F Application, Proper Use and Care of Orthoses G Application, Proper Use and Care of Prosthesis H Home Management	E Orthosis F Assistive, Adaptive, Supportive or Protective U Prosthesis Z None	Z None
Z None	J Communication Skills	K Audiovisual L Assistive Listening M Augmentative / Alternative Communication P Computer Z None	Z None

Section		F	Physical Rehabilitation and Diagnostic Audiology		
Section Qualifier		1	Diagnostic Audiology		
Type		3	Hearing Assessment: Measurement of hearing and related functions		

Body System/Region (Character 4)	Type Qualifier (Character 5)	Equipment (Character 6)	Qualifier (Character 7)
Z None	0 Hearing Screening	0 Occupational Hearing 1 Audiometer 2 Sound Field / Booth 3 Tympanometer 8 Vestibular / Balance 9 Cochlear Implant Z None	Z None
Z None	1 Pure Tone Audiometry, Air 2 Pure Tone Audiometry, Air and Bone	0 Occupational Hearing 1 Audiometer 2 Sound Field / Booth Z None	Z None
Z None	3 Bekesy Audiometry 6 Visual Reinforcement Audiometry 9 Short Increment Sensitivity Index B Stenger C Pure Tone Stenger	1 Audiometer 2 Sound Field / Booth Z None	Z None
Z None	4 Conditioned Play Audiometry 5 Select Picture Audiometry	1 Audiometer 2 Sound Field / Booth K Audiovisual Z None	Z None
Z None	7 Alternate Binaural or Monaural Loudness Balance	1 Audiometer K Audiovisual Z None	Z None
Z None	8 Tone Decay D Tympanometry F Eustachian Tube Function G Acoustic Reflex Patterns H Acoustic Reflex Threshold J Acoustic Reflex Decay	3 Tympanometer 4 Electroacoustic Immittance / Acoustic Reflex Z None	Z None
Z None	K Electrocochleography L Auditory Evoked Potentials	7 Electrophysiologic Z None	Z None
Z None	M Evoked Otoacoustic Emissions, Screening N Evoked Otoacoustic Emissions, Diagnostic	6 Otoacoustic Emission (OAE) Z None	Z None

Section		F	Physical Rehabilitation and Diagnostic Audiology		
Section Qualifier		1	Diagnostic Audiology		
Type		3	Hearing Assessment: Measurement of hearing and related functions		

Body System/Region (Character 4)	Type Qualifier (Character 5)	Equipment (Character 6)	Qualifier (Character 7)
Z None	P Aural Rehabilitation Status	1 Audiometer 2 Sound Field / Booth 4 Electroacoustic Immittance / Acoustic Reflex 9 Cochlear Implant K Audiovisual L Assistive Listening P Computer Z None	Z None
Z None	Q Auditory Processing	K Audiovisual P Computer Y Other Equipment Z None	Z None

Section	F	Physical Rehabilitation and Diagnostic Audiology
Section Qualifier	1	Diagnostic Audiology
Type	4	Hearing Aid Assessment: Measurement of the appropriateness and/or effectiveness of a hearing device

Body System/Region (Character 4)	Type Qualifier (Character 5)	Equipment (Character 6)	Qualifier (Character 7)
Z None	0 Cochlear Implant	1 Audiometer 2 Sound Field / Booth 3 Tympanometer 4 Electroacoustic Immittance / Acoustic Reflex 5 Hearing Aid Selection / Fitting / Test 7 Electrophysiologic 9 Cochlear Implant K Audiovisual L Assistive Listening P Computer Y Other Equipment Z None	Z None
Z None	1 Ear Canal Probe Microphone 6 Binaural Electroacoustic Hearing Aid Check 8 Monaural Electroacoustic Hearing Aid Check	5 Hearing Aid Selection / Fitting / Test Z None	Z None
Z None	2 Monaural Hearing Aid 3 Binaural Hearing Aid	1 Audiometer 2 Sound Field / Booth 3 Tympanometer 4 Electroacoustic Immittance / Acoustic Reflex 5 Hearing Aid Selection / Fitting / Test K Audiovisual L Assistive Listening P Computer Z None	Z None
Z None	4 Assistive Listening System/Device Selection	1 Audiometer 2 Sound Field / Booth 3 Tympanometer 4 Electroacoustic Immittance / Acoustic Reflex K Audiovisual L Assistive Listening Z None	Z None

Section	F	Physical Rehabilitation and Diagnostic Audiology
Section Qualifier	1	Diagnostic Audiology
Type	4	Hearing Aid Assessment: Measurement of the appropriateness and/or effectiveness of a hearing device

Body System/Region (Character 4)	Type Qualifier (Character 5)	Equipment (Character 6)	Qualifier (Character 7)
Z None	5 Sensory Aids	1 Audiometer 2 Sound Field / Booth 3 Tympanometer 4 Electroacoustic Immittance / Acoustic Reflex 5 Hearing Aid Selection / Fitting / Test K Audiovisual L Assistive Listening Z None	Z None
Z None	7 Ear Protector Attenuation	0 Occupational Hearing Z None	Z None

Section	F	Physical Rehabilitation and Diagnostic Audiology		
Section Qualifier	1	Diagnostic Audiology		
Type	5	Vestibular Assessment: Measurement of the vestibular system and related functions		

Body System/Region (Character 4)	Type Qualifier (Character 5)	Equipment (Character 6)	Qualifier (Character 7)
Z None	**0** Bithermal, Binaural Caloric Irrigation **1** Bithermal, Monaural Caloric Irrigation **2** Unithermal Binaural Screen **3** Oscillating Tracking **4** Sinusoidal Vertical Axis Rotational **5** Dix-Hallpike Dynamic **6** Computerized Dynamic Posturography	**8** Vestibular / Balance **Z** None	**Z** None
Z None	**7** Tinnitus Masker	**5** Hearing Aid Selection / Fitting / Test **Z** None	**Z** None

Section	G	Mental Health		
Body System	Z	None		
Type	1	Psychological Tests: The administration and interpretation of standardized psychological tests and measurement instruments for the assessment of psychological function		
Qualifier (Character 4)		**Qualifier (Character 5)**	**Qualifier (Character 6)**	**Qualifier (Character 7)**
0 Developmental **1** Personality and Behavioral **2** Intellectual and Psychoeducational **3** Neuropsychological **4** Neurobehavioral and Cognitive Status		**Z** None	**Z** None	**Z** None

Section	G	Mental Health		
Body System	Z	None		
Type	2	Crisis Intervention: Treatment of a traumatized, acutely disturbed or distressed individual for the purpose of short-term stabilization		
Qualifier (Character 4)		**Qualifier (Character 5)**	**Qualifier (Character 6)**	**Qualifier (Character 7)**
Z None		**Z** None	**Z** None	**Z** None

Section	G	Mental Health		
Body System	Z	None		
Type	3	Medication Management: Monitoring and adjusting the use of medications for the treatment of a mental health disorder		
Qualifier (Character 4)		**Qualifier (Character 5)**	**Qualifier (Character 6)**	**Qualifier (Character 7)**
Z None		**Z** None	**Z** None	**Z** None

Section	G	Mental Health		
Body System	Z	None		
Type	5	Individual Psychotherapy: Treatment of an individual with a mental health disorder by behavioral, cognitive, psychoanalytic, psychodynamic or psychophysiological means to improve functioning or well-being		
Qualifier (Character 4)		**Qualifier (Character 5)**	**Qualifier (Character 6)**	**Qualifier (Character 7)**
0 Interactive **1** Behavioral **2** Cognitive **3** Interpersonal **4** Psychoanalysis **5** Psychodynamic **6** Supportive **8** Cognitive-Behavioral **9** Psychophysiological		**Z** None	**Z** None	**Z** None

Section	G	Mental Health		
Body System	Z	None		
Type	6	Counseling: The application of psychological methods to treat an individual with normal developmental issues and psychological problems in order to increase function, improve well-being, alleviate distress, maladjustment or resolve crises		
Qualifier (Character 4)		**Qualifier (Character 5)**	**Qualifier (Character 6)**	**Qualifier (Character 7)**
0 Educational				
1 Vocational		**Z** None	**Z** None	**Z** None
3 Other Counseling				

Section	G	Mental Health		
Body System	Z	None		
Type	7	Family Psychotherapy: Treatment that includes one or more family members of an individual with a mental health disorder by behavioral, cognitive, psychoanalytic, psychodynamic or psychophysiological means to improve functioning or well-being		
Qualifier (Character 4)		**Qualifier (Character 5)**	**Qualifier (Character 6)**	**Qualifier (Character 7)**
2 Other Family Psychotherapy		**Z** None	**Z** None	**Z** None

Section	G	Mental Health		
Body System	Z	None		
Type	B	Electroconvulsive Therapy: The application of controlled electrical voltages to treat a mental health disorder		
Qualifier (Character 4)		**Qualifier (Character 5)**	**Qualifier (Character 6)**	**Qualifier (Character 7)**
0 Unilateral-Single Seizure **1** Unilateral-Multiple Seizure **2** Bilateral-Single Seizure **3** Bilateral-Multiple Seizure **4** Other Electroconvulsive Therapy		**Z** None	**Z** None	**Z** None

Section	G	Mental Health			
Body System	Z	None			
Type	C	Biofeedback: Provision of information from the monitoring and regulating of physiological processes in conjunction with cognitive-behavioral techniques to improve patient functioning or well-being			

Qualifier (Character 4)	Qualifier (Character 5)	Qualifier (Character 6)	Qualifier (Character 7)
9 Other Biofeedback	Z None	Z None	Z None

Section	G	Mental Health			
Body System	Z	None			
Type	F	Hypnosis: Induction of a state of heightened suggestibility by auditory, visual and tactile techniques to elicit an emotional or behavioral response			

Qualifier (Character 4)	Qualifier (Character 5)	Qualifier (Character 6)	Qualifier (Character 7)
Z None	Z None	Z None	Z None

Section	G	Mental Health			
Body System	Z	None			
Type	G	Narcosynthesis: Administration of intravenous barbiturates in order to release suppressed or repressed thoughts			

Qualifier (Character 4)	Qualifier (Character 5)	Qualifier (Character 6)	Qualifier (Character 7)
Z None	Z None	Z None	Z None

Section	G	Mental Health			
Body System	Z	None			
Type	H	Group Psychotherapy: Treatment of two or more individuals with a mental health disorder by behavioral, cognitive, psychoanalytic, psychodynamic or psychophysiological means to improve functioning or well-being			

Qualifier (Character 4)	Qualifier (Character 5)	Qualifier (Character 6)	Qualifier (Character 7)
Z None	Z None	Z None	Z None

Section	G	Mental Health			
Body System	Z	None			
Type	J	Light Therapy: Application of specialized light treatments to improve functioning or well-being			

Qualifier (Character 4)	Qualifier (Character 5)	Qualifier (Character 6)	Qualifier (Character 7)
Z None	Z None	Z None	Z None

Section	H	Substance Abuse Treatment			
Body System	Z	None			
Type	2	Detoxification Services: Detoxification from alcohol and/or drugs			
Qualifier (Character 4)		**Qualifier (Character 5)**	**Qualifier (Character 6)**		**Qualifier (Character 7)**
Z None		Z None	Z None		Z None

Section	H	Substance Abuse Treatment			
Body System	Z	None			
Type	3	Individual Counseling: The application of psychological methods to treat an individual with addictive behavior			
Qualifier (Character 4)		**Qualifier (Character 5)**	**Qualifier (Character 6)**		**Qualifier (Character 7)**
0 Cognitive 1 Behavioral 2 Cognitive-Behavioral 3 12-Step 4 Interpersonal 5 Vocational 6 Psychoeducation 7 Motivational Enhancement 8 Confrontational 9 Continuing Care B Spiritual C Pre/Post-Test Infectious Disease		Z None	Z None		Z None

Section	H	Substance Abuse Treatment			
Body System	Z	None			
Type	4	Group Counseling: The application of psychological methods to treat two or more individuals with addictive behavior			
Qualifier (Character 4)		**Qualifier (Character 5)**	**Qualifier (Character 6)**		**Qualifier (Character 7)**
0 Cognitive 1 Behavioral 2 Cognitive-Behavioral 3 12-Step 4 Interpersonal 5 Vocational 6 Psychoeducation 7 Motivational Enhancement 8 Confrontational 9 Continuing Care B Spiritual C Pre/Post-Test Infectious Disease		Z None	Z None		Z None

Section	H	Substance Abuse Treatment			
Body System	Z	None			
Type	5	Individual Psychotherapy: Treatment of an individual with addictive behavior by behavioral, cognitive, psychoanalytic, psychodynamic or psychophysiological means			
Qualifier (Character 4)		**Qualifier (Character 5)**	**Qualifier (Character 6)**		**Qualifier (Character 7)**
0 Cognitive 1 Behavioral 2 Cognitive-Behavioral 3 12-Step 4 Interpersonal 5 Interactive 6 Psychoeducation 7 Motivational Enhancement 8 Confrontational 9 Supportive B Psychoanalysis C Psychodynamic D Psychophysiological		Z None	Z None		Z None

Section	H	Substance Abuse Treatment			
Body System	Z	None			
Type	6	Family Counseling: The application of psychological methods that includes one or more family members to treat an individual with addictive behavior			
Qualifier (Character 4)		**Qualifier (Character 5)**	**Qualifier (Character 6)**		**Qualifier (Character 7)**
3 Other Family Counseling		Z None	Z None		Z None

Section	H	Substance Abuse Treatment		
Body System	Z	None		
Type	8	Medication Management: Monitoring and adjusting the use of replacement medications for the treatment of addiction		

Qualifier (Character 4)	Qualifier (Character 5)	Qualifier (Character 6)	Qualifier (Character 7)
0 Nicotine Replacement 1 Methadone Maintenance 2 Levo-alpha-acetyl-methadol (LAAM) 3 Antabuse 4 Naltrexone 5 Naloxone 6 Clonidine 7 Bupropion 8 Psychiatric Medication 9 Other Replacement Medication	Z None	Z None	Z None

Section	H	Substance Abuse Treatment		
Body System	Z	None		
Type	9	Pharmacotherapy: The use of replacement medications for the treatment of addiction		

Qualifier (Character 4)	Qualifier (Character 5)	Qualifier (Character 6)	Qualifier (Character 7)
0 Nicotine Replacement 1 Methadone Maintenance 2 Levo-alpha-acetyl-methadol (LAAM) 3 Antabuse 4 Naltrexone 5 Naloxone 6 Clonidine 7 Bupropion 8 Psychiatric Medication 9 Other Replacement Medication	Z None	Z None	Z None

A

Abdominal aortic plexus *use* Nerve, Abdominal Sympathetic

Abdominal esophagus *use* Esophagus, Lower

Abdominohysterectomy
  see Excision, Uterus **0UB9**
  see Resection, Uterus **0UT9**

Abdominoplasty
  see Alteration, Abdominal Wall **0W0F**
  see Repair, Abdominal Wall **0WQF**
  see Supplement, Abdominal Wall **0WUF**

Abductor hallucis muscle
  use Muscle, Foot, Right
  use Muscle, Foot, Left

AbioCor® Total Replacement Heart *use* Synthetic Substitute

Ablation *see* Destruction

Abortion
  Products of Conception **10A0**
  Abortifacient **10A07ZX**
  Laminaria **10A07ZW**
  Vacuum **10A07Z6**

Abrasion *see* Extraction

Accessory cephalic vein
  use Vein, Cephalic, Right
  use Vein, Cephalic, Left

Accessory obturator nerve *use* Nerve, Lumbar Plexus

Accessory phrenic nerve *use* Nerve, Phrenic

Accessory spleen *use* Spleen

Acellular Hydrated Dermis *use* Nonautologous Tissue Substitute

Acetabulectomy
  see Excision, Lower Bones **0QB**
  see Resection, Lower Bones **0QT**

Acetabulofemoral joint
  use Joint, Hip, Right
  use Joint, Hip, Left

Acetabuloplasty
  see Repair, Lower Bones **0QQ**
  see Replacement, Lower Bones **0QR**
  see Supplement, Lower Bones **0QU**

Achilles tendon
  use Tendon, Lower Leg, Left
  use Tendon, Lower Leg, Right

Achillorrhaphy *see* Repair, Tendons **0LQ**

Achillotenotomy, achillotomy
  see Division, Tendons **0L8**
  see Drainage, Tendons **0L9**

Acromioclavicular ligament
  use Bursa and Ligament, Shoulder, Right
  use Bursa and Ligament, Shoulder, Left

Acromion (process)
  use Scapula, Left
  use Scapula, Right

Acromionectomy
  see Excision, Upper Joints **0RB**
  see Resection, Upper Joints **0RT**

Acromioplasty
  see Repair, Upper Joints **0RQ**
  see Replacement, Upper Joints **0RR**
  see Supplement, Upper Joints **0RU**

Activa PC neurostimulator *use* Stimulator Generator, Multiple Array in **0JH**

Activa RC neurostimulator *use* Stimulator Generator, Multiple Array Rechargeable in **0JH**

Activa SC neurostimulator *use* Stimulator Generator, Single Array in **0JH**

Activities of Daily Living Assessment F02

Activities of Daily Living Treatment F08

ACUITY™ Steerable Lead
  use Cardiac Lead, Defibrillator in **02H**
  use Cardiac Lead, Pacemaker in **02H**

Acupuncture
  Breast
    Anesthesia **8E0H300**
    No Qualifier **8E0H30Z**
  Integumentary System
    Anesthesia **8E0H300**
    No Qualifier **8E0H30Z**

Adductor brevis muscle
  use Muscle, Upper Leg, Left
  use Muscle, Upper Leg, Right

Adductor hallucis muscle
  use Muscle, Foot, Left
  use Muscle, Foot, Right

Adductor longus muscle
  use Muscle, Upper Leg, Right
  use Muscle, Upper Leg, Left

Adductor magnus muscle
  use Muscle, Upper Leg, Right
  use Muscle, Upper Leg, Left

Adenohypophysis *use* Gland, Pituitary

Adenoidectomy
  see Excision, Adenoids **0CBQ**
  see Resection, Adenoids **0CTQ**

Adenoidotomy *see* Drainage, Adenoids **0C9Q**

Adhesiolysis *see* Release

Administration
  Blood products *see* Transfusion
  Other substance *see* Introduction of substance in or on

Adrenalectomy
  see Excision, Endocrine System **0GB**
  see Resection, Endocrine System **0GT**

Adrenalorrhaphy *see* Repair, Endocrine System **0GQ**

Adrenalotomy *see* Drainage, Endocrine System **0G9**

Advancement
  see Reposition
  see Transfer

Alar ligament of axis *use* Bursa and Ligament, Head and Neck

Alimentation *see* Introduction of substance in or on

Alteration
  Abdominal Wall **0W0F**
  Ankle Region
    Left **0Y0L**
    Right **0Y0K**
  Arm
    Lower
      Left **0X0F**
      Right **0X0D**
    Upper
      Left **0X09**
      Right **0X08**
  Axilla
    Left **0X05**
    Right **0X04**
  Back
    Lower **0W0L**
    Upper **0W0K**
  Breast
    Bilateral **0H0V**
    Left **0H0U**
    Right **0H0T**
  Buttock
    Left **0Y01**
    Right **0Y00**
  Chest Wall **0W08**

Alteration - *continued*
  Ear
    Bilateral **0902**
    Left **0901**
    Right **0900**
  Elbow Region
    Left **0X0C**
    Right **0X0B**
  Extremity
    Lower
      Left **0Y0B**
      Right **0Y09**
    Upper
      Left **0X07**
      Right **0X06**
  Eyelid
    Lower
      Left **080R**
      Right **080Q**
    Upper
      Left **080P**
      Right **080N**
  Face **0W02**
  Head **0W00**
  Jaw
    Lower **0W05**
    Upper **0W04**
  Knee Region
    Left **0Y0G**
    Right **0Y0F**
  Leg
    Lower
      Left **0Y0J**
      Right **0Y0H**
    Upper
      Left **0Y0D**
      Right **0Y0C**
  Lip
    Lower **0C01X**
    Upper **0C00X**
  Neck **0W06**
  Nose **090K**
  Perineum
    Female **0W0N**
    Male **0W0M**
  Shoulder Region
    Left **0X03**
    Right **0X02**
  Subcutaneous Tissue and Fascia
    Abdomen **0J08**
    Back **0J07**
    Buttock **0J09**
    Chest **0J06**
    Face **0J01**
    Lower Arm
      Left **0J0H**
      Right **0J0G**
    Lower Leg
      Left **0J0P**
      Right **0J0N**
    Neck
      Anterior **0J04**
      Posterior **0J05**
    Upper Arm
      Left **0J0F**
      Right **0J0D**
    Upper Leg
      Left **0J0M**
      Right **0J0L**
  Wrist Region
    Left **0X0H**
    Right **0X0G**

Alveolar process of mandible
  use Mandible, Left
  use Mandible, Right
Alveolar process of maxilla
  use Maxilla, Right
  use Maxilla, Left
Alveolectomy
  see Excision, Head and Facial Bones **0NB**
  see Resection, Head and Facial Bones **0NT**
Alveoloplasty
  see Repair, Head and Facial Bones **0NQ**
  see Replacement, Head and Facial Bones
  0NR
  see Supplement, Head and Facial Bones **0NU**
Alveolotomy
  see Division, Head and Facial Bones **0N8**
  see Drainage, Head and Facial Bones **0N9**
Ambulatory cardiac monitoring 4A12X45
Amniocentesis *see* Drainage, Products of
  Conception **1090**
Amnioinfusion *see* Introduction of substance in
  or on, Products of Conception **3E0E**
Amnioscopy 10J08ZZ
Amniotomy *see* Drainage, Products of
  Conception **1090**
AMPLATZER® Muscular VSD Occluder *use*
  Synthetic Substitute
Amputation *see* Detachment
AMS 800® Urinary Control System *use*
  Artificial Sphincter in Urinary System
Anal orifice *use* Anus
Analog radiography *see* Plain Radiography
Analog radiology *see* Plain Radiography
Anastomosis *see* Bypass
Anatomical snuffbox
  use Muscle, Lower Arm and Wrist, Left
  use Muscle, Lower Arm and Wrist, Right
AneuRx® AAA Advantage® *use* Intraluminal
  Device
Angiectomy
  see Excision, Heart and Great Vessels **02B**
  see Excision, Upper Arteries **03B**
  see Excision, Lower Arteries **04B**
  see Excision, Upper Veins **05B**
  see Excision, Lower Veins **06B**
Angiocardiography
  Combined right and left heart *see*
  Fluoroscopy, Heart, Right and Left **B216**
  Left Heart *see* Fluoroscopy, Heart, Left **B215**
  Right Heart *see* Fluoroscopy, Heart, Right
  B214
  SPY *see* Fluoroscopy, Heart **B21**
Angiography
  see Plain Radiography, Heart **B20**
  see Fluoroscopy, Heart **B21**
Angioplasty
  see Dilation, Heart and Great Vessels **027**
  see Repair, Heart and Great Vessels **02Q**
  see Replacement, Heart and Great Vessels
  02R
  see Dilation, Upper Arteries **037**
  see Repair, Upper Arteries **03Q**
  see Replacement, Upper Arteries **03R**
  see Dilation, Lower Arteries **047**
  see Repair, Lower Arteries **04Q**
  see Replacement, Lower Arteries **04R**
  see Supplement, Heart and Great Vessels **02U**
  see Supplement, Upper Arteries **03U**
  see Supplement, Lower Arteries **04U**
Angiorrhaphy
  see Repair, Heart and Great Vessels **02Q**
  see Repair, Upper Arteries **03Q**
  see Repair, Lower Arteries **04Q**

Angioscopy
  02JY4ZZ
  03JY4ZZ
  04JY4ZZ
Angiotripsy
  see Occlusion, Upper Arteries **03L**
  see Occlusion, Lower Arteries **04L**
Angular artery *use* Artery, Face
Angular vein
  use Vein, Face, Left
  use Vein, Face, Right
Annular ligament
  use Bursa and Ligament, Elbow, Left
  use Bursa and Ligament, Elbow, Right
Annuloplasty
  see Repair, Heart and Great Vessels **02Q**
  see Supplement, Heart and Great Vessels **02U**
Annuloplasty ring *use* Synthetic Substitute
Anoplasty
  see Repair, Anus **0DQQ**
  see Supplement, Anus **0DUQ**
Anorectal junction *use* Rectum
Anoscopy 0DJD8ZZ
Ansa cervicalis *use* Nerve, Cervical Plexus
Antabuse therapy HZ93ZZZ
Antebrachial fascia
  use Subcutaneous Tissue and Fascia, Lower
  Arm, Left
  use Subcutaneous Tissue and Fascia, Lower
  Arm, Right
Anterior (pectoral) lymph node
  use Lymphatic, Axillary, Right
  use Lymphatic, Axillary, Left
Anterior cerebral artery *use* Artery,
  Intracranial
Anterior cerebral vein *use* Vein, Intracranial
Anterior choroidal artery *use* Artery,
  Intracranial
Anterior circumflex humeral artery
  use Artery, Axillary, Left
  use Artery, Axillary, Right
Anterior communicating artery *use* Artery,
  Intracranial
Anterior cruciate ligament (ACL)
  use Bursa and Ligament, Knee, Left
  use Bursa and Ligament, Knee, Right
Anterior crural nerve *use* Nerve, Femoral
Anterior facial vein
  use Vein, Face, Left
  use Vein, Face, Right
Anterior intercostal artery
  use Artery, Internal Mammary, Right
  use Artery, Internal Mammary, Left
Anterior interosseous nerve *use* Nerve, Median
Anterior lateral malleolar artery
  use Artery, Anterior Tibial, Right
  use Artery, Anterior Tibial, Left
Anterior lingual gland *use* Gland, Minor
  Salivary
Anterior medial malleolar artery
  use Artery, Anterior Tibial, Right
  use Artery, Anterior Tibial, Left
Anterior spinal artery
  use Artery, Vertebral, Right
  use Artery, Vertebral, Left
Anterior tibial recurrent artery
  use Artery, Anterior Tibial, Right
  use Artery, Anterior Tibial, Left
Anterior ulnar recurrent artery
  use Artery, Ulnar, Right
Anterior ulnar recurrent artery
  use Artery, Ulnar, Left
Anterior vagal trunk *use* Nerve, Vagus

Anterior vertebral muscle
  use Muscle, Neck, Left
  use Muscle, Neck, Right
Antihelix
  use Ear, External, Right
  use Ear, External, Left
  use Ear, External, Bilateral
Antitragus
  use Ear, External, Bilateral
  use Ear, External, Right
  use Ear, External, Left
Antrostomy *see* Drainage, Ear, Nose, Sinus **099**
Antrotomy *see* Drainage, Ear, Nose, Sinus **099**
Antrum of Highmore
  use Sinus, Maxillary, Left
  use Sinus, Maxillary, Right
Aortic annulus *use* Valve, Aortic
Aortic arch *use* Aorta, Thoracic
Aortic intercostal artery *use* Aorta, Thoracic
Aortography
  see Plain Radiography, Upper Arteries **B30**
  see Fluoroscopy, Upper Arteries **B31**
  see Plain Radiography, Lower Arteries **B40**
  see Fluoroscopy, Lower Arteries **B41**
Aortoplasty
  see Repair, Aorta, Thoracic **02QW**
  see Replacement, Aorta, Thoracic **02RW**
  see Supplement, Aorta, Thoracic **02UW**
  see Repair, Aorta, Abdominal **04Q0**
  see Replacement, Aorta, Abdominal **04R0**
  see Supplement, Aorta, Abdominal **04U0**
Apical (subclavicular) lymph node
  use Lymphatic, Axillary, Left
  use Lymphatic, Axillary, Right
Apneustic center *use* Pons
Appendectomy
  see Excision, Appendix **0DBJ**
  see Resection, Appendix **0DTJ**
Appendicolysis *see* Release, Appendix **0DNJ**
Appendicotomy *see* Drainage, Appendix **0D9J**
Application *see* Introduction of substance in or
  on
Aquapheresis 6A550Z3
Aqueduct of Sylvius *use* Cerebral Ventricle
Aqueous humor
  use Anterior Chamber, Right
  use Anterior Chamber, Left
Arachnoid mater
Arachnoid mater
  use Spinal Meninges
  use Cerebral Meninges
Arcuate artery
  use Artery, Foot, Left
  use Artery, Foot, Right
Areola
  use Nipple, Left
  use Nipple, Right
AROM (artificial rupture of membranes)
  10907ZC
Arterial canal (duct) *use* Artery, Pulmonary,
  Left
Arterial pulse tracing *see* Measurement,
  Arterial **4A03**
Arteriectomy
  see Excision, Heart and Great Vessels **02B**
  see Excision, Upper Arteries **03B**
  see Excision, Lower Arteries **04B**
Arteriography
  see Plain Radiography, Heart **B20**
  see Fluoroscopy, Heart **B21**
  see Plain Radiography, Upper Arteries **B30**
  see Fluoroscopy, Upper Arteries **B31**

Arteriography - *continued*
   see Plain Radiography, Lower Arteries **B40**
   see Fluoroscopy, Lower Arteries **B41**
Arterioplasty
   see Repair, Heart and Great Vessels **02Q**
   see Replacement, Heart and Great Vessels
   02R
   see Repair, Upper Arteries **03Q**
   see Replacement, Upper Arteries **03R**
   see Repair, Lower Arteries **04Q**
   see Replacement, Lower Arteries **04R**
   see Supplement, Upper Arteries **03U**
   see Supplement, Lower Arteries **04U**
   see Supplement, Heart and Great Vessels **02U**
Arteriorrhaphy
   see Repair, Heart and Great Vessels **02Q**
   see Repair, Upper Arteries **03Q**
   see Repair, Lower Arteries **04Q**
Arterioscopy
   02JY4ZZ
   03JY4ZZ
   04JY4ZZ
Arthrectomy
   see Excision, Upper Joints **0RB**
   see Resection, Upper Joints **0RT**
   see Excision, Lower Joints **0SB**
   see Resection, Lower Joints **0ST**
Arthrocentesis
   see Drainage, Upper Joints **0R9**
   see Drainage, Lower Joints **0S9**
Arthrodesis
Arthrodesis
   see Fusion, Upper Joints **0RG**
   see Fusion, Lower Joints **0SG**
Arthrography
   see Plain Radiography, Skull and Facial
   Bones **BN0**
   see Plain Radiography, Non-Axial Upper
   Bones **BP0**
   see Plain Radiography, Non-Axial Lower
   Bones **BQ0**
Arthrolysis
   see Release, Upper Joints **0RN**
   see Release, Lower Joints **0SN**
Arthropexy
   see Repair, Upper Joints **0RQ**
   see Reposition, Upper Joints **0RS**
   see Repair, Lower Joints **0SQ**
   see Reposition, Lower Joints **0SS**
Arthroplasty
   see Repair, Upper Joints **0RQ**
   see Replacement, Upper Joints **0RR**
   see Repair, Lower Joints **0SQ**
   see Replacement, Lower Joints **0SR**
   see Supplement, Lower Joints **0SU**
   see Supplement, Upper Joints **0RU**
Arthroscopy
   see Inspection, Upper Joints **0RJ**
   see Inspection, Lower Joints **0SJ**
Arthrotomy
   see Drainage, Upper Joints **0R9**
   see Drainage, Lower Joints **0S9**
Artificial anal sphincter (AAS) *use* Artificial
Sphincter in Gastrointestinal System
Artificial bowel sphincter (neosphincter) *use*
Artificial Sphincter in Gastrointestinal System
Artificial Sphincter
   Insertion of device in
      Anus **0DHQ**
      Bladder **0THB**
      Bladder Neck **0THC**
      Urethra **0THD**

Artificial Sphincter – *continued*
   Removal of device from
      Anus **0DPQ**
      Bladder **0TPB**
      Urethra **0TPD**
   Revision of device in
      Anus **0DWQ**
      Bladder **0TWB**
      Urethra **0TWD**
Artificial urinary sphincter (AUS) *use*
Artificial Sphincter in Urinary System
Aryepiglottic fold *use* Larynx
Arytenoid cartilage *use* Larynx
Arytenoid muscle
   use Muscle, Neck, Left
   use Muscle, Neck, Right
Arytenoidectomy *see* Excision, Larynx **0CBS**
Arytenoidopexy *see* Repair, Larynx **0CQS**
Ascending aorta *use* Aorta, Thoracic
Ascending palatine artery *use* Artery, Face
Ascending pharyngeal artery
   use Artery, External Carotid, Left
   use Artery, External Carotid, Right
Aspiration *see* Drainage
Assessment
   Activities of daily living *see* Activities of
   Daily Living Assessment, Rehabilitation **F02**
   Hearing *see* Hearing Assessment, Diagnostic
   Audiology **F13**
   Hearing aid *see* Hearing Aid Assessment,
   Diagnostic Audiology **F14**
   Motor function *see* Motor Function
   Assessment, Rehabilitation **F01**
   Nerve function *see* Motor Function
   Assessment, Rehabilitation **F01**
   Speech *see* Speech Assessment,
   Rehabilitation **F00**
   Vestibular *see* Vestibular Assessment,
   Diagnostic Audiology **F15**
   Vocational *see* Activities of Daily Living
   Treatment, Rehabilitation **F08**
Assistance
   Cardiac
      Continuous
         Balloon Pump **5A02210**
         Impeller Pump **5A0221D**
         Other Pump **5A02216**
         Pulsatile Compression **5A02215**
      Intermittent
         Balloon Pump **5A02110**
         Impeller Pump **5A0211D**
         Other Pump **5A02116**
         Pulsatile Compression **5A02115**
   Circulatory
      Continuous
         Hyperbaric **5A05221**
         Supersaturated **5A0522C**
      Intermittent
         Hyperbaric **5A05121**
         Supersaturated **5A0512C**
   Respiratory
      24-96 Consecutive Hours
         Continuous Negative Airway Pressure
         5A09459
         Continuous Positive Airway Pressure
         5A09457
         Intermittent Negative Airway Pressure
         5A0945B
         Intermittent Positive Airway Pressure
         5A09458
         No Qualifier **5A0945Z**

Assistance - *continued*
      Greater than 96 Consecutive Hours
         Continuous Negative Airway Pressure
         5A09559
         Continuous Positive Airway Pressure
         5A09557
         Intermittent Negative Airway Pressure
         5A0955B
         Intermittent Positive Airway Pressure
         5A09558
         No Qualifier **5A0955Z**
      Less than 24 Consecutive Hours
         Continuous Negative Airway Pressure
         5A09359
         Continuous Positive Airway Pressure
         5A09357
         Intermittent Negative Airway Pressure
         5A0935B
         Intermittent Positive Airway Pressure
         5A09358
         No Qualifier **5A0935Z**
Assurant (Cobalt) stent *use* Intraluminal
Device
Atherectomy
   see Extirpation, Heart and Great Vessels **02C**
   see Extirpation, Upper Arteries **03C**
   see Extirpation, Lower Arteries **04C**
Atlantoaxial joint *use* Joint, Cervical Vertebral
Atmospheric Control 6A0Z
Atrioseptoplasty
   see Repair, Heart and Great Vessels **02Q**
   see Replacement, Heart and Great Vessels
   02R
   see Supplement, Heart and Great Vessels **02U**
Atrioventricular node *use* Conduction
Mechanism
Atrium dextrum cordis *use* Atrium, Right
Atrium pulmonale *use* Atrium, Left
Attain Ability® lead
   use Cardiac Lead, Pacemaker in **02H**
   use Cardiac Lead, Defibrillator in **02H**
Attain StarFix® (OTW) lead
   use Cardiac Lead, Defibrillator in **02H**
   use Cardiac Lead, Pacemaker in **02H**
Audiology, diagnostic
   see Hearing Assessment, Diagnostic
   Audiology **F13**
   see Hearing Aid Assessment, Diagnostic
   Audiology **F14**
   see Vestibular Assessment, Diagnostic
   Audiology **F15**
Audiometry *see* Hearing Assessment,
Diagnostic Audiology **F13**
Auditory tube
   use Eustachian Tube, Right
   use Eustachian Tube, Left
Auerbach's (myenteric) plexus *use* Nerve,
Abdominal Sympathetic
Auricle
   use Ear, External, Left
   use Ear, External, Bilateral
   use Ear, External, Right
Auricularis muscle *use* Muscle, Head
Autograft *use* Autologous Tissue Substitute
Autologous artery graft
   use Autologous Arterial Tissue in Lower
   Arteries
   use Autologous Arterial Tissue in Upper
   Veins
   use Autologous Arterial Tissue in Lower
   Veins
   use Autologous Arterial Tissue in Heart and
   Great Vessels

Autologous artery graft
  use Autologous Arterial Tissue in Upper Arteries
Autologous vein graft
  use Autologous Venous Tissue in Lower Arteries
  use Autologous Venous Tissue in Upper Veins
  use Autologous Venous Tissue in Lower Veins
  use Autologous Venous Tissue in Heart and Great Vessels
  use Autologous Venous Tissue in Upper Arteries
Autotransfusion *see* Transfusion
Autotransplant
  Adrenal tissue *see* Reposition, Endocrine System **0GS**
  Kidney *see* Reposition, Urinary System **0TS**
  Pancreatic tissue *see* Reposition, Pancreas **0FSG**
  Parathyroid tissue *see* Reposition, Endocrine System **0GS**
  Thyroid tissue *see* Reposition, Endocrine System **0GS**
  Tooth *see* Reattachment, Mouth and Throat **0CM**
Avulsion *see* Extraction
Axial Lumbar Interbody Fusion System *use* Interbody Fusion Device in Lower Joints
AxiaLIF® System *use* Interbody Fusion Device in Lower Joints
Axillary fascia
  use Subcutaneous Tissue and Fascia, Upper Arm, Left
  use Subcutaneous Tissue and Fascia, Upper Arm, Right
Axillary nerve *use* Nerve, Brachial Plexus

B

BAK/C® Interbody Cervical Fusion System
  use Interbody Fusion Device in Upper Joints
BAL (bronchial alveolar lavage), diagnostic
  see Drainage, Respiratory System **0B9**
Balanoplasty
  see Repair, Penis **0VQS**
  see Supplement, Penis **0VUS**
Balloon Pump
  Continuous, Output **5A02210**
  Intermittent, Output **5A02110**
Bandage, Elastic *see* Compression
Banding *see* Restriction
Bard® Composix® (E/X)(LP) mesh *use* Synthetic Substitute
Bard® Composix® Kugel® patch *use* Synthetic Substitute
Bard® Dulex™ mesh *use* Synthetic Substitute
Bard® Ventralex™ hernia patch *use* Synthetic Substitute
Barium swallow *see* Fluoroscopy, Gastrointestinal System **BD1**
Baroreflex Activation Therapy® (BAT®) *use* Stimulator Lead in Upper Arteries
  use Cardiac Rhythm Related Device in Subcutaneous Tissue and Fascia
Bartholin's (greater vestibular) gland *use* Gland, Vestibular
Basal (internal) cerebral vein *use* Vein, Intracranial
Basal metabolic rate (BMR) *see* Measurement, Physiological Systems **4A0Z**
Basal nuclei *use* Basal Ganglia

Basilar artery *use* Artery, Intracranial
Basis pontis *use* Pons
Beam Radiation
  Abdomen **DW03**
    Intraoperative **DW033Z0**
  Adrenal Gland **DG02**
    Intraoperative **DG023Z0**
  Bile Ducts **DF02**
    Intraoperative **DF023Z0**
  Bladder **DT02**
    Intraoperative **DT023Z0**
  Bone
    Other **DP0C**
      Intraoperative **DP0C3Z0**
  Bone Marrow **D700**
    Intraoperative **D7003Z0**
  Brain **D000**
    Intraoperative **D0003Z0**
  Brain Stem **D001**
    Intraoperative **D0013Z0**
  Breast
    Left **DM00**
      Intraoperative **DM003Z0**
    Right **DM01**
      Intraoperative **DM013Z0**
  Bronchus **DB01**
    Intraoperative **DB013Z0**
  Cervix **DU01**
    Intraoperative **DU013Z0**
  Chest **DW02**
    Intraoperative **DW023Z0**
  Chest Wall **DB07**
    Intraoperative **DB073Z0**
  Colon **DD05**
    Intraoperative **DD053Z0**
  Diaphragm **DB08**
    Intraoperative **DB083Z0**
  Duodenum **DD02**
    Intraoperative **DD023Z0**
  Ear **D900**
    Intraoperative **D9003Z0**
  Esophagus **DD00**
    Intraoperative **DD003Z0**
  Eye **D800**
    Intraoperative **D8003Z0**
  Femur **DP09**
    Intraoperative **DP093Z0**
  Fibula **DP0B**
    Intraoperative **DP0B3Z0**
  Gallbladder **DF01**
    Intraoperative **DF013Z0**
  Gland
    Adrenal **DG02**
      Intraoperative **DG023Z0**
    Parathyroid **DG04**
      Intraoperative **DG043Z0**
    Pituitary **DG00**
      Intraoperative **DG003Z0**
    Thyroid **DG05**
      Intraoperative **DG053Z0**
  Glands
    Salivary **D906**
      Intraoperative **D9063Z0**
  Head and Neck **DW01**
    Intraoperative **DW013Z0**
  Hemibody **DW04**
    Intraoperative **DW043Z0**
  Humerus **DP06**
    Intraoperative **DP063Z0**
  Hypopharynx **D903**
    Intraoperative **D9033Z0**
  Ileum **DD04**
    Intraoperative **DD043Z0**

Beam Radiation - *continued*
  Jejunum **DD03**
    Intraoperative **DD033Z0**
  Kidney **DT00**
    Intraoperative **DT003Z0**
  Larynx **D90B**
    Intraoperative **D90B3Z0**
  Liver **DF00**
    Intraoperative **DF003Z0**
  Lung **DB02**
    Intraoperative **DB023Z0**
  Lymphatics
    Abdomen **D706**
      Intraoperative **D7063Z0**
    Axillary **D704**
      Intraoperative **D7043Z0**
    Inguinal **D708**
      Intraoperative **D7083Z0**
    Neck **D703**
      Intraoperative **D7033Z0**
    Pelvis **D707**
      Intraoperative **D7073Z0**
    Thorax **D705**
      Intraoperative **D7053Z0**
  Mandible **DP03**
    Intraoperative **DP033Z0**
  Maxilla **DP02**
    Intraoperative **DP023Z0**
  Mediastinum **DB06**
    Intraoperative **DB063Z0**
  Mouth **D904**
    Intraoperative **D9043Z0**
  Nasopharynx **D90D**
    Intraoperative **D90D3Z0**
  Neck and Head **DW01**
    Intraoperative **DW013Z0**
  Nerve
    Peripheral **D007**
      Intraoperative **D0073Z0**
  Nose **D901**
    Intraoperative **D9013Z0**
  Oropharynx **D90F**
    Intraoperative **D90F3Z0**
  Ovary **DU00**
    Intraoperative **DU003Z0**
  Palate
    Hard **D908**
      Intraoperative **D9083Z0**
    Soft **D909**
      Intraoperative **D9093Z0**
  Pancreas **DF03**
    Intraoperative **DF033Z0**
  Parathyroid Gland **DG04**
    Intraoperative **DG043Z0**
  Pelvic Bones **DP08**
    Intraoperative **DP083Z0**
  Pelvic Region **DW06**
    Intraoperative **DW063Z0**
  Pineal Body **DG01**
    Intraoperative **DG013Z0**
  Pituitary Gland **DG00**
    Intraoperative **DG003Z0**
  Pleura **DB05**
    Intraoperative **DB053Z0**
  Prostate **DV00**
    Intraoperative **DV003Z0**
  Radius **DP07**
    Intraoperative **DP073Z0**
  Rectum **DD07**
    Intraoperative **DD073Z0**
  Rib **DP05**
    Intraoperative **DP053Z0**
  Sinuses **D907**

Beam Radiation - *continued*
  Intraoperative **D9073Z0**
  Skin
    Abdomen **DH08**
      Intraoperative **DH083Z0**
    Arm **DH04**
      Intraoperative **DH043Z0**
    Back **DH07**
      Intraoperative **DH073Z0**
    Buttock **DH09**
      Intraoperative **DH093Z0**
    Chest **DH06**
      Intraoperative **DH063Z0**
    Face **DH02**
      Intraoperative **DH023Z0**
    Leg **DH0B**
      Intraoperative **DH0B3Z0**
    Neck **DH03**
      Intraoperative **DH033Z0**
  Skull **DP00**
    Intraoperative **DP003Z0**
  Spinal Cord **D006**
    Intraoperative **D0063Z0**
  Spleen **D702**
    Intraoperative **D7023Z0**
  Sternum **DP04**
    Intraoperative **DP043Z0**
  Stomach **DD01**
    Intraoperative **DD013Z0**
  Testis **DV01**
    Intraoperative **DV013Z0**
  Thymus **D701**
    Intraoperative **D7013Z0**
  Thyroid Gland **DG05**
    Intraoperative **DG053Z0**
  Tibia **DP0B**
    Intraoperative **DP0B3Z0**
  Tongue **D905**
    Intraoperative **D9053Z0**
  Trachea **DB00**
    Intraoperative **DB003Z0**
  Ulna **DP07**
    Intraoperative **DP073Z0**
  Ureter **DT01**
    Intraoperative **DT013Z0**
  Urethra **DT03**
    Intraoperative **DT033Z0**
  Uterus **DU02**
    Intraoperative **DU023Z0**
  Whole Body **DW05**
    Intraoperative **DW053Z0**
Berlin Heart Ventricular Assist Device *use* Implantable Heart Assist System in Heart and Great Vessels
Biceps brachii muscle
  use Muscle, Upper Arm, Right
  use Muscle, Upper Arm, Left
Biceps femoris muscle
  use Muscle, Upper Leg, Right
  use Muscle, Upper Leg, Left
Bicipital aponeurosis
  use Subcutaneous Tissue and Fascia, Lower Arm, Left
  use Subcutaneous Tissue and Fascia, Lower Arm, Right
Bicuspid valve *use* Valve, Mitral
Bililite therapy *see* Ultraviolet Light Therapy, Skin **6A80**
Bioactive embolization coil(s) *use* Intraluminal Device, Bioactive in Upper Arteries
Biofeedback GZC9ZZZ

Biopsy
  see Drainage with qualifier Diagnostic
  see Excision with qualifier Diagnostic
  Bone Marrow *see* Extraction with qualifier Diagnostic
BiPAP *see* Assistance, Respiratory **5A09**
Bisection *see* Division
Biventricular external heart assist system *use* External Heart Assist System in Heart and Great Vessels
Blepharectomy
  see Excision, Eye **08B**
  see Resection, Eye **08T**
Blepharoplasty
  see Repair, Eye **08Q**
  see Replacement, Eye **08R**
  see Supplement, Eye **08U**
  see Reposition, Eye **08S**
Blepharorrhaphy *see* Repair, Eye **08Q**
Blepharotomy *see* Drainage, Eye **089**
Block, Nerve, anesthetic injection 3E0T3CZ
Blood glucose monitoring system *use* Monitoring Device
Blood pressure *see* Measurement, Arterial **4A03**
BMR (basal metabolic rate) *see* Measurement, Physiological Systems **4A0Z**
Body of femur
  use Femoral Shaft, Right
  use Femoral Shaft, Left
Body of fibula
  use Fibula, Right
  use Fibula, Left
Bone anchored hearing device
  use Hearing Device, Bone Conduction in **09H**
  use Hearing Device in Head and Facial Bones
Bone bank bone graft *use* Nonautologous Tissue Substitute
Bone Growth Stimulator
  Insertion of device in
    Bone
      Facial **0NHW**
      Lower **0QHY**
      Nasal **0NHB**
      Upper **0PHY**
      Skull **0NH0**
  Removal of device from
    Bone
      Facial **0NPW**
      Lower **0QPY**
      Nasal **0NPB**
      Upper **0PPY**
      Skull **0NP0**
  Revision of device in
      Facial **0NWW**
      Lower **0QWY**
      Nasal **0NWB**
      Upper **0PWY**
      Skull **0NW0**
Bone marrow transplant *see* Transfusion
Bone screw
  (interlocking)(lag)(pedicle)(recessed)
  use Internal Fixation Device in Head and Facial Bones
  use Internal Fixation Device in Upper Bones
  use Internal Fixation Device in Lower Bones
Bony labyrinth
  use Ear, Inner, Left
  use Ear, Inner, Right
Bony orbit
  use Orbit, Right
  use Orbit, Left

Bony vestibule
  use Ear, Inner, Right
  use Ear, Inner, Left
Botallo's duct *use* Artery, Pulmonary, Left
Bovine pericardial valve *use* Zooplastic Tissue in Heart and Great Vessels
Bovine pericardium graft *use* Zooplastic Tissue in Heart and Great Vessels
BP (blood pressure) *see* Measurement, Arterial **4A03**
Brachial (lateral) lymph node
  use Lymphatic, Axillary, Left
  use Lymphatic, Axillary, Right
Brachialis muscle
  use Muscle, Upper Arm, Right
  use Muscle, Upper Arm, Left
Brachiocephalic artery *use* Artery, Innominate
Brachiocephalic trunk *use* Artery, Innominate
Brachiocephalic vein
  use Vein, Innominate, Right
  use Vein, Innominate, Left
Brachioradialis muscle
  use Muscle, Lower Arm and Wrist, Right
  use Muscle, Lower Arm and Wrist, Left
Brachytherapy
  Abdomen **DW13**
  Adrenal Gland **DG12**
  Bile Ducts **DF12**
  Bladder **DT12**
  Bone Marrow **D710**
  Brain **D010**
  Brain Stem **D011**
  Breast
    Left **DM10**
    Right **DM11**
  Bronchus **DB11**
  Cervix **DU11**
  Chest **DW12**
  Chest Wall **DB17**
  Colon **DD15**
  Diaphragm **DB18**
  Duodenum **DD12**
  Ear **D910**
  Esophagus **DD10**
  Eye **D810**
  Gallbladder **DF11**
  Gland
    Adrenal **DG12**
    Parathyroid **DG14**
    Pituitary **DG10**
    Thyroid **DG15**
  Glands, Salivary **D916**
  Head and Neck **DW11**
  Hypopharynx **D913**
  Ileum **DD14**
  Jejunum **DD13**
  Kidney **DT10**
  Larynx **D91B**
  Liver **DF10**
  Lung **DB12**
  Lymphatics
    Abdomen **D716**
    Axillary **D714**
    Inguinal **D718**
    Neck **D713**
    Pelvis **D717**
    Thorax **D715**
  Mediastinum **DB16**
  Mouth **D914**
  Nasopharynx **D91D**
  Neck and Head **DW11**
  Nerve, Peripheral **D017**
  Nose **D911**

Brachytherapy - *continued*
  Oropharynx **D91F**
  Ovary **DU10**
  Palate
    Hard **D918**
    Soft **D919**
  Pancreas **DF13**
  Parathyroid Gland **DG14**
  Pelvic Region **DW16**
  Pineal Body **DG11**
  Pituitary Gland **DG10**
  Pleura **DB15**
  Prostate **DV10**
  Rectum **DD17**
  Sinuses **D917**
  Spinal Cord **D016**
  Spleen **D712**
  Stomach **DD11**
  Testis **DV11**
  Thymus **D711**
  Thyroid Gland **DG15**
  Tongue **D915**
  Trachea **DB10**
  Ureter **DT11**
  Urethra **DT13**
  Uterus **DU12**
Brachytherapy seeds *use* Radioactive Element
Broad ligament *use* Uterine Supporting
  Structure
Bronchial artery *use* Aorta, Thoracic
Bronchography
  see Plain Radiography, Respiratory System
  BB0
  see Fluoroscopy, Respiratory System **BB1**
Bronchoplasty
  see Repair, Respiratory System **0BQ**
  see Supplement, Respiratory System **0BU**
Bronchorrhaphy *see* Repair, Respiratory
  System **0BQ**
Bronchoscopy 0BJ08ZZ
Bronchotomy *see* Drainage, Respiratory System
  0B9
BRYAN® Cervical Disc System *use* Synthetic
  Substitute
Buccal gland *use* Buccal Mucosa
Buccinator lymph node *use* Lymphatic, Head
Buccinator muscle *use* Muscle, Facial
Buckling, scleral with implant *see* Supplement,
  Eye **08U**
Bulbospongiosus muscle *use* Muscle, Perineum
Bulbourethral (Cowper's) gland *use* Urethra
Bundle of His *use* Conduction Mechanism
Bundle of Kent *use* Conduction Mechanism
Bunionectomy *see* Excision, Lower Bones **0QB**
Bursectomy
  see Excision, Bursae and Ligaments **0MB**
  see Resection, Bursae and Ligaments **0MT**
Bursocentesis *see* Drainage, Bursae and
  Ligaments **0M9**
Bursography
  see Plain Radiography, Non-Axial Upper
  Bones **BP0**
  see Plain Radiography, Non-Axial Lower
  Bones **BQ0**
Bursotomy
  see Division, Bursae and Ligaments **0M8**
  see Drainage, Bursae and Ligaments **0M9**
BVS 5000 Ventricular Assist Device *use*
  External Heart Assist System in Heart and
  Great Vessels

Bypass
  Anterior Chamber
    Left **08133**
    Right **08123**
  Aorta
    Abdominal **0410**
    Thoracic **021W**
  Artery
    Axillary
      Left **03160**
      Right **03150**
    Brachial
      Left **03180**
      Right **03170**
    Common Carotid
      Left **031J0**
      Right **031H0**
    Common Iliac
      Left **041D**
      Right **041C**
    Coronary
      Four or More Sites **0213**
      One Site **0210**
      Three Sites **0212**
      Two Sites **0211**
    External Carotid
      Left **031N0**
      Right **031M0**
    External Iliac
      Left **041J**
      Right **041H**
    Femoral
      Left **041L**
      Right **041K**
    Innominate **03120**
    Internal Carotid
      Left **031L0**
      Right **031K0**
    Internal Iliac
      Left **041F**
      Right **041E**
    Intracranial **031G0**
    Popliteal
      Left **041N**
      Right **041M**
    Radial
      Left **031C0**
      Right **031B0**
    Splenic **0414**
    Subclavian
      Left **03140**
      Right **03130**
    Temporal
      Left **031T0**
      Right **031S0**
    Ulnar
      Left **031A0**
      Right **03190**
  Atrium
    Left **0217**
    Right **0216**
  Bladder **0T1B**
  Cavity, Cranial **0W110J**
  Cecum **0D1H**
  Cerebral Ventricle **0016**
  Colon
    Ascending **0D1K**
    Descending **0D1M**
    Sigmoid **0D1N**
    Transverse **0D1L**
  Duct
    Common Bile **0F19**
    Cystic **0F18**

Bypass - *continued*
    Hepatic
      Left **0F16**
      Right **0F15**
    Lacrimal
      Left **081Y**
      Right **081X**
    Pancreatic **0F1D**
      Accessory **0F1F**
  Duodenum **0D19**
  Ear
    Left **091E0**
    Right **091D0**
  Esophagus **0D15**
    Lower **0D13**
    Middle **0D12**
    Upper **0D11**
  Fallopian Tube
    Left **0U16**
    Right **0U15**
  Gallbladder **0F14**
  Ileum **0D1B**
  Jejunum **0D1A**
  Kidney Pelvis
    Left **0T14**
    Right **0T13**
  Pancreas **0F1G**
  Pelvic Cavity **0W1J**
  Peritoneal Cavity **0W1G**
  Pleural Cavity
    Left **0W1B**
    Right **0W19**
  Spinal Canal **001U**
  Stomach **0D16**
  Trachea **0B11**
  Ureter
    Left **0T17**
    Right **0T16**
  Ureters, Bilateral **0T18**
  Vas Deferens
    Bilateral **0V1Q**
    Left **0V1P**
    Right **0V1N**
  Vein
    Axillary
      Left **0518**
      Right **0517**
    Azygos **0510**
    Basilic
      Left **051C**
      Right **051B**
    Brachial
      Left **051A**
      Right **0519**
    Cephalic
      Left **051F**
      Right **051D**
    Colic **0617**
    Common Iliac
      Left **061D**
      Right **061C**
    Esophageal **0613**
    External Iliac
      Left **061G**
      Right **061F**
    External Jugular
      Left **051Q**
      Right **051P**
    Face
      Left **051V**
      Right **051T**
    Femoral
      Left **061N**

Bypass - *continued*
    Right **061M**
    Foot
        Left **061V**
        Right **061T**
    Gastric **0612**
    Greater Saphenous
        Left **061Q**
        Right **061P**
    Hand
        Left **051H**
        Right **051G**
    Hemiazygos **0511**
    Hepatic **0614**
    Hypogastric
        Left **061J**
        Right **061H**
    Inferior Mesenteric **0616**
    Innominate
        Left **0514**
        Right **0513**
    Internal Jugular
        Left **051N**
        Right **051M**
    Intracranial **051L**
    Lesser Saphenous
        Left **061S**
        Right **061R**
    Portal **0618**
    Renal
        Left **061B**
        Right **0619**
    Splenic **0611**
    Subclavian
        Left **0516**
        Right **0515**
    Superior Mesenteric **0615**
    Vertebral
        Left **051S**
        Right **051R**
    Vena Cava
        Inferior **0610**
        Superior **021V**
    Ventricle
        Left **021L**
        Right **021K**
Bypass, cardiopulmonary 5A1221Z

C

Caesarean section *see* Extraction, Products of Conception **10D0**
Calcaneocuboid joint
  use Joint, Tarsal, Left
  use Joint, Tarsal, Right
Calcaneocuboid ligament
  use Bursa and Ligament, Foot, Right
  use Bursa and Ligament, Foot, Left
Calcaneofibular ligament
  use Bursa and Ligament, Ankle, Left
  use Bursa and Ligament, Ankle, Right
Calcaneus
  use Tarsal, Right
  use Tarsal, Left
Cannulation
  see Bypass
  see Dilation
  see Drainage
  see Irrigation
Canthorrhaphy *see* Repair, Eye **08Q**
Canthotomy *see* Release, Eye **08N**

Capitate bone
  use Carpal, Left
  use Carpal, Right
Capsulectomy, lens *see* Excision, Eye **08B**
Capsulorrhaphy, joint
  see Repair, Upper Joints **0RQ**
  see Repair, Lower Joints **0SQ**
Cardia *use* Esophagogastric Junction
Cardiac contractility modulation lead *use* Cardiac Lead in Heart and Great Vessels
Cardiac event recorder *use* Monitoring Device
Cardiac Lead
  Defibrillator
    Atrium
      Left **02H7**
      Right **02H6**
    Pericardium **02HN**
    Vein, Coronary **02H4**
    Ventricle
      Left **02HL**
      Right **02HK**
  Insertion of device in
    Atrium
      Left **02H7**
      Right **02H6**
    Pericardium **02HN**
    Vein, Coronary **02H4**
    Ventricle
      Left **02HL**
      Right **02HK**
  Pacemaker
    Atrium
      Left **02H7**
      Right **02H6**
    Pericardium **02HN**
    Vein, Coronary **02H4**
    Ventricle
      Left **02HL**
      Right **02HK**
  Removal of device from, Heart **02PA**
  Revision of device in, Heart **02WA**
Cardiac plexus *use* Nerve, Thoracic Sympathetic
Cardiac Resynchronization Defibrillator Pulse Generator
  Abdomen **0JH8**
  Chest **0JH6**
Cardiac Resynchronization Pacemaker Pulse Generator
  Abdomen **0JH8**
  Chest **0JH6**
Cardiac resynchronization therapy (CRT) lead
  use Cardiac Lead, Pacemaker in **02H**
  use Cardiac Lead, Defibrillator in **02H**
Cardiac Rhythm Related Device
  Insertion of device in
    Abdomen **0JH8**
    Chest **0JH6**
  Removal of device from, Subcutaneous Tissue and Fascia, Trunk **0JPT**
  Revision of device in, Subcutaneous Tissue and Fascia, Trunk **0JWT**
Cardiocentesis *see* Drainage, Pericardial Cavity **0W9D**
Cardioesophageal junction *use* Esophagogastric Junction
Cardiolysis *see* Release, Heart and Great Vessels **02N**
CardioMEMS® pressure sensor *use* Monitoring Device, Pressure Sensor in **02H**
Cardiomyotomy *see* Division, Esophagogastric Junction **0D84**

Cardioplegia *see* Introduction of substance in or on, Heart **3E08**
Cardiorrhaphy *see* Repair, Heart and Great Vessels **02Q**
Cardioversion 5A2204Z
Caregiver Training F0FZ
Caroticotympanic artery
  use Artery, Internal Carotid, Right
  use Artery, Internal Carotid, Left
Carotid (artery) sinus (baroreceptor) lead *use* Stimulator Lead in Upper Arteries
Carotid glomus
  use Carotid Bodies, Bilateral
  use Carotid Body, Right
  use Carotid Body, Left
Carotid sinus
  use Artery, Internal Carotid, Left
  use Artery, Internal Carotid, Right
Carotid sinus nerve *use* Nerve, Glossopharyngeal
Carotid WALLSTENT® Monorail® Endoprosthesis *use* Intraluminal Device
Carpectomy
  see Excision, Upper Bones **0PB**
  see Resection, Upper Bones **0PT**
Carpometacarpal (CMC) joint
  use Joint, Metacarpocarpal, Left
  use Joint, Metacarpocarpal, Right
Carpometacarpal ligament
  use Bursa and Ligament, Hand, Left
  use Bursa and Ligament, Hand, Right
Casting *see* Immobilization
CAT scan *see* Computerized Tomography (CT Scan)
Catheterization
  see Dilation
  see Drainage
  see Irrigation
  see Insertion of device in
  Heart *see* Measurement, Cardiac **4A02**
  Umbilical vein, for infusion **06H033T**
Cauda equina *use* Spinal Cord, Lumbar
Cauterization
  see Destruction
  see Repair
Cavernous plexus *use* Nerve, Head and Neck Sympathetic
Cecectomy
  see Excision, Cecum **0DBH**
  see Resection, Cecum **0DTH**
Cecocolostomy
  see Bypass, Gastrointestinal System **0D1**
  see Drainage, Gastrointestinal System **0D9**
Cecopexy
  see Repair, Cecum **0DQH**
  see Reposition, Cecum **0DSH**
Cecoplication *see* Restriction, Cecum **0DVH**
Cecorrhaphy *see* Repair, Cecum **0DQH**
Cecostomy
  see Bypass, Cecum **0D1H**
  see Drainage, Cecum **0D9H**
Cecotomy *see* Drainage, Cecum **0D9H**
Celiac (solar) plexus *use* Nerve, Abdominal Sympathetic
Celiac ganglion *use* Nerve, Abdominal Sympathetic
Celiac lymph node *use* Lymphatic, Aortic
Celiac trunk *use* Artery, Celiac
Central axillary lymph node
  use Lymphatic, Axillary, Left
  use Lymphatic, Axillary, Right
Central venous pressure *see* Measurement, Venous **4A04**

Centrimag® Blood Pump *use* Intraluminal
Device
Cephalogram BN00ZZZ
Cerclage *see* Restriction
Cerebral aqueduct (Sylvius) *use* Cerebral
Ventricle
Cerebrum *use* Brain
Cervical esophagus *use* Esophagus, Upper
Cervical facet joint
   use Joint, Cervical Vertebral
   use Joint, Cervical Vertebral, 2 or more
Cervical ganglion *use* Nerve, Head and Neck
Sympathetic
Cervical interspinous ligament *use* Bursa and
Ligament, Head and Neck
Cervical intertransverse ligament *use* Bursa
and Ligament, Head and Neck
Cervical ligamentum flavum *use* Bursa and
Ligament, Head and Neck
Cervical lymph node
   use Lymphatic, Neck, Right
   use Lymphatic, Neck, Left
Cervicectomy
   see Excision, Cervix 0UBC
   see Resection, Cervix 0UTC
Cervicothoracic facet joint *use* Joint,
Cervicothoracic Vertebral
Cesarean section *see* Extraction, Products of
Conception 10D0
Change device in
  Abdominal Wall **0W2FX**
  Back
    Lower **0W2LX**
    Upper **0W2KX**
  Bladder **0T2BX**
  Bone
    Facial **0N2WX**
    Lower **0Q2YX**
    Nasal **0N2BX**
    Upper **0P2YX**
  Bone Marrow **072TX**
  Brain **0020X**
  Breast
    Left **0H2UX**
    Right **0H2TX**
  Bursa and Ligament
    Lower **0M2YX**
    Upper **0M2XX**
  Cavity, Cranial **0W21X**
  Chest Wall **0W28X**
  Cisterna Chyli **072LX**
  Diaphragm **0B2TX**
  Duct
    Hepatobiliary **0F2BX**
    Pancreatic **0F2DX**
  Ear
    Left **092JX**
    Right **092HX**
  Epididymis and Spermatic Cord **0V2MX**
  Extremity
    Lower
      Left **0Y2BX**
      Right **0Y29X**
    Upper
      Left **0X27X**
      Right **0X26X**
  Eye
    Left **0821X**
    Right **0820X**
  Face **0W22X**
  Fallopian Tube **0U28X**
  Gallbladder **0F24X**

Change device in – *continued*
  Gland
    Adrenal **0G25X**
    Endocrine **0G2SX**
    Pituitary **0G20X**
    Salivary **0C2AX**
  Head **0W20X**
  Intestinal Tract
    Lower **0D2DXUZ**
    Upper **0D20XUZ**
  Jaw
    Lower **0W25X**
    Upper **0W24X**
  Joint
    Lower **0S2YX**
    Upper **0R2YX**
  Kidney **0T25X**
  Larynx **0C2SX**
  Liver **0F20X**
  Lung
    Left **0B2LX**
    Right **0B2KX**
  Lymphatic **072NX**
    Thoracic Duct **072KX**
  Mediastinum **0W2CX**
  Mesentery **0D2VX**
  Mouth and Throat **0C2YX**
  Muscle
    Lower **0K2YX**
    Upper **0K2XX**
  Neck **0W26X**
  Nerve
    Cranial **002EX**
    Peripheral **012YX**
  Nose **092KX**
  Omentum **0D2UX**
  Ovary **0U23X**
  Pancreas **0F2GX**
  Parathyroid Gland **0G2RX**
  Pelvic Cavity **0W2JX**
  Penis **0V2SX**
  Pericardial Cavity **0W2DX**
  Perineum
    Female **0W2NX**
    Male **0W2MX**
  Peritoneal Cavity **0W2GX**
  Peritoneum **0D2WX**
  Pineal Body **0G21X**
  Pleura **0B2QX**
  Pleural Cavity
    Left **0W2BX**
    Right **0W29X**
  Products of Conception **10207**
  Prostate and Seminal Vesicles **0V24X**
  Retroperitoneum **0W2HX**
  Scrotum and Tunica Vaginalis **0V28X**
  Sinus **092YX**
  Skin **0H2PX**
  Skull **0N20X**
  Spinal Canal **002UX**
  Spleen **072PX**
  Subcutaneous Tissue and Fascia
    Head and Neck **0J2SX**
    Lower Extremity **0J2WX**
    Trunk **0J2TX**
    Upper Extremity **0J2VX**
  Tendon
    Lower **0L2YX**
    Upper **0L2XX**
  Testis **0V2DX**
  Thymus **072MX**
  Thyroid Gland **0G2KX**
  Trachea **0B21**

Change device in – *continued*
  Tracheobronchial Tree **0B20X**
  Ureter **0T29X**
  Urethra **0T2DX**
  Uterus and Cervix **0U2DXHZ**
  Vagina and Cul-de-sac **0U2HXGZ**
  Vas Deferens **0V2RX**
  Vulva **0U2MX**
Change device in or on
  Abdominal Wall **2W03X**
  Anorectal **2Y03X5Z**
  Arm
    Lower
      Left **2W0DX**
      Right **2W0CX**
    Upper
      Left **2W0BX**
      Right **2W0AX**
  Back **2W05X**
  Chest Wall **2W04X**
  Ear **2Y02X5Z**
  Extremity
    Lower
      Left **2W0MX**
      Right **2W0LX**
    Upper
      Left **2W09X**
      Right **2W08X**
  Face **2W01X**
  Finger
    Left **2W0KX**
    Right **2W0JX**
  Foot
    Left **2W0TX**
    Right **2W0SX**
  Genital Tract, Female **2Y04X5Z**
  Hand
    Left **2W0FX**
    Right **2W0EX**
  Head **2W00X**
  Inguinal Region
    Left **2W07X**
    Right **2W06X**
  Leg
    Lower
      Left **2W0RX**
      Right **2W0QX**
    Upper
      Left **2W0PX**
      Right **2W0NX**
  Mouth and Pharynx **2Y00X5Z**
  Nasal **2Y01X5Z**
  Neck **2W02X**
  Thumb
    Left **2W0HX**
    Right **2W0GX**
  Toe
    Left **2W0VX**
    Right **2W0UX**
  Urethra **2Y05X5Z**
Chemoembolization *see* Introduction of
substance in or on
Chemosurgery, Skin 3E00XTZ
Chemothalamectomy *see* Destruction,
Thalamus 0059
Chemotherapy, Infusion for cancer *see*
Introduction of substance in or on
Chest x-ray *see* Plain Radiography, Chest
BW03
Chiropractic Manipulation
  Abdomen **9WB9X**
  Cervical **9WB1X**

Chiropractic manipulation – *continued*
  Extremities
    Lower **9WB6X**
    Upper **9WB7X**
  Head **9WB0X**
  Lumbar **9WB3X**
  Pelvis **9WB5X**
  Rib Cage **9WB8X**
  Sacrum **9WB4X**
  Thoracic **9WB2X**
Choana *use* Nasopharynx
Cholangiogram
  see Plain Radiography, Hepatobiliary System and Pancreas **BF0**
  see Fluoroscopy, Hepatobiliary System and Pancreas **BF1**
Cholecystectomy
  see Excision, Gallbladder **0FB4**
  see Resection, Gallbladder **0FT4**
Cholecystojejunostomy
  see Bypass, Hepatobiliary System and Pancreas **0F1**
  see Drainage, Hepatobiliary System and Pancreas **0F9**
Cholecystopexy
  see Repair, Gallbladder **0FQ4**
  see Reposition, Gallbladder **0FS4**
Cholecystoscopy 0FJ44ZZ
Cholecystostomy
  see Drainage, Gallbladder **0F94**
  see Bypass, Gallbladder **0F14**
Cholecystotomy *see* Drainage, Gallbladder **0F94**
Choledochectomy
  see Excision, Hepatobiliary System and Pancreas **0FB**
  see Resection, Hepatobiliary System and Pancreas **0FT**
Choledocholithotomy *see* Extirpation, Duct, Common Bile **0FC9**
Choledochoplasty
  see Repair, Hepatobiliary System and Pancreas **0FQ**
  see Replacement, Hepatobiliary System and Pancreas **0FR**
  see Supplement, Hepatobiliary System and Pancreas **0FU**
Choledochoscopy 0FJB8ZZ
Choledochotomy *see* Drainage, Hepatobiliary System and Pancreas **0F9**
Cholelithotomy *see* Extirpation, Hepatobiliary System and Pancreas **0FC**
Chondrectomy
  see Excision, Upper Joints **0RB**
  see Excision, Lower Joints **0SB**
  Knee *see* Excision, Lower Joints **0SB**
  Semilunar cartilage *see* Excision, Lower Joints **0SB**
Chondroglossus muscle *use* Muscle, Tongue, Palate, Pharynx
Chorda tympani *use* Nerve, Facial
Chordotomy *see* Division, Central Nervous System **008**
Choroid plexus *use* Cerebral Ventricle
Choroidectomy
  see Excision, Eye **08B**
  see Resection, Eye **08T**
Ciliary body
  use Eye, Right
  use Eye, Left
Ciliary ganglion *use* Nerve, Head and Neck Sympathetic
Circle of Willis *use* Artery, Intracranial

Circumflex iliac artery
  use Artery, Femoral, Right
  use Artery, Femoral, Left
Clamp and rod internal fixation system (CRIF)
  use Internal Fixation Device in Upper Bones
  use Internal Fixation Device in Lower Bones
Clamping *see* Occlusion
Claustrum *use* Basal Ganglia
Claviculectomy
  see Excision, Upper Bones **0PB**
  see Resection, Upper Bones **0PT**
Claviculotomy
  see Division, Upper Bones **0P8**
  see Drainage, Upper Bones **0P9**
Clipping, aneurysm *see* Restriction using Extraluminal Device
Clitorectomy, clitoridectomy
  see Excision, Clitoris **0UBJ**
  see Resection, Clitoris **0UTJ**
Closure
  see Occlusion
  see Repair
Clysis *see* Introduction of substance in or on
Coagulation *see* Destruction
CoAxia NeuroFlo catheter *use* Intraluminal Device
Cobalt/chromium head and polyethylene socket *use* Synthetic Substitute, Metal on Polyethylene in **0SR**
Cobalt/chromium head and socket *use* Synthetic Substitute, Metal in **0SR**
Coccygeal body *use* Coccygeal Glomus
Coccygeus muscle
  use Muscle, Trunk, Left
  use Muscle, Trunk, Right
Cochlea
  use Ear, Inner, Left
  use Ear, Inner, Right
Cochlear implant (CI), multiple channel (electrode) *use* Hearing Device, Multiple Channel Cochlear Prosthesis in **09H**
Cochlear implant (CI), single channel (electrode) *use* Hearing Device, Single Channel Cochlear Prosthesis in **09H**
Cochlear Implant Treatment F0BZ0
Cochlear nerve *use* Nerve, Acoustic
COGNIS® CRT-D *use* Cardiac Resynchronization Defibrillator Pulse Generator in **0JH**
Colectomy
  see Excision, Gastrointestinal System **0DB**
  see Resection, Gastrointestinal System **0DT**
Collapse *see* Occlusion
Collection from
  Breast, Breast Milk **8E0HX62**
  Indwelling Device
    Circulatory System
      Blood **8C02X6K**
      Other Fluid **8C02X6L**
    Nervous System
      Cerebrospinal Fluid **8C01X6J**
      Other Fluid **8C01X6L**
  Integumentary System, Breast Milk **8E0HX62**
  Reproductive System, Male, Sperm **8E0VX63**
Colocentesis *see* Drainage, Gastrointestinal System **0D9**
Colofixation
  see Repair, Gastrointestinal System **0DQ**
  see Reposition, Gastrointestinal System **0DS**
Cololysis *see* Release, Gastrointestinal System **0DN**

Colonic Z-Stent® *use* Intraluminal Device
Colonoscopy 0DJD8ZZ
Colopexy
  see Repair, Gastrointestinal System **0DQ**
  see Reposition, Gastrointestinal System **0DS**
Coloplication *see* Restriction, Gastrointestinal System **0DV**
Coloproctectomy
  see Excision, Gastrointestinal System **0DB**
  see Resection, Gastrointestinal System **0DT**
Coloproctostomy
  see Bypass, Gastrointestinal System **0D1**
  see Drainage, Gastrointestinal System **0D9**
Colopuncture *see* Drainage, Gastrointestinal System **0D9**
Colorrhaphy *see* Repair, Gastrointestinal System **0DQ**
Colostomy
  see Bypass, Gastrointestinal System **0D1**
  see Drainage, Gastrointestinal System **0D9**
Colpectomy
  see Excision, Vagina **0UBG**
  see Resection, Vagina **0UTG**
Colpocentesis *see* Drainage, Vagina **0U9G**
Colpopexy
  see Repair, Vagina **0UQG**
  see Reposition, Vagina **0USG**
Colpoplasty
  see Repair, Vagina **0UQG**
  see Supplement, Vagina **0UUG**
Colporrhaphy *see* Repair, Vagina **0UQG**
Colposcopy 0UJH8ZZ
Columella *use* Nose
Common digital vein
  use Vein, Foot, Right
  use Vein, Foot, Left
Common facial vein
  use Vein, Face, Left
  use Vein, Face, Right
Common fibular nerve *use* Nerve, Peroneal
Common hepatic artery *use* Artery, Hepatic
Common iliac (subaortic) lymph node *use* Lymphatic, Pelvis
Common interosseous artery
  use Artery, Ulnar, Left
  use Artery, Ulnar, Right
Common peroneal nerve *use* Nerve, Peroneal
Complete (SE) stent *use* Intraluminal Device
Compression
  see Restriction
  Abdominal Wall **2W13X**
  Arm
    Lower
      Left **2W1DX**
      Right **2W1CX**
    Upper
      Left **2W1BX**
      Right **2W1AX**
  Back **2W15X**
  Chest Wall **2W14X**
  Extremity
    Lower
      Left **2W1MX**
      Right **2W1LX**
    Upper
      Left **2W19X**
      Right **2W18X**
  Face **2W11X**
  Finger
    Left **2W1KX**
    Right **2W1JX**

Compression - *continued*
  Foot
    Left **2W1TX**
    Right **2W1SX**
  Hand
    Left **2W1FX**
    Right **2W1EX**
  Head **2W10X**
  Inguinal Region
    Left **2W17X**
    Right **2W16X**
  Leg
    Lower
      Left **2W1RX**
      Right **2W1QX**
    Upper
      Left **2W1PX**
      Right **2W1NX**
  Neck **2W12X**
  Thumb
    Left **2W1HX**
    Right **2W1GX**
  Toe
    Left **2W1VX**
    Right **2W1UX**
Computer Assisted Procedure
  Extremity
    Lower
      No Qualifier **8E0YXBZ**
      With Computerized Tomography
        8E0YXBG
      With Fluoroscopy **8E0YXBF**
      With Magnetic Resonance Imaging
        8E0YXBH
    Upper
      No Qualifier **8E0XXBZ**
      With Computerized Tomography
        8E0XXBG
      With Fluoroscopy **8E0XXBF**
      With Magnetic Resonance Imaging
        8E0XXBH
  Head and Neck Region
    No Qualifier **8E09XBZ**
    With Computerized Tomography
      8E09XBG
    With Fluoroscopy **8E09XBF**
    With Magnetic Resonance Imaging
      8E09XBH
  Trunk Region
    No Qualifier **8E0WXBZ**
    With Computerized Tomography
      8E0WXBG
    With Fluoroscopy **8E0WXBF**
    With Magnetic Resonance Imaging
      8E0WXBH
Computerized Tomography (CT Scan)
  Abdomen **BW20**
    Chest and Pelvis **BW25**
  Abdomen and Chest **BW24**
  Abdomen and Pelvis **BW21**
  Airway, Trachea **BB2F**
  Ankle
    Left **BQ2H**
    Right **BQ2G**
  Aorta
    Abdominal **B420**
      Intravascular Optical Coherence
        B420Z2Z
    Thoracic **B320**
      Intravascular Optical Coherence
        B320Z2Z

Computerized Tomography - *continued*
  Arm
    Left **BP2F**
    Right **BP2E**
  Artery
    Celiac **B421**
      Intravascular Optical Coherence
        B421Z2Z
    Common Carotid
      Bilateral **B325**
      Intravascular Optical Coherence
        B325Z2Z
    Coronary
      Bypass Graft
        Multiple **B223**
        Intravascular Optical Coherence
          B223Z2Z
      Multiple **B221**
        Intravascular Optical Coherence
        B221Z2Z
    Internal Carotid
      Bilateral **B328**
      Intravascular Optical Coherence
        B328Z2Z
    Intracranial **B32R**
      Intravascular Optical Coherence
        B32RZ2Z
    Lower Extremity
      Bilateral **B42H**
        Intravascular Optical Coherence
        B42HZ2Z
      Left **B42G**
        Intravascular Optical Coherence
        B42GZ2Z
      Right **B42F**
        Intravascular Optical Coherence
        B42FZ2Z
    Pelvic **B42C**
      Intravascular Optical Coherence
        B42CZ2Z
    Pulmonary
      Left **B32T**
      Intravascular Optical Coherence
        B32TZ2Z
      Right **B32S**
      Intravascular Optical Coherence
        B32SZ2Z
    Renal
      Bilateral **B428**
      Intravascular Optical Coherence
        B428Z2Z
      Transplant **B42M**
      Intravascular Optical Coherence
        B42MZ2Z
    Superior Mesenteric **B424**
      Intravascular Optical Coherence
        B424Z2Z
    Vertebral
      Bilateral **B32G**
      Intravascular Optical Coherence
        B32GZ2Z
  Bladder **BT20**
  Bone
    Facial **BN25**
    Temporal **BN2F**
  Brain **B020**
  Calcaneus
    Left **BQ2K**
    Right **BQ2J**
  Cerebral Ventricle **B028**
  Chest, Abdomen and Pelvis **BW25**
  Chest and Abdomen **BW24**
  Cisterna **B027**

Computerized Tomography - *continued*
  Clavicle
    Left **BP25**
    Right **BP24**
  Coccyx **BR2F**
  Colon **BD24**
  Ear **B920**
  Elbow
    Left **BP2H**
    Right **BP2G**
  Extremity
    Lower
      Left **BQ2S**
      Right **BQ2R**
    Upper
      Bilateral **BP2V**
      Left **BP2U**
      Right **BP2T**
  Eye
    Bilateral **B827**
    Left **B826**
    Right **B825**
  Femur
    Left **BQ24**
    Right **BQ23**
  Fibula
    Left **BQ2C**
    Right **BQ2B**
  Finger
    Left **BP2S**
    Right **BP2R**
  Foot
    Left **BQ2M**
    Right **BQ2L**
  Forearm
    Left **BP2K**
    Right **BP2J**
  Gland
    Adrenal, Bilateral **BG22**
    Parathyroid **BG23**
    Parotid, Bilateral **B926**
    Salivary, Bilateral **B92D**
    Submandibular, Bilateral **B929**
    Thyroid **BG24**
  Hand
    Left **BP2P**
    Right **BP2N**
  Hands and Wrists, Bilateral **BP2Q**
  Head **BW28**
  Head and Neck **BW29**
  Heart
    Right and Left **B226**
    Intravascular Optical Coherence **B226Z2Z**
  Hepatobiliary System, All **BF2C**
  Hip
    Left **BQ21**
    Right **BQ20**
  Humerus
    Left **BP2B**
    Right **BP2A**
  Intracranial Sinus **B522**
    Intravascular Optical Coherence **B522Z2Z**
  Joint
    Acromioclavicular, Bilateral **BP23**
    Finger
      Left **BP2DZZZ**
      Right **BP2CZZZ**
    Foot
      Left **BQ2Y**
      Right **BQ2X**
    Hand
      Left **BP2DZZZ**
      Right **BP2CZZZ**

Computerized Tomography - *continued*
  Sacroiliac **BR2D**
  Sternoclavicular
    Bilateral **BP22**
    Left **BP21**
    Right **BP20**
  Temporomandibular, Bilateral **BN29**
  Toe
    Left **BQ2Y**
    Right **BQ2X**
  Kidney
    Bilateral **BT23**
    Left **BT22**
    Right **BT21**
    Transplant **BT29**
  Knee
    Left **BQ28**
    Right **BQ27**
  Larynx **B92J**
  Leg
    Left **BQ2F**
    Right **BQ2D**
  Liver **BF25**
  Liver and Spleen **BF26**
  Lung, Bilateral **BB24**
  Mandible **BN26**
  Nasopharynx **B92F**
  Neck **BW2F**
  Neck and Head **BW29**
  Orbit, Bilateral **BN23**
  Oropharynx **B92F**
  Pancreas **BF27**
  Patella
    Left **BQ2W**
    Right **BQ2V**
  Pelvic Region **BW2G**
  Pelvis **BR2C**
    Chest and Abdomen **BW25**
  Pelvis and Abdomen **BW21**
  Pituitary Gland **B029**
  Prostate **BV23**
  Ribs
    Left **BP2Y**
    Right **BP2X**
  Sacrum **BR2F**
  Scapula
    Left **BP27**
    Right **BP26**
  Sella Turcica **B029**
  Shoulder
    Left **BP29**
    Right **BP28**
  Sinus
    Intracranial **B522**
      Intravascular Optical Coherence
        B522Z2Z
    Paranasal **B922**
  Skull **BN20**
  Spinal Cord **B02B**
  Spine
    Cervical **BR20**
    Lumbar **BR29**
    Thoracic **BR27**
  Spleen and Liver **BF26**
  Thorax **BP2W**
  Tibia
    Left **BQ2C**
    Right **BQ2B**
  Toe
    Left **BQ2Q**
    Right **BQ2P**
  Trachea **BB2F**

Computerized Tomography - *continued*
  Tracheobronchial Tree
    Bilateral **BB29**
    Left **BB28**
    Right **BB27**
  Vein
    Pelvic (Iliac)
      Left **B52G**
        Intravascular Optical Coherence
          B52GZ2Z
      Right **B52F**
        Intravascular Optical Coherence
          B52FZ2Z
    Pelvic (Iliac) Bilateral **B52H**
      Intravascular Optical Coherence
        B52HZ2Z
    Portal **B52T**
      Intravascular Optical Coherence
        B52TZ2Z
    Pulmonary
      Bilateral **B52S**
        Intravascular Optical Coherence
          B52SZ2Z
      Left **B52R**
        Intravascular Optical Coherence
          B52RZ2Z
      Right **B52Q**
        Intravascular Optical Coherence
          B52QZ2Z
    Renal
      Bilateral **B52L**
        Intravascular Optical Coherence
          B52LZ2Z
      Left **B52K**
        Intravascular Optical Coherence
          B52KZ2Z
      Right **B52J**
        Intravascular Optical Coherence
          B52JZ2Z
    Splanchnic **B52T**
      Intravascular Optical Coherence
        B52TZ2Z
  Vena Cava
    Inferior **B529**
      Intravascular Optical Coherence
        B529Z2Z
    Superior **B528**
      Intravascular Optical Coherence
        B528Z2Z
  Ventricle, Cerebral **B028**
  Wrist
    Left **BP2M**
    Right **BP2L Concerto II CRT-D** *use*
Cardiac Resynchronization Defibrillator Pulse
Generator in **0JH Condylectomy**
  see Excision, Head and Facial Bones **0NB**
  see Excision, Upper Bones **0PB**
  see Excision, Lower Bones **0QB**
Condyloid process
  use Mandible, Left
  use Mandible, Right
Condylotomy
  see Division, Head and Facial Bones **0N8**
  see Drainage, Head and Facial Bones **0N9**
  see Division, Upper Bones **0P8**
  see Drainage, Upper Bones **0P9**
  see Division, Lower Bones **0Q8**
  see Drainage, Lower Bones **0Q9**
Condylysis
  see Release, Head and Facial Bones **0NN**
  see Release, Upper Bones **0PN**
  see Release, Lower Bones **0QN**
Conization, cervix *see* Excision, Uterus **0UB9**

Conjunctivoplasty
  see Repair, Eye **08Q**
  see Replacement, Eye **08R**
CONSERVE® PLUS Total Resurfacing Hip
  System *use* Resurfacing Device in Lower
  Joints
Construction
  Auricle, ear *see* Replacement, Ear, Nose,
  Sinus **09R**
  Ileal conduit *see* Bypass, Urinary System **0T1**
Consulta CRT-D *use* Cardiac
  Resynchronization Defibrillator Pulse
  Generator in **0JH**
Consulta CRT-P *use* Cardiac
  Resynchronization Pacemaker Pulse
  Generator in **0JH**
Contact Radiation
  Abdomen **DWY37ZZ**
  Adrenal Gland **DGY27ZZ**
  Bile Ducts **DFY27ZZ**
  Bladder **DTY27ZZ**
  Bone, Other **DPYC7ZZ**
  Brain **D0Y07ZZ**
  Brain Stem **D0Y17ZZ**
  Breast
    Left **DMY07ZZ**
    Right **DMY17ZZ**
  Bronchus **DBY17ZZ**
  Cervix **DUY17ZZ**
  Chest **DWY27ZZ**
  Chest Wall **DBY77ZZ**
  Colon **DDY57ZZ**
  Diaphragm **DBY87ZZ**
  Duodenum **DDY27ZZ**
  Ear **D9Y07ZZ**
  Esophagus **DDY07ZZ**
  Eye **D8Y07ZZ**
  Femur **DPY97ZZ**
  Fibula **DPYB7ZZ**
  Gallbladder **DFY17ZZ**
  Gland
    Adrenal **DGY27ZZ**
    Parathyroid **DGY47ZZ**
    Pituitary **DGY07ZZ**
    Thyroid **DGY57ZZ**
  Glands, Salivary **D9Y67ZZ**
  Head and Neck **DWY17ZZ**
  Hemibody **DWY47ZZ**
  Humerus **DPY67ZZ**
  Hypopharynx **D9Y37ZZ**
  Ileum **DDY47ZZ**
  Jejunum **DDY37ZZ**
  Kidney **DTY07ZZ**
  Larynx **D9YB7ZZ**
  Liver **DFY07ZZ**
  Lung **DBY27ZZ**
  Mandible **DPY37ZZ**
  Maxilla **DPY27ZZ**
  Mediastinum **DBY67ZZ**
  Mouth **D9Y47ZZ**
  Nasopharynx **D9YD7ZZ**
  Neck and Head **DWY17ZZ**
  Nerve, Peripheral **D0Y77ZZ**
  Nose **D9Y17ZZ**
  Oropharynx **D9YF7ZZ**
  Ovary **DUY07ZZ**
  Palate
    Hard **D9Y87ZZ**
    Soft **D9Y97ZZ**
  Pancreas **DFY37ZZ**
  Parathyroid Gland **DGY47ZZ**
  Pelvic Bones **DPY87ZZ**
  Pelvic Region **DWY67ZZ**

Contact Radiation - *continued*
  Pineal Body **DGY17ZZ**
  Pituitary Gland **DGY07ZZ**
  Pleura **DBY57ZZ**
  Prostate **DVY07ZZ**
  Radius **DPY77ZZ**
  Rectum **DDY77ZZ**
  Rib **DPY57ZZ**
  Sinuses **D9Y77ZZ**
  Skin
    Abdomen **DHY87ZZ**
    Arm **DHY47ZZ**
    Back **DHY77ZZ**
    Buttock **DHY97ZZ**
    Chest **DHY67ZZ**
    Face **DHY27ZZ**
    Leg **DHYB7ZZ**
    Neck **DHY37ZZ**
  Skull **DPY07ZZ**
  Spinal Cord **D0Y67ZZ**
  Sternum **DPY47ZZ**
  Stomach **DDY17ZZ**
  Testis **DVY17ZZ**
  Thyroid Gland **DGY57ZZ**
  Tibia **DPYB7ZZ**
  Tongue **D9Y57ZZ**
  Trachea **DBY07ZZ**
  Ulna **DPY77ZZ**
  Ureter **DTY17ZZ**
  Urethra **DTY37ZZ**
  Uterus **DUY27ZZ**
  Whole Body **DWY57ZZ**
CONTAK RENEWAL® 3 RF (HE) CRT-D
  use Cardiac Resynchronization Defibrillator
  Pulse Generator in **0JH**
Contegra Pulmonary Valved Conduit *use*
  Zooplastic Tissue in Heart and Great Vessels
Continuous Glucose Monitoring (CGM)
  device *use* Monitoring Device
Continuous Negative Airway Pressure
  24-96 Consecutive Hours, Ventilation
    5A09459
  Greater than 96 Consecutive Hours,
    Ventilation **5A09559**
  Less than 24 Consecutive Hours, Ventilation
    5A09359
Continuous Positive Airway Pressure
  24-96 Consecutive Hours, Ventilation
    5A09457
  Greater than 96 Consecutive Hours,
    Ventilation **5A09557**
  Less than 24 Consecutive Hours, Ventilation
    5A09357
Contraceptive Device
  Change device in, Uterus and Cervix
    0U2DXHZ
  Insertion of device in
    Cervix **0UHC**
    Subcutaneous Tissue and Fascia
      Abdomen **0JH8**
      Chest **0JH6**
      Lower Arm
        Left **0JHH**
        Right **0JHG**
      Lower Leg
        Left **0JHP**
        Right **0JHN**
      Upper Arm
        Left **0JHF**
        Right **0JHD**
      Upper Leg
        Left **0JHM**
        Right **0JHL**

Contraceptive Device - *continued*
    Uterus **0UH9**
  Removal of device from
    Subcutaneous Tissue and Fascia
      Lower Extremity **0JPW**
      Trunk **0JPT**
      Upper Extremity **0JPV**
    Uterus and Cervix **0UPD**
  Revision of device in
    Subcutaneous Tissue and Fascia
      Lower Extremity **0JWW**
      Trunk **0JWT**
      Upper Extremity **0JWV**
    Uterus and Cervix **0UWD**
Contractility Modulation Device
  Abdomen **0JH8**
  Chest **0JH6**
Control postprocedural bleeding in
  Abdominal Wall **0W3F**
  Ankle Region
    Left **0Y3L**
    Right **0Y3K**
  Arm
    Lower
      Left **0X3F**
      Right **0X3D**
    Upper
      Left **0X39**
      Right **0X38**
  Axilla
    Left **0X35**
    Right **0X34**
  Back
    Lower **0W3L**
    Upper **0W3K**
  Buttock
    Left **0Y31**
    Right **0Y30**
  Cavity, Cranial **0W31**
  Chest Wall **0W38**
  Elbow Region
    Left **0X3C**
    Right **0X3B**
  Extremity
    Lower
      Left **0Y3B**
      Right **0Y39**
    Upper
      Left **0X37**
      Right **0X36**
  Face **0W32**
  Femoral Region
    Left **0Y38**
    Right **0Y37**
  Foot
    Left **0Y3N**
    Right **0Y3M**
  Gastrointestinal Tract **0W3P**
  Genitourinary Tract **0W3R**
  Hand
    Left **0X3K**
    Right **0X3J**
  Head **0W30**
  Inguinal Region
    Left **0Y36**
    Right **0Y35**
  Jaw
    Lower **0W35**
    Upper **0W34**
  Knee Region
    Left **0Y3G**
    Right **0Y3F**

Control postprocedural bleeding - *continued*
  Leg
    Lower
      Left **0Y3J**
      Right **0Y3H**
    Upper
      Left **0Y3D**
      Right **0Y3C**
  Mediastinum **0W3C**
  Neck **0W36**
  Oral Cavity and Throat **0W33**
  Pelvic Cavity **0W3J**
  Pericardial Cavity **0W3D**
  Perineum
    Female **0W3N**
    Male **0W3M**
  Peritoneal Cavity **0W3G**
  Pleural Cavity
    Left **0W3B**
    Right **0W39**
  Respiratory Tract **0W3Q**
  Retroperitoneum **0W3H**
  Shoulder Region
    Left **0X33**
    Right **0X32**
  Wrist Region
    Left **0X3H**
    Right **0X3G**
Conus arteriosus *use* Ventricle, Right
Conus medullaris *use* Spinal Cord, Lumbar
Conversion
  Cardiac rhythm **5A2204Z**
  Gastrostomy to jejunostomy feeding device
  see Insertion of device in, Jejunum **0DHA**
Coracoacromial ligament
  use Bursa and Ligament, Shoulder, Right
  use Bursa and Ligament, Shoulder, Left
Coracobrachialis muscle
  use Muscle, Upper Arm, Left
  use Muscle, Upper Arm, Right
Coracoclavicular ligament
  use Bursa and Ligament, Shoulder, Left
  use Bursa and Ligament, Shoulder, Right
Coracohumeral ligament
  use Bursa and Ligament, Shoulder, Left
  use Bursa and Ligament, Shoulder, Right
Coracoid process
  use Scapula, Right
  use Scapula, Left
Cordotomy *see* Division, Central Nervous
  System **008**
Core needle biopsy *see* Excision with qualifier
  Diagnostic
CoreValve transcatheter aortic valve *use*
  Zooplastic Tissue in Heart and Great Vessels
Cormet Hip Resurfacing System *use*
  Resurfacing Device in Lower Joints
Corniculate cartilage *use* Larynx
CoRoent® XL *use* Interbody Fusion Device in
  Lower Joints
Coronary arteriography
  see Plain Radiography, Heart **B20**
  see Fluoroscopy, Heart **B21**
Corox (OTW) Bipolar Lead
  use Cardiac Lead, Pacemaker in **02H**
  use Cardiac Lead, Defibrillator in **02H**
Corpus callosum *use* Brain
Corpus cavernosum *use* Penis
Corpus spongiosum *use* Penis
Corpus striatum *use* Basal Ganglia
Corrugator supercilii muscle *use* Muscle,
  Facial

Cortical strip neurostimulator lead *use*
Neurostimulator Lead in Central Nervous
System
Costatectomy
see Excision, Upper Bones **0PB**
see Resection, Upper Bones **0PT**
Costectomy
see Excision, Upper Bones **0PB**
see Resection, Upper Bones **0PT**
Costocervical trunk
use Artery, Subclavian, Left
use Artery, Subclavian, Right
Costochondrectomy
see Excision, Upper Bones **0PB**
see Resection, Upper Bones **0PT**
Costoclavicular ligament
use Bursa and Ligament, Shoulder, Left
use Bursa and Ligament, Shoulder, Right
Costosternoplasty
see Repair, Upper Bones **0PQ**
see Replacement, Upper Bones **0PR**
see Supplement, Upper Bones **0PU**
Costotomy
see Division, Upper Bones **0P8**
see Drainage, Upper Bones **0P9**
Costotransverse joint
use Joint, Thoracic Vertebral
use Joint, Thoracic Vertebral, 2 to 7
use Joint, Thoracic Vertebral, 8 or more
Costotransverse ligament
use Bursa and Ligament, Thorax, Right
use Bursa and Ligament, Thorax, Left
Costovertebral joint
use Joint, Thoracic Vertebral, 8 or more
use Joint, Thoracic Vertebral, 2 to 7
use Joint, Thoracic Vertebral
Costoxiphoid ligament
use Bursa and Ligament, Thorax, Right
use Bursa and Ligament, Thorax, Left
Counseling
Family, for substance abuse, Other Family
Counseling **HZ63ZZZ**
Group
12-Step **HZ43ZZZ**
Behavioral **HZ41ZZZ**
Cognitive **HZ40ZZZ**
Cognitive-Behavioral **HZ42ZZZ**
Confrontational **HZ48ZZZ**
Continuing Care **HZ49ZZZ**
Infectious Disease
Post-Test **HZ4CZZZ**
Pre-Test **HZ4CZZZ**
Interpersonal **HZ44ZZZ**
Motivational Enhancement **HZ47ZZZ**
Psychoeducation **HZ46ZZZ**
Spiritual **HZ4BZZZ**
Vocational **HZ45ZZZ**
Individual
12-Step **HZ33ZZZ**
Behavioral **HZ31ZZZ**
Cognitive **HZ30ZZZ**
Cognitive-Behavioral **HZ32ZZZ**
Confrontational **HZ38ZZZ**
Continuing Care **HZ39ZZZ**
Infectious Disease
Post-Test **HZ3CZZZ**
Pre-Test **HZ3CZZZ**
Interpersonal **HZ34ZZZ**
Motivational Enhancement **HZ37ZZZ**
Psychoeducation **HZ36ZZZ**
Spiritual **HZ3BZZZ**
Vocational **HZ35ZZZ**

Counseling – *continued*
Mental Health Services
Educational **GZ60ZZZ**
Other Counseling **GZ63ZZZ**
Vocational **GZ61ZZZ**
Countershock, cardiac 5A2204Z
Cowper's (bulbourethral) gland *use* Urethra
CPAP (continuous positive airway pressure)
see Assistance, Respiratory **5A09**
Cranial dura mater *use* Dura Mater
Cranial epidural space *use* Epidural Space
Cranial subarachnoid space *use* Subarachnoid
Space
Cranial subdural space *use* Subdural Space
Craniectomy
see Excision, Head and Facial Bones **0NB**
see Resection, Head and Facial Bones **0NT**
Cranioplasty
see Repair, Head and Facial Bones **0NQ**
see Replacement, Head and Facial Bones
0NR
see Supplement, Head and Facial Bones **0NU**
Craniotomy
see Drainage, Central Nervous System **009**
see Division, Head and Facial Bones **0N8**
see Drainage, Head and Facial Bones **0N9**
Creation
Female **0W4N0**
Male **0W4M0**
Cremaster muscle *use* Muscle, Perineum
Cribriform plate
use Bone, Ethmoid, Left
use Bone, Ethmoid, Right
Cricoid cartilage *use* Larynx
Cricoidectomy *see* Excision, Larynx **0CBS**
Cricothyroid artery
use Artery, Thyroid, Left
use Artery, Thyroid, Right
Cricothyroid muscle
use Muscle, Neck, Right
use Muscle, Neck, Left
Crisis Intervention GZ2ZZZZ
Crural fascia
use Subcutaneous Tissue and Fascia, Upper
Leg, Right
use Subcutaneous Tissue and Fascia, Upper
Leg, Left
Crushing, nerve
Cranial *see* Destruction, Central Nervous
System **005**
Peripheral *see* Destruction, Peripheral
Nervous System **015**
Cryoablation *see* Destruction
Cryotherapy *see* Destruction
Cryptorchidectomy
see Excision, Male Reproductive System **0VB**
see Resection, Male Reproductive System
0VT
Cryptorchiectomy
see Excision, Male Reproductive System **0VB**
see Resection, Male Reproductive System
0VT
Cryptotomy
see Division, Gastrointestinal System **0D8**
see Drainage, Gastrointestinal System **0D9**
CT scan *see* Computerized Tomography (CT
Scan)
CT sialogram *see* Computerized Tomography
(CT Scan), Ear, Nose, Mouth and Throat **B92**
Cubital lymph node
use Lymphatic, Upper Extremity, Left
use Lymphatic, Upper Extremity, Right
Cubital nerve *use* Nerve, Ulnar

Cuboid bone
use Tarsal, Left
use Tarsal, Right
Cuboideonavicular joint
use Joint, Tarsal, Right
use Joint, Tarsal, Left
Culdocentesis *see* Drainage, Cul-de-sac **0U9F**
Culdoplasty
see Repair, Cul-de-sac **0UQF**
see Supplement, Cul-de-sac **0UUF**
Culdoscopy 0UJH8ZZ
Culdotomy *see* Drainage, Cul-de-sac **0U9F**
Culmen *use* Cerebellum
Cultured epidermal cell autograft *use*
Autologous Tissue Substitute
Cuneiform cartilage *use* Larynx
Cuneonavicular joint
use Joint, Tarsal, Left
use Joint, Tarsal, Right
Cuneonavicular ligament
use Bursa and Ligament, Foot, Left
use Bursa and Ligament, Foot, Right
Curettage
see Excision
see Extraction
Cutaneous (transverse) cervical nerve *use*
Nerve, Cervical Plexus
CVP (central venous pressure) *see*
Measurement, Venous **4A04**
Cyclodiathermy *see* Destruction, Eye **085**
Cyclophotocoagulation *see* Destruction, Eye
085
CYPHER® Stent *use* Intraluminal Device,
Drug-eluting in Heart and Great Vessels
Cystectomy
see Excision, Bladder **0TBB**
see Resection, Bladder **0TTB**
Cystocele repair *see* Repair, Subcutaneous
Tissue and Fascia, Pelvic Region **0JQC**
Cystography
see Plain Radiography, Urinary System **BT0**
see Fluoroscopy, Urinary System **BT1**
Cystolithotomy *see* Extirpation, Bladder **0TCB**
Cystopexy
see Repair, Bladder **0TQB**
see Reposition, Bladder **0TSB**
Cystoplasty
see Repair, Bladder **0TQB**
see Replacement, Bladder **0TRB**
see Supplement, Bladder **0TUB**
Cystorrhaphy *see* Repair, Bladder **0TQB**
Cystoscopy 0TJB8ZZ
Cystostomy *see* Bypass, Bladder **0T1B**
Cystostomy tube *use* Drainage Device
Cystotomy *see* Drainage, Bladder **0T9B**
Cystourethrography
see Plain Radiography, Urinary System **BT0**
see Fluoroscopy, Urinary System **BT1**
Cystourethroplasty
see Repair, Urinary System **0TQ**
see Replacement, Urinary System **0TR**
see Supplement, Urinary System **0TU**

D

DBS lead *use* Neurostimulator Lead in Central
Nervous System
DeBakey Left Ventricular Assist Device *use*
Implantable Heart Assist System in Heart and
Great Vessels
Debridement
Excisional *see* Excision
Non-excisional *see* Extraction

Decompression, Circulatory 6A15
Decortication, lung *see* Extraction, Respiratory System **0BD**
Deep brain neurostimulator lead *use* Neurostimulator Lead in Central Nervous System
Deep cervical fascia *use* Subcutaneous Tissue and Fascia, Neck, Anterior
Deep cervical vein
   use Vein, Vertebral, Left
   use Vein, Vertebral, Right
Deep circumflex iliac artery
   use Artery, External Iliac, Left
   use Artery, External Iliac, Right
Deep facial vein
   use Vein, Face, Left
   use Vein, Face, Right
Deep femoral (profunda femoris) vein
   use Vein, Femoral, Left
   use Vein, Femoral, Right
Deep femoral artery
   use Artery, Femoral, Right
   use Artery, Femoral, Left
Deep Inferior Epigastric Artery Perforator Flap
   Bilateral **0HRV077**
   Left **0HRU077**
   Right **0HRT077**
Deep palmar arch
   use Artery, Hand, Left
   use Artery, Hand, Right
Deep transverse perineal muscle *use* Muscle, Perineum
Deferential artery
   use Artery, Internal Iliac, Right
   use Artery, Internal Iliac, Left
Defibrillator Generator
   Abdomen **0JH8**
   Chest **0JH6**
Delivery
   Cesarean *see* Extraction, Products of Conception **10D0**
   Forceps *see* Extraction, Products of Conception **10D0**
   Manually assisted **10E0XZZ**
   Products of Conception **10E0XZZ**
   Vacuum assisted *see* Extraction, Products of Conception **10D0**
Delta frame external fixator
   use External Fixation Device, Hybrid in **0PH**
   use External Fixation Device, Hybrid in **0PS**
   use External Fixation Device, Hybrid in **0QH**
   use External Fixation Device, Hybrid in **0QS**
Delta III Reverse shoulder prosthesis *use* Synthetic Substitute, Reverse Ball and Socket in **0RR**
Deltoid fascia
   use Subcutaneous Tissue and Fascia, Upper Arm, Right
   use Subcutaneous Tissue and Fascia, Upper Arm, Left
Deltoid ligament
   use Bursa and Ligament, Ankle, Left
   use Bursa and Ligament, Ankle, Right
Deltoid muscle
   use Muscle, Shoulder, Left
   use Muscle, Shoulder, Right
Deltopectoral (infraclavicular) lymph node
   use Lymphatic, Upper Extremity, Right
   use Lymphatic, Upper Extremity, Left

Denervation
   Cranial nerve *see* Destruction, Central Nervous System **005**
   Peripheral nerve *see* Destruction, Peripheral Nervous System **015**
Densitometry
   Plain Radiography
     Femur
       Left **BQ04ZZ1**
       Right **BQ03ZZ1**
     Hip
       Left **BQ01ZZ1**
       Right **BQ00ZZ1**
     Spine
       Cervical **BR00ZZ1**
       Lumbar **BR09ZZ1**
       Thoracic **BR07ZZ1**
       Whole **BR0GZZ1**
   Ultrasonography
     Elbow
       Left **BP4HZZ1**
       Right **BP4GZZ1**
     Hand
       Left **BP4PZZ1**
       Right **BP4NZZ1**
     Shoulder
       Left **BP49ZZ1**
       Right **BP48ZZ1**
     Wrist
       Left **BP4MZZ1**
       Right **BP4LZZ1**
Dentate ligament *use* Dura Mater
Denticulate ligament *use* Spinal Meninges
Depressor anguli oris muscle *use* Muscle, Facial
Depressor labii inferioris muscle *use* Muscle, Facial
Depressor septi nasi muscle *use* Muscle, Facial
Depressor supercilii muscle *use* Muscle, Facial
Dermabrasion *see* Extraction, Skin and Breast **0HD**
Dermis *use* Skin
Descending genicular artery
   use Artery, Femoral, Right
   use Artery, Femoral, Left
Destruction
   Acetabulum
     Left **0Q55**
     Right **0Q54**
   Adenoids **0C5Q**
   Ampulla of Vater **0F5C**
   Anal Sphincter **0D5R**
   Anterior Chamber
     Left **08533ZZ**
     Right **08523ZZ**
   Anus **0D5Q**
   Aorta
     Abdominal **0450**
     Thoracic **025W**
   Aortic Body **0G5D**
   Appendix **0D5J**
   Artery
     Anterior Tibial
       Left **045Q**
       Right **045P**
     Axillary
       Left **0356**
       Right **0355**
     Brachial
       Left **0358**
       Right **0357**
     Celiac **0451**

Destruction – *continued*
   Colic
     Left **0457**
     Middle **0458**
     Right **0456**
   Common Carotid
     Left **035J**
     Right **035H**
   Common Iliac
     Left **045D**
     Right **045C**
   External Carotid
     Left **035N**
     Right **035M**
   External Iliac
     Left **045J**
     Right **045H**
   Face **035R**
   Femoral
     Left **045L**
     Right **045K**
   Foot
     Left **045W**
     Right **045V**
   Gastric **0452**
   Hand
     Left **035F**
     Right **035D**
   Hepatic **0453**
   Inferior Mesenteric **045B**
   Innominate **0352**
   Internal Carotid
     Left **035L**
     Right **035K**
   Internal Iliac
     Left **045F**
     Right **045E**
   Internal Mammary
     Left **0351**
     Right **0350**
   Intracranial **035G**
   Lower **045Y**
   Peroneal
     Left **045U**
     Right **045T**
   Popliteal
     Left **045N**
     Right **045M**
   Posterior Tibial
     Left **045S**
     Right **045R**
   Pulmonary
     Left **025R**
     Right **025Q**
   Pulmonary Trunk **025P**
   Radial
     Left **035C**
     Right **035B**
   Renal
     Left **045A**
     Right **0459**
   Splenic **0454**
   Subclavian
     Left **0354**
     Right **0353**
   Superior Mesenteric **0455**
   Temporal
     Left **035T**
     Right **035S**
   Thyroid
     Left **035V**
     Right **035U**

Destruction - *continued*
Ulnar
Left **035A**
Right **0359**
Upper **035Y**
Vertebral
Left **035Q**
Right **035P**
Atrium
Left **0257**
Right **0256**
Auditory Ossicle
Left **095A0ZZ**
Right **09590ZZ**
Basal Ganglia **0058**
Bladder **0T5B**
Bladder Neck **0T5C**
Bone
Ethmoid
Left **0N5G**
Right **0N5F**
Frontal
Left **0N52**
Right **0N51**
Hyoid **0N5X**
Lacrimal
Left **0N5J**
Right **0N5H**
Nasal **0N5B**
Occipital
Left **0N58**
Right **0N57**
Palatine
Left **0N5L**
Right **0N5K**
Parietal
Left **0N54**
Right **0N53**
Pelvic
Left **0Q53**
Right **0Q52**
Sphenoid
Left **0N5D**
Right **0N5C**
Temporal
Left **0N56**
Right **0N55**
Zygomatic
Left **0N5N**
Right **0N5M**
Brain **0050**
Breast
Bilateral **0H5V**
Left **0H5U**
Right **0H5T**
Bronchus
Lingula **0B59**
Lower Lobe
Left **0B5B**
Right **0B56**
Main
Left **0B57**
Right **0B53**
Middle Lobe, Right **0B55**
Upper Lobe
Left **0B58**
Right **0B54**
Buccal Mucosa **0C54**
Bursa and Ligament
Abdomen
Left **0M5J**
Right **0M5H**

Destruction - *continued*
Ankle
Left **0M5R**
Right **0M5Q**
Elbow
Left **0M54**
Right **0M53**
Foot
Left **0M5T**
Right **0M5S**
Hand
Left **0M58**
Right **0M57**
Head and Neck **0M50**
Hip
Left **0M5M**
Right **0M5L**
Knee
Left **0M5P**
Right **0M5N**
Lower Extremity
Left **0M5W**
Right **0M5V**
Perineum **0M5K**
Shoulder
Left **0M52**
Right **0M51**
Thorax
Left **0M5G**
Right **0M5F**
Trunk
Left **0M5D**
Right **0M5C**
Upper Extremity
Left **0M5B**
Right **0M59**
Wrist
Left **0M56**
Right **0M55**
Carina **0B52**
Carotid Bodies, Bilateral **0G58**
Carotid Body
Left **0G56**
Right **0G57**
Carpal
Left **0P5N**
Right **0P5M**
Cecum **0D5H**
Cerebellum **005C**
Cerebral Hemisphere **0057**
Cerebral Meninges **0051**
Cerebral Ventricle **0056**
Cervix **0U5C**
Chordae Tendineae **0259**
Choroid
Left **085B**
Right **085A**
Cisterna Chyli **075L**
Clavicle
Left **0P5B**
Right **0P59**
Clitoris **0U5J**
Coccygeal Glomus **0G5B**
Coccyx **0Q5S**
Colon
Ascending **0D5K**
Descending **0D5M**
Sigmoid **0D5N**
Transverse **0D5L**
Conduction Mechanism **0258**

Destruction - *continued*
Conjunctiva
Left **085TXZZ**
Right **085SXZZ**
Cord
Bilateral **0V5H**
Left **0V5G**
Right **0V5F**
Cornea
Left **0859XZZ**
Right **0858XZZ**
Cul-de-sac **0U5F**
Diaphragm
Left **0B5S**
Right **0B5R**
Disc
Cervical Vertebral **0R53**
Cervicothoracic Vertebral **0R55**
Lumbar Vertebral **0S52**
Lumbosacral **0S54**
Thoracic Vertebral **0R59**
Thoracolumbar Vertebral **0R5B**
Duct
Common Bile **0F59**
Cystic **0F58**
Hepatic
Left **0F56**
Right **0F55**
Lacrimal
Left **085Y**
Right **085X**
Pancreatic **0F5D**
Accessory **0F5F**
Parotid
Left **0C5C**
Right **0C5B**
Duodenum **0D59**
Dura Mater **0052**
Ear
External
Left **0951**
Right **0950**
External Auditory Canal
Left **0954**
Right **0953**
Inner
Left **095E0ZZ**
Right **095D0ZZ**
Middle
Left **09560ZZ**
Right **09550ZZ**
Endometrium **0U5B**
Epididymis
Bilateral **0V5L**
Left **0V5K**
Right **0V5J**
Epiglottis **0C5R**
Esophagogastric Junction **0D54**
Esophagus **0D55**
Lower **0D53**
Middle **0D52**
Upper **0D51**
Eustachian Tube
Left **095G**
Right **095F**
Eye
Left **0851XZZ**
Right **0850XZZ**
Eyelid
Lower
Left **085R**
Right **085Q**

Destruction - *continued*

Upper
Left **085P**
Right **085N**
Fallopian Tube
Left **0U56**
Right **0U55**
Fallopian Tubes, Bilateral **0U57**
Femoral Shaft
Left **0Q59**
Right **0Q58**
Femur
Lower
Left **0Q5C**
Right **0Q5B**
Upper
Left **0Q57**
Right **0Q56**
Fibula
Left **0Q5K**
Right **0Q5J**
Finger Nail **0H5QXZZ**
Gallbladder **0F54**
Gingiva
Lower **0C56**
Upper **0C55**
Gland
Adrenal
Bilateral **0G54**
Left **0G52**
Right **0G53**
Lacrimal
Left **085W**
Right **085V**
Minor Salivary **0C5J**
Parotid
Left **0C59**
Right **0C58**
Pituitary **0G50**
Sublingual
Left **0C5F**
Right **0C5D**
Submaxillary
Left **0C5H**
Right **0C5G**
Vestibular **0U5L**
Glenoid Cavity
Left **0P58**
Right **0P57**
Glomus Jugulare **0G5C**
Humeral Head
Left **0P5D**
Right **0P5C**
Humeral Shaft
Left **0P5G**
Right **0P5F**
Hymen **0U5K**
Hypothalamus **005A**
Ileocecal Valve **0D5C**
Ileum **0D5B**
Intestine
Large **0D5E**
Left **0D5G**
Right **0D5F**
Small **0D58**
Iris
Left **085D3ZZ**
Right **085C3ZZ**
Jejunum **0D5A**

Destruction - *continued*

Joint
Acromioclavicular
Left **0R5H**
Right **0R5G**
Ankle
Left **0S5G**
Right **0S5F**
Carpal
Left **0R5R**
Right **0R5Q**
Cervical Vertebral **0R51**
Cervicothoracic Vertebral **0R54**
Coccygeal **0S56**
Elbow
Left **0R5M**
Right **0R5L**
Finger Phalangeal
Left **0R5X**
Right **0R5W**
Hip
Left **0S5B**
Right **0S59**
Knee
Left **0S5D**
Right **0S5C**
Lumbar Vertebral **0S50**
Lumbosacral **0S53**
Metacarpocarpal
Left **0R5T**
Right **0R5S**
Metacarpophalangeal
Left **0R5V**
Right **0R5U**
Metatarsal-Phalangeal
Left **0S5N**
Right **0S5M**
Metatarsal-Tarsal
Left **0S5L**
Right **0S5K**
Occipital-cervical **0R50**
Sacrococcygeal **0S55**
Sacroiliac
Left **0S58**
Right **0S57**
Shoulder
Left **0R5K**
Right **0R5J**
Sternoclavicular
Left **0R5F**
Right **0R5E**
Tarsal
Left **0S5J**
Right **0S5H**
Temporomandibular
Left **0R5D**
Right **0R5C**
Thoracic Vertebral **0R56**
Thoracolumbar Vertebral **0R5A**
Toe Phalangeal
Left **0S5Q**
Right **0S5P**
Wrist
Left **0R5P**
Right **0R5N**
Kidney
Left **0T51**
Right **0T50**
Kidney Pelvis
Left **0T54**
Right **0T53**
Larynx **0C5S**

Destruction - *continued*

Lens
Left **085K3ZZ**
Right **085J3ZZ**
Lip
Lower **0C51**
Upper **0C50**
Liver **0F50**
Left Lobe **0F52**
Right Lobe **0F51**
Lung
Bilateral **0B5M**
Left **0B5L**
Lower Lobe
Left **0B5J**
Right **0B5F**
Middle Lobe, Right **0B5D**
Right **0B5K**
Upper Lobe
Left **0B5G**
Right **0B5C**
Lung Lingula **0B5H**
Lymphatic
Aortic **075D**
Axillary
Left **0756**
Right **0755**
Head **0750**
Inguinal
Left **075J**
Right **075H**
Internal Mammary
Left **0759**
Right **0758**
Lower Extremity
Left **075G**
Right **075F**
Mesenteric **075B**
Neck
Left **0752**
Right **0751**
Pelvis **075C**
Thoracic Duct **075K**
Thorax **0757**
Upper Extremity
Left **0754**
Right **0753**
Mandible
Left **0N5V**
Right **0N5T**
Maxilla
Left **0N5S**
Right **0N5R**
Medulla Oblongata **005D**
Mesentery **0D5V**
Metacarpal
Left **0P5Q**
Right **0P5P**
Metatarsal
Left **0Q5P**
Right **0Q5N**
Muscle
Abdomen
Left **0K5L**
Right **0K5K**
Extraocular
Left **085M**
Right **085L**
Facial **0K51**
Foot
Left **0K5W**
Right **0K5V**

Destruction - *continued*
- Hand
  - Left **0K5D**
  - Right **0K5C**
- Head **0K50**
- Hip
  - Left **0K5P**
  - Right **0K5N**
- Lower Arm and Wrist
  - Left **0K5B**
  - Right **0K59**
- Lower Leg
  - Left **0K5T**
  - Right **0K5S**
- Neck
  - Left **0K53**
  - Right **0K52**
- Papillary **025D**
- Perineum **0K5M**
- Shoulder
  - Left **0K56**
  - Right **0K55**
- Thorax
  - Left **0K5J**
  - Right **0K5H**
- Tongue, Palate, Pharynx **0K54**
- Trunk
  - Left **0K5G**
  - Right **0K5F**
- Upper Arm
  - Left **0K58**
  - Right **0K57**
- Upper Leg
  - Left **0K5R**
  - Right **0K5Q**
- Nasopharynx **095N**
- Nerve
  - Abdominal Sympathetic **015M**
  - Abducens **005L**
  - Accessory **005R**
  - Acoustic **005N**
  - Brachial Plexus **0153**
  - Cervical **0151**
  - Cervical Plexus **0150**
  - Facial **005M**
  - Femoral **015D**
  - Glossopharyngeal **005P**
  - Head and Neck Sympathetic **015K**
  - Hypoglossal **005S**
  - Lumbar **015B**
  - Lumbar Plexus **0159**
  - Lumbar Sympathetic **015N**
  - Lumbosacral Plexus **015A**
  - Median **0155**
  - Oculomotor **005H**
  - Olfactory **005F**
  - Optic **005G**
  - Peroneal **015H**
  - Phrenic **0152**
  - Pudendal **015C**
  - Radial **0156**
  - Sacral **015R**
  - Sacral Plexus **015Q**
  - Sacral Sympathetic **015P**
  - Sciatic **015F**
  - Thoracic **0158**
  - Thoracic Sympathetic **015L**
  - Tibial **015G**
  - Trigeminal **005K**
  - Trochlear **005J**
  - Ulnar **0154**
  - Vagus **005Q**

Destruction - *continued*
- Nipple
  - Left **0H5X**
  - Right **0H5W**
- Nose **095K**
- Omentum
  - Greater **0D5S**
  - Lesser **0D5T**
- Orbit
  - Left **0N5Q**
  - Right **0N5P**
- Ovary
  - Bilateral **0U52**
  - Left **0U51**
  - Right **0U50**
- Palate
  - Hard **0C52**
  - Soft **0C53**
- Pancreas **0F5G**
- Para-aortic Body **0G59**
- Paraganglion Extremity **0G5F**
- Parathyroid Gland **0G5R**
  - Inferior
    - Left **0G5P**
    - Right **0G5N**
  - Multiple **0G5Q**
  - Superior
    - Left **0G5M**
    - Right **0G5L**
- Patella
  - Left **0Q5F**
  - Right **0Q5D**
- Penis **0V5S**
- Pericardium **025N**
- Peritoneum **0D5W**
- Phalanx
  - Finger
    - Left **0P5V**
    - Right **0P5T**
  - Thumb
    - Left **0P5S**
    - Right **0P5R**
  - Toe
    - Left **0Q5R**
    - Right **0Q5Q**
- Pharynx **0C5M**
- Pineal Body **0G51**
- Pleura
  - Left **0B5P**
  - Right **0B5N**
- Pons **005B**
- Prepuce **0V5T**
- Prostate **0V50**
- Radius
  - Left **0P5J**
  - Right **0P5H**
- Rectum **0D5P**
- Retina
  - Left **085F3ZZ**
  - Right **085E3ZZ**
- Retinal Vessel
  - Left **085H3ZZ**
  - Right **085G3ZZ**
- Rib
  - Left **0P52**
  - Right **0P51**
- Sacrum **0Q51**
- Scapula
  - Left **0P56**
  - Right **0P55**

Destruction - *continued*
- Sclera
  - Left **0857XZZ**
  - Right **0856XZZ**
- Scrotum **0V55**
- Septum
  - Atrial **0255**
  - Nasal **095M**
  - Ventricular **025M**
- Sinus
  - Accessory **095P**
  - Ethmoid
    - Left **095V**
    - Right **095U**
  - Frontal
    - Left **095T**
    - Right **095S**
  - Mastoid
    - Left **095C**
    - Right **095B**
  - Maxillary
    - Left **095R**
    - Right **095Q**
  - Sphenoid
    - Left **095X**
    - Right **095W**
- Skin
  - Abdomen **0H57XZ**
  - Back **0H56XZ**
  - Buttock **0H58XZ**
  - Chest **0H55XZ**
  - Ear
    - Left **0H53XZ**
    - Right **0H52XZ**
  - Face **0H51XZ**
  - Foot
    - Left **0H5NXZ**
    - Right **0H5MXZ**
  - Genitalia **0H5AXZ**
  - Hand
    - Left **0H5GXZ**
    - Right **0H5FXZ**
  - Lower Arm
    - Left **0H5EXZ**
    - Right **0H5DXZ**
  - Lower Leg
    - Left **0H5LXZ**
    - Right **0H5KXZ**
  - Neck **0H54XZ**
  - Perineum **0H59XZ**
  - Scalp **0H50XZ**
  - Upper Arm
    - Left **0H5CXZ**
    - Right **0H5BXZ**
  - Upper Leg
    - Left **0H5JXZ**
    - Right **0H5HXZ**
- Skull **0N50**
- Spinal Cord
  - Cervical **005W**
  - Lumbar **005Y**
  - Thoracic **005X**
- Spinal Meninges **005T**
- Spleen **075P**
- Sternum **0P50**
- Stomach **0D56**
  - Pylorus **0D57**
- Subcutaneous Tissue and Fascia
  - Abdomen **0J58**
  - Back **0J57**
  - Buttock **0J59**
  - Chest **0J56**
  - Face **0J51**

Destruction - *continued*
- Foot
  - Left **0J5R**
  - Right **0J5Q**
- Hand
  - Left **0J5K**
  - Right **0J5J**
- Lower Arm
  - Left **0J5H**
  - Right **0J5G**
- Lower Leg
  - Left **0J5P**
  - Right **0J5N**
- Neck
  - Anterior **0J54**
  - Posterior **0J55**
- Pelvic Region **0J5C**
- Perineum **0J5B**
- Scalp **0J50**
- Upper Arm
  - Left **0J5F**
  - Right **0J5D**
- Upper Leg
  - Left **0J5M**
  - Right **0J5L**
- Tarsal
  - Left **0Q5M**
  - Right **0Q5L**
- Tendon
  - Abdomen
    - Left **0L5G**
    - Right **0L5F**
  - Ankle
    - Left **0L5T**
    - Right **0L5S**
  - Foot
    - Left **0L5W**
    - Right **0L5V**
  - Hand
    - Left **0L58**
    - Right **0L57**
  - Head and Neck **0L50**
  - Hip
    - Left **0L5K**
    - Right **0L5J**
  - Knee
    - Left **0L5R**
    - Right **0L5Q**
  - Lower Arm and Wrist
    - Left **0L56**
    - Right **0L55**
  - Lower Leg
    - Left **0L5P**
    - Right **0L5N**
  - Perineum **0L5H**
  - Shoulder
    - Left **0L52**
    - Right **0L51**
  - Thorax
    - Left **0L5D**
    - Right **0L5C**
  - Trunk
    - Left **0L5B**
    - Right **0L59**
  - Upper Arm
    - Left **0L54**
    - Right **0L53**
  - Upper Leg
    - Left **0L5M**
    - Right **0L5L**

Destruction - *continued*
- Testis
  - Bilateral **0V5C**
  - Left **0V5B**
  - Right **0V59**
- Thalamus **0059**
- Thymus **075M**
- Thyroid Gland **0G5K**
  - Left Lobe **0G5G**
  - Right Lobe **0G5H**
- Tibia
  - Left **0Q5H**
  - Right **0Q5G**
- Toe Nail **0H5RXZZ**
- Tongue **0C57**
- Tonsils **0C5P**
- Tooth
  - Lower **0C5X**
  - Upper **0C5W**
- Trachea **0B51**
- Tunica Vaginalis
  - Left **0V57**
  - Right **0V56**
- Turbinate, Nasal **095L**
- Tympanic Membrane
  - Left **0958**
  - Right **0957**
- Ulna
  - Left **0P5L**
  - Right **0P5K**
- Ureter
  - Left **0T57**
  - Right **0T56**
- Urethra **0T5D**
- Uterine Supporting Structure **0U54**
- Uterus **0U59**
- Uvula **0C5N**
- Vagina **0U5G**
- Valve
  - Aortic **025F**
  - Mitral **025G**
  - Pulmonary **025H**
  - Tricuspid **025J**
- Vas Deferens
  - Bilateral **0V5Q**
  - Left **0V5P**
  - Right **0V5N**
- Vein
  - Axillary
    - Left **0558**
    - Right **0557**
  - Azygos **0550**
  - Basilic
    - Left **055C**
    - Right **055B**
  - Brachial
    - Left **055A**
    - Right **0559**
  - Cephalic
    - Left **055F**
    - Right **055D**
  - Colic **0657**
  - Common Iliac
    - Left **065D**
    - Right **065C**
  - Coronary **0254**
  - Esophageal **0653**
  - External Iliac
    - Left **065G**
    - Right **065F**

Destruction - *continued*
- External Jugular
  - Left **055Q**
  - Right **055P**
- Face
  - Left **055V**
  - Right **055T**
- Femoral
  - Left **065N**
  - Right **065M**
- Foot
  - Left **065V**
  - Right **065T**
- Gastric **0652**
- Greater Saphenous
  - Left **065Q**
  - Right **065P**
- Hand
  - Left **055H**
  - Right **055G**
- Hemiazygos **0551**
- Hepatic **0654**
- Hypogastric
  - Left **065J**
  - Right **065H**
- Inferior Mesenteric **0656**
- Innominate
  - Left **0554**
  - Right **0553**
- Internal Jugular
  - Left **055N**
  - Right **055M**
- Intracranial **055L**
- Lesser Saphenous
  - Left **065S**
  - Right **065R**
- Lower **065Y**
- Portal **0658**
- Pulmonary
  - Left **025T**
  - Right **025S**
- Renal
  - Left **065B**
  - Right **0659**
- Splenic **0651**
- Subclavian
  - Left **0556**
  - Right **0555**
- Superior Mesenteric **0655**
- Upper **055Y**
- Vertebral
  - Left **055S**
  - Right **055R**
- Vena Cava
  - Inferior **0650**
  - Superior **025V**
- Ventricle
  - Left **025L**
  - Right **025K**
- Vertebra
  - Cervical **0P53**
  - Lumbar **0Q50**
  - Thoracic **0P54**
- Vesicle
  - Bilateral **0V53**
  - Left **0V52**
  - Right **0V51**
- Vitreous
  - Left **08553ZZ**
  - Right **08543ZZ**

Destruction - *continued*
- Vocal Cord
  - Left **0C5V**
  - Right **0C5T**
- Vulva **0U5M**

Detachment
- Arm
  - Lower
    - Left **0X6F0Z**
    - Right **0X6D0Z**
  - Upper
    - Left **0X690Z**
    - Right **0X680Z**
- Elbow Region
  - Left **0X6C0ZZ**
  - Right **0X6B0ZZ**
- Femoral Region
  - Left **0Y680ZZ**
  - Right **0Y670ZZ**
- Finger
  - Index
    - Left **0X6P0Z**
    - Right **0X6N0Z**
  - Little
    - Left **0X6W0Z**
    - Right **0X6V0Z**
  - Middle
    - Left **0X6R0Z**
    - Right **0X6Q0Z**
  - Ring
    - Left **0X6T0Z**
    - Right **0X6S0Z**
- Foot
  - Left **0Y6N0Z**
  - Right **0Y6M0Z**
- Forequarter
  - Left **0X610ZZ**
  - Right **0X600ZZ**
- Hand
  - Left **0X6K0Z**
  - Right **0X6J0Z**
- Hindquarter
  - Bilateral **0Y640ZZ**
  - Left **0Y630ZZ**
  - Right **0Y620ZZ**
- Knee Region
  - Left **0Y6G0ZZ**
  - Right **0Y6F0ZZ**
- Leg
  - Lower
    - Left **0Y6J0Z**
    - Right **0Y6H0Z**
  - Upper
    - Left **0Y6D0Z**
    - Right **0Y6C0Z**
- Shoulder Region
  - Left **0X630ZZ**
  - Right **0X620ZZ**
- Thumb
  - Left **0X6M0Z**
  - Right **0X6L0Z**
- Toe
  - 1st
    - Left **0Y6Q0Z**
    - Right **0Y6P0Z**
  - 2nd
    - Left **0Y6S0Z**
    - Right **0Y6R0Z**
  - 3rd
    - Left **0Y6U0Z**
    - Right **0Y6T0Z**

Detachment – *continued*
- 4th
  - Left **0Y6W0Z**
  - Right **0Y6V0Z**
- 5th
  - Left **0Y6Y0Z**
  - Right **0Y6X0Z**

Determination, Mental status GZ14ZZZ

Detorsion
- *see* Release
- *see* Reposition

Detoxification Services, for substance abuse HZ2ZZZZ

Device Fitting F0DZ

Diagnostic Audiology *see* Audiology, Diagnostic

Diagnostic imaging *see* Imaging, Diagnostic

Diagnostic radiology *see* Imaging, Diagnostic

Dialysis
- Hemodialysis **5A1D00Z**
- Peritoneal **3E1M39Z**

Diaphragma sellae *use* Dura Mater

Diaphragmatic pacemaker generator *use* Stimulator Generator in Subcutaneous Tissue and Fascia

Diaphragmatic Pacemaker Lead
- Insertion of device in
  - Left **0BHS**
  - Right **0BHR**
- Removal of device from, Diaphragm **0BPT**
- Revision of device in, Diaphragm **0BWT**

Digital radiography, plain *see* Plain Radiography

Dilation
- Ampulla of Vater **0F7C**
- Anus **0D7Q**
- Aorta
  - Abdominal **0470**
  - Thoracic **027W**
- Artery
  - Anterior Tibial
    - Left **047Q**
    - Right **047P**
  - Axillary
    - Left **0376**
    - Right **0375**
  - Brachial
    - Left **0378**
    - Right **0377**
  - Celiac **0471**
  - Colic
    - Left **0477**
    - Middle **0478**
    - Right **0476**
  - Common Carotid
    - Left **037J**
    - Right **037H**
  - Common Iliac
    - Left **047D**
    - Right **047C**
  - Coronary
    - Four or More Sites **0273**
    - One Site **0270**
    - Three Sites **0272**
    - Two Sites **0271**
  - External Carotid
    - Left **037N**
    - Right **037M**
  - External Iliac
    - Left **047J**
    - Right **047H**
  - Face **037R**

Dilation – *continued*
- Femoral
  - Left **047L**
  - Right **047K**
- Foot
  - Left **047W**
  - Right **047V**
- Gastric **0472**
- Hand
  - Left **037F**
  - Right **037D**
- Hepatic **0473**
- Inferior Mesenteric **047B**
- Innominate **0372**
- Internal Carotid
  - Left **037L**
  - Right **037K**
- Internal Iliac
  - Left **047F**
  - Right **047E**
- Internal Mammary
  - Left **0371**
  - Right **0370**
- Intracranial **037G**
- Lower **047Y**
- Peroneal
  - Left **047U**
  - Right **047T**
- Popliteal
  - Left **047N**
  - Right **047M**
- Posterior Tibial
  - Left **047S**
  - Right **047R**
- Pulmonary
  - Left **027R**
  - Right **027Q**
- Pulmonary Trunk **027P**
- Radial
  - Left **037C**
  - Right **037B**
- Renal
  - Left **047A**
  - Right **0479**
- Splenic **0474**
- Subclavian
  - Left **0374**
  - Right **0373**
- Superior Mesenteric **0475**
- Temporal
  - Left **037T**
  - Right **037S**
- Thyroid
  - Left **037V**
  - Right **037U**
- Ulnar
  - Left **037A**
  - Right **0379**
- Upper **037Y**
- Vertebral
  - Left **037Q**
  - Right **037P**
- Bladder **0T7B**
- Bladder Neck **0T7C**
- Bronchus
  - Lingula **0B79**
  - Lower Lobe
    - Left **0B7B**
    - Right **0B76**
  - Main
    - Left **0B77**
    - Right **0B73**

Dilation - *continued*
    Middle Lobe, Right **0B75**
    Upper Lobe
      Left **0B78**
      Right **0B74**
  Carina **0B72**
  Cecum **0D7H**
  Cervix **0U7C**
  Colon
    Ascending **0D7K**
    Descending **0D7M**
    Sigmoid **0D7N**
    Transverse **0D7L**
  Duct
    Common Bile **0F79**
    Cystic **0F78**
    Hepatic
      Left **0F76**
      Right **0F75**
    Lacrimal
      Left **087Y**
      Right **087X**
    Pancreatic **0F7D**
      Accessory **0F7F**
    Parotid
      Left **0C7C**
      Right **0C7B**
  Duodenum **0D79**
  Esophagogastric Junction **0D74**
  Esophagus **0D75**
    Lower **0D73**
    Middle **0D72**
    Upper **0D71**
  Eustachian Tube
    Left **097G**
    Right **097F**
  Fallopian Tube
    Left **0U76**
    Right **0U75**
  Fallopian Tubes, Bilateral **0U77**
  Hymen **0U7K**
  Ileocecal Valve **0D7C**
  Ileum **0D7B**
  Intestine
    Large **0D7E**
      Left **0D7G**
      Right **0D7F**
    Small **0D78**
  Jejunum **0D7A**
  Kidney Pelvis
    Left **0T74**
    Right **0T73**
  Larynx **0C7S**
  Pharynx **0C7M**
  Rectum **0D7P**
  Stomach **0D76**
    Pylorus **0D77**
  Trachea **0B71**
  Ureter
    Left **0T77**
    Right **0T76**
  Ureters, Bilateral **0T78**
  Urethra **0T7D**
  Uterus **0U79**
  Vagina **0U7G**
  Valve
    Aortic **027F**
    Mitral **027G**
    Pulmonary **027H**
    Tricuspid **027J**

Dilation – *continued*
  Vas Deferens
    Bilateral **0V7Q**
    Left **0V7P**
    Right **0V7N**
  Vein
    Axillary
      Left **0578**
      Right **0577**
    Azygos **0570**
    Basilic
      Left **057C**
      Right **057B**
    Brachial
      Left **057A**
      Right **0579**
    Cephalic
      Left **057F**
      Right **057D**
    Colic **0677**
    Common Iliac
      Left **067D**
      Right **067C**
    Esophageal **0673**
    External Iliac
      Left **067G**
      Right **067F**
    External Jugular
      Left **057Q**
      Right **057P**
    Face
      Left **057V**
      Right **057T**
    Femoral
      Left **067N**
      Right **067M**
    Foot
      Left **067V**
      Right **067T**
    Gastric **0672**
    Greater Saphenous
      Left **067Q**
      Right **067P**
    Hand
      Left **057H**
      Right **057G**
    Hemiazygos **0571**
    Hepatic **0674**
    Hypogastric
      Left **067J**
      Right **067H**
    Inferior Mesenteric **0676**
    Innominate
      Left **0574**
      Right **0573**
    Internal Jugular
      Left **057N**
      Right **057M**
    Intracranial **057L**
    Lesser Saphenous
      Left **067S**
      Right **067R**
    Lower **067Y**
    Portal **0678**
    Pulmonary
      Left **027T**
      Right **027S**
    Renal
      Left **067B**
      Right **0679**
    Splenic **0671**

Dilation – *continued*
    Subclavian
      Left **0576**
      Right **0575**
    Superior Mesenteric **0675**
    Upper **057Y**
    Vertebral
      Left **057S**
      Right **057R**
  Vena Cava
    Inferior **0670**
    Superior **027V**
  Ventricle, Right **027K**
Direct Lateral Interbody Fusion (DLIF)
  device *use* Interbody Fusion Device in Lower
    Joints
Disarticulation *see* Detachment
Discectomy, diskectomy
  see Excision, Upper Joints **0RB**
  see Resection, Upper Joints **0RT**
  see Excision, Lower Joints **0SB**
  see Resection, Lower Joints **0ST**
Discography
  see Plain Radiography, Axial Skeleton,
    Except Skull and Facial Bones **BR0**
  see Fluoroscopy, Axial Skeleton, Except Skull
    and Facial Bones **BR1**
Distal humerus
  use Humeral Shaft, Right
  use Humeral Shaft, Left
Distal humerus, involving joint
  use Joint, Elbow, Right
  use Joint, Elbow, Left
Distal radioulnar joint
  use Joint, Wrist, Right
  use Joint, Wrist, Left
Diversion *see* Bypass
Diverticulectomy *see* Excision, Gastrointestinal
  System **0DB**
Division
  Acetabulum
    Left **0Q85**
    Right **0Q84**
  Anal Sphincter **0D8R**
  Basal Ganglia **0088**
  Bladder Neck **0T8C**
  Bone
    Ethmoid
      Left **0N8G**
      Right **0N8F**
    Frontal
      Left **0N82**
      Right **0N81**
    Hyoid **0N8X**
    Lacrimal
      Left **0N8J**
      Right **0N8H**
    Nasal **0N8B**
    Occipital
      Left **0N88**
      Right **0N87**
    Palatine
      Left **0N8L**
      Right **0N8K**
    Parietal
      Left **0N84**
      Right **0N83**
    Pelvic
      Left **0Q83**
      Right **0Q82**
    Sphenoid
      Left **0N8D**
      Right **0N8C**

Division - *continued*
  Temporal
    Left **0N86**
    Right **0N85**
  Zygomatic
    Left **0N8N**
    Right **0N8M**
  Brain **0080**
  Bursa and Ligament
    Abdomen
      Left **0M8J**
      Right **0M8H**
    Ankle
      Left **0M8R**
      Right **0M8Q**
    Elbow
      Left **0M84**
      Right **0M83**
    Foot
      Left **0M8T**
      Right **0M8S**
    Hand
      Left **0M88**
      Right **0M87**
    Head and Neck **0M80**
    Hip
      Left **0M8M**
      Right **0M8L**
    Knee
      Left **0M8P**
      Right **0M8N**
    Lower Extremity
      Left **0M8W**
      Right **0M8V**
    Perineum **0M8K**
    Shoulder
      Left **0M82**
      Right **0M81**
    Thorax
      Left **0M8G**
      Right **0M8F**
    Trunk
      Left **0M8D**
      Right **0M8C**
    Upper Extremity
      Left **0M8B**
      Right **0M89**
    Wrist
      Left **0M86**
      Right **0M85**
  Carpal
    Left **0P8N**
    Right **0P8M**
  Cerebral Hemisphere **0087**
  Chordae Tendineae **0289**
  Clavicle
    Left **0P8B**
    Right **0P89**
  Coccyx **0Q8S**
  Conduction Mechanism **0288**
  Esophagogastric Junction **0D84**
  Femoral Shaft
    Left **0Q89**
    Right **0Q88**
  Femur
    Lower
      Left **0Q8C**
      Right **0Q8B**
    Upper
      Left **0Q87**
      Right **0Q86**

  Fibula
    Left **0Q8K**
    Right **0Q8J**
  Gland, Pituitary **0G80**
  Glenoid Cavity
    Left **0P88**
    Right **0P87**
  Humeral Head
    Left **0P8D**
    Right **0P8C**
  Humeral Shaft
    Left **0P8G**
    Right **0P8F**
  Hymen **0U8K**
  Kidneys, Bilateral **0T82**
  Mandible
    Left **0N8V**
    Right **0N8T**
  Maxilla
    Left **0N8S**
    Right **0N8R**
  Metacarpal
    Left **0P8Q**
    Right **0P8P**
  Metatarsal
    Left **0Q8P**
    Right **0Q8N**
  Muscle
    Abdomen
      Left **0K8L**
      Right **0K8K**
    Facial **0K81**
    Foot
      Left **0K8W**
      Right **0K8V**
    Hand
      Left **0K8D**
      Right **0K8C**
    Head **0K80**
    Hip
      Left **0K8P**
      Right **0K8N**
    Lower Arm and Wrist
      Left **0K8B**
      Right **0K89**
    Lower Leg
      Left **0K8T**
      Right **0K8S**
    Neck
      Left **0K83**
      Right **0K82**
    Papillary **028D**
    Perineum **0K8M**
    Shoulder
      Left **0K86**
      Right **0K85**
    Thorax
      Left **0K8J**
      Right **0K8H**
    Tongue, Palate, Pharynx **0K84**
    Trunk
      Left **0K8G**
      Right **0K8F**
    Upper Arm
      Left **0K88**
      Right **0K87**
    Upper Leg
      Left **0K8R**
      Right **0K8Q**

  Nerve
    Abdominal Sympathetic **018M**
    Abducens **008L**
    Accessory **008R**
    Acoustic **008N**
    Brachial Plexus **0183**
    Cervical **0181**
    Cervical Plexus **0180**
    Facial **008M**
    Femoral **018D**
    Glossopharyngeal **008P**
    Head and Neck Sympathetic **018K**
    Hypoglossal **008S**
    Lumbar **018B**
    Lumbar Plexus **0189**
    Lumbar Sympathetic **018N**
    Lumbosacral Plexus **018A**
    Median **0185**
    Oculomotor **008H**
    Olfactory **008F**
    Optic **008G**
    Peroneal **018H**
    Phrenic **0182**
    Pudendal **018C**
    Radial **0186**
    Sacral **018R**
    Sacral Plexus **018Q**
    Sacral Sympathetic **018P**
    Sciatic **018F**
    Thoracic **0188**
    Thoracic Sympathetic **018L**
    Tibial **018G**
    Trigeminal **008K**
    Trochlear **008J**
    Ulnar **0184**
    Vagus **008Q**
  Orbit
    Left **0N8Q**
    Right **0N8P**
  Ovary
    Bilateral **0U82**
    Left **0U81**
    Right **0U80**
  Pancreas **0F8G**
  Patella
    Left **0Q8F**
    Right **0Q8D**
  Perineum, Female **0W8NXZZ**
  Phalanx
    Finger
      Left **0P8V**
      Right **0P8T**
    Thumb
      Left **0P8S**
      Right **0P8R**
    Toe
      Left **0Q8R**
      Right **0Q8Q**
  Radius
    Left **0P8J**
    Right **0P8H**
  Rib
    Left **0P82**
    Right **0P81**
  Sacrum **0Q81**
  Scapula
    Left **0P86**
    Right **0P85**
  Skin
    Abdomen **0H87XZZ**
    Back **0H86XZZ**
    Buttock **0H88XZZ**

Division - *continued*
- Chest **0H85XZZ**
- Ear
  - Left **0H83XZZ**
  - Right **0H82XZZ**
- Face **0H81XZZ**
- Foot
  - Left **0H8NXZZ**
  - Right **0H8MXZZ**
- Genitalia **0H8AXZZ**
- Hand
  - Left **0H8GXZZ**
  - Right **0H8FXZZ**
- Lower Arm
  - Left **0H8EXZZ**
  - Right **0H8DXZZ**
- Lower Leg
  - Left **0H8LXZZ**
  - Right **0H8KXZZ**
- Neck **0H84XZZ**
- Perineum **0H89XZZ**
- Scalp **0H80XZZ**
- Upper Arm
  - Left **0H8CXZZ**
  - Right **0H8BXZZ**
- Upper Leg
  - Left **0H8JXZZ**
  - Right **0H8HXZZ**
- Skull **0N80**
- Spinal Cord
  - Cervical **008W**
  - Lumbar **008Y**
  - Thoracic **008X**
- Sternum **0P80**
- Stomach, Pylorus **0D87**
- Subcutaneous Tissue and Fascia
  - Abdomen **0J88**
  - Back **0J87**
  - Buttock **0J89**
  - Chest **0J86**
  - Face **0J81**
  - Foot
    - Left **0J8R**
    - Right **0J8Q**
  - Hand
    - Left **0J8K**
    - Right **0J8J**
  - Head and Neck **0J8S**
  - Lower Arm
    - Left **0J8H**
    - Right **0J8G**
  - Lower Extremity **0J8W**
  - Lower Leg
    - Left **0J8P**
    - Right **0J8N**
  - Neck
    - Anterior **0J84**
    - Posterior **0J85**
  - Pelvic Region **0J8C**
  - Perineum **0J8B**
  - Scalp **0J80**
  - Trunk **0J8T**
  - Upper Arm
    - Left **0J8F**
    - Right **0J8D**
  - Upper Extremity **0J8V**
  - Upper Leg
    - Left **0J8M**
    - Right **0J8L**
- Tarsal
  - Left **0Q8M**
  - Right **0Q8L**

Division - *continued*
- Tendon
  - Abdomen
    - Left **0L8G**
    - Right **0L8F**
  - Ankle
    - Left **0L8T**
    - Right **0L8S**
  - Foot
    - Left **0L8W**
    - Right **0L8V**
  - Hand
    - Left **0L88**
    - Right **0L87**
  - Head and Neck **0L80**
  - Hip
    - Left **0L8K**
    - Right **0L8J**
  - Knee
    - Left **0L8R**
    - Right **0L8Q**
  - Lower Arm and Wrist
    - Left **0L86**
    - Right **0L85**
  - Lower Leg
    - Left **0L8P**
    - Right **0L8N**
  - Perineum **0L8H**
  - Shoulder
    - Left **0L82**
    - Right **0L81**
  - Thorax
    - Left **0L8D**
    - Right **0L8C**
  - Trunk
    - Left **0L8B**
    - Right **0L89**
  - Upper Arm
    - Left **0L84**
    - Right **0L83**
  - Upper Leg
    - Left **0L8M**
    - Right **0L8L**
- Thyroid Gland Isthmus **0G8J**
- Tibia
  - Left **0Q8H**
  - Right **0Q8G**
- Turbinate, Nasal **098L**
- Ulna
  - Left **0P8L**
  - Right **0P8K**
- Uterine Supporting Structure **0U84**
- Vertebra
  - Cervical **0P83**
  - Lumbar **0Q80**
  - Thoracic **0P84**

Doppler study *see* Ultrasonography
Dorsal digital nerve *use* Nerve, Radial
Dorsal metacarpal vein
- *use* Vein, Hand, Left
- *use* Vein, Hand, Right
Dorsal metatarsal artery
- *use* Artery, Foot, Left
- *use* Artery, Foot, Right
Dorsal metatarsal vein
- *use* Vein, Foot, Right
- *use* Vein, Foot, Left
Dorsal scapular artery
- *use* Artery, Subclavian, Right
- *use* Artery, Subclavian, Left
Dorsal scapular nerve *use* Nerve, Brachial
Plexus

Dorsal venous arch
- *use* Vein, Foot, Right
- *use* Vein, Foot, Left
Dorsalis pedis artery
- *use* Artery, Anterior Tibial, Right
- *use* Artery, Anterior Tibial, Left
Drainage
- Abdominal Wall **0W9F**
- Acetabulum
  - Left **0Q95**
  - Right **0Q94**
- Adenoids **0C9Q**
- Ampulla of Vater **0F9C**
- Anal Sphincter **0D9R**
- Ankle Region
  - Left **0Y9L**
  - Right **0Y9K**
- Anterior Chamber
  - Left **0893**
  - Right **0892**
- Anus **0D9Q**
- Aorta, Abdominal **0490**
- Aortic Body **0G9D**
- Appendix **0D9J**
- Arm
  - Lower
    - Left **0X9F**
    - Right **0X9D**
  - Upper
    - Left **0X99**
    - Right **0X98**
- Artery
  - Anterior Tibial
    - Left **049Q**
    - Right **049P**
  - Axillary
    - Left **0396**
    - Right **0395**
  - Brachial
    - Left **0398**
    - Right **0397**
  - Celiac **0491**
  - Colic
    - Left **0497**
    - Middle **0498**
    - Right **0496**
  - Common Carotid
    - Left **039J**
    - Right **039H**
  - Common Iliac
    - Left **049D**
    - Right **049C**
  - External Carotid
    - Left **039N**
    - Right **039M**
  - External Iliac
    - Left **049J**
    - Right **049H**
  - Face **039R**
  - Femoral
    - Left **049L**
    - Right **049K**
  - Foot
    - Left **049W**
    - Right **049V**
  - Gastric **0492**
  - Hand
    - Left **039F**
    - Right **039D**
  - Hepatic **0493**
  - Inferior Mesenteric **049B**
  - Innominate **0392**

Drainage - *continued*
  Internal Carotid
    Left **039L**
    Right **039K**
  Internal Iliac
    Left **049F**
    Right **049E**
  Internal Mammary
    Left **0391**
    Right **0390**
  Intracranial **039G**
  Lower **049Y**
  Peroneal
    Left **049U**
    Right **049T**
  Popliteal
    Left **049N**
    Right **049M**
  Posterior Tibial
    Left **049S**
    Right **049R**
  Radial
    Left **039C**
    Right **039B**
  Renal
    Left **049A**
    Right **0499**
  Splenic **0494**
  Subclavian
    Left **0394**
    Right **0393**
  Superior Mesenteric **0495**
  Temporal
    Left **039T**
    Right **039S**
  Thyroid
    Left **039V**
    Right **039U**
  Ulnar
    Left **039A**
    Right **0399**
  Upper **039Y**
  Vertebral
    Left **039Q**
    Right **039P**
 Auditory Ossicle
    Left **099A**
    Right **0999**
 Axilla
    Left **0X95**
    Right **0X94**
 Back
    Lower **0W9L**
    Upper **0W9K**
 Basal Ganglia **0098**
 Bladder **0T9B**
 Bladder Neck **0T9C**
 Bone
  Ethmoid
    Left **0N9G**
    Right **0N9F**
  Frontal
    Left **0N92**
    Right **0N91**
  Hyoid **0N9X**
  Lacrimal
    Left **0N9J**
    Right **0N9H**
  Nasal **0N9B**
  Occipital
    Left **0N98**
    Right **0N97**

Drainage - *continued*
  Palatine
    Left **0N9L**
    Right **0N9K**
  Parietal
    Left **0N94**
    Right **0N93**
  Pelvic
    Left **0Q93**
    Right **0Q92**
  Sphenoid
    Left **0N9D**
    Right **0N9C**
  Temporal
    Left **0N96**
    Right **0N95**
  Zygomatic
    Left **0N9N**
    Right **0N9M**
 Bone Marrow **079T**
 Brain **0090**
 Breast
    Bilateral **0H9V**
    Left **0H9U**
    Right **0H9T**
 Bronchus
  Lingula **0B99**
  Lower Lobe
    Left **0B9B**
    Right **0B96**
  Main
    Left **0B97**
    Right **0B93**
  Middle Lobe, Right **0B95**
  Upper Lobe
    Left **0B98**
    Right **0B94**
 Buccal Mucosa **0C94**
 Bursa and Ligament
  Abdomen
    Left **0M9J**
    Right **0M9H**
  Ankle
    Left **0M9R**
    Right **0M9Q**
  Elbow
    Left **0M94**
    Right **0M93**
  Foot
    Left **0M9T**
    Right **0M9S**
  Hand
    Left **0M98**
    Right **0M97**
  Head and Neck **0M90**
  Hip
    Left **0M9M**
    Right **0M9L**
  Knee
    Left **0M9P**
    Right **0M9N**
  Lower Extremity
    Left **0M9W**
    Right **0M9V**
  Perineum **0M9K**
  Shoulder
    Left **0M92**
    Right **0M91**
  Thorax
    Left **0M9G**
    Right **0M9F**

Drainage - *continued*
  Trunk
    Left **0M9D**
    Right **0M9C**
  Upper Extremity
    Left **0M9B**
    Right **0M99**
  Wrist
    Left **0M96**
    Right **0M95**
 Buttock
    Left **0Y91**
    Right **0Y90**
 Carina **0B92**
 Carotid Bodies, Bilateral **0G98**
 Carotid Body
    Left **0G96**
    Right **0G97**
 Carpal
    Left **0P9N**
    Right **0P9M**
 Cavity, Cranial **0W91**
 Cecum **0D9H**
 Cerebellum **009C**
 Cerebral Hemisphere **0097**
 Cerebral Meninges **0091**
 Cerebral Ventricle **0096**
 Cervix **0U9C**
 Chest Wall **0W98**
 Choroid
    Left **089B**
    Right **089A**
 Cisterna Chyli **079L**
 Clavicle
    Left **0P9B**
    Right **0P99**
 Clitoris **0U9J**
 Coccygeal Glomus **0G9B**
 Coccyx **0Q9S**
 Colon
    Ascending **0D9K**
    Descending **0D9M**
    Sigmoid **0D9N**
    Transverse **0D9L**
 Conjunctiva
    Left **089T**
    Right **089S**
 Cord
    Bilateral **0V9H**
    Left **0V9G**
    Right **0V9F**
 Cornea
    Left **0899**
    Right **0898**
 Cul-de-sac **0U9F**
 Diaphragm
    Left **0B9S**
    Right **0B9R**
 Disc
    Cervical Vertebral **0R93**
    Cervicothoracic Vertebral **0R95**
    Lumbar Vertebral **0S92**
    Lumbosacral **0S94**
    Thoracic Vertebral **0R99**
    Thoracolumbar Vertebral **0R9B**
 Duct
    Common Bile **0F99**
    Cystic **0F98**
  Hepatic
    Left **0F96**
    Right **0F95**

Drainage - *continued*
- Lacrimal
  - Left **089Y**
  - Right **089X**
- Pancreatic **0F9D**
  - Accessory **0F9F**
- Parotid
  - Left **0C9C**
  - Right **0C9B**
- Duodenum **0D99**
- Dura Mater **0092**
- Ear
  - External
    - Left **0991**
    - Right **0990**
  - External Auditory Canal
    - Left **0994**
    - Right **0993**
  - Inner
    - Left **099E**
    - Right **099D**
  - Middle
    - Left **0996**
    - Right **0995**
- Elbow Region
  - Left **0X9C**
  - Right **0X9B**
- Epididymis
  - Bilateral **0V9L**
  - Left **0V9K**
  - Right **0V9J**
- Epidural Space **0093**
- Epiglottis **0C9R**
- Esophagogastric Junction **0D94**
- Esophagus **0D95**
  - Lower **0D93**
  - Middle **0D92**
  - Upper **0D91**
- Eustachian Tube
  - Left **099G**
  - Right **099F**
- Extremity
  - Lower
    - Left **0Y9B**
    - Right **0Y99**
  - Upper
    - Left **0X97**
    - Right **0X96**
- Eye
  - Left **0891**
  - Right **0890**
- Eyelid
  - Lower
    - Left **089R**
    - Right **089Q**
  - Upper
    - Left **089P**
    - Right **089N**
- Face **0W92**
- Fallopian Tube
  - Left **0U96**
  - Right **0U95**
- Fallopian Tubes, Bilateral **0U97**
- Femoral Region
  - Left **0Y98**
  - Right **0Y97**
- Femoral Shaft
  - Left **0Q99**
  - Right **0Q98**

- Femur
  - Lower
    - Left **0Q9C**
    - Right **0Q9B**
  - Upper
    - Left **0Q97**
    - Right **0Q96**
- Fibula
  - Left **0Q9K**
  - Right **0Q9J**
- Finger Nail **0H9Q**
- Foot
  - Left **0Y9N**
  - Right **0Y9M**
- Gallbladder **0F94**
- Gingiva
  - Lower **0C96**
  - Upper **0C95**
- Gland
  - Adrenal
    - Bilateral **0G94**
    - Left **0G92**
    - Right **0G93**
  - Lacrimal
    - Left **089W**
    - Right **089V**
  - Minor Salivary **0C9J**
  - Parotid
    - Left **0C99**
    - Right **0C98**
  - Pituitary **0G90**
  - Sublingual
    - Left **0C9F**
    - Right **0C9D**
  - Submaxillary
    - Left **0C9H**
    - Right **0C9G**
  - Vestibular **0U9L**
- Glenoid Cavity
  - Left **0P98**
  - Right **0P97**
- Glomus Jugulare **0G9C**
- Hand
  - Left **0X9K**
  - Right **0X9J**
- Head **0W90**
- Humeral Head
  - Left **0P9D**
  - Right **0P9C**
- Humeral Shaft
  - Left **0P9G**
  - Right **0P9F**
- Hymen **0U9K**
- Hypothalamus **009A**
- Ileocecal Valve **0D9C**
- Ileum **0D9B**
- Inguinal Region
  - Left **0Y96**
  - Right **0Y95**
- Intestine
  - Large **0D9E**
    - Left **0D9G**
    - Right **0D9F**
  - Small **0D98**
- Iris
  - Left **089D**
  - Right **089C**
- Jaw
  - Lower **0W95**
  - Upper **0W94**
- Jejunum **0D9A**

- Joint
  - Acromioclavicular
    - Left **0R9H**
    - Right **0R9G**
  - Ankle
    - Left **0S9G**
    - Right **0S9F**
  - Carpal
    - Left **0R9R**
    - Right **0R9Q**
  - Cervical Vertebral **0R91**
  - Cervicothoracic Vertebral **0R94**
  - Coccygeal **0S96**
  - Elbow
    - Left **0R9M**
    - Right **0R9L**
  - Finger Phalangeal
    - Left **0R9X**
    - Right **0R9W**
  - Hip
    - Left **0S9B**
    - Right **0S99**
  - Knee
    - Left **0S9D**
    - Right **0S9C**
  - Lumbar Vertebral **0S90**
  - Lumbosacral **0S93**
  - Metacarpocarpal
    - Left **0R9T**
    - Right **0R9S**
  - Metacarpophalangeal
    - Left **0R9V**
    - Right **0R9U**
  - Metatarsal-Phalangeal
    - Left **0S9N**
    - Right **0S9M**
  - Metatarsal-Tarsal
    - Left **0S9L**
    - Right **0S9K**
  - Occipital-cervical **0R90**
  - Sacrococcygeal **0S95**
  - Sacroiliac
    - Left **0S98**
    - Right **0S97**
  - Shoulder
    - Left **0R9K**
    - Right **0R9J**
  - Sternoclavicular
    - Left **0R9F**
    - Right **0R9E**
  - Tarsal
    - Left **0S9J**
    - Right **0S9H**
  - Temporomandibular
    - Left **0R9D**
    - Right **0R9C**
  - Thoracic Vertebral **0R96**
  - Thoracolumbar Vertebral **0R9A**
  - Toe Phalangeal
    - Left **0S9Q**
    - Right **0S9P**
  - Wrist
    - Left **0R9P**
    - Right **0R9N**
- Kidney
  - Left **0T91**
  - Right **0T90**
- Kidney Pelvis
  - Left **0T94**
  - Right **0T93**

Drainage - *continued*
- Knee Region
  - Left **0Y9G**
  - Right **0Y9F**
- Larynx **0C9S**
- Leg
  - Lower
    - Left **0Y9J**
    - Right **0Y9H**
  - Upper
    - Left **0Y9D**
    - Right **0Y9C**
- Lens
  - Left **089K**
  - Right **089J**
- Lip
  - Lower **0C91**
  - Upper **0C90**
- Liver **0F90**
  - Left Lobe **0F92**
  - Right Lobe **0F91**
- Lung
  - Bilateral **0B9M**
  - Left **0B9L**
  - Lower Lobe
    - Left **0B9J**
    - Right **0B9F**
  - Middle Lobe, Right **0B9D**
  - Right **0B9K**
  - Upper Lobe
    - Left **0B9G**
    - Right **0B9C**
- Lung Lingula **0B9H**
- Lymphatic
  - Aortic **079D**
  - Axillary
    - Left **0796**
    - Right **0795**
  - Head **0790**
  - Inguinal
    - Left **079J**
    - Right **079H**
  - Internal Mammary
    - Left **0799**
    - Right **0798**
  - Lower Extremity
    - Left **079G**
    - Right **079F**
  - Mesenteric **079B**
  - Neck
    - Left **0792**
    - Right **0791**
  - Pelvis **079C**
  - Thoracic Duct **079K**
  - Thorax **0797**
  - Upper Extremity
    - Left **0794**
    - Right **0793**
- Mandible
  - Left **0N9V**
  - Right **0N9T**
- Maxilla
  - Left **0N9S**
  - Right **0N9R**
- Mediastinum **0W9C**
- Medulla Oblongata **009D**
- Mesentery **0D9V**
- Metacarpal
  - Left **0P9Q**
  - Right **0P9P**
- Metatarsal
  - Left **0Q9P**
  - Right **0Q9N**

Drainage - *continued*
- Muscle
  - Abdomen
    - Left **0K9L**
    - Right **0K9K**
  - Extraocular
    - Left **089M**
    - Right **089L**
  - Facial **0K91**
  - Foot
    - Left **0K9W**
    - Right **0K9V**
  - Hand
    - Left **0K9D**
    - Right **0K9C**
  - Head **0K90**
  - Hip
    - Left **0K9P**
    - Right **0K9N**
  - Lower Arm and Wrist
    - Left **0K9B**
    - Right **0K99**
  - Lower Leg
    - Left **0K9T**
    - Right **0K9S**
  - Neck
    - Left **0K93**
    - Right **0K92**
  - Perineum **0K9M**
  - Shoulder
    - Left **0K96**
    - Right **0K95**
  - Thorax
    - Left **0K9J**
    - Right **0K9H**
  - Tongue, Palate, Pharynx **0K94**
  - Trunk
    - Left **0K9G**
    - Right **0K9F**
  - Upper Arm
    - Left **0K98**
    - Right **0K97**
  - Upper Leg
    - Left **0K9R**
    - Right **0K9Q**
- Nasopharynx **099N**
- Neck **0W96**
- Nerve
  - Abdominal Sympathetic **019M**
  - Abducens **009L**
  - Accessory **009R**
  - Acoustic **009N**
  - Brachial Plexus **0193**
  - Cervical **0191**
  - Cervical Plexus **0190**
  - Facial **009M**
  - Femoral **019D**
  - Glossopharyngeal **009P**
  - Head and Neck Sympathetic **019K**
  - Hypoglossal **009S**
  - Lumbar **019B**
  - Lumbar Plexus **0199**
  - Lumbar Sympathetic **019N**
  - Lumbosacral Plexus **019A**
  - Median **0195**
  - Oculomotor **009H**
  - Olfactory **009F**
  - Optic **009G**
  - Peroneal **019H**
  - Phrenic **0192**
  - Pudendal **019C**
  - Radial **0196**

Drainage - *continued*
- Sacral **019R**
- Sacral Plexus **019Q**
- Sacral Sympathetic **019P**
- Sciatic **019F**
- Thoracic **0198**
- Thoracic Sympathetic **019L**
- Tibial **019G**
- Trigeminal **009K**
- Trochlear **009J**
- Ulnar **0194**
- Vagus **009Q**
- Nipple
  - Left **0H9X**
  - Right **0H9W**
- Nose **099K**
- Omentum
  - Greater **0D9S**
  - Lesser **0D9T**
- Oral Cavity and Throat **0W93**
- Orbit
  - Left **0N9Q**
  - Right **0N9P**
- Ovary
  - Bilateral **0U92**
  - Left **0U91**
  - Right **0U90**
- Palate
  - Hard **0C92**
  - Soft **0C93**
- Pancreas **0F9G**
- Para-aortic Body **0G99**
- Paraganglion Extremity **0G9F**
- Parathyroid Gland **0G9R**
  - Inferior
    - Left **0G9P**
    - Right **0G9N**
  - Multiple **0G9Q**
  - Superior
    - Left **0G9M**
    - Right **0G9L**
- Patella
  - Left **0Q9F**
  - Right **0Q9D**
- Pelvic Cavity **0W9J**
- Penis **0V9S**
- Pericardial Cavity **0W9D**
- Perineum
  - Female **0W9N**
  - Male **0W9M**
- Peritoneal Cavity **0W9G**
- Peritoneum **0D9W**
- Phalanx
  - Finger
    - Left **0P9V**
    - Right **0P9T**
  - Thumb
    - Left **0P9S**
    - Right **0P9R**
  - Toe
    - Left **0Q9R**
    - Right **0Q9Q**
- Pharynx **0C9M**
- Pineal Body **0G91**
- Pleura
  - Left **0B9P**
  - Right **0B9N**
- Pleural Cavity
  - Left **0W9B**
  - Right **0W99**
- Pons **009B**
- Prepuce **0V9T**

Drainage - *continued*
  Products of Conception
    Amniotic Fluid
      Diagnostic **1090**
      Therapeutic **1090**
    Fetal Blood **1090**
    Fetal Cerebrospinal Fluid **1090**
    Fetal Fluid, Other **1090**
    Fluid, Other **1090**
  Prostate **0V90**
  Radius
    Left **0P9J**
    Right **0P9H**
  Rectum **0D9P**
  Retina
    Left **089F**
    Right **089E**
  Retinal Vessel
    Left **089H**
    Right **089G**
  Retroperitoneum **0W9H**
  Rib
    Left **0P92**
    Right **0P91**
  Sacrum **0Q91**
  Scapula
    Left **0P96**
    Right **0P95**
  Sclera
    Left **0897**
    Right **0896**
  Scrotum **0V95**
  Septum, Nasal **099M**
  Shoulder Region
    Left **0X93**
    Right **0X92**
  Sinus
    Accessory **099P**
    Ethmoid
      Left **099V**
      Right **099U**
    Frontal
      Left **099T**
      Right **099S**
    Mastoid
      Left **099C**
      Right **099B**
    Maxillary
      Left **099R**
      Right **099Q**
    Sphenoid
      Left **099X**
      Right **099W**
  Skin
    Abdomen **0H97**
    Back **0H96**
    Buttock **0H98**
    Chest **0H95**
    Ear
      Left **0H93**
      Right **0H92**
    Face **0H91**
    Foot
      Left **0H9N**
      Right **0H9M**
    Genitalia **0H9A**
    Hand
      Left **0H9G**
      Right **0H9F**
    Lower Arm
      Left **0H9E**
      Right **0H9D**

    Lower Leg
      Left **0H9L**
      Right **0H9K**
    Neck **0H94**
    Perineum **0H99**
    Scalp **0H90**
    Upper Arm
      Left **0H9C**
      Right **0H9B**
    Upper Leg
      Left **0H9J**
      Right **0H9H**
  Skull **0N90**
  Spinal Canal **009U**
  Spinal Cord
    Cervical **009W**
    Lumbar **009Y**
    Thoracic **009X**
  Spinal Meninges **009T**
  Spleen **079P**
  Sternum **0P90**
  Stomach **0D96**
    Pylorus **0D97**
  Subarachnoid Space **0095**
  Subcutaneous Tissue and Fascia
    Abdomen **0J98**
    Back **0J97**
    Buttock **0J99**
    Chest **0J96**
    Face **0J91**
    Foot
      Left **0J9R**
      Right **0J9Q**
    Hand
      Left **0J9K**
      Right **0J9J**
    Lower Arm
      Left **0J9H**
      Right **0J9G**
    Lower Leg
      Left **0J9P**
      Right **0J9N**
    Neck
      Anterior **0J94**
      Posterior **0J95**
    Pelvic Region **0J9C**
    Perineum **0J9B**
    Scalp **0J90**
    Upper Arm
      Left **0J9F**
      Right **0J9D**
    Upper Leg
      Left **0J9M**
      Right **0J9L**
  Subdural Space **0094**
  Tarsal
    Left **0Q9M**
    Right **0Q9L**
  Tendon
    Abdomen
      Left **0L9G**
      Right **0L9F**
    Ankle
      Left **0L9T**
      Right **0L9S**
    Foot
      Left **0L9W**
      Right **0L9V**
    Hand
      Left **0L98**
      Right **0L97**

    Head and Neck **0L90**
    Hip
      Left **0L9K**
      Right **0L9J**
    Knee
      Left **0L9R**
      Right **0L9Q**
    Lower Arm and Wrist
      Left **0L96**
      Right **0L95**
    Lower Leg
      Left **0L9P**
      Right **0L9N**
    Perineum **0L9H**
    Shoulder
      Left **0L92**
      Right **0L91**
    Thorax
      Left **0L9D**
      Right **0L9C**
    Trunk
      Left **0L9B**
      Right **0L99**
    Upper Arm
      Left **0L94**
      Right **0L93**
    Upper Leg
      Left **0L9M**
      Right **0L9L**
  Testis
    Bilateral **0V9C**
    Left **0V9B**
    Right **0V99**
  Thalamus **0099**
  Thymus **079M**
  Thyroid Gland **0G9K**
    Left Lobe **0G9G**
    Right Lobe **0G9H**
  Tibia
    Left **0Q9H**
    Right **0Q9G**
  Toe Nail **0H9R**
  Tongue **0C97**
  Tonsils **0C9P**
  Tooth
    Lower **0C9X**
    Upper **0C9W**
  Trachea **0B91**
  Tunica Vaginalis
    Left **0V97**
    Right **0V96**
  Turbinate, Nasal **099L**
  Tympanic Membrane
    Left **0998**
    Right **0997**
  Ulna
    Left **0P9L**
    Right **0P9K**
  Ureter
    Left **0T97**
    Right **0T96**
  Ureters, Bilateral **0T98**
  Urethra **0T9D**
  Uterine Supporting Structure **0U94**
  Uterus **0U99**
  Uvula **0C9N**
  Vagina **0U9G**
  Vas Deferens
    Bilateral **0V9Q**
    Left **0V9P**
    Right **0V9N**

Drainage - *continued*
- Vein
  - Axillary
    - Left **0598**
    - Right **0597**
  - Azygos **0590**
  - Basilic
    - Left **059C**
    - Right **059B**
  - Brachial
    - Left **059A**
    - Right **0599**
  - Cephalic
    - Left **059F**
    - Right **059D**
  - Colic **0697**
  - Common Iliac
    - Left **069D**
    - Right **069C**
  - Esophageal **0693**
  - External Iliac
    - Left **069G**
    - Right **069F**
  - External Jugular
    - Left **059Q**
    - Right **059P**
  - Face
    - Left **059V**
    - Right **059T**
  - Femoral
    - Left **069N**
    - Right **069M**
  - Foot
    - Left **069V**
    - Right **069T**
  - Gastric **0692**
  - Greater Saphenous
    - Left **069Q**
    - Right **069P**
  - Hand
    - Left **059H**
    - Right **059G**
  - Hemiazygos **0591**
  - Hepatic **0694**
  - Hypogastric
    - Left **069J**
    - Right **069H**
  - Inferior Mesenteric **0696**
  - Innominate
    - Left **0594**
    - Right **0593**
  - Internal Jugular
    - Left **059N**
    - Right **059M**
  - Intracranial **059L**
  - Lesser Saphenous
    - Left **069S**
    - Right **069R**
  - Lower **069Y**
  - Portal **0698**
  - Renal
    - Left **069B**
    - Right **0699**
  - Splenic **0691**
  - Subclavian
    - Left **0596**
    - Right **0595**
  - Superior Mesenteric **0695**
  - Upper **059Y**
  - Vertebral
    - Left **059S**
    - Right **059R**

Drainage - *continued*
- Vena Cava, Inferior **0690**
- Vertebra
  - Cervical **0P93**
  - Lumbar **0Q90**
  - Thoracic **0P94**
- Vesicle
  - Bilateral **0V93**
  - Left **0V92**
  - Right **0V91**
- Vitreous
  - Left **0895**
  - Right **0894**
- Vocal Cord
  - Left **0C9V**
  - Right **0C9T**
- Vulva **0U9M**
- Wrist Region
  - Left **0X9H**
  - Right **0X9G**

Dressing
- Abdominal Wall **2W23X4Z**
- Arm
  - Lower
    - Left **2W2DX4Z**
    - Right **2W2CX4Z**
  - Upper
    - Left **2W2BX4Z**
    - Right **2W2AX4Z**
- Back **2W25X4Z**
- Chest Wall **2W24X4Z**
- Extremity
  - Lower
    - Left **2W2MX4Z**
    - Right **2W2LX4Z**
  - Upper
    - Left **2W29X4Z**
    - Right **2W28X4Z**
- Face **2W21X4Z**
- Finger
  - Left **2W2KX4Z**
  - Right **2W2JX4Z**
- Foot
  - Left **2W2TX4Z**
  - Right **2W2SX4Z**
- Hand
  - Left **2W2FX4Z**
  - Right **2W2EX4Z**
- Head **2W20X4Z**
- Inguinal Region
  - Left **2W27X4Z**
  - Right **2W26X4Z**
- Leg
  - Lower
    - Left **2W2RX4Z**
    - Right **2W2QX4Z**
  - Upper
    - Left **2W2PX4Z**
    - Right **2W2NX4Z**
- Neck **2W22X4Z**
- Thumb
  - Left **2W2HX4Z**
  - Right **2W2GX4Z**
- Toe
  - Left **2W2VX4Z**
  - Right **2W2UX4Z**

Driver stent (RX) (OTW) *use* Intraluminal Device
Drotrecogin alfa *see* Introduction of Recombinant Human-activated Protein C
Duct of Santorini *use* Duct, Pancreatic, Accessory
Duct of Wirsung *use* Duct, Pancreatic

Ductogram, mammary *see* Plain Radiography, Skin, Subcutaneous Tissue and Breast **BH0**
Ductography, mammary *see* Plain Radiography, Skin, Subcutaneous Tissue and Breast **BH0**
Ductus deferens
  use Vas Deferens, Left
  use Vas Deferens, Right
  use Vas Deferens
  use Vas Deferens, Bilateral
Duodenal ampulla *use* Ampulla of Vater
Duodenectomy
  see Excision, Duodenum **0DB9**
  see Resection, Duodenum **0DT9**
Duodenocholedochotomy *see* Drainage, Gallbladder **0F94**
Duodenocystostomy
  see Bypass, Gallbladder **0F14**
  see Drainage, Gallbladder **0F94**
Duodenoenterostomy
  see Bypass, Gastrointestinal System **0D1**
  see Drainage, Gastrointestinal System **0D9**
Duodenojejunal flexure *use* Jejunum
Duodenolysis *see* Release, Duodenum **0DN9**
Duodenorrhaphy *see* Repair, Duodenum **0DQ9**
Duodenostomy
  see Bypass, Duodenum **0D19**
  see Drainage, Duodenum **0D99**
Duodenotomy *see* Drainage, Duodenum **0D99**
DuraHeart Left Ventricular Assist System *use* Implantable Heart Assist System in Heart and Great Vessels
Dural venous sinus *use* Vein, Intracranial
Durata® Defibrillation Lead *use* Cardiac Lead, Defibrillator in **02H**
Dynesys® Dynamic Stabilization System
  use Spinal Stabilization Device, Pedicle-Based in **0RH**
  use Spinal Stabilization Device, Pedicle-Based in **0SH**

E

E-Luminexx™ (Biliary)(Vascular) Stent *use* Intraluminal Device
Earlobe
  use Ear, External, Left
  use Ear, External, Bilateral
  use Ear, External, Right
Echocardiogram *see* Ultrasonography, Heart **B24**
Echography *see* Ultrasonography
ECMO *see* Performance, Circulatory **5A15**
EEG (electroencephalogram) *see* Measurement, Central Nervous **4A00**
EGD (esophagogastroduodenoscopy) 0DJ08ZZ
Eighth cranial nerve *use* Nerve, Acoustic
Ejaculatory duct
  use Vas Deferens, Bilateral
  use Vas Deferens, Left
  use Vas Deferens, Right
  use Vas Deferens
EKG (electrocardiogram) *see* Measurement, Cardiac **4A02**
Electrical bone growth stimulator (EBGS)
  use Bone Growth Stimulator in Head and Facial Bones
  use Bone Growth Stimulator in Upper Bones
  use Bone Growth Stimulator in Lower Bones
Electrical muscle stimulation (EMS) lead *use* Stimulator Lead in Muscles

Electrocautery
  Destruction *see* Destruction
  Repair *see* Repair
Electroconvulsive Therapy
  Bilateral-Multiple Seizure **GZB3ZZZ**
  Bilateral-Single Seizure **GZB2ZZZ**
  Electroconvulsive Therapy, Other **GZB4ZZZ**
  Unilateral-Multiple Seizure **GZB1ZZZ**
  Unilateral-Single Seizure **GZB0ZZZ**
Electroencephalogram (EEG) *see*
  Measurement, Central Nervous **4A00**
Electromagnetic Therapy
  Central Nervous **6A22**
  Urinary **6A21**
Electronic muscle stimulator lead *use*
  Stimulator Lead in Muscles
Electrophysiologic stimulation (EPS) *see*
  Measurement, Cardiac **4A02**
Electroshock therapy *see* Electroconvulsive
  Therapy
Elevation, bone fragments, skull *see*
  Reposition, Head and Facial Bones **0NS**
Eleventh cranial nerve *use* Nerve, Accessory
Embolectomy *see* Extirpation
Embolization
  see Occlusion
  see Restriction
Embolization coil(s) *use* Intraluminal Device
EMG (electromyogram) *see* Measurement,
  Musculoskeletal **4A0F**
Encephalon *use* Brain
Endarterectomy
  see Extirpation, Upper Arteries **03C**
  see Extirpation, Lower Arteries **04C**
**Endeavor® (III)(IV) (Sprint) Zotarolimus-
  eluting Coronary Stent System** *use*
  Intraluminal Device, Drug-eluting in Heart
  and Great Vessels
EndoSure® sensor *use* Monitoring Device,
  Pressure Sensor in **02H**
**ENDOTAK RELIANCE® (G) Defibrillation
  Lead** *use* Cardiac Lead, Defibrillator in **02H**
Endotracheal tube (cuffed)(double-lumen) *use*
  Intraluminal Device, Endotracheal Airway in
  Respiratory System
Endurant® Endovascular Stent Graft *use*
  Intraluminal Device
Enlargement
  see Dilation
  see Repair
EnRhythm *use* Pacemaker, Dual Chamber in
  0JH
Enterorrhaphy *see* Repair, Gastrointestinal
  System **0DQ**
Enterra gastric neurostimulator *use* Stimulator
  Generator, Multiple Array in **0JH**
Enucleation
  Eyeball *see* Resection, Eye **08T**
  Eyeball with prosthetic implant *see*
  Replacement, Eye **08R**
Ependyma *use* Cerebral Ventricle
Epicel® cultured epidermal autograft *use*
  Autologous Tissue Substitute
Epic™ Stented Tissue Valve (aortic) *use*
  Zooplastic Tissue in Heart and Great Vessels
Epidermis *use* Skin
Epididymectomy
  see Excision, Male Reproductive System **0VB**
  see Resection, Male Reproductive System
  0VT

Epididymoplasty
  see Repair, Male Reproductive System **0VQ**
  see Supplement, Male Reproductive System
  0VU
Epididymorrhaphy *see* Repair, Male
  Reproductive System **0VQ**
Epididymotomy *see* Drainage, Male
  Reproductive System **0V9**
Epiphysiodesis
  see Fusion, Upper Joints **0RG**
  see Fusion, Lower Joints **0SG**
Epiploic foramen *use* Peritoneum
Epiretinal Visual Prosthesis
  use Epiretinal Visual Prosthesis in Eye
  Insertion of device in
    Left **08H105Z**
    Right **08H005Z**
Episiorrhaphy *see* Repair, Perineum, Female
  0WQN
Episiotomy *see* Division, Perineum, Female
  0W8N
Epithalamus *use* Thalamus
Epitrochlear lymph node
  use Lymphatic, Upper Extremity, Left
  use Lymphatic, Upper Extremity, Right
EPS (electrophysiologic stimulation) *see*
  Measurement, Cardiac **4A02**
Eptifibatide, infusion *see* Introduction of
  Platelet Inhibitor
**ERCP (endoscopic retrograde
  cholangiopancreatography)** *see*
  Fluoroscopy, Hepatobiliary System and
  Pancreas **BF1**
Erector spinae muscle
  use Muscle, Trunk, Left
  use Muscle, Trunk, Right
Esophageal artery *use* Aorta, Thoracic
Esophageal obturator airway (EOA) *use*
  Intraluminal Device, Airway in
  Gastrointestinal System
Esophageal plexus *use* Nerve, Thoracic
  Sympathetic
Esophagectomy
  see Excision, Gastrointestinal System **0DB**
  see Resection, Gastrointestinal System **0DT**
Esophagocoloplasty
  see Repair, Gastrointestinal System **0DQ**
  see Supplement, Gastrointestinal System **0DU**
Esophagoenterostomy
  see Bypass, Gastrointestinal System **0D1**
  see Drainage, Gastrointestinal System **0D9**
Esophagoesophagostomy
  see Bypass, Gastrointestinal System **0D1**
  see Drainage, Gastrointestinal System **0D9**
Esophagogastrectomy
  see Excision, Gastrointestinal System **0DB**
  see Resection, Gastrointestinal System **0DT**
Esophagogastroduodenoscopy (EGD)
  0DJ08ZZ
Esophagogastroplasty
  see Repair, Gastrointestinal System **0DQ**
  see Supplement, Gastrointestinal System **0DU**
Esophagogastroscopy 0DJ68ZZ
Esophagogastrostomy
  see Bypass, Gastrointestinal System **0D1**
  see Drainage, Gastrointestinal System **0D9**
Esophagojejunoplasty *see* Supplement,
  Gastrointestinal System **0DU**
Esophagojejunostomy
  see Drainage, Gastrointestinal System **0D9**
  see Bypass, Gastrointestinal System **0D1**
Esophagomyotomy *see* Division,
  Esophagogastric Junction **0D84**

Esophagoplasty
  see Repair, Gastrointestinal System **0DQ**
  see Replacement, Esophagus **0DR5**
  see Supplement, Gastrointestinal System **0DU**
Esophagoplication *see* Restriction,
  Gastrointestinal System **0DV**
Esophagorrhaphy *see* Repair, Gastrointestinal
  System **0DQ**
Esophagoscopy 0DJ08ZZ
Esophagotomy *see* Drainage, Gastrointestinal
  System **0D9**
Esteem® implantable hearing system *use*
  Hearing Device in Ear, Nose, Sinus
**ESWL (extracorporeal shock wave
  lithotripsy)** *see* Fragmentation
Ethmoidal air cell
  use Sinus, Ethmoid, Left
  use Sinus, Ethmoid, Right
Ethmoidectomy
  see Excision, Ear, Nose, Sinus **09B**
  see Resection, Ear, Nose, Sinus **09T**
  see Excision, Head and Facial Bones **0NB**
  see Resection, Head and Facial Bones **0NT**
Ethmoidotomy *see* Drainage, Ear, Nose, Sinus
  099
Evacuation
  Hematoma *see* Extirpation
  Other Fluid *see* Drainage
Everolimus-eluting coronary stent *use*
  Intraluminal Device, Drug-eluting in Heart
  and Great Vessels
Evisceration
  Eyeball *see* Resection, Eye **08T**
  Eyeball with prosthetic implant *see*
  Replacement, Eye **08R**
Ex-PRESS™ mini glaucoma shunt *use*
  Synthetic Substitute
Examination *see* Inspection
Exchange *see* Change device in
Excision
  Abdominal Wall **0WBF**
  Acetabulum
    Left **0QB5**
    Right **0QB4**
  Adenoids **0CBQ**
  Ampulla of Vater **0FBC**
  Anal Sphincter **0DBR**
  Ankle Region
    Left **0YBL**
    Right **0YBK**
  Anus **0DBQ**
  Aorta
    Abdominal **04B0**
    Thoracic **02BW**
  Aortic Body **0GBD**
  Appendix **0DBJ**
  Arm
    Lower
      Left **0XBF**
      Right **0XBD**
    Upper
      Left **0XB9**
      Right **0XB8**
  Artery
    Anterior Tibial
      Left **04BQ**
      Right **04BP**
    Axillary
      Left **03B6**
      Right **03B5**
    Brachial
      Left **03B8**
      Right **03B7**

Excision - *continued*
   Celiac **04B1**
   Colic
      Left **04B7**
      Middle **04B8**
      Right **04B6**
   Common Carotid
      Left **03BJ**
      Right **03BH**
   Common Iliac
      Left **04BD**
      Right **04BC**
   External Carotid
      Left **03BN**
      Right **03BM**
   External Iliac
      Left **04BJ**
      Right **04BH**
   Face **03BR**
   Femoral
      Left **04BL**
      Right **04BK**
   Foot
      Left **04BW**
      Right **04BV**
   Gastric **04B2**
   Hand
      Left **03BF**
      Right **03BD**
   Hepatic **04B3**
   Inferior Mesenteric **04BB**
   Innominate **03B2**
   Internal Carotid
      Left **03BL**
      Right **03BK**
   Internal Iliac
      Left **04BF**
      Right **04BE**
   Internal Mammary
      Left **03B1**
      Right **03B0**
   Intracranial **03BG**
   Lower **04BY**
   Peroneal
      Left **04BU**
      Right **04BT**
   Popliteal
      Left **04BN**
      Right **04BM**
   Posterior Tibial
      Left **04BS**
      Right **04BR**
   Pulmonary
      Left **02BR**
      Right **02BQ**
   Pulmonary Trunk **02BP**
   Radial
      Left **03BC**
      Right **03BB**
   Renal
      Left **04BA**
      Right **04B9**
   Splenic **04B4**
   Subclavian
      Left **03B4**
      Right **03B3**
   Superior Mesenteric **04B5**
   Temporal
      Left **03BT**
      Right **03BS**

Excision - *continued*
   Thyroid
      Left **03BV**
      Right **03BU**
   Ulnar
      Left **03BA**
      Right **03B9**
   Upper **03BY**
   Vertebral
      Left **03BQ**
      Right **03BP**
  Atrium
      Left **02B7**
      Right **02B6**
  Auditory Ossicle
      Left **09BA0Z**
      Right **09B90Z**
  Axilla
      Left **0XB5**
      Right **0XB4**
  Back
      Lower **0WBL**
      Upper **0WBK**
  Basal Ganglia **00B8**
  Bladder **0TBB**
  Bladder Neck **0TBC**
  Bone
    Ethmoid
      Left **0NBG**
      Right **0NBF**
    Frontal
      Left **0NB2**
      Right **0NB1**
    Hyoid **0NBX**
    Lacrimal
      Left **0NBJ**
      Right **0NBH**
    Nasal **0NBB**
    Occipital
      Left **0NB8**
      Right **0NB7**
    Palatine
      Left **0NBL**
      Right **0NBK**
    Parietal
      Left **0NB4**
      Right **0NB3**
    Pelvic
      Left **0QB3**
      Right **0QB2**
    Sphenoid
      Left **0NBD**
      Right **0NBC**
    Temporal
      Left **0NB6**
      Right **0NB5**
    Zygomatic
      Left **0NBN**
      Right **0NBM**
  Brain **00B0**
  Breast
      Bilateral **0HBV**
      Left **0HBU**
      Right **0HBT**
      Supernumerary **0HBY**
  Bronchus
    Lingula **0BB9**
    Lower Lobe
      Left **0BBB**
      Right **0BB6**

Excision - *continued*
    Main
      Left **0BB7**
      Right **0BB3**
    Middle Lobe, Right **0BB5**
    Upper Lobe
      Left **0BB8**
      Right **0BB4**
  Buccal Mucosa **0CB4**
  Bursa and Ligament
    Abdomen
      Left **0MBJ**
      Right **0MBH**
    Ankle
      Left **0MBR**
      Right **0MBQ**
    Elbow
      Left **0MB4**
      Right **0MB3**
    Foot
      Left **0MBT**
      Right **0MBS**
    Hand
      Left **0MB8**
      Right **0MB7**
    Head and Neck **0MB0**
    Hip
      Left **0MBM**
      Right **0MBL**
    Knee
      Left **0MBP**
      Right **0MBN**
    Lower Extremity
      Left **0MBW**
      Right **0MBV**
    Perineum **0MBK**
    Shoulder
      Left **0MB2**
      Right **0MB1**
    Thorax
      Left **0MBG**
      Right **0MBF**
    Trunk
      Left **0MBD**
      Right **0MBC**
    Upper Extremity
      Left **0MBB**
      Right **0MB9**
    Wrist
      Left **0MB6**
      Right **0MB5**
  Buttock
      Left **0YB1**
      Right **0YB0**
  Carina **0BB2**
  Carotid Bodies, Bilateral **0GB8**
  Carotid Body
      Left **0GB6**
      Right **0GB7**
  Carpal
      Left **0PBN**
      Right **0PBM**
  Cecum **0DBH**
  Cerebellum **00BC**
  Cerebral Hemisphere **00B7**
  Cerebral Meninges **00B1**
  Cerebral Ventricle **00B6**
  Cervix **0UBC**
  Chest Wall **0WB8**
  Chordae Tendineae **02B9**

Choroid
   Left **08BB**
   Right **08BA**
Cisterna Chyli **07BL**
Clavicle
   Left **0PBB**
   Right **0PB9**
Clitoris **0UBJ**
Coccygeal Glomus **0GBB**
Coccyx **0QBS**
Colon
   Ascending **0DBK**
   Descending **0DBM**
   Sigmoid **0DBN**
   Transverse **0DBL**
Conduction Mechanism **02B8**
Conjunctiva
   Left **08BTXZ**
   Right **08BSXZ**
Cord
   Bilateral **0VBH**
   Left **0VBG**
   Right **0VBF**
Cornea
   Left **08B9XZ**
   Right **08B8XZ**
Cul-de-sac **0UBF**
Diaphragm
   Left **0BBS**
   Right **0BBR**
Disc
   Cervical Vertebral **0RB3**
   Cervicothoracic Vertebral **0RB5**
   Lumbar Vertebral **0SB2**
   Lumbosacral **0SB4**
   Thoracic Vertebral **0RB9**
   Thoracolumbar Vertebral **0RBB**
Duct
   Common Bile **0FB9**
   Cystic **0FB8**
   Hepatic
      Left **0FB6**
      Right **0FB5**
   Lacrimal
      Left **08BY**
      Right **08BX**
   Pancreatic **0FBD**
      Accessory **0FBF**
   Parotid
      Left **0CBC**
      Right **0CBB**
Duodenum **0DB9**
Dura Mater **00B2**
Ear
   External
      Left **09B1**
      Right **09B0**
   External Auditory Canal
      Left **09B4**
      Right **09B3**
   Inner
      Left **09BE0Z**
      Right **09BD0Z**
   Middle
      Left **09B60Z**
      Right **09B50Z**
Elbow Region
   Left **0XBC**
   Right **0XBB**

Epididymis
   Bilateral **0VBL**
   Left **0VBK**
   Right **0VBJ**
Epiglottis **0CBR**
Esophagogastric Junction **0DB4**
Esophagus **0DB5**
   Lower **0DB3**
   Middle **0DB2**
   Upper **0DB1**
Eustachian Tube
   Left **09BG**
   Right **09BF**
Extremity
   Lower
      Left **0YBB**
      Right **0YB9**
   Upper
      Left **0XB7**
      Right **0XB6**
Eye
   Left **08B1**
   Right **08B0**
Eyelid
   Lower
      Left **08BR**
      Right **08BQ**
   Upper
      Left **08BP**
      Right **08BN**
Face **0WB2**
Fallopian Tube
   Left **0UB6**
   Right **0UB5**
Fallopian Tubes, Bilateral **0UB7**
Femoral Region
   Left **0YB8**
   Right **0YB7**
Femoral Shaft
   Left **0QB9**
   Right **0QB8**
Femur
   Lower
      Left **0QBC**
      Right **0QBB**
   Upper
      Left **0QB7**
      Right **0QB6**
Fibula
   Left **0QBK**
   Right **0QBJ**
Finger Nail **0HBQXZ**
Foot
   Left **0YBN**
   Right **0YBM**
Gallbladder **0FB4**
Gingiva
   Lower **0CB6**
   Upper **0CB5**
Gland
   Adrenal
      Bilateral **0GB4**
      Left **0GB2**
      Right **0GB3**
   Lacrimal
      Left **08BW**
      Right **08BV**
   Minor Salivary **0CBJ**
   Parotid
      Left **0CB9**
      Right **0CB8**

   Pituitary **0GB0**
   Sublingual
      Left **0CBF**
      Right **0CBD**
   Submaxillary
      Left **0CBH**
      Right **0CBG**
   Vestibular **0UBL**
Glenoid Cavity
   Left **0PB8**
   Right **0PB7**
Glomus Jugulare **0GBC**
Hand
   Left **0XBK**
   Right **0XBJ**
Head **0WB0**
Humeral Head
   Left **0PBD**
   Right **0PBC**
Humeral Shaft
   Left **0PBG**
   Right **0PBF**
Hymen **0UBK**
Hypothalamus **00BA**
Ileocecal Valve **0DBC**
Ileum **0DBB**
Inguinal Region
   Left **0YB6**
   Right **0YB5**
Intestine
   Large **0DBE**
      Left **0DBG**
      Right **0DBF**
   Small **0DB8**
Iris
   Left **08BD3Z**
   Right **08BC3Z**
Jaw
   Lower **0WB5**
   Upper **0WB4**
Jejunum **0DBA**
Joint
   Acromioclavicular
      Left **0RBH**
      Right **0RBG**
   Ankle
      Left **0SBG**
      Right **0SBF**
   Carpal
      Left **0RBR**
      Right **0RBQ**
   Cervical Vertebral **0RB1**
   Cervicothoracic Vertebral **0RB4**
   Coccygeal **0SB6**
   Elbow
      Left **0RBM**
      Right **0RBL**
   Finger Phalangeal
      Left **0RBX**
      Right **0RBW**
   Hip
      Left **0SBB**
      Right **0SB9**
   Knee
      Left **0SBD**
      Right **0SBC**
   Lumbar Vertebral **0SB0**
   Lumbosacral **0SB3**
   Metacarpocarpal
      Left **0RBT**
      Right **0RBS**

Excision - *continued*
- Pancreas **0FBG**
- Para-aortic Body **0GB9**
- Paraganglion Extremity **0GBF**
- Parathyroid Gland **0GBR**
  - Inferior
    - Left **0GBP**
    - Right **0GBN**
  - Multiple **0GBQ**
  - Superior
    - Left **0GBM**
    - Right **0GBL**
- Patella
  - Left **0QBF**
  - Right **0QBD**
- Penis **0VBS**
- Pericardium **02BN**
- Perineum
  - Female **0WBN**
  - Male **0WBM**
- Peritoneum **0DBW**
- Phalanx
  - Finger
    - Left **0PBV**
    - Right **0PBT**
  - Thumb
    - Left **0PBS**
    - Right **0PBR**
  - Toe
    - Left **0QBR**
    - Right **0QBQ**
- Pharynx **0CBM**
- Pineal Body **0GB1**
- Pleura
  - Left **0BBP**
  - Right **0BBN**
- Pons **00BB**
- Prepuce **0VBT**
- Prostate **0VB0**
- Radius
  - Left **0PBJ**
  - Right **0PBH**
- Rectum **0DBP**
- Retina
  - Left **08BF3Z**
  - Right **08BE3Z**
- Retroperitoneum **0WBH**
- Rib
  - Left **0PB2**
  - Right **0PB1**
- Sacrum **0QB1**
- Scapula
  - Left **0PB6**
  - Right **0PB5**
- Sclera
  - Left **08B7XZ**
  - Right **08B6XZ**
- Scrotum **0VB5**
- Septum
  - Atrial **02B5**
  - Nasal **09BM**
  - Ventricular **02BM**
- Shoulder Region
  - Left **0XB3**
  - Right **0XB2**
- Sinus
  - Accessory **09BP**
  - Ethmoid
    - Left **09BV**
    - Right **09BU**
  - Frontal
    - Left **09BT**

Excision - *continued*
- Right **09BS**
- Mastoid
  - Left **09BC**
  - Right **09BB**
- Maxillary
  - Left **09BR**
  - Right **09BQ**
- Sphenoid
  - Left **09BX**
  - Right **09BW**
- Skin
  - Abdomen **0HB7XZ**
  - Back **0HB6XZ**
  - Buttock **0HB8XZ**
  - Chest **0HB5XZ**
  - Ear
    - Left **0HB3XZ**
    - Right **0HB2XZ**
  - Face **0HB1XZ**
  - Foot
    - Left **0HBNXZ**
    - Right **0HBMXZ**
  - Genitalia **0HBAXZ**
  - Hand
    - Left **0HBGXZ**
    - Right **0HBFXZ**
  - Lower Arm
    - Left **0HBEXZ**
    - Right **0HBDXZ**
  - Lower Leg
    - Left **0HBLXZ**
    - Right **0HBKXZ**
  - Neck **0HB4XZ**
  - Perineum **0HB9XZ**
  - Scalp **0HB0XZ**
  - Upper Arm
    - Left **0HBCXZ**
    - Right **0HBBXZ**
  - Upper Leg
    - Left **0HBJXZ**
    - Right **0HBHXZ**
- Skull **0NB0**
- Spinal Cord
  - Cervical **00BW**
  - Lumbar **00BY**
  - Thoracic **00BX**
- Spinal Meninges **00BT**
- Spleen **07BP**
- Sternum **0PB0**
- Stomach **0DB6**
  - Pylorus **0DB7**
- Subcutaneous Tissue and Fascia
  - Abdomen **0JB8**
  - Back **0JB7**
  - Buttock **0JB9**
  - Chest **0JB6**
  - Face **0JB1**
  - Foot
    - Left **0JBR**
    - Right **0JBQ**
  - Hand
    - Left **0JBK**
    - Right **0JBJ**
  - Lower Arm
    - Left **0JBH**
    - Right **0JBG**
  - Lower Leg
    - Left **0JBP**
    - Right **0JBN**

Excision - *continued*
- Neck
  - Anterior **0JB4**
  - Posterior **0JB5**
- Pelvic Region **0JBC**
- Perineum **0JBB**
- Scalp **0JB0**
- Upper Arm
  - Left **0JBF**
  - Right **0JBD**
- Upper Leg
  - Left **0JBM**
  - Right **0JBL**
- Tarsal
  - Left **0QBM**
  - Right **0QBL**
- Tendon
  - Abdomen
    - Left **0LBG**
    - Right **0LBF**
  - Ankle
    - Left **0LBT**
    - Right **0LBS**
  - Foot
    - Left **0LBW**
    - Right **0LBV**
  - Hand
    - Left **0LB8**
    - Right **0LB7**
  - Head and Neck **0LB0**
  - Hip
    - Left **0LBK**
    - Right **0LBJ**
  - Knee
    - Left **0LBR**
    - Right **0LBQ**
  - Lower Arm and Wrist
    - Left **0LB6**
    - Right **0LB5**
  - Lower Leg
    - Left **0LBP**
    - Right **0LBN**
  - Perineum **0LBH**
  - Shoulder
    - Left **0LB2**
    - Right **0LB1**
  - Thorax
    - Left **0LBD**
    - Right **0LBC**
  - Trunk
    - Left **0LBB**
    - Right **0LB9**
  - Upper Arm
    - Left **0LB4**
    - Right **0LB3**
  - Upper Leg
    - Left **0LBM**
    - Right **0LBL**
- Testis
  - Bilateral **0VBC**
  - Left **0VBB**
  - Right **0VB9**
- Thalamus **00B9**
- Thymus **07BM**
- Thyroid Gland
  - Left Lobe **0GBG**
  - Right Lobe **0GBH**
- Tibia
  - Left **0QBH**
  - Right **0QBG**
- Toe Nail **0HBRXZ**
- Tongue **0CB7**

Excision - *continued*
  Tonsils **0CBP**
  Tooth
    Lower **0CBX**
    Upper **0CBW**
  Trachea **0BB1**
  Tunica Vaginalis
    Left **0VB7**
    Right **0VB6**
  Turbinate, Nasal **09BL**
  Tympanic Membrane
    Left **09B8**
    Right **09B7**
  Ulna
    Left **0PBL**
    Right **0PBK**
  Ureter
    Left **0TB7**
    Right **0TB6**
  Urethra **0TBD**
  Uterine Supporting Structure **0UB4**
  Uterus **0UB9**
  Uvula **0CBN**
  Vagina **0UBG**
  Valve
    Aortic **02BF**
    Mitral **02BG**
    Pulmonary **02BH**
    Tricuspid **02BJ**
  Vas Deferens
    Bilateral **0VBQ**
    Left **0VBP**
    Right **0VBN**
  Vein
    Axillary
      Left **05B8**
      Right **05B7**
    Azygos **05B0**
    Basilic
      Left **05BC**
      Right **05BB**
    Brachial
      Left **05BA**
      Right **05B9**
    Cephalic
      Left **05BF**
      Right **05BD**
    Colic **06B7**
    Common Iliac
      Left **06BD**
      Right **06BC**
    Coronary **02B4**
    Esophageal **06B3**
    External Iliac
      Left **06BG**
      Right **06BF**
    External Jugular
      Left **05BQ**
      Right **05BP**
    Face
      Left **05BV**
      Right **05BT**
    Femoral
      Left **06BN**
      Right **06BM**
    Foot
      Left **06BV**
      Right **06BT**
    Gastric **06B2**
    Greater Saphenous
      Left **06BQ**
      Right **06BP**

Excision - *continued*
  Hand
    Left **05BH**
    Right **05BG**
  Hemiazygos **05B1**
  Hepatic **06B4**
  Hypogastric
    Left **06BJ**
    Right **06BH**
  Inferior Mesenteric **06B6**
  Innominate
    Left **05B4**
    Right **05B3**
  Internal Jugular
    Left **05BN**
    Right **05BM**
  Intracranial **05BL**
  Lesser Saphenous
    Left **06BS**
    Right **06BR**
  Lower **06BY**
  Portal **06B8**
  Pulmonary
    Left **02BT**
    Right **02BS**
  Renal
    Left **06BB**
    Right **06B9**
  Splenic **06B1**
  Subclavian
    Left **05B6**
    Right **05B5**
  Superior Mesenteric **06B5**
  Upper **05BY**
  Vertebral
    Left **05BS**
    Right **05BR**
  Vena Cava
    Inferior **06B0**
    Superior **02BV**
  Ventricle
    Left **02BL**
    Right **02BK**
  Vertebra
    Cervical **0PB3**
    Lumbar **0QB0**
    Thoracic **0PB4**
  Vesicle
    Bilateral **0VB3**
    Left **0VB2**
    Right **0VB1**
  Vitreous
    Left **08B53Z**
    Right **08B43Z**
  Vocal Cord
    Left **0CBV**
    Right **0CBT**
  Vulva **0UBM**
  Wrist Region
    Left **0XBH**
    Right **0XBG**
Exclusion, Left atrial appendage (LAA) *see*
  Occlusion, Atrium, Left **02L7**
Exercise, rehabilitation *see* Motor Treatment,
  Rehabilitation **F07**
Exploration *see* Inspection
Express® (LD) Premounted Stent System *use*
  Intraluminal Device
Express® Biliary SD Monorail® Premounted
  Stent System *use* Intraluminal Device
Express® SD Renal Monorail® Premounted
  Stent System *use* Intraluminal Device

Extensor carpi radialis muscle
  use Muscle, Lower Arm and Wrist, Left
  use Muscle, Lower Arm and Wrist, Right
Extensor carpi ulnaris muscle
  use Muscle, Lower Arm and Wrist, Left
  use Muscle, Lower Arm and Wrist, Right
Extensor digitorum brevis muscle
  use Muscle, Foot, Right
  use Muscle, Foot, Left
Extensor digitorum longus muscle
  use Muscle, Lower Leg, Left
  use Muscle, Lower Leg, Right
Extensor hallucis brevis muscle
  use Muscle, Foot, Right
  use Muscle, Foot, Left
Extensor hallucis longus muscle
  use Muscle, Lower Leg, Right
  use Muscle, Lower Leg, Left
External anal sphincter *use* Anal Sphincter
External auditory meatus
  use Ear, External Auditory Canal, Left
  use Ear, External Auditory Canal, Right
External fixator
  use External Fixation Device in Head and
  Facial Bones
  use External Fixation Device in Upper Bones
  use External Fixation Device in Lower Bones
  use External Fixation Device in Upper Joints
  use External Fixation Device in Lower Joints
External maxillary artery *use* Artery, Face
External naris *use* Nose
External oblique aponeurosis *use*
  Subcutaneous Tissue and Fascia, Trunk
External oblique muscle
  use Muscle, Abdomen, Left
  use Muscle, Abdomen, Right
External popliteal nerve *use* Nerve, Peroneal
External pudendal artery
  use Artery, Femoral, Right
  use Artery, Femoral, Left
External pudendal vein
  use Vein, Greater Saphenous, Right
  use Vein, Greater Saphenous, Left
External urethral sphincter *use* Urethra
Extirpation
  Acetabulum
    Left **0QC5**
    Right **0QC4**
  Adenoids **0CCQ**
  Ampulla of Vater **0FCC**
  Anal Sphincter **0DCR**
  Anterior Chamber
    Left **08C3**
    Right **08C2**
  Anus **0DCQ**
  Aorta
    Abdominal **04C0**
    Thoracic **02CW**
  Aortic Body **0GCD**
  Appendix **0DCJ**
  Artery
    Anterior Tibial
      Left **04CQ**
      Right **04CP**
    Axillary
      Left **03C6**
      Right **03C5**
    Brachial
      Left **03C8**
      Right **03C7**
    Celiac **04C1**

Extirpation- *continued*
- Coccyx **0QCS**
- Colon
  - Ascending **0DCK**
  - Descending **0DCM**
  - Sigmoid **0DCN**
  - Transverse **0DCL**
- Conduction Mechanism **02C8**
- Conjunctiva
  - Left **08CTXZZ**
  - Right **08CSXZZ**
- Cord
  - Bilateral **0VCH**
  - Left **0VCG**
  - Right **0VCF**
- Cornea
  - Left **08C9XZZ**
  - Right **08C8XZZ**
- Cul-de-sac **0UCF**
- Diaphragm
  - Left **0BCS**
  - Right **0BCR**
- Disc
  - Cervical Vertebral **0RC3**
  - Cervicothoracic Vertebral **0RC5**
  - Lumbar Vertebral **0SC2**
  - Lumbosacral **0SC4**
  - Thoracic Vertebral **0RC9**
  - Thoracolumbar Vertebral **0RCB**
- Duct
  - Common Bile **0FC9**
  - Cystic **0FC8**
  - Hepatic
    - Left **0FC6**
    - Right **0FC5**
  - Lacrimal
    - Left **08CY**
    - Right **08CX**
  - Pancreatic **0FCD**
    - Accessory **0FCF**
  - Parotid
    - Left **0CCC**
    - Right **0CCB**
- Duodenum **0DC9**
- Dura Mater **00C2**
- Ear
  - External
    - Left **09C1**
    - Right **09C0**
  - External Auditory Canal
    - Left **09C4**
    - Right **09C3**
  - Inner
    - Left **09CE0ZZ**
    - Right **09CD0ZZ**
  - Middle
    - Left **09C60ZZ**
    - Right **09C50ZZ**
- Endometrium **0UCB**
- Epididymis
  - Bilateral **0VCL**
  - Left **0VCK**
  - Right **0VCJ**
- Epidural Space **00C3**
- Epiglottis **0CCR**
- Esophagogastric Junction **0DC4**
- Esophagus **0DC5**
  - Lower **0DC3**
  - Middle **0DC2**
  - Upper **0DC1**

Extirpation- *continued*
- Eustachian Tube
  - Left **09CG**
  - Right **09CF**
- Eye
  - Left **08C1XZZ**
  - Right **08C0XZZ**
- Eyelid
  - Lower
    - Left **08CR**
    - Right **08CQ**
  - Upper
    - Left **08CP**
    - Right **08CN**
- Fallopian Tube
  - Left **0UC6**
  - Right **0UC5**
- Fallopian Tubes, Bilateral **0UC7**
- Femoral Shaft
  - Left **0QC9**
  - Right **0QC8**
- Femur
  - Lower
    - Left **0QCC**
    - Right **0QCB**
  - Upper
    - Left **0QC7**
    - Right **0QC6**
- Fibula
  - Left **0QCK**
  - Right **0QCJ**
- Finger Nail **0HCQXZZ**
- Gallbladder **0FC4**
- Gastrointestinal Tract **0WCP**
- Genitourinary Tract **0WCR**
- Gingiva
  - Lower **0CC6**
  - Upper **0CC5**
- Gland
  - Adrenal
    - Bilateral **0GC4**
    - Left **0GC2**
    - Right **0GC3**
  - Lacrimal
    - Left **08CW**
    - Right **08CV**
  - Minor Salivary **0CCJ**
  - Parotid
    - Left **0CC9**
    - Right **0CC8**
  - Pituitary **0GC0**
  - Sublingual
    - Left **0CCF**
    - Right **0CCD**
  - Submaxillary
    - Left **0CCH**
    - Right **0CCG**
  - Vestibular **0UCL**
- Glenoid Cavity
  - Left **0PC8**
  - Right **0PC7**
- Glomus Jugulare **0GCC**
- Humeral Head
  - Left **0PCD**
  - Right **0PCC**
- Humeral Shaft
  - Left **0PCG**
  - Right **0PCF**
- Hymen **0UCK**
- Hypothalamus **00CA**
- Ileocecal Valve **0DCC**
- Ileum **0DCB**

Extirpation- *continued*
- Intestine
  - Large **0DCE**
    - Left **0DCG**
    - Right **0DCF**
  - Small **0DC8**
- Iris
  - Left **08CD**
  - Right **08CC**
- Jejunum **0DCA**
- Joint
  - Acromioclavicular
    - Left **0RCH**
    - Right **0RCG**
  - Ankle
    - Left **0SCG**
    - Right **0SCF**
  - Carpal
    - Left **0RCR**
    - Right **0RCQ**
  - Cervical Vertebral **0RC1**
  - Cervicothoracic Vertebral **0RC4**
  - Coccygeal **0SC6**
  - Elbow
    - Left **0RCM**
    - Right **0RCL**
  - Finger Phalangeal
    - Left **0RCX**
    - Right **0RCW**
  - Hip
    - Left **0SCB**
    - Right **0SC9**
  - Knee
    - Left **0SCD**
    - Right **0SCC**
  - Lumbar Vertebral **0SC0**
  - Lumbosacral **0SC3**
  - Metacarpocarpal
    - Left **0RCT**
    - Right **0RCS**
  - Metacarpophalangeal
    - Left **0RCV**
    - Right **0RCU**
  - Metatarsal-Phalangeal
    - Left **0SCN**
    - Right **0SCM**
  - Metatarsal-Tarsal
    - Left **0SCL**
    - Right **0SCK**
  - Occipital-cervical **0RC0**
  - Sacrococcygeal **0SC5**
  - Sacroiliac
    - Left **0SC8**
    - Right **0SC7**
  - Shoulder
    - Left **0RCK**
    - Right **0RCJ**
  - Sternoclavicular
    - Left **0RCF**
    - Right **0RCE**
  - Tarsal
    - Left **0SCJ**
    - Right **0SCH**
  - Temporomandibular
    - Left **0RCD**
    - Right **0RCC**
  - Thoracic Vertebral **0RC6**
  - Thoracolumbar Vertebral **0RCA**
  - Toe Phalangeal
    - Left **0SCQ**
    - Right **0SCP**

Extirpation- *continued*
- Wrist
  - Left **0RCP**
  - Right **0RCN**
- Kidney
  - Left **0TC1**
  - Right **0TC0**
- Kidney Pelvis
  - Left **0TC4**
  - Right **0TC3**
- Larynx **0CCS**
- Lens
  - Left **08CK**
  - Right **08CJ**
- Lip
  - Lower **0CC1**
  - Upper **0CC0**
- Liver **0FC0**
  - Left Lobe **0FC2**
  - Right Lobe **0FC1**
- Lung
  - Bilateral **0BCM**
  - Left **0BCL**
  - Lower Lobe
    - Left **0BCJ**
    - Right **0BCF**
  - Middle Lobe, Right **0BCD**
  - Right **0BCK**
  - Upper Lobe
    - Left **0BCG**
    - Right **0BCC**
- Lung Lingula **0BCH**
- Lymphatic
  - Aortic **07CD**
  - Axillary
    - Left **07C6**
    - Right **07C5**
  - Head **07C0**
  - Inguinal
    - Left **07CJ**
    - Right **07CH**
  - Internal Mammary
    - Left **07C9**
    - Right **07C8**
  - Lower Extremity
    - Left **07CG**
    - Right **07CF**
  - Mesenteric **07CB**
  - Neck
    - Left **07C2**
    - Right **07C1**
  - Pelvis **07CC**
  - Thoracic Duct **07CK**
  - Thorax **07C7**
  - Upper Extremity
    - Left **07C4**
    - Right **07C3**
- Mandible
  - Left **0NCV**
  - Right **0NCT**
- Maxilla
  - Left **0NCS**
  - Right **0NCR**
- Mediastinum **0WCC**
- Medulla Oblongata **00CD**
- Mesentery **0DCV**
- Metacarpal
  - Left **0PCQ**
  - Right **0PCP**
- Metatarsal
  - Left **0QCP**
  - Right **0QCN**

Extirpation- *continued*
- Muscle
  - Abdomen
    - Left **0KCL**
    - Right **0KCK**
  - Extraocular
    - Left **08CM**
    - Right **08CL**
  - Facial **0KC1**
  - Foot
    - Left **0KCW**
    - Right **0KCV**
  - Hand
    - Left **0KCD**
    - Right **0KCC**
  - Head **0KC0**
  - Hip
    - Left **0KCP**
    - Right **0KCN**
  - Lower Arm and Wrist
    - Left **0KCB**
    - Right **0KC9**
  - Lower Leg
    - Left **0KCT**
    - Right **0KCS**
  - Neck
    - Left **0KC3**
    - Right **0KC2**
  - Papillary **02CD**
  - Perineum **0KCM**
  - Shoulder
    - Left **0KC6**
    - Right **0KC5**
  - Thorax
    - Left **0KCJ**
    - Right **0KCH**
  - Tongue, Palate, Pharynx **0KC4**
  - Trunk
    - Left **0KCG**
    - Right **0KCF**
  - Upper Arm
    - Left **0KC8**
    - Right **0KC7**
  - Upper Leg
    - Left **0KCR**
    - Right **0KCQ**
- Nasopharynx **09CN**
- Nerve
  - Abdominal Sympathetic **01CM**
  - Abducens **00CL**
  - Accessory **00CR**
  - Acoustic **00CN**
  - Brachial Plexus **01C3**
  - Cervical **01C1**
  - Cervical Plexus **01C0**
  - Facial **00CM**
  - Femoral **01CD**
  - Glossopharyngeal **00CP**
  - Head and Neck Sympathetic **01CK**
  - Hypoglossal **00CS**
  - Lumbar **01CB**
  - Lumbar Plexus **01C9**
  - Lumbar Sympathetic **01CN**
  - Lumbosacral Plexus **01CA**
  - Median **01C5**
  - Oculomotor **00CH**
  - Olfactory **00CF**
  - Optic **00CG**
  - Peroneal **01CH**
  - Phrenic **01C2**
  - Pudendal **01CC**
  - Radial **01C6**

Extirpation- *continued*
- Sacral **01CR**
- Sacral Plexus **01CQ**
- Sacral Sympathetic **01CP**
- Sciatic **01CF**
- Thoracic **01C8**
- Thoracic Sympathetic **01CL**
- Tibial **01CG**
- Trigeminal **00CK**
- Trochlear **00CJ**
- Ulnar **01C4**
- Vagus **00CQ**
- Nipple
  - Left **0HCX**
  - Right **0HCW**
- Nose **09CK**
- Omentum
  - Greater **0DCS**
  - Lesser **0DCT**
- Oral Cavity and Throat **0WC3**
- Orbit
  - Left **0NCQ**
  - Right **0NCP**
- Ovary
  - Bilateral **0UC2**
  - Left **0UC1**
  - Right **0UC0**
- Palate
  - Hard **0CC2**
  - Soft **0CC3**
- Pancreas **0FCG**
- Para-aortic Body **0GC9**
- Paraganglion Extremity **0GCF**
- Parathyroid Gland **0GCR**
  - Inferior
    - Left **0GCP**
    - Right **0GCN**
  - Multiple **0GCQ**
  - Superior
    - Left **0GCM**
    - Right **0GCL**
- Patella
  - Left **0QCF**
  - Right **0QCD**
- Pelvic Cavity **0WCJ**
- Penis **0VCS**
- Pericardial Cavity **0WCD**
- Pericardium **02CN**
- Peritoneal Cavity **0WCG**
- Peritoneum **0DCW**
- Phalanx
  - Finger
    - Left **0PCV**
    - Right **0PCT**
  - Thumb
    - Left **0PCS**
    - Right **0PCR**
  - Toe
    - Left **0QCR**
    - Right **0QCQ**
- Pharynx **0CCM**
- Pineal Body **0GC1**
- Pleura
  - Left **0BCP**
  - Right **0BCN**
- Pleural Cavity
  - Left **0WCB**
  - Right **0WC9**
- Pons **00CB**
- Prepuce **0VCT**
- Prostate **0VC0**

Extirpation- *continued*
Radius
  Left **0PCJ**
  Right **0PCH**
Rectum **0DCP**
Respiratory Tract **0WCQ**
Retina
  Left **08CF**
  Right **08CE**
Retinal Vessel
  Left **08CH**
  Right **08CG**
Rib
  Left **0PC2**
  Right **0PC1**
Sacrum **0QC1**
Scapula
  Left **0PC6**
  Right **0PC5**
Sclera
  Left **08C7XZZ**
  Right **08C6XZZ**
Scrotum **0VC5**
Septum
  Atrial **02C5**
  Nasal **09CM**
  Ventricular **02CM**
Sinus
  Accessory **09CP**
  Ethmoid
    Left **09CV**
    Right **09CU**
  Frontal
    Left **09CT**
    Right **09CS**
  Mastoid
    Left **09CC**
    Right **09CB**
  Maxillary
    Left **09CR**
    Right **09CQ**
  Sphenoid
    Left **09CX**
    Right **09CW**
Skin
  Abdomen **0HC7XZZ**
  Back **0HC6XZZ**
  Buttock **0HC8XZZ**
  Chest **0HC5XZZ**
  Ear
    Left **0HC3XZZ**
    Right **0HC2XZZ**
  Face **0HC1XZZ**
  Foot
    Left **0HCNXZZ**
    Right **0HCMXZZ**
  Genitalia **0HCAXZZ**
  Hand
    Left **0HCGXZZ**
    Right **0HCFXZZ**
  Lower Arm
    Left **0HCEXZZ**
    Right **0HCDXZZ**
  Lower Leg
    Left **0HCLXZZ**
    Right **0HCKXZZ**
  Neck **0HC4XZZ**
  Perineum **0HC9XZZ**
  Scalp **0HC0XZZ**
  Upper Arm
    Left **0HCCXZZ**
    Right **0HCBXZZ**

Extirpation- *continued*
Upper Leg
  Left **0HCJXZZ**
  Right **0HCHXZZ**
Spinal Cord
  Cervical **00CW**
  Lumbar **00CY**
  Thoracic **00CX**
Spinal Meninges **00CT**
Spleen **07CP**
Sternum **0PC0**
Stomach **0DC6**
  Pylorus **0DC7**
Subarachnoid Space **00C5**
Subcutaneous Tissue and Fascia
  Abdomen **0JC8**
  Back **0JC7**
  Buttock **0JC9**
  Chest **0JC6**
  Face **0JC1**
  Foot
    Left **0JCR**
    Right **0JCQ**
  Hand
    Left **0JCK**
    Right **0JCJ**
  Lower Arm
    Left **0JCH**
    Right **0JCG**
  Lower Leg
    Left **0JCP**
    Right **0JCN**
  Neck
    Anterior **0JC4**
    Posterior **0JC5**
  Pelvic Region **0JCC**
  Perineum **0JCB**
  Scalp **0JC0**
  Upper Arm
    Left **0JCF**
    Right **0JCD**
  Upper Leg
    Left **0JCM**
    Right **0JCL**
Subdural Space **00C4**
Tarsal
  Left **0QCM**
  Right **0QCL**
Tendon
  Abdomen
    Left **0LCG**
    Right **0LCF**
  Ankle
    Left **0LCT**
    Right **0LCS**
  Foot
    Left **0LCW**
    Right **0LCV**
  Hand
    Left **0LC8**
    Right **0LC7**
  Head and Neck **0LC0**
  Hip
    Left **0LCK**
    Right **0LCJ**
  Knee
    Left **0LCR**
    Right **0LCQ**
  Lower Arm and Wrist
    Left **0LC6**
    Right **0LC5**

Extirpation- *continued*
Lower Leg
  Left **0LCP**
  Right **0LCN**
Perineum **0LCH**
Shoulder
  Left **0LC2**
  Right **0LC1**
Thorax
  Left **0LCD**
  Right **0LCC**
Trunk
  Left **0LCB**
  Right **0LC9**
Upper Arm
  Left **0LC4**
  Right **0LC3**
Upper Leg
  Left **0LCM**
  Right **0LCL**
Testis
  Bilateral **0VCC**
  Left **0VCB**
  Right **0VC9**
Thalamus **00C9**
Thymus **07CM**
Thyroid Gland **0GCK**
  Left Lobe **0GCG**
  Right Lobe **0GCH**
Tibia
  Left **0QCH**
  Right **0QCG**
Toe Nail **0HCRXZZ**
Tongue **0CC7**
Tonsils **0CCP**
Tooth
  Lower **0CCX**
  Upper **0CCW**
Trachea **0BC1**
Tunica Vaginalis
  Left **0VC7**
  Right **0VC6**
Turbinate, Nasal **09CL**
Tympanic Membrane
  Left **09C8**
  Right **09C7**
Ulna
  Left **0PCL**
  Right **0PCK**
Ureter
  Left **0TC7**
  Right **0TC6**
Urethra **0TCD**
Uterine Supporting Structure **0UC4**
Uterus **0UC9**
Uvula **0CCN**
Vagina **0UCG**
Valve
  Aortic **02CF**
  Mitral **02CG**
  Pulmonary **02CH**
  Tricuspid **02CJ**
Vas Deferens
  Bilateral **0VCQ**
  Left **0VCP**
  Right **0VCN**
Vein
  Axillary
    Left **05C8**
    Right **05C7**
  Azygos **05C0**

Extirpation- *continued*
- Basilic
  - Left **05CC**
  - Right **05CB**
- Brachial
  - Left **05CA**
  - Right **05C9**
- Cephalic
  - Left **05CF**
  - Right **05CD**
- Colic **06C7**
- Common Iliac
  - Left **06CD**
  - Right **06CC**
- Coronary **02C4**
- Esophageal **06C3**
- External Iliac
  - Left **06CG**
  - Right **06CF**
- External Jugular
  - Left **05CQ**
  - Right **05CP**
- Face
  - Left **05CV**
  - Right **05CT**
- Femoral
  - Left **06CN**
  - Right **06CM**
- Foot
  - Left **06CV**
  - Right **06CT**
- Gastric **06C2**
- Greater Saphenous
  - Left **06CQ**
  - Right **06CP**
- Hand
  - Left **05CH**
  - Right **05CG**
- Hemiazygos **05C1**
- Hepatic **06C4**
- Hypogastric
  - Left **06CJ**
  - Right **06CH**
- Inferior Mesenteric **06C6**
- Innominate
  - Left **05C4**
  - Right **05C3**
- Internal Jugular
  - Left **05CN**
  - Right **05CM**
- Intracranial **05CL**
- Lesser Saphenous
  - Left **06CS**
  - Right **06CR**
- Lower **06CY**
- Portal **06C8**
- Pulmonary
  - Left **02CT**
  - Right **02CS**
- Renal
  - Left **06CB**
  - Right **06C9**
- Splenic **06C1**
- Subclavian
  - Left **05C6**
  - Right **05C5**
- Superior Mesenteric **06C5**
- Upper **05CY**
- Vertebral
  - Left **05CS**
  - Right **05CR**

Extirpation- *continued*
- Vena Cava
  - Inferior **06C0**
  - Superior **02CV**
- Ventricle
  - Left **02CL**
  - Right **02CK**
- Vertebra
  - Cervical **0PC3**
  - Lumbar **0QC0**
  - Thoracic **0PC4**
- Vesicle
  - Bilateral **0VC3**
  - Left **0VC2**
  - Right **0VC1**
- Vitreous
  - Left **08C5**
  - Right **08C4**
- Vocal Cord
  - Left **0CCV**
  - Right **0CCT**
- Vulva **0UCM**

Extracorporeal shock wave lithotripsy *see*
Fragmentation

Extracranial-intracranial bypass (EC-IC) *see*
Bypass, Upper Arteries **031**

Extraction
- Auditory Ossicle
  - Left **09DA0ZZ**
  - Right **09D90ZZ**
- Bone Marrow
  - Iliac **07DR**
  - Sternum **07DQ**
  - Vertebral **07DS**
- Bursa and Ligament
  - Abdomen
    - Left **0MDJ**
    - Right **0MDH**
  - Ankle
    - Left **0MDR**
    - Right **0MDQ**
  - Elbow
    - Left **0MD4**
    - Right **0MD3**
  - Foot
    - Left **0MDT**
    - Right **0MDS**
  - Hand
    - Left **0MD8**
    - Right **0MD7**
  - Head and Neck **0MD0**
  - Hip
    - Left **0MDM**
    - Right **0MDL**
  - Knee
    - Left **0MDP**
    - Right **0MDN**
  - Lower Extremity
    - Left **0MDW**
    - Right **0MDV**
  - Perineum **0MDK**
  - Shoulder
    - Left **0MD2**
    - Right **0MD1**
  - Thorax
    - Left **0MDG**
    - Right **0MDF**
  - Trunk
    - Left **0MDD**
    - Right **0MDC**

Extraction – *continued*
- Upper Extremity
  - Left **0MDB**
  - Right **0MD9**
- Wrist
  - Left **0MD6**
  - Right **0MD5**
- Cerebral Meninges **00D1**
- Cornea
  - Left **08D9XZ**
  - Right **08D8XZ**
- Dura Mater **00D2**
- Endometrium **0UDB**
- Finger Nail **0HDQXZZ**
- Hair **0HDSXZZ**
- Kidney
  - Left **0TD1**
  - Right **0TD0**
- Lens
  - Left **08DK3ZZ**
  - Right **08DJ3ZZ**
- Nerve
  - Abdominal Sympathetic **01DM**
  - Abducens **00DL**
  - Accessory **00DR**
  - Acoustic **00DN**
  - Brachial Plexus **01D3**
  - Cervical **01D1**
  - Cervical Plexus **01D0**
  - Facial **00DM**
  - Femoral **01DD**
  - Glossopharyngeal **00DP**
  - Head and Neck Sympathetic **01DK**
  - Hypoglossal **00DS**
  - Lumbar **01DB**
  - Lumbar Plexus **01D9**
  - Lumbar Sympathetic **01DN**
  - Lumbosacral Plexus **01DA**
  - Median **01D5**
  - Oculomotor **00DH**
  - Olfactory **00DF**
  - Optic **00DG**
  - Peroneal **01DH**
  - Phrenic **01D2**
  - Pudendal **01DC**
  - Radial **01D6**
  - Sacral **01DR**
  - Sacral Plexus **01DQ**
  - Sacral Sympathetic **01DP**
  - Sciatic **01DF**
  - Thoracic **01D8**
  - Thoracic Sympathetic **01DL**
  - Tibial **01DG**
  - Trigeminal **00DK**
  - Trochlear **00DJ**
  - Ulnar **01D4**
  - Vagus **00DQ**
- Ova **0UDN**
- Pleura
  - Left **0BDP**
  - Right **0BDN**
- Products of Conception
  - Classical **10D00Z0**
  - Ectopic **10D2**
  - Extraperitoneal **10D00Z2**
  - High Forceps **10D07Z5**
  - Internal Version **10D07Z7**
  - Low Cervical **10D00Z1**
  - Low Forceps **10D07Z3**
  - Mid Forceps **10D07Z4**
  - Other **10D07Z8**
  - Retained **10D1**
  - Vacuum **10D07Z6**

Extraction – *continued*
Septum, Nasal **09DM**
Sinus
Accessory **09DP**
Ethmoid
Left **09DV**
Right **09DU**
Frontal
Left **09DT**
Right **09DS**
Mastoid
Left **09DC**
Right **09DB**
Maxillary
Left **09DR**
Right **09DQ**
Sphenoid
Left **09DX**
Right **09DW**
Skin
Abdomen **0HD7XZZ**
Back **0HD6XZZ**
Buttock **0HD8XZZ**
Chest **0HD5XZZ**
Ear
Left **0HD3XZZ**
Right **0HD2XZZ**
Face **0HD1XZZ**
Foot
Left **0HDNXZZ**
Right **0HDMXZZ**
Genitalia **0HDAXZZ**
Hand
Left **0HDGXZZ**
Right **0HDFXZZ**
Lower Arm
Left **0HDEXZZ**
Right **0HDDXZZ**
Lower Leg
Left **0HDLXZZ**
Right **0HDKXZZ**
Neck **0HD4XZZ**
Perineum **0HD9XZZ**
Scalp **0HD0XZZ**
Upper Arm
Left **0HDCXZZ**
Right **0HDBXZZ**
Upper Leg
Left **0HDJXZZ**
Right **0HDHXZZ**
Spinal Meninges **00DT**
Subcutaneous Tissue and Fascia
Abdomen **0JD8**
Back **0JD7**
Buttock **0JD9**
Chest **0JD6**
Face **0JD1**
Foot
Left **0JDR**
Right **0JDQ**
Hand
Left **0JDK**
Right **0JDJ**
Lower Arm
Left **0JDH**
Right **0JDG**
Lower Leg
Left **0JDP**
Right **0JDN**
Neck
Anterior **0JD4**
Posterior **0JD5**

Extraction – *continued*
Pelvic Region **0JDC**
Perineum **0JDB**
Scalp **0JD0**
Upper Arm
Left **0JDF**
Right **0JDD**
Upper Leg
Left **0JDM**
Right **0JDL**
Toe Nail **0HDRXZZ**
Tooth
Lower **0CDXXZ**
Upper **0CDWXZ**
Turbinate, Nasal **09DL**
Tympanic Membrane
Left **09D8**
Right **09D7**
Vein
Basilic
Left **05DC**
Right **05DB**
Brachial
Left **05DA**
Right **05D9**
Cephalic
Left **05DF**
Right **05DD**
Femoral
Left **06DN**
Right **06DM**
Foot
Left **06DV**
Right **06DT**
Greater Saphenous
Left **06DQ**
Right **06DP**
Hand
Left **05DH**
Right **05DG**
Lesser Saphenous
Left **06DS**
Right **06DR**
Lower **06DY**
Upper **05DY**
Vocal Cord
Left **0CDV**
Right **0CDT**
Extradural space *use* Epidural Space
**EXtreme Lateral Interbody Fusion (XLIF)
device** *use* Interbody Fusion Device in Lower
Joints

F

Face lift *see* Alteration, Face **0W02**
Facet replacement spinal stabilization device
use Spinal Stabilization Device, Facet
Replacement in **0RH**
use Spinal Stabilization Device, Facet
Replacement in **0SH**
Facial artery *use* Artery, Face
False vocal cord *use* Larynx
Falx cerebri *use* Dura Mater
Fascia lata
use Subcutaneous Tissue and Fascia, Upper
Leg, Left
use Subcutaneous Tissue and Fascia, Upper
Leg, Right

Fasciaplasty, fascioplasty
see Repair, Subcutaneous Tissue and Fascia
0JQ
see Replacement, Subcutaneous Tissue and
Fascia **0JR**
Fasciectomy *see* Excision, Subcutaneous Tissue
and Fascia **0JB**
Fasciorrhaphy *see* Repair, Subcutaneous Tissue
and Fascia **0JQ**
Fasciotomy
see Division, Subcutaneous Tissue and Fascia
0J8
see Drainage, Subcutaneous Tissue and Fascia
0J9
Feeding Device
Change device in
Lower **0D2DXUZ**
Upper **0D20XUZ**
Insertion of device in
Duodenum **0DH9**
Esophagus **0DH5**
Ileum **0DHB**
Intestine, Small **0DH8**
Jejunum **0DHA**
Stomach **0DH6**
Removal of device from
Esophagus **0DP5**
Intestinal Tract
Lower **0DPD**
Upper **0DP0**
Stomach **0DP6**
Revision of device in
Intestinal Tract
Lower **0DWD**
Upper **0DW0**
Stomach **0DW6**
Femoral head
use Femur, Upper, Right
use Femur, Upper, Left
Femoral lymph node
use Lymphatic, Lower Extremity, Left
use Lymphatic, Lower Extremity, Right
Femoropatellar joint
use Joint, Knee, Right
use Joint, Knee, Right, Femoral Surface
use Joint, Knee, Left
use Joint, Knee, Left, Femoral Surface
Femorotibial joint
use Joint, Knee, Right
use Joint, Knee, Right, Tibial Surface
use Joint, Knee, Left
use Joint, Knee, Left, Tibial Surface
Fibular artery
use Artery, Peroneal, Right
use Artery, Peroneal, Left
Fibularis brevis muscle
use Muscle, Lower Leg, Left
use Muscle, Lower Leg, Right
Fibularis longus muscle
use Muscle, Lower Leg, Left
use Muscle, Lower Leg, Right
Fifth cranial nerve *use* Nerve, Trigeminal
Fimbriectomy
see Excision, Female Reproductive System
0UB
see Resection, Female Reproductive System
0UT
First cranial nerve *use* Nerve, Olfactory
First intercostal nerve *use* Nerve, Brachial
Plexus

Fistulization
  see Bypass
  see Drainage
  see Repair
Fitting
  Arch bars, for fracture reduction *see*
  Reposition, Mouth and Throat **0CS**
  Arch bars, for immobilization *see*
  Immobilization, Face **2W31**
  Artificial limb *see* Device Fitting,
  Rehabilitation **F0D**
  Hearing aid *see* Device Fitting, Rehabilitation
  F0D
  Ocular prosthesis **F0DZ8UZ**
  Prosthesis, limb *see* Device Fitting,
  Rehabilitation **F0D**
  Prosthesis, ocular **F0DZ8UZ Fixation, bone**
    External, with fracture reduction *see*
    Reposition
    External, without fracture reduction *see*
    Insertion
    Internal, with fracture reduction *see*
    Reposition
    Internal, without fracture reduction *see*
    Insertion
FLAIR® Endovascular Stent Graft *use*
  Intraluminal Device
Flexible Composite Mesh *use* Synthetic
  Substitute
Flexor carpi radialis muscle
  use Muscle, Lower Arm and Wrist, Right
  use Muscle, Lower Arm and Wrist, Left
Flexor carpi ulnaris muscle
  use Muscle, Lower Arm and Wrist, Right
  use Muscle, Lower Arm and Wrist, Left
Flexor digitorum brevis muscle
  use Muscle, Foot, Left
  use Muscle, Foot, Right
Flexor digitorum longus muscle
  use Muscle, Lower Leg, Left
  use Muscle, Lower Leg, Right
Flexor hallucis brevis muscle
  use Muscle, Foot, Left
  use Muscle, Foot, Right
Flexor hallucis longus muscle
  use Muscle, Lower Leg, Right
  use Muscle, Lower Leg, Left
Flexor pollicis longus muscle
  use Muscle, Lower Arm and Wrist, Left
  use Muscle, Lower Arm and Wrist, Right
Fluoroscopy
  Abdomen and Pelvis **BW11**
  Airway, Upper **BB1DZZZ**
  Ankle
    Left **BQ1H**
    Right **BQ1G**
  Aorta
    Abdominal **B410**
      Laser, Intraoperative **B410**
    Thoracic **B310**
      Laser, Intraoperative **B310**
    Thoraco-Abdominal **B31P**
      Laser, Intraoperative **B31P**
  Aorta and Bilateral Lower Extremity Arteries
  B41D
    Laser, Intraoperative **B41D**
  Arm
    Left **BP1FZZZ**
    Right **BP1EZZZ**

Fluoroscopy - *continued*
  Artery
    Brachiocephalic-Subclavian
      Right **B311**
      Laser, Intraoperative **B311**
    Bronchial **B31L**
      Laser, Intraoperative **B31L**
    Bypass Graft, Other **B21F**
    Cervico-Cerebral Arch **B31Q**
      Laser, Intraoperative **B31Q**
    Common Carotid
      Bilateral **B315**
        Laser, Intraoperative **B315**
      Left **B314**
        Laser, Intraoperative **B314**
      Right **B313**
        Laser, Intraoperative **B313**
    Coronary
      Bypass Graft
        Multiple **B213**

      Laser, Intraoperative **B213**
        Single **B212**
      Laser, Intraoperative **B212**
        Multiple **B211**
          Laser, Intraoperative **B211**
        Single **B210**
          Laser, Intraoperative **B210**
    External Carotid
      Bilateral **B31C**
        Laser, Intraoperative **B31C**
      Left **B31B**
        Laser, Intraoperative **B31B**
      Right **B319**
        Laser, Intraoperative **B319**
    Hepatic **B412**
      Laser, Intraoperative **B412**
    Inferior Mesenteric **B415**
      Laser, Intraoperative **B415**
    Intercostal **B31L**
      Laser, Intraoperative **B31L**
    Internal Carotid
      Bilateral **B318**
        Laser, Intraoperative **B318**
      Left **B317**
        Laser, Intraoperative **B317**
      Right **B316**
        Laser, Intraoperative **B316**
    Internal Mammary Bypass Graft
      Left **B218**
      Right **B217**
    Intra-Abdominal
      Other **B41B**
      Laser, Intraoperative **B41B**
    Intracranial **B31R**
      Laser, Intraoperative **B31R**
    Lower
      Other **B41J**
      Laser, Intraoperative **B41J**
    Lower Extremity
      Bilateral and Aorta **B41D**
        Laser, Intraoperative **B41D**
      Left **B41G**
        Laser, Intraoperative **B41G**
      Right **B41F**
        Laser, Intraoperative **B41F**
    Lumbar **B419**
      Laser, Intraoperative **B419**
    Pelvic **B41C**
      Laser, Intraoperative **B41C**

Fluoroscopy - *continued*
    Pulmonary
      Left **B31T**
        Laser, Intraoperative **B31T**
      Right **B31S**
        Laser, Intraoperative **B31S**
    Renal
      Bilateral **B418**
        Laser, Intraoperative **B418**
      Left **B417**
        Laser, Intraoperative **B417**
      Right **B416**
        Laser, Intraoperative **B416**
    Spinal **B31M**
      Laser, Intraoperative **B31M**
    Splenic **B413**
      Laser, Intraoperative **B413**
    Subclavian
      Left **B312**
      Laser, Intraoperative **B312**
    Superior Mesenteric **B414**
      Laser, Intraoperative **B414**
    Upper
      Other **B31N**
      Laser, Intraoperative **B31N**
    Upper Extremity
      Bilateral **B31K**
        Laser, Intraoperative **B31K**
      Left **B31J**
        Laser, Intraoperative **B31J**
      Right **B31H**
        Laser, Intraoperative **B31H**
    Vertebral
      Bilateral **B31G**
        Laser, Intraoperative **B31G**
      Left **B31F**
        Laser, Intraoperative **B31F**
      Right **B31D**
        Laser, Intraoperative **B31D**
  Bile Duct **BF10**
    Pancreatic Duct and Gallbladder **BF14**
  Bile Duct and Gallbladder **BF13**
  Biliary Duct **BF11**
  Bladder **BT10**
    Kidney and Ureter **BT14**
    Left **BT1F**
    Right **BT1D**
  Bladder and Urethra **BT1B**
  Bowel, Small **BD1**
  Calcaneus
    Left **BQ1KZZZ**
    Right **BQ1JZZZ**
  Clavicle
    Left **BP15ZZZ**
    Right **BP14ZZZ**
  Coccyx **BR1F**
  Colon **BD14**
  Corpora Cavernosa **BV10**
  Dialysis Fistula **B51W**
  Dialysis Shunt **B51W**
  Diaphragm **BB16ZZZ**
  Disc
    Cervical **BR11**
    Lumbar **BR13**
    Thoracic **BR12**
  Duodenum **BD19**
  Elbow
    Left **BP1H**
    Right **BP1G**
  Epiglottis **B91G**
  Esophagus **BD11**

Fluoroscopy - *continued*
- Extremity
  - Lower **BW1C**
  - Upper **BW1J**
- Facet Joint
  - Cervical **BR14**
  - Lumbar **BR16**
  - Thoracic **BR15**
- Fallopian Tube
  - Bilateral **BU12**
  - Left **BU11**
  - Right **BU10**
- Fallopian Tube and Uterus **BU18**
- Femur
  - Left **BQ14ZZZ**
  - Right **BQ13ZZZ**
- Finger
  - Left **BP1SZZZ**
  - Right **BP1RZZZ**
- Foot
  - Left **BQ1MZZZ**
  - Right **BQ1LZZZ**
- Forearm
  - Left **BP1KZZZ**
  - Right **BP1JZZZ**
- Gallbladder **BF12**
  - Bile Duct and Pancreatic Duct **BF14**
- Gallbladder and Bile Duct **BF13**
- Gastrointestinal, Upper **BD1**
- Hand
  - Left **BP1PZZZ**
  - Right **BP1NZZZ**
- Head and Neck **BW19**
- Heart
  - Left **B215**
  - Right **B214**
  - Right and Left **B216**
- Hip
  - Left **BQ11**
  - Right **BQ10**
- Humerus
  - Left **BP1BZZZ**
  - Right **BP1AZZZ**
- Ileal Diversion Loop **BT1C**
- Ileal Loop, Ureters and Kidney **BT1G**
- Intracranial Sinus **B512**
- Joint
  - Acromioclavicular, Bilateral **BP13ZZZ**
  - Finger
    - Left **BP1D**
    - Right **BP1C**
  - Foot
    - Left **BQ1Y**
    - Right **BQ1X**
  - Hand
    - Left **BP1D**
    - Right **BP1C**
  - Lumbosacral **BR1B**
  - Sacroiliac **BR1D**
  - Sternoclavicular
    - Bilateral **BP12ZZZ**
    - Left **BP11ZZZ**
    - Right **BP10ZZZ**
  - Temporomandibular
    - Bilateral **BN19**
    - Left **BN18**
    - Right **BN17**
  - Thoracolumbar **BR18**
  - Toe
    - Left **BQ1Y**
    - Right **BQ1X**

Fluoroscopy - *continued*
- Kidney
  - Bilateral **BT13**
  - Ileal Loop and Ureter **BT1G**
  - Left **BT12**
  - Right **BT11**
  - Ureter and Bladder **BT14**
    - Left **BT1F**
    - Right **BT1D**
- Knee
  - Left **BQ18**
  - Right **BQ17**
- Larynx **B91J**
- Leg
  - Left **BQ1FZZZ**
  - Right **BQ1DZZZ**
- Lung
  - Bilateral **BB14ZZZ**
  - Left **BB13ZZZ**
  - Right **BB12ZZZ**
- Mediastinum **BB1CZZZ**
- Mouth **BD1B**
- Neck and Head **BW19**
- Oropharynx **BD1B**
- Pancreatic Duct **BF1**
  - Gallbladder and Bile Duct **BF14**
- Patella
  - Left **BQ1WZZZ**
  - Right **BQ1VZZZ**
- Pelvis **BR1C**
- Pelvis and Abdomen **BW11**
- Pharynx **B91G**
- Ribs
  - Left **BP1YZZZ**
  - Right **BP1XZZZ**
- Sacrum **BR1F**
- Scapula
  - Left **BP17ZZZ**
  - Right **BP16ZZZ**
- Shoulder
  - Left **BP19**
  - Right **BP18**
- Sinus, Intracranial **B512**
- Spinal Cord **B01B**
- Spine
  - Cervical **BR10**
  - Lumbar **BR19**
  - Thoracic **BR17**
  - Whole **BR1G**
- Sternum **BR1H**
- Stomach **BD12**
- Toe
  - Left **BQ1QZZZ**
  - Right **BQ1PZZZ**
- Tracheobronchial Tree
  - Bilateral **BB19YZZ**
  - Left **BB18YZZ**
  - Right **BB17YZZ**
- Ureter
  - Ileal Loop and Kidney **BT1G**
  - Kidney and Bladder **BT14**
    - Left **BT1F**
    - Right **BT1D**
  - Left **BT17**
  - Right **BT16**
- Urethra **BT15**
- Urethra and Bladder **BT1B**
- Uterus **BU16**
- Uterus and Fallopian Tube **BU18**
- Vagina **BU19**
- Vasa Vasorum **BV18**

Fluoroscopy - *continued*
- Vein
  - Cerebellar **B511**
  - Cerebral **B511**
  - Epidural **B510**
  - Jugular
    - Bilateral **B515**
    - Left **B514**
    - Right **B513**
  - Lower Extremity
    - Bilateral **B51D**
    - Left **B51C**
    - Right **B51B**
  - Other **B51V**
  - Pelvic (Iliac)
    - Left **B51G**
    - Right **B51F**
  - Pelvic (Iliac) Bilateral **B51H**
  - Portal **B51T**
  - Pulmonary
    - Bilateral **B51S**
    - Left **B51R**
    - Right **B51Q**
  - Renal
    - Bilateral **B51L**
    - Left **B51K**
    - Right **B51J**
  - Splanchnic **B51T**
  - Subclavian
    - Left **B517**
    - Right **B516**
  - Upper Extremity
    - Bilateral **B51P**
    - Left **B51N**
    - Right **B51M**
  - Vena Cava
    - Inferior **B519**
    - Superior **B518**
  - Wrist
    - Left **BP1M**
    - Right **BP1L**
- **Flushing** *see* Irrigation
- **Foley catheter** *use* Drainage Device
- **Foramen magnum**
  - *use* Bone, Occipital, Right
  - *use* Bone, Occipital, Left
- **Foramen of Monro (intraventricular)** *use* Cerebral Ventricle
- **Foreskin** *use* Prepuce
- **Formula™ Balloon-Expandable Renal Stent System** *use* Intraluminal Device
- **Fossa of Rosenmüller** *use* Nasopharynx
- **Fourth cranial nerve** *use* Nerve, Trochlear
- **Fourth ventricle** *use* Cerebral Ventricle
- **Fovea**
  - *use* Retina, Right
  - *use* Retina, Left
- **Fragmentation**
  - Ampulla of Vater **0FFC**
  - Anus **0DFQ**
  - Appendix **0DFJ**
  - Bladder **0TFB**
  - Bladder Neck **0TFC**
  - Bronchus
    - Lingula **0BF9**
    - Lower Lobe
      - Left **0BFB**
      - Right **0BF6**
    - Main
      - Left **0BF7**
      - Right **0BF3**
    - Middle Lobe, Right **0BF5**

Fragmentation - *continued*
  Upper Lobe
    Left **0BF8**
    Right **0BF4**
  Carina **0BF2**
  Cavity, Cranial **0WF1**
  Cecum **0DFH**
  Cerebral Ventricle **00F6**
  Colon
    Ascending **0DFK**
    Descending **0DFM**
    Sigmoid **0DFN**
    Transverse **0DFL**
  Duct
    Common Bile **0FF9**
    Cystic **0FF8**
    Hepatic
      Left **0FF6**
      Right **0FF5**
    Pancreatic **0FFD**
      Accessory **0FFF**
    Parotid
      Left **0CFC**
      Right **0CFB**
  Duodenum **0DF9**
  Epidural Space **00F3**
  Esophagus **0DF5**
  Fallopian Tube
    Left **0UF6**
    Right **0UF5**
  Fallopian Tubes, Bilateral **0UF7**
  Gallbladder **0FF4**
  Gastrointestinal Tract **0WFP**
  Genitourinary Tract **0WFR**
  Ileum **0DFB**
  Intestine
    Large **0DFE**
      Left **0DFG**
      Right **0DFF**
    Small **0DF8**
  Jejunum **0DFA**
  Kidney Pelvis
    Left **0TF4**
    Right **0TF3**
  Mediastinum **0WFC**
  Oral Cavity and Throat **0WF3**
  Pelvic Cavity **0WFJ**
  Pericardial Cavity **0WFD**
  Pericardium **02FN**
  Peritoneal Cavity **0WFG**
  Pleural Cavity
    Left **0WFB**
    Right **0WF9**
  Rectum **0DFP**
  Respiratory Tract **0WFQ**
  Spinal Canal **00FU**
  Stomach **0DF6**
  Subarachnoid Space **00F5**
  Subdural Space **00F4**
  Trachea **0BF1**
  Ureter
    Left **0TF7**
    Right **0TF6**
  Urethra **0TFD**
  Uterus **0UF9**
  Vitreous
    Left **08F5**
    Right **08F4**
Freestyle (Stentless) Aortic Root Bioprosthesis
use Zooplastic Tissue in Heart and Great
  Vessels

Frenectomy
  see Excision, Mouth and Throat **0CB**
  see Resection, Mouth and Throat **0CT**
Frenoplasty, frenuloplasty
  see Repair, Mouth and Throat **0CQ**
  see Replacement, Mouth and Throat **0CR**
  see Supplement, Mouth and Throat **0CU**
Frenotomy
  see Drainage, Mouth and Throat **0C9**
  see Release, Mouth and Throat **0CN**
Frenulotomy
  see Drainage, Mouth and Throat **0C9**
  see Release, Mouth and Throat **0CN**
Frenulum labii inferioris *use* Lip, Lower
Frenulum labii superioris *use* Lip, Upper
Frenulum linguae *use* Tongue
Frenulumectomy
  see Excision, Mouth and Throat **0CB**
  see Resection, Mouth and Throat **0CT**
Frontal lobe *use* Cerebral Hemisphere
Frontal vein
  use Vein, Face, Right
  use Vein, Face, Left
Fulguration *see* Destruction
Fundoplication, gastroesophageal *see*
  Restriction, Esophagastric Junction **0DV4**
Fundus uteri *use* Uterus
Fusion
  Acromioclavicular
    Left **0RGH**
    Right **0RGG**
  Ankle
    Left **0SGG**
    Right **0SGF**
  Carpal
    Left **0RGR**
    Right **0RGQ**
  Cervical Vertebral **0RG1**
    2 or more **0RG2**
  Cervicothoracic Vertebral **0RG4**
  Coccygeal **0SG6**
  Elbow
    Left **0RGM**
    Right **0RGL**
  Finger Phalangeal
    Left **0RGX**
    Right **0RGW**
  Hip
    Left **0SGB**
    Right **0SG9**
  Knee
    Left **0SGD**
    Right **0SGC**
  Lumbar Vertebral **0SG0**
    2 or more **0SG1**
  Lumbosacral **0SG3**
  Metacarpocarpal
    Left **0RGT**
    Right **0RGS**
  Metacarpophalangeal
    Left **0RGV**
    Right **0RGU**
  Metatarsal-Phalangeal
    Left **0SGN**
    Right **0SGM**
  Metatarsal-Tarsal
    Left **0SGL**
    Right **0SGK**
  Occipital-cervical **0RG0**
  Sacrococcygeal **0SG5**
  Sacroiliac
    Left **0SG8**
    Right **0SG7**

Fusion - *continued*
  Shoulder
    Left **0RGK**
    Right **0RGJ**
  Sternoclavicular
    Left **0RGF**
    Right **0RGE**
  Tarsal
    Left **0SGJ**
    Right **0SGH**
  Temporomandibular
    Left **0RGD**
    Right **0RGC**
  Thoracic Vertebral **0RG6**
    2 to 7 **0RG7**
    8 or more **0RG8**
  Thoracolumbar Vertebral **0RGA**
  Toe Phalangeal
    Left **0SGQ**
    Right **0SGP**
  Wrist
    Left **0RGP**
    Right **0RGN Fusion screw**
(compression)(lag)(locking)
  use Internal Fixation Device in Upper Joints
  use Internal Fixation Device in Lower Joints

G

Gait training *see* Motor Treatment,
  Rehabilitation **F07**
Galea aponeurotica *use* Subcutaneous Tissue
  and Fascia, Scalp
Ganglion impar (ganglion of Walther) *use*
  Nerve, Sacral Sympathetic
Ganglionectomy
  Destruction of lesion *see* Destruction
  Excision of lesion *see* Excision
Gasserian ganglion *use* Nerve, Trigeminal
Gastrectomy
  Partial *see* Excision, Stomach **0DB6**
  Total *see* Resection, Stomach **0DT6**
  Vertical (sleeve) *see* Excision, Stomach **0DB6**
Gastric electrical stimulation (GES) lead *use*
  Stimulator Lead in Gastrointestinal System
Gastric lymph node *use* Lymphatic, Aortic
Gastric pacemaker lead *use* Stimulator Lead in
  Gastrointestinal System
Gastric plexus *use* Nerve, Abdominal
  Sympathetic
Gastrocnemius muscle
  use Muscle, Lower Leg, Left
  use Muscle, Lower Leg, Right
Gastrocolic ligament *use* Omentum, Greater
Gastrocolic omentum *use* Omentum, Greater
Gastrocolostomy
  see Bypass, Gastrointestinal System **0D1**
  see Drainage, Gastrointestinal System **0D9**
Gastroduodenal artery *use* Artery, Hepatic
Gastroduodenectomy
  see Excision, Gastrointestinal System **0DB**
  see Resection, Gastrointestinal System **0DT**
Gastroduodenoscopy 0DJ08ZZ
Gastroenteroplasty
  see Repair, Gastrointestinal System **0DQ**
  see Supplement, Gastrointestinal System **0DU**
Gastroenterostomy
  see Bypass, Gastrointestinal System **0D1**
  see Drainage, Gastrointestinal System **0D9**
Gastroesophageal (GE) junction *use*
  Esophagogastric Junction

Gastrogastrostomy
  see Bypass, Stomach **0D16**
  see Drainage, Stomach **0D96**
Gastrohepatic omentum *use* Omentum, Lesser
Gastrojejunostomy
  see Bypass, Stomach **0D16**
  see Drainage, Stomach **0D96**
Gastrolysis *see* Release, Stomach **0DN6**
Gastropexy
  see Repair, Stomach **0DQ6**
  see Reposition, Stomach **0DS6**
Gastrophrenic ligament *use* Omentum, Greater
Gastroplasty
  see Repair, Stomach **0DQ6**
  see Supplement, Stomach **0DU6**
Gastroplication *see* Restriction, Stomach **0DV6**
Gastropylorectomy *see* Excision,
  Gastrointestinal System **0DB**
Gastrorrhaphy *see* Repair, Stomach **0DQ6**
Gastroscopy 0DJ68ZZ
Gastrosplenic ligament *use* Omentum, Greater
Gastrostomy
  see Bypass, Stomach **0D16**
  see Drainage, Stomach **0D96**
Gastrotomy *see* Drainage, Stomach **0D96**
Gemellus muscle
  use Muscle, Hip, Left
  use Muscle, Hip, Right
Geniculate ganglion *use* Nerve, Facial
Geniculate nucleus *use* Thalamus
Genioglossus muscle *use* Muscle, Tongue,
  Palate, Pharynx
Genioplasty *see* Alteration, Jaw, Lower **0W05**
Genitofemoral nerve *use* Nerve, Lumbar Plexus
Gingivectomy *see* Excision, Mouth and Throat
  0CB
Gingivoplasty
  see Repair, Mouth and Throat **0CQ**
  see Replacement, Mouth and Throat **0CR**
  see Supplement, Mouth and Throat **0CU**
Glans penis *use* Prepuce
Glenohumeral joint
  use Joint, Shoulder, Left
  use Joint, Shoulder, Right
Glenohumeral ligament
  use Bursa and Ligament, Shoulder, Right
  use Bursa and Ligament, Shoulder, Left
Glenoid fossa (of scapula)
  use Glenoid Cavity, Left
  use Glenoid Cavity, Right
Glenoid ligament (labrum)
  use Bursa and Ligament, Shoulder, Right
  use Bursa and Ligament, Shoulder, Left
Globus pallidus *use* Basal Ganglia
Glomectomy
  see Excision, Endocrine System **0GB**
  see Resection, Endocrine System **0GT**
Glossectomy
  see Excision, Tongue **0CB7**
  see Resection, Tongue **0CT7**
Glossoepiglottic fold *use* Epiglottis
Glossopexy
  see Repair, Tongue **0CQ7**
  see Reposition, Tongue **0CS7**
Glossoplasty
  see Repair, Tongue **0CQ7**
  see Replacement, Tongue **0CR7**
  see Supplement, Tongue **0CU7**
Glossorrhaphy *see* Repair, Tongue **0CQ7**
Glossotomy *see* Drainage, Tongue **0C97**
Glottis *use* Larynx

Gluteal Artery Perforator Flap
  Bilateral **0HRV079**
  Left **0HRU079**
  Right **0HRT079**
Gluteal lymph node *use* Lymphatic, Pelvis
Gluteal vein
  use Vein, Hypogastric, Right
  use Vein, Hypogastric, Left
Gluteus maximus muscle
  use Muscle, Hip, Right
  use Muscle, Hip, Left
Gluteus medius muscle
  use Muscle, Hip, Right
  use Muscle, Hip, Left
Gluteus minimus muscle
  use Muscle, Hip, Left
  use Muscle, Hip, Right
GORE® DUALMESH® *use* Synthetic
  Substitute
Gracilis muscle
  use Muscle, Upper Leg, Left
  use Muscle, Upper Leg, Right
Graft
  see Replacement
  see Supplement
Great auricular nerve *use* Nerve, Cervical
  Plexus
Great cerebral vein *use* Vein, Intracranial
Great saphenous vein
  use Vein, Greater Saphenous, Left
  use Vein, Greater Saphenous, Right
Greater alar cartilage *use* Nose
Greater occipital nerve *use* Nerve, Cervical
Greater splanchnic nerve *use* Nerve, Thoracic
  Sympathetic
Greater superficial petrosal nerve *use* Nerve,
  Facial
Greater trochanter
  use Femur, Upper, Left
  use Femur, Upper, Right
Greater tuberosity
  use Humeral Head, Right
  use Humeral Head, Left
Greater vestibular (Bartholin's) gland *use*
  Gland, Vestibular
Greater wing
  use Bone, Sphenoid, Left
  use Bone, Sphenoid, Right
Guedel airway *use* Intraluminal Device, Airway
  in Mouth and Throat
Guidance, catheter placement
  EKG *see* Measurement, Physiological
  Systems **4A0**
  Fluoroscopy *see* Fluoroscopy, Veins **B51**
  Ultrasound *see* Ultrasonography, Veins **B54**

H

Hallux
  use Toe, 1st, Right
  use Toe, 1st, Left
Hamate bone
  use Carpal, Right
  use Carpal, Left
Hancock Bioprosthesis (aortic) (mitral) valve
  use Zooplastic Tissue in Heart and Great
  Vessels
Hancock Bioprosthetic Valved Conduit *use*
  Zooplastic Tissue in Heart and Great Vessels
Harvesting, stem cells *see* Pheresis, Circulatory
  6A55

Head of fibula
  use Fibula, Right
  use Fibula, Left
Hearing Aid Assessment F14Z
Hearing Assessment F13Z
Hearing Device
  Bone Conduction
    Left **09HE**
    Right **09HD**
  Insertion of device in
    Left **0NH6[034]SZ**
    Right **0NH5[034]SZ**
  Multiple Channel Cochlear Prosthesis
    Left **09HE**
    Right **09HD**
  Removal of device from, Skull **0NP0**
  Revision of device in, Skull **0NW0**
  Single Channel Cochlear Prosthesis
    Left **09HE**
    Right **09HD Hearing Treatment F09Z**
Heart Assist System
  External
    Insertion of device in, Heart **02HA**
    Removal of device from, Heart **02PA**
    Revision of device in, Heart **02WA**
  Implantable
    Insertion of device in, Heart **02HA**
    Removal of device from, Heart **02PA**
    Revision of device in, Heart **02WA**
**HeartMate II® Left Ventricular Assist Device
(LVAD)** *use* Implantable Heart Assist System
in Heart and Great Vessels
**HeartMate XVE® Left Ventricular Assist
Device (LVAD)** *use* Implantable Heart Assist
System in Heart and Great Vessels
HeartMate® implantable heart assist system
  see Insertion of device in, Heart **02HA**
Helix
  use Ear, External, Bilateral
  use Ear, External, Right
  use Ear, External, Left
Hemicolectomy *see* Resection, Gastrointestinal
  System **0DT**
Hemicystectomy *see* Excision, Urinary System
  0TB
Hemigastrectomy *see* Excision, Gastrointestinal
  System **0DB**
Hemiglossectomy *see* Excision, Mouth and
  Throat **0CB**
Hemilaminectomy
  see Excision, Upper Bones **0PB**
  see Excision, Lower Bones **0QB**
Hemilaryngectomy *see* Excision, Larynx **0CBS**
Hemimandibulectomy *see* Excision, Head and
  Facial Bones **0NB**
Hemimaxillectomy *see* Excision, Head and
  Facial Bones **0NB**
Hemipylorectomy *see* Excision, Gastrointestinal
  System **0DB**
Hemispherectomy
  see Excision, Central Nervous System **00B**
  see Resection, Central Nervous System **00T**
Hemithyroidectomy
  see Resection, Endocrine System **0GT**
  see Excision, Endocrine System **0GB**
Hemodialysis 5A1D00Z
Hepatectomy
  see Excision, Hepatobiliary System and
  Pancreas **0FB**
  see Resection, Hepatobiliary System and
  Pancreas **0FT**
Hepatic artery proper *use* Artery, Hepatic

Hepatic flexure *use* Colon, Ascending
Hepatic lymph node *use* Lymphatic, Aortic
Hepatic plexus *use* Nerve, Abdominal
  Sympathetic
Hepatic portal vein *use* Vein, Portal
Hepaticoduodenostomy
  see Bypass, Hepatobiliary System and
  Pancreas 0F1
  see Drainage, Hepatobiliary System and
  Pancreas 0F9
Hepaticotomy *see* Drainage, Hepatobiliary
  System and Pancreas 0F9
Hepatocholedochostomy *see* Drainage, Duct,
  Common Bile 0F99
Hepatogastric ligament *use* Omentum, Lesser
Hepatopancreatic ampulla *use* Ampulla of
  Vater
Hepatopexy
  see Repair, Hepatobiliary System and
  Pancreas 0FQ
  see Reposition, Hepatobiliary System and
  Pancreas 0FS
Hepatorrhaphy *see* Repair, Hepatobiliary
  System and Pancreas 0FQ
Hepatotomy *see* Drainage, Hepatobiliary
  System and Pancreas 0F9
Herniorrhaphy
  see Repair, Anatomical Regions, General
  0WQ
  see Repair, Anatomical Regions, Lower
  Extremities 0YQ
  with synthetic substitute
    see Supplement, Anatomical Regions,
    General 0WU
    see Supplement, Anatomical Regions,
    Lower Extremities 0YU
Hip (joint) liner *use* Liner in Lower Joints
Holter monitoring 4A12X45
Holter valve ventricular shunt *use* Synthetic
  Substitute
Humeroradial joint
  use Joint, Elbow, Right
  use Joint, Elbow, Left
Humeroulnar joint
  use Joint, Elbow, Left
  use Joint, Elbow, Right
Humerus, distal
  use Humeral Shaft, Right
  use Humeral Shaft, Left
Hydrocelectomy *see* Excision, Male
  Reproductive System 0VB
Hydrotherapy
  Assisted exercise in pool *see* Motor
  Treatment, Rehabilitation F07
  Whirlpool *see* Activities of Daily Living
  Treatment, Rehabilitation F08
Hymenectomy
  see Excision, Hymen 0UBK
  see Resection, Hymen 0UTK
Hymenoplasty
  see Repair, Hymen 0UQK
  see Supplement, Hymen 0UUK
Hymenorrhaphy *see* Repair, Hymen 0UQK
Hymenotomy
  see Division, Hymen 0U8K
  see Drainage, Hymen 0U9K
Hyoglossus muscle *use* Muscle, Tongue, Palate,
  Pharynx
Hyoid artery
  use Artery, Thyroid, Right
  use Artery, Thyroid, Left
Hyperalimentation *see* Introduction of
  substance in or on

Hyperbaric oxygenation
  Decompression sickness treatment *see*
  Decompression, Circulatory 6A15
  Wound treatment *see* Assistance, Circulatory
  5A05
Hyperthermia
  Radiation Therapy
    Abdomen **DWY38ZZ**
    Adrenal Gland **DGY28ZZ**
    Bile Ducts **DFY28ZZ**
    Bladder **DTY28ZZ**
    Bone, Other **DPYC8ZZ**
    Bone Marrow **D7Y08ZZ**
    Brain **D0Y08ZZ**
    Brain Stem **D0Y18ZZ**
    Breast
      Left **DMY08ZZ**
      Right **DMY18ZZ**
    Bronchus **DBY18ZZ**
    Cervix **DUY18ZZ**
    Chest **DWY28ZZ**
    Chest Wall **DBY78ZZ**
    Colon **DDY58ZZ**
    Diaphragm **DBY88ZZ**
    Duodenum **DDY28ZZ**
    Ear **D9Y08ZZ**
    Esophagus **DDY08ZZ**
    Eye **D8Y08ZZ**
    Femur **DPY98ZZ**
    Fibula **DPYB8ZZ**
    Gallbladder **DFY18ZZ**
    Gland
      Adrenal **DGY28ZZ**
      Parathyroid **DGY48ZZ**
      Pituitary **DGY08ZZ**
      Thyroid **DGY58ZZ**
    Glands, Salivary **D9Y68ZZ**
    Head and Neck **DWY18ZZ**
    Hemibody **DWY48ZZ**
    Humerus **DPY68ZZ**
    Hypopharynx **D9Y38ZZ**
    Ileum **DDY48ZZ**
    Jejunum **DDY38ZZ**
    Kidney **DTY08ZZ**
    Larynx **D9YB8ZZ**
    Liver **DFY08ZZ**
    Lung **DBY28ZZ**
    Lymphatics
      Abdomen **D7Y68ZZ**
      Axillary **D7Y48ZZ**
      Inguinal **D7Y88ZZ**
      Neck **D7Y38ZZ**
      Pelvis **D7Y78ZZ**
      Thorax **D7Y58ZZ**
    Mandible **DPY38ZZ**
    Maxilla **DPY28ZZ**
    Mediastinum **DBY68ZZ**
    Mouth **D9Y48ZZ**
    Nasopharynx **D9YD8ZZ**
    Neck and Head **DWY18ZZ**
    Nerve, Peripheral **D0Y78ZZ**
    Nose **D9Y18ZZ**
    Oropharynx **D9YF8ZZ**
    Ovary **DUY08ZZ**
    Palate
      Hard **D9Y88ZZ**
      Soft **D9Y98ZZ**
    Pancreas **DFY38ZZ**
    Parathyroid Gland **DGY48ZZ**
    Pelvic Bones **DPY88ZZ**
    Pelvic Region **DWY68ZZ**
    Pineal Body **DGY18ZZ**
    Pituitary Gland **DGY08ZZ**

Hyperthermia - *continued*
  Pleura **DBY58ZZ**
  Prostate **DVY08ZZ**
  Radius **DPY78ZZ**
  Rectum **DDY78ZZ**
  Rib **DPY58ZZ**
  Sinuses **D9Y78ZZ**
  Skin
    Abdomen **DHY88ZZ**
    Arm **DHY48ZZ**
    Back **DHY78ZZ**
    Buttock **DHY98ZZ**
    Chest **DHY68ZZ**
    Face **DHY28ZZ**
    Leg **DHYB8ZZ**
    Neck **DHY38ZZ**
  Skull **DPY08ZZ**
  Spinal Cord **D0Y68ZZ**
  Spleen **D7Y28ZZ**
  Sternum **DPY48ZZ**
  Stomach **DDY18ZZ**
  Testis **DVY18ZZ**
  Thymus **D7Y18ZZ**
  Thyroid Gland **DGY58ZZ**
  Tibia **DPYB8ZZ**
  Tongue **D9Y58ZZ**
  Trachea **DBY08ZZ**
  Ulna **DPY78ZZ**
  Ureter **DTY18ZZ**
  Urethra **DTY38ZZ**
  Uterus **DUY28ZZ**
  Whole Body **DWY58ZZ**
  Whole Body **6A3Z**
Hypnosis GZFZZZZ
Hypogastric artery
  use Artery, Internal Iliac, Right
  use Artery, Internal Iliac, Left
Hypopharynx *use* Pharynx
Hypophysectomy
  see Excision, Gland, Pituitary 0GB0
  see Resection, Gland, Pituitary 0GT0
Hypophysis *use* Gland, Pituitary
Hypothalamotomy *see* Destruction, Thalamus
  0059
Hypothenar muscle
  use Muscle, Hand, Right
  use Muscle, Hand, Left
Hypothermia, Whole Body 6A4Z
Hysterectomy
  see Excision, Uterus 0UB9
  see Resection, Uterus 0UT9
Hysterolysis *see* Release, Uterus 0UN9
Hysteropexy
  see Repair, Uterus 0UQ9
  see Reposition, Uterus 0US9
Hysteroplasty *see* Repair, Uterus 0UQ9
Hysterorrhaphy *see* Repair, Uterus 0UQ9
Hysteroscopy 0UJD8ZZ
Hysterotomy *see* Drainage, Uterus 0U99
Hysterotrachelectomy *see* Resection, Uterus
  0UT9
Hysterotracheloplasty *see* Repair, Uterus
  0UQ9
Hysterotrachelorrhaphy *see* Repair, Uterus
  0UQ9

I

IABP (Intra-aortic balloon pump) *see*
  Assistance, Cardiac 5A02
**IAEMT (Intraoperative anesthetic effect
  monitoring and titration)** *see* Monitoring,
  Central Nervous 4A10

Ileal artery *use* Artery, Superior Mesenteric
Ileectomy
    see Excision, Ileum **0DBB**
    see Resection, Ileum **0DTB**
Ileocolic artery *use* Artery, Superior Mesenteric
Ileocolic vein *use* Vein, Colic
Ileopexy
    see Repair, Ileum **0DQB**
    see Reposition, Ileum **0DSB**
Ileorrhaphy *see* Repair, Ileum **0DQB**
Ileoscopy 0DJD8ZZ
Ileostomy
    see Bypass, Ileum **0D1B**
    see Drainage, Ileum **0D9B**
Ileotomy *see* Drainage, Ileum **0D9B**
Ileoureterostomy *see* Bypass, Urinary System **0T1**
Iliac crest
    use Bone, Pelvic, Left
    use Bone, Pelvic, Right
Iliac fascia
    use Subcutaneous Tissue and Fascia, Upper Leg, Left
    use Subcutaneous Tissue and Fascia, Upper Leg, Right
Iliac lymph node *use* Lymphatic, Pelvis
Iliacus muscle
    use Muscle, Hip, Right
    use Muscle, Hip, Left
Iliofemoral ligament
    use Bursa and Ligament, Hip, Left
    use Bursa and Ligament, Hip, Right
Iliohypogastric nerve *use* Nerve, Lumbar Plexus
Ilioinguinal nerve *use* Nerve, Lumbar Plexus
Iliolumbar artery
    use Artery, Internal Iliac, Left
    use Artery, Internal Iliac, Right
Iliolumbar ligament
    use Bursa and Ligament, Trunk, Left
    use Bursa and Ligament, Trunk, Right
Iliotibial tract (band)
    use Subcutaneous Tissue and Fascia, Upper Leg, Right
    use Subcutaneous Tissue and Fascia, Upper Leg, Left
Ilium
    use Bone, Pelvic, Left
    use Bone, Pelvic, Right
Ilizarov external fixator
    use External Fixation Device, Ring in **0PH**
    use External Fixation Device, Ring in **0PS**
    use External Fixation Device, Ring in **0QH**
    use External Fixation Device, Ring in **0QS**
Ilizarov-Vecklich device
    use External Fixation Device, Limb Lengthening in **0PH**
    use External Fixation Device, Limb Lengthening in **0QH**
Imaging, diagnostic
    see Plain Radiography
    see Fluoroscopy
    see Computerized Tomography (CT Scan)
    see Magnetic Resonance Imaging (MRI)
    see Ultrasonography
Immobilization
    Abdominal Wall **2W33X**
    Arm
        Lower
            Left **2W3DX**
            Right **2W3CX**

Immobilization - *continued*
    Upper
        Left **2W3BX**
        Right **2W3AX**
    Back **2W35X**
    Chest Wall **2W34X**
    Extremity
        Lower
            Left **2W3MX**
            Right **2W3LX**
        Upper
            Left **2W39X**
            Right **2W38X**
    Face **2W31X**
    Finger
        Left **2W3KX**
        Right **2W3JX**
    Foot
        Left **2W3TX**
        Right **2W3SX**
    Hand
        Left **2W3FX**
        Right **2W3EX**
    Head **2W30X**
    Inguinal Region
        Left **2W37X**
        Right **2W36X**
    Leg
        Lower
            Left **2W3RX**
            Right **2W3QX**
        Upper
            Left **2W3PX**
            Right **2W3NX**
    Neck **2W32X**
    Thumb
        Left **2W3HX**
        Right **2W3GX**
    Toe
        Left **2W3VX**
        Right **2W3UX**
Immunization *see* Introduction of Serum, Toxoid, and Vaccine
Immunotherapy *see* Introduction of Immunotherapeutic Substance
Immunotherapy, antineoplastic
    Interferon *see* Introduction of Low-dose Interleukin-2
    Interleukin-2, high-dose *see* Introduction of High-dose Interleukin-2
    Interleukin-2, low-dose *see* Introduction of Low-dose Interleukin-2
    Monoclonal antibody *see* Introduction of Monoclonal Antibody
    Proleukin, high-dose *see* Introduction of High-dose Interleukin-2
    Proleukin, low-dose *see* Introduction of Low-dose Interleukin-2
Impella® (2.5) (5.0) (LD) cardiac assist device *use* Intraluminal Device
Impeller Pump
    Continuous, Output **5A0221D**
    Intermittent, Output **5A0211D**
Implantable cardioverter-defibrillator (ICD) *use* Defibrillator Generator in **0JH**
Implantable drug infusion pump (anti-spasmodic)(chemotherapy)(pain) *use* Infusion Device, Pump in Subcutaneous Tissue and Fascia
Implantable glucose monitoring device *use* Monitoring Device
Implantable hemodynamic monitor (IHM) *use* Monitoring Device, Hemodynamic in **0JH**

Implantable hemodynamic monitoring system (IHMS) *use* Monitoring Device, Hemodynamic in **0JH**
Implantable Miniature Telescope™ (IMT) *use* Synthetic Substitute, Intraocular Telescope in **08R**
Implantation
    see Insertion
    see Replacement
Implanted (venous)(access) port *use* Vascular Access Device, Reservoir in Subcutaneous Tissue and Fascia
IMV (intermittent mandatory ventilation) *see* Assistance, Respiratory **5A09**
In Vitro Fertilization 8E0ZXY1
Incision, abscess *see* Drainage
Incudectomy
    see Excision, Ear, Nose, Sinus **09B**
    see Resection, Ear, Nose, Sinus **09T**
Incudopexy
    see Reposition, Ear, Nose, Sinus **09S**
    see Repair, Ear, Nose, Sinus **09Q**
Incus
    use Auditory Ossicle, Left
    use Auditory Ossicle, Right
Induction of labor
    Artificial rupture of membranes *see* Drainage, Pregnancy **109**
    Oxytocin *see* Introduction of Hormone
InDura, intrathecal catheter (1P) (spinal) *use* Infusion Device
Inferior cardiac nerve *use* Nerve, Thoracic Sympathetic
Inferior cerebellar vein *use* Vein, Intracranial
Inferior cerebral vein *use* Vein, Intracranial
Inferior epigastric artery
    use Artery, External Iliac, Right
    use Artery, External Iliac, Left
Inferior epigastric lymph node *use* Lymphatic, Pelvis
Inferior genicular artery
    use Artery, Popliteal, Left
    use Artery, Popliteal, Right
Inferior gluteal artery
    use Artery, Internal Iliac, Right
    use Artery, Internal Iliac, Left
Inferior gluteal nerve *use* Nerve, Sacral Plexus
Inferior hypogastric plexus *use* Nerve, Abdominal Sympathetic
Inferior labial artery *use* Artery, Face
Inferior longitudinal muscle *use* Muscle, Tongue, Palate, Pharynx
Inferior mesenteric ganglion *use* Nerve, Abdominal Sympathetic
Inferior mesenteric lymph node *use* Lymphatic, Mesenteric
Inferior mesenteric plexus *use* Nerve, Abdominal Sympathetic
Inferior oblique muscle
    use Muscle, Extraocular, Right
    use Muscle, Extraocular, Left
Inferior pancreaticoduodenal artery *use* Artery, Superior Mesenteric
Inferior phrenic artery *use* Aorta, Abdominal
Inferior rectus muscle
    use Muscle, Extraocular, Right
    use Muscle, Extraocular, Left
Inferior suprarenal artery
    use Artery, Renal, Left
    use Artery, Renal, Right
Inferior tarsal plate
    use Eyelid, Lower, Right
    use Eyelid, Lower, Left

Inferior thyroid vein
   use Vein, Innominate, Left
   use Vein, Innominate, Right
Inferior tibiofibular joint
   use Joint, Ankle, Right
   use Joint, Ankle, Left
Inferior turbinate *use* Turbinate, Nasal
Inferior ulnar collateral artery
   use Artery, Brachial, Right
   use Artery, Brachial, Left
Inferior vesical artery
   use Artery, Internal Iliac, Right
   use Artery, Internal Iliac, Left
Infraauricular lymph node *use* Lymphatic,
   Head
Infraclavicular (deltopectoral) lymph node
   use Lymphatic, Upper Extremity, Left
   use Lymphatic, Upper Extremity, Right
Infrahyoid muscle
   use Muscle, Neck, Left
   use Muscle, Neck, Right
Infraparotid lymph node *use* Lymphatic, Head
Infraspinatus fascia
   use Subcutaneous Tissue and Fascia, Upper
   Arm, Right
   use Subcutaneous Tissue and Fascia, Upper
   Arm, Left
Infraspinatus muscle
   use Muscle, Shoulder, Right
   use Muscle, Shoulder, Left
Infundibulopelvic ligament *use* Uterine
   Supporting Structure
Infusion *see* Introduction of substance in or on
Infusion Device
   Insertion of device in
     Abdomen **0JH8**
     Back **0JH7**
     Chest **0JH6**
     Lower Arm
       Left **0JHH**
       Right **0JHG**
     Lower Leg
       Left **0JHP**
       Right **0JHN**
     Trunk **0JHT**
     Upper Arm
       Left **0JHF**
       Right **0JHD**
     Upper Leg
       Left **0JHM**
       Right **0JHL**
   Removal of device from
     Lower Extremity **0JPW**
     Trunk **0JPT**
     Upper Extremity **0JPV**
   Revision of device in
     Lower Extremity **0JWW**
     Trunk **0JWT**
     Upper Extremity **0JWV**
Infusion, glucarpidase
   Central vein **3E043GQ**
   Peripheral vein **3E033GQ**
Inguinal canal
   use Inguinal Region, Right
   use Inguinal Region, Left
   use Inguinal Region, Bilateral
Inguinal triangle
   use Inguinal Region, Right
   use Inguinal Region, Bilateral
   use Inguinal Region, Left
Injection *see* Introduction of substance in or on

Injection reservoir, port *use* Vascular Access
   Device, Reservoir in Subcutaneous Tissue and
   Fascia
Injection reservoir, pump *use* Infusion Device,
   Pump in Subcutaneous Tissue and Fascia
Insemination, artificial 3E0P7LZ
Insertion
   Antimicrobial envelope *see* Introduction of
   Anti-infective
   Aqueous drainage shunt
     see Bypass, Eye **081**
     see Drainage, Eye **089**
   Products of Conception **10H0**
   Spinal Stabilization Device
     see Insertion of device in, Upper Joints
   0RH
     see Insertion of device in, Lower Joints
   0SH
Insertion of device in
   Abdominal Wall **0WHF**
   Acetabulum
     Left **0QH5**
     Right **0QH4**
   Anal Sphincter **0DHR**
   Ankle Region
     Left **0YHL**
     Right **0YHK**
   Anus **0DHQ**
   Aorta
     Abdominal **04H0**
     Thoracic **02HW**
   Arm
     Lower
       Left **0XHF**
       Right **0XHD**
     Upper
       Left **0XH9**
       Right **0XH8**
   Artery
     Anterior Tibial
       Left **04HQ**
       Right **04HP**
     Axillary
       Left **03H6**
       Right **03H5**
     Brachial
       Left **03H8**
       Right **03H7**
     Celiac **04H1**
     Colic
       Left **04H7**
       Middle **04H8**
       Right **04H6**
     Common Carotid
       Left **03HJ**
       Right **03HH**
     Common Iliac
       Left **04HD**
       Right **04HC**
     External Carotid
       Left **03HN**
       Right **03HM**
     External Iliac
       Left **04HJ**
       Right **04HH**
     Face **03HR**
     Femoral
       Left **04HL**
       Right **04HK**
     Foot
       Left **04HW**
       Right **04HV**

Insertion of device – *continued*
     Gastric **04H2**
     Hand
       Left **03HF**
       Right **03HD**
     Hepatic **04H3**
     Inferior Mesenteric **04HB**
     Innominate **03H2**
     Internal Carotid
       Left **03HL**
       Right **03HK**
     Internal Iliac
       Left **04HF**
       Right **04HE**
     Internal Mammary
       Left **03H1**
       Right **03H0**
     Intracranial **03HG**
     Lower **04HY**
     Peroneal
       Left **04HU**
       Right **04HT**
     Popliteal
       Left **04HN**
       Right **04HM**
     Posterior Tibial
       Left **04HS**
       Right **04HR**
     Pulmonary
       Left **02HR**
       Right **02HQ**
     Pulmonary Trunk **02HP**
     Radial
       Left **03HC**
       Right **03HB**
     Renal
       Left **04HA**
       Right **04H9**
     Splenic **04H4**
     Subclavian
       Left **03H4**
       Right **03H3**
     Superior Mesenteric **04H5**
     Temporal
       Left **03HT**
       Right **03HS**
     Thyroid
       Left **03HV**
       Right **03HU**
     Ulnar
       Left **03HA**
       Right **03H9**
     Upper **03HY**
     Vertebral
       Left **03HQ**
       Right **03HP**
   Atrium
     Left **02H7**
     Right **02H6**
   Axilla
     Left **0XH5**
     Right **0XH4**
   Back
     Lower **0WHL**
     Upper **0WHK**
   Bladder **0THB**
   Bladder Neck **0THC**
   Bone
     Ethmoid
       Left **0NHG**
       Right **0NHF**
     Facial **0NHW**

Insertion of device – *continued*
 Pulmonary
  Left **02HT**
  Right **02HS**
 Renal
  Left **06HB**
  Right **06H9**
 Splenic **06H1**
 Subclavian
  Left **05H6**
  Right **05H5**
 Superior Mesenteric **06H5**
 Upper **05HY**
 Vertebral
  Left **05HS**
  Right **05HR**
 Vena Cava
  Inferior **06H0**
  Superior **02HV**
 Ventricle
  Left **02HL**
  Right **02HK**
 Vertebra
  Cervical **0PH3**
  Lumbar **0QH0**
  Thoracic **0PH4**
 Wrist Region
  Left **0XHH**
  Right **0XHG**
Inspection
 Abdominal Wall **0WJF**
 Ankle Region
  Left **0YJL**
  Right **0YJK**
 Arm
  Lower
   Left **0XJF**
   Right **0XJD**
  Upper
   Left **0XJ9**
   Right **0XJ8**
 Artery
  Lower **04JY**
  Upper **03JY**
 Axilla
  Left **0XJ5**
  Right **0XJ4**
 Back
  Lower **0WJL**
  Upper **0WJK**
 Bladder **0TJB**
 Bone
  Facial **0NJW**
  Lower **0QJY**
  Nasal **0NJB**
  Upper **0PJY**
 Bone Marrow **07JT**
 Brain **00J0**
 Breast
  Left **0HJU**
  Right **0HJT**
 Bursa and Ligament
  Lower **0MJY**
  Upper **0MJX**
 Buttock
  Left **0YJ1**
  Right **0YJ0**
 Cavity, Cranial **0WJ1**
 Chest Wall **0WJ8**
 Cisterna Chyli **07JL**
 Diaphragm **0BJT**

 Disc
  Cervical Vertebral **0RJ3**
  Cervicothoracic Vertebral **0RJ5**
  Lumbar Vertebral **0SJ2**
  Lumbosacral **0SJ4**
  Thoracic Vertebral **0RJ9**
  Thoracolumbar Vertebral **0RJB**
 Duct
  Hepatobiliary **0FJB**
  Pancreatic **0FJD**
 Ear
  Inner
   Left **09JE**
   Right **09JD**
  Left **09JJ**
  Right **09JH**
 Elbow Region
  Left **0XJC**
  Right **0XJB**
 Epididymis and Spermatic Cord **0VJM**
 Extremity
  Lower
   Left **0YJB**
   Right **0YJ9**
  Upper
   Left **0XJ7**
   Right **0XJ6**
 Eye
  Left **08J1XZZ**
  Right **08J0XZZ**
 Face **0WJ2**
 Fallopian Tube **0UJ8**
 Femoral Region
  Bilateral **0YJE**
  Left **0YJ8**
  Right **0YJ7**
 Finger Nail **0HJQXZZ**
 Foot
  Left **0YJN**
  Right **0YJM**
 Gallbladder **0FJ4**
 Gastrointestinal Tract **0WJP**
 Genitourinary Tract **0WJR**
 Gland
  Adrenal **0GJ5**
  Endocrine **0GJS**
  Pituitary **0GJ0**
  Salivary **0CJA**
 Great Vessel **02JY**
 Hand
  Left **0XJK**
  Right **0XJJ**
 Head **0WJ0**
 Heart **02JA**
 Inguinal Region
  Bilateral **0YJA**
  Left **0YJ6**
  Right **0YJ5**
 Intestinal Tract
  Lower **0DJD**
  Upper **0DJ0**
 Jaw
  Lower **0WJ5**
  Upper **0WJ4**
 Joint
  Acromioclavicular
   Left **0RJH**
   Right **0RJG**
  Ankle
   Left **0SJG**
   Right **0SJF**

  Carpal
   Left **0RJR**
   Right **0RJQ**
  Cervical Vertebral **0RJ1**
  Cervicothoracic Vertebral **0RJ4**
  Coccygeal **0SJ6**
  Elbow
   Left **0RJM**
   Right **0RJL**
  Finger Phalangeal
   Left **0RJX**
   Right **0RJW**
  Hip
   Left **0SJB**
   Right **0SJ9**
  Knee
   Left **0SJD**
   Right **0SJC**
  Lumbar Vertebral **0SJ0**
  Lumbosacral **0SJ3**
  Metacarpocarpal
   Left **0RJT**
   Right **0RJS**
  Metacarpophalangeal
   Left **0RJV**
   Right **0RJU**
  Metatarsal-Phalangeal
   Left **0SJN**
   Right **0SJM**
  Metatarsal-Tarsal
   Left **0SJL**
   Right **0SJK**
  Occipital-cervical **0RJ0**
  Sacrococcygeal **0SJ5**
  Sacroiliac
   Left **0SJ8**
   Right **0SJ7**
  Shoulder
   Left **0RJK**
   Right **0RJJ**
  Sternoclavicular
   Left **0RJF**
   Right **0RJE**
  Tarsal
   Left **0SJJ**
   Right **0SJH**
  Temporomandibular
   Left **0RJD**
   Right **0RJC**
  Thoracic Vertebral **0RJ6**
  Thoracolumbar Vertebral **0RJA**
  Toe Phalangeal
   Left **0SJQ**
   Right **0SJP**
  Wrist
   Left **0RJP**
   Right **0RJN**
 Kidney **0TJ5**
 Knee Region
  Left **0YJG**
  Right **0YJF**
 Larynx **0CJS**
 Leg
  Lower
   Left **0YJJ**
   Right **0YJH**
  Upper
   Left **0YJD**
   Right **0YJC**
 Lens
  Left **08JKXZZ**
  Right **08JJXZZ**

Inspection - *continued*
Liver **0FJ0**
Lung
Left **0BJL**
Right **0BJK**
Lymphatic **07JN**
Thoracic Duct **07JK**
Mediastinum **0WJC**
Mesentery **0DJV**
Mouth and Throat **0CJY**
Muscle
Extraocular
Left **08JM**
Right **08JL**
Lower **0KJY**
Upper **0KJX**
Neck **0WJ6**
Nerve
Cranial **00JE**
Peripheral **01JY**
Nose **09JK**
Omentum **0DJU**
Oral Cavity and Throat **0WJ3**
Ovary **0UJ3**
Pancreas **0FJG**
Parathyroid Gland **0GJR**
Pelvic Cavity **0WJJ**
Penis **0VJS**
Pericardial Cavity **0WJD**
Perineum
Female **0WJN**
Male **0WJM**
Peritoneal Cavity **0WJG**
Peritoneum **0DJW**
Pineal Body **0GJ1**
Pleura **0BJQ**
Pleural Cavity
Left **0WJB**
Right **0WJ9**
Products of Conception **10J0**
Ectopic **10J2**
Retained **10J1**
Prostate and Seminal Vesicles **0VJ4**
Respiratory Tract **0WJQ**
Retroperitoneum **0WJH**
Scrotum and Tunica Vaginalis **0VJ8**
Shoulder Region
Left **0XJ3**
Right **0XJ2**
Sinus **09JY**
Skin **0HJPXZZ**
Skull **0NJ0**
Spinal Canal **00JU**
Spinal Cord **00JV**
Spleen **07JP**
Stomach **0DJ6**
Subcutaneous Tissue and Fascia
Head and Neck **0JJS**
Lower Extremity **0JJW**
Trunk **0JJT**
Upper Extremity **0JJV**
Tendon
Lower **0LJY**
Upper **0LJX**
Testis **0VJD**
Thymus **07JM**
Thyroid Gland **0GJK**
Toe Nail **0HJRXZZ**
Trachea **0BJ1**
Tracheobronchial Tree **0BJ0**

Inspection - *continued*
Tympanic Membrane
Left **09J8**
Right **09J7**
Ureter **0TJ9**
Urethra **0TJD**
Uterus and Cervix **0UJD**
Vagina and Cul-de-sac **0UJH**
Vas Deferens **0VJR**
Vein
Lower **06JY**
Upper **05JY**
Vulva **0UJM**
Wrist Region
Left **0XJH**
Right **0XJG**
Instillation *see* Introduction of substance in or on
Insufflation *see* Introduction of substance in or on
Interatrial septum *use* Septum, Atrial
Interbody fusion (spine) cage
use Interbody Fusion Device in Upper Joints
use Interbody Fusion Device in Lower Joints
Intercarpal joint
use Joint, Carpal, Right
use Joint, Carpal, Left
Intercarpal ligament
use Bursa and Ligament, Hand, Right
use Bursa and Ligament, Hand, Left
Interclavicular ligament
use Bursa and Ligament, Shoulder, Right
use Bursa and Ligament, Shoulder, Left
Intercostal lymph node *use* Lymphatic, Thorax
Intercostal muscle
use Muscle, Thorax, Right
use Muscle, Thorax, Left
Intercostal nerve *use* Nerve, Thoracic
Intercostobrachial nerve *use* Nerve, Thoracic
Intercuneiform joint
use Joint, Tarsal, Right
use Joint, Tarsal, Left
Intercuneiform ligament
use Bursa and Ligament, Foot, Left
use Bursa and Ligament, Foot, Right
Intermediate cuneiform bone
use Tarsal, Right
use Tarsal, Left
Intermittent mandatory ventilation *see* Assistance, Respiratory **5A09**
Intermittent Negative Airway Pressure
24-96 Consecutive Hours, Ventilation **5A0945B**
Greater than 96 Consecutive Hours, Ventilation **5A0955B**
Less than 24 Consecutive Hours, Ventilation **5A0935B**
Intermittent Positive Airway Pressure
24-96 Consecutive Hours, Ventilation **5A09458**
Greater than 96 Consecutive Hours, Ventilation **5A09558**
Less than 24 Consecutive Hours, Ventilation **5A09358**
Intermittent positive pressure breathing *see* Assistance, Respiratory **5A09**
Internal (basal) cerebral vein *use* Vein, Intracranial
Internal anal sphincter *use* Anal Sphincter
Internal carotid plexus *use* Nerve, Head and Neck Sympathetic

Internal iliac vein
use Vein, Hypogastric, Right
use Vein, Hypogastric, Left
Internal maxillary artery
use Artery, External Carotid, Left
use Artery, External Carotid, Right
Internal naris *use* Nose
Internal oblique muscle
use Muscle, Abdomen, Right
use Muscle, Abdomen, Left
Internal pudendal artery
use Artery, Internal Iliac, Right
use Artery, Internal Iliac, Left
Internal pudendal vein
use Vein, Hypogastric, Right
use Vein, Hypogastric, Left
Internal thoracic artery
use Artery, Subclavian, Right
use Artery, Subclavian, Left
use Artery, Internal Mammary, Left
use Artery, Internal Mammary, Right
Internal urethral sphincter *use* Urethra
Interphalangeal (IP) joint
use Joint, Finger Phalangeal, Left
use Joint, Toe Phalangeal, Right
use Joint, Toe Phalangeal, Left
use Joint, Finger Phalangeal, Right
Interphalangeal ligament
use Bursa and Ligament, Hand, Left
use Bursa and Ligament, Hand, Right
use Bursa and Ligament, Foot, Right
use Bursa and Ligament, Foot, Left
Interrogation, cardiac rhythm related device
Interrogation only *see* Measurement, Cardiac **4B02**
With cardiac function testing *see* Measurement, Cardiac **4A02**
Interruption *see* Occlusion
Interspinalis muscle
use Muscle, Trunk, Right
use Muscle, Trunk, Left
Interspinous ligament
use Bursa and Ligament, Trunk, Right
use Bursa and Ligament, Trunk, Left
Interspinous process spinal stabilization device
use Spinal Stabilization Device, Interspinous Process in **0RH**
use Spinal Stabilization Device, Interspinous Process in **0SH**
InterStim® Therapy lead *use* Neurostimulator Lead in Peripheral Nervous System
InterStim® Therapy neurostimulator *use* Stimulator Generator, Single Array in **0JH**
Intertransversarius muscle
use Muscle, Trunk, Left
use Muscle, Trunk, Right
Intertransverse ligament
use Bursa and Ligament, Trunk, Right
use Bursa and Ligament, Trunk, Left
Interventricular foramen (Monro) *use* Cerebral Ventricle
Interventricular septum *use* Septum, Ventricular
Intestinal lymphatic trunk *use* Cisterna Chyli
Intraluminal Device
Airway
Esophagus **0DH5**
Mouth and Throat **0CHY**
Nasopharynx **09HN**

Intraluminal Device - *continued*
  Bioactive
    Occlusion
      Common Carotid
        Left **03LJ**
        Right **03LH**
      External Carotid
        Left **03LN**
        Right **03LM**
      Internal Carotid
        Left **03LL**
        Right **03LK**
      Intracranial **03LG**
      Vertebral
        Left **03LQ**
        Right **03LP**
    Restriction
      Common Carotid
        Left **03VJ**
        Right **03VH**
      External Carotid
        Left **03VN**
        Right **03VM**
      Internal Carotid
        Left **03VL**
        Right **03VK**
      Intracranial **03VG**
      Vertebral
        Left **03VQ**
        Right **03VP**
  Endobronchial Valve
    Lingula **0BH9**
    Lower Lobe
      Left **0BHB**
      Right **0BH6**
    Main
      Left **0BH7**
      Right **0BH3**
    Middle Lobe, Right **0BH5**
    Upper Lobe
      Left **0BH8**
      Right **0BH4**
  Endotracheal Airway
    Change device in, Trachea **0B21XEZ**
    Insertion of device in, Trachea **0BH1**
  Pessary
    Change device in, Vagina and Cul-de-sac
    0U2HXGZ
    Insertion of device in
      Cul-de-sac **0UHF**
      Vagina **0UHG**
Intramedullary (IM) rod (nail)
  use Internal Fixation Device, Intramedullary
  in Upper Bones
  use Internal Fixation Device, Intramedullary
  in Lower Bones
Intramedullary skeletal kinetic distractor
  (ISKD)
  use Internal Fixation Device, Intramedullary
  in Upper Bones
  use Internal Fixation Device, Intramedullary
  in Lower Bones
Intraocular Telescope
  Left **08RK30Z**
  Right **08RJ30Z**
Intraoperative Radiation Therapy (IORT)
  Anus **DDY8CZZ**
  Bile Ducts **DFY2CZZ**
  Bladder **DTY2CZZ**
  Cervix **DUY1CZZ**
  Colon **DDY5CZZ**
  Duodenum **DDY2CZZ**
  Gallbladder **DFY1CZZ**

Intraoperative Radiation Therapy - *continued*
  Ileum **DDY4CZZ**
  Jejunum **DDY3CZZ**
  Kidney **DTY0CZZ**
  Larynx **D9YBCZZ**
  Liver **DFY0CZZ**
  Mouth **D9Y4CZZ**
  Nasopharynx **D9YDCZZ**
  Ovary **DUY0CZZ**
  Pancreas **DFY3CZZ**
  Pharynx **D9YCCZZ**
  Prostate **DVY0CZZ**
  Rectum **DDY7CZZ**
  Stomach **DDY1CZZ**
  Ureter **DTY1CZZ**
  Urethra **DTY3CZZ**
  Uterus **DUY2CZZ**
Intrauterine device (IUD) *use* Contraceptive
  Device in Female Reproductive System
Introduction of substance in or on
  Artery
    Central **3E06**
      Analgesics **3E06**
      Anesthetic, Intracirculatory **3E06**
      Anti-infective **3E06**
      Anti-inflammatory **3E06**
      Antiarrhythmic **3E06**
      Antineoplastic **3E06**
      Destructive Agent **3E06**
      Diagnostic Substance, Other **3E06**
      Electrolytic Substance **3E06**
      Hormone **3E06**
      Hypnotics **3E06**
      Immunotherapeutic **3E06**
      Nutritional Substance **3E06**
      Platelet Inhibitor **3E06**
      Radioactive Substance **3E06**
      Sedatives **3E06**
      Serum **3E06**
      Thrombolytic **3E06**
      Toxoid **3E06**
      Vaccine **3E06**
      Vasopressor **3E06**
      Water Balance Substance **3E06**
    Coronary **3E07**
      Diagnostic Substance, Other **3E07**
      Platelet Inhibitor **3E07**
      Thrombolytic **3E07**
    Peripheral **3E05**
      Analgesics **3E05**
      Anesthetic, Intracirculatory **3E05**
      Anti-infective **3E05**
      Anti-inflammatory **3E05**
      Antiarrhythmic **3E05**
      Antineoplastic **3E05**
      Destructive Agent **3E05**
      Diagnostic Substance, Other **3E05**
      Electrolytic Substance **3E05**
      Hormone **3E05**
      Hypnotics **3E05**
      Immunotherapeutic **3E05**
      Nutritional Substance **3E05**
      Platelet Inhibitor **3E05**
      Radioactive Substance **3E05**
      Sedatives **3E05**
      Serum **3E05**
      Thrombolytic **3E05**
      Toxoid **3E05**
      Vaccine **3E05**
      Vasopressor **3E05**
      Water Balance Substance **3E05**

Introduction of substance – *continued*
  Biliary Tract **3E0J**
    Analgesics **3E0J**
    Anesthetic, Local **3E0J**
    Anti-infective **3E0J**
    Anti-inflammatory **3E0J**
    Antineoplastic **3E0J**
    Destructive Agent **3E0J**
    Diagnostic Substance, Other **3E0J**
    Electrolytic Substance **3E0J**
    Gas **3E0J**
    Hypnotics **3E0J**
    Islet Cells, Pancreatic **3E0J**
    Nutritional Substance **3E0J**
    Radioactive Substance **3E0J**
    Sedatives **3E0J**
    Water Balance Substance **3E0J**
  Bone **3E0V**
    Analgesics **3E0V3NZ**
    Anesthetic, Local **3E0V3BZ**
    Anti-infective **3E0V32**
    Anti-inflammatory **3E0V33Z**
    Antineoplastic **3E0V30**
    Destructive Agent **3E0V3TZ**
    Diagnostic Substance, Other **3E0V3KZ**
    Electrolytic Substance **3E0V37Z**
    Hypnotics **3E0V3NZ**
    Nutritional Substance **3E0V36Z**
    Radioactive Substance **3E0V3HZ**
    Sedatives **3E0V3NZ**
    Water Balance Substance **3E0V37Z**
  Bone Marrow **3E0A3GC**
    Antineoplastic **3E0A30**
  Brain **3E0Q3GC**
    Analgesics **3E0Q3NZ**
    Anesthetic, Local **3E0Q3BZ**
    Anti-infective **3E0Q32**
    Anti-inflammatory **3E0Q33Z**
    Antineoplastic **3E0Q**
    Destructive Agent **3E0Q3TZ**
    Diagnostic Substance, Other **3E0Q3KZ**
    Electrolytic Substance **3E0Q37Z**
    Gas **3E0Q**
    Hypnotics **3E0Q3NZ**
    Nutritional Substance **3E0Q36Z**
    Radioactive Substance **3E0Q3HZ**
    Sedatives **3E0Q3NZ**
    Stem Cells
      Embryonic **3E0Q**
      Somatic **3E0Q**
    Water Balance Substance **3E0Q37Z**
  Cranial Cavity **3E0Q3GC**
    Analgesics **3E0Q3NZ**
    Anesthetic, Local **3E0Q3BZ**
    Anti-infective **3E0Q32**
    Anti-inflammatory **3E0Q33Z**
    Antineoplastic **3E0Q**
    Destructive Agent **3E0Q3TZ**
    Diagnostic Substance, Other **3E0Q3KZ**
    Electrolytic Substance **3E0Q37Z**
    Gas **3E0Q**
    Hypnotics **3E0Q3NZ**
    Nutritional Substance **3E0Q36Z**
    Radioactive Substance **3E0Q3HZ**
    Sedatives **3E0Q3NZ**
    Stem Cells
      Embryonic **3E0Q**
      Somatic **3E0Q**
    Water Balance Substance **3E0Q37Z**
  Ear **3E0B**
    Analgesics **3E0B**
    Anesthetic, Local **3E0B**

Anti-infective **3E0B**
Anti-inflammatory **3E0B**
Antineoplastic **3E0B**
Destructive Agent **3E0B**
Diagnostic Substance, Other **3E0B**
Hypnotics **3E0B**
Radioactive Substance **3E0B**
Sedatives **3E0B**
Epidural Space **3E0S3GC**
Analgesics **3E0S3NZ**
Anesthetic
Local **3E0S3BZ**
Regional **3E0S3CZ**
Anti-infective **3E0S32**
Anti-inflammatory **3E0S33Z**
Antineoplastic **3E0S30**
Destructive Agent **3E0S3TZ**
Diagnostic Substance, Other **3E0S3KZ**
Electrolytic Substance **3E0S37Z**
Gas **3E0S**
Hypnotics **3E0S3NZ**
Nutritional Substance **3E0S36Z**
Radioactive Substance **3E0S3HZ**
Sedatives **3E0S3NZ**
Water Balance Substance **3E0S37Z**
Eye **3E0C**
Analgesics **3E0C**
Anesthetic, Local **3E0C**
Anti-infective **3E0C**
Anti-inflammatory **3E0C**
Antineoplastic **3E0C**
Destructive Agent **3E0C**
Diagnostic Substance, Other **3E0C**
Gas **3E0C**
Hypnotics **3E0C**
Pigment **3E0C**
Radioactive Substance **3E0C**
Sedatives **3E0C**
Gastrointestinal Tract
Lower **3E0H**
Analgesics **3E0H**
Anesthetic, Local **3E0H**
Anti-infective **3E0H**
Anti-inflammatory **3E0H**
Antineoplastic **3E0H**
Destructive Agent **3E0H**
Diagnostic Substance, Other **3E0H**
Electrolytic Substance **3E0H**
Gas **3E0H**
Hypnotics **3E0H**
Nutritional Substance **3E0H**
Radioactive Substance **3E0H**
Sedatives **3E0H**
Water Balance Substance **3E0H**
Upper **3E0G**
Analgesics **3E0G**
Anesthetic, Local **3E0G**
Anti-infective **3E0G**
Anti-inflammatory **3E0G**
Antineoplastic **3E0G**
Destructive Agent **3E0G**
Diagnostic Substance, Other **3E0G**
Electrolytic Substance **3E0G**
Gas **3E0G**
Hypnotics **3E0G**
Nutritional Substance **3E0G**
Radioactive Substance **3E0G**
Sedatives **3E0G**
Water Balance Substance **3E0G**
Genitourinary Tract **3E0K**
Analgesics **3E0K**

Anesthetic, Local **3E0K**
Anti-infective **3E0K**
Anti-inflammatory **3E0K**
Antineoplastic **3E0K**
Destructive Agent **3E0K**
Diagnostic Substance, Other **3E0K**
Electrolytic Substance **3E0K**
Gas **3E0K**
Hypnotics **3E0K**
Nutritional Substance **3E0K**
Radioactive Substance **3E0K**
Sedatives **3E0K**
Water Balance Substance **3E0K**
Heart **3E08**
Diagnostic Substance, Other **3E08**
Platelet Inhibitor **3E08**
Thrombolytic **3E08**
Joint **3E0U**
Analgesics **3E0U3NZ**
Anesthetic, Local **3E0U3BZ**
Anti-infective **3E0U**
Anti-inflammatory **3E0U33Z**
Antineoplastic **3E0U30**
Destructive Agent **3E0U3TZ**
Diagnostic Substance, Other **3E0U3KZ**
Electrolytic Substance **3E0U37Z**
Gas **3E0U3SF**
Hypnotics **3E0U3NZ**
Nutritional Substance **3E0U36Z**
Radioactive Substance **3E0U3HZ**
Sedatives **3E0U3NZ**
Water Balance Substance **3E0U37Z**
Lymphatic **3E0W3GC**
Analgesics **3E0W3NZ**
Anesthetic, Local **3E0W3BZ**
Anti-infective **3E0W32**
Anti-inflammatory **3E0W33Z**
Antineoplastic **3E0W30**
Destructive Agent **3E0W3TZ**
Diagnostic Substance, Other   **3E0W3KZ**
Electrolytic Substance **3E0W37Z**
Hypnotics **3E0W3NZ**
Nutritional Substance **3E0W36Z**
Radioactive Substance **3E0W3HZ**
Sedatives **3E0W3NZ**
Water Balance Substance **3E0W37Z**
Mouth **3E0D**
Analgesics **3E0D**
Anesthetic, Local **3E0D**
Anti-infective **3E0D**
Anti-inflammatory **3E0D**
Antiarrhythmic **3E0D**
Antineoplastic **3E0D**
Destructive Agent **3E0D**
Diagnostic Substance, Other **3E0D**
Electrolytic Substance **3E0D**
Hypnotics **3E0D**
Nutritional Substance **3E0D**
Radioactive Substance **3E0D**
Sedatives **3E0D**
Serum **3E0D**
Toxoid **3E0D**
Vaccine **3E0D**
Water Balance Substance **3E0D**
Mucous Membrane **3E00XGC**
Analgesics **3E00XNZ**
Anesthetic, Local **3E00XBZ**
Anti-infective **3E00X2**
Anti-inflammatory **3E00X3Z**
Antineoplastic **3E00X0**
Destructive Agent **3E00XTZ**

Diagnostic Substance, Other **3E00XKZ**
Hypnotics **3E00XNZ**
Pigment **3E00XMZ**
Sedatives **3E00XNZ**
Serum **3E00X4Z**
Toxoid **3E00X4Z**
Vaccine **3E00X4Z**
Muscle **3E023GC**
Analgesics **3E023NZ**
Anesthetic, Local **3E023BZ**
Anti-infective **3E0232**
Anti-inflammatory **3E0233Z**
Antineoplastic **3E0230**
Destructive Agent **3E023TZ**
Diagnostic Substance, Other **3E023KZ**
Electrolytic Substance **3E0237Z**
Hypnotics **3E023NZ**
Nutritional Substance **3E0236Z**
Radioactive Substance **3E023HZ**
Sedatives **3E023NZ**
Serum **3E0234Z**
Toxoid **3E0234Z**
Vaccine **3E0234Z**
Water Balance Substance **3E0237Z**
Nerve
Cranial **3E0X3GC**
Anesthetic
Local **3E0X3BZ**
Regional **3E0X3CZ**
Anti-inflammatory **3E0X33Z**
Destructive Agent **3E0X3TZ**
Peripheral **3E0T3GC**
Anesthetic
Local **3E0T3BZ**
Regional **3E0T3CZ**
Anti-inflammatory **3E0T33Z**
Destructive Agent **3E0T3TZ**
Plexus **3E0T3GC**
Anesthetic
Local **3E0T3BZ**
Regional **3E0T3CZ**
Anti-inflammatory **3E0T33Z**
Destructive Agent **3E0T3TZ**
Nose **3E09**
Analgesics **3E09**
Anesthetic, Local **3E09**
Anti-infective **3E09**
Anti-inflammatory **3E09**
Antineoplastic **3E09**
Destructive Agent **3E09**
Diagnostic Substance, Other **3E09**
Hypnotics **3E09**
Radioactive Substance **3E09**
Sedatives **3E09**
Serum **3E09**
Toxoid **3E09**
Vaccine **3E09**
Pancreatic Tract **3E0J**
Analgesics **3E0J**
Anesthetic, Local **3E0J**
Anti-infective **3E0J**
Anti-inflammatory **3E0J**
Antineoplastic **3E0J**
Destructive Agent **3E0J**
Diagnostic Substance, Other **3E0J**
Electrolytic Substance **3E0J**
Gas **3E0J**
Hypnotics **3E0J**
Islet Cells, Pancreatic **3E0J**
Nutritional Substance **3E0J**
Radioactive Substance **3E0J**
Sedatives **3E0J**

Introduction of substance – *continued*
    Antineoplastic **3E03**
    Destructive Agent **3E03**
    Diagnostic Substance, Other **3E03**
    Electrolytic Substance **3E03**
    Hormone **3E03**
    Hypnotics **3E03**
    Immunotherapeutic **3E03**
    Islet Cells, Pancreatic **3E03**
    Nutritional Substance **3E03**
    Platelet Inhibitor **3E03**
    Radioactive Substance **3E03**
    Sedatives **3E03**
    Serum **3E03**
    Thrombolytic **3E03**
    Toxoid **3E03**
    Vaccine **3E03**
    Vasopressor **3E03**
    Water Balance Substance **3E03**
Intubation
    Airway
      see Insertion of device in, Trachea **0BH1**
      see Insertion of device in, Mouth and
    Throat **0CHY**
      see Insertion of device in, Esophagus
    0DH5
    Drainage device *see* Drainage
    Feeding Device *see* Insertion of device in,
    Gastrointestinal System **0DH**
IPPB (intermittent positive pressure
  breathing) *see* Assistance, Respiratory **5A09**
Iridectomy
    see Excision, Eye **08B**
    see Resection, Eye **08T**
Iridoplasty
    see Repair, Eye **08Q**
    see Replacement, Eye **08R**
    see Supplement, Eye **08U**
Iridotomy *see* Drainage, Eye **089**
Irrigation
    Biliary Tract, Irrigating Substance **3E1J**
    Brain, Irrigating Substance **3E1Q38Z**
    Cranial Cavity, Irrigating Substance
    3E1Q38Z
    Ear, Irrigating Substance **3E1B**
    Epidural Space, Irrigating Substance
    3E1S38Z
    Eye, Irrigating Substance **3E1C**
    Gastrointestinal Tract
      Lower, Irrigating Substance **3E1H**
      Upper, Irrigating Substance **3E1G**
    Genitourinary Tract, Irrigating Substance
    3E1K
    Irrigating Substance **3C1ZX8Z**
    Joint, Irrigating Substance **3E1U38Z**
    Mucous Membrane, Irrigating Substance
    3E10
    Nose, Irrigating Substance **3E19**
    Pancreatic Tract, Irrigating Substance **3E1J**
    Pericardial Cavity, Irrigating Substance
    3E1Y38Z
    Peritoneal Cavity
      Dialysate **3E1M39Z**
      Irrigating Substance **3E1M38Z**
    Pleural Cavity, Irrigating Substance **3E1L38Z**
    Reproductive
      Female, Irrigating Substance **3E1P**
      Male, Irrigating Substance **3E1N**
    Respiratory Tract, Irrigating Substance **3E1F**
    Skin, Irrigating Substance **3E10**
    Spinal Canal, Irrigating Substance **3E1R38Z**
Ischiatic nerve *use* Nerve, Sciatic
Ischiocavernosus muscle *use* Muscle, Perineum

Ischiofemoral ligament
    use Bursa and Ligament, Hip, Left
    use Bursa and Ligament, Hip, Right
Ischium
    use Bone, Pelvic, Right
    use Bone, Pelvic, Left
Isolation 8E0ZXY6
Isotope Administration, Whole Body DWY5G
Itrel (3)(4) neurostimulator *use* Stimulator
  Generator, Single Array in **0JH**

J

Jejunal artery *use* Artery, Superior Mesenteric
Jejunectomy
    see Excision, Jejunum **0DBA**
    see Resection, Jejunum **0DTA**
Jejunocolostomy
    see Bypass, Gastrointestinal System **0D1**
    see Drainage, Gastrointestinal System **0D9**
Jejunopexy
    see Repair, Jejunum **0DQA**
    see Reposition, Jejunum **0DSA**
Jejunostomy
    see Bypass, Jejunum **0D1A**
    see Drainage, Jejunum **0D9A**
Jejunotomy *see* Drainage, Jejunum **0D9A**
Joint fixation plate
    use Internal Fixation Device in Upper Joints
    use Internal Fixation Device in Lower Joints
Joint liner (insert) *use* Liner in Lower Joints
Joint spacer (antibiotic)
    use Spacer in Upper Joints
    use Spacer in Lower Joints
Jugular body *use* Glomus Jugulare
Jugular lymph node
    use Lymphatic, Neck, Left
    use Lymphatic, Neck, Right

K

Kappa *use* Pacemaker, Dual Chamber in **0JH**
Keratectomy, kerectomy
    see Excision, Eye **08B**
    see Resection, Eye **08T**
Keratocentesis *see* Drainage, Eye **089**
Keratoplasty
    see Repair, Eye **08Q**
    see Replacement, Eye **08R**
    see Supplement, Eye **08U**
Keratotomy
    see Drainage, Eye **089**
    see Repair, Eye **08Q**
Kinetra® neurostimulator *use* Stimulator
  Generator, Multiple Array in **0JH**
Kirschner wire (K-wire)
    use Internal Fixation Device in Head and
    Facial Bones
    use Internal Fixation Device in Upper Bones
    use Internal Fixation Device in Lower Bones
    use Internal Fixation Device in Upper Joints
    use Internal Fixation Device in Lower Joints
Knee (implant) insert *use* Liner in Lower Joints
KUB x-ray *see* Plain Radiography, Kidney,
  Ureter and Bladder **BT04**
Küntscher nail
    use Internal Fixation Device, Intramedullary
    in Upper Bones
    use Internal Fixation Device, Intramedullary
    in Lower Bones

L

Labia majora *use* Vulva
Labia minora *use* Vulva
Labial gland
    use Lip, Upper
    use Lip, Lower
Labiectomy
    see Excision, Female Reproductive System
    0UB
    see Resection, Female Reproductive System
    0UT
Lacrimal canaliculus
    use Duct, Lacrimal, Left
    use Duct, Lacrimal, Right
Lacrimal punctum
    use Duct, Lacrimal, Right
    use Duct, Lacrimal, Left
Lacrimal sac
    use Duct, Lacrimal, Right
    use Duct, Lacrimal, Left
Laminectomy
    see Excision, Upper Bones **0PB**
    see Excision, Lower Bones **0QB**
Laminotomy
    see Drainage, Upper Joints **0R9**
    see Drainage, Lower Joints **0S9**
    see Release, Central Nervous System **00N**
    see Release, Peripheral Nervous System **01N**
    see Release, Upper Joints **0RN**
    see Release, Lower Joints **0SN**
LAP-BAND® adjustable gastric banding
  system *use* Extraluminal Device
Laparoscopy *See* Inspection
Laparotomy
    Drainage *see* Drainage, Peritoneal Cavity
    0W9G
    Exploratory *see* Inspection, Peritoneal Cavity
    0WJG
Laryngectomy
    see Excision, Larynx **0CBS**
    see Resection, Larynx **0CTS**
Laryngocentesis *see* Drainage, Larynx **0C9S**
Laryngogram *see* Fluoroscopy, Larynx **B91J**
Laryngopexy *see* Repair, Larynx **0CQS**
Laryngopharynx *use* Pharynx
Laryngoplasty
    see Repair, Larynx **0CQS**
    see Replacement, Larynx **0CRS**
    see Supplement, Larynx **0CUS**
Laryngorrhaphy *see* Repair, Larynx **0CQS**
Laryngoscopy 0CJS8ZZ
Laryngotomy *see* Drainage, Larynx **0C9S**
Laser Interstitial Thermal Therapy
    Adrenal Gland **DGY2KZZ**
    Anus **DDY8KZZ**
    Bile Ducts **DFY2KZZ**
    Brain **D0Y0KZZ**
    Brain Stem **D0Y1KZZ**
    Breast
      Left **DMY0KZZ**
      Right **DMY1KZZ**
    Bronchus **DBY1KZZ**
    Chest Wall **DBY7KZZ**
    Colon **DDY5KZZ**
    Diaphragm **DBY8KZZ**
    Duodenum **DDY2KZZ**
    Esophagus **DDY0KZZ**
    Gallbladder **DFY1KZZ**
    Gland
      Adrenal **DGY2KZZ**
      Parathyroid **DGY4KZZ**
      Pituitary **DGY0KZZ**

Laser Interstitial Thermal - *continued*
    Thyroid **DGY5KZZ**
    Ileum **DDY4KZZ**
    Jejunum **DDY3KZZ**
    Liver **DFY0KZZ**
    Lung **DBY2KZZ**
    Mediastinum **DBY6KZZ**
    Nerve, Peripheral **D0Y7KZZ**
    Pancreas **DFY3KZZ**
    Parathyroid Gland **DGY4KZZ**
    Pineal Body **DGY1KZZ**
    Pituitary Gland **DGY0KZZ**
    Pleura **DBY5KZZ**
    Prostate **DVY0KZZ**
    Rectum **DDY7KZZ**
    Spinal Cord **D0Y6KZZ**
    Stomach **DDY1KZZ**
    Thyroid Gland **DGY5KZZ**
    Trachea **DBY0KZZ**
Lateral (brachial) lymph node
  use Lymphatic, Axillary, Left
  use Lymphatic, Axillary, Right
Lateral canthus
  use Eyelid, Upper, Right
  use Eyelid, Upper, Left
Lateral collateral ligament (LCL)
  use Bursa and Ligament, Knee, Right
  use Bursa and Ligament, Knee, Left
Lateral condyle of femur
  use Femur, Lower, Right
  use Femur, Lower, Left
Lateral condyle of tibia
  use Tibia, Left
  use Tibia, Right
Lateral cuneiform bone
  use Tarsal, Right
  use Tarsal, Left
Lateral epicondyle of femur
  use Femur, Lower, Left
  use Femur, Lower, Right
Lateral epicondyle of humerus
  use Humeral Shaft, Right
  use Humeral Shaft, Left
Lateral femoral cutaneous nerve *use* Nerve, Lumbar Plexus
Lateral malleolus
  use Fibula, Right
  use Fibula, Left
Lateral meniscus
  use Joint, Knee, Left
  use Joint, Knee, Right
Lateral nasal cartilage *use* Nose
Lateral plantar artery
  use Artery, Foot, Left
  use Artery, Foot, Right
Lateral plantar nerve *use* Nerve, Tibial
Lateral rectus muscle
  use Muscle, Extraocular, Left
  use Muscle, Extraocular, Right
Lateral sacral artery
  use Artery, Internal Iliac, Left
  use Artery, Internal Iliac, Right
Lateral sacral vein
  use Vein, Hypogastric, Left
  use Vein, Hypogastric, Right
Lateral sural cutaneous nerve *use* Nerve, Peroneal
Lateral tarsal artery
  use Artery, Foot, Right
  use Artery, Foot, Left
Lateral temporomandibular ligament *use* Bursa and Ligament, Head and Neck

Lateral thoracic artery
  use Artery, Axillary, Left
  use Artery, Axillary, Right
Latissimus dorsi muscle
  use Muscle, Trunk, Left
  use Muscle, Trunk, Right
Latissimus Dorsi Myocutaneous Flap
  Bilateral **0HRV075**
  Left **0HRU075**
  Right **0HRT075**
Lavage
  see Irrigation
  bronchial alveolar, diagnostic *see* Drainage, Respiratory System **0B9**
Least splanchnic nerve *use* Nerve, Thoracic Sympathetic
Left ascending lumbar vein *use* Vein, Hemiazygos
Left atrioventricular valve *use* Valve, Mitral
Left auricular appendix *use* Atrium, Left
Left colic vein *use* Vein, Colic
Left coronary sulcus *use* Heart, Left
Left gastric artery *use* Artery, Gastric
Left gastroepiploic artery *use* Artery, Splenic
Left gastroepiploic vein *use* Vein, Splenic
Left inferior phrenic vein *use* Vein, Renal, Left
Left inferior pulmonary vein *use* Vein, Pulmonary, Left
Left jugular trunk *use* Lymphatic, Thoracic Duct
Left lateral ventricle *use* Cerebral Ventricle
Left ovarian vein *use* Vein, Renal, Left
Left second lumbar vein *use* Vein, Renal, Left
Left subclavian trunk *use* Lymphatic, Thoracic Duct
Left subcostal vein *use* Vein, Hemiazygos
Left superior pulmonary vein *use* Vein, Pulmonary, Left
Left suprarenal vein *use* Vein, Renal, Left
Left testicular vein *use* Vein, Renal, Left
Lengthening
  Bone, with device *see* Insertion of Limb Lengthening Device
  Muscle, by incision *see* Division, Muscles **0K8**
  Tendon, by incision *see* Division, Tendons **0L8**
Leptomeninges
  use Cerebral Meninges
  use Spinal Meninges
Lesser alar cartilage *use* Nose
Lesser occipital nerve *use* Nerve, Cervical Plexus
Lesser splanchnic nerve *use* Nerve, Thoracic Sympathetic
Lesser trochanter
  use Femur, Upper, Right
  use Femur, Upper, Left
Lesser tuberosity
  use Humeral Head, Left
  use Humeral Head, Right
Lesser wing
  use Bone, Sphenoid, Right
  use Bone, Sphenoid, Left
Leukopheresis, therapeutic *see* Pheresis, Circulatory **6A55**
Levator anguli oris muscle *use* Muscle, Facial
Levator ani muscle
  use Muscle, Trunk, Left
  use Muscle, Trunk, Right
Levator labii superioris alaeque nasi muscle
  use Muscle, Facial

Levator labii superioris muscle *use* Muscle, Facial
Levator palpebrae superioris muscle
  use Eyelid, Upper, Left
  use Eyelid, Upper, Right
Levator scapulae muscle
  use Muscle, Neck, Left
  use Muscle, Neck, Right
Levator veli palatini muscle *use* Muscle, Tongue, Palate, Pharynx
Levatores costarum muscle
  use Muscle, Thorax, Left
  use Muscle, Thorax, Right
LifeStent® (Flexstar)(XL) Vascular Stent System *use* Intraluminal Device
Ligament of head of fibula
  use Bursa and Ligament, Knee, Right
  use Bursa and Ligament, Knee, Left
Ligament of the lateral malleolus
  use Bursa and Ligament, Ankle, Left
  use Bursa and Ligament, Ankle, Right
Ligamentum flavum
  use Bursa and Ligament, Trunk, Left
  use Bursa and Ligament, Trunk, Right
Ligation *see* Occlusion
Ligation, hemorrhoid *see* Occlusion, Lower Veins, Hemorrhoidal Plexus
Light Therapy GZJZZZZ
Liner
  Removal of device from
    Hip
      Left **0SPB09Z**
      Right **0SP909Z**
    Knee
      Left **0SPD09Z**
      Right **0SPC09Z**
  Revision of device in
    Hip
      Left **0SWB09Z**
      Right **0SW909Z**
    Knee
      Left **0SWD09Z**
      Right **0SWC09Z**
  Supplement
    Hip
      Left **0SUB09Z**
        Acetabular Surface **0SUE09Z**
        Femoral Surface **0SUS09Z**
      Right **0SU909Z**
        Acetabular Surface **0SUA09Z**
        Femoral Surface **0SUR09Z**
    Knee
      Left **0SUD09**
        Femoral Surface **0SUU09Z**
        Tibial Surface **0SUW09Z**
      Right **0SUC09**
        Femoral Surface **0SUT09Z**
        Tibial Surface **0SUV09Z**
Lingual artery
  use Artery, External Carotid, Right
  use Artery, External Carotid, Left
Lingual tonsil *use* Tongue
Lingulectomy, lung
  see Excision, Lung Lingula **0BBH**
  see Resection, Lung Lingula **0BTH**
Lithotripsy
  see Fragmentation
  with removal of fragments *see* Extirpation
LIVIAN™ CRT-D *use* Cardiac Resynchronization Defibrillator Pulse Generator in **0JH**

Lobectomy
- see Excision, Central Nervous System **00B**
- see Excision, Respiratory System **0BB**
- see Resection, Respiratory System **0BT**
- see Excision, Hepatobiliary System and Pancreas **0FB**
- see Resection, Hepatobiliary System and Pancreas **0FT**
- see Excision, Endocrine System **0GB**
- see Resection, Endocrine System **0GT**

Lobotomy see Division, Brain **0080**

Localization
- see Map
- see Imaging

Locus ceruleus use Pons

Long thoracic nerve use Nerve, Brachial Plexus

Loop ileostomy see Bypass, Ileum **0D1B**

Loop recorder, implantable use Monitoring Device

Lower GI series see Fluoroscopy, Colon **BD14**

Lumbar artery use Aorta, Abdominal

Lumbar facet joint
- use Joint, Lumbar Vertebral, 2 or more
- use Joint, Lumbar Vertebral

Lumbar ganglion use Nerve, Lumbar Sympathetic

Lumbar lymph node use Lymphatic, Aortic

Lumbar lymphatic trunk use Cisterna Chyli

Lumbar splanchnic nerve use Nerve, Lumbar Sympathetic

Lumbosacral facet joint use Joint, Lumbosacral

Lumbosacral trunk use Nerve, Lumbar

Lumpectomy see Excision

Lunate bone
- use Carpal, Left
- use Carpal, Right

Lunotriquetral ligament
- use Bursa and Ligament, Hand, Left
- use Bursa and Ligament, Hand, Right

Lymphadenectomy
- see Excision, Lymphatic and Hemic Systems **07B**
- see Resection, Lymphatic and Hemic Systems **07T**

Lymphadenotomy see Drainage, Lymphatic and Hemic Systems **079**

Lymphangiectomy
- see Excision, Lymphatic and Hemic Systems **07B**
- see Resection, Lymphatic and Hemic Systems **07T**

Lymphangiogram see Plain Radiography, Lymphatic System **B70**

Lymphangioplasty
- see Repair, Lymphatic and Hemic Systems **07Q**
- see Supplement, Lymphatic and Hemic Systems **07U**

Lymphangiorrhaphy see Repair, Lymphatic and Hemic Systems **07Q**

Lymphangiotomy see Drainage, Lymphatic and Hemic Systems **079**

Lysis see Release

M

Macula
- use Retina, Right
- use Retina, Left

Magnet extraction, ocular foreign body see Extirpation, Eye **08C**

Magnetic Resonance Imaging (MRI)
- Abdomen **BW30**
- Ankle
  - Left **BQ3H**
  - Right **BQ3G**
- Aorta
  - Abdominal **B430**
  - Thoracic **B330**
- Arm
  - Left **BP3F**
  - Right **BP3E**
- Artery
  - Celiac **B431**
  - Cervico-Cerebral Arch **B33Q**
  - Common Carotid, Bilateral **B335**
  - Coronary
    - Bypass Graft, Multiple **B233**
    - Multiple **B231**
  - Internal Carotid, Bilateral **B338**
  - Intracranial **B33R**
  - Lower Extremity
    - Bilateral **B43H**
    - Left **B43G**
    - Right **B43F**
  - Pelvic **B43C**
  - Renal, Bilateral **B438**
  - Spinal **B33M**
  - Superior Mesenteric **B434**
  - Upper Extremity
    - Bilateral **B33K**
    - Left **B33J**
    - Right **B33H**
  - Vertebral, Bilateral **B33G**
- Bladder **BT30**
- Brachial Plexus **BW3P**
- Brain **B030**
- Breast
  - Bilateral **BH32**
  - Left **BH31**
  - Right **BH30**
- Calcaneus
  - Left **BQ3K**
  - Right **BQ3J**
- Chest **BW33Y**
- Coccyx **BR3F**
- Connective Tissue
  - Lower Extremity **BL31**
  - Upper Extremity **BL30**
- Corpora Cavernosa **BV30**
- Disc
  - Cervical **BR31**
  - Lumbar **BR33**
  - Thoracic **BR32**
- Ear **B930**
- Elbow
  - Left **BP3H**
  - Right **BP3G**
- Eye
  - Bilateral **B837**
  - Left **B836**
  - Right **B835**
- Femur
  - Left **BQ34**
  - Right **BQ33**
- Fetal Abdomen **BY33**
- Fetal Extremity **BY35**
- Fetal Head **BY30**
- Fetal Heart **BY31**
- Fetal Spine **BY34**
- Fetal Thorax **BY32**
- Fetus, Whole **BY36**

Magnetic Resonance Imaging – *continued*
- Foot
  - Left **BQ3M**
  - Right **BQ3L**
- Forearm
  - Left **BP3K**
  - Right **BP3J**
- Gland
  - Adrenal, Bilateral **BG32**
  - Parathyroid **BG33**
  - Parotid, Bilateral **B936**
  - Salivary, Bilateral **B93D**
  - Submandibular, Bilateral **B939**
  - Thyroid **BG34**
- Head **BW38**
- Heart, Right and Left **B236**
- Hip
  - Left **BQ31**
  - Right **BQ30**
- Intracranial Sinus **B532**
- Joint
  - Finger
    - Left **BP3D**
    - Right **BP3C**
  - Hand
    - Left **BP3D**
    - Right **BP3C**
  - Temporomandibular, Bilateral **BN39**
- Kidney
  - Bilateral **BT33**
  - Left **BT32**
  - Right **BT31**
  - Transplant **BT39**
- Knee
  - Left **BQ38**
  - Right **BQ37**
- Larynx **B93J**
- Leg
  - Left **BQ3F**
  - Right **BQ3D**
- Liver **BF35**
- Liver and Spleen **BF36**
- Lung Apices **BB3G**
- Nasopharynx **B93F**
- Neck **BW3F**
- Nerve
  - Acoustic **B03C**
  - Brachial Plexus **BW3P**
- Oropharynx **B93F**
- Ovary
  - Bilateral **BU35**
  - Left **BU34**
  - Right **BU33**
- Ovary and Uterus **BU3C**
- Pancreas **BF37**
- Patella
  - Left **BQ3W**
  - Right **BQ3V**
- Pelvic Region **BW3G**
- Pelvis **BR3C**
- Pituitary Gland **B039**
- Plexus, Brachial **BW3P**
- Prostate **BV33**
- Retroperitoneum **BW3H**
- Sacrum **BR3F**
- Scrotum **BV34**
- Sella Turcica **B039**
- Shoulder
  - Left **BP39**
  - Right **BP38**
- Sinus
  - Intracranial **B532**
  - Paranasal **B932**

Magnetic Resonance Imaging – *continued*
  Spinal Cord **B03B**
  Spine
    Cervical **BR30**
    Lumbar **BR39**
    Thoracic **BR37**
  Spleen and Liver **BF36**
  Subcutaneous Tissue
    Abdomen **BH3H**
    Extremity
      Lower **BH3J**
      Upper **BH3F**
    Head **BH3D**
    Neck **BH3D**
    Pelvis **BH3H**
    Thorax **BH3G**
  Tendon
    Lower Extremity **BL33**
    Upper Extremity **BL32**
  Testicle
    Bilateral **BV37**
    Left **BV36**
    Right **BV35**
  Toe
    Left **BQ3Q**
    Right **BQ3P**
  Uterus **BU36**
    Pregnant **BU3B**
  Uterus and Ovary **BU3C**
  Vagina **BU39**
  Vein
    Cerebellar **B531**
    Cerebral **B531**
    Jugular, Bilateral **B535**
    Lower Extremity
      Bilateral **B53D**
      Left **B53C**
      Right **B53B**
    Other **B53V**
    Pelvic (Iliac) Bilateral **B53H**
    Portal **B53T**
    Pulmonary, Bilateral **B53S**
    Renal, Bilateral **B53L**
    Splanchnic **B53T**
    Upper Extremity
      Bilateral **B53P**
      Left **B53N**
      Right **B53M**
  Vena Cava
    Inferior **B539**
    Superior **B538**
  Wrist
    Left **BP3M**
    Right **BP3L**
Malleotomy *see* Drainage, Ear, Nose, Sinus **099**
Malleus
  use Auditory Ossicle, Right
  use Auditory Ossicle, Left
Mammaplasty, mammoplasty
  see Alteration, Skin and Breast **0H0**
  see Repair, Skin and Breast **0HQ**
  see Replacement, Skin and Breast **0HR**
  see Supplement, Skin and Breast **0HU**
Mammary duct
  use Breast, Bilateral
  use Breast, Right
  use Breast, Left
Mammary gland
  use Breast, Bilateral
  use Breast, Right
  use Breast, Left

Mammectomy
  see Excision, Skin and Breast **0HB**
  see Resection, Skin and Breast **0HT**
Mammillary body *use* Hypothalamus
Mammography *see* Plain Radiography, Skin, Subcutaneous Tissue and Breast **BH0**
Mammotomy *see* Drainage, Skin and Breast **0H9**
Mandibular nerve *use* Nerve, Trigeminal
Mandibular notch
  use Mandible, Right
  use Mandible, Left
Mandibulectomy
  see Excision, Head and Facial Bones **0NB**
  see Resection, Head and Facial Bones **0NT**
Manipulation
  Adhesions *see* Release
  Chiropractic *see* Chiropractic Manipulation
Manubrium *use* Sternum **Map**
  Basal Ganglia **00K8**
  Brain **00K0**
  Cerebellum **00KC**
  Cerebral Hemisphere **00K7**
  Conduction Mechanism **02K8**
  Hypothalamus **00KA**
  Medulla Oblongata **00KD**
  Pons **00KB**
  Thalamus **00K9**
Mapping
  Doppler ultrasound *see* Ultrasonography
  Electrocardiogram only *see* Measurement, Cardiac **4A02**
Mark IV Breathing Pacemaker System *use* Stimulator Generator in Subcutaneous Tissue and Fascia
Marsupialization
  see Drainage
  see Excision
Massage, cardiac
  External **5A12012**
  Open **02QA0ZZ**
Masseter muscle *use* Muscle, Head
Masseteric fascia *use* Subcutaneous Tissue and Fascia, Face
Mastectomy
  see Excision, Skin and Breast **0HB**
  see Resection, Skin and Breast **0HT**
Mastoid (postauricular) lymph node
  use Lymphatic, Neck, Left
  use Lymphatic, Neck, Right
Mastoid air cells
  use Sinus, Mastoid, Left
  use Sinus, Mastoid, Right
Mastoid process
  use Bone, Temporal, Right
  use Bone, Temporal, Left
Mastoidectomy
  see Excision, Ear, Nose, Sinus **09B**
  see Resection, Ear, Nose, Sinus **09T**
Mastoidotomy *see* Drainage, Ear, Nose, Sinus **099**
Mastopexy
  see Reposition, Skin and Breast **0HS**
  see Repair, Skin and Breast **0HQ**
Mastotomy *see* Drainage, Skin and Breast **0H9**
Maxillary artery
  use Artery, External Carotid, Right
  use Artery, External Carotid, Left
Maxillary nerve *use* Nerve, Trigeminal
Maximo II DR (VR) *use* Defibrillator Generator in **0JH**

Maximo II DR CRT-D *use* Cardiac Resynchronization Defibrillator Pulse Generator in **0JH**
Measurement
  Arterial
    Flow
      Coronary **4A03**
      Peripheral **4A03**
      Pulmonary **4A03**
    Pressure
      Coronary **4A03**
      Peripheral **4A03**
      Pulmonary **4A03**
      Thoracic, Other **4A03**
    Pulse
      Coronary **4A03**
      Peripheral **4A03**
      Pulmonary **4A03**
    Saturation, Peripheral **4A03**
    Sound, Peripheral **4A03**
  Biliary
    Flow **4A0C**
    Pressure **4A0C**
  Cardiac
    Action Currents **4A02**
    Defibrillator **4B02XTZ**
    Electrical Activity **4A02**
      Guidance **4A02X4A**
      No Qualifier **4A02X4Z**
    Output **4A02**
    Pacemaker **4B02XSZ**
    Rate **4A02**
    Rhythm **4A02**
    Sampling and Pressure
      Bilateral **4A02**
      Left Heart **4A02**
      Right Heart **4A02**
    Sound **4A02**
    Total Activity, Stress **4A02XM4**
  Central Nervous
    Conductivity **4A00**
    Electrical Activity **4A00**
    Pressure **4A000BZ**
      Intracranial **4A00**
    Saturation, Intracranial **4A00**
    Stimulator **4B00XVZ**
    Temperature, Intracranial **4A00**
  Circulatory, Volume **4A05XLZ**
  Gastrointestinal
    Motility **4A0B**
    Pressure **4A0B**
    Secretion **4A0B**
  Lymphatic
    Flow **4A06**
    Pressure **4A06**
  Metabolism **4A0Z**
  Musculoskeletal
    Contractility **4A0F**
    Stimulator **4B0FXVZ**
  Olfactory, Acuity **4A08X0Z**
  Peripheral Nervous
    Conductivity
      Motor **4A01**
      Sensory **4A01**
    Electrical Activity **4A01**
    Stimulator **4B01XVZ**
  Products of Conception
    Cardiac
      Electrical Activity **4A0H**
      Rate **4A0H**
      Rhythm **4A0H**
      Sound **4A0H**

Measurement - *continued*
  Nervous
    Conductivity **4A0J**
    Electrical Activity **4A0J**
    Pressure **4A0J**
  Respiratory
    Capacity **4A09**
    Flow **4A09**
    Pacemaker **4B09XSZ**
    Rate **4A09**
    Resistance **4A09**
    Total Activity **4A09**
    Volume **4A09**
  Sleep **4A0ZXQZ**
  Temperature **4A0Z**
  Urinary
    Contractility **4A0D73Z**
    Flow **4A0D75Z**
    Pressure **4A0D7BZ**
    Resistance **4A0D7DZ**
    Volume **4A0D7LZ**
  Venous
    Flow
      Central **4A04**
      Peripheral **4A04**
      Portal **4A04**
      Pulmonary **4A04**
    Pressure
      Central **4A04**
      Peripheral **4A04**
      Portal **4A04**
      Pulmonary **4A04**
    Pulse
      Central **4A04**
      Peripheral **4A04**
      Portal **4A04**
      Pulmonary **4A04**
    Saturation, Peripheral **4A04**
  Visual
    Acuity **4A07X0Z**
    Mobility **4A07X7Z**
    Pressure **4A07XBZ**
Meatoplasty, urethra *see* Repair, Urethra **0TQD**
Meatotomy *see* Drainage, Urinary System **0T9**
Mechanical ventilation *see* Performance, Respiratory **5A19**
Medial canthus
  use Eyelid, Lower, Left
  use Eyelid, Lower, Right
Medial collateral ligament (MCL)
  use Bursa and Ligament, Knee, Left
  use Bursa and Ligament, Knee, Right
Medial condyle of femur
  use Femur, Lower, Right
  use Femur, Lower, Left
Medial condyle of tibia
  use Tibia, Left
  use Tibia, Right
Medial cuneiform bone
  use Tarsal, Right
  use Tarsal, Left
Medial epicondyle of femur
  use Femur, Lower, Right
  use Femur, Lower, Left
Medial epicondyle of humerus
  use Humeral Shaft, Left
  use Humeral Shaft, Right
Medial malleolus
  use Tibia, Right
  use Tibia, Left

Medial meniscus
  use Joint, Knee, Right
  use Joint, Knee, Left
Medial plantar artery
  use Artery, Foot, Right
  use Artery, Foot, Left
Medial plantar nerve *use* Nerve, Tibial
Medial popliteal nerve *use* Nerve, Tibial
Medial rectus muscle
  use Muscle, Extraocular, Right
  use Muscle, Extraocular, Left
Medial sural cutaneous nerve *use* Nerve, Tibial
Median antebrachial vein
  use Vein, Basilic, Left
  use Vein, Basilic, Right
Median cubital vein
  use Vein, Basilic, Left
  use Vein, Basilic, Right
Median sacral artery *use* Aorta, Abdominal
Mediastinal lymph node *use* Lymphatic, Thorax
Mediastinoscopy 0WJC4ZZ
Medication Management GZ3ZZZZ
  for substance abuse
    Antabuse **HZ83ZZZ**
    Bupropion **HZ87ZZZ**
    Clonidine **HZ86ZZZ**
    Levo-alpha-acetyl-methadol (LAAM) **HZ82ZZZ**
    Methadone Maintenance **HZ81ZZZ**
    Naloxone **HZ85ZZZ**
    Naltrexone **HZ84ZZZ**
    Nicotine Replacement **HZ80ZZZ**
    Other Replacement Medication **HZ89ZZZ**
    Psychiatric Medication **HZ88ZZZ**
Meditation 8E0ZXY5
Meissner's (submucous) plexus *use* Nerve, Abdominal Sympathetic
Melody® transcatheter pulmonary valve *use* Zooplastic Tissue in Heart and Great Vessels
Membranous urethra *use* Urethra
Meningeorrhaphy
  see Repair, Cerebral Meninges **00Q1**
  see Repair, Spinal Meninges **00QT**
Meniscectomy
  see Excision, Lower Joints **0SB**
  see Resection, Lower Joints **0ST**
Mental foramen
  use Mandible, Left
  use Mandible, Right
Mentalis muscle *use* Muscle, Facial
Mentoplasty *see* Alteration, Jaw, Lower **0W05**
Mesenterectomy *see* Excision, Mesentery **0DBV**
Mesenteriorrhaphy, mesenterorrhaphy *see* Repair, Mesentery **0DQV**
Mesenteriplication *see* Repair, Mesentery **0DQV**
Mesoappendix *use* Mesentery
Mesocolon *use* Mesentery
Metacarpal ligament
  use Bursa and Ligament, Hand, Left
  use Bursa and Ligament, Hand, Right
Metacarpophalangeal ligament
  use Bursa and Ligament, Hand, Right
  use Bursa and Ligament, Hand, Left
Metatarsal ligament
  use Bursa and Ligament, Foot, Right
  use Bursa and Ligament, Foot, Left
Metatarsectomy
  see Excision, Lower Bones **0QB**
  see Resection, Lower Bones **0QT**

Metatarsophalangeal (MTP) joint
  use Joint, Metatarsal-Phalangeal, Left
  use Joint, Metatarsal-Phalangeal, Right
Metatarsophalangeal ligament
  use Bursa and Ligament, Foot, Right
  use Bursa and Ligament, Foot, Left
Metathalamus *use* Thalamus
Micro-Driver stent (RX) (OTW) *use* Intraluminal Device
MicroMed Heart Assist *use* Implantable Heart Assist System in Heart and Great Vessels
Micrus CERECYTE microcoil *use* Intraluminal Device, Bioactive in Upper Arteries
Midcarpal joint
  use Joint, Carpal, Right
  use Joint, Carpal, Left
Middle cardiac nerve *use* Nerve, Thoracic Sympathetic
Middle cerebral artery *use* Artery, Intracranial
Middle cerebral vein *use* Vein, Intracranial
Middle colic vein *use* Vein, Colic
Middle genicular artery
  use Artery, Popliteal, Left
  use Artery, Popliteal, Right
Middle hemorrhoidal vein
  use Vein, Hypogastric, Left
  use Vein, Hypogastric, Right
Middle rectal artery
  use Artery, Internal Iliac, Right
  use Artery, Internal Iliac, Left
Middle suprarenal artery *use* Aorta, Abdominal
Middle temporal artery
  use Artery, Temporal, Left
  use Artery, Temporal, Right
Middle turbinate *use* Turbinate, Nasal
MitraClip valve repair system *use* Synthetic Substitute
Mitral annulus *use* Valve, Mitral
Mitroflow® Aortic Pericardial Heart Valve *use* Zooplastic Tissue in Heart and Great Vessels
Mobilization, adhesions *see* Release
Molar gland *use* Buccal Mucosa
Monitoring
  Arterial
    Flow
      Coronary **4A13**
      Peripheral **4A13**
      Pulmonary **4A13**
    Pressure
      Coronary **4A13**
      Peripheral **4A13**
      Pulmonary **4A13**
    Pulse
      Coronary **4A13**
      Peripheral **4A13**
      Pulmonary **4A13**
    Saturation, Peripheral **4A13**
    Sound, Peripheral **4A13**
  Cardiac
    Electrical Activity **4A12**
      Ambulatory **4A12X45**
      No Qualifier **4A12X4Z**
    Output **4A12**
    Rate **4A12**
    Rhythm **4A12**
    Sound **4A12**
    Total Activity, Stress **4A12XM4**
  Central Nervous
    Conductivity **4A10**

Monitoring - *continued*
  Electrical Activity
    Intraoperative **4A10**
    No Qualifier **4A10**
    Pressure **4A100BZ**
    Intracranial **4A10**
    Saturation, Intracranial **4A10**
    Temperature, Intracranial **4A10**
  Gastrointestinal
    Motility **4A1B**
    Pressure **4A1B**
    Secretion **4A1B**
  Lymphatic
    Flow **4A16**
    Pressure **4A16**
  Peripheral Nervous
    Conductivity
      Motor **4A11**
      Sensory **4A11**
    Electrical Activity
      Intraoperative **4A11**
      No Qualifier **4A11**
  Products of Conception
    Cardiac
      Electrical Activity **4A1H**
      Rate **4A1H**
      Rhythm **4A1H**
      Sound **4A1H**
    Nervous
      Conductivity **4A1J**
      Electrical Activity **4A1J**
      Pressure **4A1J**
  Respiratory
    Capacity **4A19**
    Flow **4A19**
    Rate **4A19**
    Resistance **4A19**
    Volume **4A19**
  Sleep **4A1ZXQZ**
  Temperature **4A1Z**
  Urinary
    Contractility **4A1D73Z**
    Flow **4A1D75Z**
    Pressure **4A1D7BZ**
    Resistance **4A1D7DZ**
    Volume **4A1D7LZ**
  Venous
    Flow
      Central **4A14**
      Peripheral **4A14**
      Portal **4A14**
      Pulmonary **4A14**
    Pressure
      Central **4A14**
      Peripheral **4A14**
      Portal **4A14**
      Pulmonary **4A14**
    Pulse
      Central **4A14**
      Peripheral **4A14**
      Portal **4A14**
      Pulmonary **4A14**
    Saturation
      Central **4A14**
      Portal **4A14**
      Pulmonary **4A14**
Monitoring Device
  Abdomen **0JH8**
  Chest **0JH6**
Motor Function Assessment F01
Motor Treatment F07

MR Angiography
  see Magnetic Resonance Imaging (MRI), Heart **B23**
  see Magnetic Resonance Imaging (MRI), Upper Arteries **B33**
  see Magnetic Resonance Imaging (MRI), Lower Arteries **B43**
Multiple sleep latency test 4A0ZXQZ
Musculocutaneous nerve *use* Nerve, Brachial Plexus
Musculopexy
  see Repair, Muscles **0KQ**
  see Reposition, Muscles **0KS**
Musculophrenic artery
  use Artery, Internal Mammary, Left
  use Artery, Internal Mammary, Right
Musculoplasty
  see Repair, Muscles **0KQ**
  see Supplement, Muscles **0KU**
Musculorrhaphy *see* Repair, Muscles **0KQ**
Musculospiral nerve *use* Nerve, Radial
Myectomy
  see Excision, Muscles **0KB**
  see Resection, Muscles **0KT**
Myelencephalon *use* Medulla Oblongata
Myelogram
  CT *see* Computerized Tomography (CT Scan), Central Nervous System **B02**
  MRI *see* Magnetic Resonance Imaging (MRI), Central Nervous System **B03**
Myenteric (Auerbach's) plexus *use* Nerve, Abdominal Sympathetic
Myomectomy *see* Excision, Female Reproductive System **0UB**
Myometrium *use* Uterus
Myopexy
  see Repair, Muscles **0KQ**
  see Reposition, Muscles **0KS**
Myoplasty
  see Repair, Muscles **0KQ**
  see Supplement, Muscles **0KU**
Myorrhaphy *see* Repair, Muscles **0KQ**
Myoscopy *see* Inspection, Muscles **0KJ**
Myotomy
  see Division, Muscles **0K8**
  see Drainage, Muscles **0K9**
Myringectomy
  see Excision, Ear, Nose, Sinus **09B**
  see Resection, Ear, Nose, Sinus **09T**
Myringoplasty
  see Repair, Ear, Nose, Sinus **09Q**
  see Replacement, Ear, Nose, Sinus **09R**
  see Supplement, Ear, Nose, Sinus **09U**
Myringostomy *see* Drainage, Ear, Nose, Sinus **099**
Myringotomy *see* Drainage, Ear, Nose, Sinus **099**

N

Nail bed
  use Finger Nail
  use Toe Nail
Nail plate
  use Finger Nail
  use Toe Nail
Narcosynthesis GZGZZZZ
Nasal cavity *use* Nose
Nasal concha *use* Turbinate, Nasal
Nasalis muscle *use* Muscle, Facial
Nasolacrimal duct
  use Duct, Lacrimal, Right
  use Duct, Lacrimal, Left

Nasopharyngeal airway (NPA) *use* Intraluminal Device, Airway in Ear, Nose, Sinus
Navicular bone
  use Tarsal, Left
  use Tarsal, Right
Near Infrared Spectroscopy, Circulatory System 8E023DZ
Neck of femur
  use Femur, Upper, Right
  use Femur, Upper, Left
Neck of humerus (anatomical)(surgical)
  use Humeral Head, Right
  use Humeral Head, Left
Nephrectomy
  see Excision, Urinary System **0TB**
  see Resection, Urinary System **0TT**
Nephrolithotomy *see* Extirpation, Urinary System **0TC**
Nephrolysis *see* Release, Urinary System **0TN**
Nephropexy
  see Repair, Urinary System **0TQ**
  see Reposition, Urinary System **0TS**
Nephroplasty
  see Repair, Urinary System **0TQ**
  see Supplement, Urinary System **0TU**
Nephropyeloureterostomy
  see Bypass, Urinary System **0T1**
  see Drainage, Urinary System **0T9**
Nephrorrhaphy *see* Repair, Urinary System **0TQ**
Nephroscopy, transurethral 0TJ58ZZ
Nephrostomy
  see Bypass, Urinary System **0T1**
  see Drainage, Urinary System **0T9**
Nephrotomography
  see Plain Radiography, Urinary System **BT0**
  see Fluoroscopy, Urinary System **BT1**
Nephrotomy
  see Drainage, Urinary System **0T9**
  see Division, Urinary System **0T8**
Nerve conduction study
  see Measurement, Central Nervous **4A00**
  see Measurement, Peripheral Nervous **4A01**
Nerve Function Assessment F01
Nerve to the stapedius *use* Nerve, Facial
Neurectomy
  see Excision, Central Nervous System **00B**
  see Excision, Peripheral Nervous System **01B**
Neurexeresis
  see Extraction, Central Nervous System **00D**
  see Extraction, Peripheral Nervous System **01D**
Neurohypophysis *use* Gland, Pituitary
Neurolysis
  see Release, Central Nervous System **00N**
  see Release, Peripheral Nervous System **01N**
Neuromuscular electrical stimulation (NEMS) lead *use* Stimulator Lead in Muscles
Neurophysiologic monitoring *see* Monitoring, Central Nervous **4A10**
Neuroplasty
  see Repair, Central Nervous System **00Q**
  see Repair, Peripheral Nervous System **01Q**
  see Supplement, Central Nervous System **00U**
  see Supplement, Peripheral Nervous System **01U**
Neurorrhaphy
  see Repair, Central Nervous System **00Q**
  see Repair, Peripheral Nervous System **01Q**

Neurostimulator Generator
  Insertion of device in, Skull **0NH00NZ**
  Removal of device from, Skull **0NP00NZ**
  Revision of device in, Skull **0NW00NZ**
Neurostimulator generator, multiple channel
  use Stimulator Generator, Multiple Array in
  0JH
Neurostimulator generator, multiple channel
  rechargeable *use* Stimulator Generator,
  Multiple Array Rechargeable in **0JH**
Neurostimulator generator, single channel *use*
  Stimulator Generator, Single Array in **0JH**
Neurostimulator generator, single channel
  rechargeable *use* Stimulator Generator,
  Single Array Rechargeable in **0JH**
Neurostimulator Lead
  Insertion of device in
    Brain **00H0**
    Cerebral Ventricle **00H6**
    Nerve
      Cranial **00HE**
      Peripheral **01HY**
    Spinal Canal **00HU**
    Spinal Cord **00HV**
  Removal of device from
    Brain **00P0**
    Cerebral Ventricle **00P6**
    Nerve
      Cranial **00PE**
      Peripheral **01PY**
    Spinal Canal **00PU**
    Spinal Cord **00PV**
  Revision of device in
    Brain **00W0**
    Cerebral Ventricle **00W6**
    Nerve
      Cranial **00WE**
      Peripheral **01WY**
    Spinal Canal **00WU**
    Spinal Cord **00WV**
Neurotomy
  see Division, Central Nervous System **008**
  see Division, Peripheral Nervous System **018**
Neurotripsy
  see Destruction, Central Nervous System **005**
  see Destruction, Peripheral Nervous System
  015
Neutralization plate
  use Internal Fixation Device in Head and
  Facial Bones
  use Internal Fixation Device in Upper Bones
  use Internal Fixation Device in Lower Bones
Ninth cranial nerve *use* Nerve,
  Glossopharyngeal
Nitinol framed polymer mesh *use* Synthetic
  Substitute
Non-tunneled central venous catheter *use*
  Infusion Device
Nonimaging Nuclear Medicine Assay
  Bladder, Kidneys and Ureters **CT63**
  Blood **C763**
  Kidneys, Ureters and Bladder **CT63**
  Lymphatics and Hematologic System
  C76YYZZ
  Ureters, Kidneys and Bladder **CT63**
  Urinary System **CT6YYZZ**
Nonimaging Nuclear Medicine Probe
  CP5YYZZ
  Abdomen **CW50**
  Abdomen and Chest **CW54**
  Abdomen and Pelvis **CW51**
  Brain **C050**

Nonimaging Nuclear Medicine Probe -
  continued
  Central Nervous System **C05YYZZ**
  Chest **CW53**
  Chest and Abdomen **CW54**
  Chest and Neck **CW56**
  Extremity
    Lower **CP5**
    Upper **CP5**
  Head and Neck **CW5B**
  Heart **C25YYZZ**
    Right and Left **C256**
  Lymphatics
    Head **C75J**
    Head and Neck **C755**
    Lower Extremity **C75P**
    Neck **C75K**
    Pelvic **C75D**
    Trunk **C75M**
    Upper Chest **C75L**
    Upper Extremity **C75N**
  Lymphatics and Hematologic System
  C75YYZZ
  Neck and Chest **CW56**
  Neck and Head **CW5B**
  Pelvic Region **CW5J**
  Pelvis and Abdomen **CW51**
  Spine **CP55ZZZ**
Nonimaging Nuclear Medicine Uptake
  Endocrine System **CG4YYZZ**
  Gland, Thyroid **CG42**
Nostril *use* Nose
Novacor Left Ventricular Assist Device *use*
  Implantable Heart Assist System in Heart and
  Great Vessels
Novation® Ceramic AHS® (Articulation Hip
  System) *use* Synthetic Substitute, Ceramic in
  0SR
Nuclear medicine
  see Planar Nuclear Medicine Imaging
  see Tomographic (Tomo) Nuclear Medicine
  Imaging
  see Positron Emission Tomographic (PET)
  Imaging
  see Nonimaging Nuclear Medicine Uptake
  see Nonimaging Nuclear Medicine Probe
  see Nonimaging Nuclear Medicine Assay
  see Systemic Nuclear Medicine Therapy
Nuclear scintigraphy *see* Nuclear Medicine
Nutrition, concentrated substances
  Enteral infusion **3E0G36Z**
  Parenteral (peripheral) infusion *see*
  Introduction of Nutritional Substance

O

Obliteration *see* Destruction
Obturator artery
  use Artery, Internal Iliac, Left
  use Artery, Internal Iliac, Right
Obturator lymph node *use* Lymphatic, Pelvis
Obturator muscle
  use Muscle, Hip, Left
  use Muscle, Hip, Right
Obturator nerve *use* Nerve, Lumbar Plexus
Obturator vein
  use Vein, Hypogastric, Right
  use Vein, Hypogastric, Left
Obtuse margin *use* Heart, Left
Occipital artery
  use Artery, External Carotid, Right
  use Artery, External Carotid, Left
Occipital lobe *use* Cerebral Hemisphere

Occipital lymph node
  use Lymphatic, Neck, Left
  use Lymphatic, Neck, Right
Occipitofrontalis muscle *use* Muscle, Facial
Occlusion
  Ampulla of Vater **0FLC**
  Anus **0DLQ**
  Aorta, Abdominal **04L0**
  Artery
    Anterior Tibial
      Left **04LQ**
      Right **04LP**
    Axillary
      Left **03L6**
      Right **03L5**
    Brachial
      Left **03L8**
      Right **03L7**
    Celiac **04L1**
    Colic
      Left **04L7**
      Middle **04L8**
      Right **04L6**
    Common Carotid
      Left **03LJ**
      Right **03LH**
    Common Iliac
      Left **04LD**
      Right **04LC**
    External Carotid
      Left **03LN**
      Right **03LM**
    External Iliac
      Left **04LJ**
      Right **04LH**
    Face **03LR**
    Femoral
      Left **04LL**
      Right **04LK**
    Foot
      Left **04LW**
      Right **04LV**
    Gastric **04L2**
    Hand
      Left **03LF**
      Right **03LD**
    Hepatic **04L3**
    Inferior Mesenteric **04LB**
    Innominate **03L2**
    Internal Carotid
      Left **03LL**
      Right **03LK**
    Internal Iliac
      Left, Uterine Artery, Left **04LF**
      Right, Uterine Artery, Right **04LE**
    Internal Mammary
      Left **03L1**
      Right **03L0**
    Intracranial **03LG**
    Lower **04LY**
    Peroneal
      Left **04LU**
      Right **04LT**
    Popliteal
      Left **04LN**
      Right **04LM**
    Posterior Tibial
      Left **04LS**
      Right **04LR**
    Pulmonary, Left **02LR**
    Radial
      Left **03LC**
      Right **03LB**

Occlusion - *continued*
Renal
Left **04LA**
Right **04L9**
Splenic **04L4**
Subclavian
Left **03L4**
Right **03L3**
Superior Mesenteric **04L5**
Temporal
Left **03LT**
Right **03LS**
Thyroid
Left **03LV**
Right **03LU**
Ulnar
Left **03LA**
Right **03L9**
Upper **03LY**
Vertebral
Left **03LQ**
Right **03LP**
Atrium, Left **02L7**
Bladder **0TLB**
Bladder Neck **0TLC**
Bronchus
Lingula **0BL9**
Lower Lobe
Left **0BLB**
Right **0BL6**
Main
Left **0BL7**
Right **0BL3**
Middle Lobe, Right **0BL5**
Upper Lobe
Left **0BL8**
Right **0BL4**
Carina **0BL2**
Cecum **0DLH**
Cisterna Chyli **07LL**
Colon
Ascending **0DLK**
Descending **0DLM**
Sigmoid **0DLN**
Transverse **0DLL**
Cord
Bilateral **0VLH**
Left **0VLG**
Right **0VLF**
Cul-de-sac **0ULF**
Duct
Common Bile **0FL9**
Cystic **0FL8**
Hepatic
Left **0FL6**
Right **0FL5**
Lacrimal
Left **08LY**
Right **08LX**
Pancreatic **0FLD**
Accessory **0FLF**
Parotid
Left **0CLC**
Right **0CLB**
Duodenum **0DL9**
Esophagogastric Junction **0DL4**
Esophagus **0DL5**
Lower **0DL3**
Middle **0DL2**
Upper **0DL1**

Occlusion - *continued*
Fallopian Tube
Left **0UL6**
Right **0UL5**
Fallopian Tubes, Bilateral **0UL7**
Ileocecal Valve **0DLC**
Ileum **0DLB**
Intestine
Large **0DLE**
Left **0DLG**
Right **0DLF**
Small **0DL8**
Jejunum **0DLA**
Kidney Pelvis
Left **0TL4**
Right **0TL3**
Left atrial appendage (LAA) *see* Occlusion,
Atrium, Left **02L7**
Lymphatic
Aortic **07LD**
Axillary
Left **07L6**
Right **07L5**
Head **07L0**
Inguinal
Left **07LJ**
Right **07LH**
Internal Mammary
Left **07L9**
Right **07L8**
Lower Extremity
Left **07LG**
Right **07LF**
Mesenteric **07LB**
Neck
Left **07L2**
Right **07L1**
Pelvis **07LC**
Thoracic Duct **07LK**
Thorax **07L7**
Upper Extremity
Left **07L4**
Right **07L3**
Rectum **0DLP**
Stomach **0DL6**
Pylorus **0DL7**
Trachea **0BL1**
Ureter
Left **0TL7**
Right **0TL6**
Urethra **0TLD**
Vagina **0ULG**
Vas Deferens
Bilateral **0VLQ**
Left **0VLP**
Right **0VLN**
Vein
Axillary
Left **05L8**
Right **05L7**
Azygos **05L0**
Basilic
Left **05LC**
Right **05LB**
Brachial
Left **05LA**
Right **05L9**
Cephalic
Left **05LF**
Right **05LD**
Colic **06L7**

Occlusion - *continued*
Common Iliac
Left **06LD**
Right **06LC**
Esophageal **06L3**
External Iliac
Left **06LG**
Right **06LF**
External Jugular
Left **05LQ**
Right **05LP**
Face
Left **05LV**
Right **05LT**
Femoral
Left **06LN**
Right **06LM**
Foot
Left **06LV**
Right **06LT**
Gastric **06L2**
Greater Saphenous
Left **06LQ**
Right **06LP**
Hand
Left **05LH**
Right **05LG**
Hemiazygos **05L1**
Hepatic **06L4**
Hypogastric
Left **06LJ**
Right **06LH**
Inferior Mesenteric **06L6**
Innominate
Left **05L4**
Right **05L3**
Internal Jugular
Left **05LN**
Right **05LM**
Intracranial **05LL**
Lesser Saphenous
Left **06LS**
Right **06LR**
Lower **06LY**
Portal **06L8**
Pulmonary
Left **02LT**
Right **02LS**
Renal
Left **06LB**
Right **06L9**
Splenic **06L1**
Subclavian
Left **05L6**
Right **05L5**
Superior Mesenteric **06L5**
Upper **05LY**
Vertebral
Left **05LS**
Right **05LR**
Vena Cava
Inferior **06L0**
Superior **02LV**
Occupational therapy *see* Activities of Daily
Living Treatment, Rehabilitation **F08**
Odontectomy
see Excision, Mouth and Throat **0CB**
see Resection, Mouth and Throat **0CT**
Olecranon bursa
use Bursa and Ligament, Elbow, Left
use Bursa and Ligament, Elbow, Right

Olecranon process
  use Ulna, Left
  use Ulna, Right
Olfactory bulb *use* Nerve, Olfactory
Omentectomy, omentumectomy
  see Excision, Gastrointestinal System **0DB**
  see Resection, Gastrointestinal System **0DT**
Omentofixation *see* Repair, Gastrointestinal
  System **0DQ**
Omentoplasty
  see Repair, Gastrointestinal System **0DQ**
  see Replacement, Gastrointestinal System
  0DR
  see Supplement, Gastrointestinal System **0DU**
Omentorrhaphy *see* Repair, Gastrointestinal
  System **0DQ**
Omentotomy *see* Drainage, Gastrointestinal
  System **0D9**
Onychectomy
  see Excision, Skin and Breast **0HB**
  see Resection, Skin and Breast **0HT**
Onychoplasty
  see Repair, Skin and Breast **0HQ**
  see Replacement, Skin and Breast **0HR**
Onychotomy *see* Drainage, Skin and Breast
  0H9
Oophorectomy
  see Excision, Female Reproductive System
  0UB
  see Resection, Female Reproductive System
  0UT
Oophoropexy
  see Repair, Female Reproductive System
  0UQ
  see Reposition, Female Reproductive System
  0US
Oophoroplasty
  see Repair, Female Reproductive System
  0UQ
  see Supplement, Female Reproductive System
  0UU
Oophororrhaphy *see* Repair, Female
  Reproductive System **0UQ**
Oophorostomy *see* Drainage, Female
  Reproductive System **0U9**
Oophorotomy
  see Drainage, Female Reproductive System
  0U9
  see Division, Female Reproductive System
  0U8
Oophorrhaphy *see* Repair, Female
  Reproductive System **0UQ**
Ophthalmic artery
  use Artery, Internal Carotid, Right
  use Artery, Internal Carotid, Left
Ophthalmic nerve *use* Nerve, Trigeminal
Ophthalmic vein *use* Vein, Intracranial
Opponensplasty
  Tendon replacement *see* Replacement,
  Tendons **0LR**
  Tendon transfer *see* Transfer, Tendons **0LX**
Optic chiasma *use* Nerve, Optic
Optic disc
  use Retina, Left
  use Retina, Right
Optic foramen
  use Bone, Sphenoid, Right
  use Bone, Sphenoid, Left
Optical coherence tomography, intravascular
  see Computerized Tomography (CT Scan)
Optimizer™ III implantable pulse generator
  use Contractility Modulation Device in **0JH**

Orbicularis oculi muscle
  use Eyelid, Upper, Left
  use Eyelid, Upper, Right
Orbicularis oris muscle *use* Muscle, Facial
Orbital fascia *use* Subcutaneous Tissue and
  Fascia, Face
Orbital portion of ethmoid bone
  use Orbit, Left
  use Orbit, Right
Orbital portion of frontal bone
  use Orbit, Right
  use Orbit, Left
Orbital portion of lacrimal bone
  use Orbit, Left
  use Orbit, Right
Orbital portion of maxilla
  use Orbit, Left
  use Orbit, Right
Orbital portion of palatine bone
  use Orbit, Right
  use Orbit, Left
Orbital portion of sphenoid bone
  use Orbit, Right
  use Orbit, Left
Orbital portion of zygomatic bone
  use Orbit, Left
  use Orbit, Right
Orchectomy, orchidectomy, orchiectomy
  see Excision, Male Reproductive System **0VB**
  see Resection, Male Reproductive System
  0VT
Orchidoplasty, orchioplasty
  see Repair, Male Reproductive System **0VQ**
  see Replacement, Male Reproductive System
  0VR
  see Supplement, Male Reproductive System
  0VU
Orchidorrhaphy, orchiorrhaphy *see* Repair,
  Male Reproductive System **0VQ**
Orchidotomy, orchiotomy, orchotomy *see*
  Drainage, Male Reproductive System **0V9**
Orchiopexy
  see Repair, Male Reproductive System **0VQ**
  see Reposition, Male Reproductive System
  0VS
Oropharyngeal airway (OPA) *use* Intraluminal
  Device, Airway in Mouth and Throat
Oropharynx *use* Pharynx
Ossicular chain
  use Auditory Ossicle, Left
  use Auditory Ossicle, Right
Ossiculectomy
  see Excision, Ear, Nose, Sinus **09B**
  see Resection, Ear, Nose, Sinus **09T**
Ossiculotomy *see* Drainage, Ear, Nose, Sinus
  099
Ostectomy
  see Excision, Head and Facial Bones **0NB**
  see Resection, Head and Facial Bones **0NT**
  see Excision, Upper Bones **0PB**
  see Resection, Upper Bones **0PT**
  see Excision, Lower Bones **0QB**
  see Resection, Lower Bones **0QT**
Osteoclasis
  see Division, Head and Facial Bones **0N8**
  see Division, Upper Bones **0P8**
  see Division, Lower Bones **0Q8**
Osteolysis
  see Release, Head and Facial Bones **0NN**
  see Release, Upper Bones **0PN**
  see Release, Lower Bones **0QN**

Osteopathic Treatment
  Abdomen **7W09X**
  Cervical **7W01X**
  Extremity
    Lower **7W06X**
    Upper **7W07X**
  Head **7W00X**
  Lumbar **7W03X**
  Pelvis **7W05X**
  Rib Cage **7W08X**
  Sacrum **7W04X**
  Thoracic **7W02X**
Osteopexy
  see Repair, Head and Facial Bones **0NQ**
  see Reposition, Head and Facial Bones **0NS**
  see Repair, Upper Bones **0PQ**
  see Reposition, Upper Bones **0PS**
  see Repair, Lower Bones **0QQ**
  see Reposition, Lower Bones **0QS**
Osteoplasty
  see Repair, Head and Facial Bones **0NQ**
  see Replacement, Head and Facial Bones
  0NR
  see Repair, Upper Bones **0PQ**
  see Replacement, Upper Bones **0PR**
  see Repair, Lower Bones **0QQ**
  see Replacement, Lower Bones **0QR**
  see Supplement, Lower Bones **0QU**
  see Supplement, Head and Facial Bones **0NU**
  see Supplement, Upper Bones **0PU**
Osteorrhaphy
  see Repair, Head and Facial Bones **0NQ**
  see Repair, Upper Bones **0PQ**
  see Repair, Lower Bones **0QQ**
Osteotomy, ostotomy
  see Division, Head and Facial Bones **0N8**
  see Drainage, Head and Facial Bones **0N9**
  see Division, Upper Bones **0P8**
  see Drainage, Upper Bones **0P9**
  see Division, Lower Bones **0Q8**
  see Drainage, Lower Bones **0Q9**
Otic ganglion *use* Nerve, Head and Neck
  Sympathetic
Otoplasty
  see Repair, Ear, Nose, Sinus **09Q**
  see Replacement, Ear, Nose, Sinus **09R**
  see Supplement, Ear, Nose, Sinus **09U**
Otoscopy *see* Inspection, Ear, Nose, Sinus **09J**
Oval window
  use Ear, Middle, Left
  use Ear, Middle, Right
Ovarian artery *use* Aorta, Abdominal
Ovarian ligament *use* Uterine Supporting
  Structure
Ovariectomy
  see Excision, Female Reproductive System
  0UB
  see Resection, Female Reproductive System
  0UT
Ovariocentesis *see* Drainage, Female
  Reproductive System **0U9**
Ovariopexy
  see Repair, Female Reproductive System
  0UQ
  see Reposition, Female Reproductive System
  0US
Ovariotomy
  see Drainage, Female Reproductive System
  0U9
  see Division, Female Reproductive System
  0U8

Ovatio™ CRT-D *use* Cardiac Resynchronization Defibrillator Pulse Generator in **0JH**

Oversewing
Gastrointestinal ulcer *see* Repair, Gastrointestinal System **0DQ**
Pleural bleb *see* Repair, Respiratory System **0BQ**

Oviduct
use Fallopian Tube, Right
use Fallopian Tube, Left

Oxidized zirconium ceramic hip bearing surface *use* Synthetic Substitute, Ceramic on Polyethylene in **0SR**

Oximetry, Fetal pulse 10H073Z

Oxygenation
Extracorporeal membrane (ECMO) *see* Assistance, Circulatory **5A05**
Hyperbaric *see* Assistance, Circulatory **5A05**
Supersaturated *see* Assistance, Circulatory **5A05**

P

Pacemaker
Dual Chamber
Abdomen **0JH8**
Chest **0JH6**
Single Chamber
Abdomen **0JH8**
Chest **0JH6**
Single Chamber Rate Responsive
Abdomen **0JH8**
Chest **0JH6**

Packing
Abdominal Wall **2W43X5Z**
Anorectal **2Y43X5Z**
Arm
Lower
Left **2W4DX5Z**
Right **2W4CX5Z**
Upper
Left **2W4BX5Z**
Right **2W4AX5Z**
Back **2W45X5Z**
Chest Wall **2W44X5Z**
Ear **2Y42X5Z**
Extremity
Lower
Left **2W4MX5Z**
Right **2W4LX5Z**
Upper
Left **2W49X5Z**
Right **2W48X5Z**
Face **2W41X5Z**
Finger
Left **2W4KX5Z**
Right **2W4JX5Z**
Foot
Left **2W4TX5Z**
Right **2W4SX5Z**
Genital Tract, Female **2Y44X5Z**
Hand
Left **2W4FX5Z**
Right **2W4EX5Z**
Head **2W40X5Z**
Inguinal Region
Left **2W47X5Z**
Right **2W46X5Z**

Packing - *continued*
Leg
Lower
Left **2W4RX5Z**
Right **2W4QX5Z**
Upper
Left **2W4PX5Z**
Right **2W4NX5Z**
Mouth and Pharynx **2Y40X5Z**
Nasal **2Y41X5Z**
Neck **2W42X5Z**
Thumb
Left **2W4HX5Z**
Right **2W4GX5Z**
Toe
Left **2W4VX5Z**
Right **2W4UX5Z**
Urethra **2Y45X5Z**

Paclitaxel-eluting coronary stent *use* Intraluminal Device, Drug-eluting in Heart and Great Vessels

Paclitaxel-eluting peripheral stent
use Intraluminal Device, Drug-eluting in Upper Arteries
use Intraluminal Device, Drug-eluting in Lower Arteries

Palatine gland *use* Buccal Mucosa
Palatine tonsil *use* Tonsils
Palatine uvula *use* Uvula
Palatoglossal muscle *use* Muscle, Tongue, Palate, Pharynx
Palatopharyngeal muscle *use* Muscle, Tongue, Palate, Pharynx

Palatoplasty
see Repair, Mouth and Throat **0CQ**
see Replacement, Mouth and Throat **0CR**
see Supplement, Mouth and Throat **0CU**

Palatorrhaphy *see* Repair, Mouth and Throat **0CQ**

Palmar (volar) digital vein
use Vein, Hand, Right
use Vein, Hand, Left

Palmar (volar) metacarpal vein
use Vein, Hand, Left
use Vein, Hand, Right

Palmar cutaneous nerve
use Nerve, Radial
use Nerve, Median

Palmar fascia (aponeurosis)
use Subcutaneous Tissue and Fascia, Hand, Left
use Subcutaneous Tissue and Fascia, Hand, Right

Palmar interosseous muscle
use Muscle, Hand, Left
use Muscle, Hand, Right

Palmar ulnocarpal ligament
use Bursa and Ligament, Wrist, Right
use Bursa and Ligament, Wrist, Left

Palmaris longus muscle
use Muscle, Lower Arm and Wrist, Left
use Muscle, Lower Arm and Wrist, Right

Pancreatectomy
see Excision, Pancreas **0FBG**
see Resection, Pancreas **0FTG**

Pancreatic artery *use* Artery, Splenic
Pancreatic plexus *use* Nerve, Abdominal Sympathetic
Pancreatic vein *use* Vein, Splenic
Pancreaticoduodenostomy *see* Bypass, Hepatobiliary System and Pancreas **0F1**
Pancreaticosplenic lymph node *use* Lymphatic, Aortic

Pancreatogram, endoscopic retrograde *see* Fluoroscopy, Pancreatic Duct **BF18**
Pancreatolithotomy *see* Extirpation, Pancreas **0FCG**

Pancreatotomy
see Drainage, Pancreas **0F9G**
see Division, Pancreas **0F8G**

Panniculectomy
see Excision, Skin, Abdomen **0HB7**
see Excision, Abdominal Wall **0WBF**

Paraaortic lymph node *use* Lymphatic, Aortic

Paracentesis
Eye *see* Drainage, Eye **089**
Peritoneal Cavity *see* Drainage, Peritoneal Cavity **0W9G**
Tympanum *see* Drainage, Ear, Nose, Sinus **099**

Pararectal lymph node *use* Lymphatic, Mesenteric
Parasternal lymph node *use* Lymphatic, Thorax

Parathyroidectomy
see Excision, Endocrine System **0GB**
see Resection, Endocrine System **0GT**

Paratracheal lymph node *use* Lymphatic, Thorax
Paraurethral (Skene's) gland *use* Gland, Vestibular
Parenteral nutrition, total *see* Introduction of Nutritional Substance
Parietal lobe *use* Cerebral Hemisphere
Parotid lymph node *use* Lymphatic, Head
Parotid plexus *use* Nerve, Facial

Parotidectomy
see Excision, Mouth and Throat **0CB**
see Resection, Mouth and Throat **0CT**

Pars flaccida
use Tympanic Membrane, Right
use Tympanic Membrane, Left

Partial joint replacement
Hip *see* Replacement, Lower Joints **0SR**
Knee *see* Replacement, Lower Joints **0SR**
Shoulder *see* Replacement, Upper Joints **0RR**

Partially absorbable mesh *use* Synthetic Substitute
Patch, blood, spinal 3E0S3GC

Patellapexy
see Repair, Lower Bones **0QQ**
see Reposition, Lower Bones **0QS**

Patellofemoral joint
use Joint, Knee, Right
use Joint, Knee, Left
use Joint, Knee, Right, Femoral Surface
use Joint, Knee, Left, Femoral Surface

Patelloplasty
see Repair, Lower Bones **0QQ**
see Replacement, Lower Bones **0QR**
see Supplement, Lower Bones **0QU**

Patellar ligament
use Bursa and Ligament, Knee, Right
use Bursa and Ligament, Knee, Left

Patellar tendon
use Tendon, Knee, Left
use Tendon, Knee, Right

Patellectomy
see Excision, Lower Bones **0QB**
see Resection, Lower Bones **0QT**

Pectineus muscle
use Muscle, Upper Leg, Left
use Muscle, Upper Leg, Right

Pectoral (anterior) lymph node
use Lymphatic, Axillary, Right
use Lymphatic, Axillary, Left

Pectoral fascia *use* Subcutaneous Tissue and
Fascia, Chest
Pectoralis major muscle
use Muscle, Thorax, Left
use Muscle, Thorax, Right
Pectoralis minor muscle
use Muscle, Thorax, Right
use Muscle, Thorax, Left
Pedicle-based dynamic stabilization device
use Spinal Stabilization Device, Pedicle-
Based in **0RH**
use Spinal Stabilization Device, Pedicle-
Based in **0SH**
PEEP (positive end expiratory pressure) *see*
Assistance, Respiratory **5A09**
PEG (percutaneous endoscopic gastrostomy)
0DH64UZ
PEJ (percutaneous endoscopic jejunostomy)
0DHA4UZ
Pelvic splanchnic nerve
use Nerve, Abdominal Sympathetic
use Nerve, Sacral Sympathetic
Penectomy
see Excision, Male Reproductive System **0VB**
see Resection, Male Reproductive System
0VT
Penile urethra *use* Urethra
Percutaneous endoscopic gastrojejunostomy
(PEG/J) tube *use* Feeding Device in
Gastrointestinal System
Percutaneous endoscopic gastrostomy (PEG)
tube *use* Feeding Device in Gastrointestinal
System
Percutaneous nephrostomy catheter *use*
Drainage Device
Percutaneous transluminal coronary
angioplasty (PTCA) *see* Dilation, Heart and
Great Vessels **027**
Performance
Biliary
Multiple, Filtration **5A1C60Z**
Single, Filtration **5A1C00Z**
Cardiac
Continuous
Output **5A1221Z**
Pacing **5A1223Z**
Intermittent, Pacing **5A1213Z**
Single, Output, Manual **5A12012**
Circulatory, Continuous, Oxygenation,
Membrane **5A15223**
Respiratory
24-96 Consecutive Hours, Ventilation
5A1945Z
Greater than 96 Consecutive Hours,
Ventilation **5A1955Z**
Less than 24 Consecutive Hours,
Ventilation **5A1935Z**
Single, Ventilation, Nonmechanical
5A19054
Urinary
Multiple, Filtration **5A1D60Z**
Single, Filtration **5A1D00Z**
Perfusion *see* Introduction of substance in or on
Pericardiectomy
see Excision, Pericardium **02BN**
see Resection, Pericardium **02TN**
Pericardiocentesis *see* Drainage, Pericardial
Cavity **0W9D**
Pericardiolysis *see* Release, Pericardium **02NN**
Pericardiophrenic artery
use Artery, Internal Mammary, Left
use Artery, Internal Mammary, Right

Pericardioplasty
see Repair, Pericardium **02QN**
see Replacement, Pericardium **02RN**
see Supplement, Pericardium **02UN**
Pericardiorrhaphy *see* Repair, Pericardium
02QN
Pericardiostomy *see* Drainage, Pericardial
Cavity **0W9D**
Pericardiotomy *see* Drainage, Pericardial
Cavity **0W9D**
Perimetrium *use* Uterus
Peripheral parenteral nutrition *see*
Introduction of Nutritional Substance
Peripherally inserted central catheter (PICC)
use Infusion Device
Peritoneal dialysis 3E1M39Z
Peritoneocentesis
see Drainage, Peritoneum **0D9W**
see Drainage, Peritoneal Cavity **0W9G**
Peritoneoplasty
see Repair, Peritoneum **0DQW**
see Replacement, Peritoneum **0DRW**
see Supplement, Peritoneum **0DUW**
Peritoneoscopy 0DJW4ZZ
Peritoneotomy *see* Drainage, Peritoneum **0D9W**
Peritoneumectomy *see* Excision, Peritoneum
0DBW
Peroneus brevis muscle
use Muscle, Lower Leg, Left
use Muscle, Lower Leg, Right
Peroneus longus muscle
use Muscle, Lower Leg, Right
use Muscle, Lower Leg, Left
Pessary ring *use* Intraluminal Device, Pessary in
Female Reproductive System
PET scan *see* Positron Emission Tomographic
(PET) Imaging
Petrous part of temporal bone
use Bone, Temporal, Right
use Bone, Temporal, Left
Phacoemulsification, lens
With IOL implant *see* Replacement, Eye **08R**
Without IOL implant *see* Extraction, Eye **08D**
Phalangectomy
see Excision, Upper Bones **0PB**
see Resection, Upper Bones **0PT**
see Excision, Lower Bones **0QB**
see Resection, Lower Bones **0QT**
Phallectomy
see Excision, Penis **0VBS**
see Resection, Penis **0VTS**
Phalloplasty
see Repair, Penis **0VQS**
see Supplement, Penis **0VUS**
Phallotomy *see* Drainage, Penis **0V9S**
Pharmacotherapy
Antabuse **HZ93ZZZ**
Bupropion **HZ97ZZZ**
Clonidine **HZ96ZZZ**
Levo-alpha-acetyl-methadol (LAAM)
HZ92ZZZ
Methadone Maintenance **HZ91ZZZ**
Naloxone **HZ95ZZZ**
Naltrexone **HZ94ZZZ**
Nicotine Replacement **HZ90ZZZ**
Psychiatric Medication **HZ98ZZZ**
Replacement Medication, Other **HZ99ZZZ**
Pharyngeal constrictor muscle *use* Muscle,
Tongue, Palate, Pharynx
Pharyngeal plexus *use* Nerve, Vagus
Pharyngeal recess *use* Nasopharynx
Pharyngeal tonsil *use* Adenoids
Pharyngogram *see* Fluoroscopy, Pharynx **B91G**

Pharyngoplasty
see Repair, Mouth and Throat **0CQ**
see Replacement, Mouth and Throat **0CR**
see Supplement, Mouth and Throat **0CU**
Pharyngorrhaphy *see* Repair, Mouth and
Throat **0CQ**
Pharyngotomy *see* Drainage, Mouth and Throat
0C9
Pharyngotympanic tube
use Eustachian Tube, Right
use Eustachian Tube, Left
Pheresis
Erythrocytes **6A55**
Leukocytes **6A55**
Plasma **6A55**
Platelets **6A55**
Stem Cells
Cord Blood **6A55**
Hematopoietic **6A55**
Phlebectomy
see Excision, Upper Veins **05B**
see Extraction, Upper Veins **05D**
see Excision, Lower Veins **06B**
see Extraction, Lower Veins **06D**
Phlebography
see Plain Radiography, Veins **B50**
Impedance **4A04X51**
Phleborrhaphy
see Repair, Upper Veins **05Q**
see Repair, Lower Veins **06Q**
Phlebotomy
see Drainage, Upper Veins **059**
see Drainage, Lower Veins **069**
Photocoagulation
for Destruction *see* Destruction
for Repair *see* Repair
Photopheresis, therapeutic *see* Phototherapy,
Circulatory **6A65**
Phototherapy
Circulatory **6A65**
Skin **6A60**
Phrenectomy, phrenoneurectomy *see*
Excision, Nerve, Phrenic **01B2**
Phrenemphraxis *see* Destruction, Nerve,
Phrenic **0152**
Phrenic nerve stimulator generator *use*
Stimulator Generator in Subcutaneous Tissue
and Fascia
Phrenic nerve stimulator lead *use*
Diaphragmatic Pacemaker Lead in
Respiratory System
Phreniclasis *see* Destruction, Nerve, Phrenic
0152
Phrenicoexeresis *see* Extraction, Nerve, Phrenic
01D2
Phrenicotomy *see* Division, Nerve, Phrenic
0182
Phrenicotripsy *see* Destruction, Nerve, Phrenic
0152
Phrenoplasty
see Repair, Respiratory System **0BQ**
see Supplement, Respiratory System **0BU**
Phrenotomy *see* Drainage, Respiratory System
0B9
Physiatry *see* Motor Treatment, Rehabilitation
F07
Physical medicine *see* Motor Treatment,
Rehabilitation **F07**
Physical therapy *see* Motor Treatment,
Rehabilitation **F07**
PHYSIOMESH™ Flexible Composite Mesh
use Synthetic Substitute

Pia mater
 use Spinal Meninges
 use Cerebral Meninges
Pinealectomy
 see Excision, Pineal Body **0GB1**
 see Resection, Pineal Body **0GT1**
Pinealoscopy 0GJ14ZZ
Pinealotomy *see* Drainage, Pineal Body **0G91**
Pinna
 use Ear, External, Left
 use Ear, External, Bilateral
 use Ear, External, Right
Pipeline™ Embolization device (PED) *use*
 Intraluminal Device
Piriform recess (sinus) *use* Pharynx
Piriformis muscle
 use Muscle, Hip, Left
 use Muscle, Hip, Right
Pisiform bone
 use Carpal, Left
 use Carpal, Right
Pisohamate ligament
 use Bursa and Ligament, Hand, Right
 use Bursa and Ligament, Hand, Left
Pisometacarpal ligament
 use Bursa and Ligament, Hand, Left
 use Bursa and Ligament, Hand, Right
Pituitectomy
 see Excision, Gland, Pituitary **0GB0**
 see Resection, Gland, Pituitary **0GT0**
Plain film radiology *see* Plain Radiography
Plain Radiography
 Abdomen **BW00ZZZ**
 Abdomen and Pelvis **BW01ZZZ**
 Abdominal Lymphatic
  Bilateral **B701**
  Unilateral **B700**
 Airway, Upper **BB0DZZZ**
 Ankle
  Left **BQ0H**
  Right **BQ0G**
 Aorta
  Abdominal **B400**
  Thoracic **B300**
  Thoraco-Abdominal **B30P**
 Aorta and Bilateral Lower Extremity Arteries
  B40D
 Arch
  Bilateral **BN0DZZZ**
  Left **BN0CZZZ**
  Right **BN0BZZZ**
 Arm
  Left **BP0FZZZ**
  Right **BP0EZZZ**
 Artery
  Brachiocephalic-Subclavian, Right **B301**
  Bronchial **B30L**
  Bypass Graft, Other **B20F**
  Cervico-Cerebral Arch **B30Q**
  Common Carotid
   Bilateral **B305**
   Left **B304**
   Right **B303**
  Coronary
   Bypass Graft
    Multiple **B203**
    Single **B202**
   Multiple **B201**
   Single **B200**
  External Carotid
   Bilateral **B30C**
   Left **B30B**
   Right **B309**

Plain Radiography - *continued*
 Hepatic **B402**
 Inferior Mesenteric **B405**
 Intercostal **B30L**
 Internal Carotid
  Bilateral **B308**
  Left **B307**
  Right **B306**
 Internal Mammary Bypass Graft
  Left **B208**
  Right **B207**
 Intra-Abdominal, Other **B40B**
 Intracranial **B30R**
 Lower, Other **B40J**
 Lower Extremity
  Bilateral and Aorta **B40D**
  Left **B40G**
  Right **B40F**
 Lumbar **B409**
 Pelvic **B40C**
 Pulmonary
  Left **B30T**
  Right **B30S**
 Renal
  Bilateral **B408**
  Left **B407**
  Right **B406**
  Transplant **B40M**
 Spinal **B30M**
 Splenic **B403**
 Subclavian, Left **B302**
 Superior Mesenteric **B404**
 Upper, Other **B30N**
 Upper Extremity
  Bilateral **B30K**
  Left **B30J**
  Right **B30H**
 Vertebral
  Bilateral **B30G**
  Left **B30F**
  Right **B30D**
 Bile Duct **BF00**
 Bile Duct and Gallbladder **BF03**
 Bladder **BT00**
  Kidney and Ureter **BT04**
 Bladder and Urethra **BT0B**
 Bone
  Facial **BN05ZZZ**
  Nasal **BN04ZZZ**
 Bones, Long, All **BW0BZZZ**
 Breast
  Bilateral **BH02ZZZ**
  Left **BH01ZZZ**
  Right **BH00ZZZ**
 Calcaneus
  Left **BQ0KZZZ**
  Right **BQ0JZZZ**
 Chest **BW03ZZZ**
 Clavicle
  Left **BP05ZZZ**
  Right **BP04ZZZ**
 Coccyx **BR0FZZZ**
 Corpora Cavernosa **BV00**
 Dialysis Fistula **B50W**
 Dialysis Shunt **B50W**
 Disc
  Cervical **BR01**
  Lumbar **BR03**
  Thoracic **BR02**
 Duct
  Lacrimal
   Bilateral **B802**

Plain Radiography - *continued*
 Left **B801**
 Right **B800**
 Mammary
  Multiple
   Left **BH06**
   Right **BH05**
  Single
   Left **BH04**
   Right **BH03**
 Elbow
  Left **BP0H**
  Right **BP0G**
 Epididymis
  Left **BV02**
  Right **BV01**
 Extremity
  Lower **BW0CZZZ**
  Upper **BW0JZZZ**
 Eye
  Bilateral **B807ZZZ**
  Left **B806ZZZ**
  Right **B805ZZZ**
 Facet Joint
  Cervical **BR04**
  Lumbar **BR06**
  Thoracic **BR05**
 Fallopian Tube
  Bilateral **BU02**
  Left **BU01**
  Right **BU00**
 Fallopian Tube and Uterus **BU08**
 Femur
  Left, Densitometry **BQ04ZZ1**
  Right, Densitometry **BQ03ZZ1**
 Finger
  Left **BP0SZZZ**
  Right **BP0RZZZ**
 Foot
  Left **BQ0MZZZ**
  Right **BQ0LZZZ**
 Forearm
  Left **BP0KZZZ**
  Right **BP0JZZZ**
 Gallbladder and Bile Duct **BF03**
 Gland
  Parotid
   Bilateral **B906**
   Left **B905**
   Right **B904**
  Salivary
   Bilateral **B90D**
   Left **B90C**
   Right **B90B**
  Submandibular
   Bilateral **B909**
   Left **B908**
   Right **B907**
 Hand
  Left **BP0PZZZ**
  Right **BP0NZZZ**
 Heart
  Left **B205**
  Right **B204**
  Right and Left **B206**
 Hepatobiliary System, All **BF0C**
 Hip
  Left **BQ01**
   Densitometry **BQ01ZZ1**
  Right **BQ00**
   Densitometry **BQ00ZZ1**

Plain Radiography - *continued*
- Humerus
  - Left **BP0BZZZ**
  - Right **BP0AZZZ**
- Ileal Diversion Loop **BT0C**
- Intracranial Sinus **B502**
- Joint
  - Acromioclavicular, Bilateral **BP03ZZZ**
  - Finger
    - Left **BP0D**
    - Right **BP0C**
  - Foot
    - Left **BQ0Y**
    - Right **BQ0X**
  - Hand
    - Left **BP0D**
    - Right **BP0C**
  - Lumbosacral **BR0BZZZ**
  - Sacroiliac **BR0D**
  - Sternoclavicular
    - Bilateral **BP02ZZZ**
    - Left **BP01ZZZ**
    - Right **BP00ZZZ**
  - Temporomandibular
    - Bilateral **BN09**
    - Left **BN08**
    - Right **BN07**
  - Thoracolumbar **BR08ZZZ**
  - Toe
    - Left **BQ0Y**
    - Right **BQ0X**
- Kidney
  - Bilateral **BT03**
  - Left **BT02**
  - Right **BT01**
  - Ureter and Bladder **BT04**
- Knee
  - Left **BQ08**
  - Right **BQ07**
- Leg
  - Left **BQ0FZZZ**
  - Right **BQ0DZZZ**
- Lymphatic
  - Head **B704**
  - Lower Extremity
    - Bilateral **B70B**
    - Left **B709**
    - Right **B708**
  - Neck **B704**
  - Pelvic **B70C**
  - Upper Extremity
    - Bilateral **B707**
    - Left **B706**
    - Right **B705**
- Mandible **BN06ZZZ**
- Mastoid **B90HZZZ**
- Nasopharynx **B90FZZZ**
- Optic Foramina
  - Left **B804ZZZ**
  - Right **B803ZZZ**
- Orbit
  - Bilateral **BN03ZZZ**
  - Left **BN02ZZZ**
  - Right **BN01ZZZ**
- Oropharynx **B90FZZZ**
- Patella
  - Left **BQ0WZZZ**
  - Right **BQ0VZZZ**
- Pelvis **BR0CZZZ**
- Pelvis and Abdomen **BW01ZZZ**
- Prostate **BV03**

Plain Radiography - *continued*
- Retroperitoneal Lymphatic
  - Bilateral **B701**
- Ribs
  - Left **BP0YZZZ**
  - Right **BP0XZZZ**
- Sacrum **BR0FZZZ**
- Scapula
  - Left **BP07ZZZ**
  - Right **BP06ZZZ**
- Shoulder
  - Left **BP09**
  - Right **BP08**
- Sinus
  - Intracranial **B502**
  - Paranasal **B902ZZZ**
- Skull **BN00ZZZ**
- Spinal Cord **B00B**
- Spine
  - Cervical, Densitometry **BR00ZZ1**
  - Lumbar, Densitometry **BR09ZZ1**
  - Thoracic, Densitometry **BR07ZZ1**
  - Whole, Densitometry **BR0GZZ1**
- Sternum **BR0HZZZ**
- Teeth
  - All **BN0JZZZ**
  - Multiple **BN0HZZZ**
- Testicle
  - Left **BV06**
  - Right **BV05**
- Toe
  - Left **BQ0QZZZ**
  - Right **BQ0PZZZ**
- Tooth, Single **BN0GZZZ**
- Tracheobronchial Tree
  - Bilateral **BB09YZZ**
  - Left **BB08YZZ**
  - Right **BB07YZZ**
- Ureter
  - Bilateral **BT08**
  - Kidney and Bladder **BT04**
  - Left **BT07**
  - Right **BT06**
- Urethra **BT05**
- Urethra and Bladder **BT0B**
- Uterus **BU06**
- Uterus and Fallopian Tube **BU08**
- Vagina **BU09**
- Vasa Vasorum **BV08**
- Vein
  - Cerebellar **B501**
  - Cerebral **B501**
  - Epidural **B500**
  - Jugular
    - Bilateral **B505**
    - Left **B504**
    - Right **B503**
  - Lower Extremity
    - Bilateral **B50D**
    - Left **B50C**
    - Right **B50B**
  - Other **B50V**
  - Pelvic (Iliac)
    - Left **B50G**
    - Right **B50F**
  - Pelvic (Iliac) Bilateral **B50H**
  - Portal **B50T**
  - Pulmonary
    - Bilateral **B50S**
    - Left **B50R**
    - Right **B50Q**

Plain Radiography - *continued*
- Renal
  - Bilateral **B50L**
  - Left **B50K**
  - Right **B50J**
- Splanchnic **B50T**
- Subclavian
  - Left **B507**
  - Right **B506**
- Upper Extremity
  - Bilateral **B50P**
  - Left **B50N**
  - Right **B50M**
- Vena Cava
  - Inferior **B509**
  - Superior **B508**
- Whole Body **BW0KZZZ**
  - Infant **BW0MZZZ**
- Whole Skeleton **BW0LZZZ**
- Wrist
  - Left **BP0M**
  - Right **BP0L**

Planar Nuclear Medicine Imaging CP1
- Abdomen **CW10**
- Abdomen and Chest **CW14**
- Abdomen and Pelvis **CW11**
- Anatomical Regions, Multiple **CW1YYZZ**
- Bladder, Kidneys and Ureters **CT13**
- Bladder and Ureters **CT1H**
- Blood **C713**
- Bone Marrow **C710**
- Brain **C010**
- Breast **CH1YYZZ**
  - Bilateral **CH12**
  - Left **CH11**
  - Right **CH10**
- Bronchi and Lungs **CB12**
- Central Nervous System **C01YYZZ**
- Cerebrospinal Fluid **C015**
- Chest **CW13**
- Chest and Abdomen **CW14**
- Chest and Neck **CW16**
- Digestive System **CD1YYZZ**
- Ducts, Lacrimal, Bilateral **C819**
- Ear, Nose, Mouth and Throat **C91YYZZ**
- Endocrine System **CG1YYZZ**
- Extremity
  - Lower **CW1D**
    - Bilateral **CP1F**
    - Left **CP1D**
    - Right **CP1C**
  - Upper **CW1M**
    - Bilateral **CP1B**
    - Left **CP19**
    - Right **CP18**
- Eye **C81YYZZ**
- Gallbladder **CF14**
- Gastrointestinal Tract **CD17**
  - Upper **CD15**
- Gland
  - Adrenal, Bilateral **CG14**
  - Parathyroid **CG11**
  - Thyroid **CG12**
- Glands, Salivary, Bilateral **C91B**
- Head and Neck **CW1B**
- Heart **C21YYZZ**
  - Right and Left **C216**
- Hepatobiliary System, All **CF1C**
- Hepatobiliary System and Pancreas **CF1YYZZ**
- Kidneys, Ureters and Bladder **CT13**
- Liver **CF15**

Planar Nuclear Medicine - *continued*
  Liver and Spleen **CF16**
  Lungs and Bronchi **CB12**
  Lymphatics
    Head **C71J**
    Head and Neck **C715**
    Lower Extremity **C71P**
    Neck **C71K**
    Pelvic **C71D**
    Trunk **C71M**
    Upper Chest **C71L**
    Upper Extremity **C71N**
  Lymphatics and Hematologic System
  C71YYZZ
  Musculoskeletal System, All **CP1Z**
  Myocardium **C21G**
  Neck and Chest **CW16**
  Neck and Head **CW1B**
  Pancreas and Hepatobiliary System
  CF1YYZZ
  Pelvic Region **CW1J**
  Pelvis **CP16**
  Pelvis and Abdomen **CW11**
  Pelvis and Spine **CP17**
  Reproductive System, Male **CV1YYZZ**
  Respiratory System **CB1YYZZ**
  Skin **CH1YYZZ**
  Skull **CP11**
  Spine **CP15**
  Spine and Pelvis **CP17**
  Spleen **C712**
  Spleen and Liver **CF16**
  Subcutaneous Tissue **CH1YYZZ**
  Testicles, Bilateral **CV19**
  Thorax **CP14**
  Ureters, Kidneys and Bladder **CT13**
  Ureters and Bladder **CT1H**
  Urinary System **CT1YYZZ**
  Veins **C51YYZZ**
    Central **C51R**
    Lower Extremity
      Bilateral **C51D**
      Left **C51C**
      Right **C51B**
    Upper Extremity
      Bilateral **C51Q**
      Left **C51P**
      Right **C51N**
  Whole Body **CW1N Plantar digital vein**
  use Vein, Foot, Right
  use Vein, Foot, Left
Plantar fascia (aponeurosis)
  use Subcutaneous Tissue and Fascia, Foot,
  Right
  use Subcutaneous Tissue and Fascia, Foot,
  Left
Plantar metatarsal vein
  use Vein, Foot, Right
  use Vein, Foot, Left
Plantar venous arch
  use Vein, Foot, Right
  use Vein, Foot, Left
Plaque Radiation
  Abdomen **DWY3FZZ**
  Adrenal Gland **DGY2FZZ**
  Anus **DDY8FZZ**
  Bile Ducts **DFY2FZZ**
  Bladder **DTY2FZZ**
  Bone, Other **DPYCFZZ**
  Bone Marrow **D7Y0FZZ**
  Brain **D0Y0FZZ**
  Brain Stem **D0Y1FZZ**

Plaque Radiation - *continued*
  Breast
    Left **DMY0FZZ**
    Right **DMY1FZZ**
  Bronchus **DBY1FZZ**
  Cervix **DUY1FZZ**
  Chest **DWY2FZZ**
  Chest Wall **DBY7FZZ**
  Colon **DDY5FZZ**
  Diaphragm **DBY8FZZ**
  Duodenum **DDY2FZZ**
  Ear **D9Y0FZZ**
  Esophagus **DDY0FZZ**
  Eye **D8Y0FZZ**
  Femur **DPY9FZZ**
  Fibula **DPYBFZZ**
  Gallbladder **DFY1FZZ**
  Gland
    Adrenal **DGY2FZZ**
    Parathyroid **DGY4FZZ**
    Pituitary **DGY0FZZ**
    Thyroid **DGY5FZZ**
  Glands, Salivary **D9Y6FZZ**
  Head and Neck **DWY1FZZ**
  Hemibody **DWY4FZZ**
  Humerus **DPY6FZZ**
  Ileum **DDY4FZZ**
  Jejunum **DDY3FZZ**
  Kidney **DTY0FZZ**
  Larynx **D9YBFZZ**
  Liver **DFY0FZZ**
  Lung **DBY2FZZ**
  Lymphatics
    Abdomen **D7Y6FZZ**
    Axillary **D7Y4FZZ**
    Inguinal **D7Y8FZZ**
    Neck **D7Y3FZZ**
    Pelvis **D7Y7FZZ**
    Thorax **D7Y5FZZ**
  Mandible **DPY3FZZ**
  Maxilla **DPY2FZZ**
  Mediastinum **DBY6FZZ**
  Mouth **D9Y4FZZ**
  Nasopharynx **D9YDFZZ**
  Neck and Head **DWY1FZZ**
  Nerve, Peripheral **D0Y7FZZ**
  Nose **D9Y1FZZ**
  Ovary **DUY0FZZ**
  Palate
    Hard **D9Y8FZZ**
    Soft **D9Y9FZZ**
  Pancreas **DFY3FZZ**
  Parathyroid Gland **DGY4FZZ**
  Pelvic Bones **DPY8FZZ**
  Pelvic Region **DWY6FZZ**
  Pharynx **D9YCFZZ**
  Pineal Body **DGY1FZZ**
  Pituitary Gland **DGY0FZZ**
  Pleura **DBY5FZZ**
  Prostate **DVY0FZZ**
  Radius **DPY7FZZ**
  Rectum **DDY7FZZ**
  Rib **DPY5FZZ**
  Sinuses **D9Y7FZZ**
  Skin
    Abdomen **DHY8FZZ**
    Arm **DHY4FZZ**
    Back **DHY7FZZ**
    Buttock **DHY9FZZ**
    Chest **DHY6FZZ**
    Face **DHY2FZZ**
    Foot **DHYCFZZ**
    Hand **DHY5FZZ**

Plaque Radiation - *continued*
  Leg **DHYBFZZ**
  Neck **DHY3FZZ**
  Skull **DPY0FZZ**
  Spinal Cord **D0Y6FZZ**
  Spleen **D7Y2FZZ**
  Sternum **DPY4FZZ**
  Stomach **DDY1FZZ**
  Testis **DVY1FZZ**
  Thymus **D7Y1FZZ**
  Thyroid Gland **DGY5FZZ**
  Tibia **DPYBFZZ**
  Tongue **D9Y5FZZ**
  Trachea **DBY0FZZ**
  Ulna **DPY7FZZ**
  Ureter **DTY1FZZ**
  Urethra **DTY3FZZ**
  Uterus **DUY2FZZ**
  Whole Body **DWY5FZZ**
Plasmapheresis, therapeutic 6A550Z3
Plateletpheresis, therapeutic 6A550Z2
Platysma muscle
  use Muscle, Neck, Left
  use Muscle, Neck, Right
Pleurectomy
  see Excision, Respiratory System **0BB**
  see Resection, Respiratory System **0BT**
Pleurocentesis *see* Drainage, Anatomical
  Regions, General **0W9**
Pleurodesis, pleurosclerosis
  Chemical injection *see* Introduction of
  substance in or on, Pleural Cavity **3E0L**
  Surgical *see* Destruction, Respiratory System
  0B5
Pleurolysis *see* Release, Respiratory System
  0BN
Pleuroscopy 0BJQ4ZZ
Pleurotomy *see* Drainage, Respiratory System
  0B9
Plica semilunaris
  use Conjunctiva, Left
  use Conjunctiva, Right
Plication *see* Restriction
Pneumectomy
  see Excision, Respiratory System **0BB**
  see Resection, Respiratory System **0BT**
Pneumocentesis *see* Drainage, Respiratory
  System **0B9**
Pneumogastric nerve *use* Nerve, Vagus
Pneumolysis *see* Release, Respiratory System
  0BN
Pneumonectomy *see* Resection, Respiratory
  System **0BT**
Pneumonolysis *see* Release, Respiratory System
  0BN
Pneumonopexy
  see Repair, Respiratory System **0BQ**
  see Reposition, Respiratory System **0BS**
Pneumonorrhaphy *see* Repair, Respiratory
  System **0BQ**
Pneumonotomy *see* Drainage, Respiratory
  System **0B9**
Pneumotaxic center *use* Pons
Pneumotomy *see* Drainage, Respiratory System
  0B9
Pollicization *see* Transfer, Anatomical Regions,
  Upper Extremities **0XX**
Polyethylene socket *use* Synthetic Substitute,
  Polyethylene in **0SR**
Polymethylmethacrylate (PMMA) *use*
  Synthetic Substitute
Polypectomy, gastrointestinal *see* Excision,
  Gastrointestinal System **0DB**

Polypropylene mesh *use* Synthetic Substitute
Polysomnogram 4A1ZXQZ
Pontine tegmentum *use* Pons
Popliteal ligament
   use Bursa and Ligament, Knee, Right
   use Bursa and Ligament, Knee, Left
Popliteal lymph node
   use Lymphatic, Lower Extremity, Right
   use Lymphatic, Lower Extremity, Left
Popliteal vein
   use Vein, Femoral, Right
   use Vein, Femoral, Left
Popliteus muscle
   use Muscle, Lower Leg, Right
   use Muscle, Lower Leg, Left
Porcine (bioprosthetic) valve *use* Zooplastic
   Tissue in Heart and Great Vessels
Positive end expiratory pressure *see*
   Performance, Respiratory **5A19**
Positron Emission Tomographic (PET)
   Imaging
   Brain **C030**
   Bronchi and Lungs **CB32**
   Central Nervous System **C03YYZZ**
   Heart **C23YYZZ**
   Lungs and Bronchi **CB32**
   Myocardium **C23G**
   Respiratory System **CB3YYZZ**
   Whole Body **CW3NYZZ**
Positron emission tomography *see* Positron
   Emission Tomographic (PET) Imaging
Postauricular (mastoid) lymph node
   use Lymphatic, Neck, Right
   use Lymphatic, Neck, Left
Postcava *use* Vena Cava, Inferior
Posterior (subscapular) lymph node
   use Lymphatic, Axillary, Left
   use Lymphatic, Axillary, Right
Posterior auricular artery
   use Artery, External Carotid, Right
   use Artery, External Carotid, Left
Posterior auricular nerve *use* Nerve, Facial
Posterior auricular vein
   use Vein, External Jugular, Left
   use Vein, External Jugular, Right
Posterior cerebral artery *use* Artery,
   Intracranial
Posterior chamber
   use Eye, Right
   use Eye, Left
Posterior circumflex humeral artery
   use Artery, Axillary, Right
   use Artery, Axillary, Left
Posterior communicating artery *use* Artery,
   Intracranial
Posterior cruciate ligament (PCL)
   use Bursa and Ligament, Knee, Right
   use Bursa and Ligament, Knee, Left
Posterior facial (retromandibular) vein
   use Vein, Face, Right
   use Vein, Face, Left
Posterior femoral cutaneous nerve *use* Nerve,
   Sacral Plexus
Posterior inferior cerebellar artery (PICA)
   use Artery, Intracranial
Posterior interosseous nerve *use* Nerve, Radial
Posterior labial nerve *use* Nerve, Pudendal
Posterior scrotal nerve *use* Nerve, Pudendal
Posterior spinal artery
   use Artery, Vertebral, Left
   use Artery, Vertebral, Right

Posterior tibial recurrent artery
   use Artery, Anterior Tibial, Right
   use Artery, Anterior Tibial, Left
Posterior ulnar recurrent artery
   use Artery, Ulnar, Left
   use Artery, Ulnar, Right
Posterior vagal trunk *use* Nerve, Vagus
PPN (peripheral parenteral nutrition) *see*
   Introduction of Nutritional Substance
Preauricular lymph node *use* Lymphatic, Head
Precava *use* Vena Cava, Superior
Prepatellar bursa
   use Bursa and Ligament, Knee, Right
   use Bursa and Ligament, Knee, Left
Preputiotomy *see* Drainage, Male Reproductive
   System **0V9**
Pressure support ventilation *see* Performance,
   Respiratory **5A19**
PRESTIGE® Cervical Disc *use* Synthetic
   Substitute
Pretracheal fascia *use* Subcutaneous Tissue and
   Fascia, Neck, Anterior
Prevertebral fascia *use* Subcutaneous Tissue
   and Fascia, Neck, Posterior
PrimeAdvanced neurostimulator *use*
   Stimulator Generator, Multiple Array in **0JH**
Princeps pollicis artery
   use Artery, Hand, Left
   use Artery, Hand, Right
Probing, duct
   Diagnostic *see* Inspection
   Dilation *see* Dilation
PROCEED™ Ventral Patch *use* Synthetic
   Substitute
Procerus muscle *use* Muscle, Facial
Proctectomy
   see Excision, Rectum **0DBP**
   see Resection, Rectum **0DTP**
Proctoclysis *see* Introduction of substance in or
   on, Gastrointestinal Tract, Lower **3E0H**
Proctocolectomy
   see Excision, Gastrointestinal System **0DB**
   see Resection, Gastrointestinal System **0DT**
Proctocolpoplasty
   see Repair, Gastrointestinal System **0DQ**
   see Supplement, Gastrointestinal System **0DU**
Proctoperineoplasty
   see Repair, Gastrointestinal System **0DQ**
   see Supplement, Gastrointestinal System **0DU**
Proctoperineorrhaphy *see* Repair,
   Gastrointestinal System **0DQ**
Proctopexy
   see Repair, Rectum **0DQP**
   see Reposition, Rectum **0DSP**
Proctoplasty
   see Repair, Rectum **0DQP**
   see Supplement, Rectum **0DUP**
Proctorrhaphy *see* Repair, Rectum **0DQP**
Proctoscopy 0DJD8ZZ
Proctosigmoidectomy
   see Excision, Gastrointestinal System **0DB**
   see Resection, Gastrointestinal System **0DT**
Proctosigmoidoscopy 0DJD8ZZ
Proctostomy *see* Drainage, Rectum **0D9P**
Proctotomy *see* Drainage, Rectum **0D9P**
Prodisc-C *use* Synthetic Substitute **Prodisc-L**
   use Synthetic Substitute
Production, atrial septal defect *see* Excision,
   Septum, Atrial **02B5**
Profunda brachii
   use Artery, Brachial, Right
   use Artery, Brachial, Left

Profunda femoris (deep femoral) vein
   use Vein, Femoral, Right
   use Vein, Femoral, Left
PROLENE Polypropylene Hernia System
   (PHS) *use* Synthetic Substitute
Pronator quadratus muscle
   use Muscle, Lower Arm and Wrist, Left
   use Muscle, Lower Arm and Wrist, Right
Pronator teres muscle
   use Muscle, Lower Arm and Wrist, Right
   use Muscle, Lower Arm and Wrist, Left
Prostatectomy
   see Excision, Prostate **0VB0**
   see Resection, Prostate **0VT0**
Prostatic urethra *use* Urethra
Prostatomy, prostatotomy *see* Drainage,
   Prostate **0V90**
Protecta XT CRT-D *use* Cardiac
   Resynchronization Defibrillator Pulse
   Generator in **0JH**
Protecta XT DR (XT VR) *use* Defibrillator
   Generator in **0JH**
Protégé® RX Carotid Stent System *use*
   Intraluminal Device
Proximal radioulnar joint
   use Joint, Elbow, Left
   use Joint, Elbow, Right
Psoas muscle
   use Muscle, Hip, Right
   use Muscle, Hip, Left
PSV (pressure support ventilation) *see*
   Performance, Respiratory **5A19**
Psychoanalysis GZ54ZZZ
Psychological Tests
   Cognitive Status **GZ14ZZZ**
   Developmental **GZ10ZZZ**
   Intellectual and Psychoeducational **GZ12ZZZ**
   Neurobehavioral Status **GZ14ZZZ**
   Neuropsychological **GZ13ZZZ**
   Personality and Behavioral **GZ11ZZZ**
Psychotherapy
   Family, Mental Health Services **GZ72ZZZ**
   Group
     GZHZZZZ
     Mental Health Services **GZHZZZZ**
   Individual
     see Psychotherapy, Individual, Mental
   Health Services
     for substance abuse
       12-Step **HZ53ZZZ**
       Behavioral **HZ51ZZZ**
       Cognitive **HZ50ZZZ**
       Cognitive-Behavioral **HZ52ZZZ**
       Confrontational **HZ58ZZZ**
       Interactive **HZ55ZZZ**
       Interpersonal **HZ54ZZZ**
       Motivational Enhancement **HZ57ZZZ**
       Psychoanalysis **HZ5BZZZ**
       Psychodynamic **HZ5CZZZ**
       Psychoeducation **HZ56ZZZ**
       Psychophysiological **HZ5DZZZ**
       Supportive **HZ59ZZZ**
     Mental Health Services
       Behavioral **GZ51ZZZ**
       Cognitive **GZ52ZZZ**
       Cognitive-Behavioral **GZ58ZZZ**
       Interactive **GZ50ZZZ**
       Interpersonal **GZ53ZZZ**
       Psychoanalysis **GZ54ZZZ**
       Psychodynamic **GZ55ZZZ**
       Psychophysiological **GZ59ZZZ**
       Supportive **GZ56ZZZ**

PTCA (percutaneous transluminal coronary angioplasty) *see* Dilation, Heart and Great Vessels **027**
Pterygoid muscle *use* Muscle, Head
Pterygoid process
  use Bone, Sphenoid, Right
  use Bone, Sphenoid, Left
Pterygopalatine (sphenopalatine) ganglion *use* Nerve, Head and Neck Sympathetic
Pubic ligament
  use Bursa and Ligament, Trunk, Right
  use Bursa and Ligament, Trunk, Left
Pubis
  use Bone, Pelvic, Right
  use Bone, Pelvic, Left
Pubofemoral ligament
  use Bursa and Ligament, Hip, Left
  use Bursa and Ligament, Hip, Right
Pudendal nerve *use* Nerve, Sacral Plexus
Pull-through, rectal *see* Resection, Rectum **0DTP**
Pulmoaortic canal *use* Artery, Pulmonary, Left
Pulmonary annulus *use* Valve, Pulmonary
Pulmonary artery wedge monitoring *see* Monitoring, Arterial **4A13**
Pulmonary plexus
  use Nerve, Vagus
  use Nerve, Thoracic Sympathetic
Pulmonic valve *use* Valve, Pulmonary
Pulpectomy *see* Excision, Mouth and Throat **0CB**
Pulverization *see* Fragmentation
Pulvinar *use* Thalamus
Pump reservoir *use* Infusion Device, Pump in Subcutaneous Tissue and Fascia
Punch biopsy *see* Excision with qualifier Diagnostic
Puncture *see* Drainage
Puncture, lumbar *see* Drainage, Spinal Canal **009U**
Pyelography
  see Plain Radiography, Urinary System **BT0**
  see Fluoroscopy, Urinary System **BT1**
Pyeloileostomy, urinary diversion *see* Bypass, Urinary System **0T1**
Pyeloplasty
  see Repair, Urinary System **0TQ**
  see Replacement, Urinary System **0TR**
  see Supplement, Urinary System **0TU**
Pyelorrhaphy *see* Repair, Urinary System **0TQ**
Pyeloscopy 0TJ58ZZ
Pyelostomy
  see Drainage, Urinary System **0T9**
  see Bypass, Urinary System **0T1**
Pyelotomy *see* Drainage, Urinary System **0T9**
Pylorectomy
  see Excision, Stomach, Pylorus **0DB7**
  see Resection, Stomach, Pylorus **0DT7**
Pyloric antrum *use* Stomach, Pylorus
Pyloric canal *use* Stomach, Pylorus
Pyloric sphincter *use* Stomach, Pylorus
Pylorodiosis *see* Dilation, Stomach, Pylorus **0D77**
Pylorogastrectomy
  see Excision, Gastrointestinal System **0DB**
  see Resection, Gastrointestinal System **0DT**
Pyloroplasty
  see Repair, Stomach, Pylorus **0DQ7**
  see Supplement, Stomach, Pylorus **0DU7**
Pyloroscopy 0DJ68ZZ
Pylorotomy *see* Drainage, Stomach, Pylorus **0D97**

Pyramidalis muscle
  use Muscle, Abdomen, Left
  use Muscle, Abdomen, Right

Q

Quadrangular cartilage *use* Septum, Nasal
Quadrant resection of breast *see* Excision, Skin and Breast **0HB**
Quadrate lobe *use* Liver
Quadratus femoris muscle
  use Muscle, Hip, Left
  use Muscle, Hip, Right
Quadratus lumborum muscle
  use Muscle, Trunk, Left
  use Muscle, Trunk, Right
Quadratus plantae muscle
  use Muscle, Foot, Left
  use Muscle, Foot, Right
Quadriceps (femoris)
  use Muscle, Upper Leg, Left
  use Muscle, Upper Leg, Right
Quarantine 8E0ZXY6

R

Radial collateral carpal ligament
  use Bursa and Ligament, Wrist, Right
  use Bursa and Ligament, Wrist, Left
Radial collateral ligament
  use Bursa and Ligament, Elbow, Left
  use Bursa and Ligament, Elbow, Right
Radial notch
  use Ulna, Left
  use Ulna, Right
Radial recurrent artery
  use Artery, Radial, Right
  use Artery, Radial, Left
Radial vein
  use Vein, Brachial, Right
  use Vein, Brachial, Left
Radialis indicis
  use Artery, Hand, Right
  use Artery, Hand, Left
Radiation Therapy
  see Beam Radiation
  see Brachytherapy
Radiation treatment *see* Radiation Oncology
Radiocarpal joint
  use Joint, Wrist, Left
  use Joint, Wrist, Right
Radiocarpal ligament
  use Bursa and Ligament, Wrist, Left
  use Bursa and Ligament, Wrist, Right
Radiography *see* Plain Radiography
Radiology, analog *see* Plain Radiography
Radiology, diagnostic *see* Imaging, Diagnostic
Radioulnar ligament
  use Bursa and Ligament, Wrist, Right
  use Bursa and Ligament, Wrist, Left
Range of motion testing *see* Motor Function Assessment, Rehabilitation **F01**
REALIZE® Adjustable Gastric Band *use* Extraluminal Device
Reattachment
  Abdominal Wall **0WMF0ZZ**
  Ampulla of Vater **0FMC**
  Ankle Region
    Left **0YML0ZZ**
    Right **0YMK0ZZ**

Reattachment - *continued*
  Arm
    Lower
      Left **0XMF0ZZ**
      Right **0XMD0ZZ**
    Upper
      Left **0XM90ZZ**
      Right **0XM80ZZ**
  Axilla
    Left **0XM50ZZ**
    Right **0XM40ZZ**
  Back
    Lower **0WML0ZZ**
    Upper **0WMK0ZZ**
  Bladder **0TMB**
  Bladder Neck **0TMC**
  Breast
    Bilateral **0HMVXZZ**
    Left **0HMUXZZ**
    Right **0HMTXZZ**
  Bronchus
    Lingula **0BM90ZZ**
    Lower Lobe
      Left **0BMB0ZZ**
      Right **0BM60ZZ**
    Main
      Left **0BM70ZZ**
      Right **0BM30ZZ**
    Middle Lobe, Right **0BM50ZZ**
    Upper Lobe
      Left **0BM80ZZ**
      Right **0BM40ZZ**
  Bursa and Ligament
    Abdomen
      Left **0MMJ**
      Right **0MMH**
    Ankle
      Left **0MMR**
      Right **0MMQ**
    Elbow
      Left **0MM4**
      Right **0MM3**
    Foot
      Left **0MMT**
      Right **0MMS**
    Hand
      Left **0MM8**
      Right **0MM7**
    Head and Neck **0MM0**
    Hip
      Left **0MMM**
      Right **0MML**
    Knee
      Left **0MMP**
      Right **0MMN**
    Lower Extremity
      Left **0MMW**
      Right **0MMV**
    Perineum **0MMK**
    Shoulder
      Left **0MM2**
      Right **0MM1**
    Thorax
      Left **0MMG**
      Right **0MMF**
    Trunk
      Left **0MMD**
      Right **0MMC**
    Upper Extremity
      Left **0MMB**
      Right **0MM9**

Reattachment - *continued*
- Wrist
  - Left **0MM6**
  - Right **0MM5**
- Buttock
  - Left **0YM10ZZ**
  - Right **0YM00ZZ**
- Carina **0BM20ZZ**
- Cecum **0DMH**
- Cervix **0UMC**
- Chest Wall **0WM80ZZ**
- Clitoris **0UMJXZZ**
- Colon
  - Ascending **0DMK**
  - Descending **0DMM**
  - Sigmoid **0DMN**
  - Transverse **0DML**
- Cord
  - Bilateral **0VMH**
  - Left **0VMG**
  - Right **0VMF**
- Cul-de-sac **0UMF**
- Diaphragm
  - Left **0BMS0ZZ**
  - Right **0BMR0ZZ**
- Duct
  - Common Bile **0FM9**
  - Cystic **0FM8**
  - Hepatic
    - Left **0FM6**
    - Right **0FM5**
  - Pancreatic **0FMD**
    - Accessory **0FMF**
- Duodenum **0DM9**
- Ear
  - Left **09M1XZZ**
  - Right **09M0XZZ**
- Elbow Region
  - Left **0XMC0ZZ**
  - Right **0XMB0ZZ**
- Esophagus **0DM5**
- Extremity
  - Lower
    - Left **0YMB0ZZ**
    - Right **0YM90ZZ**
  - Upper
    - Left **0XM70ZZ**
    - Right **0XM60ZZ**
- Eyelid
  - Lower
    - Left **08MRXZZ**
    - Right **08MQXZZ**
  - Upper
    - Left **08MPXZZ**
    - Right **08MNXZZ**
- Face **0WM20ZZ**
- Fallopian Tube
  - Left **0UM6**
  - Right **0UM5**
- Fallopian Tubes, Bilateral **0UM7**
- Femoral Region
  - Left **0YM80ZZ**
  - Right **0YM70ZZ**
- Finger
  - Index
    - Left **0XMP0ZZ**
    - Right **0XMN0ZZ**
  - Little
    - Left **0XMW0ZZ**
    - Right **0XMV0ZZ**
  - Middle
    - Left **0XMR0ZZ**

Reattachment - *continued*
- Right **0XMQ0ZZ**
- Ring
  - Left **0XMT0ZZ**
  - Right **0XMS0ZZ**
- Foot
  - Left **0YMN0ZZ**
  - Right **0YMM0ZZ**
- Forequarter
  - Left **0XM10ZZ**
  - Right **0XM00ZZ**
- Gallbladder **0FM4**
- Gland
  - Left **0GM2**
  - Right **0GM3**
- Hand
  - Left **0XMK0ZZ**
  - Right **0XMJ0ZZ**
- Hindquarter
  - Bilateral **0YM40ZZ**
  - Left **0YM30ZZ**
  - Right **0YM20ZZ**
- Hymen **0UMK**
- Ileum **0DMB**
- Inguinal Region
  - Left **0YM60ZZ**
  - Right **0YM50ZZ**
- Intestine
  - Large **0DME**
    - Left **0DMG**
    - Right **0DMF**
  - Small **0DM8**
- Jaw
  - Lower **0WM50ZZ**
  - Upper **0WM40ZZ**
- Jejunum **0DMA**
- Kidney
  - Left **0TM1**
  - Right **0TM0**
- Kidney Pelvis
  - Left **0TM4**
  - Right **0TM3**
- Kidneys, Bilateral **0TM2**
- Knee Region
  - Left **0YMG0ZZ**
  - Right **0YMF0ZZ**
- Leg
  - Lower
    - Left **0YMJ0ZZ**
    - Right **0YMH0ZZ**
  - Upper
    - Left **0YMD0ZZ**
    - Right **0YMC0ZZ**
- Lip
  - Lower **0CM10ZZ**
  - Upper **0CM00ZZ**
- Liver **0FM0**
  - Left Lobe **0FM2**
  - Right Lobe **0FM1**
- Lung
  - Left **0BML0ZZ**
  - Lower Lobe
    - Left **0BMJ0ZZ**
    - Right **0BMF0ZZ**
  - Middle Lobe, Right **0BMD0ZZ**
  - Right **0BMK0ZZ**
  - Upper Lobe
    - Left **0BMG0ZZ**
    - Right **0BMC0ZZ**
- Lung Lingula **0BMH0ZZ**

Reattachment - *continued*
- Muscle
  - Abdomen
    - Left **0KML**
    - Right **0KMK**
  - Facial **0KM1**
  - Foot
    - Left **0KMW**
    - Right **0KMV**
  - Hand
    - Left **0KMD**
    - Right **0KMC**
  - Head **0KM0**
  - Hip
    - Left **0KMP**
    - Right **0KMN**
  - Lower Arm and Wrist
    - Left **0KMB**
    - Right **0KM9**
  - Lower Leg
    - Left **0KMT**
    - Right **0KMS**
  - Neck
    - Left **0KM3**
    - Right **0KM2**
  - Perineum **0KMM**
  - Shoulder
    - Left **0KM6**
    - Right **0KM5**
  - Thorax
    - Left **0KMJ**
    - Right **0KMH**
  - Tongue, Palate, Pharynx **0KM4**
  - Trunk
    - Left **0KMG**
    - Right **0KMF**
  - Upper Arm
    - Left **0KM8**
    - Right **0KM7**
  - Upper Leg
    - Left **0KMR**
    - Right **0KMQ**
- Neck **0WM60ZZ**
- Nipple
  - Left **0HMXXZZ**
  - Right **0HMWXZZ**
- Nose **09MKXZZ**
- Ovary
  - Bilateral **0UM2**
  - Left **0UM1**
  - Right **0UM0**
- Palate, Soft **0CM30ZZ**
- Pancreas **0FMG**
- Parathyroid Gland **0GMR**
  - Inferior
    - Left **0GMP**
    - Right **0GMN**
  - Multiple **0GMQ**
  - Superior
    - Left **0GMM**
    - Right **0GML**
- Penis **0VMSXZZ**
- Perineum
  - Female **0WMN0ZZ**
  - Male **0WMM0ZZ**
- Rectum **0DMP**
- Scrotum **0VM5XZZ**
- Shoulder Region
  - Left **0XM30ZZ**
  - Right **0XM20ZZ**

Reattachment - *continued*
  Skin
    Abdomen 0HM7XZZ
    Back 0HM6XZZ
    Buttock 0HM8XZZ
    Chest 0HM5XZZ
    Ear
      Left 0HM3XZZ
      Right 0HM2XZZ
    Face 0HM1XZZ
    Foot
      Left 0HMNXZZ
      Right 0HMMXZZ
    Genitalia 0HMAXZZ
    Hand
      Left 0HMGXZZ
      Right 0HMFXZZ
    Lower Arm
      Left 0HMEXZZ
      Right 0HMDXZZ
    Lower Leg
      Left 0HMLXZZ
      Right 0HMKXZZ
    Neck 0HM4XZZ
    Perineum 0HM9XZZ
    Scalp 0HM0XZZ
    Upper Arm
      Left 0HMCXZZ
      Right 0HMBXZZ
    Upper Leg
      Left 0HMJXZZ
      Right 0HMHXZZ
  Stomach 0DM6
  Tendon
    Abdomen
      Left 0LMG
      Right 0LMF
    Ankle
      Left 0LMT
      Right 0LMS
    Foot
      Left 0LMW
      Right 0LMV
    Hand
      Left 0LM8
      Right 0LM7
    Head and Neck 0LM0
    Hip
      Left 0LMK
      Right 0LMJ
    Knee
      Left 0LMR
      Right 0LMQ
    Lower Arm and Wrist
      Left 0LM6
      Right 0LM5
    Lower Leg
      Left 0LMP
      Right 0LMN
    Perineum 0LMH
    Shoulder
      Left 0LM2
      Right 0LM1
    Thorax
      Left 0LMD
      Right 0LMC
    Trunk
      Left 0LMB
      Right 0LM9
    Upper Arm
      Left 0LM4
      Right 0LM3

Reattachment - *continued*
  Upper Leg
    Left 0LMM
    Right 0LML
  Testis
    Bilateral 0VMC
    Left 0VMB
    Right 0VM9
  Thumb
    Left 0XMM0ZZ
    Right 0XML0ZZ
  Thyroid Gland
    Left Lobe 0GMG
    Right Lobe 0GMH
  Toe
    1st
      Left 0YMQ0ZZ
      Right 0YMP0ZZ
    2nd
      Left 0YMS0ZZ
      Right 0YMR0ZZ
    3rd
      Left 0YMU0ZZ
      Right 0YMT0ZZ
    4th
      Left 0YMW0ZZ
      Right 0YMV0ZZ
    5th
      Left 0YMY0ZZ
      Right 0YMX0ZZ
  Tongue 0CM70ZZ
  Tooth
    Lower 0CMX
    Upper 0CMW
  Trachea 0BM10ZZ
  Tunica Vaginalis
    Left 0VM7
    Right 0VM6
  Ureter
    Left 0TM7
    Right 0TM6
  Ureters, Bilateral 0TM8
  Urethra 0TMD
  Uterine Supporting Structure 0UM4
  Uterus 0UM9
  Uvula 0CMN0ZZ
  Vagina 0UMG
  Vulva 0UMMXZZ
  Wrist Region
    Left 0XMH0ZZ
    Right 0XMG0ZZ
Rebound HRD® (Hernia Repair Device) *use*
  Synthetic Substitute
Recession
  see Repair
  see Reposition
Reclosure, disrupted abdominal wall
  0WQFXZZ
Reconstruction
  see Repair
  see Replacement
  see Supplement
Rectectomy
  see Excision, Rectum 0DBP
  see Resection, Rectum 0DTP
Rectocele repair *see* Repair, Subcutaneous
  Tissue and Fascia, Pelvic Region 0JQC
Rectopexy
  see Repair, Gastrointestinal System 0DQ
  see Reposition, Gastrointestinal System 0DS
Rectoplasty
  see Repair, Gastrointestinal System 0DQ
  see Supplement, Gastrointestinal System 0DU

Rectorrhaphy *see* Repair, Gastrointestinal
  System 0DQ
Rectoscopy 0DJD8ZZ
Rectosigmoid junction *use* Colon, Sigmoid
Rectosigmoidectomy
  see Excision, Gastrointestinal System 0DB
  see Resection, Gastrointestinal System 0DT
Rectostomy *see* Drainage, Rectum 0D9P
Rectotomy *see* Drainage, Rectum 0D9P
Rectus abdominis muscle
  use Muscle, Abdomen, Left
  use Muscle, Abdomen, Right
Rectus femoris muscle
  use Muscle, Upper Leg, Left
  use Muscle, Upper Leg, Right
Recurrent laryngeal nerve *use* Nerve, Vagus
Reduction
  Dislocation *see* Reposition
  Fracture *see* Reposition
  Intussusception, intestinal *see* Reposition,
    Gastrointestinal System 0DS
  Mammoplasty *see* Excision, Skin and Breast
    0HB
  Prolapse *see* Reposition
  Torsion *see* Reposition
  Volvulus, gastrointestinal *see* Reposition,
    Gastrointestinal System 0DS
Refusion *see* Fusion
Reimplantation
  see Reposition
  see Transfer
  see Reattachment
Reinforcement
  see Repair
  see Supplement
Relaxation, scar tissue *see* Release
Release
  Acetabulum
    Left 0QN5
    Right 0QN4
  Adenoids 0CNQ
  Ampulla of Vater 0FNC
  Anal Sphincter 0DNR
  Anterior Chamber
    Left 08N33ZZ
    Right 08N23ZZ
  Anus 0DNQ
  Aorta
    Abdominal 04N0
    Thoracic 02NW
  Aortic Body 0GND
  Appendix 0DNJ
  Artery
    Anterior Tibial
      Left 04NQ
      Right 04NP
    Axillary
      Left 03N6
      Right 03N5
    Brachial
      Left 03N8
      Right 03N7
    Celiac 04N1
    Colic
      Left 04N7
      Middle 04N8
      Right 04N6
    Common Carotid
      Left 03NJ
      Right 03NH
    Common Iliac
      Left 04ND
      Right 04NC

Release - *continued*
- External Carotid
  - Left **03NN**
  - Right **03NM**
- External Iliac
  - Left **04NJ**
  - Right **04NH**
- Face **03NR**
- Femoral
  - Left **04NL**
  - Right **04NK**
- Foot
  - Left **04NW**
  - Right **04NV**
- Gastric **04N2**
- Hand
  - Left **03NF**
  - Right **03ND**
- Hepatic **04N3**
- Inferior Mesenteric **04NB**
- Innominate **03N2**
- Internal Carotid
  - Left **03NL**
  - Right **03NK**
- Internal Iliac
  - Left **04NF**
  - Right **04NE**
- Internal Mammary
  - Left **03N1**
  - Right **03N0**
- Intracranial **03NG**
- Lower **04NY**
- Peroneal
  - Left **04NU**
  - Right **04NT**
- Popliteal
  - Left **04NN**
  - Right **04NM**
- Posterior Tibial
  - Left **04NS**
  - Right **04NR**
- Pulmonary
  - Left **02NR**
  - Right **02NQ**
- Pulmonary Trunk **02NP**
- Radial
  - Left **03NC**
  - Right **03NB**
- Renal
  - Left **04NA**
  - Right **04N9**
- Splenic **04N4**
- Subclavian
  - Left **03N4**
  - Right **03N3**
- Superior Mesenteric **04N5**
- Temporal
  - Left **03NT**
  - Right **03NS**
- Thyroid
  - Left **03NV**
  - Right **03NU**
- Ulnar
  - Left **03NA**
  - Right **03N9**
- Upper **03NY**
- Vertebral
  - Left **03NQ**
  - Right **03NP**
- Atrium
  - Left **02N7**
  - Right **02N6**

Release - *continued*
- Auditory Ossicle
  - Left **09NA0ZZ**
  - Right **09N90ZZ**
- Basal Ganglia **00N8**
- Bladder **0TNB**
- Bladder Neck **0TNC**
- Bone
  - Ethmoid
    - Left **0NNG**
    - Right **0NNF**
  - Frontal
    - Left **0NN2**
    - Right **0NN1**
  - Hyoid **0NNX**
  - Lacrimal
    - Left **0NNJ**
    - Right **0NNH**
  - Nasal **0NNB**
  - Occipital
    - Left **0NN8**
    - Right **0NN7**
  - Palatine
    - Left **0NNL**
    - Right **0NNK**
  - Parietal
    - Left **0NN4**
    - Right **0NN3**
  - Pelvic
    - Left **0QN3**
    - Right **0QN2**
  - Sphenoid
    - Left **0NND**
    - Right **0NNC**
  - Temporal
    - Left **0NN6**
    - Right **0NN5**
  - Zygomatic
    - Left **0NNN**
    - Right **0NNM**
- Brain **00N0**
- Breast
  - Bilateral **0HNV**
  - Left **0HNU**
  - Right **0HNT**
- Bronchus
  - Lingula **0BN9**
  - Lower Lobe
    - Left **0BNB**
    - Right **0BN6**
  - Main
    - Left **0BN7**
    - Right **0BN3**
  - Middle Lobe, Right **0BN5**
  - Upper Lobe
    - Left **0BN8**
    - Right **0BN4**
- Buccal Mucosa **0CN4**
- Bursa and Ligament
  - Abdomen
    - Left **0MNJ**
    - Right **0MNH**
  - Ankle
    - Left **0MNR**
    - Right **0MNQ**
  - Elbow
    - Left **0MN4**
    - Right **0MN3**
  - Foot
    - Left **0MNT**
    - Right **0MNS**

Release - *continued*
- Hand
  - Left **0MN8**
  - Right **0MN7**
- Head and Neck **0MN0**
- Hip
  - Left **0MNM**
  - Right **0MNL**
- Knee
  - Left **0MNP**
  - Right **0MNN**
- Lower Extremity
  - Left **0MNW**
  - Right **0MNV**
- Perineum **0MNK**
- Shoulder
  - Left **0MN2**
  - Right **0MN1**
- Thorax
  - Left **0MNG**
  - Right **0MNF**
- Trunk
  - Left **0MND**
  - Right **0MNC**
- Upper Extremity
  - Left **0MNB**
  - Right **0MN9**
- Wrist
  - Left **0MN6**
  - Right **0MN5**
- Carina **0BN2**
- Carotid Bodies, Bilateral **0GN8**
- Carotid Body
  - Left **0GN6**
  - Right **0GN7**
- Carpal
  - Left **0PNN**
  - Right **0PNM**
- Cecum **0DNH**
- Cerebellum **00NC**
- Cerebral Hemisphere **00N7**
- Cerebral Meninges **00N1**
- Cerebral Ventricle **00N6**
- Cervix **0UNC**
- Chordae Tendineae **02N9**
- Choroid
  - Left **08NB**
  - Right **08NA**
- Cisterna Chyli **07NL**
- Clavicle
  - Left **0PNB**
  - Right **0PN9**
- Clitoris **0UNJ**
- Coccygeal Glomus **0GNB**
- Coccyx **0QNS**
- Colon
  - Ascending **0DNK**
  - Descending **0DNM**
  - Sigmoid **0DNN**
  - Transverse **0DNL**
- Conduction Mechanism **02N8**
- Conjunctiva
  - Left **08NTXZZ**
  - Right **08NSXZZ**
- Cord
  - Bilateral **0VNH**
  - Left **0VNG**
  - Right **0VNF**
- Cornea
  - Left **08N9XZZ**
  - Right **08N8XZZ**
- Cul-de-sac **0UNF**

Release - *continued*
  Diaphragm
    Left **0BNS**
    Right **0BNR**
  Disc
    Cervical Vertebral **0RN3**
    Cervicothoracic Vertebral **0RN5**
    Lumbar Vertebral **0SN2**
    Lumbosacral **0SN4**
    Thoracic Vertebral **0RN9**
    Thoracolumbar Vertebral **0RNB**
  Duct
    Common Bile **0FN9**
    Cystic **0FN8**
    Hepatic
      Left **0FN6**
      Right **0FN5**
    Lacrimal
      Left **08NY**
      Right **08NX**
    Pancreatic **0FND**
      Accessory **0FNF**
    Parotid
      Left **0CNC**
      Right **0CNB**
  Duodenum **0DN9**
  Dura Mater **00N2**
  Ear
    External
      Left **09N1**
      Right **09N0**
    External Auditory Canal
      Left **09N4**
      Right **09N3**
    Inner
      Left **09NE0ZZ**
      Right **09ND0ZZ**
    Middle
      Left **09N60ZZ**
      Right **09N50ZZ**
  Epididymis
    Bilateral **0VNL**
    Left **0VNK**
    Right **0VNJ**
  Epiglottis **0CNR**
  Esophagogastric Junction **0DN4**
  Esophagus **0DN5**
    Lower **0DN3**
    Middle **0DN2**
    Upper **0DN1**
  Eustachian Tube
    Left **09NG**
    Right **09NF**
  Eye
    Left **08N1XZZ**
    Right **08N0XZZ**
  Eyelid
    Lower
      Left **08NR**
      Right **08NQ**
    Upper
      Left **08NP**
      Right **08NN**
  Fallopian Tube
    Left **0UN6**
    Right **0UN5**
  Fallopian Tubes, Bilateral **0UN7**
  Femoral Shaft
    Left **0QN9**
    Right **0QN8**

Release - *continued*
  Femur
    Lower
      Left **0QNC**
      Right **0QNB**
    Upper
      Left **0QN7**
      Right **0QN6**
  Fibula
    Left **0QNK**
    Right **0QNJ**
  Finger Nail **0HNQXZZ**
  Gallbladder **0FN4**
  Gingiva
    Lower **0CN6**
    Upper **0CN5**
  Gland
    Adrenal
      Bilateral **0GN4**
      Left **0GN2**
      Right **0GN3**
    Lacrimal
      Left **08NW**
      Right **08NV**
    Minor Salivary **0CNJ**
    Parotid
      Left **0CN9**
      Right **0CN8**
    Pituitary **0GN0**
    Sublingual
      Left **0CNF**
      Right **0CND**
    Submaxillary
      Left **0CNH**
      Right **0CNG**
    Vestibular **0UNL**
  Glenoid Cavity
    Left **0PN8**
    Right **0PN7**
  Glomus Jugulare **0GNC**
  Humeral Head
    Left **0PND**
    Right **0PNC**
  Humeral Shaft
    Left **0PNG**
    Right **0PNF**
  Hymen **0UNK**
  Hypothalamus **00NA**
  Ileocecal Valve **0DNC**
  Ileum **0DNB**
  Intestine
    Large **0DNE**
      Left **0DNG**
      Right **0DNF**
    Small **0DN8**
  Iris
    Left **08ND3ZZ**
    Right **08NC3ZZ**
  Jejunum **0DNA**
  Joint
    Acromioclavicular
      Left **0RNH**
      Right **0RNG**
    Ankle
      Left **0SNG**
      Right **0SNF**
    Carpal
      Left **0RNR**
      Right **0RNQ**
    Cervical Vertebral **0RN1**
    Cervicothoracic Vertebral **0RN4**
    Coccygeal **0SN6**

Release - *continued*
  Elbow
    Left **0RNM**
    Right **0RNL**
    Finger Phalangeal
      Left **0RNX**
      Right **0RNW**
    Hip
      Left **0SNB**
      Right **0SN9**
    Knee
      Left **0SND**
      Right **0SNC**
    Lumbar Vertebral **0SN0**
    Lumbosacral **0SN3**
    Metacarpocarpal
      Left **0RNT**
      Right **0RNS**
    Metacarpophalangeal
      Left **0RNV**
      Right **0RNU**
    Metatarsal-Phalangeal
      Left **0SNN**
      Right **0SNM**
    Metatarsal-Tarsal
      Left **0SNL**
      Right **0SNK**
    Occipital-cervical **0RN0**
    Sacrococcygeal **0SN5**
    Sacroiliac
      Left **0SN8**
      Right **0SN7**
    Shoulder
      Left **0RNK**
      Right **0RNJ**
    Sternoclavicular
      Left **0RNF**
      Right **0RNE**
    Tarsal
      Left **0SNJ**
      Right **0SNH**
    Temporomandibular
      Left **0RND**
      Right **0RNC**
    Thoracic Vertebral **0RN6**
    Thoracolumbar Vertebral **0RNA**
    Toe Phalangeal
      Left **0SNQ**
      Right **0SNP**
    Wrist
      Left **0RNP**
      Right **0RNN**
  Kidney
    Left **0TN1**
    Right **0TN0**
  Kidney Pelvis
    Left **0TN4**
    Right **0TN3**
  Larynx **0CNS**
  Lens
    Left **08NK3ZZ**
    Right **08NJ3ZZ**
  Lip
    Lower **0CN1**
    Upper **0CN0**
  Liver **0FN0**
    Left Lobe **0FN2**
    Right Lobe **0FN1**
  Lung
    Bilateral **0BNM**
    Left **0BNL**

Lower Lobe
  Left **0BNJ**
  Right **0BNF**
Middle Lobe, Right **0BND**
Right **0BNK**
Upper Lobe
  Left **0BNG**
  Right **0BNC**
Lung Lingula **0BNH**
Lymphatic
  Aortic **07ND**
  Axillary
    Left **07N6**
    Right **07N5**
  Head **07N0**
  Inguinal
    Left **07NJ**
    Right **07NH**
  Internal Mammary
    Left **07N9**
    Right **07N8**
  Lower Extremity
    Left **07NG**
    Right **07NF**
  Mesenteric **07NB**
  Neck
    Left **07N2**
    Right **07N1**
  Pelvis **07NC**
  Thoracic Duct **07NK**
  Thorax **07N7**
  Upper Extremity
    Left **07N4**
    Right **07N3**
Mandible
  Left **0NNV**
  Right **0NNT**
Maxilla
  Left **0NNS**
  Right **0NNR**
Medulla Oblongata **00ND**
Mesentery **0DNV**
Metacarpal
  Left **0PNQ**
  Right **0PNP**
Metatarsal
  Left **0QNP**
  Right **0QNN**
Muscle
  Abdomen
    Left **0KNL**
    Right **0KNK**
  Extraocular
    Left **08NM**
    Right **08NL**
  Facial **0KN1**
  Foot
    Left **0KNW**
    Right **0KNV**
  Hand
    Left **0KND**
    Right **0KNC**
  Head **0KN0**
  Hip
    Left **0KNP**
    Right **0KNN**
  Lower Arm and Wrist
    Left **0KNB**
    Right **0KN9**

  Lower Leg
    Left **0KNT**
    Right **0KNS**
  Neck
    Left **0KN3**
    Right **0KN2**
  Papillary **02ND**
  Perineum **0KNM**
  Shoulder
    Left **0KN6**
    Right **0KN5**
  Thorax
    Left **0KNJ**
    Right **0KNH**
  Tongue, Palate, Pharynx **0KN4**
  Trunk
    Left **0KNG**
    Right **0KNF**
  Upper Arm
    Left **0KN8**
    Right **0KN7**
  Upper Leg
    Left **0KNR**
    Right **0KNQ**
Nasopharynx **09NN**
Nerve
  Abdominal Sympathetic **01NM**
  Abducens **00NL**
  Accessory **00NR**
  Acoustic **00NN**
  Brachial Plexus **01N3**
  Cervical **01N1**
  Cervical Plexus **01N0**
  Facial **00NM**
  Femoral **01ND**
  Glossopharyngeal **00NP**
  Head and Neck Sympathetic **01NK**
  Hypoglossal **00NS**
  Lumbar **01NB**
  Lumbar Plexus **01N9**
  Lumbar Sympathetic **01NN**
  Lumbosacral Plexus **01NA**
  Median **01N5**
  Oculomotor **00NH**
  Olfactory **00NF**
  Optic **00NG**
  Peroneal **01NH**
  Phrenic **01N2**
  Pudendal **01NC**
  Radial **01N6**
  Sacral **01NR**
  Sacral Plexus **01NQ**
  Sacral Sympathetic **01NP**
  Sciatic **01NF**
  Thoracic **01N8**
  Thoracic Sympathetic **01NL**
  Tibial **01NG**
  Trigeminal **00NK**
  Trochlear **00NJ**
  Ulnar **01N4**
  Vagus **00NQ**
Nipple
  Left **0HNX**
  Right **0HNW**
Nose **09NK**
Omentum
  Greater **0DNS**
  Lesser **0DNT**
Orbit
  Left **0NNQ**
  Right **0NNP**

Ovary
  Bilateral **0UN2**
  Left **0UN1**
  Right **0UN0**
Palate
  Hard **0CN2**
  Soft **0CN3**
Pancreas **0FNG**
Para-aortic Body **0GN9**
Paraganglion Extremity **0GNF**
Parathyroid Gland **0GNR**
  Inferior
    Left **0GNP**
    Right **0GNN**
  Multiple **0GNQ**
  Superior
    Left **0GNM**
    Right **0GNL**
Patella
  Left **0QNF**
  Right **0QND**
Penis **0VNS**
Pericardium **02NN**
Peritoneum **0DNW**
Phalanx
  Finger
    Left **0PNV**
    Right **0PNT**
  Thumb
    Left **0PNS**
    Right **0PNR**
  Toe
    Left **0QNR**
    Right **0QNQ**
Pharynx **0CNM**
Pineal Body **0GN1**
Pleura
  Left **0BNP**
  Right **0BNN**
Pons **00NB**
Prepuce **0VNT**
Prostate **0VN0**
Radius
  Left **0PNJ**
  Right **0PNH**
Rectum **0DNP**
Retina
  Left **08NF3ZZ**
  Right **08NE3ZZ**
Retinal Vessel
  Left **08NH3ZZ**
  Right **08NG3ZZ**
Rib
  Left **0PN2**
  Right **0PN1**
Sacrum **0QN1**
Scapula
  Left **0PN6**
  Right **0PN5**
Sclera
  Left **08N7XZZ**
  Right **08N6XZZ**
Scrotum **0VN5**
Septum
  Atrial **02N5**
  Nasal **09NM**
  Ventricular **02NM**
Sinus
  Accessory **09NP**
  Ethmoid
    Left **09NV**
    Right **09NU**

Destruction - *continued*
  Vocal Cord
    Left **0C5V**
    Right **0C5T**
  Vulva **0U5M**
Detachment
  Arm
    Lower
      Left **0X6F0Z**
      Right **0X6D0Z**
    Upper
      Left **0X690Z**
      Right **0X680Z**
  Elbow Region
    Left **0X6C0ZZ**
    Right **0X6B0ZZ**
  Femoral Region
    Left **0Y680ZZ**
    Right **0Y670ZZ**
  Finger
    Index
      Left **0X6P0Z**
      Right **0X6N0Z**
    Little
      Left **0X6W0Z**
      Right **0X6V0Z**
    Middle
      Left **0X6R0Z**
      Right **0X6Q0Z**
    Ring
      Left **0X6T0Z**
      Right **0X6S0Z**
  Foot
    Left **0Y6N0Z**
    Right **0Y6M0Z**
  Forequarter
    Left **0X610ZZ**
    Right **0X600ZZ**
  Hand
    Left **0X6K0Z**
    Right **0X6J0Z**
  Hindquarter
    Bilateral **0Y640ZZ**
    Left **0Y630ZZ**
    Right **0Y620ZZ**
  Knee Region
    Left **0Y6G0ZZ**
    Right **0Y6F0ZZ**
  Leg
    Lower
      Left **0Y6J0Z**
      Right **0Y6H0Z**
    Upper
      Left **0Y6D0Z**
      Right **0Y6C0Z**
  Shoulder Region
    Left **0X630ZZ**
    Right **0X620ZZ**
  Thumb
    Left **0X6M0Z**
    Right **0X6L0Z**
  Toe
    1st
      Left **0Y6Q0Z**
      Right **0Y6P0Z**
    2nd
      Left **0Y6S0Z**
      Right **0Y6R0Z**
    3rd
      Left **0Y6U0Z**
      Right **0Y6T0Z**

Detachment – *continued*
  4th
    Left **0Y6W0Z**
    Right **0Y6V0Z**
  5th
    Left **0Y6Y0Z**
    Right **0Y6X0Z**
Determination, Mental status GZ14ZZZ
Detorsion
  see Release
  see Reposition
Detoxification Services, for substance abuse
  HZ2ZZZZ
Device Fitting F0DZ
Diagnostic Audiology *see* Audiology,
  Diagnostic
Diagnostic imaging *see* Imaging, Diagnostic
Diagnostic radiology *see* Imaging, Diagnostic
Dialysis
  Hemodialysis **5A1D00Z**
  Peritoneal **3E1M39Z**
Diaphragma sellae *use* Dura Mater
Diaphragmatic pacemaker generator *use*
  Stimulator Generator in Subcutaneous Tissue
  and Fascia
Diaphragmatic Pacemaker Lead
  Insertion of device in
    Left **0BHS**
    Right **0BHR**
  Removal of device from, Diaphragm **0BPT**
  Revision of device in, Diaphragm **0BWT**
Digital radiography, plain *see* Plain
  Radiography
Dilation
  Ampulla of Vater **0F7C**
  Anus **0D7Q**
  Aorta
    Abdominal **0470**
    Thoracic **027W**
  Artery
    Anterior Tibial
      Left **047Q**
      Right **047P**
    Axillary
      Left **0376**
      Right **0375**
    Brachial
      Left **0378**
      Right **0377**
    Celiac **0471**
    Colic
      Left **0477**
      Middle **0478**
      Right **0476**
    Common Carotid
      Left **037J**
      Right **037H**
    Common Iliac
      Left **047D**
      Right **047C**
    Coronary
      Four or More Sites **0273**
      One Site **0270**
      Three Sites **0272**
      Two Sites **0271**
    External Carotid
      Left **037N**
      Right **037M**
    External Iliac
      Left **047J**
      Right **047H**
    Face **037R**

Dilation – *continued*
  Femoral
    Left **047L**
    Right **047K**
  Foot
    Left **047W**
    Right **047V**
  Gastric **0472**
  Hand
    Left **037F**
    Right **037D**
  Hepatic **0473**
  Inferior Mesenteric **047B**
  Innominate **0372**
  Internal Carotid
    Left **037L**
    Right **037K**
  Internal Iliac
    Left **047F**
    Right **047E**
  Internal Mammary
    Left **0371**
    Right **0370**
  Intracranial **037G**
  Lower **047Y**
  Peroneal
    Left **047U**
    Right **047T**
  Popliteal
    Left **047N**
    Right **047M**
  Posterior Tibial
    Left **047S**
    Right **047R**
  Pulmonary
    Left **027R**
    Right **027Q**
  Pulmonary Trunk **027P**
  Radial
    Left **037C**
    Right **037B**
  Renal
    Left **047A**
    Right **0479**
  Splenic **0474**
  Subclavian
    Left **0374**
    Right **0373**
  Superior Mesenteric **0475**
  Temporal
    Left **037T**
    Right **037S**
  Thyroid
    Left **037V**
    Right **037U**
  Ulnar
    Left **037A**
    Right **0379**
  Upper **037Y**
  Vertebral
    Left **037Q**
    Right **037P**
Bladder **0T7B**
Bladder Neck **0T7C**
Bronchus
  Lingula **0B79**
  Lower Lobe
    Left **0B7B**
    Right **0B76**
  Main
    Left **0B77**
    Right **0B73**

Frontal
Left **09NT**
Right **09NS**
Mastoid
Left **09NC**
Right **09NB**
Maxillary
Left **09NR**
Right **09NQ**
Sphenoid
Left **09NX**
Right **09NW**
Skin
Abdomen **0HN7XZZ**
Back **0HN6XZZ**
Buttock **0HN8XZZ**
Chest **0HN5XZZ**
Ear
Left **0HN3XZZ**
Right **0HN2XZZ**
Face **0HN1XZZ**
Foot
Left **0HNNXZZ**
Right **0HNMXZZ**
Genitalia **0HNAXZZ**
Hand
Left **0HNGXZZ**
Right **0HNFXZZ**
Lower Arm
Left **0HNEXZZ**
Right **0HNDXZZ**
Lower Leg
Left **0HNLXZZ**
Right **0HNKXZZ**
Neck **0HN4XZZ**
Perineum **0HN9XZZ**
Scalp **0HN0XZZ**
Upper Arm
Left **0HNCXZZ**
Right **0HNBXZZ**
Upper Leg
Left **0HNJXZZ**
Right **0HNHXZZ**
Spinal Cord
Cervical **00NW**
Lumbar **00NY**
Thoracic **00NX**
Spinal Meninges **00NT**
Spleen **07NP**
Sternum **0PN0**
Stomach **0DN6**
Pylorus **0DN7**
Subcutaneous Tissue and Fascia
Abdomen **0JN8**
Back **0JN7**
Buttock **0JN9**
Chest **0JN6**
Face **0JN1**
Foot
Left **0JNR**
Right **0JNQ**
Hand
Left **0JNK**
Right **0JNJ**
Lower Arm
Left **0JNH**
Right **0JNG**
Lower Leg
Left **0JNP**
Right **0JNN**

Neck
Anterior **0JN4**
Posterior **0JN5**
Pelvic Region **0JNC**
Perineum **0JNB**
Scalp **0JN0**
Upper Arm
Left **0JNF**
Right **0JND**
Upper Leg
Left **0JNM**
Right **0JNL**
Tarsal
Left **0QNM**
Right **0QNL**
Tendon
Abdomen
Left **0LNG**
Right **0LNF**
Ankle
Left **0LNT**
Right **0LNS**
Foot
Left **0LNW**
Right **0LNV**
Hand
Left **0LN8**
Right **0LN7**
Head and Neck **0LN0**
Hip
Left **0LNK**
Right **0LNJ**
Knee
Left **0LNR**
Right **0LNQ**
Lower Arm and Wrist
Left **0LN6**
Right **0LN5**
Lower Leg
Left **0LNP**
Right **0LNN**
Perineum **0LNH**
Shoulder
Left **0LN2**
Right **0LN1**
Thorax
Left **0LND**
Right **0LNC**
Trunk
Left **0LNB**
Right **0LN9**
Upper Arm
Left **0LN4**
Right **0LN3**
Upper Leg
Left **0LNM**
Right **0LNL**
Testis
Bilateral **0VNC**
Left **0VNB**
Right **0VN9**
Thalamus **00N9**
Thymus **07NM**
Thyroid Gland **0GNK**
Left Lobe **0GNG**
Right Lobe **0GNH**
Tibia
Left **0QNH**
Right **0QNG**
Toe Nail **0HNRXZZ**
Tongue **0CN7**

Tonsils **0CNP**
Tooth
Lower **0CNX**
Upper **0CNW**
Trachea **0BN1**
Tunica Vaginalis
Left **0VN7**
Right **0VN6**
Turbinate, Nasal **09NL**
Tympanic Membrane
Left **09N8**
Right **09N7**
Ulna
Left **0PNL**
Right **0PNK**
Ureter
Left **0TN7**
Right **0TN6**
Urethra **0TND**
Uterine Supporting Structure **0UN4**
Uterus **0UN9**
Uvula **0CNN**
Vagina **0UNG**
Valve
Aortic **02NF**
Mitral **02NG**
Pulmonary **02NH**
Tricuspid **02NJ**
Vas Deferens
Bilateral **0VNQ**
Left **0VNP**
Right **0VNN**
Vein
Axillary
Left **05N8**
Right **05N7**
Azygos **05N0**
Basilic
Left **05NC**
Right **05NB**
Brachial
Left **05NA**
Right **05N9**
Cephalic
Left **05NF**
Right **05ND**
Colic **06N7**
Common Iliac
Left **06ND**
Right **06NC**
Coronary **02N4**
Esophageal **06N3**
External Iliac
Left **06NG**
Right **06NF**
External Jugular
Left **05NQ**
Right **05NP**
Face
Left **05NV**
Right **05NT**
Femoral
Left **06NN**
Right **06NM**
Foot
Left **06NV**
Right **06NT**
Gastric **06N2**
Greater Saphenous
Left **06NQ**
Right **06NP**

Release - *continued*
- Hand
  - Left **05NH**
  - Right **05NG**
- Hemiazygos **05N1**
- Hepatic **06N4**
- Hypogastric
  - Left **06NJ**
  - Right **06NH**
- Inferior Mesenteric **06N6**
- Innominate
  - Left **05N4**
  - Right **05N3**
- Internal Jugular
  - Left **05NN**
  - Right **05NM**
- Intracranial **05NL**
- Lesser Saphenous
  - Left **06NS**
  - Right **06NR**
- Lower **06NY**
- Portal **06N8**
- Pulmonary
  - Left **02NT**
  - Right **02NS**
- Renal
  - Left **06NB**
  - Right **06N9**
- Splenic **06N1**
- Subclavian
  - Left **05N6**
  - Right **05N5**
- Superior Mesenteric **06N5**
- Upper **05NY**
- Vertebral
  - Left **05NS**
  - Right **05NR**
- Vena Cava
  - Inferior **06N0**
  - Superior **02NV**
- Ventricle
  - Left **02NL**
  - Right **02NK**
- Vertebra
  - Cervical **0PN3**
  - Lumbar **0QN0**
  - Thoracic **0PN4**
- Vesicle
  - Bilateral **0VN3**
  - Left **0VN2**
  - Right **0VN1**
- Vitreous
  - Left **08N53ZZ**
  - Right **08N43ZZ**
- Vocal Cord
  - Left **0CNV**
  - Right **0CNT**
- Vulva **0UNM**

Relocation *see* Reposition

Removal
- Abdominal Wall **2W53X**
- Anorectal **2Y53X5Z**
- Arm
  - Lower
    - Left **2W5DX**
    - Right **2W5CX**
  - Upper
    - Left **2W5BX**
    - Right **2W5AX**
- Back **2W55X**
- Chest Wall **2W54X**
- Ear **2Y52X5Z**

Removal - *continued*
- Extremity
  - Lower
    - Left **2W5MX**
    - Right **2W5LX**
  - Upper
    - Left **2W59X**
    - Right **2W58X**
- Face **2W51X**
- Finger
  - Left **2W5KX**
  - Right **2W5JX**
- Foot
  - Left **2W5TX**
  - Right **2W5SX**
- Genital Tract, Female **2Y54X5Z**
- Hand
  - Left **2W5FX**
  - Right **2W5EX**
- Head **2W50X**
- Inguinal Region
  - Left **2W57X**
  - Right **2W56X**
- Leg
  - Lower
    - Left **2W5RX**
    - Right **2W5QX**
  - Upper
    - Left **2W5PX**
    - Right **2W5NX**
- Mouth and Pharynx **2Y50X5Z**
- Nasal **2Y51X5Z**
- Neck **2W52X**
- Thumb
  - Left **2W5HX**
  - Right **2W5GX**
- Toe
  - Left **2W5VX**
  - Right **2W5UX**
- Urethra **2Y55X5Z**

Removal of device from
- Abdominal Wall **0WPF**
- Acetabulum
  - Left **0QP5**
  - Right **0QP4**
- Anal Sphincter **0DPR**
- Anus **0DPQ**
- Artery
  - Lower **04PY**
  - Upper **03PY**
- Back
  - Lower **0WPL**
  - Upper **0WPK**
- Bladder **0TPB**
- Bone
  - Facial **0NPW**
  - Lower **0QPY**
  - Nasal **0NPB**
  - Pelvic
    - Left **0QP3**
    - Right **0QP2**
  - Upper **0PPY**
- Bone Marrow **07PT**
- Brain **00P0**
- Breast
  - Left **0HPU**
  - Right **0HPT**
- Bursa and Ligament
  - Lower **0MPY**
  - Upper **0MPX**
- Carpal
  - Left **0PPN**
  - Right **0PPM**

Removal of device from - *continued*
- Cavity, Cranial **0WP1**
- Cerebral Ventricle **00P6**
- Chest Wall **0WP8**
- Cisterna Chyli **07PL**
- Clavicle
  - Left **0PPB**
  - Right **0PP9**
- Coccyx **0QPS**
- Diaphragm **0BPT**
- Disc
  - Cervical Vertebral **0RP3**
  - Cervicothoracic Vertebral **0RP5**
  - Lumbar Vertebral **0SP2**
  - Lumbosacral **0SP4**
  - Thoracic Vertebral **0RP9**
  - Thoracolumbar Vertebral **0RPB**
- Duct
  - Hepatobiliary **0FPB**
  - Pancreatic **0FPD**
- Ear
  - Inner
    - Left **09PE**
    - Right **09PD**
  - Left **09PJ**
  - Right **09PH**
- Epididymis and Spermatic Cord **0VPM**
- Esophagus **0DP5**
- Extremity
  - Lower
    - Left **0YPB**
    - Right **0YP9**
  - Upper
    - Left **0XP7**
    - Right **0XP6**
- Eye
  - Left **08P1**
  - Right **08P0**
- Face **0WP2**
- Fallopian Tube **0UP8**
- Femoral Shaft
  - Left **0QP9**
  - Right **0QP8**
- Femur
  - Lower
    - Left **0QPC**
    - Right **0QPB**
  - Upper
    - Left **0QP7**
    - Right **0QP6**
- Fibula
  - Left **0QPK**
  - Right **0QPJ**
- Finger Nail **0HPQX**
- Gallbladder **0FP4**
- Gastrointestinal Tract **0WPP**
- Genitourinary Tract **0WPR**
- Gland
  - Adrenal **0GP5**
  - Endocrine **0GPS**
  - Pituitary **0GP0**
  - Salivary **0CPA**
- Glenoid Cavity
  - Left **0PP8**
  - Right **0PP7**
- Great Vessel **02PY**
- Hair **0HPSX**
- Head **0WP0**
- Heart **02PA**
- Humeral Head
  - Left **0PPD**
  - Right **0PPC**

Removal of device from - *continued*
  Humeral Shaft
    Left **0PPG**
    Right **0PPF**
  Intestinal Tract
    Lower **0DPD**
    Upper **0DP0**
  Jaw
    Lower **0WP5**
    Upper **0WP4**
  Joint
    Acromioclavicular
      Left **0RPH**
      Right **0RPG**
    Ankle
      Left **0SPG**
      Right **0SPF**
    Carpal
      Left **0RPR**
      Right **0RPQ**
    Cervical Vertebral **0RP1**
    Cervicothoracic Vertebral **0RP4**
    Coccygeal **0SP6**
    Elbow
      Left **0RPM**
      Right **0RPL**
    Finger Phalangeal
      Left **0RPX**
      Right **0RPW**
    Hip
      Left **0SPB**
      Right **0SP9**
    Knee
      Left **0SPD**
      Right **0SPC**
    Lumbar Vertebral **0SP0**
    Lumbosacral **0SP3**
    Metacarpocarpal
      Left **0RPT**
      Right **0RPS**
    Metacarpophalangeal
      Left **0RPV**
      Right **0RPU**
    Metatarsal-Phalangeal
      Left **0SPN**
      Right **0SPM**
    Metatarsal-Tarsal
      Left **0SPL**
      Right **0SPK**
    Occipital-cervical **0RP0**
    Sacrococcygeal **0SP5**
    Sacroiliac
      Left **0SP8**
      Right **0SP7**
    Shoulder
      Left **0RPK**
      Right **0RPJ**
    Sternoclavicular
      Left **0RPF**
      Right **0RPE**
    Tarsal
      Left **0SPJ**
      Right **0SPH**
    Temporomandibular
      Left **0RPD**
      Right **0RPC**
    Thoracic Vertebral **0RP6**
    Thoracolumbar Vertebral **0RPA**
    Toe Phalangeal
      Left **0SPQ**
      Right **0SPP**

Removal of device from - *continued*
  Wrist
    Left **0RPP**
    Right **0RPN**
  Kidney **0TP5**
  Larynx **0CPS**
  Lens
    Left **08PK3JZ**
    Right **08PJ3JZ**
  Liver **0FP0**
  Lung
    Left **0BPL**
    Right **0BPK**
  Lymphatic **07PN**
    Thoracic Duct **07PK**
  Mediastinum **0WPC**
  Mesentery **0DPV**
  Metacarpal
    Left **0PPQ**
    Right **0PPP**
  Metatarsal
    Left **0QPP**
    Right **0QPN**
  Mouth and Throat **0CPY**
  Muscle
    Extraocular
      Left **08PM**
      Right **08PL**
    Lower **0KPY**
    Upper **0KPX**
  Neck **0WP6**
  Nerve
    Cranial **00PE**
    Peripheral **01PY**
  Nose **09PK**
  Omentum **0DPU**
  Ovary **0UP3**
  Pancreas **0FPG**
  Parathyroid Gland **0GPR**
  Patella
    Left **0QPF**
    Right **0QPD**
  Pelvic Cavity **0WPJ**
  Penis **0VPS**
  Pericardial Cavity **0WPD**
  Perineum
    Female **0WPN**
    Male **0WPM**
  Peritoneal Cavity **0WPG**
  Peritoneum **0DPW**
  Phalanx
    Finger
      Left **0PPV**
      Right **0PPT**
    Thumb
      Left **0PPS**
      Right **0PPR**
    Toe
      Left **0QPR**
      Right **0QPQ**
  Pineal Body **0GP1**
  Pleura **0BPQ**
  Pleural Cavity
    Left **0WPB**
    Right **0WP9**
  Products of Conception **10P0**
  Prostate and Seminal Vesicles **0VP4**
  Radius
    Left **0PPJ**
    Right **0PPH**
  Rectum **0DPP**
  Respiratory Tract **0WPQ**

Removal of device from - *continued*
  Retroperitoneum **0WPH**
  Rib
    Left **0PP2**
    Right **0PP1**
  Sacrum **0QP1**
  Scapula
    Left **0PP6**
    Right **0PP5**
  Scrotum and Tunica Vaginalis **0VP8**
  Sinus **09PY**
  Skin **0HPPX**
  Skull **0NP0**
  Spinal Canal **00PU**
  Spinal Cord **00PV**
  Spleen **07PP**
  Sternum **0PP0**
  Stomach **0DP6**
  Subcutaneous Tissue and Fascia
    Head and Neck **0JPS**
    Lower Extremity **0JPW**
    Trunk **0JPT**
    Upper Extremity **0JPV**
  Tarsal
    Left **0QPM**
    Right **0QPL**
  Tendon
    Lower **0LPY**
    Upper **0LPX**
  Testis **0VPD**
  Thymus **07PM**
  Thyroid Gland **0GPK**
  Tibia
    Left **0QPH**
    Right **0QPG**
  Toe Nail **0HPRX**
  Trachea **0BP1**
  Tracheobronchial Tree **0BP0**
  Tympanic Membrane
    Left **09P8**
    Right **09P7**
  Ulna
    Left **0PPL**
    Right **0PPK**
  Ureter **0TP9**
  Urethra **0TPD**
  Uterus and Cervix **0UPD**
  Vagina and Cul-de-sac **0UPH**
  Vas Deferens **0VPR**
  Vein
    Lower **06PY**
    Upper **05PY**
  Vertebra
    Cervical **0PP3**
    Lumbar **0QP0**
    Thoracic **0PP4**
  Vulva **0UPM**
Renal calyx
  use Kidney
  use Kidneys, Bilateral
  use Kidney, Left
  use Kidney, Right
Renal capsule
  use Kidney, Left
  use Kidney
  use Kidney, Right
  use Kidneys, Bilateral
Renal cortex
  use Kidneys, Bilateral
  use Kidney, Left
  use Kidney, Right
  use Kidney

Renal dialysis *see* Performance, Urinary **5A1D**
Renal plexus *use* Nerve, Abdominal
  Sympathetic
Renal segment
  use Kidney
  use Kidney, Left
  use Kidney, Right
  use Kidneys, Bilateral
Renal segmental artery
  use Artery, Renal, Left
  use Artery, Renal, Right
Reopening, operative site
  Control of bleeding *see* Control
  postprocedural bleeding in
  Inspection only *see* Inspection
Repair
  Abdominal Wall **0WQF**
  Acetabulum
    Left **0QQ5**
    Right **0QQ4**
  Adenoids **0CQQ**
  Ampulla of Vater **0FQC**
  Anal Sphincter **0DQR**
  Ankle Region
    Left **0YQL**
    Right **0YQK**
  Anterior Chamber
    Left **08Q33ZZ**
    Right **08Q23ZZ**
  Anus **0DQQ**
  Aorta
    Abdominal **04Q0**
    Thoracic **02QW**
  Aortic Body **0GQD**
  Appendix **0DQJ**
  Arm
    Lower
      Left **0XQF**
      Right **0XQD**
    Upper
      Left **0XQ9**
      Right **0XQ8**
  Artery
    Anterior Tibial
      Left **04QQ**
      Right **04QP**
    Axillary
      Left **03Q6**
      Right **03Q5**
    Brachial
      Left **03Q8**
      Right **03Q7**
    Celiac **04Q1**
    Colic
      Left **04Q7**
      Middle **04Q8**
      Right **04Q6**
    Common Carotid
      Left **03QJ**
      Right **03QH**
    Common Iliac
      Left **04QD**
      Right **04QC**
    Coronary
      Four or More Sites **02Q3**
      One Site **02Q0**
      Three Sites **02Q2**
      Two Sites **02Q1**
    External Carotid
      Left **03QN**
      Right **03QM**

Repair - *continued*
    External Iliac
      Left **04QJ**
      Right **04QH**
    Face **03QR**
    Femoral
      Left **04QL**
      Right **04QK**
    Foot
      Left **04QW**
      Right **04QV**
    Gastric **04Q2**
    Hand
      Left **03QF**
      Right **03QD**
    Hepatic **04Q3**
    Inferior Mesenteric **04QB**
    Innominate **03Q2**
    Internal Carotid
      Left **03QL**
      Right **03QK**
    Internal Iliac
      Left **04QF**
      Right **04QE**
    Internal Mammary
      Left **03Q1**
      Right **03Q0**
    Intracranial **03QG**
    Lower **04QY**
    Peroneal
      Left **04QU**
      Right **04QT**
    Popliteal
      Left **04QN**
      Right **04QM**
    Posterior Tibial
      Left **04QS**
      Right **04QR**
    Pulmonary
      Left **02QR**
      Right **02QQ**
    Pulmonary Trunk **02QP**
    Radial
      Left **03QC**
      Right **03QB**
    Renal
      Left **04QA**
      Right **04Q9**
    Splenic **04Q4**
    Subclavian
      Left **03Q4**
      Right **03Q3**
    Superior Mesenteric **04Q5**
    Temporal
      Left **03QT**
      Right **03QS**
    Thyroid
      Left **03QV**
      Right **03QU**
    Ulnar
      Left **03QA**
      Right **03Q9**
    Upper **03QY**
    Vertebral
      Left **03QQ**
      Right **03QP**
  Atrium
    Left **02Q7**
    Right **02Q6**
  Auditory Ossicle
    Left **09QA0ZZ**
    Right **09Q90ZZ**

Repair - *continued*
  Axilla
    Left **0XQ5**
    Right **0XQ4**
  Back
    Lower **0WQL**
    Upper **0WQK**
  Basal Ganglia **00Q8**
  Bladder **0TQB**
  Bladder Neck **0TQC**
  Bone
    Ethmoid
      Left **0NQG**
      Right **0NQF**
    Frontal
      Left **0NQ2**
      Right **0NQ1**
    Hyoid **0NQX**
    Lacrimal
      Left **0NQJ**
      Right **0NQH**
    Nasal **0NQB**
    Occipital
      Left **0NQ8**
      Right **0NQ7**
    Palatine
      Left **0NQL**
      Right **0NQK**
    Parietal
      Left **0NQ4**
      Right **0NQ3**
    Pelvic
      Left **0QQ3**
      Right **0QQ2**
    Sphenoid
      Left **0NQD**
      Right **0NQC**
    Temporal
      Left **0NQ6**
      Right **0NQ5**
    Zygomatic
      Left **0NQN**
      Right **0NQM**
  Brain **00Q0**
  Breast
    Bilateral **0HQV**
    Left **0HQU**
    Right **0HQT**
    Supernumerary **0HQY**
  Bronchus
    Lingula **0BQ9**
    Lower Lobe
      Left **0BQB**
      Right **0BQ6**
    Main
      Left **0BQ7**
      Right **0BQ3**
    Middle Lobe, Right **0BQ5**
    Upper Lobe
      Left **0BQ8**
      Right **0BQ4**
  Buccal Mucosa **0CQ4**
  Bursa and Ligament
    Abdomen
      Left **0MQJ**
      Right **0MQH**
    Ankle
      Left **0MQR**
      Right **0MQQ**
    Elbow
      Left **0MQ4**
      Right **0MQ3**

Repair - *continued*
   Foot
      Left **0MQT**
      Right **0MQS**
   Hand
      Left **0MQ8**
      Right **0MQ7**
   Head and Neck **0MQ0**
   Hip
      Left **0MQM**
      Right **0MQL**
   Knee
      Left **0MQP**
      Right **0MQN**
   Lower Extremity
      Left **0MQW**
      Right **0MQV**
   Perineum **0MQK**
   Shoulder
      Left **0MQ2**
      Right **0MQ1**
   Thorax
      Left **0MQG**
      Right **0MQF**
   Trunk
      Left **0MQD**
      Right **0MQC**
   Upper Extremity
      Left **0MQB**
      Right **0MQ9**
   Wrist
      Left **0MQ6**
      Right **0MQ5**
  Buttock
      Left **0YQ1**
      Right **0YQ0**
  Carina **0BQ2**
  Carotid Bodies, Bilateral **0GQ8**
  Carotid Body
      Left **0GQ6**
      Right **0GQ7**
  Carpal
      Left **0PQN**
      Right **0PQM**
  Cecum **0DQH**
  Cerebellum **00QC**
  Cerebral Hemisphere **00Q7**
  Cerebral Meninges **00Q1**
  Cerebral Ventricle **00Q6**
  Cervix **0UQC**
  Chest Wall **0WQ8**
  Chordae Tendineae **02Q9**
  Choroid
      Left **08QB**
      Right **08QA**
  Cisterna Chyli **07QL**
  Clavicle
      Left **0PQB**
      Right **0PQ9**
  Clitoris **0UQJ**
  Coccygeal Glomus **0GQB**
  Coccyx **0QQS**
  Colon
      Ascending **0DQK**
      Descending **0DQM**
      Sigmoid **0DQN**
      Transverse **0DQL**
  Conduction Mechanism **02Q8**
  Conjunctiva
      Left **08QTXZZ**
      Right **08QSXZZ**

Repair - *continued*
  Cord
      Bilateral **0VQH**
      Left **0VQG**
      Right **0VQF**
  Cornea
      Left **08Q9XZZ**
      Right **08Q8XZZ**
  Cul-de-sac **0UQF**
  Diaphragm
      Left **0BQS**
      Right **0BQR**
  Disc
      Cervical Vertebral **0RQ3**
      Cervicothoracic Vertebral **0RQ5**
      Lumbar Vertebral **0SQ2**
      Lumbosacral **0SQ4**
      Thoracic Vertebral **0RQ9**
      Thoracolumbar Vertebral **0RQB**
  Duct
      Common Bile **0FQ9**
      Cystic **0FQ8**
      Hepatic
         Left **0FQ6**
         Right **0FQ5**
      Lacrimal
         Left **08QY**
         Right **08QX**
      Pancreatic **0FQD**
         Accessory **0FQF**
      Parotid
         Left **0CQC**
         Right **0CQB**
  Duodenum **0DQ9**
  Dura Mater **00Q2**
  Ear
      External
         Bilateral **09Q2**
         Left **09Q1**
         Right **09Q0**
      External Auditory Canal
         Left **09Q4**
         Right **09Q3**
      Inner
         Left **09QE0ZZ**
         Right **09QD0ZZ**
      Middle
         Left **09Q60ZZ**
         Right **09Q50ZZ**
  Elbow Region
      Left **0XQC**
      Right **0XQB**
  Epididymis
      Bilateral **0VQL**
      Left **0VQK**
      Right **0VQJ**
  Epiglottis **0CQR**
  Esophagogastric Junction **0DQ4**
  Esophagus **0DQ5**
      Lower **0DQ3**
      Middle **0DQ2**
      Upper **0DQ1**
  Eustachian Tube
      Left **09QG**
      Right **09QF**
  Extremity
      Lower
         Left **0YQB**
         Right **0YQ9**
      Upper
         Left **0XQ7**
         Right **0XQ6**

Repair - *continued*
  Eye
      Left **08Q1XZZ**
      Right **08Q0XZZ**
  Eyelid
      Lower
         Left **08QR**
         Right **08QQ**
      Upper
         Left **08QP**
         Right **08QN**
  Face **0WQ2**
  Fallopian Tube
      Left **0UQ6**
      Right **0UQ5**
  Fallopian Tubes, Bilateral **0UQ7**
  Femoral Region
      Bilateral **0YQE**
      Left **0YQ8**
      Right **0YQ7**
  Femoral Shaft
      Left **0QQ9**
      Right **0QQ8**
  Femur
      Lower
         Left **0QQC**
         Right **0QQB**
      Upper
         Left **0QQ7**
         Right **0QQ6**
  Fibula
      Left **0QQK**
      Right **0QQJ**
  Finger
      Index
         Left **0XQP**
         Right **0XQN**
      Little
         Left **0XQW**
         Right **0XQV**
      Middle
         Left **0XQR**
         Right **0XQQ**
      Ring
         Left **0XQT**
         Right **0XQS**
  Finger Nail **0HQQXZZ**
  Foot
      Left **0YQN**
      Right **0YQM**
  Gallbladder **0FQ4**
  Gingiva
      Lower **0CQ6**
      Upper **0CQ5**
  Gland
      Adrenal
         Bilateral **0GQ4**
         Left **0GQ2**
         Right **0GQ3**
      Lacrimal
         Left **08QW**
         Right **08QV**
      Minor Salivary **0CQJ**
      Parotid
         Left **0CQ9**
         Right **0CQ8**
      Pituitary **0GQ0**
      Sublingual
         Left **0CQF**
         Right **0CQD**
      Submaxillary
         Left **0CQH**
         Right **0CQG**

Repair - *continued*
- Vestibular **0UQL**
- Glenoid Cavity
  - Left **0PQ8**
  - Right **0PQ7**
- Glomus Jugulare **0GQC**
- Hand
  - Left **0XQK**
  - Right **0XQJ**
- Head **0WQ0**
- Heart **02QA**
  - Left **02QC**
  - Right **02QB**
- Humeral Head
  - Left **0PQD**
  - Right **0PQC**
- Humeral Shaft
  - Left **0PQG**
  - Right **0PQF**
- Hymen **0UQK**
- Hypothalamus **00QA**
- Ileocecal Valve **0DQC**
- Ileum **0DQB**
- Inguinal Region
  - Bilateral **0YQA**
  - Left **0YQ6**
  - Right **0YQ5**
- Intestine
  - Large **0DQE**
    - Left **0DQG**
    - Right **0DQF**
  - Small **0DQ8**
- Iris
  - Left **08QD3ZZ**
  - Right **08QC3ZZ**
- Jaw
  - Lower **0WQ5**
  - Upper **0WQ4**
- Jejunum **0DQA**
- Joint
  - Acromioclavicular
    - Left **0RQH**
    - Right **0RQG**
  - Ankle
    - Left **0SQG**
    - Right **0SQF**
  - Carpal
    - Left **0RQR**
    - Right **0RQQ**
  - Cervical Vertebral **0RQ1**
  - Cervicothoracic Vertebral **0RQ4**
  - Coccygeal **0SQ6**
  - Elbow
    - Left **0RQM**
    - Right **0RQL**
  - Finger Phalangeal
    - Left **0RQX**
    - Right **0RQW**
  - Hip
    - Left **0SQB**
    - Right **0SQ9**
  - Knee
    - Left **0SQD**
    - Right **0SQC**
  - Lumbar Vertebral **0SQ0**
  - Lumbosacral **0SQ3**
  - Metacarpocarpal
    - Left **0RQT**
    - Right **0RQS**
  - Metacarpophalangeal
    - Left **0RQV**
    - Right **0RQU**

Repair - *continued*
- Metatarsal-Phalangeal
  - Left **0SQN**
  - Right **0SQM**
- Metatarsal-Tarsal
  - Left **0SQL**
  - Right **0SQK**
- Occipital-cervical **0RQ0**
- Sacrococcygeal **0SQ5**
- Sacroiliac
  - Left **0SQ8**
  - Right **0SQ7**
- Shoulder
  - Left **0RQK**
  - Right **0RQJ**
- Sternoclavicular
  - Left **0RQF**
  - Right **0RQE**
- Tarsal
  - Left **0SQJ**
  - Right **0SQH**
- Temporomandibular
  - Left **0RQD**
  - Right **0RQC**
- Thoracic Vertebral **0RQ6**
- Thoracolumbar Vertebral **0RQA**
- Toe Phalangeal
  - Left **0SQQ**
  - Right **0SQP**
- Wrist
  - Left **0RQP**
  - Right **0RQN**
- Kidney
  - Left **0TQ1**
  - Right **0TQ0**
- Kidney Pelvis
  - Left **0TQ4**
  - Right **0TQ3**
- Knee Region
  - Left **0YQG**
  - Right **0YQF**
- Larynx **0CQS**
- Leg
  - Lower
    - Left **0YQJ**
    - Right **0YQH**
  - Upper
    - Left **0YQD**
    - Right **0YQC**
- Lens
  - Left **08QK3ZZ**
  - Right **08QJ3ZZ**
- Lip
  - Lower **0CQ1**
  - Upper **0CQ0**
- Liver **0FQ0**
  - Left Lobe **0FQ2**
  - Right Lobe **0FQ1**
- Lung
  - Bilateral **0BQM**
  - Left **0BQL**
  - Lower Lobe
    - Left **0BQJ**
    - Right **0BQF**
  - Middle Lobe, Right **0BQD**
  - Right **0BQK**
  - Upper Lobe
    - Left **0BQG**
    - Right **0BQC**
- Lung Lingula **0BQH**
- Lymphatic
  - Aortic **07QD**

Repair - *continued*
- Axillary
  - Left **07Q6**
  - Right **07Q5**
- Head **07Q0**
- Inguinal
  - Left **07QJ**
  - Right **07QH**
- Internal Mammary
  - Left **07Q9**
  - Right **07Q8**
- Lower Extremity
  - Left **07QG**
  - Right **07QF**
- Mesenteric **07QB**
- Neck
  - Left **07Q2**
  - Right **07Q1**
- Pelvis **07QC**
- Thoracic Duct **07QK**
- Thorax **07Q7**
- Upper Extremity
  - Left **07Q4**
  - Right **07Q3**
- Mandible
  - Left **0NQV**
  - Right **0NQT**
- Maxilla
  - Left **0NQS**
  - Right **0NQR**
- Mediastinum **0WQC**
- Medulla Oblongata **00QD**
- Mesentery **0DQV**
- Metacarpal
  - Left **0PQQ**
  - Right **0PQP**
- Metatarsal
  - Left **0QQP**
  - Right **0QQN**
- Muscle
  - Abdomen
    - Left **0KQL**
    - Right **0KQK**
  - Extraocular
    - Left **08QM**
    - Right **08QL**
  - Facial **0KQ1**
  - Foot
    - Left **0KQW**
    - Right **0KQV**
  - Hand
    - Left **0KQD**
    - Right **0KQC**
  - Head **0KQ0**
  - Hip
    - Left **0KQP**
    - Right **0KQN**
  - Lower Arm and Wrist
    - Left **0KQB**
    - Right **0KQ9**
  - Lower Leg
    - Left **0KQT**
    - Right **0KQS**
  - Neck
    - Left **0KQ3**
    - Right **0KQ2**
  - Papillary **02QD**
  - Perineum **0KQM**
  - Shoulder
    - Left **0KQ6**
    - Right **0KQ5**

Repair - *continued*
- Thorax
  - Left **0KQJ**
  - Right **0KQH**
- Tongue, Palate, Pharynx **0KQ4**
- Trunk
  - Left **0KQG**
  - Right **0KQF**
- Upper Arm
  - Left **0KQ8**
  - Right **0KQ7**
- Upper Leg
  - Left **0KQR**
  - Right **0KQQ**
- Nasopharynx **09QN**
- Neck **0WQ6**
- Nerve
  - Abdominal Sympathetic **01QM**
  - Abducens **00QL**
  - Accessory **00QR**
  - Acoustic **00QN**
  - Brachial Plexus **01Q3**
  - Cervical **01Q1**
  - Cervical Plexus **01Q0**
  - Facial **00QM**
  - Femoral **01QD**
  - Glossopharyngeal **00QP**
  - Head and Neck Sympathetic **01QK**
  - Hypoglossal **00QS**
  - Lumbar **01QB**
  - Lumbar Plexus **01Q9**
  - Lumbar Sympathetic **01QN**
  - Lumbosacral Plexus **01QA**
  - Median **01Q5**
  - Oculomotor **00QH**
  - Olfactory **00QF**
  - Optic **00QG**
  - Peroneal **01QH**
  - Phrenic **01Q2**
  - Pudendal **01QC**
  - Radial **01Q6**
  - Sacral **01QR**
  - Sacral Plexus **01QQ**
  - Sacral Sympathetic **01QP**
  - Sciatic **01QF**
  - Thoracic **01Q8**
  - Thoracic Sympathetic **01QL**
  - Tibial **01QG**
  - Trigeminal **00QK**
  - Trochlear **00QJ**
  - Ulnar **01Q4**
  - Vagus **00QQ**
- Nipple
  - Left **0HQX**
  - Right **0HQW**
- Nose **09QK**
- Omentum
  - Greater **0DQS**
  - Lesser **0DQT**
- Orbit
  - Left **0NQQ**
  - Right **0NQP**
- Ovary
  - Bilateral **0UQ2**
  - Left **0UQ1**
  - Right **0UQ0**
- Palate
  - Hard **0CQ2**
  - Soft **0CQ3**
- Pancreas **0FQG**
- Para-aortic Body **0GQ9**
- Paraganglion Extremity **0GQF**

Repair - *continued*
- Parathyroid Gland **0GQR**
  - Inferior
    - Left **0GQP**
    - Right **0GQN**
  - Multiple **0GQQ**
  - Superior
    - Left **0GQM**
    - Right **0GQL**
- Patella
  - Left **0QQF**
  - Right **0QQD**
- Penis **0VQS**
- Pericardium **02QN**
- Perineum
  - Female **0WQN**
  - Male **0WQM**
- Peritoneum **0DQW**
- Phalanx
  - Finger
    - Left **0PQV**
    - Right **0PQT**
  - Thumb
    - Left **0PQS**
    - Right **0PQR**
  - Toe
    - Left **0QQR**
    - Right **0QQQ**
- Pharynx **0CQM**
- Pineal Body **0GQ1**
- Pleura
  - Left **0BQP**
  - Right **0BQN**
- Pons **00QB**
- Prepuce **0VQT**
- Products of Conception **10Q0**
- Prostate **0VQ0**
- Radius
  - Left **0PQJ**
  - Right **0PQH**
- Rectum **0DQP**
- Retina
  - Left **08QF3ZZ**
  - Right **08QE3ZZ**
- Retinal Vessel
  - Left **08QH3ZZ**
  - Right **08QG3ZZ**
- Rib
  - Left **0PQ2**
  - Right **0PQ1**
- Sacrum **0QQ1**
- Scapula
  - Left **0PQ6**
  - Right **0PQ5**
- Sclera
  - Left **08Q7XZZ**
  - Right **08Q6XZZ**
- Scrotum **0VQ5**
- Septum
  - Atrial **02Q5**
  - Nasal **09QM**
  - Ventricular **02QM**
- Shoulder Region
  - Left **0XQ3**
  - Right **0XQ2**
- Sinus
  - Accessory **09QP**
  - Ethmoid
    - Left **09QV**
    - Right **09QU**

Repair - *continued*
- Frontal
  - Left **09QT**
  - Right **09QS**
- Mastoid
  - Left **09QC**
  - Right **09QB**
- Maxillary
  - Left **09QR**
  - Right **09QQ**
- Sphenoid
  - Left **09QX**
  - Right **09QW**
- Skin
  - Abdomen **0HQ7XZZ**
  - Back **0HQ6XZZ**
  - Buttock **0HQ8XZZ**
  - Chest **0HQ5XZZ**
  - Ear
    - Left **0HQ3XZZ**
    - Right **0HQ2XZZ**
  - Face **0HQ1XZZ**
  - Foot
    - Left **0HQNXZZ**
    - Right **0HQMXZZ**
  - Genitalia **0HQAXZZ**
  - Hand
    - Left **0HQGXZZ**
    - Right **0HQFXZZ**
  - Lower Arm
    - Left **0HQEXZZ**
    - Right **0HQDXZZ**
  - Lower Leg
    - Left **0HQLXZZ**
    - Right **0HQKXZZ**
  - Neck **0HQ4XZZ**
  - Perineum **0HQ9XZZ**
  - Scalp **0HQ0XZZ**
  - Upper Arm
    - Left **0HQCXZZ**
    - Right **0HQBXZZ**
  - Upper Leg
    - Left **0HQJXZZ**
    - Right **0HQHXZZ**
- Skull **0NQ0**
- Spinal Cord
  - Cervical **00QW**
  - Lumbar **00QY**
  - Thoracic **00QX**
- Spinal Meninges **00QT**
- Spleen **07QP**
- Sternum **0PQ0**
- Stomach **0DQ6**
  - Pylorus **0DQ7**
- Subcutaneous Tissue and Fascia
  - Abdomen **0JQ8**
  - Back **0JQ7**
  - Buttock **0JQ9**
  - Chest **0JQ6**
  - Face **0JQ1**
  - Foot
    - Left **0JQR**
    - Right **0JQQ**
  - Hand
    - Left **0JQK**
    - Right **0JQJ**
  - Lower Arm
    - Left **0JQH**
    - Right **0JQG**
  - Lower Leg
    - Left **0JQP**
    - Right **0JQN**

Repair - *continued*
- Neck
    - Anterior **0JQ4**
    - Posterior **0JQ5**
    - Pelvic Region **0JQC**
    - Perineum **0JQB**
    - Scalp **0JQ0**
    - Upper Arm
        - Left **0JQF**
        - Right **0JQD**
    - Upper Leg
        - Left **0JQM**
        - Right **0JQL**
- Tarsal
    - Left **0QQM**
    - Right **0QQL**
- Tendon
    - Abdomen
        - Left **0LQG**
        - Right **0LQF**
    - Ankle
        - Left **0LQT**
        - Right **0LQS**
    - Foot
        - Left **0LQW**
        - Right **0LQV**
    - Hand
        - Left **0LQ8**
        - Right **0LQ7**
    - Head and Neck **0LQ0**
    - Hip
        - Left **0LQK**
        - Right **0LQJ**
    - Knee
        - Left **0LQR**
        - Right **0LQQ**
    - Lower Arm and Wrist
        - Left **0LQ6**
        - Right **0LQ5**
    - Lower Leg
        - Left **0LQP**
        - Right **0LQN**
    - Perineum **0LQH**
    - Shoulder
        - Left **0LQ2**
        - Right **0LQ1**
    - Thorax
        - Left **0LQD**
        - Right **0LQC**
    - Trunk
        - Left **0LQB**
        - Right **0LQ9**
    - Upper Arm
        - Left **0LQ4**
        - Right **0LQ3**
    - Upper Leg
        - Left **0LQM**
        - Right **0LQL**
- Testis
    - Bilateral **0VQC**
    - Left **0VQB**
    - Right **0VQ9**
- Thalamus **00Q9**
- Thumb
    - Left **0XQM**
    - Right **0XQL**
- Thymus **07QM**
- Thyroid Gland **0GQK**
    - Left Lobe **0GQG**
    - Right Lobe **0GQH**
- Thyroid Gland Isthmus **0GQJ**

Repair - *continued*
- Tibia
    - Left **0QQH**
    - Right **0QQG**
- Toe
    - 1st
        - Left **0YQQ**
        - Right **0YQP**
    - 2nd
        - Left **0YQS**
        - Right **0YQR**
    - 3rd
        - Left **0YQU**
        - Right **0YQT**
    - 4th
        - Left **0YQW**
        - Right **0YQV**
    - 5th
        - Left **0YQY**
        - Right **0YQX**
- Toe Nail **0HQRXZZ**
- Tongue **0CQ7**
- Tonsils **0CQP**
- Tooth
    - Lower **0CQX**
    - Upper **0CQW**
- Trachea **0BQ1**
- Tunica Vaginalis
    - Left **0VQ7**
    - Right **0VQ6**
- Turbinate, Nasal **09QL**
- Tympanic Membrane
    - Left **09Q8**
    - Right **09Q7**
- Ulna
    - Left **0PQL**
    - Right **0PQK**
- Ureter
    - Left **0TQ7**
    - Right **0TQ6**
- Urethra **0TQD**
- Uterine Supporting Structure **0UQ4**
- Uterus **0UQ9**
- Uvula **0CQN**
- Vagina **0UQG**
- Valve
    - Aortic **02QF**
    - Mitral **02QG**
    - Pulmonary **02QH**
    - Tricuspid **02QJ**
- Vas Deferens
    - Bilateral **0VQQ**
    - Left **0VQP**
    - Right **0VQN**
- Vein
    - Axillary
        - Left **05Q8**
        - Right **05Q7**
    - Azygos **05Q0**
    - Basilic
        - Left **05QC**
        - Right **05QB**
    - Brachial
        - Left **05QA**
        - Right **05Q9**
    - Cephalic
        - Left **05QF**
        - Right **05QD**
    - Colic **06Q7**
    - Common Iliac
        - Left **06QD**
        - Right **06QC**

Repair - *continued*
- Coronary **02Q4**
- Esophageal **06Q3**
- External Iliac
    - Left **06QG**
    - Right **06QF**
- External Jugular
    - Left **05QQ**
    - Right **05QP**
- Face
    - Left **05QV**
    - Right **05QT**
- Femoral
    - Left **06QN**
    - Right **06QM**
- Foot
    - Left **06QV**
    - Right **06QT**
- Gastric **06Q2**
- Greater Saphenous
    - Left **06QQ**
    - Right **06QP**
- Hand
    - Left **05QH**
    - Right **05QG**
- Hemiazygos **05Q1**
- Hepatic **06Q4**
- Hypogastric
    - Left **06QJ**
    - Right **06QH**
- Inferior Mesenteric **06Q6**
- Innominate
    - Left **05Q4**
    - Right **05Q3**
- Internal Jugular
    - Left **05QN**
    - Right **05QM**
- Intracranial **05QL**
- Lesser Saphenous
    - Left **06QS**
    - Right **06QR**
- Lower **06QY**
- Portal **06Q8**
- Pulmonary
    - Left **02QT**
    - Right **02QS**
- Renal
    - Left **06QB**
    - Right **06Q9**
- Splenic **06Q1**
- Subclavian
    - Left **05Q6**
    - Right **05Q5**
- Superior Mesenteric **06Q5**
- Upper **05QY**
- Vertebral
    - Left **05QS**
    - Right **05QR**
- Vena Cava
    - Inferior **06Q0**
    - Superior **02QV**
- Ventricle
    - Left **02QL**
    - Right **02QK**
- Vertebra
    - Cervical **0PQ3**
    - Lumbar **0QQ0**
    - Thoracic **0PQ4**
- Vesicle
    - Bilateral **0VQ3**
    - Left **0VQ2**
    - Right **0VQ1**

Replacement - *continued*
- Femoral Shaft
  - Left **0QR9**
  - Right **0QR8**
- Femur
  - Lower
    - Left **0QRC**
    - Right **0QRB**
  - Upper
    - Left **0QR7**
    - Right **0QR6**
- Fibula
  - Left **0QRK**
  - Right **0QRJ**
- Finger Nail **0HRQX**
- Gingiva
  - Lower **0CR6**
  - Upper **0CR5**
- Glenoid Cavity
  - Left **0PR8**
  - Right **0PR7**
- Hair **0HRSX**
- Humeral Head
  - Left **0PRD**
  - Right **0PRC**
- Humeral Shaft
  - Left **0PRG**
  - Right **0PRF**
- Iris
  - Left **08RD3**
  - Right **08RC3**
- Joint
  - Acromioclavicular
    - Left **0RRH0**
    - Right **0RRG0**
  - Ankle
    - Left **0SRG**
    - Right **0SRF**
  - Carpal
    - Left **0RRR0**
    - Right **0RRQ0**
  - Cervical Vertebral **0RR10**
  - Cervicothoracic Vertebral **0RR40**
  - Coccygeal **0SR60**
  - Elbow
    - Left **0RRM0**
    - Right **0RRL0**
  - Finger Phalangeal
    - Left **0RRX0**
    - Right **0RRW0**
  - Hip
    - Left **0SRB**
      - Acetabular Surface **0SRE**
      - Femoral Surface **0SRS**
    - Right **0SR9**
      - Acetabular Surface **0SRA**
      - Femoral Surface **0SRR**
  - Knee
    - Left **0SRD**
      - Femoral Surface **0SRU**
      - Tibial Surface **0SRW**
    - Right **0SRC**
      - Femoral Surface **0SRT**
      - Tibial Surface **0SRV**
  - Lumbar Vertebral **0SR00**
  - Lumbosacral **0SR30**
  - Metacarpocarpal
    - Left **0RRT0**
    - Right **0RRS0**
  - Metacarpophalangeal
    - Left **0RRV0**
    - Right **0RRU0**

  - Metatarsal-Phalangeal
    - Left **0SRN0**
    - Right **0SRM0**
  - Metatarsal-Tarsal
    - Left **0SRL0**
    - Right **0SRK0**
  - Occipital-cervical **0RR00**
  - Sacrococcygeal **0SR50**
  - Sacroiliac
    - Left **0SR80**
    - Right **0SR70**
  - Shoulder
    - Left **0RRK**
    - Right **0RRJ**
  - Sternoclavicular
    - Left **0RRF0**
    - Right **0RRE0**
  - Tarsal
    - Left **0SRJ0**
    - Right **0SRH0**
  - Temporomandibular
    - Left **0RRD0**
    - Right **0RRC0**
  - Thoracic Vertebral **0RR60**
  - Thoracolumbar Vertebral **0RRA0**
  - Toe Phalangeal
    - Left **0SRQ0**
    - Right **0SRP0**
  - Wrist
    - Left **0RRP0**
    - Right **0RRN0**
- Kidney Pelvis
  - Left **0TR4**
  - Right **0TR3**
- Larynx **0CRS**
- Lens
  - Left **08RK30Z**
  - Right **08RJ30Z**
- Lip
  - Lower **0CR1**
  - Upper **0CR0**
- Mandible
  - Left **0NRV**
  - Right **0NRT**
- Maxilla
  - Left **0NRS**
  - Right **0NRR**
- Mesentery **0DRV**
- Metacarpal
  - Left **0PRQ**
  - Right **0PRP**
- Metatarsal
  - Left **0QRP**
  - Right **0QRN**
- Muscle, Papillary **02RD**
- Nasopharynx **09RN**
- Nipple
  - Left **0HRX**
  - Right **0HRW**
- Nose **09RK**
- Omentum
  - Greater **0DRS**
  - Lesser **0DRT**
- Orbit
  - Left **0NRQ**
  - Right **0NRP**
- Palate
  - Hard **0CR2**
  - Soft **0CR3**

- Patella
  - Left **0QRF**
  - Right **0QRD**
- Pericardium **02RN**
- Peritoneum **0DRW**
- Phalanx
  - Finger
    - Left **0PRV**
    - Right **0PRT**
  - Thumb
    - Left **0PRS**
    - Right **0PRR**
  - Toe
    - Left **0QRR**
    - Right **0QRQ**
- Pharynx **0CRM**
- Radius
  - Left **0PRJ**
  - Right **0PRH**
- Retinal Vessel
  - Left **08RH3**
  - Right **08RG3**
- Rib
  - Left **0PR2**
  - Right **0PR1**
- Sacrum **0QR1**
- Scapula
  - Left **0PR6**
  - Right **0PR5**
- Sclera
  - Left **08R7X**
  - Right **08R6X**
- Septum
  - Atrial **02R5**
  - Nasal **09RM**
  - Ventricular **02RM**
- Skin
  - Abdomen **0HR7**
  - Back **0HR6**
  - Buttock **0HR8**
  - Chest **0HR5**
  - Ear
    - Left **0HR3**
    - Right **0HR2**
  - Face **0HR1**
  - Foot
    - Left **0HRN**
    - Right **0HRM**
  - Genitalia **0HRA**
  - Hand
    - Left **0HRG**
    - Right **0HRF**
  - Lower Arm
    - Left **0HRE**
    - Right **0HRD**
  - Lower Leg
    - Left **0HRL**
    - Right **0HRK**
  - Neck **0HR4**
  - Perineum **0HR9**
  - Scalp **0HR0**
  - Upper Arm
    - Left **0HRC**
    - Right **0HRB**
  - Upper Leg
    - Left **0HRJ**
    - Right **0HRH**
- Skull **0NR0**
- Sternum **0PR0**

Replacement - *continued*
  Subcutaneous Tissue and Fascia
    Abdomen **0JR8**
    Back **0JR7**
    Buttock **0JR9**
    Chest **0JR6**
    Face **0JR1**
    Foot
      Left **0JRR**
      Right **0JRQ**
    Hand
      Left **0JRK**
      Right **0JRJ**
    Lower Arm
      Left **0JRH**
      Right **0JRG**
    Lower Leg
      Left **0JRP**
      Right **0JRN**
    Neck
      Anterior **0JR4**
      Posterior **0JR5**
    Pelvic Region **0JRC**
    Perineum **0JRB**
    Scalp **0JR0**
    Upper Arm
      Left **0JRF**
      Right **0JRD**
    Upper Leg
      Left **0JRM**
      Right **0JRL**
  Tarsal
    Left **0QRM**
    Right **0QRL**
  Tendon
    Abdomen
      Left **0LRG**
      Right **0LRF**
    Ankle
      Left **0LRT**
      Right **0LRS**
    Foot
      Left **0LRW**
      Right **0LRV**
    Hand
      Left **0LR8**
      Right **0LR7**
    Head and Neck **0LR0**
    Hip
      Left **0LRK**
      Right **0LRJ**
    Knee
      Left **0LRR**
      Right **0LRQ**
    Lower Arm and Wrist
      Left **0LR6**
      Right **0LR5**
    Lower Leg
      Left **0LRP**
      Right **0LRN**
    Perineum **0LRH**
    Shoulder
      Left **0LR2**
      Right **0LR1**
    Thorax
      Left **0LRD**
      Right **0LRC**
    Trunk
      Left **0LRB**
      Right **0LR9**

Replacement - *continued*
  Upper Arm
    Left **0LR4**
    Right **0LR3**
  Upper Leg
    Left **0LRM**
    Right **0LRL**
  Testis
    Bilateral **0VRC0JZ**
    Left **0VRB0JZ**
    Right **0VR90JZ**
  Thumb
    Left **0XRM**
    Right **0XRL**
  Tibia
    Left **0QRH**
    Right **0QRG**
  Toe Nail **0HRRX**
  Tongue **0CR7**
  Tooth
    Lower **0CRX**
    Upper **0CRW**
  Turbinate, Nasal **09RL**
  Tympanic Membrane
    Left **09R8**
    Right **09R7**
  Ulna
    Left **0PRL**
    Right **0PRK**
  Ureter
    Left **0TR7**
    Right **0TR6**
  Urethra **0TRD**
  Uvula **0CRN**
  Valve
    Aortic **02RF**
    Mitral **02RG**
    Pulmonary **02RH**
    Tricuspid **02RJ**
  Vein
    Axillary
      Left **05R8**
      Right **05R7**
    Azygos **05R0**
    Basilic
      Left **05RC**
      Right **05RB**
    Brachial
      Left **05RA**
      Right **05R9**
    Cephalic
      Left **05RF**
      Right **05RD**
    Colic **06R7**
    Common Iliac
      Left **06RD**
      Right **06RC**
    Esophageal **06R3**
    External Iliac
      Left **06RG**
      Right **06RF**
    External Jugular
      Left **05RQ**
      Right **05RP**
    Face
      Left **05RV**
      Right **05RT**
    Femoral
      Left **06RN**
      Right **06RM**

Replacement - *continued*
  Foot
    Left **06RV**
    Right **06RT**
  Gastric **06R2**
  Greater Saphenous
    Left **06RQ**
    Right **06RP**
  Hand
    Left **05RH**
    Right **05RG**
  Hemiazygos **05R1**
  Hepatic **06R4**
  Hypogastric
    Left **06RJ**
    Right **06RH**
  Inferior Mesenteric **06R6**
  Innominate
    Left **05R4**
    Right **05R3**
  Internal Jugular
    Left **05RN**
    Right **05RM**
  Intracranial **05RL**
  Lesser Saphenous
    Left **06RS**
    Right **06RR**
  Lower **06RY**
  Portal **06R8**
  Pulmonary
    Left **02RT**
    Right **02RS**
  Renal
    Left **06RB**
    Right **06R9**
  Splenic **06R1**
  Subclavian
    Left **05R6**
    Right **05R5**
  Superior Mesenteric **06R5**
  Upper **05RY**
  Vertebral
    Left **05RS**
    Right **05RR**
  Vena Cava
    Inferior **06R0**
    Superior **02RV**
  Ventricle
    Left **02RL**
    Right **02RK**
  Vertebra
    Cervical **0PR3**
    Lumbar **0QR0**
    Thoracic **0PR4**
  Vitreous
    Left **08R53**
    Right **08R43**
  Vocal Cord
    Left **0CRV**
    Right **0CRT**
Replantation *see* Reposition
Replantation, scalp *see* Reattachment, Skin, Scalp **0HM0**
Reposition
  Acetabulum
    Left **0QS5**
    Right **0QS4**
  Ampulla of Vater **0FSC**
  Anus **0DSQ**
  Aorta
    Abdominal **04S0**
    Thoracic **02SW0ZZ**

Artery
  Anterior Tibial
    Left **04SQ**
    Right **04SP**
  Axillary
    Left **03S6**
    Right **03S5**
  Brachial
    Left **03S8**
    Right **03S7**
  Celiac **04S1**
  Colic
    Left **04S7**
    Middle **04S8**
    Right **04S6**
  Common Carotid
    Left **03SJ**
    Right **03SH**
  Common Iliac
    Left **04SD**
    Right **04SC**
  External Carotid
    Left **03SN**
    Right **03SM**
  External Iliac
    Left **04SJ**
    Right **04SH**
  Face **03SR**
  Femoral
    Left **04SL**
    Right **04SK**
  Foot
    Left **04SW**
    Right **04SV**
  Gastric **04S2**
  Hand
    Left **03SF**
    Right **03SD**
  Hepatic **04S3**
  Inferior Mesenteric **04SB**
  Innominate **03S2**
    Left **03SL**
    Right **03SK**
  Internal Iliac
    Left **04SF**
    Right **04SE**
  Internal Mammary
    Left **03S1**
    Right **03S0**
  Intracranial **03SG**
  Lower **04SY**
  Peroneal
    Left **04SU**
    Right **04ST**
  Popliteal
    Left **04SN**
    Right **04SM**
  Posterior Tibial
    Left **04SS**
    Right **04SR**
  Pulmonary
    Left **02SR0ZZ**
    Right **02SQ0ZZ**
  Pulmonary Trunk **02SP0ZZ**
  Radial
    Left **03SC**
    Right **03SB**
  Renal
    Left **04SA**
    Right **04S9**
  Splenic **04S4**

  Subclavian
    Left **03S4**
    Right **03S3**
  Superior Mesenteric **04S5**
  Temporal
    Left **03ST**
    Right **03SS**
  Thyroid
    Left **03SV**
    Right **03SU**
  Ulnar
    Left **03SA**
    Right **03S9**
  Upper **03SY**
  Vertebral
    Left **03SQ**
    Right **03SP**
Auditory Ossicle
  Left **09SA**
  Right **09S9**
Bladder **0TSB**
Bladder Neck **0TSC**
Bone
  Ethmoid
    Left **0NSG**
    Right **0NSF**
  Frontal
    Left **0NS2**
    Right **0NS1**
  Hyoid **0NSX**
  Lacrimal
    Left **0NSJ**
    Right **0NSH**
  Nasal **0NSB**
  Occipital
    Left **0NS8**
    Right **0NS7**
  Palatine
    Left **0NSL**
    Right **0NSK**
  Parietal
    Left **0NS4**
    Right **0NS3**
  Pelvic
    Left **0QS3**
    Right **0QS2**
  Sphenoid
    Left **0NSD**
    Right **0NSC**
  Temporal
    Left **0NS6**
    Right **0NS5**
  Zygomatic
    Left **0NSN**
    Right **0NSM**
Breast
  Bilateral **0HSV0ZZ**
  Left **0HSU0ZZ**
  Right **0HST0ZZ**
Bronchus
  Lingula **0BS90ZZ**
  Lower Lobe
    Left **0BSB0ZZ**
    Right **0BS60ZZ**
  Main
    Left **0BS70ZZ**
    Right **0BS30ZZ**
  Middle Lobe, Right **0BS50ZZ**
  Upper Lobe
    Left **0BS80ZZ**
    Right **0BS40ZZ**

Bursa and Ligament
  Abdomen
    Left **0MSJ**
    Right **0MSH**
  Ankle
    Left **0MSR**
    Right **0MSQ**
  Elbow
    Left **0MS4**
    Right **0MS3**
  Foot
    Left **0MST**
    Right **0MSS**
  Hand
    Left **0MS8**
    Right **0MS7**
  Head and Neck **0MS0**
  Hip
    Left **0MSM**
    Right **0MSL**
  Knee
    Left **0MSP**
    Right **0MSN**
  Lower Extremity
    Left **0MSW**
    Right **0MSV**
  Perineum **0MSK**
  Shoulder
    Left **0MS2**
    Right **0MS1**
  Thorax
    Left **0MSG**
    Right **0MSF**
  Trunk
    Left **0MSD**
    Right **0MSC**
  Upper Extremity
    Left **0MSB**
    Right **0MS9**
  Wrist
    Left **0MS6**
    Right **0MS5**
Carina **0BS20ZZ**
Carpal
  Left **0PSN**
  Right **0PSM**
Cecum **0DSH**
Cervix **0USC**
Clavicle
  Left **0PSB**
  Right **0PS9**
Coccyx **0QSS**
Colon
  Ascending **0DSK**
  Descending **0DSM**
  Sigmoid **0DSN**
  Transverse **0DSL**
Cord
  Bilateral **0VSH**
  Left **0VSG**
  Right **0VSF**
Cul-de-sac **0USF**
Diaphragm
  Left **0BSS0ZZ**
  Right **0BSR0ZZ**
Duct
  Common Bile **0FS9**
  Cystic **0FS8**
  Hepatic
    Left **0FS6**
    Right **0FS5**

Reposition - *continued*
- Lacrimal
    - Left **08SY**
    - Right **08SX**
- Pancreatic **0FSD**
    - Accessory **0FSF**
- Parotid
    - Left **0CSC**
    - Right **0CSB**
- Duodenum **0DS9**
- Ear
    - Bilateral **09S2**
    - Left **09S1**
    - Right **09S0**
- Epiglottis **0CSR**
- Esophagus **0DS5**
- Eustachian Tube
    - Left **09SG**
    - Right **09SF**
- Eyelid
    - Lower
        - Left **08SR**
        - Right **08SQ**
    - Upper
        - Left **08SP**
        - Right **08SN**
- Fallopian Tube
    - Left **0US6**
    - Right **0US5**
- Fallopian Tubes, Bilateral **0US7**
- Femoral Shaft
    - Left **0QS9**
    - Right **0QS8**
- Femur
    - Lower
        - Left **0QSC**
        - Right **0QSB**
    - Upper
        - Left **0QS7**
        - Right **0QS6**
- Fibula
    - Left **0QSK**
    - Right **0QSJ**
- Gallbladder **0FS4**
- Gland
    - Adrenal
        - Left **0GS2**
        - Right **0GS3**
    - Lacrimal
        - Left **08SW**
        - Right **08SV**
- Glenoid Cavity
    - Left **0PS8**
    - Right **0PS7**
- Hair **0HSSXZZ**
- Humeral Head
    - Left **0PSD**
    - Right **0PSC**
- Humeral Shaft
    - Left **0PSG**
    - Right **0PSF**
- Ileum **0DSB**
- Iris
    - Left **08SD3ZZ**
    - Right **08SC3ZZ**
- Jejunum **0DSA**
- Joint
    - Acromioclavicular
        - Left **0RSH**
        - Right **0RSG**

Reposition - *continued*
- Ankle
    - Left **0SSG**
    - Right **0SSF**
- Carpal
    - Left **0RSR**
    - Right **0RSQ**
- Cervical Vertebral **0RS1**
- Cervicothoracic Vertebral **0RS4**
- Coccygeal **0SS6**
- Elbow
    - Left **0RSM**
    - Right **0RSL**
- Finger Phalangeal
    - Left **0RSX**
    - Right **0RSW**
- Hip
    - Left **0SSB**
    - Right **0SS9**
- Knee
    - Left **0SSD**
    - Right **0SSC**
- Lumbar Vertebral **0SS0**
- Lumbosacral **0SS3**
- Metacarpocarpal
    - Left **0RST**
    - Right **0RSS**
- Metacarpophalangeal
    - Left **0RSV**
    - Right **0RSU**
- Metatarsal-Phalangeal
    - Left **0SSN**
    - Right **0SSM**
- Metatarsal-Tarsal
    - Left **0SSL**
    - Right **0SSK**
- Occipital-cervical **0RS0**
- Sacrococcygeal **0SS5**
- Sacroiliac
    - Left **0SS8**
    - Right **0SS7**
- Shoulder
    - Left **0RSK**
    - Right **0RSJ**
- Sternoclavicular
    - Left **0RSF**
    - Right **0RSE**
- Tarsal
    - Left **0SSJ**
    - Right **0SSH**
- Temporomandibular
    - Left **0RSD**
    - Right **0RSC**
- Thoracic Vertebral **0RS6**
- Thoracolumbar Vertebral **0RSA**
- Toe Phalangeal
    - Left **0SSQ**
    - Right **0SSP**
- Wrist
    - Left **0RSP**
    - Right **0RSN**
- Kidney
    - Left **0TS1**
    - Right **0TS0**
- Kidney Pelvis
    - Left **0TS4**
    - Right **0TS3**
- Kidneys, Bilateral **0TS2**
- Lens
    - Left **08SK3ZZ**
    - Right **08SJ3ZZ**

Reposition - *continued*
- Lip
    - Lower **0CS1**
    - Upper **0CS0**
- Liver **0FS0**
- Lung
    - Left **0BSL0ZZ**
    - Lower Lobe
        - Left **0BSJ0ZZ**
        - Right **0BSF0ZZ**
    - Middle Lobe, Right **0BSD0ZZ**
    - Right **0BSK0ZZ**
    - Upper Lobe
        - Left **0BSG0ZZ**
        - Right **0BSC0ZZ**
- Lung Lingula **0BSH0ZZ**
- Mandible
    - Left **0NSV**
    - Right **0NST**
- Maxilla
    - Left **0NSS**
    - Right **0NSR**
- Metacarpal
    - Left **0PSQ**
    - Right **0PSP**
- Metatarsal
    - Left **0QSP**
    - Right **0QSN**
- Muscle
    - Abdomen
        - Left **0KSL**
        - Right **0KSK**
    - Extraocular
        - Left **08SM**
        - Right **08SL**
    - Facial **0KS1**
    - Foot
        - Left **0KSW**
        - Right **0KSV**
    - Hand
        - Left **0KSD**
        - Right **0KSC**
    - Head **0KS0**
    - Hip
        - Left **0KSP**
        - Right **0KSN**
    - Lower Arm and Wrist
        - Left **0KSB**
        - Right **0KS9**
    - Lower Leg
        - Left **0KST**
        - Right **0KSS**
    - Neck
        - Left **0KS3**
        - Right **0KS2**
    - Perineum **0KSM**
    - Shoulder
        - Left **0KS6**
        - Right **0KS5**
    - Thorax
        - Left **0KSJ**
        - Right **0KSH**
    - Tongue, Palate, Pharynx **0KS4**
    - Trunk
        - Left **0KSG**
        - Right **0KSF**
    - Upper Arm
        - Left **0KS8**
        - Right **0KS7**
    - Upper Leg
        - Left **0KSR**
        - Right **0KSQ**

Reposition - *continued*
- Nerve
  - Abducens **00SL**
  - Accessory **00SR**
  - Acoustic **00SN**
  - Brachial Plexus **01S3**
  - Cervical **01S1**
  - Cervical Plexus **01S0**
  - Facial **00SM**
  - Femoral **01SD**
  - Glossopharyngeal **00SP**
  - Hypoglossal **00SS**
  - Lumbar **01SB**
  - Lumbar Plexus **01S9**
  - Lumbosacral Plexus **01SA**
  - Median **01S5**
  - Oculomotor **00SH**
  - Olfactory **00SF**
  - Optic **00SG**
  - Peroneal **01SH**
  - Phrenic **01S2**
  - Pudendal **01SC**
  - Radial **01S6**
  - Sacral **01SR**
  - Sacral Plexus **01SQ**
  - Sciatic **01SF**
  - Thoracic **01S8**
  - Tibial **01SG**
  - Trigeminal **00SK**
  - Trochlear **00SJ**
  - Ulnar **01S4**
  - Vagus **00SQ**
- Nipple
  - Left **0HSXXZZ**
  - Right **0HSWXZZ**
- Nose **09SK**
- Orbit
  - Left **0NSQ**
  - Right **0NSP**
- Ovary
  - Bilateral **0US2**
  - Left **0US1**
  - Right **0US0**
- Palate
  - Hard **0CS2**
  - Soft **0CS3**
- Pancreas **0FSG**
- Parathyroid Gland **0GSR**
  - Inferior
    - Left **0GSP**
    - Right **0GSN**
  - Multiple **0GSQ**
  - Superior
    - Left **0GSM**
    - Right **0GSL**
- Patella
  - Left **0QSF**
  - Right **0QSD**
- Phalanx
  - Finger
    - Left **0PSV**
    - Right **0PST**
  - Thumb
    - Left **0PSS**
    - Right **0PSR**
  - Toe
    - Left **0QSR**
    - Right **0QSQ**
- Products of Conception **10S0**
  - Ectopic **10S2**

Reposition - *continued*
- Radius
  - Left **0PSJ**
  - Right **0PSH**
- Rectum **0DSP**
- Retinal Vessel
  - Left **08SH3ZZ**
  - Right **08SG3ZZ**
- Rib
  - Left **0PS2**
  - Right **0PS1**
- Sacrum **0QS1**
- Scapula
  - Left **0PS6**
  - Right **0PS5**
- Septum, Nasal **09SM**
- Skull **0NS0**
- Spinal Cord
  - Cervical **00SW**
  - Lumbar **00SY**
  - Thoracic **00SX**
- Spleen **07SP0ZZ**
- Sternum **0PS0**
- Stomach **0DS6**
- Tarsal
  - Left **0QSM**
  - Right **0QSL**
- Tendon
  - Abdomen
    - Left **0LSG**
    - Right **0LSF**
  - Ankle
    - Left **0LST**
    - Right **0LSS**
  - Foot
    - Left **0LSW**
    - Right **0LSV**
  - Hand
    - Left **0LS8**
    - Right **0LS7**
  - Head and Neck **0LS0**
  - Hip
    - Left **0LSK**
    - Right **0LSJ**
  - Knee
    - Left **0LSR**
    - Right **0LSQ**
  - Lower Arm and Wrist
    - Left **0LS6**
    - Right **0LS5**
  - Lower Leg
    - Left **0LSP**
    - Right **0LSN**
  - Perineum **0LSH**
  - Shoulder
    - Left **0LS2**
    - Right **0LS1**
  - Thorax
    - Left **0LSD**
    - Right **0LSC**
  - Trunk
    - Left **0LSB**
    - Right **0LS9**
  - Upper Arm
    - Left **0LS4**
    - Right **0LS3**
  - Upper Leg
    - Left **0LSM**
    - Right **0LSL**

Reposition - *continued*
- Testis
  - Bilateral **0VSC**
  - Left **0VSB**
  - Right **0VS9**
- Thymus **07SM0ZZ**
- Thyroid Gland
  - Left Lobe **0GSG**
  - Right Lobe **0GSH**
- Tibia
  - Left **0QSH**
  - Right **0QSG**
- Tongue **0CS7**
- Tooth
  - Lower **0CSX**
  - Upper **0CSW**
- Trachea **0BS10ZZ**
- Turbinate, Nasal **09SL**
- Tympanic Membrane
  - Left **09S8**
  - Right **09S7**
- Ulna
  - Left **0PSL**
  - Right **0PSK**
- Ureter
  - Left **0TS7**
  - Right **0TS6**
- Ureters, Bilateral **0TS8**
- Urethra **0TSD**
- Uterine Supporting Structure **0US4**
- Uterus **0US9**
- Uvula **0CSN**
- Vagina **0USG**
- Vein
  - Axillary
    - Left **05S8**
    - Right **05S7**
  - Azygos **05S0**
  - Basilic
    - Left **05SC**
    - Right **05SB**
  - Brachial
    - Left **05SA**
    - Right **05S9**
  - Cephalic
    - Left **05SF**
    - Right **05SD**
  - Colic **06S7**
  - Common Iliac
    - Left **06SD**
    - Right **06SC**
  - Esophageal **06S3**
  - External Iliac
    - Left **06SG**
    - Right **06SF**
  - External Jugular
    - Left **05SQ**
    - Right **05SP**
  - Face
    - Left **05SV**
    - Right **05ST**
  - Femoral
    - Left **06SN**
    - Right **06SM**
  - Foot
    - Left **06SV**
    - Right **06ST**
  - Gastric **06S2**
  - Greater Saphenous
    - Left **06SQ**
    - Right **06SP**

Reposition - *continued*
- Hand
  - Left **05SH**
  - Right **05SG**
- Hemiazygos **05S1**
- Hepatic **06S4**
- Hypogastric
  - Left **06SJ**
  - Right **06SH**
- Inferior Mesenteric **06S6**
- Innominate
  - Left **05S4**
  - Right **05S3**
- Internal Jugular
  - Left **05SN**
  - Right **05SM**
- Intracranial **05SL**
- Lesser Saphenous
  - Left **06SS**
  - Right **06SR**
- Lower **06SY**
- Portal **06S8**
- Pulmonary
  - Left **02ST0ZZ**
  - Right **02SS0ZZ**
- Renal
  - Left **06SB**
  - Right **06S9**
- Splenic **06S1**
- Subclavian
  - Left **05S6**
  - Right **05S5**
- Superior Mesenteric **06S5**
- Upper **05SY**
- Vertebral
  - Left **05SS**
  - Right **05SR**
- Vena Cava
  - Inferior **06S0**
  - Superior **02SV0ZZ**
- Vertebra
  - Cervical **0PS3**
  - Lumbar **0QS0**
  - Thoracic **0PS4**
- Vocal Cord
  - Left **0CSV**
  - Right **0CST**

Resection
- Acetabulum
  - Left **0QT50ZZ**
  - Right **0QT40ZZ**
- Adenoids **0CTQ**
- Ampulla of Vater **0FTC**
- Anal Sphincter **0DTR**
- Anus **0DTQ**
- Aortic Body **0GTD**
- Appendix **0DTJ**
- Auditory Ossicle
  - Left **09TA0ZZ**
  - Right **09T90ZZ**
- Bladder **0TTB**
- Bladder Neck **0TTC**
- Bone
  - Ethmoid
    - Left **0NTG0ZZ**
    - Right **0NTF0ZZ**
  - Frontal
    - Left **0NT20ZZ**
    - Right **0NT10ZZ**
  - Hyoid **0NTX0ZZ**

Resection - *continued*
- Lacrimal
  - Left **0NTJ0ZZ**
  - Right **0NTH0ZZ**
- Nasal **0NTB0ZZ**
- Occipital
  - Left **0NT80ZZ**
  - Right **0NT70ZZ**
- Palatine
  - Left **0NTL0ZZ**
  - Right **0NTK0ZZ**
- Parietal
  - Left **0NT40ZZ**
  - Right **0NT30ZZ**
- Pelvic
  - Left **0QT30ZZ**
  - Right **0QT20ZZ**
- Sphenoid
  - Left **0NTD0ZZ**
  - Right **0NTC0ZZ**
- Temporal
  - Left **0NT60ZZ**
  - Right **0NT50ZZ**
- Zygomatic
  - Left **0NTN0ZZ**
  - Right **0NTM0ZZ**
- Breast
  - Bilateral **0HTV0ZZ**
  - Left **0HTU0ZZ**
  - Right **0HTT0ZZ**
  - Supernumerary **0HTY0ZZ**
- Bronchus
  - Lingula **0BT9**
  - Lower Lobe
    - Left **0BTB**
    - Right **0BT6**
  - Main
    - Left **0BT7**
    - Right **0BT3**
  - Middle Lobe, Right **0BT5**
  - Upper Lobe
    - Left **0BT8**
    - Right **0BT4**
- Bursa and Ligament
  - Abdomen
    - Left **0MTJ**
    - Right **0MTH**
  - Ankle
    - Left **0MTR**
    - Right **0MTQ**
  - Elbow
    - Left **0MT4**
    - Right **0MT3**
  - Foot
    - Left **0MTT**
    - Right **0MTS**
  - Hand
    - Left **0MT8**
    - Right **0MT7**
  - Head and Neck **0MT0**
  - Hip
    - Left **0MTM**
    - Right **0MTL**
  - Knee
    - Left **0MTP**
    - Right **0MTN**
  - Lower Extremity
    - Left **0MTW**
    - Right **0MTV**
  - Perineum **0MTK**
  - Shoulder
    - Left **0MT2**
    - Right **0MT1**

Resection - *continued*
- Thorax
  - Left **0MTG**
  - Right **0MTF**
- Trunk
  - Left **0MTD**
  - Right **0MTC**
- Upper Extremity
  - Left **0MTB**
  - Right **0MT9**
- Wrist
  - Left **0MT6**
  - Right **0MT5**
- Carina **0BT2**
- Carotid Bodies, Bilateral **0GT8**
- Carotid Body
  - Left **0GT6**
  - Right **0GT7**
- Carpal
  - Left **0PTN0ZZ**
  - Right **0PTM0ZZ**
- Cecum **0DTH**
- Cerebral Hemisphere **00T7**
- Cervix **0UTC**
- Chordae Tendineae **02T9**
- Cisterna Chyli **07TL**
- Clavicle
  - Left **0PTB0ZZ**
  - Right **0PT90ZZ**
- Clitoris **0UTJ**
- Coccygeal Glomus **0GTB**
- Coccyx **0QTS0ZZ**
- Colon
  - Ascending **0DTK**
  - Descending **0DTM**
  - Sigmoid **0DTN**
  - Transverse **0DTL**
- Conduction Mechanism **02T8**
- Cord
  - Bilateral **0VTH**
  - Left **0VTG**
  - Right **0VTF**
- Cornea
  - Left **08T9XZZ**
  - Right **08T8XZZ**
- Cul-de-sac **0UTF**
- Diaphragm
  - Left **0BTS**
  - Right **0BTR**
- Disc
  - Cervical Vertebral **0RT30ZZ**
  - Cervicothoracic Vertebral **0RT50ZZ**
  - Lumbar Vertebral **0ST20ZZ**
  - Lumbosacral **0ST40ZZ**
  - Thoracic Vertebral **0RT90ZZ**
  - Thoracolumbar Vertebral **0RTB0ZZ**
- Duct
  - Common Bile **0FT9**
  - Cystic **0FT8**
  - Hepatic
    - Left **0FT6**
    - Right **0FT5**
  - Lacrimal
    - Left **08TY**
    - Right **08TX**
  - Pancreatic **0FTD**
    - Accessory **0FTF**
  - Parotid
    - Left **0CTC0ZZ**
    - Right **0CTB0ZZ**
- Duodenum **0DT9**

Resection - *continued*
- Ear
  - External
    - Left **09T1**
    - Right **09T0**
  - Inner
    - Left **09TE0ZZ**
    - Right **09TD0ZZ**
  - Middle
    - Left **09T60ZZ**
    - Right **09T50ZZ**
- Epididymis
  - Bilateral **0VTL**
  - Left **0VTK**
  - Right **0VTJ**
- Epiglottis **0CTR**
- Esophagogastric Junction **0DT4**
- Esophagus **0DT5**
  - Lower **0DT3**
  - Middle **0DT2**
  - Upper **0DT1**
- Eustachian Tube
  - Left **09TG**
  - Right **09TF**
- Eye
  - Left **08T1XZZ**
  - Right **08T0XZZ**
- Eyelid
  - Lower
    - Left **08TR**
    - Right **08TQ**
  - Upper
    - Left **08TP**
    - Right **08TN**
- Fallopian Tube
  - Left **0UT6**
  - Right **0UT5**
- Fallopian Tubes, Bilateral **0UT7**
- Femoral Shaft
  - Left **0QT90ZZ**
  - Right **0QT80ZZ**
- Femur
  - Lower
    - Left **0QTC0ZZ**
    - Right **0QTB0ZZ**
  - Upper
    - Left **0QT70ZZ**
    - Right **0QT60ZZ**
- Fibula
  - Left **0QTK0ZZ**
  - Right **0QTJ0ZZ**
- Finger Nail **0HTQXZZ**
- Gallbladder **0FT4**
- Gland
  - Adrenal
    - Bilateral **0GT4**
    - Left **0GT2**
    - Right **0GT3**
  - Lacrimal
    - Left **08TW**
    - Right **08TV**
  - Minor Salivary **0CTJ0ZZ**
  - Parotid
    - Left **0CT90ZZ**
    - Right **0CT80ZZ**
  - Pituitary **0GT0**
  - Sublingual
    - Left **0CTF0ZZ**
    - Right **0CTD0ZZ**
  - Submaxillary
    - Left **0CTH0ZZ**
    - Right **0CTG0ZZ**

Resection - *continued*
- Vestibular **0UTL**
- Glenoid Cavity
  - Left **0PT80ZZ**
  - Right **0PT70ZZ**
- Glomus Jugulare **0GTC**
- Humeral Head
  - Left **0PTD0ZZ**
  - Right **0PTC0ZZ**
- Humeral Shaft
  - Left **0PTG0ZZ**
  - Right **0PTF0ZZ**
- Hymen **0UTK**
- Ileocecal Valve **0DTC**
- Ileum **0DTB**
- Intestine
  - Large **0DTE**
    - Left **0DTG**
    - Right **0DTF**
  - Small **0DT8**
- Iris
  - Left **08TD3ZZ**
  - Right **08TC3ZZ**
- Jejunum **0DTA**
- Joint
  - Acromioclavicular
    - Left **0RTH0ZZ**
    - Right **0RTG0ZZ**
  - Ankle
    - Left **0STG0ZZ**
    - Right **0STF0ZZ**
  - Carpal
    - Left **0RTR0ZZ**
    - Right **0RTQ0ZZ**
  - Cervicothoracic Vertebral **0RT40ZZ**
  - Coccygeal **0ST60ZZ**
  - Elbow
    - Left **0RTM0ZZ**
    - Right **0RTL0ZZ**
  - Finger Phalangeal
    - Left **0RTX0ZZ**
    - Right **0RTW0ZZ**
  - Hip
    - Left **0STB0ZZ**
    - Right **0ST90ZZ**
  - Knee
    - Left **0STD0ZZ**
    - Right **0STC0ZZ**
  - Metacarpocarpal
    - Left **0RTT0ZZ**
    - Right **0RTS0ZZ**
  - Metacarpophalangeal
    - Left **0RTV0ZZ**
    - Right **0RTU0ZZ**
  - Metatarsal-Phalangeal
    - Left **0STN0ZZ**
    - Right **0STM0ZZ**
  - Metatarsal-Tarsal
    - Left **0STL0ZZ**
    - Right **0STK0ZZ**
  - Sacrococcygeal **0ST50ZZ**
  - Sacroiliac
    - Left **0ST80ZZ**
    - Right **0ST70ZZ**
  - Shoulder
    - Left **0RTK0ZZ**
    - Right **0RTJ0ZZ**
  - Sternoclavicular
    - Left **0RTF0ZZ**
    - Right **0RTE0ZZ**
  - Tarsal
    - Left **0STJ0ZZ**

Resection - *continued*
- Right **0STH0ZZ**
  - Temporomandibular
    - Left **0RTD0ZZ**
    - Right **0RTC0ZZ**
  - Toe Phalangeal
    - Left **0STQ0ZZ**
    - Right **0STP0ZZ**
  - Wrist
    - Left **0RTP0ZZ**
    - Right **0RTN0ZZ**
- Kidney
  - Left **0TT1**
  - Right **0TT0**
- Kidney Pelvis
  - Left **0TT4**
  - Right **0TT3**
- Kidneys, Bilateral **0TT2**
- Larynx **0CTS**
- Lens
  - Left **08TK3ZZ**
  - Right **08TJ3ZZ**
- Lip
  - Lower **0CT1**
  - Upper **0CT0**
- Liver **0FT0**
  - Left Lobe **0FT2**
  - Right Lobe **0FT1**
- Lung
  - Bilateral **0BTM**
  - Left **0BTL**
  - Lower Lobe
    - Left **0BTJ**
    - Right **0BTF**
  - Middle Lobe, Right **0BTD**
  - Right **0BTK**
  - Upper Lobe
    - Left **0BTG**
    - Right **0BTC**
- Lung Lingula **0BTH**
- Lymphatic
  - Aortic **07TD**
  - Axillary
    - Left **07T6**
    - Right **07T5**
  - Head **07T0**
  - Inguinal
    - Left **07TJ**
    - Right **07TH**
  - Internal Mammary
    - Left **07T9**
    - Right **07T8**
  - Lower Extremity
    - Left **07TG**
    - Right **07TF**
  - Mesenteric **07TB**
  - Neck
    - Left **07T2**
    - Right **07T1**
  - Pelvis **07TC**
  - Thoracic Duct **07TK**
  - Thorax **07T7**
  - Upper Extremity
    - Left **07T4**
    - Right **07T3**
- Mandible
  - Left **0NTV0ZZ**
  - Right **0NTT0ZZ**
- Maxilla
  - Left **0NTS0ZZ**
  - Right **0NTR0ZZ**

Resection - *continued*
  Metacarpal
    Left **0PTQ0ZZ**
    Right **0PTP0ZZ**
  Metatarsal
    Left **0QTP0ZZ**
    Right **0QTN0ZZ**
  Muscle
    Abdomen
      Left **0KTL**
      Right **0KTK**
    Extraocular
      Left **08TM**
      Right **08TL**
    Facial **0KT1**
    Foot
      Left **0KTW**
      Right **0KTV**
    Hand
      Left **0KTD**
      Right **0KTC**
    Head **0KT0**
    Hip
      Left **0KTP**
      Right **0KTN**
    Lower Arm and Wrist
      Left **0KTB**
      Right **0KT9**
    Lower Leg
      Left **0KTT**
      Right **0KTS**
    Neck
      Left **0KT3**
      Right **0KT2**
    Papillary **02TD**
    Perineum **0KTM**
    Shoulder
      Left **0KT6**
      Right **0KT5**
    Thorax
      Left **0KTJ**
      Right **0KTH**
    Tongue, Palate, Pharynx **0KT4**
    Trunk
      Left **0KTG**
      Right **0KTF**
    Upper Arm
      Left **0KT8**
      Right **0KT7**
    Upper Leg
      Left **0KTR**
      Right **0KTQ**
  Nasopharynx **09TN**
  Nipple
    Left **0HTXXZZ**
    Right **0HTWXZZ**
  Nose **09TK**
  Omentum
    Greater **0DTS**
    Lesser **0DTT**
  Orbit
    Left **0NTQ0ZZ**
    Right **0NTP0ZZ**
  Ovary
    Bilateral **0UT2**
    Left **0UT1**
    Right **0UT0**
  Palate
    Hard **0CT2**
    Soft **0CT3**
  Pancreas **0FTG**
  Para-aortic Body **0GT9**

Resection - *continued*
  Paraganglion Extremity **0GTF**
  Parathyroid Gland **0GTR**
    Inferior
      Left **0GTP**
      Right **0GTN**
    Multiple **0GTQ**
    Superior
      Left **0GTM**
      Right **0GTL**
  Patella
    Left **0QTF0ZZ**
    Right **0QTD0ZZ**
  Penis **0VTS**
  Pericardium **02TN**
  Phalanx
    Finger
      Left **0PTV0ZZ**
      Right **0PTT0ZZ**
    Thumb
      Left **0PTS0ZZ**
      Right **0PTR0ZZ**
    Toe
      Left **0QTR0ZZ**
      Right **0QTQ0ZZ**
  Pharynx **0CTM**
  Pineal Body **0GT1**
  Prepuce **0VTT**
  Products of Conception, Ectopic **10T2**
  Prostate **0VT0**
  Radius
    Left **0PTJ0ZZ**
    Right **0PTH0ZZ**
  Rectum **0DTP**
  Rib
    Left **0PT20ZZ**
    Right **0PT10ZZ**
  Scapula
    Left **0PT60ZZ**
    Right **0PT50ZZ**
  Scrotum **0VT5**
  Septum
    Atrial **02T5**
    Nasal **09TM**
    Ventricular **02TM**
  Sinus
    Accessory **09TP**
    Ethmoid
      Left **09TV**
      Right **09TU**
    Frontal
      Left **09TT**
      Right **09TS**
    Mastoid
      Left **09TC**
      Right **09TB**
    Maxillary
      Left **09TR**
      Right **09TQ**
    Sphenoid
      Left **09TX**
      Right **09TW**
  Spleen **07TP**
  Sternum **0PT00ZZ**
  Stomach **0DT6**
    Pylorus **0DT7**
  Tarsal
    Left **0QTM0ZZ**
    Right **0QTL0ZZ**

Resection - *continued*
  Tendon
    Abdomen
      Left **0LTG**
      Right **0LTF**
    Ankle
      Left **0LTT**
      Right **0LTS**
    Foot
      Left **0LTW**
      Right **0LTV**
    Hand
      Left **0LT8**
      Right **0LT7**
    Head and Neck **0LT0**
    Hip
      Left **0LTK**
      Right **0LTJ**
    Knee
      Left **0LTR**
      Right **0LTQ**
    Lower Arm and Wrist
      Left **0LT6**
      Right **0LT5**
    Lower Leg
      Left **0LTP**
      Right **0LTN**
    Perineum **0LTH**
    Shoulder
      Left **0LT2**
      Right **0LT1**
    Thorax
      Left **0LTD**
      Right **0LTC**
    Trunk
      Left **0LTB**
      Right **0LT9**
    Upper Arm
      Left **0LT4**
      Right **0LT3**
    Upper Leg
      Left **0LTM**
      Right **0LTL**
  Testis
    Bilateral **0VTC**
    Left **0VTB**
    Right **0VT9**
  Thymus **07TM**
  Thyroid Gland **0GTK**
    Left Lobe **0GTG**
    Right Lobe **0GTH**
  Tibia
    Left **0QTH0ZZ**
    Right **0QTG0ZZ**
  Toe Nail **0HTRXZZ**
  Tongue **0CT7**
  Tonsils **0CTP**
  Tooth
    Lower **0CTX0Z**
    Upper **0CTW0Z**
  Trachea **0BT1**
  Tunica Vaginalis
    Left **0VT7**
    Right **0VT6**
  Turbinate, Nasal **09TL**
  Tympanic Membrane
    Left **09T8**
    Right **09T7**
  Ulna
    Left **0PTL0ZZ**
    Right **0PTK0ZZ**

Resection - *continued*
Ureter
    Left **0TT7**
    Right **0TT6**
Urethra **0TTD**
Uterine Supporting Structure **0UT4**
Uterus **0UT9**
Uvula **0CTN**
Vagina **0UTG**
Valve, Pulmonary **02TH**
Vas Deferens
    Bilateral **0VTQ**
    Left **0VTP**
    Right **0VTN**
Vesicle
    Bilateral **0VT3**
    Left **0VT2**
    Right **0VT1**
Vitreous
    Left **08T53ZZ**
    Right **08T43ZZ**
Vocal Cord
    Left **0CTV**
    Right **0CTT**
Vulva **0UTM**
Restoration, Cardiac, Single, Rhythm 5A2204Z
RestoreAdvanced neurostimulator *use* Stimulator Generator, Multiple Array Rechargeable in **0JH**
RestoreSensor neurostimulator *use* Stimulator Generator, Multiple Array Rechargeable in **0JH**
RestoreUltra neurostimulator *use* Stimulator Generator, Multiple Array Rechargeable in **0JH**
Restriction
Ampulla of Vater **0FVC**
Anus **0DVQ**
Aorta
    Abdominal **04V0**
    Thoracic **02VW[034][CDZ]Z**
Artery
    Anterior Tibial
        Left **04VQ**
        Right **04VP**
    Axillary
        Left **03V6**
        Right **03V5**
    Brachial
        Left **03V8**
        Right **03V7**
    Celiac **04V1**
    Colic
        Left **04V7**
        Middle **04V8**
        Right **04V6**
    Common Carotid
        Left **03VJ**
        Right **03VH**
    Common Iliac
        Left **04VD**
        Right **04VC**
    External Carotid
        Left **03VN**
        Right **03VM**
    External Iliac
        Left **04VJ**
        Right **04VH**
    Face **03VR**

Restriction - *continued*
Femoral
    Left **04VL**
    Right **04VK**
Foot
    Left **04VW**
    Right **04VV**
Gastric **04V2**
Hand
    Left **03VF**
    Right **03VD**
Hepatic **04V3**
Inferior Mesenteric **04VB**
Innominate **03V2**
Internal Carotid
    Left **03VL**
    Right **03VK**
Internal Iliac
    Left **04VF**
    Right **04VE**
Internal Mammary
    Left **03V1**
    Right **03V0**
Intracranial **03VG**
Lower **04VY**
Peroneal
    Left **04VU**
    Right **04VT**
Popliteal
    Left **04VN**
    Right **04VM**
Posterior Tibial
    Left **04VS**
    Right **04VR**
Pulmonary
    Left **02VR**
    Right **02VQ**
Pulmonary Trunk **02VP**
Radial
    Left **03VC**
    Right **03VB**
Renal
    Left **04VA**
    Right **04V9**
Splenic **04V4**
Subclavian
    Left **03V4**
    Right **03V3**
Superior Mesenteric **04V5**
Temporal
    Left **03VT**
    Right **03VS**
Thyroid
    Left **03VV**
    Right **03VU**
Ulnar
    Left **03VA**
    Right **03V9**
Upper **03VY**
Vertebral
    Left **03VQ**
    Right **03VP**
Bladder **0TVB**
Bladder Neck **0TVC**
Bronchus
    Lingula **0BV9**
    Lower Lobe
        Left **0BVB**
        Right **0BV6**
    Main
        Left **0BV7**
        Right **0BV3**

Restriction - *continued*
    Middle Lobe, Right **0BV5**
    Upper Lobe
        Left **0BV8**
        Right **0BV4**
Carina **0BV2**
Cecum **0DVH**
Cervix **0UVC**
Cisterna Chyli **07VL**
Colon
    Ascending **0DVK**
    Descending **0DVM**
    Sigmoid **0DVN**
    Transverse **0DVL**
Duct
    Common Bile **0FV9**
    Cystic **0FV8**
    Hepatic
        Left **0FV6**
        Right **0FV5**
    Lacrimal
        Left **08VY**
        Right **08VX**
    Pancreatic **0FVD**
        Accessory **0FVF**
    Parotid
        Left **0CVC**
        Right **0CVB**
Duodenum **0DV9**
Esophagogastric Junction **0DV4**
Esophagus **0DV5**
    Lower **0DV3**
    Middle **0DV2**
    Upper **0DV1**
Heart **02VA**
Ileocecal Valve **0DVC**
Ileum **0DVB**
Intestine
    Large **0DVE**
        Left **0DVG**
        Right **0DVF**
    Small **0DV8**
Jejunum **0DVA**
Kidney Pelvis
    Left **0TV4**
    Right **0TV3**
Lymphatic
    Aortic **07VD**
    Axillary
        Left **07V6**
        Right **07V5**
    Head **07V0**
    Inguinal
        Left **07VJ**
        Right **07VH**
    Internal Mammary
        Left **07V9**
        Right **07V8**
    Lower Extremity
        Left **07VG**
        Right **07VF**
    Mesenteric **07VB**
    Neck
        Left **07V2**
        Right **07V1**
    Pelvis **07VC**
    Thoracic Duct **07VK**
    Thorax **07V7**
    Upper Extremity
        Left **07V4**
        Right **07V3**
Rectum **0DVP**

Upper
Left **0QW7**
Right **0QW6**
Fibula
Left **0QWK**
Right **0QWJ**
Finger Nail **0HWQX**
Gallbladder **0FW4**
Gastrointestinal Tract **0WWP**
Genitourinary Tract **0WWR**
Gland
Adrenal **0GW5**
Endocrine **0GWS**
Pituitary **0GW0**
Salivary **0CWA**
Glenoid Cavity
Left **0PW8**
Right **0PW7**
Great Vessel **02WY**
Hair **0HWSX**
Head **0WW0**
Heart **02WA**
Humeral Head
Left **0PWD**
Right **0PWC**
Humeral Shaft
Left **0PWG**
Right **0PWF**
Intestinal Tract
Lower **0DWD**
Upper **0DW0**
Intestine
Large **0DWE**
Small **0DW8**
Jaw
Lower **0WW5**
Upper **0WW4**
Joint
Acromioclavicular
Left **0RWH**
Right **0RWG**
Ankle
Left **0SWG**
Right **0SWF**
Carpal
Left **0RWR**
Right **0RWQ**
Cervical Vertebral **0RW1**
Cervicothoracic Vertebral **0RW4**
Coccygeal **0SW6**
Elbow
Left **0RWM**
Right **0RWL**
Finger Phalangeal
Left **0RWX**
Right **0RWW**
Hip
Left **0SWB**
Right **0SW9**
Knee
Left **0SWD**
Right **0SWC**
Lumbar Vertebral **0SW0**
Lumbosacral **0SW3**
Metacarpocarpal
Left **0RWT**
Right **0RWS**
Metacarpophalangeal
Left **0RWV**
Right **0RWU**

Metatarsal-Phalangeal
Left **0SWN**
Right **0SWM**
Metatarsal-Tarsal
Left **0SWL**
Right **0SWK**
Occipital-cervical **0RW0**
Sacrococcygeal **0SW5**
Sacroiliac
Left **0SW8**
Right **0SW7**
Shoulder
Left **0RWK**
Right **0RWJ**
Sternoclavicular
Left **0RWF**
Right **0RWE**
Tarsal
Left **0SWJ**
Right **0SWH**
Temporomandibular
Left **0RWD**
Right **0RWC**
Thoracic Vertebral **0RW6**
Thoracolumbar Vertebral **0RWA**
Toe Phalangeal
Left **0SWQ**
Right **0SWP**
Wrist
Left **0RWP**
Right **0RWN**
Kidney **0TW5**
Larynx **0CWS**
Lens
Left **08WK**
Right **08WJ**
Liver **0FW0**
Lung
Left **0BWL**
Right **0BWK**
Lymphatic **07WN**
Thoracic Duct **07WK**
Mediastinum **0WWC**
Mesentery **0DWV**
Metacarpal
Left **0PWQ**
Right **0PWP**
Metatarsal
Left **0QWP**
Right **0QWN**
Mouth and Throat **0CWY**
Muscle
Extraocular
Left **08WM**
Right **08WL**
Lower **0KWY**
Upper **0KWX**
Neck **0WW6**
Nerve
Cranial **00WE**
Peripheral **01WY**
Nose **09WK**
Omentum **0DWU**
Ovary **0UW3**
Pancreas **0FWG**
Parathyroid Gland **0GWR**
Patella
Left **0QWF**
Right **0QWD**
Pelvic Cavity **0WWJ**
Penis **0VWS**

Pericardial Cavity **0WWD**
Perineum
Female **0WWN**
Male **0WWM**
Peritoneal Cavity **0WWG**
Peritoneum **0DWW**
Phalanx
Finger
Left **0PWV**
Right **0PWT**
Thumb
Left **0PWS**
Right **0PWR**
Toe
Left **0QWR**
Right **0QWQ**
Pineal Body **0GW1**
Pleura **0BWQ**
Pleural Cavity
Left **0WWB**
Right **0WW9**
Prostate and Seminal Vesicles **0VW4**
Radius
Left **0PWJ**
Right **0PWH**
Respiratory Tract **0WWQ**
Retroperitoneum **0WWH**
Rib
Left **0PW2**
Right **0PW1**
Sacrum **0QW1**
Scapula
Left **0PW6**
Right **0PW5**
Scrotum and Tunica Vaginalis **0VW8**
Septum
Atrial **02W5**
Ventricular **02WM**
Sinus **09WY**
Skin **0HWPX**
Skull **0NW0**
Spinal Canal **00WU**
Spinal Cord **00WV**
Spleen **07WP**
Sternum **0PW0**
Stomach **0DW6**
Subcutaneous Tissue and Fascia
Head and Neck **0JWS**
Lower Extremity **0JWW**
Trunk **0JWT**
Upper Extremity **0JWV**
Tarsal
Left **0QWM**
Right **0QWL**
Tendon
Lower **0LWY**
Upper **0LWX**
Testis **0VWD**
Thymus **07WM**
Thyroid Gland **0GWK**
Tibia
Left **0QWH**
Right **0QWG**
Toe Nail **0HWRX**
Trachea **0BW1**
Tracheobronchial Tree **0BW0**
Tympanic Membrane
Left **09W8**
Right **09W7**
Ulna
Left **0PWL**
Right **0PWK**

Revision of device – *continued*
Ureter **0TW9**
Urethra **0TWD**
Uterus and Cervix **0UWD**
Vagina and Cul-de-sac **0UWH**
Valve
Aortic **02WF**
Mitral **02WG**
Pulmonary **02WH**
Tricuspid **02WJ**
Vas Deferens **0VWR**
Vein
Lower **06WY**
Upper **05WY**
Vertebra
Cervical **0PW3**
Lumbar **0QW0**
Thoracic **0PW4**
Vulva **0UWM**
Revo MRI™ SureScan® pacemaker *use* Pacemaker, Dual Chamber in **0JH**
Rheos® System device *use* Cardiac Rhythm Related Device in Subcutaneous Tissue and Fascia
Rheos® System lead *use* Stimulator Lead in Upper Arteries
Rhinopharynx *use* Nasopharynx
Rhinoplasty
see Alteration, Nose **090K**
see Repair, Nose **09QK**
see Replacement, Nose **09RK**
see Supplement, Nose **09UK**
Rhinorrhaphy *see* Repair, Nose **09QK**
Rhinoscopy 09JKXZZ
Rhizotomy
see Division, Central Nervous System **008**
see Division, Peripheral Nervous System **018**
Rhomboid major muscle
use Muscle, Trunk, Left
use Muscle, Trunk, Right
Rhomboid minor muscle
use Muscle, Trunk, Right
use Muscle, Trunk, Left
Rhythm electrocardiogram *see* Measurement, Cardiac **4A02**
Rhytidectomy *see* Face lift
Right ascending lumbar vein *use* Vein, Azygos
Right atrioventricular valve *use* Valve, Tricuspid
Right auricular appendix *use* Atrium, Right
Right colic vein *use* Vein, Colic
Right coronary sulcus *use* Heart, Right
Right gastric artery *use* Artery, Gastric
Right gastroepiploic vein *use* Vein, Superior Mesenteric
Right inferior phrenic vein *use* Vena Cava, Inferior
Right inferior pulmonary vein *use* Vein, Pulmonary, Right
Right jugular trunk *use* Lymphatic, Neck, Right
Right lateral ventricle *use* Cerebral Ventricle
Right lymphatic duct *use* Lymphatic, Neck, Right
Right ovarian vein *use* Vena Cava, Inferior
Right second lumbar vein *use* Vena Cava, Inferior
Right subclavian trunk *use* Lymphatic, Neck, Right
Right subcostal vein *use* Vein, Azygos
Right superior pulmonary vein *use* Vein, Pulmonary, Right

Right suprarenal vein *use* Vena Cava, Inferior
Right testicular vein *use* Vena Cava, Inferior
Rima glottidis *use* Larynx
Risorius muscle *use* Muscle, Facial
RNS System lead *use* Neurostimulator Lead in Central Nervous System
RNS system neurostimulator generator *use* Neurostimulator Generator in Head and Facial Bones
Robotic Assisted Procedure
Extremity
Lower **8E0Y**
Upper **8E0X**
Head and Neck Region **8E09**
Trunk Region **8E0W**
Rotation of fetal head
Forceps **10S07ZZ**
Manual **10S0XZZ**
Round ligament of uterus *use* Uterine Supporting Structure
Round window
use Ear, Inner, Right
use Ear, Inner, Left
Roux-en-Y operation
see Bypass, Gastrointestinal System **0D1**
see Bypass, Hepatobiliary System and Pancreas **0F1**
Rupture
Adhesions *see* Release
Fluid collection *see* Drainage

S

Sacral ganglion *use* Nerve, Sacral Sympathetic
Sacral lymph node *use* Lymphatic, Pelvis
Sacral nerve modulation (SNM) lead *use* Stimulator Lead in Urinary System
Sacral neuromodulation lead *use* Stimulator Lead in Urinary System
Sacral splanchnic nerve *use* Nerve, Sacral Sympathetic
Sacrectomy *see* Excision, Lower Bones **0QB**
Sacrococcygeal ligament
use Bursa and Ligament, Trunk, Right
use Bursa and Ligament, Trunk, Left
Sacrococcygeal symphysis *use* Joint, Sacrococcygeal
Sacroiliac ligament
use Bursa and Ligament, Trunk, Left
use Bursa and Ligament, Trunk, Right
Sacrospinous ligament
use Bursa and Ligament, Trunk, Left
use Bursa and Ligament, Trunk, Right
Sacrotuberous ligament
use Bursa and Ligament, Trunk, Left
use Bursa and Ligament, Trunk, Right
Salpingectomy
see Excision, Female Reproductive System **0UB**
see Resection, Female Reproductive System **0UT**
Salpingolysis *see* Release, Female Reproductive System **0UN**
Salpingopexy
see Repair, Female Reproductive System **0UQ**
see Reposition, Female Reproductive System **0US**
Salpingopharyngeus muscle *use* Muscle, Tongue, Palate, Pharynx

Salpingoplasty
see Repair, Female Reproductive System **0UQ**
see Supplement, Female Reproductive System **0UU**
Salpingorrhaphy *see* Repair, Female Reproductive System **0UQ**
Salpingoscopy 0UJ88ZZ
Salpingostomy *see* Drainage, Female Reproductive System **0U9**
Salpingotomy *see* Drainage, Female Reproductive System **0U9**
Salpinx
use Fallopian Tube, Left
use Fallopian Tube, Right
Saphenous nerve *use* Nerve, Femoral
SAPIEN transcatheter aortic valve *use* Zooplastic Tissue in Heart and Great Vessels
Sartorius muscle
use Muscle, Upper Leg, Right
use Muscle, Upper Leg, Left
Scalene muscle
use Muscle, Neck, Right
use Muscle, Neck, Left
Scan
Computerized Tomography (CT) *see* Computerized Tomography (CT Scan)
Radioisotope *see* Planar Nuclear Medicine Imaging
Scaphoid bone
use Carpal, Left
use Carpal, Right
Scapholunate ligament
use Bursa and Ligament, Hand, Right
use Bursa and Ligament, Hand, Left
Scaphotrapezium ligament
use Bursa and Ligament, Hand, Right
use Bursa and Ligament, Hand, Left
Scapulectomy
see Excision, Upper Bones **0PB**
see Resection, Upper Bones **0PT**
Scapulopexy
see Repair, Upper Bones **0PQ**
see Reposition, Upper Bones **0PS**
Scarpa's (vestibular) ganglion *use* Nerve, Acoustic
Sclerectomy *see* Excision, Eye **08B**
Sclerotherapy, mechanical *see* Destruction
Sclerotomy *see* Drainage, Eye **089**
Scrotectomy
see Excision, Male Reproductive System **0VB**
see Resection, Male Reproductive System **0VT**
Scrotoplasty
see Repair, Male Reproductive System **0VQ**
see Supplement, Male Reproductive System **0VU**
Scrotorrhaphy *see* Repair, Male Reproductive System **0VQ**
Scrototomy *see* Drainage, Male Reproductive System **0V9**
Sebaceous gland *use* Skin
Second cranial nerve *use* Nerve, Optic
Section, cesarean *see* Extraction, Pregnancy **10D**
Secura (DR) (VR) *use* Defibrillator Generator in **0JH**
Sella Turcica
use Bone, Sphenoid, Right
use Bone, Sphenoid, Left
Semicircular canal
use Ear, Inner, Right
use Ear, Inner, Left

Semimembranosus muscle
   use Muscle, Upper Leg, Left
   use Muscle, Upper Leg, Right
Semitendinosus muscle
   use Muscle, Upper Leg, Left
   use Muscle, Upper Leg, Right
Septal cartilage *use* Septum, Nasal
Septectomy
   see Excision, Heart and Great Vessels **02B**
   see Resection, Heart and Great Vessels **02T**
   see Excision, Ear, Nose, Sinus **09B**
   see Resection, Ear, Nose, Sinus **09T**
Septoplasty
   see Repair, Ear, Nose, Sinus **09Q**
   see Replacement, Ear, Nose, Sinus **09R**
   see Supplement, Ear, Nose, Sinus **09U**
   see Reposition, Ear, Nose, Sinus **09S**
   see Repair, Heart and Great Vessels **02Q**
   see Replacement, Heart and Great Vessels
   02R
   see Supplement, Heart and Great Vessels **02U**
Septotomy *see* Drainage, Ear, Nose, Sinus **099**
Sequestrectomy, bone *see* Extirpation
Serratus anterior muscle
   use Muscle, Thorax, Left
   use Muscle, Thorax, Right
Serratus posterior muscle
   use Muscle, Trunk, Left
   use Muscle, Trunk, Right
Seventh cranial nerve *use* Nerve, Facial
Sheffield hybrid external fixator
   use External Fixation Device, Hybrid in **0PH**
   use External Fixation Device, Hybrid in **0PS**
   use External Fixation Device, Hybrid in **0QH**
   use External Fixation Device, Hybrid in **0QS**
Sheffield ring external fixator
   use External Fixation Device, Ring in **0PH**
   use External Fixation Device, Ring in **0PS**
   use External Fixation Device, Ring in **0QH**
   use External Fixation Device, Ring in **0QS**
Shirodkar cervical cerclage 0UVC7ZZ
Shock Wave Therapy, Musculoskeletal 6A93
Short gastric artery *use* Artery, Splenic
Shortening
   see Excision
   see Repair
   see Reposition
Shunt creation *see* Bypass
Sialoadenectomy
   Complete *see* Resection, Mouth and Throat
   0CT
   Partial *see* Excision, Mouth and Throat **0CB**
Sialodochoplasty
   see Repair, Mouth and Throat **0CQ**
   see Replacement, Mouth and Throat **0CR**
   see Supplement, Mouth and Throat **0CU**
Sialoectomy
   see Excision, Mouth and Throat **0CB**
   see Resection, Mouth and Throat **0CT**
Sialography *see* Plain Radiography, Ear, Nose,
   Mouth and Throat **B90**
Sialolithotomy *see* Extirpation, Mouth and
   Throat **0CC**
Sigmoid artery *use* Artery, Inferior Mesenteric
Sigmoid flexure *use* Colon, Sigmoid
Sigmoid vein *use* Vein, Inferior Mesenteric
Sigmoidectomy
   see Excision, Gastrointestinal System **0DB**
   see Resection, Gastrointestinal System **0DT**
Sigmoidorrhaphy *see* Repair, Gastrointestinal
   System **0DQ**
Sigmoidoscopy 0DJD8ZZ

Sigmoidotomy *see* Drainage, Gastrointestinal
   System **0D9**
Single lead pacemaker (atrium)(ventricle) *use*
   Pacemaker, Single Chamber in **0JH**
**Single lead rate responsive pacemaker
   (atrium)(ventricle)** *use* Pacemaker, Single
   Chamber Rate Responsive in **0JH**
Sinoatrial node *use* Conduction Mechanism
Sinogram
   Abdominal Wall *see* Fluoroscopy, Abdomen
   and Pelvis **BW11**
   Chest Wall *see* Plain Radiography, Chest
   BW03
   Retroperitoneum *see* Fluoroscopy, Abdomen
   and Pelvis **BW11**
Sinus venosus *use* Atrium, Right
Sinusectomy
   see Excision, Ear, Nose, Sinus **09B**
   see Resection, Ear, Nose, Sinus **09T**
Sinusoscopy 09JY4ZZ
Sinusotomy *see* Drainage, Ear, Nose, Sinus **099**
Sirolimus-eluting coronary stent *use*
   Intraluminal Device, Drug-eluting in Heart
   and Great Vessels
Sixth cranial nerve *use* Nerve, Abducens
Size reduction, breast *see* Excision, Skin and
   Breast **0HB**
SJM Biocor®
Stented Valve System *use* Zooplastic Tissue in
   Heart and Great Vessels
Skene's (paraurethral) gland *use* Gland,
   Vestibular
Sling
   Fascial, orbicularis muscle (mouth) *see*
   Supplement, Muscle, Facial **0KU1**
   Levator muscle, for urethral suspension *see*
   Reposition, Bladder Neck **0TSC**
   Pubococcygeal, for urethral suspension *see*
   Reposition, Bladder Neck **0TSC**
   Rectum *see* Reposition, Rectum **0DSP**
Small bowel series *see* Fluoroscopy, Bowel,
   Small **BD13**
Small saphenous vein
   use Vein, Lesser Saphenous, Left
   use Vein, Lesser Saphenous, Right
Snaring, polyp, colon *see* Excision,
   Gastrointestinal System **0DB**
Solar (celiac) plexus *use* Nerve, Abdominal
   Sympathetic
Soletra® neurostimulator *use* Stimulator
   Generator, Single Array in **0JH**
Soleus muscle
   use Muscle, Lower Leg, Left
   use Muscle, Lower Leg, Right
Spacer
   Insertion of device in
     Disc
       Lumbar Vertebral **0SH2**
       Lumbosacral **0SH4**
     Joint
       Acromioclavicular
         Left **0RHH**
         Right **0RHG**
       Ankle
         Left **0SHG**
         Right **0SHF**
       Carpal
         Left **0RHR**
         Right **0RHQ**
       Cervical Vertebral **0RH1**
       Cervicothoracic Vertebral **0RH4**
       Coccygeal **0SH6**

Spacer - *continued*
       Elbow
         Left **0RHM**
         Right **0RHL**
       Finger Phalangeal
         Left **0RHX**
         Right **0RHW**
       Hip
         Left **0SHB**
         Right **0SH9**
       Knee
         Left **0SHD**
         Right **0SHC**
       Lumbar Vertebral **0SH0**
       Lumbosacral **0SH3**
       Metacarpocarpal
         Left **0RHT**
         Right **0RHS**
       Metacarpophalangeal
         Left **0RHV**
         Right **0RHU**
       Metatarsal-Phalangeal
         Left **0SHN**
         Right **0SHM**
       Metatarsal-Tarsal
         Left **0SHL**
         Right **0SHK**
       Occipital-cervical **0RH0**
       Sacrococcygeal **0SH5**
       Sacroiliac
         Left **0SH8**
         Right **0SH7**
       Shoulder
         Left **0RHK**
         Right **0RHJ**
       Sternoclavicular
         Left **0RHF**
         Right **0RHE**
       Tarsal
         Left **0SHJ**
         Right **0SHH**
       Temporomandibular
         Left **0RHD**
         Right **0RHC**
       Thoracic Vertebral **0RH6**
       Thoracolumbar Vertebral **0RHA**
       Toe Phalangeal
         Left **0SHQ**
         Right **0SHP**
       Wrist
         Left **0RHP**
         Right **0RHN**
   Removal of device from
     Acromioclavicular
       Left **0RPH**
       Right **0RPG**
     Ankle
       Left **0SPG**
       Right **0SPF**
     Carpal
       Left **0RPR**
       Right **0RPQ**
     Cervical Vertebral **0RP1**
     Cervicothoracic Vertebral **0RP4**
     Coccygeal **0SP6**
     Elbow
       Left **0RPM**
       Right **0RPL**
     Finger Phalangeal
       Left **0RPX**
       Right **0RPW**

Spacer - *continued*
Hip
Left **0SPB**
Right **0SP9**
Knee
Left **0SPD**
Right **0SPC**
Lumbar Vertebral **0SP0**
Lumbosacral **0SP3**
Metacarpocarpal
Left **0RPT**
Right **0RPS**
Metacarpophalangeal
Left **0RPV**
Right **0RPU**
Metatarsal-Phalangeal
Left **0SPN**
Right **0SPM**
Metatarsal-Tarsal
Left **0SPL**
Right **0SPK**
Occipital-cervical **0RP0**
Sacrococcygeal **0SP5**
Sacroiliac
Left **0SP8**
Right **0SP7**
Shoulder
Left **0RPK**
Right **0RPJ**
Sternoclavicular
Left **0RPF**
Right **0RPE**
Tarsal
Left **0SPJ**
Right **0SPH**
Temporomandibular
Left **0RPD**
Right **0RPC**
Thoracic Vertebral **0RP6**
Thoracolumbar Vertebral **0RPA**
Toe Phalangeal
Left **0SPQ**
Right **0SPP**
Wrist
Left **0RPP**
Right **0RPN**
Revision of device in
Acromioclavicular
Left **0RWH**
Right **0RWG**
Ankle
Left **0SWG**
Right **0SWF**
Carpal
Left **0RWR**
Right **0RWQ**
Cervical Vertebral **0RW1**
Cervicothoracic Vertebral **0RW4**
Coccygeal **0SW6**
Elbow
Left **0RWM**
Right **0RWL**
Finger Phalangeal
Left **0RWX**
Right **0RWW**
Hip
Left **0SWB**
Right **0SW9**
Knee
Left **0SWD**
Right **0SWC**

Spacer - *continued*
Lumbar Vertebral **0SW0**
Lumbosacral **0SW3**
Metacarpocarpal
Left **0RWT**
Right **0RWS**
Metacarpophalangeal
Left **0RWV**
Right **0RWU**
Metatarsal-Phalangeal
Left **0SWN**
Right **0SWM**
Metatarsal-Tarsal
Left **0SWL**
Right **0SWK**
Occipital-cervical **0RW0**
Sacrococcygeal **0SW5**
Sacroiliac
Left **0SW8**
Right **0SW7**
Shoulder
Left **0RWK**
Right **0RWJ**
Sternoclavicular
Left **0RWF**
Right **0RWE**
Tarsal
Left **0SWJ**
Right **0SWH**
Temporomandibular
Left **0RWD**
Right **0RWC**
Thoracic Vertebral **0RW6**
Thoracolumbar Vertebral **0RWA**
Toe Phalangeal
Left **0SWQ**
Right **0SWP**
Wrist
Left **0RWP**
Right **0RWN** **Spectroscopy**
Intravascular **8E023DZ**
Near infrared **8E023DZ**
Speech Assessment F00
Speech therapy *see* Speech Treatment, Rehabilitation **F06**
Speech Treatment F06
Sphenoidectomy
see Excision, Ear, Nose, Sinus **09B**
see Resection, Ear, Nose, Sinus **09T**
see Excision, Head and Facial Bones **0NB**
see Resection, Head and Facial Bones **0NT**
Sphenoidotomy *see* Drainage, Ear, Nose, Sinus **099**
Sphenomandibular ligament *use* Bursa and Ligament, Head and Neck
Sphenopalatine (pterygopalatine) ganglion *use* Nerve, Head and Neck Sympathetic
Sphincterorrhaphy, anal *see* Repair, Anal Sphincter **0DQR**
Sphincterotomy, anal
see Drainage, Anal Sphincter **0D9R**
see Division, Anal Sphincter **0D8R**
Spinal cord neurostimulator lead *use* Neurostimulator Lead in Central Nervous System
Spinal dura mater *use* Dura Mater
Spinal epidural space *use* Epidural Space
Spinal nerve
cervical *use* Nerve, Cervical
lumbar *use* Nerve, Lumbar
sacral *use* Nerve, Sacral
thoracic *use* Nerve, Thoracic

Spinal Stabilization Device
Facet Replacement
Cervical Vertebral **0RH1**
Cervicothoracic Vertebral **0RH4**
Lumbar Vertebral **0SH0**
Lumbosacral **0SH3**
Occipital-cervical **0RH0**
Thoracic Vertebral **0RH6**
Thoracolumbar Vertebral **0RHA**
Interspinous Process
Cervical Vertebral **0RH1**
Cervicothoracic Vertebral **0RH4**
Lumbar Vertebral **0SH0**
Lumbosacral **0SH3**
Occipital-cervical **0RH0**
Thoracic Vertebral **0RH6**
Thoracolumbar Vertebral **0RHA**
Pedicle-Based
Cervical Vertebral **0RH1**
Cervicothoracic Vertebral **0RH4**
Lumbar Vertebral **0SH0**
Lumbosacral **0SH3**
Occipital-cervical **0RH0**
Thoracic Vertebral **0RH6**
Thoracolumbar Vertebral **0RHA**
Spinal subarachnoid space *use* Subarachnoid Space
Spinal subdural space *use* Subdural Space
Spinous process
use Vertebra, Thoracic
use Vertebra, Lumbar
use Vertebra, Cervical
Spiral ganglion *use* Nerve, Acoustic
Spiration IBV™ Valve System *use* Intraluminal Device, Endobronchial Valve in Respiratory System
Splenectomy
see Excision, Lymphatic and Hemic Systems **07B**
see Resection, Lymphatic and Hemic Systems **07T**
Splenic flexure *use* Colon, Transverse
Splenic plexus *use* Nerve, Abdominal Sympathetic
Splenius capitis muscle *use* Muscle, Head
Splenius cervicis muscle
use Muscle, Neck, Left
use Muscle, Neck, Right
Splenolysis *see* Release, Lymphatic and Hemic Systems **07N**
Splenopexy
see Repair, Lymphatic and Hemic Systems **07Q**
see Reposition, Lymphatic and Hemic Systems **07S**
Splenoplasty *see* Repair, Lymphatic and Hemic Systems **07Q**
Splenorrhaphy *see* Repair, Lymphatic and Hemic Systems **07Q**
Splenotomy *see* Drainage, Lymphatic and Hemic Systems **079**
Splinting, musculoskeletal *see* Immobilization, Anatomical Regions **2W3**
Stapedectomy
see Excision, Ear, Nose, Sinus **09B**
see Resection, Ear, Nose, Sinus **09T**
Stapediolysis *see* Release, Ear, Nose, Sinus **09N**
Stapedioplasty
see Repair, Ear, Nose, Sinus **09Q**
see Replacement, Ear, Nose, Sinus **09R**
see Supplement, Ear, Nose, Sinus **09U**
Stapedotomy *see* Drainage, Ear, Nose, Sinus **099**

Stapes
  use Auditory Ossicle, Right
  use Auditory Ossicle, Left
Stellate ganglion *use* Nerve, Head and Neck
  Sympathetic
Stensen's duct
  use Duct, Parotid, Right
  use Duct, Parotid, Left
Stent (angioplasty)(embolization) *use*
  Intraluminal Device
Stented tissue valve *use* Zooplastic Tissue in
  Heart and Great Vessels
Stereotactic Radiosurgery
  Gamma Beam
    Abdomen **DW23JZZ**
    Adrenal Gland **DG22JZZ**
    Bile Ducts **DF22JZZ**
    Bladder **DT22JZZ**
    Bone Marrow **D720JZZ**
    Brain **D020JZZ**
    Brain Stem **D021JZZ**
    Breast
      Left **DM20JZZ**
      Right **DM21JZZ**
    Bronchus **DB21JZZ**
    Cervix **DU21JZZ**
    Chest **DW22JZZ**
    Chest Wall **DB27JZZ**
    Colon **DD25JZZ**
    Diaphragm **DB28JZZ**
    Duodenum **DD22JZZ**
    Ear **D920JZZ**
    Esophagus **DD20JZZ**
    Eye **D820JZZ**
    Gallbladder **DF21JZZ**
    Gland
      Adrenal **DG22JZZ**
      Parathyroid **DG24JZZ**
      Pituitary **DG20JZZ**
      Thyroid **DG25JZZ**
    Glands, Salivary **D926JZZ**
    Head and Neck **DW21JZZ**
    Ileum **DD24JZZ**
    Jejunum **DD23JZZ**
    Kidney **DT20JZZ**
    Larynx **D92BJZZ**
    Liver **DF20JZZ**
    Lung **DB22JZZ**
    Lymphatics
      Abdomen **D726JZZ**
      Axillary **D724JZZ**
      Inguinal **D728JZZ**
      Neck **D723JZZ**
      Pelvis **D727JZZ**
      Thorax **D725JZZ**
    Mediastinum **DB26JZZ**
    Mouth **D924JZZ**
    Nasopharynx **D92DJZZ**
    Neck and Head **DW21JZZ**
    Nerve, Peripheral **D027JZZ**
    Nose **D921JZZ**
    Ovary **DU20JZZ**
    Palate
      Hard **D928JZZ**
      Soft **D929JZZ**
    Pancreas **DF23JZZ**
    Parathyroid Gland **DG24JZZ**
    Pelvic Region **DW26JZZ**
    Pharynx **D92CJZZ**
    Pineal Body **DG21JZZ**
    Pituitary Gland **DG20JZZ**
    Pleura **DB25JZZ**

Stereotactic Radiosurgery - *continued*
    Prostate **DV20JZZ**
    Rectum **DD27JZZ**
    Sinuses **D927JZZ**
    Spinal Cord **D026JZZ**
    Spleen **D722JZZ**
    Stomach **DD21JZZ**
    Testis **DV21JZZ**
    Thymus **D721JZZ**
    Thyroid Gland **DG25JZZ**
    Tongue **D925JZZ**
    Trachea **DB20JZZ**
    Ureter **DT21JZZ**
    Urethra **DT23JZZ**
    Uterus **DU22JZZ**
  Other Photon
    Abdomen **DW23DZZ**
    Adrenal Gland **DG22DZZ**
    Bile Ducts **DF22DZZ**
    Bladder **DT22DZZ**
    Bone Marrow **D720DZZ**
    Brain **D020DZZ**
    Brain Stem **D021DZZ**
    Breast
      Left **DM20DZZ**
      Right **DM21DZZ**
    Bronchus **DB21DZZ**
    Cervix **DU21DZZ**
    Chest **DW22DZZ**
    Chest Wall **DB27DZZ**
    Colon **DD25DZZ**
    Diaphragm **DB28DZZ**
    Duodenum **DD22DZZ**
    Ear **D920DZZ**
    Esophagus **DD20DZZ**
    Eye **D820DZZ**
    Gallbladder **DF21DZZ**
    Gland
      Adrenal **DG22DZZ**
      Parathyroid **DG24DZZ**
      Pituitary **DG20DZZ**
      Thyroid **DG25DZZ**
    Glands, Salivary **D926DZZ**
    Head and Neck **DW21DZZ**
    Ileum **DD24DZZ**
    Jejunum **DD23DZZ**
    Kidney **DT20DZZ**
    Larynx **D92BDZZ**
    Liver **DF20DZZ**
    Lung **DB22DZZ**
    Lymphatics
      Abdomen **D726DZZ**
      Axillary **D724DZZ**
      Inguinal **D728DZZ**
      Neck **D723DZZ**
      Pelvis **D727DZZ**
      Thorax **D725DZZ**
    Mediastinum **DB26DZZ**
    Mouth **D924DZZ**
    Nasopharynx **D92DDZZ**
    Neck and Head **DW21DZZ**
    Nerve, Peripheral **D027DZZ**
    Nose **D921DZZ**
    Ovary **DU20DZZ**
    Palate
      Hard **D928DZZ**
      Soft **D929DZZ**
    Pancreas **DF23DZZ**
    Parathyroid Gland **DG24DZZ**
    Pelvic Region **DW26DZZ**
    Pharynx **D92CDZZ**
    Pineal Body **DG21DZZ**

Stereotactic Radiosurgery - *continued*
    Pituitary Gland **DG20DZZ**
    Pleura **DB25DZZ**
    Prostate **DV20DZZ**
    Rectum **DD27DZZ**
    Sinuses **D927DZZ**
    Spinal Cord **D026DZZ**
    Spleen **D722DZZ**
    Stomach **DD21DZZ**
    Testis **DV21DZZ**
    Thymus **D721DZZ**
    Thyroid Gland **DG25DZZ**
    Tongue **D925DZZ**
    Trachea **DB20DZZ**
    Ureter **DT21DZZ**
    Urethra **DT23DZZ**
    Uterus **DU22DZZ**
  Particulate
    Abdomen **DW23HZZ**
    Adrenal Gland **DG22HZZ**
    Bile Ducts **DF22HZZ**
    Bladder **DT22HZZ**
    Bone Marrow **D720HZZ**
    Brain **D020HZZ**
    Brain Stem **D021HZZ**
    Breast
      Left **DM20HZZ**
      Right **DM21HZZ**
    Bronchus **DB21HZZ**
    Cervix **DU21HZZ**
    Chest **DW22HZZ**
    Chest Wall **DB27HZZ**
    Colon **DD25HZZ**
    Diaphragm **DB28HZZ**
    Duodenum **DD22HZZ**
    Ear **D920HZZ**
    Esophagus **DD20HZZ**
    Eye **D820HZZ**
    Gallbladder **DF21HZZ**
    Gland
      Adrenal **DG22HZZ**
      Parathyroid **DG24HZZ**
      Pituitary **DG20HZZ**
      Thyroid **DG25HZZ**
    Glands, Salivary **D926HZZ**
    Head and Neck **DW21HZZ**
    Ileum **DD24HZZ**
    Jejunum **DD23HZZ**
    Kidney **DT20HZZ**
    Larynx **D92BHZZ**
    Liver **DF20HZZ**
    Lung **DB22HZZ**
    Lymphatics
      Abdomen **D726HZZ**
      Axillary **D724HZZ**
      Inguinal **D728HZZ**
      Neck **D723HZZ**
      Pelvis **D727HZZ**
      Thorax **D725HZZ**
    Mediastinum **DB26HZZ**
    Mouth **D924HZZ**
    Nasopharynx **D92DHZZ**
    Neck and Head **DW21HZZ**
    Nerve, Peripheral **D027HZZ**
    Nose **D921HZZ**
    Ovary **DU20HZZ**
    Palate
      Hard **D928HZZ**
      Soft **D929HZZ**
    Pancreas **DF23HZZ**
    Parathyroid Gland **DG24HZZ**
    Pelvic Region **DW26HZZ**

Stereotactic Radiosurgery - *continued*
Pharynx **D92CHZZ**
Pineal Body **DG21HZZ**
Pituitary Gland **DG20HZZ**
Pleura **DB25HZZ**
Prostate **DV20HZZ**
Rectum **DD27HZZ**
Sinuses **D927HZZ**
Spinal Cord **D026HZZ**
Spleen **D722HZZ**
Stomach **DD21HZZ**
Testis **DV21HZZ**
Thymus **D721HZZ**
Thyroid Gland **DG25HZZ**
Tongue **D925HZZ**
Trachea **DB20HZZ**
Ureter **DT21HZZ**
Urethra **DT23HZZ**
Uterus **DU22HZZ**
Sternoclavicular ligament
use Bursa and Ligament, Shoulder, Left
use Bursa and Ligament, Shoulder, Right
Sternocleidomastoid artery
use Artery, Thyroid, Left
use Artery, Thyroid, Right
Sternocleidomastoid muscle
use Muscle, Neck, Left
use Muscle, Neck, Right
Sternocostal ligament
use Bursa and Ligament, Thorax, Right
use Bursa and Ligament, Thorax, Left
Sternotomy
see Division, Sternum **0P80**
see Drainage, Sternum **0P90**
Stimulation, cardiac
Cardioversion **5A2204Z**
Electrophysiologic testing *see* Measurement,
Cardiac **4A02**
Stimulator Generator
Insertion of device in
Abdomen **0JH8**
Back **0JH7**
Chest **0JH6**
Multiple Array
Abdomen **0JH8**
Back **0JH7**
Chest **0JH6**
Multiple Array Rechargeable
Abdomen **0JH8**
Back **0JH7**
Chest **0JH6**
Removal of device from, Subcutaneous Tissue
and Fascia, Trunk **0JPT**
Revision of device in, Subcutaneous Tissue
and Fascia, Trunk **0JWT**
Single Array
Abdomen **0JH8**
Back **0JH7**
Chest **0JH6**
Single Array Rechargeable
Abdomen **0JH8**
Back **0JH7**
Chest **0JH6**
Stimulator Lead
Insertion of device in
Anal Sphincter **0DHR**
Artery
Left **03HL**
Right **03HK**
Bladder **0THB**

Stimulator Lead - *continued*
Muscle
Lower **0KHY**
Upper **0KHX**
Stomach **0DH6**
Ureter **0TH9**
Removal of device from
Anal Sphincter **0DPR**
Artery, Upper **03PY**
Bladder **0TPB**
Muscle
Lower **0KPY**
Upper **0KPX**
Stomach **0DP6**
Ureter **0TP9**
Revision of device in
Anal Sphincter **0DWR**
Artery, Upper **03WY**
Bladder **0TWB**
Muscle
Lower **0KWY**
Upper **0KWX**
Stomach **0DW6**
Ureter **0TW9**
Stoma
Excision
Abdominal Wall **0WBFXZ2**
Neck **0WB6XZ2**
Repair
Abdominal Wall **0WQFXZ2**
Neck **0WQ6XZ2**
Stomatoplasty
see Repair, Mouth and Throat **0CQ**
see Replacement, Mouth and Throat **0CR**
see Supplement, Mouth and Throat **0CU**
Stomatorrhaphy *see* Repair, Mouth and Throat
0CQ
Stratos LV *use* Cardiac Resynchronization
Pacemaker Pulse Generator in **0JH**
Stress test
4A02XM4
4A12XM4
Stripping *see* Extraction
Study
Electrophysiologic stimulation, cardiac *see*
Measurement, Cardiac **4A02**
Ocular motility **4A07X7Z**
Pulmonary airway flow measurement *see*
Measurement, Respiratory **4A09**
Visual acuity **4A07X0Z**
Styloglossus muscle *use* Muscle, Tongue,
Palate, Pharynx
Stylomandibular ligament *use* Bursa and
Ligament, Head and Neck
Stylopharyngeus muscle *use* Muscle, Tongue,
Palate, Pharynx
Subacromial bursa
use Bursa and Ligament, Shoulder, Left
use Bursa and Ligament, Shoulder, Right
Subaortic (common iliac) lymph node *use*
Lymphatic, Pelvis
Subclavicular (apical) lymph node
use Lymphatic, Axillary, Left
use Lymphatic, Axillary, Right
Subclavius muscle
use Muscle, Thorax, Left
use Muscle, Thorax, Right
Subclavius nerve *use* Nerve, Brachial Plexus
Subcostal artery *use* Aorta, Thoracic
Subcostal muscle
use Muscle, Thorax, Left
use Muscle, Thorax, Right
Subcostal nerve *use* Nerve, Thoracic

Subcutaneous injection reservoir, port *use*
Vascular Access Device, Reservoir in
Subcutaneous Tissue and Fascia \
Subcutaneous injection reservoir, pump *use*
Infusion Device, Pump in Subcutaneous
Tissue and Fascia
Subdermal progesterone implant *use*
Contraceptive Device in Subcutaneous Tissue
and Fascia
Submandibular ganglion
use Nerve, Head and Neck Sympathetic
use Nerve, Facial
Submandibular gland
use Gland, Submaxillary, Left
use Gland, Submaxillary, Right
Submandibular lymph node *use* Lymphatic,
Head
Submaxillary ganglion *use* Nerve, Head and
Neck Sympathetic
Submaxillary lymph node *use* Lymphatic,
Head
Submental artery *use* Artery, Face
Submental lymph node *use* Lymphatic, Head
Submucous (Meissner's) plexus *use* Nerve,
Abdominal Sympathetic
Suboccipital nerve *use* Nerve, Cervical
Suboccipital venous plexus
use Vein, Vertebral, Left
use Vein, Vertebral, Right
Subparotid lymph node *use* Lymphatic, Head
Subscapular (posterior) lymph node
use Lymphatic, Axillary, Left
use Lymphatic, Axillary, Right
Subscapular aponeurosis
use Subcutaneous Tissue and Fascia, Upper
Arm, Right
use Subcutaneous Tissue and Fascia, Upper
Arm, Left
Subscapular artery
use Artery, Axillary, Left
use Artery, Axillary, Right
Subscapularis muscle
use Muscle, Shoulder, Left
use Muscle, Shoulder, Right
Substance Abuse Treatment
Counseling
Family, for substance abuse, Other Family
Counseling **HZ63ZZZ**
Group
12-Step **HZ43ZZZ**
Behavioral **HZ41ZZZ**
Cognitive **HZ40ZZZ**
Cognitive-Behavioral **HZ42ZZZ**
Confrontational **HZ48ZZZ**
Continuing Care **HZ49ZZZ**
Infectious Disease
Post-Test **HZ4CZZZ**
Pre-Test **HZ4CZZZ**
Interpersonal **HZ44ZZZ**
Motivational Enhancement **HZ47ZZZ**
Psychoeducation **HZ46ZZZ**
Spiritual **HZ4BZZZ**
Vocational **HZ45ZZZ**
Individual
12-Step **HZ33ZZZ**
Behavioral **HZ31ZZZ**
Cognitive **HZ30ZZZ**
Cognitive-Behavioral **HZ32ZZZ**
Confrontational **HZ38ZZZ**
Continuing Care **HZ39ZZZ**
Infectious Disease
Post-Test **HZ3CZZZ**
Pre-Test **HZ3CZZZ**

Substance Abuse Treatment - *continued*
    Interpersonal **HZ34ZZZ**
    Motivational Enhancement **HZ37ZZZ**
    Psychoeducation **HZ36ZZZ**
    Spiritual **HZ3BZZZ**
    Vocational **HZ35ZZZ**
  Detoxification Services, for substance abuse **HZ2ZZZZ**
  Medication Management
    Antabuse **HZ83ZZZ**
    Bupropion **HZ87ZZZ**
    Clonidine **HZ86ZZZ**
    Levo-alpha-acetyl-methadol (LAAM) **HZ82ZZZ**
    Methadone Maintenance **HZ81ZZZ**
    Naloxone **HZ85ZZZ**
    Naltrexone **HZ84ZZZ**
    Nicotine Replacement **HZ80ZZZ**
    Other Replacement Medication **HZ89ZZZ**
    Psychiatric Medication **HZ88ZZZ**
  Pharmacotherapy
    Antabuse **HZ93ZZZ**
    Bupropion **HZ97ZZZ**
    Clonidine **HZ96ZZZ**
    Levo-alpha-acetyl-methadol (LAAM) **HZ92ZZZ**
    Methadone Maintenance **HZ91ZZZ**
    Naloxone **HZ95ZZZ**
    Naltrexone **HZ94ZZZ**
    Nicotine Replacement **HZ90ZZZ**
    Psychiatric Medication **HZ98ZZZ**
    Replacement Medication, Other **HZ99ZZZ**
  Psychotherapy
    12-Step **HZ53ZZZ**
    Behavioral **HZ51ZZZ**
    Cognitive **HZ50ZZZ**
    Cognitive-Behavioral **HZ52ZZZ**
    Confrontational **HZ58ZZZ**
    Interactive **HZ55ZZZ**
    Interpersonal **HZ54ZZZ**
    Motivational Enhancement **HZ57ZZZ**
    Psychoanalysis **HZ5BZZZ**
    Psychodynamic **HZ5CZZZ**
    Psychoeducation **HZ56ZZZ**
    Psychophysiological **HZ5DZZZ**
    Supportive **HZ59ZZZ**
Substantia nigra *use* Basal Ganglia
Subtalar (talocalcaneal) joint
  use Joint, Tarsal, Right
  use Joint, Tarsal, Left
Subtalar ligament
  use Bursa and Ligament, Foot, Left
  use Bursa and Ligament, Foot, Right
Subthalamic nucleus *use* Basal Ganglia
Suction *see* Drainage
Suction curettage (D&C), nonobstetric *see* Extraction, Endometrium **0UDB**
Suction curettage, obstetric post-delivery *see* Extraction, Products of Conception, Retained **10D1**
Superficial circumflex iliac vein
  use Vein, Greater Saphenous, Right
  use Vein, Greater Saphenous, Left
Superficial epigastric artery
  use Artery, Femoral, Left
  use Artery, Femoral, Right
Superficial epigastric vein
  use Vein, Greater Saphenous, Right
  use Vein, Greater Saphenous, Left
Superficial Inferior Epigastric Artery Flap
  Bilateral **0HRV078**
  Left **0HRU078**
  Right **0HRT078**

Superficial palmar arch
  use Artery, Hand, Left
  use Artery, Hand, Right
Superficial palmar venous arch
  use Vein, Hand, Left
  use Vein, Hand, Right
Superficial temporal artery
  use Artery, Temporal, Right
  use Artery, Temporal, Left
Superficial transverse perineal muscle *use* Muscle, Perineum
Superior cardiac nerve *use* Nerve, Thoracic Sympathetic
Superior cerebellar vein *use* Vein, Intracranial
Superior cerebral vein *use* Vein, Intracranial
Superior clunic (cluneal) nerve *use* Nerve, Lumbar
Superior epigastric artery
  use Artery, Internal Mammary, Right
  use Artery, Internal Mammary, Left
Superior genicular artery
  use Artery, Popliteal, Left
  use Artery, Popliteal, Right
Superior gluteal artery
  use Artery, Internal Iliac, Left
  use Artery, Internal Iliac, Right
Superior gluteal nerve *use* Nerve, Lumbar Plexus
Superior hypogastric plexus *use* Nerve, Abdominal Sympathetic
Superior labial artery *use* Artery, Face
Superior laryngeal artery
  use Artery, Thyroid, Left
  use Artery, Thyroid, Right
Superior laryngeal nerve *use* Nerve, Vagus
Superior longitudinal muscle *use* Muscle, Tongue, Palate, Pharynx
Superior mesenteric ganglion *use* Nerve, Abdominal Sympathetic
Superior mesenteric lymph node *use* Lymphatic, Mesenteric
Superior mesenteric plexus *use* Nerve, Abdominal Sympathetic
Superior oblique muscle
  use Muscle, Extraocular, Left
  use Muscle, Extraocular, Right
Superior olivary nucleus *use* Pons
Superior rectal artery *use* Artery, Inferior Mesenteric
Superior rectal vein *use* Vein, Inferior Mesenteric
Superior rectus muscle
  use Muscle, Extraocular, Left
  use Muscle, Extraocular, Right
Superior tarsal plate
  use Eyelid, Upper, Right
  use Eyelid, Upper, Left
Superior thoracic artery
  use Artery, Axillary, Left
  use Artery, Axillary, Right
Superior thyroid artery
  use Artery, Thyroid, Right
  use Artery, External Carotid, Right
  use Artery, Thyroid, Left
  use Artery, External Carotid, Left
Superior turbinate *use* Turbinate, Nasal
Superior ulnar collateral artery
  use Artery, Brachial, Right
  use Artery, Brachial, Left

Supplement
  Abdominal Wall **0WUF**
  Acetabulum
    Left **0QU5**
    Right **0QU4**
  Ampulla of Vater **0FUC**
  Anal Sphincter **0DUR**
  Ankle Region
    Left **0YUL**
    Right **0YUK**
  Anus **0DUQ**
  Aorta
    Abdominal **04U0**
    Thoracic **02UW**
  Arm
    Lower
      Left **0XUF**
      Right **0XUD**
    Upper
      Left **0XU9**
      Right **0XU8**
  Artery
    Anterior Tibial
      Left **04UQ**
      Right **04UP**
    Axillary
      Left **03U6**
      Right **03U5**
    Brachial
      Left **03U8**
      Right **03U7**
    Celiac **04U1**
    Colic
      Left **04U7**
      Middle **04U8**
      Right **04U6**
    Common Carotid
      Left **03UJ**
      Right **03UH**
    Common Iliac
      Left **04UD**
      Right **04UC**
    External Carotid
      Left **03UN**
      Right **03UM**
    External Iliac
      Left **04UJ**
      Right **04UH**
    Face **03UR**
    Femoral
      Left **04UL**
      Right **04UK**
    Foot
      Left **04UW**
      Right **04UV**
    Gastric **04U2**
    Hand
      Left **03UF**
      Right **03UD**
    Hepatic **04U3**
    Inferior Mesenteric **04UB**
    Innominate **03U2**
    Internal Carotid
      Left **03UL**
      Right **03UK**
    Internal Iliac
      Left **04UF**
      Right **04UE**
    Internal Mammary
      Left **03U1**
      Right **03U0**
    Intracranial **03UG**

Lower **04UY**
Peroneal
    Left **04UU**
    Right **04UT**
Popliteal
    Left **04UN**
    Right **04UM**
Posterior Tibial
    Left **04US**
    Right **04UR**
Pulmonary
    Left **02UR**
    Right **02UQ**
Pulmonary Trunk **02UP**
Radial
    Left **03UC**
    Right **03UB**
Renal
    Left **04UA**
    Right **04U9**
Splenic **04U4**
Subclavian
    Left **03U4**
    Right **03U3**
Superior Mesenteric **04U5**
Temporal
    Left **03UT**
    Right **03US**
Thyroid
    Left **03UV**
    Right **03UU**
Ulnar
    Left **03UA**
    Right **03U9**
Upper **03UY**
Vertebral
    Left **03UQ**
    Right **03UP**
Atrium
    Left **02U7**
    Right **02U6**
Auditory Ossicle
    Left **09UA0**
    Right **09U90**
Axilla
    Left **0XU5**
    Right **0XU4**
Back
    Lower **0WUL**
    Upper **0WUK**
Bladder **0TUB**
Bladder Neck **0TUC**
Bone
    Ethmoid
        Left **0NUG**
        Right **0NUF**
    Frontal
        Left **0NU2**
        Right **0NU1**
    Hyoid **0NUX**
    Lacrimal
        Left **0NUJ**
        Right **0NUH**
    Nasal **0NUB**
    Occipital
        Left **0NU8**
        Right **0NU7**
    Palatine
        Left **0NUL**
        Right **0NUK**

Parietal
    Left **0NU4**
    Right **0NU3**
Pelvic
    Left **0QU3**
    Right **0QU2**
Sphenoid
    Left **0NUD**
    Right **0NUC**
Temporal
    Left **0NU6**
    Right **0NU5**
Zygomatic
    Left **0NUN**
    Right **0NUM**
Breast
    Bilateral **0HUV**
    Left **0HUU**
    Right **0HUT**
Bronchus
    Lingula **0BU9**
    Lower Lobe
        Left **0BUB**
        Right **0BU6**
    Main
        Left **0BU7**
        Right **0BU3**
    Middle Lobe, Right **0BU5**
    Upper Lobe
        Left **0BU8**
        Right **0BU4**
Buccal Mucosa **0CU4**
Bursa and Ligament
    Abdomen
        Left **0MUJ**
        Right **0MUH**
    Ankle
        Left **0MUR**
        Right **0MUQ**
    Elbow
        Left **0MU4**
        Right **0MU3**
    Foot
        Left **0MUT**
        Right **0MUS**
    Hand
        Left **0MU8**
        Right **0MU7**
    Head and Neck **0MU0**
    Hip
        Left **0MUM**
        Right **0MUL**
    Knee
        Left **0MUP**
        Right **0MUN**
    Lower Extremity
        Left **0MUW**
        Right **0MUV**
    Perineum **0MUK**
    Shoulder
        Left **0MU2**
        Right **0MU1**
    Thorax
        Left **0MUG**
        Right **0MUF**
    Trunk
        Left **0MUD**
        Right **0MUC**
    Upper Extremity
        Left **0MUB**
        Right **0MU9**

Wrist
    Left **0MU6**
    Right **0MU5**
Buttock
    Left **0YU1**
    Right **0YU0**
Carina **0BU2**
Carpal
    Left **0PUN**
    Right **0PUM**
Cecum **0DUH**
Cerebral Meninges **00U1**
Chest Wall **0WU8**
Chordae Tendineae **02U9**
Cisterna Chyli **07UL**
Clavicle
    Left **0PUB**
    Right **0PU9**
Clitoris **0UUJ**
Coccyx **0QUS**
Colon
    Ascending **0DUK**
    Descending **0DUM**
    Sigmoid **0DUN**
    Transverse **0DUL**
Cord
    Bilateral **0VUH**
    Left **0VUG**
    Right **0VUF**
Cornea
    Left **08U9**
    Right **08U8**
Cul-de-sac **0UUF**
Diaphragm
    Left **0BUS**
    Right **0BUR**
Disc
    Cervical Vertebral **0RU3**
    Cervicothoracic Vertebral **0RU5**
    Lumbar Vertebral **0SU2**
    Lumbosacral **0SU4**
    Thoracic Vertebral **0RU9**
    Thoracolumbar Vertebral **0RUB**
Duct
    Common Bile **0FU9**
    Cystic **0FU8**
    Hepatic
        Left **0FU6**
        Right **0FU5**
    Lacrimal
        Left **08UY**
        Right **08UX**
    Pancreatic **0FUD**
        Accessory **0FUF**
Duodenum **0DU9**
Dura Mater **00U2**
Ear
    External
        Bilateral **09U2**
        Left **09U1**
        Right **09U0**
    Inner
        Left **09UE0**
        Right **09UD0**
    Middle
        Left **09U60**
        Right **09U50**
Elbow Region
    Left **0XUC**
    Right **0XUB**

Epididymis
   Bilateral **0VUL**
   Left **0VUK**
   Right **0VUJ**
Epiglottis **0CUR**
Esophagogastric Junction **0DU4**
Esophagus **0DU5**
   Lower **0DU3**
   Middle **0DU2**
   Upper **0DU1**
Extremity
   Lower
      Left **0YUB**
      Right **0YU9**
   Upper
      Left **0XU7**
      Right **0XU6**
Eye
   Left **08U1**
   Right **08U0**
Eyelid
   Lower
      Left **08UR**
      Right **08UQ**
   Upper
      Left **08UP**
      Right **08UN**
Face **0WU2**
Fallopian Tube
   Left **0UU6**
   Right **0UU5**
Fallopian Tubes, Bilateral **0UU7**
Femoral Region
   Bilateral **0YUE**
   Left **0YU8**
   Right **0YU7**
Femoral Shaft
   Left **0QU9**
   Right **0QU8**
Femur
   Lower
      Left **0QUC**
      Right **0QUB**
   Upper
      Left **0QU7**
      Right **0QU6**
Fibula
   Left **0QUK**
   Right **0QUJ**
Finger
   Index
      Left **0XUP**
      Right **0XUN**
   Little
      Left **0XUW**
      Right **0XUV**
   Middle
      Left **0XUR**
      Right **0XUQ**
   Ring
      Left **0XUT**
      Right **0XUS**
Foot
   Left **0YUN**
   Right **0YUM**
Gingiva
   Lower **0CU6**
   Upper **0CU5**
Glenoid Cavity
   Left **0PU8**
   Right **0PU7**

Hand
   Left **0XUK**
   Right **0XUJ**
Head **0WU0**
Heart **02UA**
Humeral Head
   Left **0PUD**
   Right **0PUC**
Humeral Shaft
   Left **0PUG**
   Right **0PUF**
Hymen **0UUK**
Ileocecal Valve **0DUC**
Ileum **0DUB**
Inguinal Region
   Bilateral **0YUA**
   Left **0YU6**
   Right **0YU5**
Intestine
   Large **0DUE**
      Left **0DUG**
      Right **0DUF**
   Small **0DU8**
Iris
   Left **08UD**
   Right **08UC**
Jaw
   Lower **0WU5**
   Upper **0WU4**
Jejunum **0DUA**
Joint
   Acromioclavicular
      Left **0RUH**
      Right **0RUG**
   Ankle
      Left **0SUG**
      Right **0SUF**
   Carpal
      Left **0RUR**
      Right **0RUQ**
   Cervical Vertebral **0RU1**
   Cervicothoracic Vertebral **0RU4**
   Coccygeal **0SU6**
   Elbow
      Left **0RUM**
      Right **0RUL**
   Finger Phalangeal
      Left **0RUX**
      Right **0RUW**
   Hip
      Left **0SUB**
         Acetabular Surface **0SUE**
         Femoral Surface **0SUS**
      Right **0SU9**
         Acetabular Surface **0SUA**
         Femoral Surface **0SUR**
   Knee
      Left **0SUD**
         Femoral Surface **0SUU09Z**
         Tibial Surface **0SUW09Z**
      Right **0SUC**
         Femoral Surface **0SUT09Z**
         Tibial Surface **0SUV09Z**
   Lumbar Vertebral **0SU0**
   Lumbosacral **0SU3**
   Metacarpocarpal
      Left **0RUT**
      Right **0RUS**
   Metacarpophalangeal
      Left **0RUV**
      Right **0RUU**

   Metatarsal-Phalangeal
      Left **0SUN**
      Right **0SUM**
   Metatarsal-Tarsal
      Left **0SUL**
      Right **0SUK**
   Occipital-cervical **0RU0**
   Sacrococcygeal **0SU5**
   Sacroiliac
      Left **0SU8**
      Right **0SU7**
   Shoulder
      Left **0RUK**
      Right **0RUJ**
   Sternoclavicular
      Left **0RUF**
      Right **0RUE**
   Tarsal
      Left **0SUJ**
      Right **0SUH**
   Temporomandibular
      Left **0RUD**
      Right **0RUC**
   Thoracic Vertebral **0RU6**
   Thoracolumbar Vertebral **0RUA**
   Toe Phalangeal
      Left **0SUQ**
      Right **0SUP**
   Wrist
      Left **0RUP**
      Right **0RUN**
Kidney Pelvis
   Left **0TU4**
   Right **0TU3**
Knee Region
   Left **0YUG**
   Right **0YUF**
Larynx **0CUS**
Leg
   Lower
      Left **0YUJ**
      Right **0YUH**
   Upper
      Left **0YUD**
      Right **0YUC**
Lip
   Lower **0CU1**
   Upper **0CU0**
Lymphatic
   Aortic **07UD**
   Axillary
      Left **07U6**
      Right **07U5**
   Head **07U0**
   Inguinal
      Left **07UJ**
      Right **07UH**
   Internal Mammary
      Left **07U9**
      Right **07U8**
   Lower Extremity
      Left **07UG**
      Right **07UF**
   Mesenteric **07UB**
   Neck
      Left **07U2**
      Right **07U1**
   Pelvis **07UC**
   Thoracic Duct **07UK**
   Thorax **07U7**

Supplement - *continued*
   Perineum **0LUH**
   Shoulder
     Left **0LU2**
     Right **0LU1**
   Thorax
     Left **0LUD**
     Right **0LUC**
   Trunk
     Left **0LUB**
     Right **0LU9**
   Upper Arm
     Left **0LU4**
     Right **0LU3**
   Upper Leg
     Left **0LUM**
     Right **0LUL**
  Testis
   Bilateral **0VUC0**
   Left **0VUB0**
   Right **0VU90**
  Thumb
   Left **0XUM**
   Right **0XUL**
  Tibia
   Left **0QUH**
   Right **0QUG**
  Toe
   1st
     Left **0YUQ**
     Right **0YUP**
   2nd
     Left **0YUS**
     Right **0YUR**
   3rd
     Left **0YUU**
     Right **0YUT**
   4th
     Left **0YUW**
     Right **0YUV**
   5th
     Left **0YUY**
     Right **0YUX**
  Tongue **0CU7**
  Trachea **0BU1**
  Tunica Vaginalis
   Left **0VU7**
   Right **0VU6**
  Turbinate, Nasal **09UL**
  Tympanic Membrane
   Left **09U8**
   Right **09U7**
  Ulna
   Left **0PUL**
   Right **0PUK**
  Ureter
   Left **0TU7**
   Right **0TU6**
  Urethra **0TUD**
  Uterine Supporting Structure **0UU4**
  Uvula **0CUN**
  Vagina **0UUG**
  Valve
   Aortic **02UF**
   Mitral **02UG**
   Pulmonary **02UH**
   Tricuspid **02UJ**
  Vas Deferens
   Bilateral **0VUQ**
   Left **0VUP**
   Right **0VUN**

Supplement - *continued*
  Vein
   Axillary
     Left **05U8**
     Right **05U7**
   Azygos **05U0**
   Basilic
     Left **05UC**
     Right **05UB**
   Brachial
     Left **05UA**
     Right **05U9**
   Cephalic
     Left **05UF**
     Right **05UD**
   Colic **06U7**
   Common Iliac
     Left **06UD**
     Right **06UC**
   Esophageal **06U3**
   External Iliac
     Left **06UG**
     Right **06UF**
   External Jugular
     Left **05UQ**
     Right **05UP**
   Face
     Left **05UV**
     Right **05UT**
   Femoral
     Left **06UN**
     Right **06UM**
   Foot
     Left **06UV**
     Right **06UT**
   Gastric **06U2**
   Greater Saphenous
     Left **06UQ**
     Right **06UP**
   Hand
     Left **05UH**
     Right **05UG**
   Hemiazygos **05U1**
   Hepatic **06U4**
   Hypogastric
     Left **06UJ**
     Right **06UH**
   Inferior Mesenteric **06U6**
   Innominate
     Left **05U4**
     Right **05U3**
   Internal Jugular
     Left **05UN**
     Right **05UM**
   Intracranial **05UL**
   Lesser Saphenous
     Left **06US**
     Right **06UR**
   Lower **06UY**
   Portal **06U8**
   Pulmonary
     Left **02UT**
     Right **02US**
   Renal
     Left **06UB**
     Right **06U9**
   Splenic **06U1**
   Subclavian
     Left **05U6**
     Right **05U5**
   Superior Mesenteric **06U5**
   Upper **05UY**

Supplement - *continued*
   Vertebral
     Left **05US**
     Right **05UR**
  Vena Cava
   Inferior **06U0**
   Superior **02UV**
  Ventricle
   Left **02UL**
   Right **02UK**
  Vertebra
   Cervical **0PU3**
   Lumbar **0QU0**
   Thoracic **0PU4**
  Vesicle
   Bilateral **0VU3**
   Left **0VU2**
   Right **0VU1**
  Vocal Cord
   Left **0CUV**
   Right **0CUT**
  Vulva **0UUM**
  Wrist Region
   Left **0XUH**
   Right **0XUG**
Supraclavicular (Virchow's) lymph node
  use Lymphatic, Neck, Left
  use Lymphatic, Neck, Right
Supraclavicular nerve *use* Nerve, Cervical
  Plexus
Suprahyoid lymph node *use* Lymphatic, Head
Suprahyoid muscle
  use Muscle, Neck, Right
  use Muscle, Neck, Left
Suprainguinal lymph node *use* Lymphatic,
  Pelvis
Supraorbital vein
  use Vein, Face, Left
  use Vein, Face, Right
Suprarenal gland
  use Gland, Adrenal, Left
  use Gland, Adrenal, Right
  use Gland, Adrenal, Bilateral
  use Gland, Adrenal
Suprarenal plexus *use* Nerve, Abdominal
  Sympathetic
Suprascapular nerve *use* Nerve, Brachial
  Plexus
Supraspinatus fascia
  use Subcutaneous Tissue and Fascia, Upper
  Arm, Right
  use Subcutaneous Tissue and Fascia, Upper
  Arm, Left
Supraspinatus muscle
  use Muscle, Shoulder, Right
  use Muscle, Shoulder, Left
Supraspinous ligament
  use Bursa and Ligament, Trunk, Right
  use Bursa and Ligament, Trunk, Left
Suprasternal notch *use* Sternum
Supratrochlear lymph node
  use Lymphatic, Upper Extremity, Right
  use Lymphatic, Upper Extremity, Left
Sural artery
  use Artery, Popliteal, Right
  use Artery, Popliteal, Left
Suspension
  Bladder Neck *see* Reposition, Bladder Neck
  0TSC
  Kidney *see* Reposition, Urinary System **0TS**
  Urethra *see* Reposition, Urinary System **0TS**
  Urethrovesical *see* Reposition, Bladder Neck
  0TSC

Suspension - *continued*
    Uterus *see* Reposition, Uterus **0US9**
    Vagina *see* Reposition, Vagina **0USG**
Suture
    Laceration repair *see* Repair
    Ligation *see* Occlusion
Suture Removal
    Extremity
        Lower **8E0YXY8**
        Upper **8E0XXY8**
    Head and Neck Region **8E09XY8**
    Trunk Region **8E0WXY8**
Sweat gland *use* Skin
Sympathectomy *see* Excision, Peripheral
    Nervous System **01B**
SynCardia Total Artificial Heart *use* Synthetic
    Substitute
Synchra CRT-P *use* Cardiac Resynchronization
    Pacemaker Pulse Generator in **0JH**
Synechiotomy, iris *see* Release, Eye **08N**
Synovectomy
    Lower joint *see* Excision, Lower Joints **0SB**
    Upper joint *see* Excision, Upper Joints **0RB**
Systemic Nuclear Medicine Therapy
    Abdomen **CW70**
    Anatomical Regions, Multiple **CW7YYZZ**
    Chest **CW73**
    Thyroid **CW7G**
    Whole Body **CW7N**

T

Takedown
    Arteriovenous shunt *see* Removal of device
    from, Upper Arteries **03P**
    Arteriovenous shunt, with creation of new
    shunt *see* Bypass, Upper Arteries **031**
    Stoma *see* Repair
Talent® Converter *use* Intraluminal Device
Talent® Occluder *use* Intraluminal Device
Talent® Stent Graft (abdominal)(thoracic)
    use Intraluminal Device
Talocalcaneal (subtalar) joint
    use Joint, Tarsal, Left
    use Joint, Tarsal, Right
Talocalcaneal ligament
    use Bursa and Ligament, Foot, Left
    use Bursa and Ligament, Foot, Right
Talocalcaneonavicular joint
    use Joint, Tarsal, Right
    use Joint, Tarsal, Left
Talocalcaneonavicular ligament
    use Bursa and Ligament, Foot, Left
    use Bursa and Ligament, Foot, Right
Talocrural joint
    use Joint, Ankle, Right
    use Joint, Ankle, Left
Talofibular ligament
    use Bursa and Ligament, Ankle, Right
    use Bursa and Ligament, Ankle, Left
Talus bone
    use Tarsal, Right
    use Tarsal, Left
TandemHeart® System *use* External Heart
    Assist System in Heart and Great Vessels
Tarsectomy
    see Excision, Lower Bones **0QB**
    see Resection, Lower Bones **0QT**
Tarsometatarsal joint
    use Joint, Metatarsal-Tarsal, Right
    use Joint, Metatarsal-Tarsal, Left

Tarsometatarsal ligament
    use Bursa and Ligament, Foot, Right
    use Bursa and Ligament, Foot, Left
Tarsorrhaphy *see* Repair, Eye **08Q**
Tattooing
    Cornea **3E0CXMZ**
    Skin *see* Introduction of substance in or on,
    Skin **3E00**
TAXUS® Liberté® Paclitaxel-eluting
    Coronary Stent System *use* Intraluminal
    Device, Drug-eluting in Heart and Great
    Vessels
TBNA (transbronchial needle aspiration) *see*
    Drainage, Respiratory System **0B9**
Telemetry
    4A12X4Z
    Ambulatory **4A12X45**
Temperature gradient study 4A0ZXKZ
Temporal lobe *use* Cerebral Hemisphere
Temporalis muscle *use* Muscle, Head
Temporoparietalis muscle *use* Muscle, Head
Tendolysis *see* Release, Tendons **0LN**
Tendonectomy
    see Excision, Tendons **0LB**
    see Resection, Tendons **0LT**
Tendonoplasty, tenoplasty
    see Repair, Tendons **0LQ**
    see Replacement, Tendons **0LR**
    see Supplement, Tendons **0LU**
Tendorrhaphy *see* Repair, Tendons **0LQ**
Tendototomy
    see Division, Tendons **0L8**
    see Drainage, Tendons **0L9**
Tenectomy, tenonectomy
    see Excision, Tendons **0LB**
    see Resection, Tendons **0LT Tenolysis** *see*
    Release, Tendons **0LN**
Tenontorrhaphy *see* Repair, Tendons **0LQ**
Tenontotomy
    see Division, Tendons **0L8**
    see Drainage, Tendons **0L9**
Tenorrhaphy *see* Repair, Tendons **0LQ**
Tenosynovectomy
    see Excision, Tendons **0LB**
    see Resection, Tendons **0LT**
Tenotomy
    see Division, Tendons **0L8**
    see Drainage, Tendons **0L9**
Tensor fasciae latae muscle
    use Muscle, Hip, Left
    use Muscle, Hip, Right
Tensor veli palatini muscle *use* Muscle,
    Tongue, Palate, Pharynx
Tenth cranial nerve *use* Nerve, Vagus
Tentorium cerebelli *use* Dura Mater
Teres major muscle
    use Muscle, Shoulder, Left
    use Muscle, Shoulder, Right
Teres minor muscle
    use Muscle, Shoulder, Right
    use Muscle, Shoulder, Left
Termination of pregnancy
    Aspiration curettage **10A07ZZ**
    Dilation and curettage **10A07ZZ**
    Hysterotomy **10A00ZZ**
    Intra-amniotic injection **10A03ZZ**
    Laminaria **10A07ZW**
    Vacuum **10A07Z6**
Testectomy
    see Excision, Male Reproductive System **0VB**
    see Resection, Male Reproductive System
    0VT
Testicular artery *use* Aorta, Abdominal

Testing
    Glaucoma **4A07XBZ**
    Hearing *see* Hearing Assessment, Diagnostic
    Audiology **F13**
    Mental health *see* Psychological Tests
    Muscle function, electromyography (EMG)
    see Measurement, Musculoskeletal **4A0F**
    Muscle function, manual *see* Motor Function
    Assessment, Rehabilitation **F01**
    Neurophysiologic monitoring, intra-operative
    see Monitoring, Physiological Systems **4A1**
    Range of motion *see* Motor Function
    Assessment, Rehabilitation **F01**
    Vestibular function *see* Vestibular
    Assessment, Diagnostic Audiology **F15**
Thalamectomy *see* Excision, Thalamus **00B9**
Thalamotomy *see* Drainage, Thalamus **0099**
Thenar muscle
    use Muscle, Hand, Right
    use Muscle, Hand, Left
Therapeutic Massage
    Musculoskeletal System **8E0KX1Z**
    Reproductive System
        Prostate **8E0VX1C**
        Rectum **8E0VX1D**
Therapeutic occlusion coil(s) *use* Intraluminal
    Device
Thermography 4A0ZXKZ
Thermotherapy, prostate *see* Destruction,
    Prostate **0V50**
Third cranial nerve *use* Nerve, Oculomotor
Third occipital nerve *use* Nerve, Cervical
Third ventricle *use* Cerebral Ventricle
Thoracectomy *see* Excision, Anatomical
    Regions, General **0WB**
Thoracentesis *see* Drainage, Anatomical
    Regions, General **0W9**
Thoracic aortic plexus *use* Nerve, Thoracic
    Sympathetic
Thoracic esophagus *use* Esophagus, Middle
Thoracic facet joint
    use Joint, Thoracic Vertebral, 2 to 7
    use Joint, Thoracic Vertebral, 8 or more
    use Joint, Thoracic Vertebral
Thoracic ganglion *use* Nerve, Thoracic
    Sympathetic
Thoracoacromial artery
    use Artery, Axillary, Right
    use Artery, Axillary, Left
Thoracocentesis *see* Drainage, Anatomical
    Regions, General **0W9**
Thoracolumbar facet joint *use* Joint,
    Thoracolumbar Vertebral
Thoracoplasty
    see Repair, Anatomical Regions, General
    0WQ
    see Supplement, Anatomical Regions, General
    0WU
Thoracostomy tube *use* Drainage Device
Thoracostomy, for lung collapse *see* Drainage,
    Respiratory System **0B9**
Thoracotomy *see* Drainage, Anatomical
    Regions, General **0W9**
Thoratec IVAD (Implantable Ventricular
    Assist Device) *use* Implantable Heart Assist
    System in Heart and Great Vessels
Thoratec Paracorporeal Ventricular Assist
    Device *use* External Heart Assist System in
    Heart and Great Vessels
Thrombectomy *see* Extirpation

Thymectomy
  see Excision, Lymphatic and Hemic Systems
  07B
  see Resection, Lymphatic and Hemic Systems
  07T
Thymopexy
  see Repair, Lymphatic and Hemic Systems
  07Q
  see Reposition, Lymphatic and Hemic
  Systems 07S
Thymus gland *use* Thymus
Thyroarytenoid muscle
  use Muscle, Neck, Right
  use Muscle, Neck, Left
Thyrocervical trunk
  use Artery, Thyroid, Right
  use Artery, Thyroid, Left
Thyroid cartilage *use* Larynx
Thyroidectomy
  see Excision, Endocrine System 0GB
  see Resection, Endocrine System 0GT
Thyroidorrhaphy *see* Repair, Endocrine
  System 0GQ
Thyroidoscopy 0GJK4ZZ
Thyroidotomy *see* Drainage, Endocrine System
  0G9
Tibialis anterior muscle
  use Muscle, Lower Leg, Right
  use Muscle, Lower Leg, Left
Tibialis posterior muscle
  use Muscle, Lower Leg, Right
  use Muscle, Lower Leg, Left
Tibiofemoral joint
  use Joint, Knee, Right, Tibial Surface
  use Joint, Knee, Left, Tibial Surface
  use Joint, Knee, Right
  use Joint, Knee, Left
**TigerPaw® system for closure of left atrial
  appendage** *use* Extraluminal Device
Tissue bank graft *use* Nonautologous Tissue
  Substitute
Tissue Expander
  Insertion of device in
    Breast
      Bilateral **0HHV**
      Left **0HHU**
      Right **0HHT**
    Nipple
      Left **0HHX**
      Right **0HHW**
    Subcutaneous Tissue and Fascia
      Abdomen **0JH8**
      Back **0JH7**
      Buttock **0JH9**
      Chest **0JH6**
      Face **0JH1**
      Foot
        Left **0JHR**
        Right **0JHQ**
      Hand
        Left **0JHK**
        Right **0JHJ**
      Lower Arm
        Left **0JHH**
        Right **0JHG**
      Lower Leg
        Left **0JHP**
        Right **0JHN**
      Neck
        Anterior **0JH4**
        Posterior **0JH5**
      Pelvic Region **0JHC**

Tissue Expander - *continued*
      Perineum **0JHB**
      Scalp **0JH0**
      Upper Arm
        Left **0JHF**
        Right **0JHD**
      Upper Leg
        Left **0JHM**
        Right **0JHL**
  Removal of device from
    Breast
      Left **0HPU**
      Right **0HPT**
    Subcutaneous Tissue and Fascia
      Head and Neck **0JPS**
      Lower Extremity **0JPW**
      Trunk **0JPT**
      Upper Extremity **0JPV**
  Revision of device in
    Breast
      Left **0HWU**
      Right **0HWT**
    Subcutaneous Tissue and Fascia
      Head and Neck **0JWS**
      Lower Extremity **0JWW**
      Trunk **0JWT**
      Upper Extremity **0JWV**
Tissue expander (inflatable)(injectable)
  use Tissue Expander in Skin and Breast
  use Tissue Expander in Subcutaneous Tissue
  and Fascia
Titanium Sternal Fixation System (TSFS)
  use Internal Fixation Device, Rigid Plate in
  0PS
  use Internal Fixation Device, Rigid Plate in
  0PH
**Tomographic (Tomo) Nuclear Medicine
  Imaging CP2YYZZ**
  Abdomen **CW20**
  Abdomen and Chest **CW24**
  Abdomen and Pelvis **CW21**
  Anatomical Regions, Multiple **CW2YYZZ**
  Bladder, Kidneys and Ureters **CT23**
  Brain **C020**
  Breast **CH2YYZZ**
    Bilateral **CH22**
    Left **CH21**
    Right **CH20**
  Bronchi and Lungs **CB22**
  Central Nervous System **C02YYZZ**
  Cerebrospinal Fluid **C025**
  Chest **CW23**
  Chest and Abdomen **CW24**
  Chest and Neck **CW26**
  Digestive System **CD2YYZZ**
  Endocrine System **CG2YYZZ**
  Extremity
    Lower **CW2D**
      Bilateral **CP2F**
      Left **CP2D**
      Right **CP2C**
    Upper **CW2M**
      Bilateral **CP2B**
      Left **CP29**
      Right **CP28**
  Gallbladder **CF24**
  Gastrointestinal Tract **CD27**
  Gland, Parathyroid **CG21**
  Head and Neck **CW2B**
  Heart **C22YYZZ**
    Right and Left **C226**
  Hepatobiliary System and Pancreas
  CF2YYZZ

Tomographic Nuclear Imaging - *continued*
  Kidneys, Ureters and Bladder **CT23**
  Liver **CF25**
  Liver and Spleen **CF26**
  Lungs and Bronchi **CB22**
  Lymphatics and Hematologic System
  C72YYZZ
  Myocardium **C22G**
  Neck and Chest **CW26**
  Neck and Head **CW2B**
  Pancreas and Hepatobiliary System
  CF2YYZZ
  Pelvic Region **CW2J**
  Pelvis **CP26**
  Pelvis and Abdomen **CW21**
  Pelvis and Spine **CP27**
  Respiratory System **CB2YYZZ**
  Skin **CH2YYZZ**
  Skull **CP21**
  Skull and Cervical Spine **CP23**
  Spine
    Cervical **CP22**
    Cervical and Skull **CP23**
    Lumbar **CP2H**
    Thoracic **CP2G**
    Thoracolumbar **CP2J**
  Spine and Pelvis **CP27**
  Spleen **C722**
  Spleen and Liver **CF26**
  Subcutaneous Tissue **CH2YYZZ**
  Thorax **CP24**
  Ureters, Kidneys and Bladder **CT23**
  Urinary System **CT2YYZZ**
Tomography, computerized *see* Computerized
  Tomography (CT Scan)
Tonometry 4A07XBZ
Tonsillectomy
  see Excision, Mouth and Throat 0CB
  see Resection, Mouth and Throat 0CT
Tonsillotomy *see* Drainage, Mouth and Throat
  0C9
Total artificial (replacement) heart *use*
  Synthetic Substitute
Total parenteral nutrition (TPN) *see*
  Introduction of Nutritional Substance
Trachectomy
  see Excision, Trachea 0BB1
  see Resection, Trachea 0BT1
Trachelectomy
  see Excision, Cervix 0UBC
  see Resection, Cervix 0UTC
Trachelopexy
  see Repair, Cervix 0UQC
  see Reposition, Cervix 0USC
Tracheloplasty *see* Repair, Cervix 0UQC
Trachelorrhaphy *see* Repair, Cervix 0UQC
Trachelotomy *see* Drainage, Cervix 0U9C
Tracheobronchial lymph node *use* Lymphatic,
  Thorax
Tracheoesophageal fistulization 0B110D6
Tracheolysis *see* Release, Respiratory System
  0BN
Tracheoplasty
  see Repair, Respiratory System 0BQ
  see Supplement, Respiratory System 0BU
Tracheorrhaphy *see* Repair, Respiratory
  System 0BQ
Tracheoscopy 0BJ18ZZ
Tracheostomy *see* Bypass, Respiratory System
  0B1

Tracheostomy Device
  Bypass, Trachea **0B11**
  Change device in, Trachea **0B21XFZ**
  Removal of device from, Trachea **0BP1**
  Revision of device in, Trachea **0BW1**
Tracheostomy tube *use* Tracheostomy Device
  in Respiratory System
Tracheotomy *see* Drainage, Respiratory System
  0B9
Traction
  Abdominal Wall **2W63X**
  Arm
    Lower
      Left **2W6DX**
      Right **2W6CX**
    Upper
      Left **2W6BX**
      Right **2W6AX**
  Back **2W65X**
  Chest Wall **2W64X**
  Extremity
    Lower
      Left **2W6MX**
      Right **2W6LX**
    Upper
      Left **2W69X**
      Right **2W68X**
  Face **2W61X**
  Finger
    Left **2W6KX**
    Right **2W6JX**
  Foot
    Left **2W6TX**
    Right **2W6SX**
  Hand
    Left **2W6FX**
    Right **2W6EX**
  Head **2W60X**
  Inguinal Region
    Left **2W67X**
    Right **2W66X**
  Leg
    Lower
      Left **2W6RX**
      Right **2W6QX**
    Upper
      Left **2W6PX**
      Right **2W6NX**
  Neck **2W62X**
  Thumb
    Left **2W6HX**
    Right **2W6GX**
  Toe
    Left **2W6VX**
    Right **2W6UX**
Tractotomy *see* Division, Central Nervous
  System **008**
Tragus
  use Ear, External, Left
  use Ear, External, Right
  use Ear, External, Bilateral
Training, caregiver *see* Caregiver Training
TRAM (transverse rectus abdominis
  myocutaneous) flap reconstruction
  Free *see* Replacement, Skin and Breast **0HR**
  Pedicled *see* Transfer, Muscles **0KX**
Transection *see* Division
Transfer
  Buccal Mucosa **0CX4**
  Bursa and Ligament
    Abdomen
      Left **0MXJ**
      Right **0MXH**

Transfer - *continued*
  Ankle
    Left **0MXR**
    Right **0MXQ**
  Elbow
    Left **0MX4**
    Right **0MX3**
  Foot
    Left **0MXT**
    Right **0MXS**
  Hand
    Left **0MX8**
    Right **0MX7**
  Head and Neck **0MX0**
  Hip
    Left **0MXM**
    Right **0MXL**
  Knee
    Left **0MXP**
    Right **0MXN**
  Lower Extremity
    Left **0MXW**
    Right **0MXV**
  Perineum **0MXK**
  Shoulder
    Left **0MX2**
    Right **0MX1**
  Thorax
    Left **0MXG**
    Right **0MXF**
  Trunk
    Left **0MXD**
    Right **0MXC**
  Upper Extremity
    Left **0MXB**
    Right **0MX9**
  Wrist
    Left **0MX6**
    Right **0MX5**
  Finger
    Left **0XXP0ZM**
    Right **0XXN0ZL**
  Gingiva
    Lower **0CX6**
    Upper **0CX5**
  Intestine
    Large **0DXE**
    Small **0DX8**
  Lip
    Lower **0CX1**
    Upper **0CX0**
  Muscle
    Abdomen
      Left **0KXL**
      Right **0KXK**
    Extraocular
      Left **08XM**
      Right **08XL**
    Facial **0KX1**
    Foot
      Left **0KXW**
      Right **0KXV**
    Hand
      Left **0KXD**
      Right **0KXC**
    Head **0KX0**
    Hip
      Left **0KXP**
      Right **0KXN**
    Lower Arm and Wrist
      Left **0KXB**
      Right **0KX9**

Transfer - *continued*
  Lower Leg
    Left **0KXT**
    Right **0KXS**
  Neck
    Left **0KX3**
    Right **0KX2**
  Perineum **0KXM**
  Shoulder
    Left **0KX6**
    Right **0KX5**
  Thorax
    Left **0KXJ**
    Right **0KXH**
  Tongue, Palate, Pharynx **0KX4**
  Trunk
    Left **0KXG**
    Right **0KXF**
  Upper Arm
    Left **0KX8**
    Right **0KX7**
  Upper Leg
    Left **0KXR**
    Right **0KXQ**
  Nerve
    Abducens **00XL**
    Accessory **00XR**
    Acoustic **00XN**
    Cervical **01X1**
    Facial **00XM**
    Femoral **01XD**
    Glossopharyngeal **00XP**
    Hypoglossal **00XS**
    Lumbar **01XB**
    Median **01X5**
    Oculomotor **00XH**
    Olfactory **00XF**
    Optic **00XG**
    Peroneal **01XH**
    Phrenic **01X2**
    Pudendal **01XC**
    Radial **01X6**
    Sciatic **01XF**
    Thoracic **01X8**
    Tibial **01XG**
    Trigeminal **00XK**
    Trochlear **00XJ**
    Ulnar **01X4**
    Vagus **00XQ**
  Palate, Soft **0CX3**
  Skin
    Abdomen **0HX7XZZ**
    Back **0HX6XZZ**
    Buttock **0HX8XZZ**
    Chest **0HX5XZZ**
    Ear
      Left **0HX3XZZ**
      Right **0HX2XZZ**
    Face **0HX1XZZ**
    Foot
      Left **0HXNXZZ**
      Right **0HXMXZZ**
    Genitalia **0HXAXZZ**
    Hand
      Left **0HXGXZZ**
      Right **0HXFXZZ**
    Lower Arm
      Left **0HXEXZZ**
      Right **0HXDXZZ**
    Lower Leg
      Left **0HXLXZZ**
      Right **0HXKXZZ**

Transfer - *continued*
    Neck 0HX4XZZ
    Perineum 0HX9XZZ
    Scalp 0HX0XZZ
    Upper Arm
        Left 0HXCXZZ
        Right 0HXBXZZ
    Upper Leg
        Left 0HXJXZZ
        Right 0HXHXZZ
  Stomach 0DX6
  Subcutaneous Tissue and Fascia
    Abdomen 0JX8
    Back 0JX7
    Buttock 0JX9
    Chest 0JX6
    Face 0JX1
    Foot
        Left 0JXR
        Right 0JXQ
    Hand
        Left 0JXK
        Right 0JXJ
    Lower Arm
        Left 0JXH
        Right 0JXG
    Lower Leg
        Left 0JXP
        Right 0JXN
    Neck
        Anterior 0JX4
        Posterior 0JX5
    Pelvic Region 0JXC
    Perineum 0JXB
    Scalp 0JX0
    Upper Arm
        Left 0JXF
        Right 0JXD
    Upper Leg
        Left 0JXM
        Right 0JXL
  Tendon
    Abdomen
        Left 0LXG
        Right 0LXF
    Ankle
        Left 0LXT
        Right 0LXS
    Foot
        Left 0LXW
        Right 0LXV
    Hand
        Left 0LX8
        Right 0LX7
    Head and Neck 0LX0
    Hip
        Left 0LXK
        Right 0LXJ
    Knee
        Left 0LXR
        Right 0LXQ
    Lower Arm and Wrist
        Left 0LX6
        Right 0LX5
    Lower Leg
        Left 0LXP
        Right 0LXN
    Perineum 0LXH
    Shoulder
        Left 0LX2
        Right 0LX1

Transfer - *continued*
    Thorax
        Left 0LXD
        Right 0LXC
    Trunk
        Left 0LXB
        Right 0LX9
    Upper Arm
        Left 0LX4
        Right 0LX3
    Upper Leg
        Left 0LXM
        Right 0LXL
  Tongue 0CX7
Transfusion
  Artery
    Central
        Antihemophilic Factors 3026
        Blood
            Platelets 3026
            Red Cells 3026
        Frozen 3026
            White Cells 3026
            Whole 3026
        Bone Marrow 3026
        Factor IX 3026
        Fibrinogen 3026
        Globulin 3026
        Plasma
            Fresh 3026
            Frozen 3026
        Plasma Cryoprecipitate 3026
        Serum Albumin 3026
        Stem Cells
            Cord Blood 3026
            Hematopoietic 3026
    Peripheral
        Antihemophilic Factors 3025
        Blood
            Platelets 3025
            Red Cells 3025
        Frozen 3025
            White Cells 3025
            Whole 3025
        Bone Marrow 3025
        Factor IX 3025
        Fibrinogen 3025
        Globulin 3025
        Plasma
            Fresh 3025
            Frozen 3025
        Plasma Cryoprecipitate 3025
        Serum Albumin 3025
        Stem Cells
            Cord Blood 3025
            Hematopoietic 3025
  Products of Conception
    Antihemophilic Factors 3027
    Blood
        Platelets 3027
        Red Cells 3027
            Frozen 3027
        White Cells 3027
        Whole 3027
    Factor IX 3027
    Fibrinogen 3027
    Globulin 3027
    Plasma
        Fresh 3027
        Frozen 3027
    Plasma Cryoprecipitate 3027
    Serum Albumin 3027

Transfusion - *continued*
  Vein
    4-Factor Prothrombin Complex
        Concentrate 3028[03]B1
    Central
        Antihemophilic Factors 3024
        Blood
            Platelets 3024
            Red Cells 3024
        Frozen 3024
            White Cells 3024
            Whole 3024
        Bone Marrow 3024
        Factor IX 3024
        Fibrinogen 3024
        Globulin 3024
        Plasma
            Fresh 3024
            Frozen 3024
        Plasma Cryoprecipitate 3024
        Serum Albumin 3024
        Stem Cells
            Cord Blood 3024
            Embryonic 3024
            Hematopoietic 3024
    Peripheral
        Antihemophilic Factors 3023
        Blood
            Platelets 3023
            Red Cells 3023
        Frozen 3023
            White Cells 3023
            Whole 3023
        Bone Marrow 3023
        Factor IX 3023
        Fibrinogen 3023
        Globulin 3023
        Plasma
            Fresh 3023
            Frozen 3023
        Plasma Cryoprecipitate 3023
        Serum Albumin 3023
        Stem Cells
            Cord Blood 3023
            Embryonic 3023
            Hematopoietic 3023
Transplantation
  Esophagus 0DY50Z
  Heart 02YA0Z
  Intestine
    Large 0DYE0Z
    Small 0DY80Z
  Kidney
    Left 0TY10Z
    Right 0TY00Z
  Liver 0FY00Z
  Lung
    Bilateral 0BYM0Z
    Left 0BYL0Z
    Lower Lobe
        Left 0BYJ0Z
        Right 0BYF0Z
    Middle Lobe, Right 0BYD0Z
    Right 0BYK0Z
    Upper Lobe
        Left 0BYG0Z
        Right 0BYC0Z
  Lung Lingula 0BYH0Z
  Ovary
    Left 0UY10Z
    Right 0UY00Z

Transplantation - *continued*
   Pancreas **0FYG0Z**
   Products of Conception **10Y0**
   Spleen **07YP0Z**
   Stomach **0DY60Z**
   Thymus **07YM0Z**
Transposition
   see Reposition
   see Transfer
Transversalis fascia *use* Subcutaneous Tissue
   and Fascia, Trunk
Transverse (cutaneous) cervical nerve *use*
   Nerve, Cervical Plexus
Transverse acetabular ligament
   use Bursa and Ligament, Hip, Left
   use Bursa and Ligament, Hip, Right
Transverse facial artery
   use Artery, Temporal, Left
   use Artery, Temporal, Right
Transverse humeral ligament
   use Bursa and Ligament, Shoulder, Left
   use Bursa and Ligament, Shoulder, Right
Transverse ligament of atlas *use* Bursa and
   Ligament, Head and Neck
Transverse Rectus Abdominis Myocutaneous
   Flap
   Replacement
      Bilateral **0HRV076**
      Left **0HRU076**
      Right **0HRT076**
   Transfer
      Left **0KXL**
      Right **0KXK**
Transverse scapular ligament
   use Bursa and Ligament, Shoulder, Left
   use Bursa and Ligament, Shoulder, Right
Transverse thoracis muscle
   use Muscle, Thorax, Right
   use Muscle, Thorax, Left
Transversospinalis muscle
   use Muscle, Trunk, Right
   use Muscle, Trunk, Left
Transversus abdominis muscle
   use Muscle, Abdomen, Left
   use Muscle, Abdomen, Right
Trapezium bone
   use Carpal, Right
   use Carpal, Left
Trapezius muscle
   use Muscle, Trunk, Right
   use Muscle, Trunk, Left
Trapezoid bone
   use Carpal, Right
   use Carpal, Left
Triceps brachii muscle
   use Muscle, Upper Arm, Right
   use Muscle, Upper Arm, Left
Tricuspid annulus *use* Valve, Tricuspid
Trifacial nerve *use* Nerve, Trigeminal
Trifecta™ Valve (aortic) *use* Zooplastic Tissue
   in Heart and Great Vessels
Trigone of bladder *use* Bladder
Trimming, excisional *see* Excision
Triquetral bone
   use Carpal, Right
   use Carpal, Left
Trochanteric bursa
   use Bursa and Ligament, Hip, Right
   use Bursa and Ligament, Hip, Left
TUMT (Transurethral microwave
   thermotherapy of prostate) 0V507ZZ
TUNA (transurethral needle ablation of
   prostate) 0V507ZZ

Tunneled central venous catheter *use* Vascular
   Access Device in Subcutaneous Tissue and
   Fascia
Tunneled spinal (intrathecal) catheter *use*
   Infusion Device
Turbinectomy
   see Excision, Ear, Nose, Sinus **09B**
   see Resection, Ear, Nose, Sinus **09T**
Turbinoplasty
   see Repair, Ear, Nose, Sinus **09Q**
   see Replacement, Ear, Nose, Sinus **09R**
   see Supplement, Ear, Nose, Sinus **09U**
Turbinotomy
   see Drainage, Ear, Nose, Sinus **099**
   see Division, Ear, Nose, Sinus **098**
TURP (transurethral resection of prostate)
   0VB07ZZ
Twelfth cranial nerve *use* Nerve, Hypoglossal
Two lead pacemaker *use* Pacemaker, Dual
   Chamber in **0JH**
Tympanic cavity
   use Ear, Middle, Left
   use Ear, Middle, Right
Tympanic nerve *use* Nerve, Glossopharyngeal
Tympanic part of temporal bone
   use Bone, Temporal, Right
   use Bone, Temporal, Left
Tympanogram *see* Hearing Assessment,
   Diagnostic Audiology **F13**
Tympanoplasty
   see Repair, Ear, Nose, Sinus **09Q**
   see Replacement, Ear, Nose, Sinus **09R**
   see Supplement, Ear, Nose, Sinus **09U**
Tympanosympathectomy *see* Excision, Nerve,
   Head and Neck Sympathetic **01BK**
Tympanotomy *see* Drainage, Ear, Nose, Sinus
   099

U

Ulnar collateral carpal ligament
   use Bursa and Ligament, Wrist, Left
   use Bursa and Ligament, Wrist, Right
Ulnar collateral ligament
   use Bursa and Ligament, Elbow, Right
   use Bursa and Ligament, Elbow, Left
Ulnar notch
   use Radius, Left
   use Radius, Right
Ulnar vein
   use Vein, Brachial, Left
   use Vein, Brachial, Right
Ultrafiltration
   Hemodialysis *see* Performance, Urinary
   5A1D
   Therapeutic plasmapheresis *see* Pheresis,
   Circulatory **6A55**
Ultraflex™ Precision Colonic Stent System
   use Intraluminal Device
ULTRAPRO Hernia System (UHS) *use*
   Synthetic Substitute
ULTRAPRO Partially Absorbable
   Lightweight Mesh *use* Synthetic Substitute
ULTRAPRO Plug *use* Synthetic Substitute
Ultrasonic osteogenic stimulator
   use Bone Growth Stimulator in Upper Bones
   use Bone Growth Stimulator in Head and
   Facial Bones
   use Bone Growth Stimulator in Lower Bones
Ultrasonography
   Abdomen **BW40ZZZ**
   Abdomen and Pelvis **BW41ZZZ**
   Abdominal Wall **BH49ZZZ**

Ultrasonography - *continued*
   Aorta
      Abdominal, Intravascular **B440ZZ3**
      Thoracic, Intravascular **B340ZZ3**
   Appendix **BD48ZZZ**
   Artery
      Brachiocephalic-Subclavian, Right,
   Intravascular **B341ZZ3**
      Celiac and Mesenteric, Intravascular
         B44KZZ3
      Common Carotid
         Bilateral, Intravascular **B345ZZ3**
         Left, Intravascular **B344ZZ3**
         Right, Intravascular **B343ZZ3**
      Coronary
         Multiple **B241YZZ**
            Intravascular **B241ZZ3**
            Transesophageal **B241ZZ4**
         Single **B240YZZ**
            Intravascular **B240ZZ3**
            Transesophageal **B240ZZ4**
      Femoral, Intravascular **B44LZZ3**
      Inferior Mesenteric, Intravascular
         B445ZZ3
      Internal Carotid
         Bilateral, Intravascular **B348ZZ3**
         Left, Intravascular **B347ZZ3**
         Right, Intravascular **B346ZZ3**
      Intra-Abdominal, Other, Intravascular
         B44BZZ3
      Intracranial, Intravascular **B34RZZ3**
      Lower Extremity
         Bilateral, Intravascular **B44HZZ3**
         Left, Intravascular **B44GZZ3**
         Right, Intravascular **B44FZZ3**
      Mesenteric and Celiac, Intravascular
         B44KZZ3
      Ophthalmic, Intravascular **B34VZZ3**
      Penile, Intravascular **B44NZZ3**
      Pulmonary
         Left, Intravascular **B34TZZ3**
         Right, Intravascular **B34SZZ3**
      Renal
         Bilateral, Intravascular **B448ZZ3**
         Left, Intravascular **B447ZZ3**
         Right, Intravascular **B446ZZ3**
      Subclavian, Left, Intravascular **B342ZZ3**
      Superior Mesenteric, Intravascular
         B444ZZ3
      Upper Extremity
         Bilateral, Intravascular **B34KZZ3**
         Left, Intravascular **B34JZZ3**
         Right, Intravascular **B34HZZ3**
   Bile Duct **BF40ZZZ**
   Bile Duct and Gallbladder **BF43ZZZ**
   Bladder **BT40ZZZ**
      and Kidney **BT4JZZZ**
   Brain **B040ZZZ**
   Breast
      Bilateral **BH42ZZZ**
      Left **BH41ZZZ**
      Right **BH40ZZZ**
   Chest Wall **BH4BZZZ**
   Coccyx **BR4FZZZ**
   Connective Tissue
      Lower Extremity **BL41ZZZ**
      Upper Extremity **BL40ZZZ**
   Duodenum **BD49ZZZ**
   Elbow
      Left, Densitometry **BP4HZZ1**
      Right, Densitometry **BP4GZZ1**
   Esophagus **BD41ZZZ**

Ultrasonography - *continued*
- Extremity
  - Lower **BH48ZZZ**
  - Upper **BH47ZZZ**
- Eye
  - Bilateral **B847ZZZ**
  - Left **B846ZZZ**
  - Right **B845ZZZ**
- Fallopian Tube
  - Bilateral **BU42**
  - Left **BU41**
  - Right **BU40**
- Fetal Umbilical Cord **BY47ZZZ**
- Fetus
  - First Trimester, Multiple Gestation **BY4BZZZ**
  - Second Trimester, Multiple Gestation **BY4DZZZ**
  - Single
    - First Trimester **BY49ZZZ**
    - Second Trimester **BY4CZZZ**
    - Third Trimester **BY4FZZZ**
  - Third Trimester, Multiple Gestation **BY4GZZZ**
- Gallbladder **BF42ZZZ**
- Gallbladder and Bile Duct **BF43ZZZ**
- Gastrointestinal Tract **BD47ZZZ**
- Gland
  - Adrenal
    - Bilateral **BG42ZZZ**
    - Left **BG41ZZZ**
    - Right **BG40ZZZ**
  - Parathyroid **BG43ZZZ**
  - Thyroid **BG44ZZZ**
- Hand
  - Left, Densitometry **BP4PZZ1**
  - Right, Densitometry **BP4NZZ1**
- Head and Neck **BH4CZZZ**
- Heart
  - Left **B245YZZ**
    - Intravascular **B245ZZ3**
    - Transesophageal **B245ZZ4**
  - Pediatric **B24DYZZ**
    - Intravascular **B24DZZ3**
    - Transesophageal **B24DZZ4**
  - Right **B244YZZ**
    - Intravascular **B244ZZ3**
    - Transesophageal **B244ZZ4**
  - Right and Left **B246YZZ**
    - Intravascular **B246ZZ3**
    - Transesophageal **B246ZZ4**
- Heart with Aorta **B24BYZZ**
  - Intravascular **B24BZZ3**
  - Transesophageal **B24BZZ4**
- Hepatobiliary System, All **BF4CZZZ**
- Hip
  - Bilateral **BQ42ZZZ**
  - Left **BQ41ZZZ**
  - Right **BQ40ZZZ**
- Kidney
  - and Bladder **BT4JZZZ**
  - Bilateral **BT43ZZZ**
  - Left **BT42ZZZ**
  - Right **BT41ZZZ**
  - Transplant **BT49ZZZ**
- Knee
  - Bilateral **BQ49ZZZ**
  - Left **BQ48ZZZ**
  - Right **BQ47ZZZ**
- Liver **BF45ZZZ**
- Liver and Spleen **BF46ZZZ**
- Mediastinum **BB4CZZZ**
- Neck **BW4FZZZ**

Ultrasonography - *continued*
- Ovary
  - Bilateral **BU45**
  - Left **BU44**
  - Right **BU43**
- Ovary and Uterus **BU4C**
- Pancreas **BF47ZZZ**
- Pelvic Region **BW4GZZZ**
- Pelvis and Abdomen **BW41ZZZ**
- Penis **BV4BZZZ**
- Pericardium **B24CYZZ**
  - Intravascular **B24CZZ3**
  - Transesophageal **B24CZZ4**
- Placenta **BY48ZZZ**
- Pleura **BB4BZZZ**
- Prostate and Seminal Vesicle **BV49ZZZ**
- Rectum **BD4CZZZ**
- Sacrum **BR4FZZZ**
- Scrotum **BV44ZZZ**
- Seminal Vesicle and Prostate **BV49ZZZ**
- Shoulder
  - Left, Densitometry **BP49ZZ1**
  - Right, Densitometry **BP48ZZ1**
- Spinal Cord **B04BZZZ**
- Spine
  - Cervical **BR40ZZZ**
  - Lumbar **BR49ZZZ**
  - Thoracic **BR47ZZZ**
- Spleen and Liver **BF46ZZZ**
- Stomach **BD42ZZZ**
- Tendon
  - Lower Extremity **BL43ZZZ**
  - Upper Extremity **BL42ZZZ**
- Ureter
  - Bilateral **BT48ZZZ**
  - Left **BT47ZZZ**
  - Right **BT46ZZZ**
- Urethra **BT45ZZZ**
- Uterus **BU46**
- Uterus and Ovary **BU4C**
- Vein
  - Jugular
    - Left, Intravascular **B544ZZ3**
    - Right, Intravascular **B543ZZ3**
  - Lower Extremity
    - Bilateral, Intravascular **B54DZZ3**
    - Left, Intravascular **B54CZZ3**
    - Right, Intravascular **B54BZZ3**
  - Portal, Intravascular **B54TZZ3**
  - Renal
    - Bilateral, Intravascular **B54LZZ3**
    - Left, Intravascular **B54KZZ3**
    - Right, Intravascular **B54JZZ3**
  - Splanchnic, Intravascular **B54TZZ3**
  - Subclavian
    - Left, Intravascular **B547ZZ3**
    - Right, Intravascular **B546ZZ3**
  - Upper Extremity
    - Bilateral, Intravascular **B54PZZ3**
    - Left, Intravascular **B54NZZ3**
    - Right, Intravascular **B54MZZ3**
- Vena Cava
  - Inferior, Intravascular **B549ZZ3**
  - Superior, Intravascular **B548ZZ3**
- Wrist
  - Left, Densitometry **BP4MZZ1**
  - Right, Densitometry **BP4LZZ1**

Ultrasound bone healing system
- *use* Bone Growth Stimulator in Upper Bones
- *use* Bone Growth Stimulator in Head and Facial Bones
- *use* Bone Growth Stimulator in Lower Bones

Ultrasound Therapy
- Heart **6A75**
- No Qualifier **6A75**
- Vessels
  - Head and Neck **6A75**
  - Other **6A75**
  - Peripheral **6A75**

Ultraviolet Light Therapy, Skin 6A80

Umbilical artery
- *use* Artery, Internal Iliac, Left
- *use* Artery, Internal Iliac, Right

Uniplanar external fixator
- *use* External Fixation Device, Monoplanar in **0PH**
- *use* External Fixation Device, Monoplanar in **0PS**
- *use* External Fixation Device, Monoplanar in **0QH**
- *use* External Fixation Device, Monoplanar in **0QS**

Upper GI series *see* Fluoroscopy, Gastrointestinal, Upper **BD15**

Ureteral orifice
- *use* Ureter, Left
- *use* Ureter
- *use* Ureter, Right
- *use* Ureters, Bilateral

Ureterectomy
- *see* Excision, Urinary System **0TB**
- *see* Resection, Urinary System **0TT**

Ureterocolostomy *see* Bypass, Urinary System **0T1**

Ureterocystostomy *see* Bypass, Urinary System **0T1**

Ureteroenterostomy *see* Bypass, Urinary System **0T1**

Ureteroileostomy *see* Bypass, Urinary System **0T1**

Ureterolithotomy *see* Extirpation, Urinary System **0TC**

Ureterolysis *see* Release, Urinary System **0TN**

Ureteroneocystostomy
- *see* Bypass, Urinary System **0T1**
- *see* Reposition, Urinary System **0TS**

Ureteropelvic junction (UPJ)
- *use* Kidney Pelvis, Right
- *use* Kidney Pelvis, Left

Ureteropexy
- *see* Repair, Urinary System **0TQ**
- *see* Reposition, Urinary System **0TS**

Ureteroplasty
- *see* Repair, Urinary System **0TQ**
- *see* Replacement, Urinary System **0TR**
- *see* Supplement, Urinary System **0TU**

Ureteroplication *see* Restriction, Urinary System **0TV**

Ureteropyelography *see* Fluoroscopy, Urinary System **BT1**

Ureterorrhaphy *see* Repair, Urinary System **0TQ**

Ureteroscopy 0TJ98ZZ

Ureterostomy
- *see* Bypass, Urinary System **0T1**
- *see* Drainage, Urinary System **0T9**

Ureterotomy *see* Drainage, Urinary System **0T9**

Ureteroureterostomy *see* Bypass, Urinary System **0T1**

Ureterovesical orifice
- *use* Ureter, Right
- *use* Ureter, Left
- *use* Ureters, Bilateral
- *use* Ureter

Urethral catheterization, indwelling 0T9B70Z

Urethrectomy
 see Excision, Urethra **0TBD**
 see Resection, Urethra **0TTD**
Urethrolithotomy *see* Extirpation, Urethra
 0TCD
Urethrolysis *see* Release, Urethra **0TND**
Urethropexy
 see Repair, Urethra **0TQD**
 see Reposition, Urethra **0TSD**
Urethroplasty
 see Repair, Urethra **0TQD**
 see Replacement, Urethra **0TRD**
 see Supplement, Urethra **0TUD**
Urethrorrhaphy *see* Repair, Urethra **0TQD**
Urethroscopy 0TJD8ZZ
Urethrotomy *see* Drainage, Urethra **0T9D**
Urinary incontinence stimulator lead *use*
 Stimulator Lead in Urinary System
Urography *see* Fluoroscopy, Urinary System
 BT1
Uterine Artery
 use Artery, Internal Iliac, Left
 use Artery, Internal Iliac, Right
 Left, Occlusion, Artery, Internal Iliac, Left
 04LF
 Right, Occlusion, Artery, Internal Iliac, Right
 04LE
Uterine artery embolization (UAE) *see*
 Occlusion, Lower Arteries **04L**
Uterine cornu *use* Uterus
Uterine tube
 use Fallopian Tube, Left
 use Fallopian Tube, Right
Uterine vein
 use Vein, Hypogastric, Left
 use Vein, Hypogastric, Right
Uvulectomy
 see Excision, Uvula **0CBN**
 see Resection, Uvula **0CTN**
Uvulorrhaphy *see* Repair, Uvula **0CQN**
Uvulotomy *see* Drainage, Uvula **0C9N**

V

Vaccination *see* Introduction of Serum, Toxoid,
 and Vaccine
Vacuum extraction, obstetric 10D07Z6
Vaginal artery
 use Artery, Internal Iliac, Right
 use Artery, Internal Iliac, Left
Vaginal pessary *use* Intraluminal Device,
 Pessary in Female Reproductive System
Vaginal vein
 use Vein, Hypogastric, Right
 use Vein, Hypogastric, Left
Vaginectomy
 see Excision, Vagina **0UBG**
 see Resection, Vagina **0UTG**
Vaginofixation
 see Repair, Vagina **0UQG**
 see Reposition, Vagina **0USG**
Vaginoplasty
 see Repair, Vagina **0UQG**
 see Supplement, Vagina **0UUG**
Vaginorrhaphy *see* Repair, Vagina **0UQG**
Vaginoscopy 0UJH8ZZ
Vaginotomy *see* Drainage, Female Reproductive
 System **0U9**
Vagotomy *see* Division, Nerve, Vagus **008Q**
Valiant Thoracic Stent Graft *use* Intraluminal
 Device

Valvotomy, valvulotomy
 see Division, Heart and Great Vessels **028**
 see Release, Heart and Great Vessels **02N**
Valvuloplasty
 see Repair, Heart and Great Vessels **02Q**
 see Replacement, Heart and Great Vessels
 02R
 see Supplement, Heart and Great Vessels **02U**
Vascular Access Device
 Insertion of device in
  Abdomen **0JH8**
  Chest **0JH6**
  Lower Arm
   Left **0JHH**
   Right **0JHG**
  Lower Leg
   Left **0JHP**
   Right **0JHN**
  Upper Arm
   Left **0JHF**
   Right **0JHD**
  Upper Leg
   Left **0JHM**
   Right **0JHL**
 Removal of device from
  Lower Extremity **0JPW**
  Trunk **0JPT**
  Upper Extremity **0JPV**
 Reservoir
  Insertion of device in
   Abdomen **0JH8**
   Chest **0JH6**
   Lower Arm
    Left **0JHH**
    Right **0JHG**
   Lower Leg
    Left **0JHP**
    Right **0JHN**
   Upper Arm
    Left **0JHF**
    Right **0JHD**
   Upper Leg
    Left **0JHM**
    Right **0JHL**
  Removal of device from
   Lower Extremity **0JPW**
   Trunk **0JPT**
   Upper Extremity **0JPV**
  Revision of device in
   Lower Extremity **0JWW**
   Trunk **0JWT**
   Upper Extremity **0JWV**
 Revision of device in
  Lower Extremity **0JWW**
  Trunk **0JWT**
  Upper Extremity **0JWV**
Vasectomy *see* Excision, Male Reproductive
 System **0VB**
Vasography
 see Plain Radiography, Male Reproductive
 System **BV0**
 see Fluoroscopy, Male Reproductive System
 BV1
Vasoligation *see* Occlusion, Male Reproductive
 System **0VL**
Vasorrhaphy *see* Repair, Male Reproductive
 System **0VQ**
Vasostomy *see* Bypass, Male Reproductive
 System **0V1**

Vasotomy
 Drainage *see* Drainage, Male Reproductive
 System **0V9**
 With ligation *see* Occlusion, Male
 Reproductive System **0VL**
Vasovasostomy *see* Repair, Male Reproductive
 System **0VQ**
Vastus intermedius muscle
 use Muscle, Upper Leg, Right
 use Muscle, Upper Leg, Left
Vastus lateralis muscle
 use Muscle, Upper Leg, Left
 use Muscle, Upper Leg, Right
Vastus medialis muscle
 use Muscle, Upper Leg, Right
 use Muscle, Upper Leg, Left
VCG (vectorcardiogram) *see* Measurement,
 Cardiac **4A02**
Vectra® Vascular Access Graft *use* Vascular
 Access Device in Subcutaneous Tissue and
 Fascia
Venectomy
 see Excision, Upper Veins **05B**
 see Excision, Lower Veins **06B**
Venography
 see Plain Radiography, Veins **B50**
 see Fluoroscopy, Veins **B51**
Venorrhaphy
 see Repair, Upper Veins **05Q**
 see Repair, Lower Veins **06Q**
Venotripsy
 see Occlusion, Upper Veins **05L**
 see Occlusion, Lower Veins **06L**
Ventricular fold *use* Larynx
Ventriculoatriostomy *see* Bypass, Central
 Nervous System **001**
Ventriculocisternostomy *see* Bypass, Central
 Nervous System **001**
Ventriculogram, cardiac
 Combined left and right heart *see*
 Fluoroscopy, Heart, Right and Left **B216**
 Left ventricle *see* Fluoroscopy, Heart, Left
 B215
 Right ventricle *see* Fluoroscopy, Heart, Right
 B214
Ventriculopuncture, through previously
 implanted catheter 8C01X6J
Ventriculoscopy 00J04ZZ
Ventriculostomy
 External drainage *see* Drainage, Cerebral
 Ventricle **0096**
 Internal shunt *see* Bypass, Cerebral Ventricle
 0016
Ventriculovenostomy *see* Bypass, Cerebral
 Ventricle **0016**
Ventrio™ Hernia Patch *use* Synthetic
 Substitute
VEP (visual evoked potential) 4A07X0Z
Vermiform appendix *use* Appendix
Vermilion border
 use Lip, Lower
 use Lip, Upper
Versa *use* Pacemaker, Dual Chamber in **0JH**
Version, obstetric
 External **10S0XZZ**
 Internal **10S07ZZ**
Vertebral arch
 use Vertebra, Thoracic
 use Vertebra, Lumbar
 use Vertebra, Cervical
Vertebral canal *use* Spinal Canal

Vertebral foramen
   use Vertebra, Thoracic
   use Vertebra, Lumbar
   use Vertebra, Cervical
Vertebral lamina
   use Vertebra, Thoracic
   use Vertebra, Cervical
   use Vertebra, Lumbar
Vertebral pedicle
   use Vertebra, Lumbar
   use Vertebra, Thoracic
   use Vertebra, Cervical
Vesical vein
   use Vein, Hypogastric, Left
   use Vein, Hypogastric, Right
Vesicotomy *see* Drainage, Urinary System **0T9**
Vesiculectomy
   see Excision, Male Reproductive System **0VB**
   see Resection, Male Reproductive System **0VT**
Vesiculogram, seminal *see* Plain Radiography, Male Reproductive System **BV0**
Vesiculotomy *see* Drainage, Male Reproductive System **0V9**
Vestibular (Scarpa's) ganglion *use* Nerve, Acoustic
Vestibular Assessment F15Z
Vestibular nerve *use* Nerve, Acoustic
Vestibular Treatment F0C
Vestibulocochlear nerve *use* Nerve, Acoustic
Virchow's (supraclavicular) lymph node
   use Lymphatic, Neck, Left
   use Lymphatic, Neck, Right
Virtuoso (II) (DR) (VR) *use* Defibrillator Generator in **0JH**
Vitrectomy
   see Excision, Eye **08B**
   see Resection, Eye **08T**
Vitreous body
   use Vitreous, Left
   use Vitreous, Right
Vocal fold
   use Vocal Cord, Left
   use Vocal Cord, Right
Vocational
   Assessment *see* Activities of Daily Living Assessment, Rehabilitation **F02**
   Retraining *see* Activities of Daily Living Treatment, Rehabilitation **F08**
Volar (palmar) digital vein
   use Vein, Hand, Left
   use Vein, Hand, Right
Volar (palmar) metacarpal vein
   use Vein, Hand, Right
   use Vein, Hand, Left
Vomer bone *use* Septum, Nasal
Vomer of nasal septum *use* Bone, Nasal
Vulvectomy
   see Excision, Female Reproductive System **0UB**
   see Resection, Female Reproductive System **0UT**

W

WALLSTENT® Endoprosthesis *use* Intraluminal Device
Washing *see* Irrigation
Wedge resection, pulmonary *see* Excision, Respiratory System **0BB**
Window *see* Drainage
Wiring, dental 2W31X9Z

X

X-ray *see* Plain Radiography
X-STOP® Spacer
   use Spinal Stabilization Device, Interspinous Process in **0RH**
   use Spinal Stabilization Device, Interspinous Process in **0SH**
Xenograft *use* Zooplastic Tissue in Heart and Great Vessels
XIENCE V Everolimus Eluting Coronary Stent System *use* Intraluminal Device, Drug-eluting in Heart and Great Vessels
Xiphoid process *use* Sternum
XLIF® System *use* Interbody Fusion Device in Lower Joints

Y

Yoga Therapy 8E0ZXY4

Z

Z-plasty, skin for scar contracture *see* Release, Skin and Breast **0HN**
Zenith Flex® AAA Endovascular Graft *use* Intraluminal Device
Zenith TX2® TAA Endovascular Graft *use* Intraluminal Device
Zenith® Renu™ AAA Ancillary Graft *use* Intraluminal Device
Zilver® PTX® (paclitaxel) Drug-Eluting Peripheral Stent
   use Intraluminal Device, Drug-eluting in Upper Arteries
   use Intraluminal Device, Drug-eluting in Lower Arteries
Zimmer® NexGen® LPS Mobile Bearing Knee *use* Synthetic Substitute
Zimmer® NexGen® LPS-Flex Mobile Knee *use* Synthetic Substitute
Zonule of Zinn
   use Lens, Left
   use Lens, Right
Zotarolimus-eluting coronary stent *use* Intraluminal Device, Drug-eluting in Heart and Great Vessels
Zygomatic process of frontal bone
   use Bone, Frontal, Left
   use Bone, Frontal, Right
Zygomatic process of temporal bone
   use Bone, Temporal, Right
   use Bone, Temporal, Left
Zygomaticus muscle *use* Muscle, Facial

APPENDIX A: DEFINITIONS

SECTION 0 - MEDICAL AND SURGICAL CHARACTER 3 – OPERATION

Alteration	**Definition:** Modifying the anatomic structure of a body part without affecting the function of the body part **Explanation:** Principal purpose is to improve appearance **Includes/Examples:** Face lift, breast augmentation
Bypass	**Definition:** Altering the route of passage of the contents of a tubular body part **Explanation:** Rerouting contents of a body part to a downstream area of the normal route, to a similar route and body part, or to an abnormal route and dissimilar body part. Includes one or more anastomoses, with or without the use of a device **Includes/Examples:** Coronary artery bypass, colostomy formation
Change	**Definition:** Taking out or off a device from a body part and putting back an identical or similar device in or on the same body part without cutting or puncturing the skin or a mucous membrane **Explanation:** All CHANGE procedures are coded using the approach EXTERNAL **Includes/Examples:** Urinary catheter change, gastrostomy tube change
Control	**Definition:** Stopping, or attempting to stop, postprocedural bleeding **Explanation:** The site of the bleeding is coded as an anatomical region and not to a specific body part **Includes/Examples:** Control of post-prostatectomy hemorrhage, control of post-tonsillectomy hemorrhage
Creation	**Definition:** Making a new genital structure that does not take over the function of a body part **Explanation:** Used only for sex change operations **Includes/Examples:** Creation of vagina in a male, creation of penis in a female
Destruction	**Definition:** Physical eradication of all or a portion of a body part by the direct use of energy, force, or a destructive agent **Explanation:** None of the body part is physically taken out **Includes/Examples:** Fulguration of rectal polyp, cautery of skin lesion
Detachment	**Definition:** Cutting off all or a portion of the upper or lower extremities **Explanation:** The body part value is the site of the detachment, with a qualifier if applicable to further specify the level where the extremity was detached **Includes/Examples:** Below knee amputation, disarticulation of shoulder
Dilation	**Definition:** Expanding an orifice or the lumen of a tubular body part **Explanation:** The orifice can be a natural orifice or an artificially created orifice. Accomplished by stretching a tubular body part using intraluminal pressure or by cutting part of the orifice or wall of the tubular body part **Includes/Examples:** Percutaneous transluminal angioplasty, pyloromyotomy
Division	**Definition:** Cutting into a body part, without draining fluids and/or gases from the body part, in order to separate or transect a body part **Explanation:** All or a portion of the body part is separated into two or more portions **Includes/Examples:** Spinal cordotomy, osteotomy
Drainage	**Definition:** Taking or letting out fluids and/or gases from a body part **Explanation:** The qualifier DIAGNOSTIC is used to identify drainage procedures that are biopsies **Includes/Examples:** Thoracentesis, incision and drainage
Excision	**Definition:** Cutting out or off, without replacement, a portion of a body part **Explanation:** The qualifier DIAGNOSTIC is used to identify excision procedures that are biopsies **Includes/Examples:** Partial nephrectomy, liver biopsy
Extirpation	**Definition:** Taking or cutting out solid matter from a body part **Explanation:** The solid matter may be an abnormal byproduct of a biological function or a foreign body; it may be imbedded in a body part or in the lumen of a tubular body part. The solid matter may or may not have been previously broken into pieces **Includes/Examples:** Thrombectomy, choledocholithotomy
Extraction	**Definition:** Pulling or stripping out or off all or a portion of a body part by the use of force **Explanation:** The qualifier DIAGNOSTIC is used to identify extraction procedures that are biopsies **Includes/Examples:** Dilation and curettage, vein stripping
Fragmentation	**Definition:** Breaking solid matter in a body part into pieces **Explanation:** Physical force (e.g., manual, ultrasonic) applied directly or indirectly is used to break the solid matter into pieces. The solid matter may be an abnormal byproduct of a biological function or a foreign body. The pieces of solid matter are not taken out **Includes/Examples:** Extracorporeal shockwave lithotripsy, transurethral lithotripsy
Fusion	**Definition:** Joining together portions of an articular body part rendering the articular body part immobile **Explanation:** The body part is joined together by fixation device, bone graft, or other means **Includes/Examples:** Spinal fusion, ankle arthrodesis
Insertion	**Definition:** Putting in a nonbiological appliance that monitors, assists, performs, or prevents a physiological function but does not physically take the place of a body part **Includes/Examples:** Insertion of radioactive implant, insertion of central venous catheter
Inspection	**Definition:** Visually and/or manually exploring a body part **Explanation:** Visual exploration may be performed with or without optical instrumentation. Manual exploration may be performed directly or through intervening body layers **Includes/Examples:** Diagnostic arthroscopy, exploratory laparotomy
Map	**Definition:** Locating the route of passage of electrical impulses and/or locating functional areas in a body part **Explanation:** Applicable only to the cardiac conduction mechanism and the central nervous system **Includes/Examples:** Cardiac mapping, cortical mapping
Occlusion	**Definition:** Completely closing an orifice or the lumen of a tubular body part **Explanation:** The orifice can be a natural orifice or an artificially created orifice **Includes/Examples:** Fallopian tube ligation, ligation of inferior vena cava
Reattachment	**Definition:** Putting back in or on all or a portion of a separated body part to its normal location or other suitable location

	Explanation: Vascular circulation and nervous pathways may or may not be reestablished Includes/Examples: Reattachment of hand, reattachment of avulsed kidney
Release	Definition: Freeing a body part from an abnormal physical constraint by cutting or by the use of force Explanation: Some of the restraining tissue may be taken out but none of the body part is taken out Includes/Examples: Adhesiolysis, carpal tunnel release
Removal	Definition: Taking out or off a device from a body part Explanation: If a device is taken out and a similar device put in without cutting or puncturing the skin or mucous membrane, the procedure is coded to the root operation CHANGE. Otherwise, the procedure for taking out a device is coded to the root operation REMOVAL Includes/Examples: Drainage tube removal, cardiac pacemaker removal
Repair	Definition: Restoring, to the extent possible, a body part to its normal anatomic structure and function Explanation: Used only when the method to accomplish the repair is not one of the other root operations Includes/Examples: Colostomy takedown, suture of laceration
Replacement	Definition: Putting in or on biological or synthetic material that physically takes the place and/or function of all or a portion of a body part Explanation: The body part may have been taken out or replaced, or may be taken out, physically eradicated, or rendered nonfunctional during the Replacement procedure. A Removal procedure is coded for taking out the device used in a previous replacement procedure Includes/Examples: Total hip replacement, bone graft, free skin graft
Reposition	Definition: Moving to its normal location, or other suitable location, all or a portion of a body part Explanation: The body part is moved to a new location from an abnormal location, or from a normal location where it is not functioning correctly. The body part may or may not be cut out or off to be moved to the new location Includes/Examples: Reposition of undescended testicle, fracture reduction
Resection	Definition: Cutting out or off, without replacement, all of a body part Includes/Examples: Total nephrectomy, total lobectomy of lung
Restriction	Definition: Partially closing an orifice or the lumen of a tubular body part Explanation: The orifice can be a natural orifice or an artificially created orifice Includes/Examples: Esophagogastric fundoplication, cervical cerclage
Revision	Definition: Correcting, to the extent possible, a portion of a malfunctioning device or the position of a displaced device Explanation: Revision can include correcting a malfunctioning or displaced device by taking out or putting in components of the device such as a screw or pin Includes/Examples: Adjustment of position of pacemaker lead, recementing of hip prosthesis
Supplement	Definition: Putting in or on biological or synthetic material that physically reinforces and/or augments the function of a portion of a body part Explanation: The biological material is non-living, or is living and from the same individual. The body part may have been previously replaced, and the Supplement procedure is performed to physically reinforce and/or augment the function of the replaced body part Includes/Examples: Herniorrhaphy using mesh, free nerve graft, mitral valve ring annuloplasty, put a new acetabular liner in a previous hip replacement
Transfer	Definition: Moving, without taking out, all or a portion of a body part to another location to take over the function of all or a portion of a body part Explanation: The body part transferred remains connected to its vascular and nervous supply Includes/Examples: Tendon transfer, skin pedicle flap transfer
Transplantation	Definition: Putting in or on all or a portion of a living body part taken from another individual or animal to physically take the place and/or function of all or a portion of a similar body part Explanation: The native body part may or may not be taken out, and the transplanted body part may take over all or a portion of its function Includes/Examples: Kidney transplant, heart transplant

SECTION 0 - MEDICAL AND SURGICAL CHARACTER 4 - BODY PART	
1st Toe, Left 1st Toe, Right	Includes: Hallux
Abdomen Muscle, Left Abdomen Muscle, Right	Includes: External oblique muscle Internal oblique muscle Pyramidalis muscle Rectus abdominis muscle Transversus abdominis muscle
Abdominal Aorta	Includes: Inferior phrenic artery Lumbar artery Median sacral artery Middle suprarenal artery Ovarian artery Testicular artery

Abdominal Sympathetic Nerve	**Includes:** Abdominal aortic plexus Auerbach's (myenteric) plexus Celiac (solar) plexus Celiac ganglion Gastric plexus Hepatic plexus Inferior hypogastric plexus Inferior mesenteric ganglion Inferior mesenteric plexus Meissner's (submucous) plexus Myenteric (Auerbach's) plexus Pancreatic plexus Pelvic splanchnic nerve Renal plexus Solar (celiac) plexus Splenic plexus Submucous (Meissner's) plexus Superior hypogastric plexus Superior mesenteric ganglion Superior mesenteric plexus Suprarenal plexus
Abducens Nerve	**Includes:** Sixth cranial nerve
Accessory Nerve	**Includes:** Eleventh cranial nerve
Acoustic Nerve	**Includes:** Cochlear nerve Eighth cranial nerve Scarpa's (vestibular) ganglion Spiral ganglion Vestibular (Scarpa's) ganglion Vestibular nerve Vestibulocochlear nerve
Adenoids	**Includes:** Pharyngeal tonsil
Adrenal Gland Adrenal Gland, Left Adrenal Gland, Right Adrenal Glands, Bilateral	**Includes:** Suprarenal gland
Ampulla of Vater	**Includes:** Duodenal ampulla Hepatopancreatic ampulla
Anal Sphincter	**Includes:** External anal sphincter Internal anal sphincter
Ankle Bursa and Ligament, Left Ankle Bursa and Ligament, Right	**Includes:** Calcaneofibular ligament Deltoid ligament Ligament of the lateral malleolus Talofibular ligament
Ankle Joint, Left Ankle Joint, Right	**Includes:** Inferior tibiofibular joint Talocrural joint
Anterior Chamber, Left Anterior Chamber, Right	**Includes:** Aqueous humor
Anterior Tibial Artery, Left Anterior Tibial Artery, Right	**Includes:** Anterior lateral malleolar artery Anterior medial malleolar artery Anterior tibial recurrent artery Dorsalis pedis artery Posterior tibial recurrent artery
Anus	**Includes:** Anal orifice
Aortic Valve	**Includes:** Aortic annulus
Appendix	**Includes:** Vermiform appendix
Ascending Colon	**Includes:** Hepatic flexure
Atrial Septum	**Includes:** Interatrial septum
Atrium, Left	**Includes:** Atrium pulmonale Left auricular appendix

Atrium, Right	**Includes:** Atrium dextrum cordis Right auricular appendix Sinus venosus
Auditory Ossicle, Left Auditory Ossicle, Right	**Includes:** Incus Malleus Ossicular chain Stapes
Axillary Artery, Left Axillary Artery, Right	**Includes:** Anterior circumflex humeral artery Lateral thoracic artery Posterior circumflex humeral artery Subscapular artery Superior thoracic artery Thoracoacromial artery
Azygos Vein	**Includes:** Right ascending lumbar vein Right subcostal vein
Basal Ganglia	**Includes:** Basal nuclei Claustrum Corpus striatum Globus pallidus Substantia nigra Subthalamic nucleus
Basilic Vein, Left Basilic Vein, Right	**Includes:** Median antebrachial vein Median cubital vein
Bladder	**Includes:** Trigone of bladder
Brachial Artery, Left Brachial Artery, Right	**Includes:** Inferior ulnar collateral artery Profunda brachii Superior ulnar collateral artery
Brachial Plexus	**Includes:** Axillary nerve Dorsal scapular nerve First intercostal nerve Long thoracic nerve Musculocutaneous nerve Subclavius nerve Suprascapular nerve
Brachial Vein, Left Brachial Vein, Right	**Includes:** Radial vein Ulnar vein
Brain	**Includes:** Cerebrum Corpus callosum Encephalon
Breast, Bilateral Breast, Left Breast, Right	**Includes:** Mammary duct Mammary gland
Buccal Mucosa	**Includes:** Buccal gland Molar gland Palatine gland
Carotid Bodies, Bilateral Carotid Body, Left Carotid Body, Right	**Includes:** Carotid glomus
Carpal Joint, Left Carpal Joint, Right	**Includes:** Intercarpal joint Midcarpal joint
Carpal, Left Carpal, Right	**Includes:** Capitate bone Hamate bone Lunate bone Pisiform bone Scaphoid bone Trapezium bone Trapezoid bone Triquetral bone
Celiac Artery	**Includes:** Celiac trunk
Cephalic Vein, Left Cephalic Vein, Right	**Includes:** Accessory cephalic vein

Cerebellum	**Includes:** Culmen
Cerebral Hemisphere	**Includes:** Frontal lobe Occipital lobe Parietal lobe Temporal lobe
Cerebral Meninges	**Includes:** Arachnoid mater Leptomeninges Pia mater
Cerebral Ventricle	**Includes:** Aqueduct of Sylvius Cerebral aqueduct (Sylvius) Choroid plexus Ependyma Foramen of Monro (intraventricular) Fourth ventricle Interventricular foramen (Monro) Left lateral ventricle Right lateral ventricle Third ventricle
Cervical Nerve	**Includes:** Greater occipital nerve Suboccipital nerve Third occipital nerve
Cervical Plexus	**Includes:** Ansa cervicalis Cutaneous (transverse) cervical nerve Great auricular nerve Lesser occipital nerve Supraclavicular nerve Transverse (cutaneous) cervical nerve
Cervical Vertebra	**Includes:** Spinous process Vertebral arch Vertebral foramen Vertebral lamina Vertebral pedicle
Cervical Vertebral Joint	**Includes:** Atlantoaxial joint Cervical facet joint
Cervical Vertebral Joints, 2 or more	**Includes:** Cervical facet joint
Cervicothoracic Vertebral Joint	**Includes:** Cervicothoracic facet joint
Cisterna Chyli	**Includes:** Intestinal lymphatic trunk Lumbar lymphatic trunk
Coccygeal Glomus	**Includes:** Coccygeal body
Colic Vein	**Includes:** Ileocolic vein Left colic vein Middle colic vein Right colic vein
Conduction Mechanism	**Includes:** Atrioventricular node Bundle of His Bundle of Kent Sinoatrial node
Conjunctiva, Left Conjunctiva, Right	**Includes:** Plica semilunaris
Dura Mater	**Includes:** Cranial dura mater Dentate ligament Diaphragma sellae Falx cerebri Spinal dura mater Tentorium cerebelli
Elbow Bursa and Ligament, Left Elbow Bursa and Ligament, Right	**Includes:** Annular ligament Olecranon bursa Radial collateral ligament Ulnar collateral ligament

Elbow Joint, Left Elbow Joint, Right	**Includes:** Distal humerus, involving joint Humeroradial joint Humeroulnar joint Proximal radioulnar joint
Epidural Space	**Includes:** Cranial epidural space Extradural space Spinal epidural space
Epiglottis	**Includes:** Glossoepiglottic fold
Esophagogastric Junction	**Includes:** Cardia Cardioesophageal junction Gastroesophageal (GE) junction
Esophagus, Lower	**Includes:** Abdominal esophagus
Esophagus, Middle	**Includes:** Thoracic esophagus
Esophagus, Upper	**Includes:** Cervical esophagus
Ethmoid Bone, Left Ethmoid Bone, Right	**Includes:** Cribriform plate
Ethmoid Sinus, Left Ethmoid Sinus, Right	**Includes:** Ethmoidal air cell
Eustachian Tube, Left Eustachian Tube, Right	**Includes:** Auditory tube Pharyngotympanic tube
External Auditory Canal, Left External Auditory Canal, Right	**Includes:** External auditory meatus
External Carotid Artery, Left External Carotid Artery, Right	**Includes:** Ascending pharyngeal artery Internal maxillary artery Lingual artery Maxillary artery Occipital artery Posterior auricular artery Superior thyroid artery
External Ear, Bilateral External Ear, Left External Ear, Right	**Includes:** Antihelix Antitragus Auricle Earlobe Helix Pinna Tragus
External Iliac Artery, Left External Iliac Artery, Right	**Includes:** Deep circumflex iliac artery Inferior epigastric artery
External Jugular Vein, Left External Jugular Vein, Right	**Includes:** Posterior auricular vein
Extraocular Muscle, Left Extraocular Muscle, Right	**Includes:** Inferior oblique muscle Inferior rectus muscle Lateral rectus muscle Medial rectus muscle Superior oblique muscle Superior rectus muscle
Eye, Left Eye, Right	**Includes:** Ciliary body Posterior chamber
Face Artery	**Includes:** Angular artery Ascending palatine artery External maxillary artery Facial artery Inferior labial artery Submental artery Superior labial artery
Face Vein, Left Face Vein, Right	**Includes:** Angular vein Anterior facial vein Common facial vein Deep facial vein Frontal vein Posterior facial (retromandibular) vein Supraorbital vein

Facial Muscle	**Includes:** Buccinator muscle Corrugator supercilii muscle Depressor anguli oris muscle Depressor labii inferioris muscle Depressor septi nasi muscle Depressor supercilii muscle Levator anguli oris muscle Levator labii superioris alaeque nasi muscle Levator labii superioris muscle Mentalis muscle Nasalis muscle Occipitofrontalis muscle Orbicularis oris muscle Procerus muscle Risorius muscle Zygomaticus muscle
Facial Nerve	**Includes:** Chorda tympani Geniculate ganglion Greater superficial petrosal nerve Nerve to the stapedius Parotid plexus Posterior auricular nerve Seventh cranial nerve Submandibular ganglion
Fallopian Tube, Left Fallopian Tube, Right	**Includes:** Oviduct Salpinx Uterine tube
Femoral Artery, Left Femoral Artery, Right	**Includes:** Circumflex iliac artery Deep femoral artery Descending genicular artery External pudendal artery Superficial epigastric artery
Femoral Nerve	**Includes:** Anterior crural nerve Saphenous nerve
Femoral Shaft, Left Femoral Shaft, Right	**Includes:** Body of femur
Femoral Vein, Left Femoral Vein, Right	**Includes:** Deep femoral (profunda femoris) vein Popliteal vein Profunda femoris (deep femoral) vein
Fibula, Left Fibula, Right	**Includes:** Body of fibula Head of fibula Lateral malleolus
Finger Nail	**Includes:** Nail bed Nail plate
Finger Phalangeal Joint, Left Finger Phalangeal Joint, Right	**Includes:** Interphalangeal (IP) joint
Foot Artery, Left Foot Artery, Right	**Includes:** Arcuate artery Dorsal metatarsal artery Lateral plantar artery Lateral tarsal artery Medial plantar artery
Foot Bursa and Ligament, Left Foot Bursa and Ligament, Right	**Includes:** Calcaneocuboid ligament Cuneonavicular ligament Intercuneiform ligament Interphalangeal ligament Metatarsal ligament Metatarsophalangeal ligament Subtalar ligament Talocalcaneal ligament Talocalcaneonavicular ligament Tarsometatarsal ligament
Foot Muscle, Left Foot Muscle, Right	**Includes:** Abductor hallucis muscle Adductor hallucis muscle Extensor digitorum brevis muscle

Foot Muscle, Left Foot Muscle, Right (continued)	Extensor hallucis brevis muscle Flexor digitorum brevis muscle Flexor hallucis brevis muscle Quadratus plantae muscle
Foot Vein, Left Foot Vein, Right	**Includes:** Common digital vein Dorsal metatarsal vein Dorsal venous arch Plantar digital vein Plantar metatarsal vein Plantar venous arch
Frontal Bone, Left Frontal Bone, Right	**Includes:** Zygomatic process of frontal bone
Gastric Artery	**Includes:** Left gastric artery Right gastric artery
Glenoid Cavity, Left Glenoid Cavity, Right	**Includes:** Glenoid fossa (of scapula)
Glomus Jugulare	**Includes:** Jugular body
Glossopharyngeal Nerve	**Includes:** Carotid sinus nerve Ninth cranial nerve Tympanic nerve
Greater Omentum	**Includes:** Gastrocolic ligament Gastrocolic omentum Gastrophrenic ligament Gastrosplenic ligament
Greater Saphenous Vein, Left Greater Saphenous Vein, Right	**Includes:** External pudendal vein Great saphenous vein Superficial circumflex iliac vein Superficial epigastric vein
Hand Artery, Left Hand Artery, Right	**Includes:** Deep palmar arch Princeps pollicis artery Radialis indicis Superficial palmar arch
Hand Bursa and Ligament, Left Hand Bursa and Ligament, Right	**Includes:** Carpometacarpal ligament Intercarpal ligament Interphalangeal ligament Lunotriquetral ligament Metacarpal ligament Metacarpophalangeal ligament Pisohamate ligament Pisometacarpal ligament Scapholunate ligament Scaphotrapezium ligament
Hand Muscle, Left Hand Muscle, Right	**Includes:** Hypothenar muscle Palmar interosseous muscle Thenar muscle
Hand Vein, Left Hand Vein, Right	**Includes:** Dorsal metacarpal vein Palmar (volar) digital vein Palmar (volar) metacarpal vein Superficial palmar venous arch Volar (palmar) digital vein Volar (palmar) metacarpal vein
Head and Neck Bursa and Ligament	**Includes:** Alar ligament of axis Cervical interspinous ligament Cervical intertransverse ligament Cervical ligamentum flavum Lateral temporomandibular ligament Sphenomandibular ligament Stylomandibular ligament Transverse ligament of atlas
Head and Neck Sympathetic Nerve	**Includes:** Cavernous plexus Cervical ganglion Ciliary ganglion Internal carotid plexus Otic ganglion

Head and Neck Sympathetic Nerve (continued)	Pterygopalatine (sphenopalatine) ganglion Sphenopalatine (pterygopalatine) ganglion Stellate ganglion Submandibular ganglion Submaxillary ganglion
Head Muscle	**Includes:** Auricularis muscle Masseter muscle Pterygoid muscle Splenius capitis muscle Temporalis muscle Temporoparietalis muscle
Heart, Left	**Includes:** Left coronary sulcus Obtuse margin
Heart, Right	**Includes:** Right coronary sulcus
Hemiazygos Vein	**Includes:** Left ascending lumbar vein Left subcostal vein
Hepatic Artery	**Includes:** Common hepatic artery Gastroduodenal artery Hepatic artery proper
Hip Bursa and Ligament, Left Hip Bursa and Ligament, Right	**Includes:** Iliofemoral ligament Ischiofemoral ligament Pubofemoral ligament Transverse acetabular ligament Trochanteric bursa
Hip Joint, Left Hip Joint, Right	**Includes:** Acetabulofemoral joint
Hip Muscle, Left Hip Muscle, Right	**Includes:** Gemellus muscle Gluteus maximus muscle Gluteus medius muscle Gluteus minimus muscle Iliacus muscle Obturator muscle Piriformis muscle Psoas muscle Quadratus femoris muscle Tensor fasciae latae muscle
Humeral Head, Left Humeral Head, Right	**Includes:** Greater tuberosity Lesser tuberosity Neck of humerus (anatomical)(surgical)
Humeral Shaft, Left Humeral Shaft, Right	**Includes:** Distal humerus Humerus, distal Lateral epicondyle of humerus Medial epicondyle of humerus
Hypogastric Vein, Left Hypogastric Vein, Right	**Includes:** Gluteal vein Internal iliac vein Internal pudendal vein Lateral sacral vein Middle hemorrhoidal vein Obturator vein Uterine vein Vaginal vein Vesical vein
Hypoglossal Nerve	**Includes:** Twelfth cranial nerve
Hypothalamus	**Includes:** Mammillary body
Inferior Mesenteric Artery	**Includes:** Sigmoid artery Superior rectal artery
Inferior Mesenteric Vein	**Includes:** Sigmoid vein Superior rectal vein
Inferior Vena Cava	**Includes:** Postcava Right inferior phrenic vein Right ovarian vein

Inferior Vena Cava (continued)	Right second lumbar vein Right suprarenal vein Right testicular vein
Inguinal Region, Bilateral Inguinal Region, Left Inguinal Region, Right	**Includes:** Inguinal canal Inguinal triangle
Inner Ear, Left Inner Ear, Right	**Includes:** Bony labyrinth Bony vestibule Cochlea Round window Semicircular canal
Innominate Artery	**Includes:** Brachiocephalic artery Brachiocephalic trunk
Innominate Vein, Left Innominate Vein, Right	**Includes:** Brachiocephalic vein Inferior thyroid vein
Internal Carotid Artery, Left Internal Carotid Artery, Right	**Includes:** Caroticotympanic artery Carotid sinus Ophthalmic artery
Internal Iliac Artery, Left Internal Iliac Artery, Right	**Includes:** Deferential artery Hypogastric artery Iliolumbar artery Inferior gluteal artery Inferior vesical artery Internal pudendal artery Lateral sacral artery Middle rectal artery Obturator artery Superior gluteal artery Umbilical artery Uterine artery Vaginal artery
Internal Mammary Artery, Left Internal Mammary Artery, Right	**Includes:** Anterior intercostal artery Internal thoracic artery Musculophrenic artery Pericardiophrenic artery Superior epigastric artery
Intracranial Artery	**Includes:** Anterior cerebral artery Anterior choroidal artery Anterior communicating artery Basilar artery Circle of Willis Middle cerebral artery Posterior cerebral artery Posterior communicating artery Posterior inferior cerebellar artery (PICA)
Intracranial Vein	**Includes:** Anterior cerebral vein Basal (internal) cerebral vein Dural venous sinus Great cerebral vein Inferior cerebellar vein Inferior cerebral vein Internal (basal) cerebral vein Middle cerebral vein Ophthalmic vein Superior cerebellar vein Superior cerebral vein
Jejunum	**Includes:** Duodenojejunal flexure
Kidney	**Includes:** Renal calyx Renal capsule Renal cortex Renal segment
Kidney Pelvis, Left Kidney Pelvis, Right	**Includes:** Ureteropelvic junction (UPJ)
Kidney, Left Kidney, Right Kidneys, Bilateral	**Includes:** Renal calyx Renal capsule Renal cortex Renal segment

Knee Bursa and Ligament, Left Knee Bursa and Ligament, Right	**Includes:** Anterior cruciate ligament (ACL) Lateral collateral ligament (LCL) Ligament of head of fibula Medial collateral ligament (MCL) Patellar ligament Popliteal ligament Posterior cruciate ligament (PCL) Prepatellar bursa
Knee Joint, Left Knee Joint, Right	**Includes:** Femoropatellar joint Femorotibial joint Lateral meniscus Medial meniscus
Knee Tendon, Left Knee Tendon, Right	**Includes:** Patellar tendon
Lacrimal Duct, Left Lacrimal Duct, Right	**Includes:** Lacrimal canaliculus Lacrimal punctum Lacrimal sac Nasolacrimal duct
Larynx	**Includes:** Aryepiglottic fold Arytenoid cartilage Corniculate cartilage Cricoid cartilage Cuneiform cartilage False vocal cord Glottis Rima glottidis Thyroid cartilage Ventricular fold
Lens, Left Lens, Right	**Includes:** Zonule of Zinn
Lesser Omentum	**Includes:** Gastrohepatic omentum Hepatogastric ligament
Lesser Saphenous Vein, Left Lesser Saphenous Vein, Right	**Includes:** Small saphenous vein
Liver	**Includes:** Quadrate lobe
Lower Arm and Wrist Muscle, Left Lower Arm and Wrist Muscle, Right	**Includes:** Anatomical snuffbox Brachioradialis muscle Extensor carpi radialis muscle Extensor carpi ulnaris muscle Flexor carpi radialis muscle Flexor carpi ulnaris muscle Flexor pollicis longus muscle Palmaris longus muscle Pronator quadratus muscle Pronator teres muscle
Lower Eyelid, Left Lower Eyelid, Right	**Includes:** Inferior tarsal plate Medial canthus
Lower Femur, Left Lower Femur, Right	**Includes:** Lateral condyle of femur Lateral epicondyle of femur Medial condyle of femur Medial epicondyle of femur
Lower Leg Muscle, Left Lower Leg Muscle, Right	**Includes:** Extensor digitorum longus muscle Extensor hallucis longus muscle Fibularis brevis muscle Fibularis longus muscle Flexor digitorum longus muscle Flexor hallucis longus muscle Gastrocnemius muscle Peroneus brevis muscle Peroneus longus muscle Popliteus muscle Soleus muscle Tibialis anterior muscle Tibialis posterior muscle

Lower Leg Tendon, Left Lower Leg Tendon, Right	**Includes:** Achilles tendon
Lower Lip	**Includes:** Frenulum labii inferioris Labial gland Vermilion border
Lumbar Nerve	**Includes:** Lumbosacral trunk Superior clunic (cluneal) nerve
Lumbar Plexus	**Includes:** Accessory obturator nerve Genitofemoral nerve Iliohypogastric nerve Ilioinguinal nerve Lateral femoral cutaneous nerve Obturator nerve Superior gluteal nerve
Lumbar Spinal Cord	**Includes:** Cauda equina Conus medullaris
Lumbar Sympathetic Nerve	**Includes:** Lumbar ganglion Lumbar splanchnic nerve
Lumbar Vertebra	**Includes:** Spinous process Vertebral arch Vertebral foramen Vertebral lamina Vertebral pedicle
Lumbar Vertebral Joint Lumbar Vertebral Joints, 2 or more	**Includes:** Lumbar facet joint
Lumbosacral Joint	**Includes:** Lumbosacral facet joint
Lymphatic, Aortic	**Includes:** Celiac lymph node Gastric lymph node Hepatic lymph node Lumbar lymph node Pancreaticosplenic lymph node Paraaortic lymph node Retroperitoneal lymph node
Lymphatic, Head	**Includes:** Buccinator lymph node Infraauricular lymph node Infraparotid lymph node Parotid lymph node Preauricular lymph node Submandibular lymph node Submaxillary lymph node Submental lymph node Subparotid lymph node Suprahyoid lymph node
Lymphatic, Left Axillary	**Includes:** Anterior (pectoral) lymph node Apical (subclavicular) lymph node Brachial (lateral) lymph node Central axillary lymph node Lateral (brachial) lymph node Pectoral (anterior) lymph node Posterior (subscapular) lymph node Subclavicular (apical) lymph node Subscapular (posterior) lymph node
Lymphatic, Left Lower Extremity	**Includes:** Femoral lymph node Popliteal lymph node
Lymphatic, Left Neck	**Includes:** Cervical lymph node Jugular lymph node Mastoid (postauricular) lymph node Occipital lymph node Postauricular (mastoid) lymph node Retropharyngeal lymph node Supraclavicular (Virchow's) lymph node Virchow's (supraclavicular) lymph node

Lymphatic, Left Upper Extremity	**Includes:** Cubital lymph node Deltopectoral (infraclavicular) lymph node Epitrochlear lymph node Infraclavicular (deltopectoral) lymph node Supratrochlear lymph node
Lymphatic, Mesenteric	**Includes:** Inferior mesenteric lymph node Pararectal lymph node Superior mesenteric lymph node
Lymphatic, Pelvis	**Includes:** Common iliac (subaortic) lymph node Gluteal lymph node Iliac lymph node Inferior epigastric lymph node Obturator lymph node Sacral lymph node Subaortic (common iliac) lymph node Suprainguinal lymph node
Lymphatic, Right Axillary	**Includes:** Anterior (pectoral) lymph node Apical (subclavicular) lymph node Brachial (lateral) lymph node Central axillary lymph node Lateral (brachial) lymph node Pectoral (anterior) lymph node Posterior (subscapular) lymph node Subclavicular (apical) lymph node Subscapular (posterior) lymph node
Lymphatic, Right Lower Extremity	**Includes:** Femoral lymph node Popliteal lymph node
Lymphatic, Right Neck	**Includes:** Cervical lymph node Jugular lymph node Mastoid (postauricular) lymph node Occipital lymph node Postauricular (mastoid) lymph node Retropharyngeal lymph node Right jugular trunk Right lymphatic duct Right subclavian trunk Supraclavicular (Virchow's) lymph node Virchow's (supraclavicular) lymph node
Lymphatic, Right Upper Extremity	**Includes:** Cubital lymph node Deltopectoral (infraclavicular) lymph node Epitrochlear lymph node Infraclavicular (deltopectoral) lymph node Supratrochlear lymph node
Lymphatic, Thorax	**Includes:** Intercostal lymph node Mediastinal lymph node Parasternal lymph node Paratracheal lymph node Tracheobronchial lymph node
Mandible, Left Mandible, Right	**Includes:** Alveolar process of mandible Condyloid process Mandibular notch Mental foramen
Mastoid Sinus, Left Mastoid Sinus, Right	**Includes:** Mastoid air cells
Maxilla, Left Maxilla, Right	**Includes:** Alveolar process of maxilla
Maxillary Sinus, Left Maxillary Sinus, Right	**Includes:** Antrum of Highmore
Median Nerve	**Includes:** Anterior interosseous nerve Palmar cutaneous nerve
Medulla Oblongata	**Includes:** Myelencephalon
Mesentery	**Includes:** Mesoappendix Mesocolon

Metacarpocarpal Joint, Left Metacarpocarpal Joint, Right	**Includes:** Carpometacarpal (CMC) joint
Metatarsal-Phalangeal Joint, Left Metatarsal-Phalangeal Joint, Right	**Includes:** Metatarsophalangeal (MTP) joint
Metatarsal-Tarsal Joint, Left Metatarsal-Tarsal Joint, Right	**Includes:** Tarsometatarsal joint
Middle Ear, Left Middle Ear, Right	**Includes:** Oval window Tympanic cavity
Minor Salivary Gland	**Includes:** Anterior lingual gland
Mitral Valve	**Includes:** Bicuspid valve Left atrioventricular valve Mitral annulus
Nasal Bone	**Includes:** Vomer of nasal septum
Nasal Septum	**Includes:** Quadrangular cartilage Septal cartilage Vomer bone
Nasal Turbinate	**Includes:** Inferior turbinate Middle turbinate Nasal concha Superior turbinate
Nasopharynx	**Includes:** Choana Fossa of Rosenmüller Pharyngeal recess Rhinopharynx
Neck Muscle, Left Neck Muscle, Right	**Includes:** Anterior vertebral muscle Arytenoid muscle Cricothyroid muscle Infrahyoid muscle Levator scapulae muscle Platysma muscle Scalene muscle Splenius cervicis muscle Sternocleidomastoid muscle Suprahyoid muscle Thyroarytenoid muscle
Nipple, Left Nipple, Right	**Includes:** Areola
Nose	**Includes:** Columella External naris Greater alar cartilage Internal naris Lateral nasal cartilage Lesser alar cartilage Nasal cavity Nostril
Occipital Bone, Left Occipital Bone, Right	**Includes:** Foramen magnum
Oculomotor Nerve	**Includes:** Third cranial nerve
Olfactory Nerve	**Includes:** First cranial nerve Olfactory bulb
Optic Nerve	**Includes:** Optic chiasma Second cranial nerve
Orbit, Left Orbit, Right	**Includes:** Bony orbit Orbital portion of ethmoid bone Orbital portion of frontal bone Orbital portion of lacrimal bone Orbital portion of maxilla Orbital portion of palatine bone Orbital portion of sphenoid bone Orbital portion of zygomatic bone

Pancreatic Duct	**Includes:** Duct of Wirsung
Pancreatic Duct, Accessory	**Includes:** Duct of Santorini
Parotid Duct, Left Parotid Duct, Right	**Includes:** Stensen's duct
Pelvic Bone, Left Pelvic Bone, Right	**Includes:** Iliac crest Ilium Ischium Pubis
Pelvic Cavity	**Includes:** Retropubic space
Penis	**Includes:** Corpus cavernosum Corpus spongiosum
Perineum Muscle	**Includes:** Bulbospongiosus muscle Cremaster muscle Deep transverse perineal muscle Ischiocavernosus muscle Superficial transverse perineal muscle
Peritoneum	**Includes:** Epiploic foramen
Peroneal Artery, Left Peroneal Artery, Right	**Includes:** Fibular artery
Peroneal Nerve	**Includes:** Common fibular nerve Common peroneal nerve External popliteal nerve Lateral sural cutaneous nerve
Pharynx	**Includes:** Hypopharynx Laryngopharynx Oropharynx Piriform recess (sinus)
Phrenic Nerve	**Includes:** Accessory phrenic nerve
Pituitary Gland	**Includes:** Adenohypophysis Hypophysis Neurohypophysis
Pons	**Includes:** Apneustic center Basis pontis Locus ceruleus Pneumotaxic center Pontine tegmentum Superior olivary nucleus
Popliteal Artery, Left Popliteal Artery, Right	**Includes:** Inferior genicular artery Middle genicular artery Superior genicular artery Sural artery
Portal Vein	**Includes:** Hepatic portal vein
Prepuce	**Includes:** Foreskin Glans penis
Pudendal Nerve	**Includes:** Posterior labial nerve Posterior scrotal nerve
Pulmonary Artery, Left	**Includes:** Arterial canal (duct) Botallo's duct Pulmoaortic canal
Pulmonary Valve	**Includes:** Pulmonary annulus Pulmonic valve
Pulmonary Vein, Left	**Includes:** Left inferior pulmonary vein Left superior pulmonary vein
Pulmonary Vein, Right	**Includes:** Right inferior pulmonary vein Right superior pulmonary vein

Radial Artery, Left Radial Artery, Right	**Includes:** Radial recurrent artery
Radial Nerve	**Includes:** Dorsal digital nerve Musculospiral nerve Palmar cutaneous nerve Posterior interosseous nerve
Radius, Left Radius, Right	**Includes:** Ulnar notch
Rectum	**Includes:** Anorectal junction
Renal Artery, Left Renal Artery, Right	**Includes:** Inferior suprarenal artery Renal segmental artery
Renal Vein, Left	**Includes:** Left inferior phrenic vein Left ovarian vein Left second lumbar vein Left suprarenal vein Left testicular vein
Retina, Left Retina, Right	**Includes:** Fovea Macula Optic disc
Retroperitoneum	**Includes:** Retroperitoneal space
Sacral Plexus	**Includes:** Inferior gluteal nerve Posterior femoral cutaneous nerve Pudendal nerve
Sacral Sympathetic Nerve	**Includes:** Ganglion impar (ganglion of Walther) Pelvic splanchnic nerve Sacral ganglion Sacral splanchnic nerve
Sacrococcygeal Joint	**Includes:** Sacrococcygeal symphysis
Scapula, Left Scapula, Right	**Includes:** Acromion (process) Coracoid process
Sciatic Nerve	**Includes:** Ischiatic nerve
Shoulder Bursa and Ligament, Left Shoulder Bursa and Ligament, Right	**Includes:** Acromioclavicular ligament Coracoacromial ligament Coracoclavicular ligament Coracohumeral ligament Costoclavicular ligament Glenohumeral ligament Glenoid ligament (labrum) Interclavicular ligament Sternoclavicular ligament Subacromial bursa Transverse humeral ligament Transverse scapular ligament
Shoulder Joint, Left Shoulder Joint, Right	**Includes:** Glenohumeral joint
Shoulder Muscle, Left Shoulder Muscle, Right	**Includes:** Deltoid muscle Infraspinatus muscle Subscapularis muscle Supraspinatus muscle Teres major muscle Teres minor muscle
Sigmoid Colon	**Includes:** Rectosigmoid junction Sigmoid flexure
Skin	**Includes:** Dermis Epidermis Sebaceous gland Sweat gland
Sphenoid Bone, Left Sphenoid Bone, Right	**Includes:** Greater wing Lesser wing
Sphenoid Bone, Left	Optic foramen

Sphenoid Bone, Right (continued)	Pterygoid process Sella turcica
Spinal Canal	**Includes:** Vertebral canal
Spinal Cord	**Includes:** Denticulate ligament
Spinal Meninges	**Includes:** Arachnoid mater Leptomeninges Pia mater
Spleen	**Includes:** Accessory spleen
Splenic Artery	**Includes:** Left gastroepiploic artery Pancreatic artery Short gastric artery
Splenic Vein	**Includes:** Left gastroepiploic vein Pancreatic vein
Sternum	**Includes:** Manubrium Suprasternal notch Xiphoid process
Stomach, Pylorus	**Includes:** Pyloric antrum Pyloric canal Pyloric sphincter
Subarachnoid Space	**Includes:** Cranial subarachnoid space Spinal subarachnoid space
Subclavian Artery, Left Subclavian Artery, Right	**Includes:** Costocervical trunk Dorsal scapular artery Internal thoracic artery
Subcutaneous Tissue and Fascia, Anterior Neck	**Includes:** Deep cervical fascia Pretracheal fascia
Subcutaneous Tissue and Fascia, Chest	**Includes:** Pectoral fascia
Subcutaneous Tissue and Fascia, Face	**Includes:** Masseteric fascia Orbital fascia
Subcutaneous Tissue and Fascia, Left Foot	**Includes:** Plantar fascia (aponeurosis)
Subcutaneous Tissue and Fascia, Left Hand	**Includes:** Palmar fascia (aponeurosis)
Subcutaneous Tissue and Fascia, Left Lower Arm	**Includes:** Antebrachial fascia Bicipital aponeurosis
Subcutaneous Tissue and Fascia, Left Upper Arm	**Includes:** Axillary fascia Deltoid fascia Infraspinatus fascia Subscapular aponeurosis Supraspinatus fascia
Subcutaneous Tissue and Fascia, Left Upper Leg	**Includes:** Crural fascia Fascia lata Iliac fascia Iliotibial tract (band)
Subcutaneous Tissue and Fascia, Posterior Neck	**Includes:** Prevertebral fascia
Subcutaneous Tissue and Fascia, Right Foot	**Includes:** Plantar fascia (aponeurosis)
Subcutaneous Tissue and Fascia, Right Hand	**Includes:** Palmar fascia (aponeurosis)
Subcutaneous Tissue and Fascia, Right Lower Arm	**Includes:** Antebrachial fascia Bicipital aponeurosis
Subcutaneous Tissue and Fascia, Right Upper Arm	**Includes:** Axillary fascia Deltoid fascia Infraspinatus fascia Subscapular aponeurosis Supraspinatus fascia
Subcutaneous Tissue and Fascia, Right Upper Leg	**Includes:** Crural fascia

	Fascia lata Iliac fascia Iliotibial tract (band)
Subcutaneous Tissue and Fascia, Scalp	**Includes:** Galea aponeurotica
Subcutaneous Tissue and Fascia, Trunk	**Includes:** External oblique aponeurosis Transversalis fascia
Subdural Space	**Includes:** Cranial subdural space Spinal subdural space
Submaxillary Gland, Left Submaxillary Gland, Right	**Includes:** Submandibular gland
Superior Mesenteric Artery	**Includes:** Ileal artery Ileocolic artery Inferior pancreaticoduodenal artery Jejunal artery
Superior Mesenteric Vein	**Includes:** Right gastroepiploic vein
Superior Vena Cava	**Includes:** Precava
Tarsal Joint, Left Tarsal Joint, Right	**Includes:** Calcaneocuboid joint Cuboideonavicular joint Cuneonavicular joint Intercuneiform joint Subtalar (talocalcaneal) joint Talocalcaneal (subtalar) joint Talocalcaneonavicular joint
Tarsal, Left Tarsal, Right	**Includes:** Calcaneus Cuboid bone Intermediate cuneiform bone Lateral cuneiform bone Medial cuneiform bone Navicular bone Talus bone
Temporal Artery, Left Temporal Artery, Right	**Includes:** Middle temporal artery Superficial temporal artery Transverse facial artery
Temporal Bone, Left Temporal Bone, Right	**Includes:** Mastoid process Petrous part of temporal bone Tympanic part of temporal bone Zygomatic process of temporal bone
Thalamus	**Includes:** Epithalamus Geniculate nucleus Metathalamus Pulvinar
Thoracic Aorta	**Includes:** Aortic arch Aortic intercostal artery Ascending aorta Bronchial artery Esophageal artery Subcostal artery
Thoracic Duct	**Includes:** Left jugular trunk Left subclavian trunk
Thoracic Nerve	**Includes:** Intercostal nerve Intercostobrachial nerve Subcostal nerve
Thoracic Sympathetic Nerve	**Includes:** Cardiac plexus Esophageal plexus Greater splanchnic nerve Inferior cardiac nerve Least splanchnic nerve Lesser splanchnic nerve Middle cardiac nerve
Thoracic Sympathetic Nerve (continued)	Pulmonary plexus Superior cardiac nerve

	Thoracic aortic plexus Thoracic ganglion
Thoracic Vertebra	**Includes:** Spinous process Vertebral arch Vertebral foramen Vertebral lamina Vertebral pedicle
Thoracic Vertebral Joint Thoracic Vertebral Joints, 2 to 7 Thoracic Vertebral Joints, 8 or more	**Includes:** Costotransverse joint Costovertebral joint Thoracic facet joint
Thoracolumbar Vertebral Joint	**Includes:** Thoracolumbar facet joint
Thorax Bursa and Ligament, Left Thorax Bursa and Ligament, Right	**Includes:** Costotransverse ligament Costoxiphoid ligament Sternocostal ligament
Thorax Muscle, Left Thorax Muscle, Right	**Includes:** Intercostal muscle Levatores costarum muscle Pectoralis major muscle Pectoralis minor muscle Serratus anterior muscle Subclavius muscle Subcostal muscle Transverse thoracis muscle
Thymus	**Includes:** Thymus gland
Thyroid Artery, Left Thyroid Artery, Right	**Includes:** Cricothyroid artery Hyoid artery Sternocleidomastoid artery Superior laryngeal artery Superior thyroid artery Thyrocervical trunk
Tibia, Left Tibia, Right	**Includes:** Lateral condyle of tibia Medial condyle of tibia Medial malleolus
Tibial Nerve	**Includes:** Lateral plantar nerve Medial plantar nerve Medial popliteal nerve Medial sural cutaneous nerve
Toe Nail	**Includes:** Nail bed Nail plate
Toe Phalangeal Joint, Left Toe Phalangeal Joint, Right	**Includes:** Interphalangeal (IP) joint
Tongue	**Includes:** Frenulum linguae Lingual tonsil
Tongue, Palate, Pharynx Muscle Tongue, Palate, Pharynx Muscle (continued)	**Includes:** Chondroglossus muscle Genioglossus muscle Hyoglossus muscle Inferior longitudinal muscle Levator veli palatini muscle Palatoglossal muscle Palatopharyngeal muscle Pharyngeal constrictor muscle Salpingopharyngeus muscle Styloglossus muscle Stylopharyngeus muscle Superior longitudinal muscle Tensor veli palatini muscle
Tonsils	**Includes:** Palatine tonsil
Transverse Colon	**Includes:** Splenic flexure
Tricuspid Valve	**Includes:** Right atrioventricular valve Tricuspid annulus
Trigeminal Nerve	**Includes:** Fifth cranial nerve

	Gasserian ganglion Mandibular nerve Maxillary nerve Ophthalmic nerve Trifacial nerve
Trochlear Nerve	**Includes:** Fourth cranial nerve
Trunk Bursa and Ligament, Left Trunk Bursa and Ligament, Right	**Includes:** Iliolumbar ligament Interspinous ligament Intertransverse ligament Ligamentum flavum Pubic ligament Sacrococcygeal ligament Sacroiliac ligament Sacrospinous ligament Sacrotuberous ligament Supraspinous ligament
Trunk Muscle, Left Trunk Muscle, Right	**Includes:** Coccygeus muscle Erector spinae muscle Interspinalis muscle Intertransversarius muscle Latissimus dorsi muscle Levator ani muscle Quadratus lumborum muscle Rhomboid major muscle Rhomboid minor muscle Serratus posterior muscle Transversospinalis muscle Trapezius muscle
Tympanic Membrane, Left Tympanic Membrane, Right	**Includes:** Pars flaccida
Ulna, Left Ulna, Right	**Includes:** Olecranon process Radial notch
Ulnar Artery, Left Ulnar Artery, Right	**Includes:** Anterior ulnar recurrent artery Common interosseous artery Posterior ulnar recurrent artery
Ulnar Nerve	**Includes:** Cubital nerve
Upper Arm Muscle, Left Upper Arm Muscle, Right	**Includes:** Biceps brachii muscle Brachialis muscle Coracobrachialis muscle Triceps brachii muscle
Upper Eyelid, Left Upper Eyelid, Right	**Includes:** Lateral canthus Levator palpebrae superioris muscle Orbicularis oculi muscle Superior tarsal plate
Upper Femur, Left Upper Femur, Right	**Includes:** Femoral head Greater trochanter Lesser trochanter Neck of femur
Upper Leg Muscle, Left Upper Leg Muscle, Right Upper Leg Muscle, Left Upper Leg Muscle, Right (continued)	**Includes:** Adductor brevis muscle Adductor longus muscle Adductor magnus muscle Biceps femoris muscle Gracilis muscle Pectineus muscle Quadriceps (femoris) Rectus femoris muscle Sartorius muscle Semimembranosus muscle Semitendinosus muscle Vastus intermedius muscle Vastus lateralis muscle Vastus medialis muscle
Upper Lip	**Includes:** Frenulum labii superioris Labial gland Vermilion border
Ureter Ureter, Left	**Includes:** Ureteral orifice

Ureter, Right Ureters, Bilateral	Ureterovesical orifice
Urethra	**Includes:** Bulbourethral (Cowper's) gland Cowper's (bulbourethral) gland External urethral sphincter Internal urethral sphincter Membranous urethra Penile urethra Prostatic urethra
Uterine Supporting Structure	**Includes:** Broad ligament Infundibulopelvic ligament Ovarian ligament Round ligament of uterus
Uterus	**Includes:** Fundus uteri Myometrium Perimetrium Uterine cornu
Uvula	**Includes:** Palatine uvula
Vagus Nerve	**Includes:** Anterior vagal trunk Pharyngeal plexus Pneumogastric nerve Posterior vagal trunk Pulmonary plexus Recurrent laryngeal nerve Superior laryngeal nerve Tenth cranial nerve
Vas Deferens Vas Deferens, Bilateral Vas Deferens, Left Vas Deferens, Right	**Includes:** Ductus deferens Ejaculatory duct
Ventricle, Right	**Includes:** Conus arteriosus
Ventricular Septum	**Includes:** Interventricular septum
Vertebral Artery, Left Vertebral Artery, Right	**Includes:** Anterior spinal artery Posterior spinal artery
Vertebral Vein, Left Vertebral Vein, Right	**Includes:** Deep cervical vein Suboccipital venous plexus
Vestibular Gland	**Includes:** Bartholin's (greater vestibular) gland Greater vestibular (Bartholin's) gland Paraurethral (Skene's) gland Skene's (paraurethral) gland
Vitreous, Left Vitreous, Right	**Includes:** Vitreous body
Vocal Cord, Left Vocal Cord, Right	**Includes:** Vocal fold
Vulva	**Includes:** Labia majora Labia minora
Wrist Bursa and Ligament, Left Wrist Bursa and Ligament, Right	**Includes:** Palmar ulnocarpal ligament Radial collateral carpal ligament Radiocarpal ligament Radioulnar ligament Ulnar collateral carpal ligament
Wrist Joint, Left Wrist Joint, Right	**Includes:** Distal radioulnar joint Radiocarpal joint

SECTION 0 - MEDICAL AND SURGICAL CHARACTER 5 - APPROACH	
External	**Definition:** Procedures performed directly on the skin or mucous membrane and procedures performed indirectly by the application of external force through the skin or mucous membrane
Open	**Definition:** Cutting through the skin or mucous membrane and any other body layers necessary to expose the site of the procedure
Percutaneous	**Definition:** Entry, by puncture or minor incision, of instrumentation through the skin or mucous membrane and any other body layers necessary to reach the site of the procedure
Percutaneous Endoscopic	**Definition:** Entry, by puncture or minor incision, of instrumentation through the skin or mucous membrane and any other body layers necessary to reach and visualize the site of the procedure

Via Natural or Artificial Opening	**Definition:** Entry of instrumentation through a natural or artificial external opening to reach the site of the procedure
Via Natural or Artificial Opening Endoscopic	**Definition:** Entry of instrumentation through a natural or artificial external opening to reach and visualize the site of the procedure
Via Natural or Artificial Opening With Percutaneous Endoscopic Assistance	**Definition:** Entry of instrumentation through a natural or artificial external opening and entry, by puncture or minor incision, of instrumentation through the skin or mucous membrane and any other body layers necessary to aid in the performance of the procedure

SECTION 0 - MEDICAL AND SURGICAL CHARACTER 6 - DEVICE

Artificial Sphincter in Gastrointestinal System	**Includes:** Artificial anal sphincter (AAS) Artificial bowel sphincter (neosphincter)
Artificial Sphincter in Urinary System	**Includes:** AMS 800® Urinary Control System Artificial urinary sphincter (AUS)
Autologous Arterial Tissue in Heart and Great Vessels	**Includes:** Autologous artery graft
Autologous Arterial Tissue in Lower Arteries	**Includes:** Autologous artery graft
Autologous Arterial Tissue in Lower Veins	**Includes:** Autologous artery graft
Autologous Arterial Tissue in Upper Arteries	**Includes:** Autologous artery graft
Autologous Arterial Tissue in Upper Veins	**Includes:** Autologous artery graft
Autologous Tissue Substitute	**Includes:** Autograft Cultured epidermal cell autograft Epicel® cultured epidermal autograft
Autologous Venous Tissue in Heart and Great Vessels	**Includes:** Autologous vein graft
Autologous Venous Tissue in Lower Arteries	**Includes:** Autologous vein graft
Autologous Venous Tissue in Lower Veins	**Includes:** Autologous vein graft
Autologous Venous Tissue in Upper Arteries	**Includes:** Autologous vein graft
Autologous Venous Tissue in Upper Veins	**Includes:** Autologous vein graft
Bone Growth Stimulator in Head and Facial Bones	**Includes:** Electrical bone growth stimulator (EBGS) Ultrasonic osteogenic stimulator Ultrasound bone healing system
Bone Growth Stimulator in Lower Bones	**Includes:** Electrical bone growth stimulator (EBGS) Ultrasonic osteogenic stimulator Ultrasound bone healing system
Bone Growth Stimulator in Upper Bones	**Includes:** Electrical bone growth stimulator (EBGS) Ultrasonic osteogenic stimulator Ultrasound bone healing system
Cardiac Lead in Heart and Great Vessels	**Includes:** Cardiac contractility modulation lead
Cardiac Lead, Defibrillator for Insertion in Heart and Great Vessels	**Includes:** ACUITY™ Steerable Lead Attain Ability® lead Attain StarFix® (OTW) lead Cardiac resynchronization therapy (CRT) lead Corox (OTW) Bipolar Lead Durata® Defibrillation Lead ENDOTAK RELIANCE® (G) Defibrillation Lead
Cardiac Lead, Pacemaker for Insertion in Heart and Great Vessels	**Includes:** ACUITY™ Steerable Lead Attain Ability® lead Attain StarFix® (OTW) lead Cardiac resynchronization therapy (CRT) lead Corox (OTW) Bipolar Lead
Cardiac Resynchronization Defibrillator Pulse Generator for Insertion in Subcutaneous Tissue and Fascia (continued)	**Includes:** COGNIS® CRT-D Concerto II CRT-D Consulta CRT-D CONTAK RENEWAL® 3 RF (HE) CRT-D LIVIAN™ CRT-D Maximo II DR CRT-D Ovatio™ CRT-D Protecta XT CRT-D
Cardiac Resynchronization	**Includes:**

Pacemaker Pulse Generator for Insertion in Subcutaneous Tissue and Fascia	Consulta CRT-P Stratos LV Synchra CRT-P
Cardiac Rhythm Related Device in Subcutaneous Tissue and Fascia	**Includes:** Baroreflex Activation Therapy® (BAT®) Rheos® System device
Contraceptive Device in Female Reproductive System	**Includes:** Intrauterine device (IUD)
Contraceptive Device in Subcutaneous Tissue and Fascia	**Includes:** Subdermal progesterone implant
Contractility Modulation Device for Insertion in Subcutaneous Tissue and Fascia	**Includes:** Optimizer™ III implantable pulse generator
Defibrillator Generator for Insertion in Subcutaneous Tissue and Fascia	**Includes:** Implantable cardioverter-defibrillator (ICD) Maximo II DR (VR) Protecta XT DR (XT VR) Secura (DR) (VR) Virtuoso (II) (DR) (VR)
Diaphragmatic Pacemaker Lead in Respiratory System	**Includes:** Phrenic nerve stimulator lead
Drainage Device	**Includes:** Cystostomy tube Foley catheter Percutaneous nephrostomy catheter Thoracostomy tube
External Fixation Device in Head and Facial Bones	**Includes:** External fixator
External Fixation Device in Lower Bones	**Includes:** External fixator
External Fixation Device in Lower Joints	**Includes:** External fixator
External Fixation Device in Upper Bones	**Includes:** External fixator
External Fixation Device in Upper Joints	**Includes:** External fixator
External Fixation Device, Hybrid for Insertion in Upper Bones	**Includes:** Delta frame external fixator Sheffield hybrid external fixator
External Fixation Device, Hybrid for Insertion in Lower Bones	**Includes:** Delta frame external fixator Sheffield hybrid external fixator
External Fixation Device, Hybrid for Reposition in Upper Bones	**Includes:** Delta frame external fixator Sheffield hybrid external fixator
External Fixation Device, Hybrid for Reposition in Lower Bones	**Includes:** Delta frame external fixator Sheffield hybrid external fixator
External Fixation Device, Limb Lengthening for Insertion in Upper Bones	**Includes:** Ilizarov-Vecklich device
External Fixation Device, Limb Lengthening for Insertion in Lower Bones	**Includes:** Ilizarov-Vecklich device
External Fixation Device, Monoplanar for Insertion in Upper Bones	**Includes:** Uniplanar external fixator
External Fixation Device, Monoplanar for Insertion in Lower Bones	**Includes:** Uniplanar external fixator
External Fixation Device, Monoplanar for Reposition in Upper Bones	**Includes:** Uniplanar external fixator
External Fixation Device, Monoplanar for Reposition in Lower Bones	**Includes:** Uniplanar external fixator
External Fixation Device, Ring for Insertion in Upper Bones	**Includes:** Ilizarov external fixator Sheffield ring external fixator
External Fixation Device, Ring for Insertion in Lower Bones	**Includes:** Ilizarov external fixator Sheffield ring external fixator
External Fixation Device,	**Includes:**

Ring for Reposition in Upper Bones	Ilizarov external fixator Sheffield ring external fixator
External Fixation Device, Ring for Reposition in Lower Bones	**Includes:** Ilizarov external fixator Sheffield ring external fixator
External Heart Assist System in Heart and Great Vessels	**Includes:** Biventricular external heart assist system BVS 5000 Ventricular Assist Device PVAD™ Ventricular Assist Device
Extraluminal Device	**Includes:** LAP-BAND® adjustable gastric banding system REALIZE® Adjustable Gastric Band TigerPaw® system for closure of left atrial appendage
Feeding Device in Gastrointestinal System	**Includes:** Percutaneous endoscopic gastrojejunostomy (PEG/J) tube Percutaneous endoscopic gastrostomy (PEG) tube
Hearing Device in Ear, Nose, Sinus	**Includes:** Esteem® implantable hearing system
Hearing Device in Head and Facial Bones	**Includes:** Bone anchored hearing device
Hearing Device, Bone Conduction for Insertion in Ear, Nose, Sinus	**Includes:** Bone anchored hearing device
Hearing Device, Multiple Channel Cochlear Prosthesis for Insertion in Ear, Nose, Sinus	**Includes:** Cochlear implant (CI), multiple channel (electrode)
Hearing Device, Single Channel Cochlear Prosthesis for Insertion in Ear, Nose, Sinus	**Includes:** Cochlear implant (CI), single channel (electrode)
Implantable Heart Assist System in Heart and Great Vessels	**Includes:** Berlin Heart Ventricular Assist Device DeBakey Left Ventricular Assist Device DuraHeart Left Ventricular Assist System HeartMate II® Left Ventricular Assist Device (LVAD) HeartMate XVE® Left Ventricular Assist Device (LVAD) Novacor Left Ventricular Assist Device Thoratec IVAD (Implantable Ventricular Assist Device)
Infusion Device	**Includes:** InDura, intrathecal catheter (1P) (spinal) Non-tunneled central venous catheter Peripherally inserted central catheter (PICC) Tunneled spinal (intrathecal) catheter
Infusion Device, Pump in Subcutaneous Tissue and Fascia	**Includes:** Implantable drug infusion pump (anti-spasmodic) (chemotherapy)(pain) Injection reservoir, pump Pump reservoir Subcutaneous injection reservoir, pump
Interbody Fusion Device in Lower Joints	**Includes:** Axial Lumbar Interbody Fusion System AxiaLIF® System CoRoent® XL Direct Lateral Interbody Fusion (DLIF) device EXtreme Lateral Interbody Fusion (XLIF) device Interbody fusion (spine) cage XLIF® System
Interbody Fusion Device in Upper Joints	**Includes:** BAK/C® Interbody Cervical Fusion System Interbody fusion (spine) cage
Internal Fixation Device in Head and Facial Bones	**Includes:** Bone screw (interlocking)(lag)(pedicle)(recessed) Kirschner wire (K-wire) Neutralization plate
Internal Fixation Device in Lower Bones	**Includes:** Bone screw (interlocking)(lag)(pedicle)(recessed) Clamp and rod internal fixation system (CRIF) Kirschner wire (K-wire) Neutralization plate
Internal Fixation Device in Lower Joints	**Includes:** Fusion screw (compression)(lag)(locking) Joint fixation plate Kirschner wire (K-wire)
Internal Fixation Device in Upper Bones	**Includes:** Bone screw (interlocking)(lag)(pedicle)(recessed) Clamp and rod internal fixation system (CRIF) Kirschner wire (K-wire)

	Neutralization plate
Internal Fixation Device in Upper Joints	**Includes:** Fusion screw (compression)(lag)(locking) Joint fixation plate Kirschner wire (K-wire)
Internal Fixation Device, Intramedullary in Lower Bones	**Includes:** Intramedullary (IM) rod (nail) Intramedullary skeletal kinetic distractor (ISKD) Küntscher nail
Internal Fixation Device, Intramedullary in Upper Bones	**Includes:** Intramedullary (IM) rod (nail) Intramedullary skeletal kinetic distractor (ISKD) Küntscher nail
Internal Fixation Device, Rigid Plate for Insertion in Upper Bones	**Includes:** Titanium Sternal Fixation System (TSFS)
Internal Fixation Device, Rigid Plate for Reposition in Upper Bones	**Includes:** Titanium Sternal Fixation System (TSFS)
Intraluminal Device	**Includes:** AneuRx® AAA Advantage® Assurant (Cobalt) stent Carotid WALLSTENT® Monorail® Endoprosthesis Centrimag® Blood Pump CoAxia NeuroFlo catheter Colonic Z-Stent® Complete (SE) stent Driver stent (RX) (OTW) E-Luminexx™ (Biliary)(Vascular) Stent Embolization coil(s) Endurant® Endovascular Stent Graft Express® (LD) Premounted Stent System Express® Biliary SD Monorail® Premounted Stent System Express® SD Renal Monorail® Premounted Stent System FLAIR® Endovascular Stent Graft Formula™ Balloon-Expandable Renal Stent System LifeStent® (Flexstar)(XL) Vascular Stent System Micro-Driver stent (RX) (OTW) Pipeline™ Embolization device (PED) Protege® RX Carotid Stent System Stent (angioplasty)(embolization) Talent® Converter Talent® Occluder Talent® Stent Graft (abdominal)(thoracic) TandemHeart® System Therapeutic occlusion coil(s) Ultraflex™ Precision Colonic Stent System Valiant Thoracic Stent Graft WALLSTENT® Endoprosthesis Zenith Flex® AAA Endovascular Graft Zenith® Renu™ AAA Ancillary Graft Zenith TX2® TAA Endovascular Graft
Intraluminal Device, Pessary in Female Reproductive System	**Includes:** Pessary ring Vaginal pessary
Intraluminal Device, Airway in Ear, Nose, Sinus	**Includes:** Nasopharyngeal airway (NPA)
Intraluminal Device, Airway in Gastrointestinal System	**Includes:** Esophageal obturator airway (EOA)
Intraluminal Device, Airway in Mouth and Throat	**Includes:** Guedel airway Oropharyngeal airway (OPA)
Intraluminal Device, Bioactive in Upper Arteries	**Includes:** Bioactive embolization coil(s) Micrus CERECYTE microcoil
Intraluminal Device, Drug-eluting in Heart and Great Vessels (continued)	**Includes:** CYPHER® Stent Endeavor® (III)(IV) (Sprint) Zotarolimus-eluting Coronary Stent System Everolimus-eluting coronary stent Paclitaxel-eluting coronary stent Sirolimus-eluting coronary stent TAXUS® Liberte® Paclitaxel-eluting Coronary Stent System XIENCE V Everolimus Eluting Coronary Stent System Zotarolimus-eluting coronary stent
Intraluminal Device, Drug-eluting in Lower Arteries	**Includes:** Paclitaxel-eluting peripheral stent

	Zilver® PTX® (paclitaxel) Drug-Eluting Peripheral Stent
Intraluminal Device, Drug-eluting in Upper Arteries	**Includes:** Paclitaxel-eluting peripheral stent Zilver® PTX® (paclitaxel) Drug-Eluting Peripheral Stent
Intraluminal Device, Endobronchial Valve in Respiratory System	**Includes:** Spiration IBV™ Valve System
Intraluminal Device, Endotracheal Airway in Respiratory System	**Includes:** Endotracheal tube (cuffed)(double-lumen)
Liner in Lower Joints	**Includes:** Hip (joint) liner Joint liner (insert) Knee (implant) insert
Monitoring Device	**Includes:** Blood glucose monitoring system Cardiac event recorder Continuous Glucose Monitoring (CGM) device Implantable glucose monitoring device Loop recorder, implantable Reveal (DX)(XT)
Monitoring Device, Hemodynamic for Insertion in Subcutaneous Tissue and Fascia	**Includes:** Implantable hemodynamic monitor (IHM) Implantable hemodynamic monitoring system (IHMS)
Monitoring Device, Pressure Sensor for Insertion in Heart and Great Vessels	**Includes:** CardioMEMS® pressure sensor EndoSure® sensor
Neurostimulator Lead in Central Nervous System	**Includes:** Cortical strip neurostimulator lead DBS lead Deep brain neurostimulator lead RNS System lead Spinal cord neurostimulator lead
Neurostimulator Lead in Peripheral Nervous System	**Includes:** InterStim® Therapy lead
Neurostimulator Generator in Head and Facial Bones	**Includes:** RNS system neurostimulator generator
Nonautologous Tissue Substitute	**Includes:** Acellular Hydrated Dermis Bone bank bone graft Tissue bank graft
Pacemaker, Dual Chamber for Insertion in Subcutaneous Tissue and Fascia	**Includes:** EnRhythm Kappa Revo MRI™ SureScan® pacemaker Two lead pacemaker Versa
Pacemaker, Single Chamber for Insertion in Subcutaneous Tissue and Fascia	**Includes:** Single lead pacemaker (atrium)(ventricle)
Pacemaker, Single Chamber Rate Responsive for Insertion in Subcutaneous Tissue and Fascia	**Includes:** Single lead rate responsive pacemaker (atrium) (ventricle)
Radioactive Element	**Includes:** Brachytherapy seeds
Resurfacing Device in Lower Joints	**Includes:** CONSERVE® PLUS Total Resurfacing Hip System Cormet Hip Resurfacing System
Spacer in Lower Joints	**Includes:** Joint spacer (antibiotic)
Spacer in Upper Joints	**Includes:** Joint spacer (antibiotic)
Spinal Stabilization Device, Facet Replacement for Insertion in Upper Joints	**Includes:** Facet replacement spinal stabilization device
Spinal Stabilization Device, Facet Replacement for Insertion in Lower Joints	**Includes:** Facet replacement spinal stabilization device
Spinal Stabilization Device, Interspinous Process for Insertion in Upper Joints	**Includes:** Interspinous process spinal stabilization device X-STOP® Spacer
Spinal Stabilization Device, Interspinous Process for Insertion in Lower Joints	**Includes:** Interspinous process spinal stabilization device X-STOP® Spacer
Spinal Stabilization Device,	**Includes:**

Pedicle-Based for Insertion in Upper Joints	Dynesys® Dynamic Stabilization System Pedicle-based dynamic stabilization device
Spinal Stabilization Device, Pedicle-Based for Insertion in Lower Joints	**Includes:** Dynesys® Dynamic Stabilization System Pedicle-based dynamic stabilization device
Stimulator Generator in Subcutaneous Tissue and Fascia	**Includes:** Diaphragmatic pacemaker generator Mark IV Breathing Pacemaker System Phrenic nerve stimulator generator
Stimulator Generator, Multiple Array for Insertion in Subcutaneous Tissue and Fascia	**Includes:** Activa PC neurostimulator Enterra gastric neurostimulator Kinetra® neurostimulator Neurostimulator generator, multiple channel PrimeAdvanced neurostimulator
Stimulator Generator, Multiple Array Rechargeable for Insertion in Subcutaneous Tissue and Fascia	**Includes:** Activa RC neurostimulator Neurostimulator generator, multiple channel rechargeable RestoreAdvanced neurostimulator RestoreSensor neurostimulator RestoreUltra neurostimulator
Stimulator Generator, Single Array for Insertion in Subcutaneous Tissue and Fascia	**Includes:** Activa SC neurostimulator InterStim® Therapy neurostimulator Itrel (3)(4) neurostimulator Neurostimulator generator, single channel Soletra® neurostimulator
Stimulator Generator, Single Array Rechargeable for Insertion in Subcutaneous Tissue and Fascia	**Includes:** Neurostimulator generator, single channel rechargeable
Stimulator Lead in Gastrointestinal System	**Includes:** Gastric electrical stimulation (GES) lead Gastric pacemaker lead
Stimulator Lead in Muscles	**Includes:** Electrical muscle stimulation (EMS) lead Electronic muscle stimulator lead Neuromuscular electrical stimulation (NEMS) lead
Stimulator Lead in Upper Arteries	**Includes:** Baroreflex Activation Therapy® (BAT®) Carotid (artery) sinus (baroreceptor) lead Rheos® System lead
Stimulator Lead in Urinary System	**Includes:** Sacral nerve modulation (SNM) lead Sacral neuromodulation lead Urinary incontinence stimulator lead
Synthetic Substitute	**Includes:** AbioCor® Total Replacement Heart AMPLATZER® Muscular VSD Occluder Annuloplasty ring Bard® Composix® (E/X)(LP) mesh Bard® Composix® Kugel® patch Bard® Dulex™ mesh Bard® Ventralex™ hernia patch BRYAN® Cervical Disc System Ex-PRESS™ mini glaucoma shunt Flexible Composite Mesh GORE® DUALMESH® Holter valve ventricular shunt MitraClip valve repair system Nitinol framed polymer mesh Partially absorbable mesh PHYSIOMESH™ Flexible Composite Mesh Polymethylmethacrylate (PMMA) Polypropylene mesh PRESTIGE® Cervical Disc PROCEED™ Ventral Patch Prodisc-C Prodisc-L PROLENE Polypropylene Hernia System (PHS) Rebound HRD® (Hernia Repair Device) SynCardia Total Artificial Heart Total artificial (replacement) heart
Synthetic Substitute (continued)	ULTRAPRO Hernia System (UHS) ULTRAPRO Partially Absorbable Lightweight Mesh ULTRAPRO Plug Ventrio™ Hernia Patch

	Zimmer® NexGen® LPS Mobile Bearing Knee Zimmer® NexGen® LPS-Flex Mobile Knee
Synthetic Substitute, Ceramic for Replacement in Lower Joints	**Includes:** Novation® Ceramic AHS® (Articulation Hip System)
Synthetic Substitute, Ceramic on Polyethylene for Replacement in Lower Joints	**Includes:** Oxidized zirconium ceramic hip bearing surface
Synthetic Substitute, Intraocular Telescope for Replacement in Eye	**Includes:** Implantable Miniature Telescope™ (IMT)
Synthetic Substitute, Metal for Replacement in Lower Joints	**Includes:** Cobalt/chromium head and socket
Synthetic Substitute, Metal on Polyethylene for Replacement in Lower Joints	**Includes:** Cobalt/chromium head and polyethylene socket
Synthetic Substitute, Polyethylene for Replacement in Lower Joints	**Includes:** Polyethylene socket
Synthetic Substitute, Reverse Ball and Socket for Replacement in Upper Joints	**Includes:** Delta III Reverse shoulder prosthesis Reverse® Shoulder Prosthesis
Tissue Expander in Skin and Breast	**Includes:** Tissue expander (inflatable)(injectable)
Tissue Expander in Subcutaneous Tissue and Fascia	**Includes:** Tissue expander (inflatable)(injectable)
Tracheostomy Device in Respiratory System	**Includes:** Tracheostomy tube
Vascular Access Device in Subcutaneous Tissue and Fascia	**Includes:** Tunneled central venous catheter Vectra® Vascular Access Graft
Vascular Access Device, Reservoir in Subcutaneous Tissue and Fascia	**Includes:** Implanted (venous)(access) port Injection reservoir, port Subcutaneous injection reservoir, port
Zooplastic Tissue in Heart and Great Vessels	**Includes:** 3f (Aortic) Bioprosthesis valve Bovine pericardial valve Bovine pericardium graft Contegra Pulmonary Valved Conduit CoreValve transcatheter aortic valve Epic™ Stented Tissue Valve (aortic) Freestyle (Stentless) Aortic Root Bioprosthesis Hancock Bioprosthesis (aortic) (mitral) valve Hancock Bioprosthetic Valved Conduit Melody® transcatheter pulmonary valve Mitroflow® Aortic Pericardial Heart Valve Porcine (bioprosthetic) valve SAPIEN transcatheter aortic valve SJM Biocor® Stented Valve System Stented tissue valve Trifecta™ Valve (aortic) Xenograft

SECTION 1 - OBSTETRICS CHARACTER 3 - OPERATION

Abortion	**Definition:** Artificially terminating a pregnancy
Change	**Definition:** Taking out or off a device from a body part and putting back an identical or similar device in or on the same body part without cutting or puncturing the skin or a mucous membrane **Explanation:** All CHANGE procedures are coded using the approach EXTERNAL
Delivery	**Definition:** Assisting the passage of the products of conception from the genital canal
Drainage	**Definition:** Taking or letting out fluids and/or gases from a body part **Explanation:** The qualifier DIAGNOSTIC is used to identify drainage procedures that are biopsies
Extraction	**Definition:** Pulling or stripping out or off all or a portion of a body part by the use of force **Explanation:** The qualifier DIAGNOSTIC is used to identify extraction procedures that are biopsies
Insertion	**Definition:** Putting in a nonbiological appliance that monitors, assists, performs, or prevents a physiological function but does not physically take the place of a body part
Inspection	**Definition:** Visually and/or manually exploring a body part **Explanation:** Visual exploration may be performed with or without optical instrumentation. Manual exploration may be performed directly or through intervening body layers
Removal	**Definition:** Taking out or off a device from a body part, region or orifice **Explanation:** If a device is taken out and a similar device put in without cutting or puncturing the skin or mucous membrane, the procedure is coded to the root operation CHANGE. Otherwise, the procedure for taking out a device is coded to the root operation REMOVAL
Repair	**Definition:** Restoring, to the extent possible, a body part to its normal anatomic structure and function

	Explanation: Used only when the method to accomplish the repair is not one of the other root operations
Reposition	**Definition:** Moving to its normal location, or other suitable location, all or a portion of a body part
	Explanation: The body part is moved to a new location from an abnormal location, or from a normal location where it is not functioning correctly. The body part may or may not be cut out or off to be moved to the new location
Resection	**Definition:** Cutting out or off, without replacement, all of a body part
Transplantation	**Definition:** Putting in or on all or a portion of a living body part taken from another individual or animal to physically take the place and/or function of all or a portion of a similar body part
	Explanation: The native body part may or may not be taken out, and the transplanted body part may take over all or a portion of its function

SECTION 1 - OBSTETRICS CHARACTER 5 - APPROACH

External	**Definition:** Procedures performed directly on the skin or mucous membrane and procedures performed indirectly by the application of external force through the skin or mucous membrane
Open	**Definition:** Cutting through the skin or mucous membrane and any other body layers necessary to expose the site of the procedure
Percutaneous	**Definition:** Entry, by puncture or minor incision, of instrumentation through the skin or mucous membrane and any other body layers necessary to reach the site of the procedure
Percutaneous Endoscopic	**Definition:** Entry, by puncture or minor incision, of instrumentation through the skin or mucous membrane and any other body layers necessary to reach and visualize the site of the procedure
Via Natural or Artificial Opening	**Definition:** Entry of instrumentation through a natural or artificial external opening to reach the site of the procedure
Via Natural or Artificial Opening Endoscopic	**Definition:** Entry of instrumentation through a natural or artificial external opening to reach and visualize the site of the procedure

SECTION 2 - PLACEMENT CHARACTER 3 - OPERATION

Change	**Definition:** Taking out or off a device from a body part and putting back an identical or similar device in or on the same body part without cutting or puncturing the skin or a mucous membrane
Compression	**Definition:** Putting pressure on a body region
Dressing	**Definition:** Putting material on a body region for protection
Immobilization	**Definition:** Limiting or preventing motion of a body region
Packing	**Definition:** Putting material in a body region or orifice
Removal	**Definition:** Taking out or off a device from a body part
Traction	**Definition:** Exerting a pulling force on a body region in a distal direction

SECTION 2 - PLACEMENT CHARACTER 5 - APPROACH

External	**Definition:** Procedures performed directly on the skin or mucous membrane and procedures performed indirectly by the application of external force through the skin or mucous membrane

SECTION 3 - ADMINISTRATION CHARACTER 3 - OPERATION

Introduction	**Definition:** Putting in or on a therapeutic, diagnostic, nutritional, physiological, or prophylactic substance except blood or blood products
Irrigation	**Definition:** Putting in or on a cleansing substance
Transfusion	**Definition:** Putting in blood or blood products

SECTION 3 - ADMINISTRATION CHARACTER 5 - APPROACH

External	**Definition:** Procedures performed directly on the skin or mucous membrane and procedures performed indirectly by the application of external force through the skin or mucous membrane
Open	**Definition:** Cutting through the skin or mucous membrane and any other body layers necessary to expose the site of the procedure
Percutaneous	**Definition:** Entry, by puncture or minor incision, of instrumentation through the skin or mucous membrane and any other body layers necessary to reach the site of the procedure
Via Natural or Artificial Opening	**Definition:** Entry of instrumentation through a natural or artificial external opening to reach the site of the procedure
Via Natural or Artificial Opening Endoscopic	**Definition:** Entry of instrumentation through a natural or artificial external opening to reach and visualize the site of the procedure

SECTION 4 - MEASUREMENT AND MONITORING CHARACTER 3 - OPERATION

Measurement	**Definition:** Determining the level of a physiological or physical function at a point in time
Monitoring	**Definition:** Determining the level of a physiological or physical function repetitively over a period of time

SECTION 4 - MEASUREMENT AND MONITORING CHARACTER 5 - APPROACH

External	**Definition:** Procedures performed directly on the skin or mucous membrane and procedures performed indirectly by the application of external force through the skin or mucous membrane
Open	**Definition:** Cutting through the skin or mucous membrane and any other body layers necessary to expose the site of the procedure
Percutaneous	**Definition:** Entry, by puncture or minor incision, of instrumentation through the skin or mucous membrane and any other body layers necessary to reach the site of the procedure
Percutaneous Endoscopic	**Definition:** Entry, by puncture or minor incision, of instrumentation through the skin or mucous membrane and any other body layers necessary to reach and visualize the site of the procedure
Via Natural or Artificial Opening	**Definition:** Entry of instrumentation through a natural or artificial external opening to reach the site of the procedure
Via Natural or Artificial Opening Endoscopic	**Definition:** Entry of instrumentation through a natural or artificial external opening to reach and visualize the site of the procedure

SECTION 5 - EXTRACORPOREAL ASSISTANCE AND PERFORMANCE CHARACTER 3 - OPERATION	
Assistance	**Definition:** Taking over a portion of a physiological function by extracorporeal means
Performance	**Definition:** Completely taking over a physiological function by extracorporeal means
Restoration	**Definition:** Returning, or attempting to return, a physiological function to its original state by extracorporeal means.

SECTION 6 - EXTRACORPOREAL THERAPIES CHARACTER 3 - OPERATION	
Atmospheric Control	**Definition:** Extracorporeal control of atmospheric pressure and composition
Decompression	**Definition:** Extracorporeal elimination of undissolved gas from body fluids
Electromagnetic Therapy	**Definition:** Extracorporeal treatment by electromagnetic rays
Hyperthermia	**Definition:** Extracorporeal raising of body temperature
Hypothermia	**Definition:** Extracorporeal lowering of body temperature
Pheresis	**Definition:** Extracorporeal separation of blood products
Phototherapy	**Definition:** Extracorporeal treatment by light rays
Shock Wave Therapy	**Definition:** Extracorporeal treatment by shock waves
Ultrasound Therapy	**Definition:** Extracorporeal treatment by ultrasound
Ultraviolet Light Therapy	**Definition:** Extracorporeal treatment by ultraviolet light

SECTION 7 - OSTEOPATHIC CHARACTER 3 - OPERATION	
Treatment	**Definition:** Manual treatment to eliminate or alleviate somatic dysfunction and related disorders

SECTION 7 - OSTEOPATHIC CHARACTER 5 - APPROACH	
External	**Definition:** Procedures performed directly on the skin or mucous membrane and procedures performed indirectly by the application of external force through the skin or mucous membrane

SECTION 8 - OTHER PROCEDURES CHARACTER 3 - OPERATION	
Other Procedures	**Definition:** Methodologies which attempt to remediate or cure a disorder or disease

SECTION 8 - OTHER PROCEDURES CHARACTER 5 - APPROACH	
External	**Definition:** Procedures performed directly on the skin or mucous membrane and procedures performed indirectly by the application of external force through the skin or mucous membrane
Percutaneous	**Definition:** Entry, by puncture or minor incision, of instrumentation through the skin or mucous membrane and any other body layers necessary to reach the site of the procedure
Percutaneous Endoscopic	**Definition:** Entry, by puncture or minor incision, of instrumentation through the skin or mucous membrane and any other body layers necessary to reach and visualize the site of the procedure
Via Natural or Artificial Opening	**Definition:** Entry of instrumentation through a natural or artificial external opening to reach the site of the procedure
Via Natural or Artificial Opening Endoscopic	**Definition:** Entry of instrumentation through a natural or artificial external opening to reach and visualize the site of the procedure

SECTION 9 - CHIROPRACTIC CHARACTER 3 - OPERATION	
Manipulation	**Definition:** Manual procedure that involves a directed thrust to move a joint past the physiological range of motion, without exceeding the anatomical limit

SECTION 9 - CHIROPRACTIC CHARACTER 5 - APPROACH	
External	Definition: Procedures performed directly on the skin or mucous membrane and procedures performed indirectly by the application of external force through the skin or mucous membrane

SECTION B - IMAGING CHARACTER 3 - TYPE	
Computerized Tomography (CT Scan)	**Definition:** Computer reformatted digital display of multiplanar images developed from the capture of multiple exposures of external ionizing radiation
Fluoroscopy	**Definition:** Single plane or bi-plane real time display of an image developed from the capture of external ionizing radiation on a fluorescent screen. The image may also be stored by either digital or analog means
Magnetic Resonance Imaging (MRI)	**Definition:** Computer reformatted digital display of multiplanar images developed from the capture of radiofrequency signals emitted by nuclei in a body site excited within a magnetic field
Plain Radiography	**Definition:** Planar display of an image developed from the capture of external ionizing radiation on photographic or photoconductive plate
Ultrasonography	**Definition:** Real time display of images of anatomy or flow information developed from the capture of reflected and attenuated high frequency sound waves

SECTION C - NUCLEAR MEDICINE CHARACTER 3 - TYPE	
Nonimaging Nuclear Medicine Assay	**Definition:** Introduction of radioactive materials into the body for the study of body fluids and blood elements, by the detection of radioactive emissions
Nonimaging Nuclear Medicine Probe	**Definition:** Introduction of radioactive materials into the body for the study of distribution and fate of certain substances by the detection of radioactive emissions; or, alternatively, measurement of absorption of radioactive emissions from an external source
Nonimaging Nuclear Medicine Uptake	**Definition:** Introduction of radioactive materials into the body for measurements of organ function, from the detection of radioactive emissions
Planar Nuclear Medicine Imaging	**Definition:** Introduction of radioactive materials into the body for single plane display of images developed from the capture of radioactive emissions
Positron Emission	**Definition:** Introduction of radioactive materials into the body for three dimensional display of images

Tomographic (PET) Imaging	developed from the simultaneous capture, 180 degrees apart, of radioactive emissions
Systemic Nuclear Medicine Therapy	**Definition:** Introduction of unsealed radioactive materials into the body for treatment
Tomographic (Tomo) Nuclear Medicine Imaging	**Definition:** Introduction of radioactive materials into the body for three dimensional display of images developed from the capture of radioactive emissions

SECTION F - PHYSICAL REHABILITATION AND DIAGNOSTIC AUDIOLOGY CHARACTER 3 - TYPE

Activities of Daily Living Assessment	**Definition:** Measurement of functional level for activities of daily living
Activities of Daily Living Treatment	**Definition:** Exercise or activities to facilitate functional competence for activities of daily living
Caregiver Training	**Definition:** Training in activities to support patient's optimal level of function
Cochlear Implant Treatment	**Definition:** Application of techniques to improve the communication abilities of individuals with cochlear implant
Device Fitting	**Definition:** Fitting of a device designed to facilitate or support achievement of a higher level of function
Hearing Aid Assessment	**Definition:** Measurement of the appropriateness and/or effectiveness of a hearing device
Hearing Assessment	**Definition:** Measurement of hearing and related functions
Hearing Treatment	**Definition:** Application of techniques to improve, augment, or compensate for hearing and related functional impairment
Motor and/or Nerve Function Assessment	**Definition:** Measurement of motor, nerve, and related functions
Motor Treatment	**Definition:** Exercise or activities to increase or facilitate motor function
Speech Assessment	**Definition:** Measurement of speech and related functions
Speech Treatment	**Definition:** Application of techniques to improve, augment, or compensate for speech and related functional impairment
Vestibular Assessment	**Definition:** Measurement of the vestibular system and related functions
Vestibular Treatment	**Definition:** Application of techniques to improve, augment, or compensate for vestibular and related functional impairment

SECTION F - PHYSICAL REHABILITATION AND DIAGNOSTIC AUDIOLOGY CHARACTER 5 - TYPE QUALIFIER

Acoustic Reflex Decay	**Definition:** Measures reduction in size/strength of acoustic reflex over time **Includes/Examples:** Includes site of lesion test
Acoustic Reflex Patterns	**Definition:** Defines site of lesion based upon presence/absence of acoustic reflexes with ipsilateral vs. contralateral stimulation
Acoustic Reflex Threshold	**Definition:** Determines minimal intensity that acoustic reflex occurs with ipsilateral and/or contralateral stimulation
Aerobic Capacity and Endurance	**Definition:** Measures autonomic responses to positional changes; perceived exertion, dyspnea or angina during activity; performance during exercise protocols; standard vital signs; and blood gas analysis or oxygen consumption
Alternate Binaural or Monaural Loudness Balance	**Definition:** Determines auditory stimulus parameter that yields the same objective sensation **Includes/Examples:** Sound intensities that yield same loudness perception
Anthropometric Characteristics	**Definition:** Measures edema, body fat composition, height, weight, length and girth
Aphasia (Assessment)	**Definition:** Measures expressive and receptive speech and language function including reading and writing
Aphasia (Treatment)	**Definition:** Applying techniques to improve, augment, or compensate for receptive/ expressive language impairments
Articulation/Phonology (Assessment)	**Definition:** Measures speech production
Articulation/Phonology (Treatment)	**Definition:** Applying techniques to correct, improve, or compensate for speech productive impairment
Assistive Listening Device	**Definition:** Assists in use of effective and appropriate assistive listening device/system
Assistive Listening System/Device Selection	**Definition:** Measures the effectiveness and appropriateness of assistive listening systems/devices
Assistive, Adaptive, Supportive or Protective Devices	**Explanation:** Devices to facilitate or support achievement of a higher level of function in wheelchair mobility; bed mobility; transfer or ambulation ability; bath and showering ability; dressing; grooming; personal hygiene; play or leisure
Auditory Evoked Potentials	**Definition:** Measures electric responses produced by the VIIIth cranial nerve and brainstem following auditory stimulation
Auditory Processing (Assessment)	**Definition:** Evaluates ability to receive and process auditory information and comprehension of spoken language
Auditory Processing (Treatment)	**Definition:** Applying techniques to improve the receiving and processing of auditory information and comprehension of spoken language
Augmentative/Alternative Communication System (Assessment)	**Definition:** Determines the appropriateness of aids, techniques, symbols, and/or strategies to augment or replace speech and enhance communication **Includes/Examples:** Includes the use of telephones, writing equipment, emergency equipment, and TDD
Augmentative/Alternative Communication System (Treatment)	**Includes/Examples:** Includes augmentative communication devices and aids
Aural Rehabilitation	**Definition:** Applying techniques to improve the communication abilities associated with hearing loss
Aural Rehabilitation Status	**Definition:** Measures impact of a hearing loss including evaluation of receptive and expressive communication skills
Bathing/Showering	**Includes/Examples:** Includes obtaining and using supplies; soaping, rinsing, and drying body parts; maintaining bathing position; and transferring to and from bathing positions
Bathing/Showering	**Definition:** Activities to facilitate obtaining and using supplies, soaping, rinsing and drying body parts,

Techniques	maintaining bathing position, and transferring to and from bathing positions
Bed Mobility (Assessment)	**Definition:** Transitional movement within bed
Bed Mobility (Treatment)	**Definition:** Exercise or activities to facilitate transitional movements within bed
Bedside Swallowing and Oral Function	**Includes/Examples:** Bedside swallowing includes assessment of sucking, masticating, coughing, and swallowing. Oral function includes assessment of musculature for controlled movements, structures and functions to determine coordination and phonation
Bekesy Audiometry	**Definition:** Uses an instrument that provides a choice of discrete or continuously varying pure tones; choice of pulsed or continuous signal
Binaural Electroacoustic Hearing Aid Check	**Definition:** Determines mechanical and electroacoustic function of bilateral hearing aids using hearing aid test box
Binaural Hearing Aid (Assessment)	**Definition:** Measures the candidacy, effectiveness, and appropriateness of a hearing aids **Explanation:** Measures bilateral fit
Binaural Hearing Aid (Treatment)	**Explanation:** Assists in achieving maximum understanding and performance
Bithermal, Binaural Caloric Irrigation	**Definition:** Measures the rhythmic eye movements stimulated by changing the temperature of the vestibular system
Bithermal, Monaural Caloric Irrigation	**Definition:** Measures the rhythmic eye movements stimulated by changing the temperature of the vestibular system in one ear
Brief Tone Stimuli	**Definition:** Measures specific central auditory process
Cerumen Management	**Definition:** Includes examination of external auditory canal and tympanic membrane and removal of cerumen from external ear canal
Cochlear Implant	**Definition:** Measures candidacy for cochlear implant
Cochlear Implant Rehabilitation	**Definition:** Applying techniques to improve the communication abilities of individuals with cochlear implant; includes programming the device, providing patients/families with information
Communicative/Cognitive Integration Skills (Assessment)	**Definition:** Measures ability to use higher cortical functions **Includes/Examples:** Includes orientation, recognition, attention span, initiation and termination of activity, memory, sequencing, categorizing, concept formation, spatial operations, judgment, problem solving, generalization and pragmatic communication
Communicative/Cognitive Integration Skills (Treatment)	**Definition:** Activities to facilitate the use of higher cortical functions **Includes/Examples:** Includes level of arousal, orientation, recognition, attention span, initiation and termination of activity, memory sequencing, judgment and problem solving, learning and generalization, and pragmatic communication
Computerized Dynamic Posturography	**Definition:** Measures the status of the peripheral and central vestibular system and the sensory/motor component of balance; evaluates the efficacy of vestibular rehabilitation
Conditioned Play Audiometry	**Definition:** Behavioral measures using nonspeech and speech stimuli to obtain frequency-specific and ear-specific information on auditory status from the patient **Explanation:** Obtains speech reception threshold by having patient point to pictures of spondaic words
Coordination/Dexterity (Assessment)	**Definition:** Measures large and small muscle groups for controlled goal-directed movements **Explanation:** Dexterity includes object manipulation
Coordination/Dexterity (Treatment)	**Definition:** Exercise or activities to facilitate gross coordination and fine coordination
Cranial Nerve Integrity	**Definition:** Measures cranial nerve sensory and motor functions, including tastes, smell and facial expression
Dichotic Stimuli	**Definition:** Measures specific central auditory process
Distorted Speech	**Definition:** Measures specific central auditory process
Dix-Hallpike Dynamic	**Definition:** Measures nystagmus following Dix-Hallpike maneuver
Dressing	**Includes/Examples:** Includes selecting clothing and accessories, obtaining clothing from storage, dressing and, fastening and adjusting clothing and shoes, and applying and removing personal devices, prosthesis or orthosis
Dressing Techniques	**Definition:** Activities to facilitate selecting clothing and accessories, dressing and undressing, adjusting clothing and shoes, applying and removing devices, prostheses or orthoses
Dynamic Orthosis	**Includes/Examples:** Includes customized and prefabricated splints, inhibitory casts, spinal and other braces, and protective devices; allows motion through transfer of movement from other body parts or by use of outside forces
Ear Canal Probe Microphone	**Definition:** Real ear measures
Ear Protector Attenuation	**Definition:** Measures ear protector fit and effectiveness
Electrocochleography	**Definition:** Measures the VIIIth cranial nerve action potential
Environmental, Home and Work Barriers	**Definition:** Measures current and potential barriers to optimal function, including safety hazards, access problems and home or office design
Ergonomics and Body Mechanics	**Definition:** Ergonomic measurement of job tasks, work hardening or work conditioning needs; functional capacity; and body mechanics
Eustachian Tube Function	**Definition:** Measures eustachian tube function and patency of eustachian tube
Evoked Otoacoustic Emissions, Diagnostic	**Definition:** Measures auditory evoked potentials in a diagnostic format
Evoked Otoacoustic Emissions, Screening	**Definition:** Measures auditory evoked potentials in a screening format
Facial Nerve Function	**Definition:** Measures electrical activity of the VIIth cranial nerve (facial nerve)
Feeding/Eating (Assessment)	**Includes/Examples:** Includes setting up food, selecting and using utensils and tableware, bringing food or drink to mouth, cleaning face, hands, and clothing, and management of alternative methods of nourishment
Feeding/Eating (Treatment)	**Definition:** Exercise or activities to facilitate setting up food, selecting and using utensils and tableware, bringing food or drink to mouth, cleaning face, hands, and clothing, and management of alternative methods of nourishment
Filtered Speech	**Definition:** Uses high or low pass filtered speech stimuli to assess central auditory processing disorders, site of lesion testing
Fluency (Assessment)	**Definition:** Measures speech fluency or stuttering

Fluency (Treatment)	**Definition:** Applying techniques to improve and augment fluent speech
Gait and/or Balance	**Definition:** Measures biomechanical, arthrokinematic and other spatial and temporal characteristics of gait and balance
Gait Training/Functional Ambulation	**Definition:** Exercise or activities to facilitate ambulation on a variety of surfaces and in a variety of environments
Grooming/Personal Hygiene (Assessment)	**Includes/Examples:** Includes ability to obtain and use supplies in a sequential fashion, general grooming, oral hygiene, toilet hygiene, personal care devices, including care for artificial airways
Grooming/Personal Hygiene (Treatment)	**Definition:** Activities to facilitate obtaining and using supplies in a sequential fashion: general grooming, oral hygiene, toilet hygiene, cleaning body, and personal care devices, including artificial airways
Hearing and Related Disorders Counseling	**Definition:** Provides patients/families/caregivers with information, support, referrals to facilitate recovery from a communication disorder **Includes/Examples:** Includes strategies for psychosocial adjustment to hearing loss for clients and families/caregivers
Hearing and Related Disorders Prevention	**Definition:** Provides patients/families/caregivers with information and support to prevent communication disorders
Hearing Screening	**Definition:** Pass/refer measures designed to identify need for further audiologic assessment
Home Management (Assessment)	**Definition:** Obtaining and maintaining personal and household possessions and environment **Includes/Examples:** Includes clothing care, cleaning, meal preparation and cleanup, shopping, money management, household maintenance, safety procedures, and childcare/parenting
Home Management (Treatment)	**Definition:** Activities to facilitate obtaining and maintaining personal household possessions and environment **Includes/Examples:** Includes clothing care, cleaning, meal preparation and clean-up, shopping, money management, household maintenance, safety procedures, childcare/parenting
Instrumental Swallowing and Oral Function	**Definition:** Measures swallowing function using instrumental diagnostic procedures **Explanation:** Methods include videofluoroscopy, ultrasound, manometry, endoscopy
Integumentary Integrity	**Includes/Examples:** Includes burns, skin conditions, ecchymosis, bleeding, blisters, scar tissue, wounds and other traumas, tissue mobility, turgor and texture
Manual Therapy Techniques	**Definition:** Techniques in which the therapist uses his/her hands to administer skilled movements **Includes/Examples:** Includes connective tissue massage, joint mobilization and manipulation, manual lymph drainage, manual traction, soft tissue mobilization and manipulation
Masking Patterns	**Definition:** Measures central auditory processing status
Monaural Electroacoustic Hearing Aid Check	**Definition:** Determines mechanical and electroacoustic function of one hearing aid using hearing aid test box
Monaural Hearing Aid (Assessment)	**Definition:** Measures the candidacy, effectiveness, and appropriateness of a hearing aid **Explanation:** Measures unilateral fit
Monaural Hearing Aid (Treatment)	**Explanation:** Assists in achieving maximum understanding and performance
Motor Function (Assessment)	**Definition:** Measures the body's functional and versatile movement patterns **Includes/Examples:** Includes motor assessment scales, analysis of head, trunk and limb movement, and assessment of motor learning
Motor Function (Treatment)	**Definition:** Exercise or activities to facilitate crossing midline, laterality, bilateral integration, praxis, neuromuscular relaxation, inhibition, facilitation, motor function and motor learning
Motor Speech (Assessment)	**Definition:** Measures neurological motor aspects of speech production
Motor Speech (Treatment)	**Definition:** Applying techniques to improve and augment the impaired neurological motor aspects of speech production
Muscle Performance (Assessment)	**Definition:** Measures muscle strength, power and endurance using manual testing, dynamometry or computer-assisted electromechanical muscle test; functional muscle strength, power and endurance; muscle pain, tone, or soreness; or pelvic-floor musculature **Explanation:** Muscle endurance refers to the ability to contract a muscle repeatedly over time
Muscle Performance (Treatment)	**Definition:** Exercise or activities to increase the capacity of a muscle to do work in terms of strength, power, and/or endurance **Explanation:** Muscle strength is the force exerted to overcome resistance in one maximal effort. Muscle power is work produced per unit of time, or the product of strength and speed. Muscle endurance is the ability to contract a muscle repeatedly over time
Neuromotor Development	**Definition:** Measures motor development, righting and equilibrium reactions, and reflex and equilibrium reactions
Neurophysiologic Intraoperative	**Definition:** Monitors neural status during surgery
Non-invasive Instrumental Status	**Definition:** Instrumental measures of oral, nasal, vocal, and velopharyngeal functions as they pertain to speech production
Nonspoken Language (Assessment)	**Definition:** Measures nonspoken language (print, sign, symbols) for communication
Nonspoken Language (Treatment)	**Definition:** Applying techniques that improve, augment, or compensate spoken communication
Oral Peripheral Mechanism	**Definition:** Structural measures of face, jaw, lips, tongue, teeth, hard and soft palate, pharynx as related to speech production
Orofacial Myofunctional (Assessment)	**Definition:** Measures orofacial myofunctional patterns for speech and related functions
Orofacial Myofunctional (Treatment)	**Definition:** Applying techniques to improve, alter, or augment impaired orofacial myofunctional patterns and related speech production errors
Oscillating Tracking	**Definition:** Measures ability to visually track
Pain	**Definition:** Measures muscle soreness, pain and soreness with joint movement, and pain perception **Includes/Examples:** Includes questionnaires, graphs, symptom magnification scales or visual analog scales
Perceptual Processing	**Definition:** Measures stereognosis, kinesthesia, body schema, right-left discrimination, form constancy,

(Assessment)	position in space, visual closure, figure-ground, depth perception, spatial relations and topographical orientation
Perceptual Processing (Treatment)	**Definition:** Exercise and activities to facilitate perceptual processing **Explanation:** Includes stereognosis, kinesthesia, body schema, right-left discrimination, form constancy, position in space, visual closure, figure-ground, depth perception, spatial relations, and topographical orientation **Includes/Examples:** Includes stereognosis, kinesthesia, body schema, right-left discrimination, form constancy, position in space, visual closure, figure-ground, depth perception, spatial relations, and topographical orientation
Performance Intensity Phonetically Balanced Speech Discrimination	**Definition:** Measures word recognition over varying intensity levels
Postural Control	**Definition:** Exercise or activities to increase postural alignment and control
Prosthesis	**Explanation:** Artificial substitutes for missing body parts that augment performance or function
Psychosocial Skills (Assessment)	**Definition:** The ability to interact in society and to process emotions **Includes/Examples:** Includes psychological (values, interests, self-concept); social (role performance, social conduct, interpersonal skills, self expression); self-management (coping skills, time management, self-control)
Psychosocial Skills (Treatment)	**Definition:** The ability to interact in society and to process emotions **Includes/Examples:** Includes psychological (values, interests, self-concept); social (role performance, social conduct, interpersonal skills, self expression); self-management (coping skills, time management, self-control)
Pure Tone Audiometry, Air	**Definition:** Air-conduction pure tone threshold measures with appropriate masking
Pure Tone Audiometry, Air and Bone	**Definition:** Air-conduction and bone-conduction pure tone threshold measures with appropriate masking
Pure Tone Stenger	**Definition:** Measures unilateral nonorganic hearing loss based on simultaneous presentation of pure tones of differing volume
Range of Motion and Joint Integrity	**Definition:** Measures quantity, quality, grade, and classification of joint movement and/or mobility **Explanation:** Range of Motion is the space, distance or angle through which movement occurs at a joint or series of joints. Joint integrity is the conformance of joints to expected anatomic, biomechanical and kinematic norms
Range of Motion and Joint Mobility	**Definition:** Exercise or activities to increase muscle length and joint mobility
Receptive/Expressive Language (Assessment)	**Definition:** Measures receptive and expressive language
Receptive/Expressive Language (Treatment)	**Definition:** Applying techniques tot improve and augment receptive/ expressive language
Reflex Integrity	**Definition:** Measures the presence, absence, or exaggeration of developmentally appropriate, pathologic or normal reflexes
Select Picture Audiometry	**Definition:** Establishes hearing threshold levels for speech using pictures
Sensorineural Acuity Level	**Definition:** Measures sensorineural acuity masking presented via bone conduction
Sensory Aids	**Definition:** Determines the appropriateness of a sensory prosthetic device, other than a hearing aid or assistive listening system/device
Sensory Awareness/ Processing/Integrity	**Includes/Examples:** Includes light touch, pressure, temperature, pain, sharp/dull, proprioception, vestibular, visual, auditory, gustatory, and olfactory
Short Increment Sensitivity Index	**Definition:** Measures the ear's ability to detect small intensity changes; site of lesion test requiring a behavioral response
Sinusoidal Vertical Axis Rotational	**Definition:** Measures nystagmus following rotation
Somatosensory Evoked Potentials	**Definition:** Measures neural activity from sites throughout the body
Speech and/or Language Screening	**Definition:** Identifies need for further speech and/or language evaluation
Speech Threshold	**Definition:** Measures minimal intensity needed to repeat spondaic words
Speech-Language Pathology and Related Disorders Counseling	**Definition:** Provides patients/families with information, support, referrals to facilitate recovery from a communication disorder
Speech-Language Pathology and Related Disorders Prevention	**Definition:** Applying techniques to avoid or minimize onset and/or development of a communication disorder
Speech/Word Recognition	**Definition:** Measures ability to repeat/identify single syllable words; scores given as a percentage; includes word recognition/ speech discrimination
Staggered Spondaic Word	**Definition:** Measures central auditory processing site of lesion based upon dichotic presentation of spondaic words
Static Orthosis	**Includes/Examples:** Includes customized and prefabricated splints, inhibitory casts, spinal and other braces, and protective devices; has no moving parts, maintains joint(s) in desired position
Stenger	**Definition:** Measures unilateral nonorganic hearing loss based on simultaneous presentation of signals of differing volume
Swallowing Dysfunction	**Definition:** Activities to improve swallowing function in coordination with respiratory function **Includes/Examples:** Includes function and coordination of sucking, mastication, coughing, swallowing
Synthetic Sentence Identification	**Definition:** Measures central auditory dysfunction using identification of third order approximations of sentences and competing messages
Temporal Ordering of Stimuli	**Definition:** Measures specific central auditory process
Therapeutic Exercise	**Definition:** Exercise or activities to facilitate sensory awareness, sensory processing, sensory integration,

	balance training, conditioning, reconditioning **Includes/Examples:** Includes developmental activities, breathing exercises, aerobic endurance activities, aquatic exercises, stretching and ventilatory muscle training
Tinnitus Masker (Assessment)	**Definition:** Determines candidacy for tinnitus masker
Tinnitus Masker (Treatment)	**Explanation:** Used to verify physical fit, acoustic appropriateness, and benefit; assists in achieving maximum benefit
Transfer	**Definition:** Transitional movement from one surface to another
Transfer Training	**Definition:** Exercise or activities to facilitate movement from one surface to another
Tympanometry	**Definition:** Measures the integrity of the middle ear; measures ease at which sound flows through the tympanic membrane while air pressure against the membrane is varied
Unithermal Binaural Screen	**Definition:** Measures the rhythmic eye movements stimulated by changing the temperature of the vestibular system in both ears using warm water, screening format
Ventilation, Respiration and Circulation	**Definition:** Measures ventilatory muscle strength, power and endurance, pulmonary function and ventilatory mechanics **Includes/Examples:** Includes ability to clear airway, activities that aggravate or relieve edema, pain, dyspnea or other symptoms, chest wall mobility, cardiopulmonary response to performance of ADL and IAD, cough and sputum, standard vital signs
Vestibular	**Definition:** Applying techniques to compensate for balance disorders; includes habituation, exercise therapy, and balance retraining
Visual Motor Integration (Assessment)	**Definition:** Coordinating the interaction of information from the eyes with body movement during activity
Visual Motor Integration (Treatment)	**Definition:** Exercise or activities to facilitate coordinating the interaction of information from eyes with body movement during activity
Visual Reinforcement Audiometry	**Definition:** Behavioral measures using nonspeech and speech stimuli to obtain frequency/ear-specific information on auditory status **Includes/Examples:** Includes a conditioned response of looking toward a visual reinforcer (e.g., lights, animated toy) every time auditory stimuli are heard
Vocational Activities and Functional Community or Work Reintegration Skills (Assessment)	**Definition:** Measures environmental, home, work (job/school/play) barriers that keep patients from functioning optimally in their environment **Includes/Examples:** Includes assessment of vocational skill and interests, environment of work (job/school/play), injury potential and injury prevention or reduction, ergonomic stressors, transportation skills, and ability to access and use community resources
Vocational Activities and Functional Community or Work Reintegration Skills (Treatment)	**Definition:** Activities to facilitate vocational exploration, body mechanics training, job acquisition, and environmental or work (job/ school/play) task adaptation **Includes/Examples:** Includes injury prevention and reduction, ergonomic stressor reduction, job coaching and simulation, work hardening and conditioning, driving training, transportation skills, and use of community resources
Voice (Assessment)	**Definition:** Measures vocal structure, function and production
Voice (Treatment)	**Definition:** Applying techniques to improve voice and vocal function
Voice Prosthetic (Assessment)	**Definition:** Determines the appropriateness of voice prosthetic/adaptive device to enhance or facilitate communication
Voice Prosthetic (Treatment)	**Includes/Examples:** Includes electrolarynx, and other assistive, adaptive, supportive devices
Wheelchair Mobility (Assessment)	**Definition:** Measures fit and functional abilities within wheelchair in a variety of environments
Wheelchair Mobility (Treatment)	**Definition:** Management, maintenance and controlled operation of a wheelchair, scooter or other device, in and on a variety of surfaces and environments
Wound Management	**Includes/Examples:** Includes non-selective and selective debridement (enzymes, autolysis, sharp debridement), dressings (wound coverings, hydrogel, vacuum-assisted closure), topical agents, etc.

SECTION G - MENTAL HEALTH CHARACTER 3 - TYPE	
Biofeedback	**Definition:** Provision of information from the monitoring and regulating of physiological processes in conjunction with cognitive-behavioral techniques to improve patient functioning or well-being **Includes/Examples:** Includes EEG, blood pressure, skin temperature or peripheral blood flow, ECG, electrooculogram, EMG, respiratory or capnometry, GSR/EDR, perineometry to monitor/regulate bowel/bladder activity, electrogastrogram to monitor/ regulate gastric motility
Counseling	**Definition:** The application of psychological methods to treat an individual with normal developmental issues and psychological problems in order to increase function, improve well-being, alleviate distress, maladjustment or resolve crises
Crisis Intervention	**Definition:** Treatment of a traumatized, acutely disturbed or distressed individual for the purpose of short-term stabilization **Includes/Examples:** Includes defusing, debriefing, counseling, psychotherapy and/ or coordination of care with other providers or agencies
Electroconvulsive Therapy	**Definition:** The application of controlled electrical voltages to treat a mental health disorder **Includes/Examples:** Includes appropriate sedation and other preparation of the individual
Family Psychotherapy	**Definition:** Treatment that includes one or more family members of an individual with a mental health disorder by behavioral, cognitive, psychoanalytic, psychodynamic or psychophysiological means to improve functioning or well-being **Explanation:** Remediation of emotional or behavioral problems presented by one or more family members in cases where psychotherapy with more than one family member is indicated
Group Psychotherapy	**Definition:** Treatment of two or more individuals with a mental health disorder by behavioral, cognitive, psychoanalytic, psychodynamic or psychophysiological means to improve functioning or well-being
Hypnosis	**Definition:** Induction of a state of heightened suggestibility by auditory, visual and tactile techniques to elicit an emotional or behavioral response
Individual Psychotherapy	**Definition:** Treatment of an individual with a mental health disorder by behavioral, cognitive, psychoanalytic, psychodynamic or psychophysiological means to improve functioning or well-being

Light Therapy	**Definition:** Application of specialized light treatments to improve functioning or well-being
Medication Management	**Definition:** Monitoring and adjusting the use of medications for the treatment of a mental health disorder
Narcosynthesis	**Definition:** Administration of intravenous barbiturates in order to release suppressed or repressed thoughts
Psychological Tests	**Definition:** The administration and interpretation of standardized psychological tests and measurement instruments for the assessment of psychological function

SECTION G - MENTAL HEALTH CHARACTER 4 - QUALIFIER

Behavioral	**Definition:** Primarily to modify behavior **Includes/Examples:** Includes modeling and role playing, positive reinforcement of target behaviors, response cost, and training of self-management skills
Cognitive	**Definition:** Primarily to correct cognitive distortions and errors
Cognitive-Behavioral	**Definition:** Combining cognitive and behavioral treatment strategies to improve functioning **Explanation:** Maladaptive responses are examined to determine how cognitions relate to behavior patterns in response to an event. Uses learning principles and information-processing models
Developmental	**Definition:** Age-normed developmental status of cognitive, social and adaptive behavior skills
Intellectual and Psychoeducational	**Definition:** Intellectual abilities, academic achievement and learning capabilities (including behaviors and emotional factors affecting learning
Interactive	**Definition:** Uses primarily physical aids and other forms of non-oral interaction with a patient who is physically, psychologically or developmentally unable to use ordinary language for communication **Includes/Examples:** Includes. the use of toys in symbolic play
Interpersonal	**Definition:** Helps an individual make changes in interpersonal behaviors to reduce psychological dysfunction **Includes/Examples:** Includes exploratory techniques, encouragement of affective expression, clarification of patient statements, analysis of communication patterns, use of therapy relationship and behavior change techniques
Neurobehavioral and Cognitive Status	**Definition:** Includes neurobehavioral status exam, interview(s), and observation for the clinical assessment of thinking, reasoning and judgment, acquired knowledge, attention, memory, visual spatial abilities, language functions, and planning
Neuropsychological	**Definition:** Thinking, reasoning and judgment, acquired knowledge, attention, memory, visual spatial abilities, language functions, planning
Personality and Behavioral	**Definition:** Mood, emotion, behavior, social functioning, psychopathological conditions, personality traits and characteristics
Psychoanalysis	**Definition:** Methods of obtaining a detailed account of past and present mental and emotional experiences to determine the source and eliminate or diminish the undesirable effects of unconscious conflicts **Explanation:** Accomplished by making the individual aware of their existence, origin, and inappropriate expression in emotions and behavior
Psychodynamic	**Definition:** Exploration of past and present emotional experiences to understand motives and drives using insight-oriented techniques to reduce the undesirable effects of internal conflicts on emotions and behavior **Explanation:** Techniques include empathetic listening, clarifying self-defeating behavior patterns, and exploring adaptive alternatives
Psychophysiological	**Definition:** Monitoring and alteration of physiological processes to help the individual associate physiological reactions combined with cognitive and behavioral strategies to gain improved control of these processes to help the individual cope more effectively
Supportive	**Definition:** Formation of therapeutic relationship primarily for providing emotional support to prevent further deterioration in functioning during periods of particular stress **Explanation:** Often used in conjunction with other therapeutic approaches
Vocational	**Definition:** Exploration of vocational interests, aptitudes and required adaptive behavior skills to develop and carry out a plan for achieving a successful vocational placement **Includes/Examples:** Includes enhancing work related adjustment and/or pursuing viable options in training education or preparation

SECTION H - SUBSTANCE ABUSE TREATMENT CHARACTER 3 - TYPE

Detoxification Services	**Definition:** Detoxification from alcohol and/or drugs **Explanation:** Not a treatment modality, but helps the patient stabilize physically and psychologically until the body becomes free of drugs and the effects of alcohol
Family Counseling	**Definition:** The application of psychological methods that includes one or more family members to treat an individual with addictive behavior **Explanation:** Provides support and education for family members of addicted individuals. Family member participation is seen as a critical area of substance abuse treatment
Group Counseling	**Definition:** The application of psychological methods to treat two or more individuals with addictive behavior **Explanation:** Provides structured group counseling sessions and healing power through the connection with others
Individual Counseling	**Definition:** The application of psychological methods to treat an individual with addictive behavior **Explanation:** Comprised of several different techniques, which apply various strategies to address drug addiction
Individual Psychotherapy	**Definition:** Treatment of an individual with addictive behavior by behavioral, cognitive, psychoanalytic, psychodynamic or psychophysiological means
Medication Management	**Definition:** Monitoring and adjusting the use of replacement medications for the treatment of addiction
Pharmacotherapy	**Definition:** The use of replacement medications for the treatment of addiction

Body Part	PCS Description
3f (Aortic) Bioprosthesis valve	Zooplastic tissue in heart and great vessels
AbioCor® Total Replacement Heart	Synthetic substitute
Abdominal aortic plexus	Abdominal Sympathetic Nerve
Abdominal esophagus	Esophagus, Lower
Abductor hallucis muscle	Foot Muscle, Right Foot Muscle, Left
Accessory cephalic vein	Cephalic Vein, Right Cephalic Vein, Left
Accessory obturator nerve	Lumbar Plexus
Accessory phrenic nerve	Phrenic Nerve
Accessory spleen	Spleen
Acetabulofemoral joint	Hip Joint, Right Hip Joint, Left
Achilles tendon	Lower Leg Tendon, Right Lower Leg Tendon, Left
Acromioclavicular ligament	Shoulder Bursa And Ligament, Right Shoulder Bursa And Ligament, Left
Acromion (process)	Scapula, Right Scapula, Left
Adductor brevis muscle	Upper Leg Muscle, Right Upper Leg Muscle, Left
Adductor hallucis muscle	Foot Muscle, Right Foot Muscle, Left
Adductor longus muscle	Upper Leg Muscle, Right Upper Leg Muscle, Left
Adductor magnus muscle	Upper Leg Muscle, Right Upper Leg Muscle, Left
Adenohypophysis	Pituitary Gland
Alar ligament of axis	Head And Neck Bursa And Ligament
Alveolar process of mandible	Mandible, Right Mandible, Left
Alveolar process of maxilla	Maxilla, Right Maxilla, Left
Anal orifice	Anus
Anatomical snuffbox	Lower Arm And Wrist Muscle, Right Lower Arm And Wrist Muscle, Left
Angular artery	Face Artery
Angular vein	Face Vein, Right Face Vein, Left
Annular ligament	Elbow Bursa And Ligament, Right Elbow Bursa And Ligament, Left
Anorectal junction	Rectum
Ansa cervicalis	Cervical Plexus
Antebrachial fascia	Subcutaneous Tissue And Fascia, Right Lower Arm Subcutaneous Tissue And Fascia, Left Lower Arm
Anterior (pectoral) lymph node	Lymphatic, Right Axillary Lymphatic, Left Axillary
Anterior cerebral artery	Intracranial Artery
Anterior cerebral vein	Intracranial Vein
Anterior choroidal artery	Intracranial Artery
Anterior circumflex humeral artery	Axillary Artery, Right Axillary Artery, Left
Anterior communicating artery	Intracranial Artery
Anterior cruciate ligament (ACL)	Knee Bursa And Ligament, Right Knee Bursa And Ligament, Left
Anterior crural nerve	Femoral Nerve

Body Part	PCS Description
Anterior facial vein	Face Vein, Right Face Vein, Left
Anterior intercostal artery	Internal Mammary Artery, Right Internal Mammary Artery, Left
Anterior interosseous nerve	Median Nerve
Anterior lateral malleolar artery	Anterior Tibial Artery, Right Anterior Tibial Artery, Left
Anterior lingual gland	Minor Salivary Gland
Anterior medial malleolar artery	Anterior Tibial Artery, Right Anterior Tibial Artery, Left
Anterior spinal artery	Vertebral Artery, Right Vertebral Artery, Left
Anterior tibial recurrent artery	Anterior Tibial Artery, Right Anterior Tibial Artery, Left
Anterior ulnar recurrent artery	Ulnar Artery, Right Ulnar Artery, Left
Anterior vagal trunk	Vagus Nerve
Anterior vertebral muscle	Neck Muscle, Right Neck Muscle, Left
Antihelix Antitragus	External Ear, Right External Ear, Left External Ear, Bilateral
Antrum of Highmore	Maxillary Sinus, Right Maxillary Sinus, Left
Aortic annulus	Aortic Valve
Aortic arch Aortic intercostal artery	Thoracic Aorta
Apical (subclavicular) lymph node	Lymphatic, Right Axillary Lymphatic, Left Axillary
Apneustic center	Pons
Aqueduct of Sylvius	Cerebral Ventricle
Aqueous humor	Anterior Chamber, Right Anterior Chamber, Left
Arachnoid mater	Cerebral Meninges Spinal Meninges
Arcuate artery	Foot Artery, Right Foot Artery, Left
Areola	Nipple, Right Nipple, Left
Arterial canal (duct)	Pulmonary Artery, Left
Aryepiglottic fold	Larynx
Arytenoid cartilage	Larynx
Arytenoid muscle	Neck Muscle, Right Neck Muscle, Left
Ascending aorta	Thoracic Aorta
Ascending palatine artery	Face Artery
Ascending pharyngeal artery	External Carotid Artery, Right External Carotid Artery, Left
Atlantoaxial joint	Cervical Vertebral Joint
Atrioventricular node	Conduction Mechanism
Atrium dextrum cordis	Atrium, Right
Atrium pulmonale	Atrium, Left
Auditory tube	Eustachian Tube, Right Eustachian Tube, Left
Auerbach's (myenteric) plexus	Abdominal Sympathetic Nerve
Auricle	External Ear, Right External Ear, Left External Ear, Bilateral
Auricularis muscle	Head Muscle
Axillary fascia	Subcutaneous Tissue And Fascia, Right Upper Arm Subcutaneous Tissue And Fascia, Left Upper Arm
Axillary nerve	Brachial Plexus
Bartholin's (greater vestibular) gland	Vestibular Gland
Basal (internal) cerebral vein	Intracranial Vein

Body Part	PCS Description
Basal nuclei	Basal Ganglia
Basilar artery	Intracranial Artery
Basis pontis	Pons
Biceps brachii muscle	Upper Arm Muscle, Right
	Upper Arm Muscle, Left
Biceps femoris muscle	Upper Leg Muscle, Right
	Upper Leg Muscle, Left
Bicipital aponeurosis	Subcutaneous Tissue And Fascia, Right Lower Arm
	Subcutaneous Tissue And Fascia, Left Lower Arm
Bicuspid valve	Mitral Valve
Body of femur	Femoral Shaft, Right
	Femoral Shaft, Left
Body of fibula	Fibula, Right
	Fibula, Left
Bony labyrinth	Inner Ear, Right
	Inner Ear, Left
Bony orbit	Orbit, Right
	Orbit, Left
Bony vestibule	Inner Ear, Right
	Inner Ear, Left
Botallo's duct	Pulmonary Artery, Left
Brachial (lateral) lymph node	Lymphatic, Right Axillary
	Lymphatic, Left Axillary
Brachialis muscle	Upper Arm Muscle, Right
	Upper Arm Muscle, Left
Brachiocephalic artery	Innominate Artery
Brachiocephalic trunk	Innominate Artery
Brachiocephalic vein	Innominate Vein, Right
	Innominate Vein, Left
Brachioradialis muscle	Lower Arm And Wrist Muscle, Right
	Lower Arm And Wrist Muscle, Left
Broad ligament	Uterine Supporting Structure
Bronchial artery	Thoracic Aorta
Buccal gland	Buccal Mucosa
Buccinator lymph node	Lymphatic, Head
Buccinator muscle	Facial Muscle
Bulbospongiosus muscle	Perineum Muscle
Bulbourethral (Cowper's) gland	Urethra
Bundle of His Bundle of Kent	Conduction Mechanism
Calcaneocuboid joint	Tarsal Joint, Right
	Tarsal Joint, Left
Calcaneocuboid ligament	Foot Bursa And Ligament, Right
	Foot Bursa And Ligament, Left
Calcaneofibular ligament	Ankle Bursa And Ligament, Right
	Ankle Bursa And Ligament, Left
Calcaneus	Tarsal, Right
	Tarsal, Left
Capitate bone	Carpal, Right
	Carpal, Left
Cardia	Esophagogastric Junction
Cardiac plexus	Thoracic Sympathetic Nerve
Cardioesophageal junction	Esophagogastric Junction
Caroticotympanic artery	Internal Carotid Artery, Right
	Internal Carotid Artery, Left
Carotid glomus	Carotid Body, Left
	Carotid Body, Right
	Carotid Bodies, Bilateral
Carotid sinus	Internal Carotid Artery, Right
	Internal Carotid Artery, Left
Carotid sinus nerve	Glossopharyngeal Nerve
Carpometacarpal (CMC) joint	Metacarpocarpal Joint, Right
	Metacarpocarpal Joint, Left

Body Part	PCS Description
Carpometacarpal ligament	Hand Bursa And Ligament, Right
	Hand Bursa And Ligament, Left
Cauda equina	Lumbar Spinal Cord
Cavernous plexus	Head And Neck Sympathetic Nerve
Celiac (solar) plexus	Abdominal Sympathetic Nerve
Celiac ganglion	Abdominal Sympathetic Nerve
Celiac lymph node	Lymphatic, Aortic
Celiac trunk	Celiac Artery
Central axillary lymph node	Lymphatic, Right Axillary
	Lymphatic, Left Axillary
Cerebral aqueduct (Sylvius)	Cerebral Ventricle
Cerebrum	Brain
Cervical esophagus	Esophagus, Upper
Cervical facet joint	Cervical Vertebral Joint
	Cervical Vertebral Joints, 2 Or More
Cervical ganglion	Head And Neck Sympathetic Nerve
Cervical interspinous ligament	Head And Neck Bursa And Ligament
Cervical intertransverse ligament	Head And Neck Bursa And Ligament
Cervical ligamentum flavum	Head And Neck Bursa And Ligament
Cervical lymph node	Lymphatic, Right Neck
	Lymphatic, Left Neck
Cervicothoracic facet joint	Cervicothoracic Vertebral Joint
Choana	Nasopharynx
Chondroglossus muscle	Tongue, Palate, Pharynx Muscle
Chorda tympani	Facial Nerve
Choroid plexus	Cerebral Ventricle
Ciliary body	Eye, Right
	Eye, Left
Ciliary ganglion	Head And Neck Sympathetic Nerve
Circle of Willis	Intracranial Artery
Circumflex iliac artery	Femoral Artery, Right
	Femoral Artery, Left
Claustrum	Basal Ganglia
Coccygeal body	Coccygeal Glomus
Coccygeus muscle	Trunk Muscle, Right
	Trunk Muscle, Left
Cochlea	Inner Ear, Right
	Inner Ear, Left
Cochlear nerve	Acoustic Nerve
Columella	Nose
Common digital vein	Foot Vein, Right
	Foot Vein, Left
Common facial vein	Face Vein, Right
	Face Vein, Left
Common fibular nerve	Peroneal Nerve
Common hepatic artery	Hepatic Artery
Common iliac (subaortic) lymph node	Lymphatic, Pelvis
Common interosseous artery	Ulnar Artery, Right
	Ulnar Artery, Left
Common peroneal nerve	Peroneal Nerve
Condyloid process	Mandible, Right
	Mandible, Left
Conus arteriosus	Ventricle, Right
Conus medullaris	Lumbar Spinal Cord
Coracoacromial ligament	Shoulder Bursa And Ligament, Right
	Shoulder Bursa And Ligament, Left
Coracobrachialis muscle	Upper Arm Muscle, Right
	Upper Arm Muscle, Left

Body Part	PCS Description
Coracoclavicular ligament	Shoulder Bursa And Ligament, Right Shoulder Bursa And Ligament, Left
Coracohumeral ligament	Shoulder Bursa And Ligament, Right Shoulder Bursa And Ligament, Left
Coracoid process	Scapula, Right Scapula, Left
Corniculate cartilage	Larynx
Corpus callosum	Brain
Corpus cavernosum Corpus spongiosum	Penis
Corpus striatum	Basal Ganglia
Corrugator supercilii muscle	Facial Muscle
Costocervical trunk	Subclavian Artery, Right Subclavian Artery, Left
Costoclavicular ligament	Shoulder Bursa And Ligament, Right Shoulder Bursa And Ligament, Left
Costotransverse joint	Thoracic Vertebral Joint Thoracic Vertebral Joints, 2 To 7 Thoracic Vertebral Joints, 8 Or More
Costotransverse ligament	Thorax Bursa And Ligament, Right Thorax Bursa And Ligament, Left
Costovertebral joint	Thoracic Vertebral Joint Thoracic Vertebral Joints, 2 To 7 Thoracic Vertebral Joints, 8 Or More
Costoxiphoid ligament	Thorax Bursa And Ligament, Right Thorax Bursa And Ligament, Left
Cowper's (bulbourethral) gland	Urethra
Cranial dura mater	Dura Mater
Cranial epidural space	Epidural Space
Cranial subarachnoid space	Subarachnoid Space
Cranial subdural space	Subdural Space
Cremaster muscle	Perineum Muscle
Cribriform plate	Ethmoid Bone, Right Ethmoid Bone, Left
Cricoid cartilage	Larynx
Cricothyroid artery	Thyroid Artery, Right Thyroid Artery, Left
Cricothyroid muscle	Neck Muscle, Right Neck Muscle, Left
Crural fascia	Subcutaneous Tissue And Fascia, Right Upper Leg Subcutaneous Tissue And Fascia, Left Upper Leg
Cubital lymph node	Lymphatic, Right Upper Extremity Lymphatic, Left Upper Extremity
Cubital nerve	Ulnar Nerve
Cuboid bone	Tarsal, Right Tarsal, Left
Cuboideonavicular joint	Tarsal Joint, Right Tarsal Joint, Left
Culmen	Cerebellum
Cuneiform cartilage	Larynx

Body Part	PCS Description
Cuneonavicular joint	Tarsal Joint, Right Tarsal Joint, Left
Cuneonavicular ligament	Foot Bursa And Ligament, Right Foot Bursa And Ligament, Left
Cutaneous (transverse) cervical nerve	Cervical Plexus
Deep cervical fascia	Subcutaneous Tissue And Fascia, Anterior Neck
Deep cervical vein	Vertebral Vein, Right Vertebral Vein, Left
Deep circumflex iliac artery	External Iliac Artery, Right External Iliac Artery, Left
Deep facial vein	Face Vein, Right Face Vein, Left
Deep femoral (profunda femoris) vein	Femoral Vein, Right Femoral Vein, Left
Deep femoral artery	Femoral Artery, Right Femoral Artery, Left
Deep palmar arch	Hand Artery, Right Hand Artery, Left
Deep transverse perineal muscle	Perineum Muscle
Deferential artery	Internal Iliac Artery, Right Internal Iliac Artery, Left
Deltoid fascia	Subcutaneous Tissue And Fascia, Right Upper Arm Subcutaneous Tissue And Fascia, Left Upper Arm
Deltoid ligament	Ankle Bursa And Ligament, Right Ankle Bursa And Ligament, Left
Deltoid muscle	Shoulder Muscle, Right Shoulder Muscle, Left
Deltopectoral (infraclavicular) lymph node	Lymphatic, Right Upper Extremity Lymphatic, Left Upper Extremity
Dentate ligament	Dura Mater
Denticulate ligament	Spinal Cord
Depressor anguli oris muscle	Facial Muscle
Depressor labii inferioris muscle	Facial Muscle
Depressor septi nasi muscle	Facial Muscle
Depressor supercilii muscle	Facial Muscle
Dermis	Skin
Descending genicular artery	Femoral Artery, Right Femoral Artery, Left
Diaphragma sellae	Dura Mater
Distal humerus	Humeral Shaft, Right Humeral Shaft, Left
Distal humerus, involving joint	Elbow Joint, Right Elbow Joint, Left
Distal radioulnar joint	Wrist Joint, Right Wrist Joint, Left
Dorsal digital nerve	Radial Nerve
Dorsal metacarpal vein	Hand Vein, Right Hand Vein, Left
Dorsal metatarsal artery	Foot Artery, Right Foot Artery, Left
Dorsal metatarsal vein	Foot Vein, Right Foot Vein, Left
Dorsal scapular artery	Subclavian Artery, Right Subclavian Artery, Left
Dorsal scapular nerve	Brachial Plexus
Dorsal venous arch	Foot Vein, Right Foot Vein, Left
Dorsalis pedis artery	Anterior Tibial Artery, Right Anterior Tibial Artery, Left
Duct of Santorini	Pancreatic Duct, Accessory

Body Part	PCS Description
Duct of Wirsung	Pancreatic Duct
Ductus deferens	Vas Deferens, Right Vas Deferens, Left Vas Deferens, Bilateral Vas Deferens
Duodenal ampulla	Ampulla Of Vater
Duodenojejunal flexure	Jejunum
Dural venous sinus	Intracranial Vein
Earlobe	External Ear, Right External Ear, Left External Ear, Bilateral
Eighth cranial nerve	Acoustic Nerve
Ejaculatory duct	Vas Deferens, Right Vas Deferens, Left Vas Deferens, Bilateral Vas Deferens
Eleventh cranial nerve	Accessory Nerve
Encephalon	Brain
Ependyma	Cerebral Ventricle
Epidermis	Skin
Epiploic foramen	Peritoneum
Epithalamus	Thalamus
Epitrochlear lymph node	Lymphatic, Right Upper Extremity Lymphatic, Left Upper Extremity
Erector spinae muscle	Trunk Muscle, Right Trunk Muscle, Left
Esophageal artery	Thoracic Aorta
Esophageal plexus	Thoracic Sympathetic Nerve
Ethmoidal air cell	Ethmoid Sinus, Right Ethmoid Sinus, Left
Extensor carpi radialis muscle	Lower Arm And Wrist Muscle, Right Lower Arm And Wrist Muscle, Left
Extensor carpi ulnaris muscle	Lower Arm And Wrist Muscle, Right Lower Arm And Wrist Muscle, Left
Extensor digitorum brevis muscle	Foot Muscle, Right Foot Muscle, Left
Extensor digitorum longus muscle	Lower Leg Muscle, Right Lower Leg Muscle, Left
Extensor hallucis brevis muscle	Foot Muscle, Right Foot Muscle, Left
Extensor hallucis longus muscle	Lower Leg Muscle, Right Lower Leg Muscle, Left
External anal sphincter	Anal Sphincter
External auditory meatus	External Auditory Canal, Right External Auditory Canal, Left
External maxillary artery	Face Artery
External naris	Nose
External oblique aponeurosis	Subcutaneous Tissue And Fascia, Trunk
External oblique muscle	Abdomen Muscle, Right Abdomen Muscle, Left
External popliteal nerve	Peroneal Nerve
External pudendal artery	Femoral Artery, Right Femoral Artery, Left
External pudendal vein	Greater Saphenous Vein, Right Greater Saphenous Vein, Left
External urethral sphincter	Urethra
Extradural space	Epidural Space
Facial artery	Face Artery
False vocal cord	Larynx
Falx cerebri	Dura Mater
Fascia lata	Subcutaneous Tissue And Fascia, Right Upper Leg Subcutaneous Tissue And Fascia,

Body Part	PCS Description
	Left Upper Leg
Femoral head	Upper Femur, Right Upper Femur, Left
Femoral lymph node	Lymphatic, Right Lower Extremity Lymphatic, Left Lower Extremity
Femoropatellar joint	Knee Joint, Right Knee Joint, Left
Femorotibial joint	Knee Joint, Right Knee Joint, Left
Fibular artery	Peroneal Artery, Right Peroneal Artery, Left
Fibularis brevis muscle	Lower Leg Muscle, Right Lower Leg Muscle, Left
Fibularis longus muscle	Lower Leg Muscle, Right Lower Leg Muscle, Left
Fifth cranial nerve	Trigeminal Nerve
First cranial nerve	Olfactory Nerve
First intercostal nerve	Brachial Plexus
Flexor carpi radialis muscle	Lower Arm And Wrist Muscle, Right Lower Arm And Wrist Muscle, Left
Flexor carpi ulnaris muscle	Lower Arm And Wrist Muscle, Right Lower Arm And Wrist Muscle, Left
Flexor digitorum brevis muscle	Foot Muscle, Right Foot Muscle, Left
Flexor digitorum longus muscle	Lower Leg Muscle, Right Lower Leg Muscle, Left
Flexor hallucis brevis muscle	Foot Muscle, Right Foot Muscle, Left
Flexor hallucis longus muscle	Lower Leg Muscle, Right Lower Leg Muscle, Left
Flexor pollicis longus muscle	Lower Arm And Wrist Muscle, Right Lower Arm And Wrist Muscle, Left
Foramen magnum	Occipital Bone, Right Occipital Bone, Left
Foramen of Monro (intraventricular)	Cerebral Ventricle
Foreskin	Prepuce
Fossa of Rosenmüller	Nasopharynx
Fourth cranial nerve	Trochlear Nerve
Fourth ventricle	Cerebral Ventricle
Fovea	Retina, Right Retina, Left
Frenulum labii inferioris	Lower Lip
Frenulum labii superioris	Upper Lip
Frenulum linguae	Tongue
Frontal lobe	Cerebral Hemisphere
Frontal vein	Face Vein, Right Face Vein, Left
Fundus uteri	Uterus
Galea aponeurotica	Subcutaneous Tissue And Fascia, Scalp
Ganglion impar (ganglion of Walther)	Sacral Sympathetic Nerve
Gasserian ganglion	Trigeminal Nerve
Gastric lymph node	Lymphatic, Aortic
Gastric plexus	Abdominal Sympathetic Nerve
Gastrocnemius muscle	Lower Leg Muscle, Right Lower Leg Muscle, Left
Gastrocolic ligament	Greater Omentum
Gastrocolic omentum	Greater Omentum
Gastroduodenal artery	Hepatic Artery
Gastroesophageal (GE) junction	Esophagogastric Junction

Body Part	PCS Description
Gastrohepatic omentum	Lesser Omentum
Gastrophrenic ligament	Greater Omentum
Gastrosplenic ligament	Greater Omentum
Gemellus muscle	Hip Muscle, Right Hip Muscle, Left
Geniculate ganglion	Facial Nerve
Geniculate nucleus	Thalamus
Genioglossus muscle	Tongue, Palate, Pharynx Muscle
Genitofemoral nerve	Lumbar Plexus
Glans penis	Prepuce
Glenohumeral joint	Shoulder Joint, Right Shoulder Joint, Left
Glenohumeral ligament	Shoulder Bursa And Ligament, Right Shoulder Bursa And Ligament, Left
Glenoid fossa (of scapula)	Glenoid Cavity, Right Glenoid Cavity, Left
Glenoid ligament (labrum)	Shoulder Bursa And Ligament, Right Shoulder Bursa And Ligament, Left
Globus pallidus	Basal Ganglia
Glossoepiglottic fold	Epiglottis
Glottis	Larynx
Gluteal lymph node	Lymphatic, Pelvis
Gluteal vein	Hypogastric Vein, Right Hypogastric Vein, Left
Gluteus maximus muscle	Hip Muscle, Right Hip Muscle, Left
Gluteus medius muscle	Hip Muscle, Right Hip Muscle, Left
Gluteus minimus muscle	Hip Muscle, Right Hip Muscle, Left
Gracilis muscle	Upper Leg Muscle, Right Upper Leg Muscle, Left
Great auricular nerve	Cervical Plexus
Great cerebral vein	Intracranial Vein
Great saphenous vein	Greater Saphenous Vein, Right Greater Saphenous Vein, Left
Greater alar cartilage	Nose
Greater occipital nerve	Cervical Nerve
Greater splanchnic nerve	Thoracic Sympathetic Nerve
Greater superficial petrosal nerve	Facial Nerve
Greater trochanter	Upper Femur, Right Upper Femur, Left
Greater tuberosity	Humeral Head, Right Humeral Head, Left
Greater vestibular (Bartholin's) gland	Vestibular Gland
Greater wing	Sphenoid Bone, Right Sphenoid Bone, Left
Hallux	1st Toe, Right 1st Toe, Left
Hamate bone	Carpal, Right Carpal, Left
Head of fibula	Fibula, Right Fibula, Left
Helix	External Ear, Right External Ear, Left External Ear, Bilateral
Hepatic artery proper	Hepatic Artery
Hepatic flexure	Ascending Colon
Hepatic lymph node	Lymphatic, Aortic
Hepatic plexus	Abdominal Sympathetic Nerve
Hepatic portal vein	Portal Vein
Hepatogastric ligament	Lesser Omentum
Hepatopancreatic ampulla	Ampulla Of Vater

Body Part	PCS Description
Humeroradial joint	Elbow Joint, Right Elbow Joint, Left
Humeroulnar joint	Elbow Joint, Right Elbow Joint, Left
Humerus, distal	Humeral Shaft, Right Humeral Shaft, Left
Hyoglossus muscle	Tongue, Palate, Pharynx Muscle
Hyoid artery	Thyroid Artery, Right Thyroid Artery, Left
Hypogastric artery	Internal Iliac Artery, Right Internal Iliac Artery, Left
Hypopharynx	Pharynx
Hypophysis	Pituitary Gland
Hypothenar muscle	Hand Muscle, Right Hand Muscle, Left
Ileal artery Ileocolic artery	Superior Mesenteric Artery
Ileocolic vein	Colic Vein
Iliac crest	Pelvic Bone, Right Pelvic Bone, Left
Iliac fascia	Subcutaneous Tissue And Fascia, Right Upper Leg Subcutaneous Tissue And Fascia, Left Upper Leg
Iliac lymph node	Lymphatic, Pelvis
Iliacus muscle	Hip Muscle, Right Hip Muscle, Left
Iliofemoral ligament	Hip Bursa And Ligament, Right Hip Bursa And Ligament, Left
Iliohypogastric nerve Ilioinguinal nerve	Lumbar Plexus
Iliolumbar artery	Internal Iliac Artery, Right Internal Iliac Artery, Left
Iliolumbar ligament	Trunk Bursa And Ligament, Right Trunk Bursa And Ligament, Left
Iliotibial tract (band)	Subcutaneous Tissue And Fascia, Right Upper Leg Subcutaneous Tissue And Fascia, Left Upper Leg
Ilium	Pelvic Bone, Right Pelvic Bone, Left
Incus	Auditory Ossicle, Right Auditory Ossicle, Left
Inferior cardiac nerve	Thoracic Sympathetic Nerve
Inferior cerebellar vein Inferior cerebral vein	Intracranial Vein
Inferior epigastric artery	External Iliac Artery, Right External Iliac Artery, Left
Inferior epigastric lymph node	Lymphatic, Pelvis
Inferior genicular artery	Popliteal Artery, Right Popliteal Artery, Left
Inferior gluteal artery	Internal Iliac Artery, Right Internal Iliac Artery, Left
Inferior gluteal nerve	Sacral Plexus
Inferior hypogastric plexus	Abdominal Sympathetic Nerve
Inferior labial artery	Face Artery
Inferior longitudinal muscle	Tongue, Palate, Pharynx Muscle
Inferior mesenteric ganglion	Abdominal Sympathetic Nerve
Inferior mesenteric lymph node	Lymphatic, Mesenteric
Inferior mesenteric plexus	Abdominal Sympathetic Nerve
Inferior oblique muscle	Extraocular Muscle, Right Extraocular Muscle, Left
Inferior pancreaticoduodenal artery	Superior Mesenteric Artery
Inferior phrenic artery	Abdominal Aorta
Inferior rectus muscle	Extraocular Muscle, Right Extraocular Muscle, Left

Body Part	PCS Description	Body Part	PCS Description
Inferior suprarenal artery	Renal Artery, Right		Subclavian Artery, Left
	Renal Artery, Left	Internal urethral sphincter	Urethra
Inferior tarsal plate	Lower Eyelid, Right	Interphalangeal (IP) joint	Finger Phalangeal Joint, Right
	Lower Eyelid, Left		Finger Phalangeal Joint, Left
Inferior thyroid vein	Innominate Vein, Right		Toe Phalangeal Joint, Right
	Innominate Vein, Left		Toe Phalangeal Joint, Left
Inferior tibiofibular joint	Ankle Joint, Right	Interphalangeal ligament	Hand Bursa And Ligament, Right
	Ankle Joint, Left		Hand Bursa And Ligament, Left
Inferior turbinate	Nasal Turbinate		Foot Bursa And Ligament, Right
Inferior ulnar collateral artery	Brachial Artery, Right		Foot Bursa And Ligament, Left
	Brachial Artery, Left	Interspinalis muscle	Trunk Muscle, Right
Inferior vesical artery	Internal Iliac Artery, Right		Trunk Muscle, Left
	Internal Iliac Artery, Left	Interspinous ligament	Trunk Bursa And Ligament, Right
Infraauricular lymph node	Lymphatic, Head		Trunk Bursa And Ligament, Left
Infraclavicular (deltopectoral) lymph node	Lymphatic, Right Upper Extremity	Intertransversarius muscle	Trunk Muscle, Right
	Lymphatic, Left Upper Extremity		Trunk Muscle, Left
Infrahyoid muscle	Neck Muscle, Right	Intertransverse ligament	Trunk Bursa And Ligament, Right
	Neck Muscle, Left		Trunk Bursa And Ligament, Left
Infraparotid lymph node	Lymphatic, Head	Interventricular foramen (Monro)	Cerebral Ventricle
Infraspinatus fascia	Subcutaneous Tissue And Fascia, Right Upper Arm	Interventricular septum	Ventricular Septum
	Subcutaneous Tissue And Fascia, Left Upper Arm	Intestinal lymphatic trunk	Cisterna Chyli
Infraspinatus muscle	Shoulder Muscle, Right	Ischiatic nerve	Sciatic Nerve
	Shoulder Muscle, Left	Ischiocavernosus muscle	Perineum Muscle
Infundibulopelvic ligament	Uterine Supporting Structure	Ischiofemoral ligament	Hip Bursa And Ligament, Right
Inguinal canal Inguinal triangle	Inguinal Region, Right		Hip Bursa And Ligament, Left
	Inguinal Region, Left	Ischium	Pelvic Bone, Right
	Inguinal Region, Bilateral		Pelvic Bone, Left
Interatrial septum	Atrial Septum	Jejunal artery	Superior Mesenteric Artery
Intercarpal joint	Carpal Joint, Right	Jugular body	Glomus Jugulare
	Carpal Joint, Left	Jugular lymph node	Lymphatic, Right
Intercarpal ligament	Hand Bursa And Ligament, Right		Neck Lymphatic, Left Neck
	Hand Bursa And Ligament, Left	Labia majora Labia minora	Vulva
Interclavicular ligament	Shoulder Bursa And Ligament, Right	Labial gland	Upper Lip Lower Lip
	Shoulder Bursa And Ligament, Left	Lacrimal canaliculus	Lacrimal Duct, Right
			Lacrimal Duct, Left
Intercostal lymph node	Lymphatic, Thorax	Lacrimal punctum	Lacrimal Duct, Right
Intercostal muscle	Thorax Muscle, Right		Lacrimal Duct, Left
	Thorax Muscle, Left	Lacrimal sac	Lacrimal Duct, Right
Intercostal nerve	Thoracic Nerve		Lacrimal Duct, Left
Intercostobrachial nerve	Thoracic Nerve	Laryngopharynx	Pharynx
Intercuneiform joint	Tarsal Joint, Right	Lateral (brachial) lymph node	Lymphatic, Right Axillary
	Tarsal Joint, Left		Lymphatic, Left Axillary
Intercuneiform ligament	Foot Bursa And Ligament, Right	Lateral canthus	Upper Eyelid, Right
	Foot Bursa And Ligament, Left		Upper Eyelid, Left
Intermediate cuneiform bone	Tarsal, Right	Lateral collateral ligament (LCL)	Knee Bursa And Ligament, Right
	Tarsal, Left		Knee Bursa And Ligament, Left
Internal (basal) cerebral vein	Intracranial Vein	Lateral condyle of femur	Lower Femur, Right
Internal anal sphincter	Anal Sphincter		Lower Femur, Left
Internal carotid plexus	Head And Neck Sympathetic Nerve	Lateral condyle of tibia	Tibia, Right
			Tibia, Left
Internal iliac vein	Hypogastric Vein, Right	Lateral cuneiform bone	Tarsal, Right
	Hypogastric Vein, Left		Tarsal, Left
Internal maxillary artery	External Carotid Artery, Right	Lateral epicondyle of femur	Lower Femur, Right
	External Carotid Artery, Left		Lower Femur, Left
Internal naris	Nose	Lateral epicondyle of humerus	Humeral Shaft, Right
Internal oblique muscle	Abdomen Muscle, Right		Humeral Shaft, Left
	Abdomen Muscle, Left	Lateral femoral cutaneous nerve	Lumbar Plexus
Internal pudendal artery	Internal Iliac Artery, Right		
	Internal Iliac Artery, Left	Lateral malleolus	Fibula, Right
Internal pudendal vein	Hypogastric Vein, Right		Fibula, Left
	Hypogastric Vein, Left	Lateral meniscus	Knee Joint, Right
Internal thoracic artery	Internal Mammary Artery, Right		Knee Joint, Left
	Internal Mammary Artery, Left	Lateral nasal cartilage	Nose
	Subclavian Artery, Right	Lateral plantar artery	Foot Artery, Right
			Foot Artery, Left

Body Part	PCS Description
Lateral plantar nerve	Tibial Nerve
Lateral rectus muscle	Extraocular Muscle, Right
	Extraocular Muscle, Left
Lateral sacral artery	Internal Iliac Artery, Right
	Internal Iliac Artery, Left
Lateral sacral vein	Hypogastric Vein, Right
	Hypogastric Vein, Left
Lateral sural cutaneous nerve	Peroneal Nerve
Lateral tarsal artery	Foot Artery, Right
	Foot Artery, Left
Lateral temporomandibular ligament	Head And Neck Bursa And Ligament
Lateral thoracic artery	Axillary Artery, Right
	Axillary Artery, Left
Latissimus dorsi muscle	Trunk Muscle, Right
	Trunk Muscle, Left
Least splanchnic nerve	Thoracic Sympathetic Nerve
Left ascending lumbar vein	Hemiazygos Vein
Left atrioventricular valve	Mitral Valve
Left auricular appendix	Atrium, Left
Left colic vein	Colic Vein
Left coronary sulcus	Heart, Left
Left gastric artery	Gastric Artery
Left gastroepiploic artery	Splenic Artery
Left gastroepiploic vein	Splenic Vein
Left inferior phrenic vein	Renal Vein, Left
Left inferior pulmonary vein	Pulmonary Vein, Left
Left jugular trunk	Thoracic Duct
Left lateral ventricle	Cerebral Ventricle
Left ovarian vein	Renal Vein, Left
Left second lumbar vein	Renal Vein, Left
Left subclavian trunk	Thoracic Duct
Left subcostal vein	Hemiazygos Vein
Left superior pulmonary vein	Pulmonary Vein, Left
Left suprarenal vein	Renal Vein, Left
Left testicular vein	Renal Vein, Left
Leptomeninges	Cerebral Meninges Spinal Meninges
Lesser alar cartilage	Nose
Lesser occipital nerve	Cervical Plexus
Lesser splanchnic nerve	Thoracic Sympathetic Nerve
Lesser trochanter	Upper Femur, Right
	Upper Femur, Left
Lesser tuberosity	Humeral Head, Right
	Humeral Head, Left
Lesser wing	Sphenoid Bone, Right
	Sphenoid Bone, Left
Levator anguli oris muscle	Facial Muscle
Levator ani muscle	Trunk Muscle, Right
	Trunk Muscle, Left
Levator labii superioris alaeque nasi muscle	Facial Muscle
Levator labii superioris muscle	Facial Muscle
Levator labii superioris muscle	Facial Muscle
Levator palpebrae superioris muscle	Upper Eyelid, Right
	Upper Eyelid, Left
Levator scapulae muscle	Neck Muscle, Right
	Neck Muscle, Left
Levator veli palatini muscle	Tongue, Palate, Pharynx Muscle
Levatores costarum muscle	Thorax Muscle, Right
	Thorax Muscle, Left
Ligament of head of fibula	Knee Bursa And Ligament, Right
	Knee Bursa And Ligament, Left

Body Part	PCS Description
Ligament of the lateral malleolus	Ankle Bursa And Ligament, Right
	Ankle Bursa And Ligament, Left
Ligamentum flavum	Trunk Bursa And Ligament, Right
	Trunk Bursa And Ligament, Left
Lingual artery	External Carotid Artery, Right
	External Carotid Artery, Left
Lingual tonsil	Tongue
Locus ceruleus	Pons
Long thoracic nerve	Brachial Plexus
Lumbar artery	Abdominal Aorta
Lumbar facet joint	Lumbar Vertebral Joint
	Lumbar Vertebral Joints, 2 Or More
Lumbar ganglion	Lumbar Sympathetic Nerve
Lumbar lymph node	Lymphatic, Aortic
Lumbar lymphatic trunk	Cisterna Chyli
Lumbar splanchnic nerve	Lumbar Sympathetic Nerve
Lumbosacral facet joint	Lumbosacral Joint
Lumbosacral trunk	Lumbar Nerve
Lunate bone	Carpal, Right
	Carpal, Left
Lunotriquetral ligament	Hand Bursa And Ligament, Right
	Hand Bursa And Ligament, Left
Macula	Retina, Right
	Retina, Left
Malleus	Auditory Ossicle, Right
	Auditory Ossicle, Left
Mammary duct	Breast, Right
	Breast, Left Breast, Bilateral
Mammary gland	Breast, Right
	Breast, Left Breast, Bilateral
Mammillary body	Hypothalamus
Mandibular nerve	Trigeminal Nerve
Mandibular notch	Mandible, Right
	Mandible, Left
Manubrium	Sternum
Masseter muscle	Head Muscle
Masseteric fascia	Subcutaneous Tissue And Fascia, Face
Mastoid (postauricular) lymph node	Lymphatic, Right
	Neck Lymphatic, Left Neck
Mastoid air cells	Mastoid Sinus, Right
	Mastoid Sinus, Left
Mastoid process	Temporal Bone, Right
	Temporal Bone, Left
Maxillary artery	External Carotid Artery, Right
	External Carotid Artery, Left
Maxillary nerve	Trigeminal Nerve
Medial canthus	Lower Eyelid, Right
	Lower Eyelid, Left
Medial collateral ligament (MCL)	Knee Bursa And Ligament, Right
	Knee Bursa And Ligament, Left
Medial condyle of femur	Lower Femur, Right
	Lower Femur, Left
Medial condyle of tibia	Tibia, Right
	Tibia, Left
Medial cuneiform bone	Tarsal, Right
	Tarsal, Left
Medial epicondyle of femur	Lower Femur, Right
	Lower Femur, Left
Medial epicondyle of humerus	Humeral Shaft, Right
	Humeral Shaft, Left
Medial malleolus	Tibia, Right
	Tibia, Left
Medial meniscus	Knee Joint, Right
	Knee Joint, Left

Body Part	PCS Description	Body Part	PCS Description
Medial plantar artery	Foot Artery, Right Foot Artery, Left	Navicular bone	Tarsal, Right Tarsal, Left
Medial plantar nerve	Tibial Nerve	Neck of femur	Upper Femur, Right Upper Femur, Left
Medial popliteal nerve	Tibial Nerve		
Medial rectus muscle	Extraocular Muscle, Right Extraocular Muscle, Left	Neck of humerus (anatomical)(surgical)	Humeral Head, Right Humeral Head, Left
Medial sural cutaneous nerve	Tibial Nerve	Nerve to the stapedius	Facial Nerve
		Neurohypophysis	Pituitary Gland
Median antebrachial vein	Basilic Vein, Right Basilic Vein, Left	Ninth cranial nerve	Glossopharyngeal Nerve
		Nostril	Nose
Median cubital vein	Basilic Vein, Right Basilic Vein, Left	Obturator artery	Internal Iliac Artery, Right Internal Iliac Artery, Left
Median sacral artery	Abdominal Aorta	Obturator lymph node	Lymphatic, Pelvis
Mediastinal lymph node	Lymphatic, Thorax	Obturator muscle	Hip Muscle, Right Hip Muscle, Left
Meissner's (submucous) plexus	Abdominal Sympathetic Nerve		
		Obturator nerve	Lumbar Plexus
Membranous urethra	Urethra	Obturator vein	Hypogastric Vein, Right Hypogastric Vein, Left
Mental foramen	Mandible, Right Mandible, Left		
		Obtuse margin	Heart, Left
Mentalis muscle	Facial Muscle	Occipital artery	External Carotid Artery, Right External Carotid Artery, Left
Mesoappendix Mesocolon	Mesentery		
Metacarpal ligament	Hand Bursa And Ligament, Right Hand Bursa And Ligament, Left	Occipital lobe	Cerebral Hemisphere
		Occipital lymph node	Lymphatic, Right Neck Lymphatic, Left Neck
Metacarpophalangeal ligament	Hand Bursa And Ligament, Right Hand Bursa And Ligament, Left	Occipitofrontalis muscle	Facial Muscle
		Olecranon bursa	Elbow Bursa And Ligament, Right Elbow Bursa And Ligament, Left
Metatarsal ligament	Foot Bursa And Ligament, Right Foot Bursa And Ligament, Left		
		Olecranon process	Ulna, Right Ulna, Left
Metatarsophalangeal (MTP) joint	Metatarsal-Phalangeal Joint, Right Metatarsal-Phalangeal Joint, Left	Olfactory bulb	Olfactory Nerve
		Ophthalmic artery	Internal Carotid Artery, Right Internal Carotid Artery, Left
Metatarsophalangeal ligament	Foot Bursa And Ligament, Right Foot Bursa And Ligament, Left	Ophthalmic nerve	Trigeminal Nerve
		Ophthalmic vein	Intracranial Vein
Metathalamus	Thalamus	Optic chiasma	Optic Nerve
Midcarpal joint	Carpal Joint, Right Carpal Joint, Left	Optic disc	Retina, Right Retina, Left
Middle cardiac nerve	Thoracic Sympathetic Nerve	Optic foramen	Sphenoid Bone, Right Sphenoid Bone, Left
Middle cerebral artery	Intracranial Artery		
Middle cerebral vein	Intracranial Vein	Orbicularis oculi muscle	Upper Eyelid, Right Upper Eyelid, Left
Middle colic vein	Colic Vein		
Middle genicular artery	Popliteal Artery, Right Popliteal Artery, Left	Orbicularis oris muscle	Facial Muscle
		Orbital fascia	Subcutaneous Tissue And Fascia, Face
Middle hemorrhoidal vein	Hypogastric Vein, Right Hypogastric Vein, Left	Orbital portion of ethmoid bone	Orbit, Right Orbit, Left
Middle rectal artery	Internal Iliac Artery, Right Internal Iliac Artery, Left	Orbital portion of frontal bone	Orbit, Right Orbit, Left
Middle suprarenal artery	Abdominal Aorta	Orbital portion of lacrimal bone	Orbit, Right Orbit, Left
Middle temporal artery	Temporal Artery, Right Temporal Artery, Left	Orbital portion of maxilla	Orbit, Right Orbit, Left
Middle turbinate	Nasal Turbinate	Orbital portion of palatine bone	Orbit, Right Orbit, Left
Mitral annulus	Mitral Valve		
Molar gland	Buccal Mucosa	Orbital portion of sphenoid bone	Orbit, Right Orbit, Left
Musculocutaneous nerve	Brachial Plexus		
Musculophrenic artery	Internal Mammary Artery, Right Internal Mammary Artery, Left	Orbital portion of zygomatic bone	Orbit, Right Orbit, Left
Musculospiral nerve	Radial Nerve	Oropharynx	Pharynx
Myelencephalon	Medulla Oblongata	Ossicular chain	Auditory Ossicle, Right Auditory Ossicle, Left
Myenteric (Auerbach's) plexus	Abdominal Sympathetic Nerve	Otic ganglion	Head And Neck Sympathetic Nerve
Myometrium	Uterus		
Nail bed Nail plate	Finger Nail Toe Nail	Oval window	Middle Ear, Right Middle Ear, Left
Nasal cavity	Nose		
Nasal concha	Nasal Turbinate	Ovarian artery	Abdominal Aorta
Nasalis muscle	Facial Muscle	Ovarian ligament	Uterine Supporting Structure
Nasolacrimal duct	Lacrimal Duct, Right Lacrimal Duct, Left		

Body Part	PCS Description
Oviduct	Fallopian Tube, Right Fallopian Tube, Left
Palatine gland	Buccal Mucosa
Palatine tonsil	Tonsils
Palatine uvula	Uvula
Palatoglossal muscle	Tongue, Palate, Pharynx Muscle
Palatopharyngeal muscle	Tongue, Palate, Pharynx Muscle
Palmar (volar) digital vein	Hand Vein, Right Hand Vein, Left
Palmar (volar) metacarpal vein	Hand Vein, Right Hand Vein, Left
Palmar cutaneous nerve	Median Nerve Radial Nerve
Palmar fascia (aponeurosis)	Subcutaneous Tissue And Fascia, Right Hand Subcutaneous Tissue And Fascia, Left Hand
Palmar interosseous muscle	Hand Muscle, Right Hand Muscle, Left
Palmar ulnocarpal ligament	Wrist Bursa And Ligament, Right Wrist Bursa And Ligament, Left
Palmaris longus muscle	Lower Arm And Wrist Muscle, Right Lower Arm And Wrist Muscle, Left
Pancreatic artery	Splenic Artery
Pancreatic plexus	Abdominal Sympathetic Nerve
Pancreatic vein	Splenic Vein
Pancreaticosplenic lymph node	Lymphatic, Aortic
Paraaortic lymph node	Lymphatic, Aortic
Pararectal lymph node	Lymphatic, Mesenteric
Parasternal lymph node	Lymphatic, Thorax
Paratracheal lymph node	Lymphatic, Thorax
Paraurethral (Skene's) gland	Vestibular Gland
Parietal lobe	Cerebral Hemisphere
Parotid lymph node	Lymphatic, Head
Parotid plexus	Facial Nerve
Pars flaccida	Tympanic Membrane, Right Tympanic Membrane, Left
Patellar ligament	Knee Bursa And Ligament, Right Knee Bursa And Ligament, Left
Patellar tendon	Knee Tendon, Right Knee Tendon, Left
Pectineus muscle	Upper Leg Muscle, Right Upper Leg Muscle, Left
Pectoral (anterior) lymph node	Lymphatic, Right Axillary Lymphatic, Left Axillary
Pectoral fascia	Subcutaneous Tissue And Fascia, Chest
Pectoralis major muscle	Thorax Muscle, Right Thorax Muscle, Left
Pectoralis minor muscle	Thorax Muscle, Right Thorax Muscle, Left
Pelvic splanchnic nerve	Abdominal Sympathetic Nerve Sacral Sympathetic Nerve
Penile urethra	Urethra
Pericardiophrenic artery	Internal Mammary Artery, Right Internal Mammary Artery, Left
Perimetrium	Uterus
Peroneus brevis muscle	Lower Leg Muscle, Right Lower Leg Muscle, Left
Peroneus longus muscle	Lower Leg Muscle, Right Lower Leg Muscle, Left
Petrous part of temporal bone	Temporal Bone, Right Temporal Bone, Left

Body Part	PCS Description
Pharyngeal constrictor muscle	Tongue, Palate, Pharynx Muscle
Pharyngeal plexus	Vagus Nerve
Pharyngeal recess	Nasopharynx
Pharyngeal tonsil	Adenoids
Pharyngotympanic tube	Eustachian Tube, Right Eustachian Tube, Left
Pia mater	Cerebral Meninges Spinal Meninges
Pinna	External Ear, Right External Ear, Left External Ear, Bilateral
Piriform recess (sinus)	Pharynx
Piriformis muscle	Hip Muscle, Right Hip Muscle, Left
Pisiform bone	Carpal, Right Carpal, Left
Pisohamate ligament	Hand Bursa And Ligament, Right Hand Bursa And Ligament, Left
Pisometacarpal ligament	Hand Bursa And Ligament, Right Hand Bursa And Ligament, Left
Plantar digital vein	Foot Vein, Right Foot Vein, Left
Plantar fascia (aponeurosis)	Subcutaneous Tissue And Fascia, Right Foot Subcutaneous Tissue And Fascia, Left Foot
Plantar metatarsal vein Plantar venous arch	Foot Vein, Right Foot Vein, Left
Platysma muscle	Neck Muscle, Right Neck Muscle, Left
Plica semilunaris	Conjunctiva, Right Conjunctiva, Left
Pneumogastric nerve	Vagus Nerve
Pneumotaxic center	Pons
Pontine tegmentum	Pons
Popliteal ligament	Knee Bursa And Ligament, Right Knee Bursa And Ligament, Left
Popliteal lymph node	Lymphatic, Right Lower Extremity Lymphatic, Left Lower Extremity
Popliteal vein	Femoral Vein, Right Femoral Vein, Left
Popliteus muscle	Lower Leg Muscle, Right Lower Leg Muscle, Left
Postauricular (mastoid) lymph node	Lymphatic, Right Neck Lymphatic, Left Neck
Postcava	Inferior Vena Cava
Posterior (subscapular) lymph node	Lymphatic, Right Axillary Lymphatic, Left Axillary
Posterior auricular artery	External Carotid Artery, Right External Carotid Artery, Left
Posterior auricular nerve	Facial Nerve
Posterior auricular vein	External Jugular Vein, Right External Jugular Vein, Left
Posterior cerebral artery	Intracranial Artery
Posterior chamber	Eye, Right Eye, Left
Posterior circumflex humeral artery	Axillary Artery, Right Axillary Artery, Left
Posterior communicating artery	Intracranial Artery
Posterior cruciate ligament (PCL)	Knee Bursa And Ligament, Right Knee Bursa And Ligament, Left
Posterior facial	Face Vein, Right

641

Body Part	PCS Description
(retromandibular) vein	Face Vein, Left
Posterior femoral cutaneous nerve	Sacral Plexus
Posterior inferior cerebellar artery (PICA)	Intracranial Artery
Posterior interosseous nerve	Radial Nerve
Posterior labial nerve	Pudendal Nerve
Posterior scrotal nerve	Pudendal Nerve
Posterior spinal artery	Vertebral Artery, Right Vertebral Artery, Left
Posterior tibial recurrent artery	Anterior Tibial Artery, Right Anterior Tibial Artery, Left
Posterior ulnar recurrent artery	Ulnar Artery, Right Ulnar Artery, Left
Posterior vagal trunk	Vagus Nerve
Preauricular lymph node	Lymphatic, Head
Precava	Superior Vena Cava
Prepatellar bursa	Knee Bursa And Ligament, Right Knee Bursa And Ligament, Left
Pretracheal fascia	Subcutaneous Tissue And Fascia, Anterior Neck
Prevertebral fascia	Subcutaneous Tissue And Fascia, Posterior Neck
Princeps pollicis artery	Hand Artery, Right Hand Artery, Left
Procerus muscle	Facial Muscle
Profunda brachii	Brachial Artery, Right Brachial Artery, Left
Profunda femoris (deep femoral) vein	Femoral Vein, Right Femoral Vein, Left
Pronator quadratus muscle	Lower Arm And Wrist Muscle, Right Lower Arm And Wrist Muscle, Left
Pronator teres muscle	Lower Arm And Wrist Muscle, Right Lower Arm And Wrist Muscle, Left
Prostatic urethra	Urethra
Proximal radioulnar joint	Elbow Joint, Right Elbow Joint, Left
Psoas muscle	Hip Muscle, Right Hip Muscle, Left
Pterygoid muscle	Head Muscle
Pterygoid process	Sphenoid Bone, Right Sphenoid Bone, Left
Pterygopalatine (sphenopalatine) ganglion	Head And Neck Sympathetic Nerve
Pubic ligament	Trunk Bursa And Ligament, Right Trunk Bursa And Ligament, Left
Pubis	Pelvic Bone, Right Pelvic Bone, Left
Pubofemoral ligament	Hip Bursa And Ligament, Right Hip Bursa And Ligament, Left
Pudendal nerve	Sacral Plexus
Pulmoaortic canal	Pulmonary Artery, Left
Pulmonary annulus	Pulmonary Valve
Pulmonary plexus	Vagus Nerve Thoracic Sympathetic Nerve
Pulmonic valve	Pulmonary Valve
Pulvinar	Thalamus
Pyloric antrum	Stomach, Pylorus
Pyloric canal	Stomach, Pylorus
Pyloric sphincter	Stomach, Pylorus
Pyramidalis muscle	Abdomen Muscle, Right Abdomen Muscle, Left
Quadrangular cartilage	Nasal Septum

Body Part	PCS Description
Quadrate lobe	Liver
Quadratus femoris muscle	Hip Muscle, Right Hip Muscle, Left
Quadratus lumborum muscle	Trunk Muscle, Right Trunk Muscle, Left
Quadratus plantae muscle	Foot Muscle, Right Foot Muscle, Left
Quadriceps (femoris)	Upper Leg Muscle, Right Upper Leg Muscle, Left
Radial collateral carpal ligament	Wrist Bursa And Ligament, Right Wrist Bursa And Ligament, Left
Radial collateral ligament	Elbow Bursa And Ligament, Right Elbow Bursa And Ligament, Left
Radial notch	Ulna, Right Ulna, Left
Radial recurrent artery	Radial Artery, Right Radial Artery, Left
Radial vein	Brachial Vein, Right Brachial Vein, Left
Radialis indicis	Hand Artery, Right Hand Artery, Left
Radiocarpal joint	Wrist Joint, Right Wrist Joint, Left
Radiocarpal ligament	Wrist Bursa And Ligament, Right Wrist Bursa And Ligament, Left
Radioulnar ligament	Wrist Bursa And Ligament, Right Wrist Bursa And Ligament, Left
Rectosigmoid junction	Sigmoid Colon
Rectus abdominis muscle	Abdomen Muscle, Right Abdomen Muscle, Left
Rectus femoris muscle	Upper Leg Muscle, Right Upper Leg Muscle, Left
Recurrent laryngeal nerve	Vagus Nerve
Renal calyx	Kidney, Right Kidney, Left Kidneys, Bilateral Kidney
Renal capsule	Kidney, Right Kidney, Left Kidneys, Bilateral Kidney
Renal cortex	Kidney, Right Kidney, Left Kidneys, Bilateral Kidney
Renal plexus	Abdominal Sympathetic Nerve
Renal segment	Kidney, Right Kidney, Left Kidneys, Bilateral Kidney
Renal segmental artery	Renal Artery, Right Renal Artery, Left
Retroperitoneal lymph node	Lymphatic, Aortic
Retroperitoneal space	Retroperitoneum
Retropharyngeal lymph node	Lymphatic, Right Neck Lymphatic, Left Neck
Retropubic space	Pelvic Cavity
Rhinopharynx	Nasopharynx
Rhomboid major muscle	Trunk Muscle, Right Trunk Muscle, Left
Rhomboid minor muscle	Trunk Muscle, Right Trunk Muscle, Left
Right ascending lumbar vein	Azygos Vein
Right atrioventricular valve	Tricuspid Valve
Right auricular appendix	Atrium, Right
Right colic vein	Colic Vein
Right coronary sulcus	Heart, Right
Right gastric artery	Gastric Artery
Right gastroepiploic vein	Superior Mesenteric Vein

Body Part	PCS Description
Right inferior phrenic vein	Inferior Vena Cava
Right inferior pulmonary vein	Pulmonary Vein, Right
Right jugular trunk	Lymphatic, Right Neck
Right lateral ventricle	Cerebral Ventricle
Right lymphatic duct	Lymphatic, Right Neck
Right ovarian vein	Inferior Vena Cava
Right second lumbar vein	Inferior Vena Cava
Right subclavian trunk	Lymphatic, Right Neck
Right subcostal vein	Azygos Vein
Right superior pulmonary vein	Pulmonary Vein, Right
Right suprarenal vein	Inferior Vena Cava
Right testicular vein	Inferior Vena Cava
Rima glottidis	Larynx
Risorius muscle	Facial Muscle
Round ligament of uterus	Uterine Supporting Structure
Round window	Inner Ear, Right Inner Ear, Left
Sacral ganglion	Sacral Sympathetic Nerve
Sacral lymph node	Lymphatic, Pelvis
Sacral splanchnic nerve	Sacral Sympathetic Nerve
Sacrococcygeal ligament	Trunk Bursa And Ligament, Right Trunk Bursa And Ligament, Left
Sacrococcygeal symphysis	Sacrococcygeal Joint
Sacroiliac ligament	Trunk Bursa And Ligament, Right Trunk Bursa And Ligament, Left
Sacrospinous ligament	Trunk Bursa And Ligament, Right Trunk Bursa And Ligament, Left
Sacrotuberous ligament	Trunk Bursa And Ligament, Right Trunk Bursa And Ligament, Left
Salpingopharyngeus muscle	Tongue, Palate, Pharynx Muscle
Salpinx	Fallopian Tube, Right Fallopian Tube, Left
Saphenous nerve	Femoral Nerve
Sartorius muscle	Upper Leg Muscle, Right Upper Leg Muscle, Left
Scalene muscle	Neck Muscle, Right Neck Muscle, Left
Scaphoid bone	Carpal, Right Carpal, Left
Scapholunate ligament	Hand Bursa And Ligament, Right Hand Bursa And Ligament, Left
Scaphotrapezium ligament	Hand Bursa And Ligament, Right Hand Bursa And Ligament, Left
Scarpa's (vestibular) ganglion	Acoustic Nerve
Sebaceous gland	Skin
Second cranial nerve	Optic Nerve
Sella turcica	Sphenoid Bone, Right Sphenoid Bone, Left
Semicircular canal	Inner Ear, Right Inner Ear, Left
Semimembranosus muscle	Upper Leg Muscle, Right Upper Leg Muscle, Left
Semitendinosus muscle	Upper Leg Muscle, Right Upper Leg Muscle, Left
Septal cartilage	Nasal Septum
Serratus anterior muscle	Thorax Muscle, Right Thorax Muscle, Left
Serratus posterior muscle	Trunk Muscle, Right Trunk Muscle, Left

Body Part	PCS Description
Seventh cranial nerve	Facial Nerve
Short gastric artery	Splenic Artery
Sigmoid artery	Inferior Mesenteric Artery
Sigmoid flexure	Sigmoid Colon
Sigmoid vein	Inferior Mesenteric Vein
Sinoatrial node	Conduction Mechanism
Sinus venosus	Atrium, Right
Sixth cranial nerve	Abducens Nerve
Skene's (paraurethral) gland	Vestibular Gland
Small saphenous vein	Lesser Saphenous Vein, Right Lesser Saphenous Vein, Left
Solar (celiac) plexus	Abdominal Sympathetic Nerve
Soleus muscle	Lower Leg Muscle, Right Lower Leg Muscle, Left
Sphenomandibular ligament	Head And Neck Bursa And Ligament
Sphenopalatine (pterygopalatine) ganglion	Head And Neck Sympathetic Nerve
Spinal dura mater	Dura Mater
Spinal epidural space	Epidural Space
Spinal subarachnoid space	Subarachnoid Space
Spinal subdural space	Subdural Space
Spinous process	Cervical Vertebra Thoracic Vertebra Lumbar Vertebra
Spiral ganglion	Acoustic Nerve
Splenic flexure	Transverse Colon
Splenic plexus	Abdominal Sympathetic Nerve
Splenius capitis muscle	Head Muscle
Splenius cervicis muscle	Neck Muscle, Right Neck Muscle, Left
Stapes	Auditory Ossicle, Right Auditory Ossicle, Left
Stellate ganglion	Head And Neck Sympathetic Nerve
Stensen's duct	Parotid Duct, Right Parotid Duct, Left
Sternoclavicular ligament	Shoulder Bursa And Ligament, Right Shoulder Bursa And Ligament, Left
Sternocleidomastoid artery	Thyroid Artery, Right Thyroid Artery, Left
Sternocleidomastoid muscle	Neck Muscle, Right Neck Muscle, Left
Sternocostal ligament	Thorax Bursa And Ligament, Right Thorax Bursa And Ligament, Left
Styloglossus muscle	Tongue, Palate, Pharynx Muscle
Stylomandibular ligament	Head And Neck Bursa And Ligament
Stylopharyngeus muscle	Tongue, Palate, Pharynx Muscle
Subacromial bursa	Shoulder Bursa And Ligament, Right Shoulder Bursa And Ligament, Left
Subaortic (common iliac) lymph node	Lymphatic, Pelvis
Subclavicular (apical) lymph node	Lymphatic, Right Axillary Lymphatic, Left Axillary
Subclavius muscle	Thorax Muscle, Right Thorax Muscle, Left
Subclavius nerve	Brachial Plexus
Subcostal artery	Thoracic Aorta
Subcostal muscle	Thorax Muscle, Right Thorax Muscle, Left
Subcostal nerve	Thoracic Nerve

Body Part	PCS Description
Submandibular ganglion	Facial Nerve Head And Neck Sympathetic Nerve
Submandibular gland	Submaxillary Gland, Right Submaxillary Gland, Left
Submandibular lymph node	Lymphatic, Head
Submaxillary ganglion	Head And Neck Sympathetic Nerve
Submaxillary lymph node	Lymphatic, Head
Submental artery	Face Artery
Submental lymph node	Lymphatic, Head
Submucous (Meissner's) plexus	Abdominal Sympathetic Nerve
Suboccipital nerve	Cervical Nerve
Suboccipital venous plexus	Vertebral Vein, Right Vertebral Vein, Left
Subparotid lymph node	Lymphatic, Head
Subscapular (posterior) lymph node	Lymphatic, Right Axillary Lymphatic, Left Axillary
Subscapular aponeurosis	Subcutaneous Tissue And Fascia, Right Upper Arm Subcutaneous Tissue And Fascia, Left Upper Arm
Subscapular artery	Axillary Artery, Right Axillary Artery, Left
Subscapularis muscle	Shoulder Muscle, Right Shoulder Muscle, Left
Substantia nigra	Basal Ganglia
Subtalar (talocalcaneal) joint	Tarsal Joint, Right Tarsal Joint, Left
Subtalar ligament	Foot Bursa And Ligament, Right Foot Bursa And Ligament, Left
Subthalamic nucleus	Basal Ganglia
Superficial circumflex iliac vein	Greater Saphenous Vein, Right Greater Saphenous Vein, Left
Superficial epigastric artery	Femoral Artery, Right Femoral Artery, Left
Superficial epigastric vein	Greater Saphenous Vein, Right Greater Saphenous Vein, Left
Superficial palmar arch	Hand Artery, Right Hand Artery, Left
Superficial palmar venous arch	Hand Vein, Right Hand Vein, Left
Superficial temporal artery	Temporal Artery, Right Temporal Artery, Left
Superficial transverse perineal muscle	Perineum Muscle
Superior cardiac nerve	Thoracic Sympathetic Nerve
Superior cerebellar vein Superior cerebral vein	Intracranial Vein
Superior clunic (cluneal) nerve	Lumbar Nerve
Superior epigastric artery	Internal Mammary Artery, Right Internal Mammary Artery, Left
Superior genicular artery	Popliteal Artery, Right Popliteal Artery, Left
Superior gluteal artery	Internal Iliac Artery, Right Internal Iliac Artery, Left
Superior gluteal nerve	Lumbar Plexus
Superior hypogastric plexus	Abdominal Sympathetic Nerve
Superior labial artery	Face Artery
Superior laryngeal artery	Thyroid Artery, Right Thyroid Artery, Left
Superior laryngeal nerve	Vagus Nerve
Superior longitudinal muscle	Tongue, Palate, Pharynx Muscle
Superior mesenteric ganglion	Abdominal Sympathetic Nerve
Superior mesenteric lymph	Lymphatic, Mesenteric

Body Part	PCS Description
node	
Superior mesenteric plexus	Abdominal Sympathetic Nerve
Superior oblique muscle	Extraocular Muscle, Right Extraocular Muscle, Left
Superior olivary nucleus	Pons
Superior rectal artery	Inferior Mesenteric Artery
Superior rectal vein	Inferior Mesenteric Vein
Superior rectus muscle	Extraocular Muscle, Right Extraocular Muscle, Left
Superior tarsal plate	Upper Eyelid, Right Upper Eyelid, Left
Superior thoracic artery	Axillary Artery, Right Axillary Artery, Left
Superior thyroid artery	External Carotid Artery, Right External Carotid Artery, Left Thyroid Artery, Right Thyroid Artery, Left
Superior turbinate	Nasal Turbinate
Superior ulnar collateral artery	Brachial Artery, Right Brachial Artery, Left
Supraclavicular (Virchow's) lymph node	Lymphatic, Right Neck Lymphatic, Left Neck
Supraclavicular nerve	Cervical Plexus
Suprahyoid lymph node	Lymphatic, Head
Suprahyoid muscle	Neck Muscle, Right Neck Muscle, Left
Suprainguinal lymph node	Lymphatic, Pelvis
Supraorbital vein	Face Vein, Right Face Vein, Left
Suprarenal gland	Adrenal Gland, Left Adrenal Gland, Right Adrenal Glands, Bilateral
Suprarenal plexus	Abdominal Sympathetic Nerve
Suprascapular nerve	Brachial Plexus
Supraspinatus fascia	Subcutaneous Tissue And Fascia, Right Upper Arm Subcutaneous Tissue And Fascia, Left Upper Arm
Supraspinatus muscle	Shoulder Muscle, Right Shoulder Muscle, Left
Supraspinous ligament	Trunk Bursa And Ligament, Right Trunk Bursa And Ligament, Left
Suprasternal notch	Sternum
Supratrochlear lymph node	Lymphatic, Right Upper Extremity Lymphatic, Left Upper Extremity
Sural artery	Popliteal Artery, Right Popliteal Artery, Left
Sweat gland	Skin
Talocalcaneal (subtalar) joint	Tarsal Joint, Right Tarsal Joint, Left
Talocalcaneal ligament	Foot Bursa And Ligament, Right Foot Bursa And Ligament, Left
Talocalcaneonavicular joint	Tarsal Joint, Right Tarsal Joint, Left
Talocalcaneonavicular ligament	Foot Bursa And Ligament, Right Foot Bursa And Ligament, Left
Talocrural joint	Ankle Joint, Right Ankle Joint, Left
Talofibular ligament	Ankle Bursa And Ligament, Right Ankle Bursa And Ligament, Left
Talus bone	Tarsal, Right Tarsal, Left
Tarsometatarsal joint	Metatarsal-Tarsal Joint, Right Metatarsal-Tarsal Joint, Left
Tarsometatarsal ligament	Foot Bursa And Ligament,

Body Part	PCS Description
	Right Foot Bursa And Ligament, Left
Temporal lobe	Cerebral Hemisphere
Temporalis muscle Temporoparietalis muscle	Head Muscle
Tensor fasciae latae muscle	Hip Muscle, Right Hip Muscle, Left
Tensor veli palatini muscle	Tongue, Palate, Pharynx Muscle
Tenth cranial nerve	Vagus Nerve
Tentorium cerebelli	Dura Mater
Teres major muscle	Shoulder Muscle, Right Shoulder Muscle, Left
Teres minor muscle	Shoulder Muscle, Right Shoulder Muscle, Left
Testicular artery	Abdominal Aorta
Thenar muscle	Hand Muscle, Right Hand Muscle, Left
Third cranial nerve	Oculomotor Nerve
Third occipital nerve	Cervical Nerve
Third ventricle	Cerebral Ventricle
Thoracic aortic plexus	Thoracic Sympathetic Nerve
Thoracic esophagus	Esophagus, Middle
Thoracic facet joint	Thoracic Vertebral Joint Thoracic Vertebral Joints, 2-7 Thoracic Vertebral Joints, 8 Or More
Thoracic ganglion	Thoracic Sympathetic Nerve
Thoracoacromial artery	Axillary Artery, Right Axillary Artery, Left
Thoracolumbar facet joint	Thoracolumbar Vertebral Joint
Thymus gland	Thymus
Thyroarytenoid muscle	Neck Muscle, Right Neck Muscle, Left
Thyrocervical trunk	Thyroid Artery, Right Thyroid Artery, Left
Thyroid cartilage	Larynx
Tibialis anterior muscle	Lower Leg Muscle, Right Lower Leg Muscle, Left
Tibialis posterior muscle	Lower Leg Muscle, Right Lower Leg Muscle, Left
Tracheobronchial lymph node	Lymphatic, Thorax
Tragus	External Ear, Right External Ear, Left External Ear, Bilateral
Transversalis fascia	Subcutaneous Tissue And Fascia, Trunk
Transverse (cutaneous) cervical nerve	Cervical Plexus
Transverse acetabular ligament	Hip Bursa And Ligament, Right Hip Bursa And Ligament, Left
Transverse facial artery	Temporal Artery, Right Temporal Artery, Left
Transverse humeral ligament	Shoulder Bursa And Ligament, Right Shoulder Bursa And Ligament, Left
Transverse ligament of atlas	Head And Neck Bursa And Ligament
Transverse scapular ligament	Shoulder Bursa And Ligament, Right Shoulder Bursa And Ligament, Left
Transverse thoracis muscle	Thorax Muscle, Right Thorax Muscle, Left
Transversospinalis muscle	Trunk Muscle, Right Trunk Muscle, Left
Transversus abdominis muscle	Abdomen Muscle, Right Abdomen Muscle, Left

Body Part	PCS Description
Trapezium bone	Carpal, Right Carpal, Left
Trapezius muscle	Trunk Muscle, Right Trunk Muscle, Left
Trapezoid bone	Carpal, Right Carpal, Left
Triceps brachii muscle	Upper Arm Muscle, Right Upper Arm Muscle, Left
Tricuspid annulus	Tricuspid Valve
Trifacial nerve	Trigeminal Nerve
Trigone of bladder	Bladder
Triquetral bone	Carpal, Right Carpal, Left
Trochanteric bursa	Hip Bursa And Ligament, Right Hip Bursa And Ligament, Left
Twelfth cranial nerve	Hypoglossal Nerve
Tympanic cavity	Middle Ear, Right Middle Ear, Left
Tympanic nerve	Glossopharyngeal Nerve
Tympanic part of temporal bone	Temporal Bone, Right Temporal Bone, Left
Ulnar collateral carpal ligament	Wrist Bursa And Ligament, Right Wrist Bursa And Ligament, Left
Ulnar collateral ligament	Elbow Bursa And Ligament, Right Elbow Bursa And Ligament, Left
Ulnar notch	Radius, Right Radius, Left
Ulnar vein	Brachial Vein, Right Brachial Vein, Left
Umbilical artery	Internal Iliac Artery, Right Internal Iliac Artery, Left
Ureteral orifice	Ureter, Right Ureter, Left Ureters, Bilateral Ureter
Ureteropelvic junction (UPJ)	Kidney Pelvis, Right Kidney Pelvis, Left
Ureterovesical orifice	Ureter, Right Ureter, Left Ureters, Bilateral Ureter
Uterine artery	Internal Iliac Artery, Right Internal Iliac Artery, Left
Uterine cornu	Uterus
Uterine tube	Fallopian Tube, Right Fallopian Tube, Left
Uterine vein	Hypogastric Vein, Right Hypogastric Vein, Left
Vaginal artery	Internal Iliac Artery, Right Internal Iliac Artery, Left
Vaginal vein	Hypogastric Vein, Right Hypogastric Vein, Left
Vastus intermedius muscle	Upper Leg Muscle, Right Upper Leg Muscle, Left
Vastus lateralis muscle	Upper Leg Muscle, Right Upper Leg Muscle, Left
Vastus medialis muscle	Upper Leg Muscle, Right Upper Leg Muscle, Left
Ventricular fold	Larynx
Vermiform appendix	Appendix
Vermilion border	Upper Lip Lower Lip
Vertebral arch	Cervical Vertebra Thoracic Vertebra Lumbar Vertebra
Vertebral canal	Spinal Canal
Vertebral foramen	Cervical Vertebra Thoracic Vertebra Lumbar Vertebra
Vertebral lamina	Cervical Vertebra Thoracic Vertebra

Body Part	PCS Description	Body Part	PCS Description
	Lumbar Vertebra		
Vertebral pedicle	Cervical Vertebra Thoracic Vertebra Lumbar Vertebra		
Vesical vein	Hypogastric Vein, Right Hypogastric Vein, Left		
Vestibular (Scarpa's) ganglion	Acoustic Nerve		
Vestibular nerve	Acoustic Nerve		
Vestibulocochlear nerve	Acoustic Nerve		
Virchow's (supraclavicular) lymph node	Lymphatic, Right Neck Lymphatic, Left Neck		
Vitreous body	Vitreous, Right Vitreous, Left		
Vocal fold	Vocal Cord, Right Vocal Cord, Left		
Volar (palmar) digital vein	Hand Vein, Right Hand Vein, Left		
Volar (palmar) metacarpal vein	Hand Vein, Right Hand Vein, Left		
Vomer bone	Nasal Septum		
Vomer of nasal septum	Nasal Bone		
Xiphoid process	Sternum		
Zonule of Zinn	Lens, Right Lens, Left		
Zygomatic process of frontal bone	Frontal Bone, Right Frontal Bone, Left		
Zygomatic process of temporal bone	Temporal Bone, Right Temporal Bone, Left		

Device Term	PCS Description
3f (Aortic) Bioprosthesis valve	Zooplastic tissue in heart and great vessels
AbioCor® Total Replacement Heart	Synthetic substitute
Acellular Hydrated Dermis	Nonautologous tissue substitute
Activa PC neurostimulator	Stimulator generator, multiple array for insertion in subcutaneous tissue and fascia
Activa RC neurostimulator	Stimulator generator, multiple array rechargeable for insertion in subcutaneous tissue and fascia
Activa SC neurostimulator	Stimulator generator, single array for insertion in subcutaneous tissue and fascia
ACUITY™ Steerable Lead	Cardiac lead, pacemaker for insertion in heart and great vessels cardiac lead, defibrillator for insertion in heart and great vessels
AMPLATZER® Muscular VSD Occluder	Synthetic substitute
AMS 800® Urinary Control System	Artificial sphincter in urinary system
AneuRx® AAA Advantage®	Intraluminal device
Annuloplasty ring	Synthetic substitute
Artificial anal sphincter (AAS)	Artificial sphincter in gastrointestinal system
Artificial bowel sphincter (neosphincter)	Artificial sphincter in gastrointestinal system
Artificial urinary sphincter (AUS)	Artificial sphincter in urinary system
Assurant (Cobalt) stent	Intraluminal device
Attain Ability® lead	Cardiac lead, pacemaker for insertion in heart and great vessels cardiac lead, defibrillator for insertion in heart and great vessels
Attain StarFix® (OTW) lead	Cardiac lead, pacemaker for insertion in heart and great vessels cardiac lead, defibrillator for insertion in heart and great vessels
Autograft	Autologous tissue substitute
Autologous artery graft	Autologous arterial tissue in heart and great vessels autologous arterial tissue in upper arteries autologous arterial tissue in lower arteries autologous arterial tissue in upper veins autologous arterial tissue in lower veins
Autologous vein graft	Autologous venous tissue in heart and great vessels autologous venous tissue in upper arteries autologous venous tissue in lower arteries autologous venous tissue in upper veins autologous venous tissue in lower veins
Axial Lumbar Interbody Fusion System	Interbody fusion device in lower joints
AxiaLIF® System	Interbody fusion device in lower joints
BAK/C® Interbody Cervical Fusion System	Interbody fusion device in upper joints
Bard® Composix® (E/X)(LP) mesh	Synthetic substitute

Device Term	PCS Description
Bard® Composix® Kugel® patch	Synthetic substitute
Bard® Dulex™ mesh	Synthetic substitute
Bard® Ventralex™ hernia patch	Synthetic substitute
Baroreflex Activation Therapy® (BAT®)	Stimulator lead in upper arteries cardiac rhythm related device in subcutaneous tissue and fascia
Berlin Heart Ventricular Assist Device	Implantable heart assist system in heart and great vessels
Bioactive embolization coil(s)	Intraluminal device, bioactive in upper arteries
Biventricular external heart assist system	External heart assist system in heart and great vessels
Blood glucose monitoring system	Monitoring device
Bone anchored hearing device	Hearing device, bone conduction for insertion in ear, nose, sinus hearing device in head and facial bones
Bone bank bone graft	Nonautologous tissue substitute
Bone screw (interlocking)(lag)(pedicle)(recessed)	Internal fixation device in head and facial bones internal fixation device in upper bones internal fixation device in lower bones
Bovine pericardial valve	Zooplastic tissue in heart and great vessels
Bovine pericardium graft	Zooplastic tissue in heart and great vessels
Brachytherapy seeds	Radioactive element
BRYAN® Cervical Disc System	Synthetic substitute
BVS 5000 Ventricular Assist Device	External heart assist system in heart and great vessels
Cardiac contractility modulation lead	Cardiac lead in heart and great vessels
Cardiac event recorder	Monitoring device
Cardiac resynchronization therapy (CRT) lead	Cardiac lead, pacemaker for insertion in heart and great vessels cardiac lead, defibrillator for insertion in heart and great vessels
CardioMEMS® pressure sensor	Monitoring device, pressure sensor for insertion in heart and great vessels
Carotid (artery) sinus (baroreceptor) lead	Stimulator lead in upper arteries
Carotid WALLSTENT® Monorail® Endoprosthesis	Intraluminal device
Centrimag® Blood Pump	Intraluminal device
Clamp and rod internal fixation system (CRIF)	Internal fixation device in upper bones internal fixation device in lower bones
CoAxia NeuroFlo catheter	Intraluminal device
Cobalt/chromium head and polyethylene socket	Synthetic substitute, metal on polyethylene for replacement in lower joints
Cobalt/chromium head and socket	Synthetic substitute, metal for replacement in lower joints
Cochlear implant (CI), multiple channel (electrode)	Hearing device, multiple channel cochlear prosthesis for insertion in ear, nose, sinus
Cochlear implant (CI), single channel (electrode)	Hearing device, single channel cochlear prosthesis for insertion in ear, nose, sinus

Anatomical Term	PCS Description	Anatomical Term	PCS Description
COGNIS® CRT-D	Cardiac resynchronization defibrillator pulse generator for insertion in subcutaneous tissue and fascia		insertion in heart and great vessels
Colonic Z-Stent®	Intraluminal device	Dynesys® Dynamic Stabilization System	Spinal stabilization device, pedicle-based for insertion in upper joints spinal stabilization device, pedicle-based for insertion in lower joints
Complete (SE) stent	Intraluminal device		
Concerto II CRT-D	Cardiac resynchronization defibrillator pulse generator for insertion in subcutaneous tissue and fascia		
		E-Luminexx™ (Biliary)(Vascular) Stent	Intraluminal device
CONSERVE® PLUS Total Resurfacing Hip System	Resurfacing device in lower joints	Electrical bone growth stimulator (EBGS)	Bone growth stimulator in head and facial bones bone growth stimulator in upper bones bone growth stimulator in lower bones
Consulta CRT-D	Cardiac resynchronization defibrillator pulse generator for insertion in subcutaneous tissue and fascia		
		Electrical muscle stimulation (EMS) lead	Stimulator lead in muscles
Consulta CRT-P	Cardiac resynchronization pacemaker pulse generator for insertion in subcutaneous tissue and fascia	Electronic muscle stimulator lead	Stimulator lead in muscles
		Embolization coil(s)	Intraluminal device
CONTAK RENEWAL® 3 RF (HE) CRT-D	Cardiac resynchronization defibrillator pulse generator for insertion in subcutaneous tissue and fascia	Endeavor® (III)(IV) (Sprint) Zotarolimus-eluting Coronary Stent System	Intraluminal device, drug-eluting in heart and great vessels
		EndoSure® sensor	Monitoring device, pressure sensor for insertion in heart and great vessels
Contegra Pulmonary Valved Conduit	Zooplastic tissue in heart and great vessels		
Continuous Glucose Monitoring (CGM) device	Monitoring device	ENDOTAK RELIANCE® (G) Defibrillation Lead	Cardiac lead, defibrillator for insertion in heart and great vessels
CoreValve transcatheter aortic valve	Zooplastic tissue in heart and great vessels		
Cormet Hip Resurfacing System	Resurfacing device in lower joints	Endotracheal tube (cuffed)(double-lumen)	Intraluminal device, endotracheal airway in respiratory system
CoRoent® XL	Interbody fusion device in lower joints	Endurant® Endovascular Stent Graft	Intraluminal device
Corox (OTW) Bipolar Lead	Cardiac lead, pacemaker for insertion in heart and great vessels cardiac lead, defibrillator for insertion in heart and great vessels	EnRhythm	Pacemaker, dual chamber for insertion in subcutaneous tissue and fascia
		Enterra gastric neurostimulator	Stimulator generator, multiple array for insertion in subcutaneous tissue and fascia
Cortical strip neurostimulator lead	Neurostimulator lead in central nervous system		
Cultured epidermal cell autograft	Autologous tissue substitute	Epicel® cultured epidermal autograft	Autologous tissue substitute
CYPHER® Stent	Intraluminal device, drug-eluting in heart and great vessels	Epic™ Stented Tissue Valve (aortic)	Zooplastic tissue in heart and great vessels
		Esophageal obturator airway (EOA)	Intraluminal device, airway in gastrointestinal system
Cystostomy tube	Drainage device		
DBS lead	Neurostimulator lead in central nervous system	Esteem® implantable hearing system	Hearing device in ear, nose, sinus
DeBakey Left Ventricular Assist Device	Implantable heart assist system in heart and great vessels	Everolimus-eluting coronary stent	Intraluminal device, drug-eluting in heart and great vessels
Deep brain neurostimulator lead	Neurostimulator lead in central nervous system		
		Ex-PRESS™ mini glaucoma shunt	Synthetic substitute
Delta frame external fixator	External fixation device, hybrid for insertion in upper bones external fixation device, hybrid for reposition in upper bones external fixation device, hybrid for insertion in lower bones external fixation device, hybrid for reposition in lower bones	Express® (LD) Premounted Stent System	Intraluminal device
		Express® Biliary SD Monorail® Premounted Stent System	Intraluminal device
		Express® SD Renal Monorail® Premounted Stent System	Intraluminal device
Delta III Reverse shoulder prosthesis	Synthetic substitute, reverse ball and socket for replacement in upper joints	External fixator	External fixation device in head and facial bones external fixation device in upper bones external fixation device in lower bones external fixation device in upper joints external fixation device in lower joints
Diaphragmatic pacemaker generator	Stimulator generator in subcutaneous tissue and fascia		
Direct Lateral Interbody Fusion (DLIF) device	Interbody fusion device in lower joints		
Driver stent (RX) (OTW)	Intraluminal device	EXtreme Lateral Interbody Fusion (XLIF) device	Interbody fusion device in lower joints
DuraHeart Left Ventricular Assist System	Implantable heart assist system in heart and great vessels		
		Facet replacement spinal stabilization device	Spinal stabilization device, facet replacement for insertion
Durata® Defibrillation Lead	Cardiac lead, defibrillator for		

Device Term	PCS Description
	in upper joints spinal stabilization device, facet replacement for insertion in lower joints
FLAIR® Endovascular Stent Graft	Intraluminal device
Flexible Composite Mesh	Synthetic substitute
Foley catheter	Drainage device
Formula™ Balloon-Expandable Renal Stent System	Intraluminal device
Freestyle (Stentless) Aortic Root Bioprosthesis	Zooplastic tissue in heart and great vessels
Fusion screw (compression)(lag)(locking)	Internal fixation device in upper joints internal fixation device in lower joints
Gastric electrical stimulation (GES) lead	Stimulator lead in gastrointestinal system
Gastric pacemaker lead	Stimulator lead in gastrointestinal system
GORE® DUALMESH®	Synthetic substitute
Guedel airway	Intraluminal device, airway in mouth and throat
Hancock Bioprosthesis (aortic) (mitral) valve	Zooplastic tissue in heart and great vessels
Hancock Bioprosthetic Valved Conduit	Zooplastic tissue in heart and great vessels
HeartMate II® Left Ventricular Assist Device (LVAD)	Implantable heart assist system in heart and great vessels
HeartMate XVE® Left Ventricular Assist Device (LVAD)	Implantable heart assist system in heart and great vessels
Hip (joint) liner	Liner in lower joints
Holter valve ventricular shunt	Synthetic substitute
Ilizarov external fixator	External fixation device, ring for insertion in upper bones external fixation device, ring for reposition in upper bones external fixation device, ring for insertion in lower bones external fixation device, ring for reposition in lower bones
Ilizarov-Vecklich device	External fixation device, limb lengthening for insertion in upper bones external fixation device, limb lengthening for insertion in lower bones
Implantable cardioverter-defibrillator (ICD)	Defibrillator generator for insertion in subcutaneous tissue and fascia
Implantable drug infusion pump (anti-spasmodic) (chemotherapy)(pain)	Infusion device, pump in subcutaneous tissue and fascia
Implantable glucose monitoring device	Monitoring device
Implantable hemodynamic monitor (IHM)	Monitoring device, hemodynamic for insertion in subcutaneous tissue and fascia
Implantable hemodynamic monitoring system (IHMS)	Monitoring device, hemodynamic for insertion in subcutaneous tissue and fascia
Implantable Miniature Telescope™ (IMT)	Synthetic substitute, intraocular telescope for replacement in eye
Implanted (venous)(access) port	Vascular access device, reservoir in subcutaneous tissue and fascia
InDura, intrathecal catheter (1P) (spinal)	Infusion device
Injection reservoir, port	Vascular access device,

Device Term	PCS Description
	reservoir in subcutaneous tissue and fascia
Injection reservoir, pump	Infusion device, pump in subcutaneous tissue and fascia
Interbody fusion (spine) cage	Interbody fusion device in upper joints interbody fusion device in lower joints
Interspinous process spinal stabilization device	Spinal stabilization device, interspinous process for insertion in upper joints spinal stabilization device, interspinous process for insertion in lower joints
InterStim® Therapy neurostimulator	Stimulator generator, single array for insertion in subcutaneous tissue and fascia
Intramedullary (IM) rod (nail)	Internal fixation device, intramedullary in upper bones internal fixation device, intramedullary in lower bones
Intramedullary skeletal kinetic distractor (ISKD)	Internal fixation device, intramedullary in upper bones internal fixation device, intramedullary in lower bones
Intrauterine device (IUD)	Contraceptive device in female reproductive system
Itrel (3)(4) neurostimulator	Stimulator generator, single array for insertion in subcutaneous tissue and fascia
Joint fixation plate	Internal fixation device in upper joints internal fixation device in lower joints
Joint liner (insert)	Liner in lower joints
Joint spacer (antibiotic)	Spacer in upper joints spacer in lower joints
Kappa	Pacemaker, dual chamber for insertion in subcutaneous tissue and fascia
Kinetra® neurostimulator	Stimulator generator, multiple array for insertion in subcutaneous tissue and fascia
Kirschner wire (K-wire)	Internal fixation device in head and facial bones internal fixation device in upper bones internal fixation device in lower bones internal fixation device in upper joints internal fixation device in lower joints
Knee (implant) insert	Liner in lower joints
Küntscher nail	Internal fixation device, intramedullary in upper bones internal fixation device, intramedullary in lower bones
LAP-BAND® adjustable gastric banding system	Extraluminal device
LifeStent® (Flexstar)(XL) Vascular Stent System	Intraluminal device
LIVIAN™ CRT-D	Cardiac resynchronization defibrillator pulse generator for insertion in subcutaneous tissue and fascia
Loop recorder, implantable	Monitoring device
Mark IV Breathing Pacemaker System	Stimulator generator in subcutaneous tissue and fascia
Maximo II DR (VR)	Defibrillator generator for insertion in subcutaneous tissue and fascia
Maximo II DR CRT-D	Cardiac resynchronization defibrillator pulse generator for insertion in subcutaneous

Anatomical Term	PCS Description	Anatomical Term	PCS Description
	tissue and fascia	Percutaneous endoscopic gastrostomy (PEG) tube	Feeding device in gastrointestinal system
Melody® transcatheter pulmonary valve	Zooplastic tissue in heart and great vessels	Percutaneous nephrostomy catheter	Drainage device
Micro-Driver stent (RX) (OTW)	Intraluminal device	Peripherally inserted central catheter (PICC)	Infusion device
Micrus CERECYTE microcoil	Intraluminal device, bioactive in upper arteries	Pessary ring	Intraluminal device, pessary in female reproductive system
MitraClip valve repair system	Synthetic substitute	Phrenic nerve stimulator generator	Stimulator generator in subcutaneous tissue and fascia
Mitroflow® Aortic Pericardial Heart Valve	Zooplastic tissue in heart and great vessels	Phrenic nerve stimulator lead	Diaphragmatic pacemaker lead in respiratory system
Nasopharyngeal airway (NPA)	Intraluminal device, airway in ear, nose, sinus	PHYSIOMESH™ Flexible Composite Mesh	Synthetic substitute
Neuromuscular electrical stimulation (NEMS) lead	Stimulator lead in muscles	Pipeline™ Embolization device (PED)	Intraluminal device
Neurostimulator generator, multiple channel	Stimulator generator, multiple array for insertion in subcutaneous tissue and fascia	Polyethylene socket	Synthetic substitute, polyethylene for replacement in lower joints
Neurostimulator generator, single channel	Stimulator generator, single array for insertion in subcutaneous tissue and fascia	Polymethylmethacrylate (PMMA)	Synthetic substitute
		Polypropylene mesh	Synthetic substitute
Neurostimulator generator, multiple channel rechargeable	Stimulator generator, multiple array rechargeable for insertion in subcutaneous tissue and fascia	Porcine (bioprosthetic) valve	Zooplastic tissue in heart and great vessels
		PRESTIGE® Cervical Disc	Synthetic substitute
Neurostimulator generator, single channel rechargeable	Stimulator generator, single array rechargeable for insertion in subcutaneous tissue and fascia	PrimeAdvanced neurostimulator	Stimulator generator, multiple array for insertion in subcutaneous tissue and fascia
		PROCEED™ Ventral Patch	Synthetic substitute
Neutralization plate	Internal fixation device in head and facial bones internal fixation device in upper bones internal fixation device in lower bones	Prodisc-C	Synthetic substitute
		Prodisc-L	Synthetic substitute
		PROLENE Polypropylene Hernia System (PHS)	Synthetic substitute
Nitinol framed polymer mesh	Synthetic substitute	Protecta XT CRT-D	Cardiac resynchronization defibrillator pulse generator for insertion in subcutaneous tissue and fascia
Non-tunneled central venous catheter	Infusion device		
Novacor Left Ventricular Assist Device	Implantable heart assist system in heart and great vessels	Protecta XT DR (XT VR)	Defibrillator generator for insertion in subcutaneous tissue and fascia
Novation® Ceramic AHS® (Articulation Hip System)	Synthetic substitute, ceramic for replacement in lower joints	Protege® RX Carotid Stent System	Intraluminal device
Optimizer™ III implantable pulse generator	Contractility modulation device for insertion in subcutaneous tissue and fascia	Pump reservoir	Infusion device, pump in subcutaneous tissue and fascia
Oropharyngeal airway (OPA)	Intraluminal device, airway in mouth and throat	PVAD™ Ventricular Assist Device	External heart assist system in heart and great vessels
Ovatio™ CRT-D	Cardiac resynchronization defibrillator pulse generator for insertion in subcutaneous tissue and fascia	REALIZE® Adjustable Gastric Band	Extraluminal device
		Rebound HRD® (Hernia Repair Device)	Synthetic substitute
Oxidized zirconium ceramic hip bearing surface	Synthetic substitute, ceramic on polyethylene for replacement in lower joints	RestoreAdvanced neurostimulator	Stimulator generator, multiple array rechargeable for insertion in subcutaneous tissue and fascia
Paclitaxel-eluting coronary stent	Intraluminal device, drug-eluting in heart and great vessels	RestoreSensor neurostimulator	Stimulator generator, multiple array rechargeable for insertion in subcutaneous tissue and fascia
Paclitaxel-eluting peripheral stent	Intraluminal device, drug-eluting in upper arteries intraluminal device, drug-eluting in lower arteries	RestoreUltra neurostimulator	Stimulator generator, multiple array rechargeable for insertion in subcutaneous tissue and fascia
Partially absorbable mesh	Synthetic substitute		
Pedicle-based dynamic stabilization device	Spinal stabilization device, pedicle-based for insertion in upper joints spinal stabilization device, pedicle-based for insertion in lower joints	Reveal (DX)(XT)	Monitoring device
		Reverse® Shoulder Prosthesis	Synthetic substitute, reverse ball and socket for replacement in upper joints
Percutaneous endoscopic gastrojejunostomy (PEG/J) tube	Feeding device in gastrointestinal system	Revo MRI™ SureScan® pacemaker	Pacemaker, dual chamber for insertion in subcutaneous tissue and fascia

Device Term	PCS Description	Device Term	PCS Description
Rheos® System device	Cardiac rhythm related device in subcutaneous tissue and fascia		pacemaker pulse generator for insertion in subcutaneous tissue and fascia
Rheos® System lead	Stimulator lead in upper arteries	Talent® Converter	Intraluminal device
RNS System lead	Neurostimulator lead in central nervous system	Talent® Occluder	Intraluminal device
RNS system neurostimulator generator	Neurostimulator generator in head and facial bones	Talent® Stent Graft (abdominal)(thoracic)	Intraluminal device
Sacral nerve modulation (SNM) lead	Stimulator lead in urinary system	TandemHeart® System	Intraluminal device
Sacral neuromodulation lead	Stimulator lead in urinary system	TAXUS® Liberte® Paclitaxel-eluting Coronary Stent System	Intraluminal device, drug-eluting in heart and great vessels
SAPIEN transcatheter aortic valve	Zooplastic tissue in heart and great vessels	Therapeutic occlusion coil(s)	Intraluminal device
Secura (DR) (VR)	Defibrillator generator for insertion in subcutaneous tissue and fascia	Thoracostomy tube	Drainage device
Sheffield hybrid external fixator	External fixation device, hybrid for insertion in upper bones external fixation device, hybrid for reposition in upper bones external fixation device, hybrid for insertion in lower bones external fixation device, hybrid for reposition in lower bones	Thoratec IVAD (Implantable Ventricular Assist Device)	Implantable heart assist system in heart and great vessels
		TigerPaw® system for closure of left atrial appendage	Extraluminal device
		Tissue bank graft	Nonautologous tissue substitute
		Tissue expander (inflatable)(injectable)	Tissue expander in skin and breast tissue expander in subcutaneous tissue and fascia
Sheffield ring external fixator	External fixation device, ring for insertion in upper bones external fixation device, ring for reposition in upper bones external fixation device, ring for insertion in lower bones external fixation device, ring for reposition in lower bones	Titanium Sternal Fixation System (TSFS)	Internal fixation device, rigid plate for insertion in upper bones internal fixation device, rigid plate for reposition in upper bones
		Total artificial (replacement) heart	Synthetic substitute
		Tracheostomy tube	Tracheostomy device in respiratory system
Single lead pacemaker (atrium)(ventricle)	Pacemaker, single chamber for insertion in subcutaneous tissue and fascia	Trifecta™ Valve (aortic)	Zooplastic tissue in heart and great vessels
Single lead rate responsive pacemaker (atrium)(ventricle)	Pacemaker, single chamber rate responsive for insertion in subcutaneous tissue and fascia	Tunneled central venous catheter	Vascular access device in subcutaneous tissue and fascia
Sirolimus-eluting coronary stent	Intraluminal device, drug-eluting in heart and great vessels	Tunneled spinal (intrathecal) catheter	Infusion device
		Two lead pacemaker	Pacemaker, dual chamber for insertion in subcutaneous tissue and fascia
SJM Biocor® Stented Valve System	Zooplastic tissue in heart and great vessels	Ultraflex™ Precision Colonic Stent System	Intraluminal device
Soletra® neurostimulator	Stimulator generator, single array for insertion in subcutaneous tissue and fascia	ULTRAPRO Hernia System (UHS)	Synthetic substitute
Spinal cord neurostimulator lead	Neurostimulator lead in central nervous system	ULTRAPRO Partially Absorbable Lightweight Mesh	Synthetic substitute
Spiration IBV™ Valve System	Intraluminal device, endobronchial valve in respiratory system	ULTRAPRO Plug	Synthetic substitute
		Ultrasonic osteogenic stimulator	Bone growth stimulator in head and facial bones bone growth stimulator in upper bones bone growth stimulator in lower bones
Stent (angioplasty)(embolization)	Intraluminal device		
Stented tissue valve	Zooplastic tissue in heart and great vessels	Ultrasound bone healing system	Bone growth stimulator in head and facial bones bone growth stimulator in upper bones bone growth stimulator in lower bones
Stratos LV	Cardiac resynchronization pacemaker pulse generator for insertion in subcutaneous tissue and fascia		
Subcutaneous injection reservoir, port	Use :vascular access device, reservoir in subcutaneous tissue and fascia	Uniplanar external fixator	External fixation device, monoplanar for insertion in upper bones external fixation device, monoplanar for reposition in upper bones external fixation device, monoplanar for insertion in lower bones external fixation device, monoplanar for reposition in lower bones
Subcutaneous injection reservoir, pump	Infusion device, pump in subcutaneous tissue and fascia		
Subdermal progesterone implant	Contraceptive device in subcutaneous tissue and fascia		
SynCardia Total Artificial Heart	Synthetic substitute	Urinary incontinence stimulator lead	Stimulator lead in urinary system
Synchra CRT-P	Cardiac resynchronization	Vaginal pessary	Intraluminal device, pessary in

Anatomical Term	PCS Description		Anatomical Term	PCS Description
	female reproductive system			
Valiant Thoracic Stent Graft	Intraluminal device			
Vectra® Vascular Access Graft	Vascular access device in subcutaneous tissue and fascia			
Ventrio™ Hernia Patch	Synthetic substitute			
Versa	Pacemaker, dual chamber for insertion in subcutaneous tissue and fascia			
Virtuoso (II) (DR) (VR)	Defibrillator generator for insertion in subcutaneous tissue and fascia			
WALLSTENT® Endoprosthesis	Intraluminal device			
X-STOP® Spacer	Spinal stabilization device, interspinous process for insertion in upper joints spinal stabilization device, interspinous process for insertion in lower joints			
Xenograft	Zooplastic tissue in heart and great vessels			
XIENCE V Everolimus Eluting Coronary Stent System	Intraluminal device, drug-eluting in heart and great vessels			
XLIF® System	Interbody fusion device in lower joints			
Zenith TX2® TAA Endovascular Graft	Intraluminal device			
Zenith® Renu™ AAA Ancillary Graft	Intraluminal device			
Zilver® PTX® (paclitaxel) Drug-Eluting Peripheral Stent	Intraluminal device, drug-eluting in upper arteries intraluminal device, drug-eluting in lower arteries			
Zimmer® NexGen® LPS Mobile Bearing Knee	Synthetic substitute			
Zimmer® NexGen® LPS-Flex Mobile Knee	Synthetic substitute			
Zotarolimus-eluting coronary stent	Intraluminal device, drug-eluting in heart and great vessels			

APPENDIX D: DEVICE KEY AND AGGREGATION TABLE

Specific Device	For Operation	In Body System	General Device
Autologous Arterial Tissue	All applicable	Heart and Great Vessels Lower Arteries Lower Veins Upper Arteries Upper Veins	**7** Autologous Tissue Substitute
Autologous Venous Tissue	All applicable	Heart and Great Vessels Lower Arteries Lower Veins Upper Arteries Upper Veins	**7** Autologous Tissue Substitute
Cardiac Lead, Defibrillator	Insertion	Heart and Great Vessels	**M** Cardiac Lead
Cardiac Lead, Pacemaker	Insertion	Heart and Great Vessels	**M** Cardiac Lead
Cardiac Resynchronization Defibrillator Pulse Generator	Insertion	Subcutaneous Tissue and Fascia	**P** Cardiac Rhythm Related Device
Cardiac Resynchronization Pacemaker Pulse Generator	Insertion	Subcutaneous Tissue and Fascia	**P** Cardiac Rhythm Related Device
Contractility Modulation Device	Insertion	Subcutaneous Tissue and Fascia	**P** Cardiac Rhythm Related Device
Defibrillator Generator	Insertion	Subcutaneous Tissue and Fascia	**P** Cardiac Rhythm Related Device
External Fixation Device, Hybrid	Insertion	Lower Bones Upper Bones	**5** External Fixation Device
External Fixation Device, Hybrid	Reposition	Lower Bones Upper Bones	**5** External Fixation Device
External Fixation Device, Limb Lengthening	Insertion	Lower Bones Upper Bones	**5** External Fixation Device
External Fixation Device, Monoplanar	Insertion	Lower Bones Upper Bones	**5** External Fixation Device
External Fixation Device, Monoplanar	Reposition	Lower Bones Upper Bones	**5** External Fixation Device
External Fixation Device, Ring	Insertion	Lower Bones Upper Bones	**5** External Fixation Device
External Fixation Device, Ring	Reposition	Lower Bones Upper Bones	**5** External Fixation Device
Hearing Device, Bone Conduction	Insertion	Ear, Nose, Sinus	**S** Hearing Device
Hearing Device, Multiple Channel Cochlear Prosthesis	Insertion	Ear, Nose, Sinus	**S** Hearing Device
Hearing Device, Single Channel Cochlear Prosthesis	Insertion	Ear, Nose, Sinus	**S** Hearing Device
Internal Fixation Device, Intramedullary	All applicable	Lower Bones Upper Bones	**4** Internal Fixation Device
Internal Fixation Device, Rigid Plate	Insertion	Upper Bones	**4** Internal Fixation Device
Internal Fixation Device, Rigid Plate	Reposition	Upper Bones	**4** Internal Fixation Device
Intraluminal Device, Pessary	All applicable	Female Reproductive System	**D** Intraluminal Device
Intraluminal Device, Airway	All applicable	Ear, Nose, Sinus Gastrointestinal System Mouth and Throat	**D** Intraluminal Device
Intraluminal Device, Bioactive	All applicable	Upper Arteries	**D** Intraluminal Device
Intraluminal Device, Drug-eluting	All applicable	Heart and Great Vessels Lower Arteries Upper Arteries	**D** Intraluminal Device
Intraluminal Device, Endobronchial Valve	All applicable	Respiratory System	**D** Intraluminal Device
Intraluminal Device, Endotracheal Airway	All applicable	Respiratory System	**D** Intraluminal Device
Intraluminal Device, Radioactive	All applicable	Heart and Great Vessels	**D** Intraluminal Device
Monitoring Device, Hemodynamic	Insertion	Subcutaneous Tissue and Fascia	**2** Monitoring Device
Monitoring Device, Pressure Sensor	Insertion	Heart and Great Vessels	**2** Monitoring Device
Pacemaker, Dual Chamber	Insertion	Subcutaneous Tissue and Fascia	**P** Cardiac Rhythm Related Device
Pacemaker, Single Chamber	Insertion	Subcutaneous Tissue and Fascia	**P** Cardiac Rhythm Related Device
Pacemaker, Single Chamber Rate Responsive	Insertion	Subcutaneous Tissue and Fascia	**P** Cardiac Rhythm Related Device
Spinal Stabilization Device, Facet Replacement	Insertion	Lower Joints Upper Joints	**4** Internal Fixation Device
Spinal Stabilization Device, Interspinous Process	Insertion	Lower Joints Upper Joints	**4** Internal Fixation Device

Specific Device	for Operation	in Body System	General Device
Spinal Stabilization Device, Pedicle-Based	Insertion	Lower Joints Upper Joints	**4** Internal Fixation Device
Stimulator Generator, Multiple Array	Insertion	Subcutaneous Tissue and Fascia	**M** Stimulator Generator
Stimulator Generator, Multiple Array Rechargeable	Insertion	Subcutaneous Tissue and Fascia	**M** Stimulator Generator
Stimulator Generator, Single Array	Insertion	Subcutaneous Tissue and Fascia	**M** Stimulator Generator
Stimulator Generator, Single Array Rechargeable	Insertion	Subcutaneous Tissue and Fascia	**M** Stimulator Generator
Synthetic Substitute, Ceramic	Replacement	Lower Joints	**J** Synthetic Substitute
Synthetic Substitute, Ceramic on Polyethylene	Replacement	Lower Joints	**J** Synthetic Substitute
Synthetic Substitute, Intraocular Telescope	Replacement	Eye	**J** Synthetic Substitute
Synthetic Substitute, Metal	Replacement	Lower Joints	**J** Synthetic Substitute
Synthetic Substitute, Metal on Polyethylene	Replacement	Lower Joints	**J** Synthetic Substitute
Synthetic Substitute, Polyethylene	Replacement	Lower Joints	**J** Synthetic Substitute
Synthetic Substitute, Reverse Ball and Socket	Replacement	Upper Joints	**J** Synthetic Substitute